a LANGE medical book

CURRENT Diagnosis & Treatment Gastroenterology, Hepatology, & Endoscopy

Editor

Norton J. Greenberger, MD
Clinical Professor of Medicine, Harvard Medical School
Senior Physician, Division of Gastroenterology, Hepatology and Endoscopy
Brigham and Women's Hospital
Boston, Massachusetts

Associate Editors

Richard S. Blumberg, MD
Professor of Medicine, Harvard Medical School
Chief, Division of Gastroenterology, Hepatology and Endoscopy
Brigham and Women's Hospital
Boston, Massachusetts

Robert Burakoff, MD, MPH
Associate Professor of Medicine, Harvard Medical School
Clinical Chief of Gastroenterology, Division of Gastroenterology and Hepatology
Brigham and Women's Hospital
Boston, Massachusetts

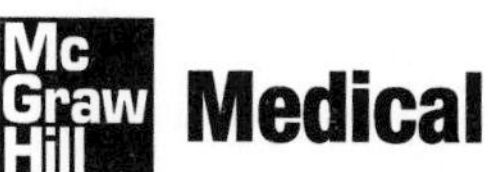

New York Chicago San Francisco Lisbon London Madrid Mexico City
Milan New Delhi San Juan Seoul Singapore Sydney Toronto

The McGraw·Hill Companies

CURRENT Diagnosis & Treatment: Gastroenterology, Hepatology, & Endoscopy, Second Edition

1 2 3 4 5 6 7 8 9 0 DOC/DOC 15 14 13 12 11

ISBN 978-0-07-176848-1
MHID 0-07-176848-3
ISSN 1946-3030

Notice

Medicine is an ever-changing science. As new research and clinical experience broaden our knowledge, changes in treatment and drug therapy are required. The authors and the publisher of this work have checked with sources believed to be reliable in their efforts to provide information that is complete and generally in accord with the standards accepted at the time of publication. However, in view of the possibility of human error or changes in medical sciences, neither the authors nor the publisher nor any other party who has been involved in the preparation or publication of this work warrants that the information contained herein is in every respect accurate or complete, and they disclaim all responsibility for any errors or omissions or for the results obtained from use of the information contained in this work. Readers are encouraged to confirm the information contained herein with other sources. For example and in particular, readers are advised to check the product information sheet included in the package of each drug they plan to administer to be certain that the information contained in this work is accurate and that changes have not been made in the recommended dose or in the contraindications for administration. This recommendation is of particular importance in connection with new or infrequently used drugs.

This book was set in Minion by Cenveo Publisher Services.
The editors were James Shanahan and Harriet Lebowitz.
The production supervisor was Catherine Saggese.
Project management was provided by Sapna Rastogi, Cenveo Publisher Services.
The text was designed by Alan Barnett Design.
The index was prepared by Cenveo Publisher Services.
RR Donnelley was printer and binder.
Cover photos: (clockwise from top left) *Helicobacter pylori* bacteria, credit: David Mack/Photo Researchers, Inc.; Endoscopic procedure, credit: David Grossman/Photo Researchers, Inc.; Endoscopic appearance of Barrett esophagus.

This book is printed on acid-free paper.

International Edition ISBN 978-0-07-178843-4; MHID 0-07-178843-3

Contents

Color insert appears between pages 402 and 403.

Authors

Jaya R. Agrawal, MD, MPH
Attending Gastroenterologist, Hampshire Gastroenterology Associates, Florence, Massachusetts
Gastrointestinal & Biliary Complications of Pregnancy

Frank A. Anania, MD, FACP, AGAF
Associate Professor of Medicine, Director of Hepatology, Division of Digestive Diseases, Department of Medicine, Emory University School of Medicine, Atlanta, Georgia
fanania@emory.edu
Nonalcoholic Fatty Liver Disease

Peter A. Banks, MD
Director of the Center for Pancreatic Disease, Division of Gastroenterology, Brigham and Women's Hospital; Professor of Medicine, Harvard Medical School, Boston, Massachusetts
pabanks@partners.org
Acute Pancreatitis; Chronic Pancreatitis

Ronald Bleday, MD
Chief, Section of Colon and Rectal Surgery, Brigham and Women's Hospital & Dana-Farber Cancer Institute; Associate Professor of Surgery, Harvard Medical School, Boston, Massachusetts
rbleday@partners.org
Inflammatory Bowel Disease: Surgical Considerations

Richard S. Blumberg, MD
Professor of Medicine, Harvard Medical School; Chief, Division of Gastroenterology, Hepatology, and Endoscopy, Brigham and Women's Hospital, Boston, Massachusetts
rblumberg@partners.org
Inflammatory Bowel Disease: Immunologic Considerations and Therapeutic Implications; Diverticular Disease of the Colon

Robert Burakoff, MD, MPH
Clinical Chief of Gastroenterology, Division of Gastroenterology and Hepatology, Brigham and Women's Hospital; Associate Professor of Medicine, Harvard Medical School, Boston, Massachusetts
rburakoff@partners.org
Inflammatory Bowel Disease: Medical Considerations; Functional (Nonulcer) Dyspepsia; Disorders of Gastric & Small Bowel Motility

David L. Carr-Locke, MA, MD, DRCOG, FRCP, FACG, FASGE
Chief, Division of Digestive Diseases, Co-Director of the Center for Digestive Health, Beth Israel Medical Center; Professor, Albert Einstein College of Medicine, New York, New York
dcarrlocke@chpnet.org
Endoscopic Retrograde Cholangiopancreatography (ERCP)

Walter W. Chan, MD, MPH
Instructor in Medicine, Harvard Medical School; Associate Physician, Division of Gastroenterology, Hepatology and Endoscopy, Brigham and Women's Hospital, Boston, Massachusetts
wwchan@partners.org
Functional (Nonulcer) Dyspepsia; Disorders of Gastric & Small Bowel Motility

Arun Chaudhury, MBBS, MD
Senior Research Fellow in Medicine, Beth Israel Deaconess Medical Center and Center for Swallowing & Motility Disorders, VA Boston Healthcare System (VABHS), West Roxbury, Massachusetts
arun_chaudhury@hms.harvard.edu
Oropharyngeal & Esophageal Motility Disorders

David E. Cohen, MD, PhD
Robert H. Ebert Associate Professor of Medicine and Health Sciences and Technology; Director of Hepatology, Division of Gastroenterology, Department of Medicine, Brigham and Women's Hospital; Director, Harvard–Massachusetts Institute of Technology Division of Health Sciences and Technology, Harvard Medical School, Boston, Massachusetts
dcohen@partners.org
Nonalcoholic Fatty Liver Disease

Darwin L. Conwell, MD, MS
Associate Professor of Medicine, Division of Gastroenterology, Center for Pancreatic Disease, Brigham and Women's Hospital, Boston, Massachusetts
dconwell@partners.org
Acute Pancreatitis; Chronic Pancreatitis

Jules L. Dienstag, MD
Carl W. Walter Professor of Medicine and Dean for Medical Education, Harvard Medical School; Physician, Massachusetts General Hospital, Boston, Massachusetts
jdienstag@partners.org
Viral Hepatitis

Sonia Friedman, MD
Assistant Professor of Medicine, Harvard Medical School; Associate Physician, Brigham and Women's Hospital, Boston, Massachusetts
sfriedman1@partners.org
Gastrointestinal & Biliary Complications of Pregnancy; Irritable Bowel Syndrome

Norman D. Grace, MD
Director of Clinical Hepatology, Division of Gastroenterology and Hepatology, Brigham and Women's Hospital; Lecturer on Medicine, Harvard Medical School; Professor of Medicine, Tufts University School of Medicine, Boston, Massachusetts
ngrace@partners.org
Hereditary Hemochromatosis; Alcoholic Liver Disease; Portal Hypertension & Esophageal Variceal Hemorrhage

Norton J. Greenberger, MD
Clinical Professor of Medicine, Harvard Medical School; Senior Physician, Division of Gastroenterology, Hepatology and Endoscopy, Brigham and Women's Hospital, Boston, Massachusetts
ngreenberger@partners.org
Acute Abdominal Pain: Basic Principles & Current Challenges; Mesenteric Ischemia; Eosinophilic Esophagitis; Treatment of Obesity: The Impact of Bariatric Surgery; Autoimmune Pancreatitis; Approach to the Patient with Jaundice & Abnormal Liver Tests; Portal Systemic Encephalopathy & Hepatic Encephalopathy; Ascites & Spontaneous Bacterial Peritonitis; Hepatorenal Syndrome; Primary Sclerosing Cholangitis; Gallstone Disease

Jennifer L. Irani, MD
Instructor in Surgery, Harvard Medical School; Staff Surgeon, Section of Colon and Rectal Surgery, Brigham and Women's Hospital, Boston, Massachusetts
jirani@partners.org
Inflammatory Bowel Disease: Surgical Considerations

Kunal Jajoo, MD
Lecturer in Medicine, Harvard Medical School; Associate Physician, Brigham and Women's Hospital, Boston, Massachusetts
kjajoo@partners.org
Barrett Esophagus; Polypectomy

Fay Kastrinos, MD, MPH
Assistant Professor in Medicine, Columbia University, College of Physicians and Surgeons, Division of Digestive and Liver Diseases, New York, New York
fk18@columbia.edu
Colorectal Cancer Screening

Sonal Kumar, MD
Gastroenterology Fellow, Division of Gastroenterology, Hepatology and Endoscopy, Brigham and Women's Hospital, Boston, Massachusetts
skumar11@partners.org
Acute Liver Failure

Timothy T. Kuo, MD
Instructor in Medicine, Harvard Medical School, Boston, Massachusetts
ttkuo@partners.org
Alcoholic Liver Disease

Linda S. Lee, MD
Assistant Professor of Medicine, Harvard Medical School; Director of Women's Health and Endoscopic Education in Gastroenterology, Brigham and Women's Hospital, Boston, Massachusetts
lslee@partners.org
Acute Lower Gastrointestinal Bleeding; Endoscopic Retrograde Cholangiopancreatography (ERCP); Endoscopic Ultrasound

Jonathan S. Levine, MD
Instructor in Medicine, Harvard Medical School; Associate Physician, Division of Gastroenterology, Hepatology and Endoscopy, Brigham and Women's Hospital, Boston, Massachusetts
jslevine@partners.org
Inflammatory Bowel Disease: Medical Considerations

Edward Lew, MD, MPH
Staff Gastroenterologist, VA Boston Healthcare System; Assistant Professor of Medicine, Harvard Medical School, Boston, Massachusetts
elew@partners.org
Peptic Ulcer Disease; Zollinger-Ellison Syndrome (Gastrinoma)

Willis C. Maddrey, MD, MACP, FRCP
Professor of Internal Medicine, The University of Texas Southwestern Medical Center, Dallas, Texas
wcmaddrey@utsouthwestern.edu
Drug-Induced Liver Disease

Frederick L. Makrauer, MD
Instructor in Medicine, Harvard Medical School; Center for Crohn's and Colitis, Brigham and Women's Hospital, Boston, Massachusetts
fmakrauer@partners.org
Acute Abdominal Pain

Hiroshi Mashimo, MD, PhD
Assistant Professor of Medicine, Harvard Medical School; Director, GI Motility Service, VA Boston Healthcare System, Boston, Massachusetts
hmashimo@hms.harvard.edu
Oropharyngeal & Esophageal Motility Disorders

Melissa A. Minor, MD, MPH
Gastroenterologist, Gastrointestinal Physicians, PC, North Shore Medical Center, Salem, Massachusetts
mminor@partners.org
Portal Hypertension & Esophageal Variceal Hemorrhage

Koenraad J. Mortele, MD
Associate Professor of Radiology, Harvard Medical School; Associate Director, Division of Abdominal Imaging and Intervention; Director, Abdominal and Pelvic MRI; Director, CME, Department of Radiology Brigham and Women's Hospital; Boston, Massachusetts
kmortele@partners.org
State-of-the-Art Imaging of the Gastrointestinal System

Gustav Paumgartner, MD, FRCP
Professor of Medicine Emeritus, University Hospital Munich-Grosshadern, Munich, Germany
Gustav.Paumgartner@med.uni-muenchen.de
Gallstone Disease

Daniel S. Pratt, MD
Assistant Professor of Medicine, Harvard Medical School; Director, Liver-Biliary-Pancreas Center, Massachusetts General Hospital, Boston, Massachusetts
dspratt@partners.org
Primary Biliary Cirrhosis

Amir A. Qamar, MD
Instructor in Medicine, Harvard Medical School and Division of Gastroenterology, Hepatology and Endoscopy, Brigham and Women's Hospital, Boston, Massachusetts
aqamar@partners.org
Acute Liver Failure; Liver Neoplasms; Liver Transplantation

Anthony Ramsanahie, MD
Specialist Registrar General Surgery, United Lincolnshire Hospitals, NHS Trust. East Midlands Deanery Training Program
aramsanahie@hotmail.com
Inflammatory Bowel Disease: Surgical Considerations

Malcolm K. Robinson, MD
Assistant Professor of Surgery, Harvard Medical School and Brigham and Women's Hospital, Boston, Massachusetts
mkrobinson@partners.org
Treatment of Obesity: The Impact of Bariatric Surgery

Anna Rutherford, MD, MPH
Instructor in Medicine, Harvard Medical School; Associate Physician, Division of Gastroenterology, Hepatology and Endoscopy, Brigham and Women's Hospital, Boston, Massachusetts
arutherford@partners.org
Viral Hepatitis

John R. Saltzman, MD
Associate Professor of Medicine, Harvard Medical School; Director of Endoscopy, Brigham and Women's Hospital, Boston, Massachusetts
jsaltzman@partners.org
Gastroesophageal Reflux Disease; Barrett Esophagus; Acute Upper Gastrointestinal Bleeding; Acute Lower Gastrointestinal Bleeding; Wireless Capsule Endoscopy & Deep Small Bowel Enteroscopy; Primary Sclerosing Cholangitis

Ashish Sharma, MD
Clinical Instructor, Harvard Medical School; Staff Physician, VA Boston Healthcare System, Boston, Massachusetts
ashish.sharma2@med.va.gov
Tumors of the Pancreas

Benjamin Smith, MD
Lecturer on Medicine, Harvard Medical School; Assistant Professor, Tufts University School of Medicine; Director of Endoscopy and Attending Physician, Faulkner Hospital; Affiliate Staff, Brigham and Women's Hospital, Boston, Massachusetts
bnsmith@partners.org
Hereditary Hemochromatosis

Scott B. Snapper, MD, PhD
Associate Professor of Medicine, Harvard Medical School; Physician, Brigham and Women's Hospital; Director, Inflammatory Bowel Disease Center, Children's Hospital, Boston, Massachusetts
ssnapper@partners.org
Inflammatory Bowel Disease: Immunologic Considerations and Therapeutic Implications

Elena M. Stoffel, MD, MPH
Assistant Professor of Medicine, Harvard Medical School, Boston, Massachusetts
estoffel@partners.org
Mesenteric Ischemia; Hereditary Gastrointestinal Cancer Syndromes

Sapna Syngal, MD, MPH
Director, Gastroenterology; Clinical Director, Cancer Genetics and Prevention Center, Dana-Farber Cancer Institute/Brigham and Women's Hospital; Associate Professor of Medicine, Harvard Medical School, Boston, Massachusetts
sapna_syngal@dfci.harvard.edu
Colorectal Cancer Screening; Hereditary Gastrointestinal Cancer Syndromes

Christopher C. Thompson, MD, MSc, FACG, FASGE
Director of Therapeutic Endoscopy, Division of Gastroenterology, Brigham and Women's Hospital; Assistant Professor of Medicine, Harvard Medical School, Boston, Massachusetts
ccthompson@partners.org
Endoscopic Management of Acute Biliary & Pancreatic Conditions; Gastrointestinal Foreign Bodies

Anne C. Travis, MD, MSc, FACG
Associate Physician, Division of Gastroenterology, Hepatology and Endoscopy, Brigham and Women's Hospital, Boston, Massachusetts
atravis@partners.org
Diverticular Disease of the Colon; Wireless Capsule Endoscopy & Deep Small Bowel Enteroscopy

Jerry S. Trier, MD
Professor of Medicine Emeritus, Harvard Medical School; Senior Physician, Division of Gastroenterology, Department of Medicine, Brigham and Women's Hospital, Boston, Massachusetts
jtrier@partners.org
Acute Diarrheal Disorders; Intestinal Malabsorption

Chinweike Ukomadu, MD, PhD
Attending Physician, Brigham and Women's Hospital; Assistant Professor of Medicine, Harvard Medical School, Boston, Massachusetts
cukomadu@partners.org
Hepatic Complications of Pregnancy; Chronic Nonviral Hepatitis; Liver Neoplasms

Bechien U. Wu, MD, MPH
Instructor in Medicine, Division of Gastroenterology, Center for Pancreatic Disease, Brigham and Women's Hospital, Boston, Massachusetts
buwu@partners.org
Acute Pancreatitis; Chronic Pancreatitis

Zhenglun Zhu, MD, PhD
Associate Physician, Brigham and Women's Hospital; Assistant Professor of Medicine, Harvard Medical School, Boston, Massachusetts
zzhu@partners.org
Gastrointestinal Manifestations of Immunodeficiency

Preface

We are pleased that the second edition of *Current Diagnosis & Treatment: Gastroenterology, Hepatology, & Endoscopy* has been published within two years of the publication of the first edition. The editors felt this timetable was especially important in order to provide up-to-date information on a number of topics in which there is rapidly accumulating information, especially with regard to therapeutic considerations. Disorders in which there have been noteworthy advances in diagnosis and therapeutics include, but are not limited to, chronic hepatitis B, chronic hepatitis C, autoimmune pancreatitis, acute pancreatitis, eosinophilic esophagitis, Barrett esophagus, inflammatory bowel disease, and nonalcoholic fatty liver disease. We have been particularly interested in incorporating important advances in therapeutics in many of the sections in the textbook. We especially want to thank Mr. Clayton R. Bemis for his fine efforts in incorporating the many changes submitted by the authors into the final revisions.

Preface to the First Edition

The fields of gastroenterology and hepatology have changed dramatically in the past ten years, partially as a result of the impressive advances in understanding the molecular and pathophysiologic basis of gastrointestinal disorders. Such advances have spawned translational research, which in turn has resulted in important new diagnostic and therapeutic modalities. In addition, the expanding knowledge base has resulted in the development of sub-subspecialties within the fields of gastroenterology and hepatology, such as liver transplantation, pancreatic disease, inflammatory bowel disease, and motility disorders. Several topics in these disciplines are discussed in detail in *Current Diagnosis & Treatment: Gastroenterology, Hepatology, & Endoscopy.* Most notably, an entire section of the book is devoted to advances in diagnostic and therapeutic endoscopy.

As a specialty, gastroenterology interfaces with other medical and surgical sub-specialties, specifically gastrointestinal surgery, gastrointestinal radiology, and gastrointestinal pathology. Accordingly, several of the chapters in this book deal with important information in these related specialties. A comprehensive chapter on gastrointestinal radiology includes over 50 images that help clarify the appropriate use of the many imaging techniques currently available. Gastrointestinal disorders that have surgical implications, such as bariatric surgery and inflammatory bowel disease, are presented in detail. The chapter on bariatric surgery highlights the advances in this field that have led to over 100,000 bariatric surgical procedures performed every year. With over 1.5 million patients in the United States with inflammatory bowel disease, surgical considerations for these disorders have become increasingly important.

This book strikes the right balance between comprehensiveness and convenience. It emphasizes the practical aspects of diagnosis of gastrointestinal and hepatic disorders, with each chapter outlining the essentials of diagnosis of various disorders. *Current Diagnosis & Treatment: Gastroenterology, Hepatology, & Endoscopy* provides concise, complete, and accessible clinical information that is up-to-date.

A unique feature of this book is that virtually all of the authors are faculty members at the Harvard Medical School and Brigham and Women's Hospital. Importantly, it has been possible for the editor and associate editors to work closely with all the authors to ensure uniformity of presentation as well as clarity and relevance. The intended audience for which this book has been written comprises gastroenterologists, general internists, family physicians, and surgeons, all of whom can derive benefit from the easily accessible, up-to-date information that this book offers on diagnosis and treatment in gastroenterology, hepatology, and endoscopy.

Norton J. Greenberger, MD
Richard S. Blumberg, MD
Robert Burakoff, MD

Acute Abdominal Pain: Basic Principles & Current Challenges

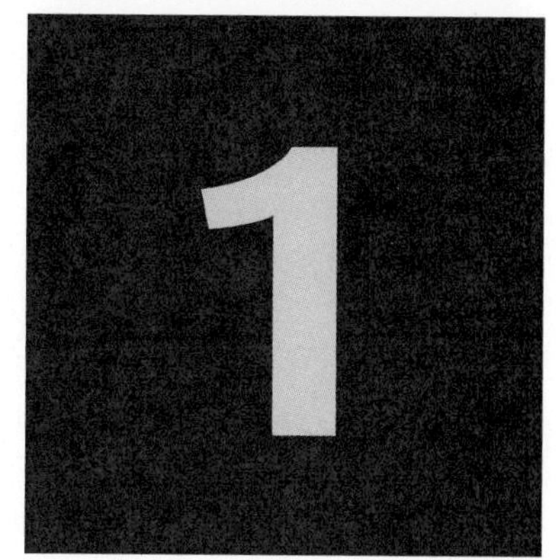

Frederick L. Makrauer, MD
Norton J. Greenberger, MD

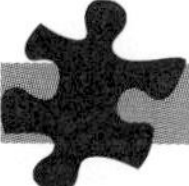

ESSENTIAL CONCEPTS

- Nonsurgical causes of acute abdominal pain simulating an acute abdomen account for up to 30% of patients requiring hospital admission.
- Multidetector-row computed tomography (MDCT) is the benchmark imaging modality in the evaluation of acute abdominal pain *except* in patients with right upper quadrant (RUQ) pain and abnormal liver function tests (LFTs) or in women who are, or may be, pregnant.
- Ultrasound is the initial imaging study of choice in patients with RUQ pain, abnormal LFTs, and suspicion of biliary tract disease.
- Ultrasound is the preferred initial imaging study for young women and those who are pregnant.
- Always perform imaging studies preoperatively in patients with a clinical diagnosis of acute appendicitis.
- Irritable bowel syndrome, functional abdominal pain syndrome, and anxiety disorder may confound accurate diagnosis and are associated with an increased rate of negative appendectomy.
- Narcotic pain medication, if indicated, should not be withheld from a patient with abdominal pain; it will not reduce the recognition of key physical findings and may improve diagnostic accuracy by relaxing the patient.
- The patient's cumulative radiation dose must always be considered before choosing an imaging study, particularly in the young and women of childbearing age.
- Prior abuse should always be considered in patients with recurrent unexplained abdominal pain, regardless of the patient's age or gender.

General Considerations

Acute abdominal pain is defined as severe pain of more than 6 hours' duration in a previously healthy person that requires timely diagnosis and aggressive treatment, usually surgical.

This chapter focuses on the basic principles and challenges in the evaluation of acute, nontraumatic abdominal pain in the adult patient. Emphasis is placed on recent advances in the medical literature and the appropriate tools currently available for improving diagnostic accuracy. The patient with acute abdominal pain remains a clinical challenge for every gastroenterologist. Successful management requires a firm grasp of the patient's history and physical examination and an understanding of appropriate current imaging technology. Clinical scores can be helpful in determining and measuring disease severity and guiding therapy, particularly in acute pancreatitis and inflammatory bowel disease. The clinician should be conditioned to "think outside of the box" and consider the atypical presentation of common disorders.

The management of acute appendicitis provides an ideal example of how the general principles outlined in this chapter can be effectively applied to the care of gastrointestinal illness and is discussed in detail below. The clinician should apply these principles in considering the other conditions discussed in subsequent chapters. It should be remembered that all information is dated and new insights and experience should always be pursued (Table 1–1).

Abdominal pain continues to be the number one complaint in U.S. emergency departments. The U.S. population is progressively aging, with the number of elderly (defined as age >64 years) projected to reach 20% by 2030. Currently the elderly account for 20% of all emergency department visits per year in the United States and more than 4% of patients with acute abdominal pain. Appendicitis, cholecystitis and choledocholithiasis, intestinal obstruction, pancreatitis, mesenteric ischemia, bowel perforation, and diverticulitis

Table 1–1. Differential diagnosis of acute abdominal pain.

Common Conditions	Key Diagnostic Test(s)
Acute appendicitis	CT scan, ultrasound
Acute cholecystitis	Ultrasound
Choledocholithiasis	Ultrasound, MRCP
Acute diverticulitis	CT scan
Acute pancreatitis	Serum amylase/lipase, CT scan
Bowel perforation	CT scan
Acute mesenteric ischemia	CT angiogram, MRI
Ischemic colitis	CT scan, colonoscopy
Intestinal obstruction	Flat and upright film, CT scan
Anterior abdominal wall pain (in rectus abdominis hematoma)	Carnett sign, Fothergill sign, CT scan
Nonsurgical disorders simulating acute abdomen	See Table 1-2
Acute abdominal pain in women:	HCG, ALT, UA, pelvic examination, pelvic ultrasound, MRI, laparoscopy
• Pelvic inflammatory disease • Ectopic pregnancy • Adnexal pathology	Pelvic examination Ultrasound
Sigmoid volvulus	Barium enema
Biliary duct or pancreatic duct rupture	MRCP, ERCP (technetium-99 sulfur colloid scan)

ALT, alanine transaminase; CT, computed tomography; ERCP, endoscopic retrograde cholangiopancreatography; HCG, human chorionic gonadotropin; MRCP, magnetic resonance cholangiopancreatography; MRI, magnetic resonance imaging; UA, urinalysis.

account for two thirds of hospital admissions for acute abdominal pain and are associated with significant morbidity and mortality. Care must be taken to recognize chronic and nonsurgical causes of abdominal pain that masquerade as surgical disorders and lead to unnecessary surgery, particularly functional disorders.

The initial diagnosis of the patient with acute abdominal pain may be challenging and is often incorrect in the elderly, the young, and women of childbearing age. The history and physical examination remain the critical first step in effective management and must be based on a thorough understanding of the anatomy and physiology of abdominal pain. Laboratory studies are of limited value. Complete blood count (CBC), urinalysis, LFTs, serum lipase, and pregnancy test are most helpful, particularly when abnormal.

Computed tomography (CT) has led to the greatest improvement in the care of patients with acute abdominal pain. Its value for any given patient depends on a given institution's experience in its application and interpretation. A patient's cumulative dose of radiation must always be considered before ordering this examination.

The role of laparoscopy in patient management, particularly in young and pregnant women, remains controversial and hotly debated.

The cause of acute abdominal pain remains unclear at the time of discharge in up to 30% of patients. A long and varied group of nonsurgical disorders must be considered in this subgroup of patients (Table 1–2). The elderly and young

Table 1–2. Nonsurgical disorders causing acute abdominal pain.

Category	Key Diagnostic Feature(s)
Metabolic/Endocrine	
Diabetic ketoacidosis	High serum glucose; ketoacidosis
Hyperthyroidism	High T_4, low TSH
Hypercalcemia	High serum calcium
Hypokalemia	Low serum potassium
Hypophosphatemia	Low serum phosphate
Addison disease	Low serum cortisol, elevated ACTH
Porphyria	High porphobilinogen and delta-ALA
Familial Mediterranean fever	Duration 1–3 days; pleuritis and peritonitis
Vascular/Cardiopulmonary	
Myocardial ischemia/infarction	Abnormal ECG, high troponin
Aortic dissection	Widened mediastinum and diagnostic CT angiogram
Median arcuate ligament syndrome	MRA or CTA
Pneumonia/pleurisy	Chest radiograph
Pulmonary embolus	Wells score, high D-dimer, pulmonary embolism CT angiography
Drug/Toxin	
Salicylate	Tinnitus, confusion, mixed respiratory alkalosis and metabolic acidosis
Anticholinergics	Confusion, dilated pupils, tachycardia, ileus, urinary retention
Tricyclic antidepressants (TCAs)	Delirium, anticholinergic symptoms, ECG changes, serum/urine TCA level
Cocaine	Tachycardia, hypertension, systemic end-organ ischemia, positive toxic screen
Heavy metals	Renal, neurologic toxicity, 24-hour urine assay
Vasculitis/Connective Tissue	
Systemic lupus erythematosus (SLE)	>4 of 11 SLE criteria
Systemic vasculitis	Multiorgan disease with positive P-ANCA and ANA, low complement

(*continued*)

Table 1–2. Nonsurgical disorders causing acute abdominal pain. (continued)

Category	Key Diagnostic Feature(s)
Scleroderma	Skin changes, Raynaud phenomenon and visceral disease, Scl-70
Hematologic/Immunologic	
Sickle cell crisis	History, periarticular pain, effusions
Henoch-Schönlein purpura	Skin biopsy: leukocytoclastic vasculitis with IgA and C3 deposition
Hemolytic uremic syndrome	ARF with schistocytes on smear
Hereditary angioneurotic edema	Low C1 esterase inhibitor level
Systemic mast cell disease	High serum tryptase, urinary histamine, and prostaglandin D_2; increased tissue mast cells; abnormal bone marrow biopsy
Mast cell activation syndrome	Serologic markers as above
Food allergy	History, increased IgE level, challenge; mucosal eosinophilia
Thrombotic thrombocytopenic purpura	Fever, confusion, thrombocytopenia, schistocytes
Infectious	
Staphylotoxin	Fever, hypotension, rash (CDC case definition)
Bornholm disease	Fever, rash, spasmodic pain, enterovirus (coxsackie/echo)
Yersinia enterocolitica	Diarrhea, fever, positive stool culture, ileal inflammation
Tuberculous mesenteritis	Fever, fatigue, diarrhea, RLQ mass and ascites, positive biopsy
Dengue fever	Fever, hemolytic anemia, myalgias/arthralgias, low platelets, high LFTs, positive serology
Malaria	Fever, chill, diaphoresis, hemolytic anemia, myalgia, cough, multiorgan disease, RBC smear
Musculoskeletal	
"Slipping rib" (lower rib margin) syndrome	Production of pain with rib compression only on affected side
Rectus sheath hematoma/neuroma	Carnett and Fothergill signs
Chronic abdominal wall pain syndrome	RUQ (mainly) tenderness and positive Carnett sign
Neuropsychiatric	
Herpes zoster	Unilateral, painful vesicular rash in dermatomal distribution, positive DFA of lesion or PCR of fluid
Abdominal migraine	Adolescents, cyclic occurrence
Temporal lobe seizures	Adolescents, aura, abnormal EEG
Radiculopathy	Mechanical pain in dermatomal distribution, positive MRI
Functional abdominal pain syndrome	See Camilleri, 2006, cited in text
Irritable bowel syndrome	Manning or Rome III criteria
Narcotic bowel syndrome	Recent acceleration or taper of chronic narcotic dose
Renal	
Nephrolithiasis/ureterolithiasis	Hematuria and positive CT
Papillary necrosis	Hematuria, obstructive uropathy, diabetes, sickle cell disease

ACTH, adrenocorticotropic hormone; ANA, antinuclear antibody; ARF, acute renal failure; CDC, Centers for Disease Control and Prevention; CT, computed tomography; CTA, CT angiography; posteroanterior; delta-ALA, delta-aminolevulinic acid (test); DFA, direct fluorescent antibody; ECG, electrocardiogram; EEG, electroencephalogram; IgA, immunoglobulin A; IgE, immunoglobulin E; LFTs, liver function tests; MRA, magnetic resonance angiography; MRI, magnetic resonance imaging; P-ANCA, perinuclear antineutrophilic cytoplasmic antibody; PCR, polymerase chain reaction (amplification); RBC, red blood cell; RLQ, right lower quadrant; RUQ, right upper quadrant; T4, thyroxine; TSH, thyroid-stimulating hormone.

women with functional abdominal pain syndrome (FAPS) represent a large portion of this patient population. A prior diagnosis of irritable bowel syndrome is associated with an increased likelihood of negative appendectomy. Careful consideration with frequent reexamination of the abdomen of patients with undiagnosed acute abdominal pain is strongly advised.

Cartwright SL, Knudson MP. Evaluation of acute abdominal pain in adults. *Am Fam Physician.* 2008;77:971–978. [PMID: 18441863]

Flasar MH, Goldberg E. Acute abdominal pain. *Med Clin North Am.* 2006;90:481–503. [PMID: 16473101]

Langell JT, Mulvihill SJ. Gastrointestinal perforation and the acute abdomen. *Med Clin North Am.* 2008;92:599–625. [PMID: 18387378]

Leschka S, Alkadhi H, Wildermuth S, et al. Multi-detector computed tomography of acute abdomen. *Euro Radiol.* 2005;15:2435–2447. [PMID: 16132914]

Pearigen PD. Unusual causes of abdominal pain. *Emerg Med Clin North Am.* 1996;14:593–613. [PMID: 8681886]

Shanley CJ, Weinberger JB. Acute abdominal vascular emergencies. *Med Clin North Am.* 2008;92:627–647. [PMID: 18387379]

Singh VK, Wu BU, Bollen TL, et al. A prospective evaluation of the bedside index for severity in acute pancreatitis score in assessing mortality and intermediate markers of severity in acute pancreatitis. *Am J Gastroenterol.* 2009;104:966–971. [PMID: 19293787]

Singh VK, Wu BU, Bollen TL, et al. Early systemic inflammatory response syndrome is associated with severe acute pancreatitis. *Clin Gastroenterol Hepatol.* 2009;7:1247–1251. [PMID: 19686869]

Turner D, Seow CH, Greenberg GR, et al. A systematic prospective comparison of noninvasive disease activity indices in ulcerative colitis. *Clin Gastroenterol Hepatol.* 2009;7:1081–1088. [PMID: 19577010]

ACUTE ABDOMINAL PAIN IN THE ELDERLY

Fifty percent of elderly patients with acute abdominal pain are admitted to the hospital, and 33% of them eventually undergo surgery. It may be very difficult to obtain an accurate history due to multiple sources of medical care, including family and friends, and to altered mental status. Physical and laboratory findings may be subtle due to the presence of malnutrition, medications such as β-blockers, physiologic hypothermia, and diminished T-cell function or leukocyte response. Altered mental status and hypotension may be the sole indicators of serious intra-abdominal disease. Upwards of 40% of the elderly do not have a clear diagnosis at discharge.

Flasar MH, Goldberg E. Acute abdominal pain. *Med Clin North Am.* 2006;90:481–503. [PMID: 16473101]

NONSURGICAL DISORDERS SIMULATING THE ACUTE ABDOMEN

A considerable number of emergency admissions for acute abdominal pain conclude without a definite diagnosis. Functional disorders occupy a large portion of this patient group. Recurrent episodes have been reported in up to 30% of patients and may signify abuse at home. Irritable bowel syndrome, when postinfectious, can demonstrate mucosal inflammatory changes. Chronic abdominal wall pain (CAWP) and FAPS may be distinguished from each other by the patient's response to food ingestion and the character of bowel movements. Constitutional symptoms are usually absent. Obstacles to proper diagnosis include experiential, psychosocial, anatomic, and pathophysiologic factors. Narcotic bowel syndrome was first described in 1984. It may appear in patients with previously normal digestive tracts and has become more common with the increasing use of narcotics for the treatment of functional abdominal pain. It is often misdiagnosed, and symptoms mimic FAPS. Imaging may suggest bowel obstruction (ie, pseudo-obstruction). Of note, a patient may be unchanged or have markedly worse pain with increase or decrease in dose of narcotic.

Adverse reactions to food (ARFs) are common, affecting up to 20% of the adult population. They may be immune mediated (immunoglobulin E [IgE]–mediated, eosinophilic syndromes) or nonimmunologic.

The diagnosis of mast cell activation syndrome (MCAS) needs to be considered in all patients with recurrent acute abdominal pain especially after negative studies for standard blood tests, upper and lower endoscopy, and imaging studies (ie, CT scan, ultrasound). The cardinal factors in addition to recurrent acute abdominal pain, are (1) female sex, (2) flushing, (3) dermatographism, (4) diarrhea, (5) alcohol intolerance, (6) episodes of mental fogginess (ie, inability to concentrate), (7) headaches, and (8) increased sweating. Eighty percent of patients have the triad of abdominal pain, flushing, and dermatographism. Confirmatory laboratory studies are elevated urine histamine and prostaglandin D_2 and increased serum tryptase. It is especially important to suspect this diagnosis in patients with the above clinical features because the response to therapy with histamine H_1 and histamine H_2 antagonists and other mast cell mediators is often quite dramatic.

Camilleri M. Management of patients with chronic abdominal pain in clinical practice. *Neurogastroenterol Motil.* 2006;18:499–506. [PMID: 16771765]

Choung RS, Locke GR 3rd, Zinsmeister AR, et al. Opioid bowel dysfunction and narcotic bowel syndrome: a population-based study. *Am J Gastroenterol.* 2009;104:1199–1204. [PMID: 19367263]

Costanza CD, Longstreth GF, Liu AL. Chronic abdominal wall pain: clinical features, health care costs, and long-term outcome. *Clin Gastroenterol Hepatol.* 2004;2:395–399. [PMID: 15118977]

Degaetani MA, Crowe SE. A 41-year-old woman with abdominal complaints: is it food allergy or food intolerance? How to tell the difference. *Clin Gastroenterol Hepatol.* 2010;8:755–759. [PMID: 20363367]

Grunkemeier DM, Cassara JE, Dalton CB, et al. The narcotic bowel syndrome: clinical features, pathophysiology, and management. *Clin Gastroenterol Hepatol.* 2007;5:1126–1139. [PMID: 17916540]

Hamilton MJ, Hornick JL, Akin C, et al. Mast cell activation syndrome—a newly recognized disorder with systemic manifestations. *J Allergy Clin Immunol.* 2011;128:147–152. [PMID: 21621255].

Longstreth GF. Avoiding unnecessary surgery in irritable bowel syndrome. *Gut.* 2007;56:608–610. [PMID: 17440179]

Marshall JK, Thabane M, Garg AX, et al. Eight year prognosis of postinfectious irritable bowel syndrome following waterborne bacterial dysentery. *Gut.* 2010;59:605–611. [PMID: 20427395]

Pearigen PD. Unusual causes of abdominal pain. *Emerg Med Clin North Am.* 1996;14:593–613. [PMID: 8681886]

Weijenborg PT, Gardien K, Toorenvliet BR, et al. Acute abdominal pain in women at an emergency department: predictors of chronicity. *Eur J Pain.* 2010;14:183–188. [PMID: 19419889]

Youssef NN, Atienza K, Langseder AL, et al. Chronic abdominal pain and depressive symptoms: analysis of the national longitudinal study of adolescent health. *Clin Gastroenterol Hepatol.* 2008;6:329–332. [PMID: 18258491]

EVALUATION OF THE ACUTE ABDOMEN

Medical History

"More errors in diagnosis are traceable to a lack of acumen in eliciting or interpreting symptoms than have ever been caused by failure to hear a murmur, feel a mass or take an electrocardiogram."—F. Dennette Adams, 1958

A proper medical history of acute abdominal pain must begin with consideration of the point of contact with the patient. A complaint of left lower quadrant (LLQ) pain and irregularity by telephone at 3 PM in the deep of winter from a 24-year-old mother of three busy at her second job most likely will represent a differential diagnosis different from that of a 75-year-old woman at 1 AM with a temperature of 101°F who has recently received outpatient chemotherapy for stage IV ovarian cancer.

The clinician can better localize the organ responsible for pain by first determining in what region of the abdomen the patient experiences distress (Figure 1–1). A distinction should first be drawn between pain from a *visceral* source and that from a *somatic* source (ie, peritoneum) by noting whether the patient describes the slow-onset, poorly localized, dull discomfort typical of the former or the sudden, sharp, well-localized, lateralizing distress of the latter. It must be remembered that *visceral* pain may be *referred* to a location distant from the affected organ, mimicking somatic pain, when its autonomic fibers enter a spinal cord segment shared by an unrelated spinothalamic pathway. Pain out of proportion to physical findings should always raise a concern for mesenteric ischemia. The patient's perception of pain represents the sum effects of the patient's age, mental status, and medications. Newly recognized physiologic moderators of pain perception include visceral hyperalgesia and impaired inhibitory nociception. Cultural experience, socioeconomic status, a history of physical and mental abuse, and prior experience with medical professionals and illness also come into play.

Physical Examination

The examination of the abdomen in a patient with acute pain remains an important tool and, with a proper history, will yield the correct diagnosis at least 50% of the time. The quality of physical examinations performed by recent trainees has been found to be deficient. There must be continued emphasis on the physical examination in training programs, particularly as reliance on imaging studies increases. Narcotic pain medication may alter the physical findings but not to a degree that will affect diagnostic accuracy or management.

The clinician can distinguish painful chest and abdominal wall disorders from intra-abdominal disease with several simple bedside maneuvers. Distress from a so-called slipping rib (also termed a lower rib margin syndrome) can be elicited by grasping the costal (usually left) margin with the fingers and then gently pulling up. Pain due to a rectus sheath hematoma, muscle tear, or postoperative neuroma can be elicited by Carnett sign and Fothergill sign. In Carnett sign, the patient who complains of an area of tenderness during conventional palpation is asked to tense the abdominal wall with neck flexion (protecting the abdominal viscera and cavity from the pressure of the examiner's hands), and the abdomen is then reexamined. If the patient's discomfort worsens, it suggests a disorder of the abdominal wall. If it lessens, an intra-abdominal process is more likely. In Fothergill sign, a rectus sheath hematoma produces a painful, tender mass that does not cross the midline and remains palpable when the rectus is contracted.

Cherry WB, Mueller PS. Rectus sheath hematoma: review of 126 cases at a single institution. *Medicine (Baltimore).* 2006;85:105–110. [PMID: 16609349]

Elsenbruch S, Rosenberger C, Bingel U, et al. Patients with irritable bowel syndrome have altered emotional modulation of neural responses to visceral stimuli. *Gastroenterology.* 2010;139:1310–1319. [PMID: 20600024]

Olesen SS, Brock C, Krarup AL, et al. Descending inhibitory pain modulation is impaired in patients with chronic pancreatitis. *Clin Gastroenterol Hepatol.* 2010;8:724–730. [PMID: 20304100]

Ranji SR, Goldman LE, Simel DL, et al. Do opiates affect the clinical evaluation of patients with acute abdominal pain? *JAMA.* 2006;296:1764–1774. [PMID: 17032990]

Laboratory Studies

The misinterpretation of basic laboratory tests can lead to errors in diagnosis and patient management, and any recommended list must be used with caution. Overinterpretation (eg, leukocytosis in a patient on corticosteroids) or underinterpretation (eg, normal white blood cell count in a patient who is elderly or undergoing chemotherapy) of results is not uncommon. White blood cell count and hematocrit may be normal in a patient with an incipient intra-abdominal catastrophe. A normal urinalysis does not exclude nephrolithiasis. Electrocardiogram and chest radiograph do not exclude cardiovascular or pulmonary disease. A pregnancy test must always be performed in a woman of childbearing age. Patients are often sicker than their laboratory studies suggest, particularly if they are elderly, immunosuppressed, or pregnant.

Imaging Studies

The role of imaging in the evaluation and management of the patient with acute abdominal pain has been revolutionized by abdominal ultrasound, multidetector-row computed tomography (MDCT), and magnetic resonance imaging (MRI). The physician's choice of imaging study must take into account the patient's likely diagnosis, clinical condition, and cumulative radiation dose. Is the study safe, available, and easy to interpret? Does it have therapeutic value? MDCT remains the "gold standard" because of its high sensitivity, its specificity in global evaluation of acute and chronic abdominal

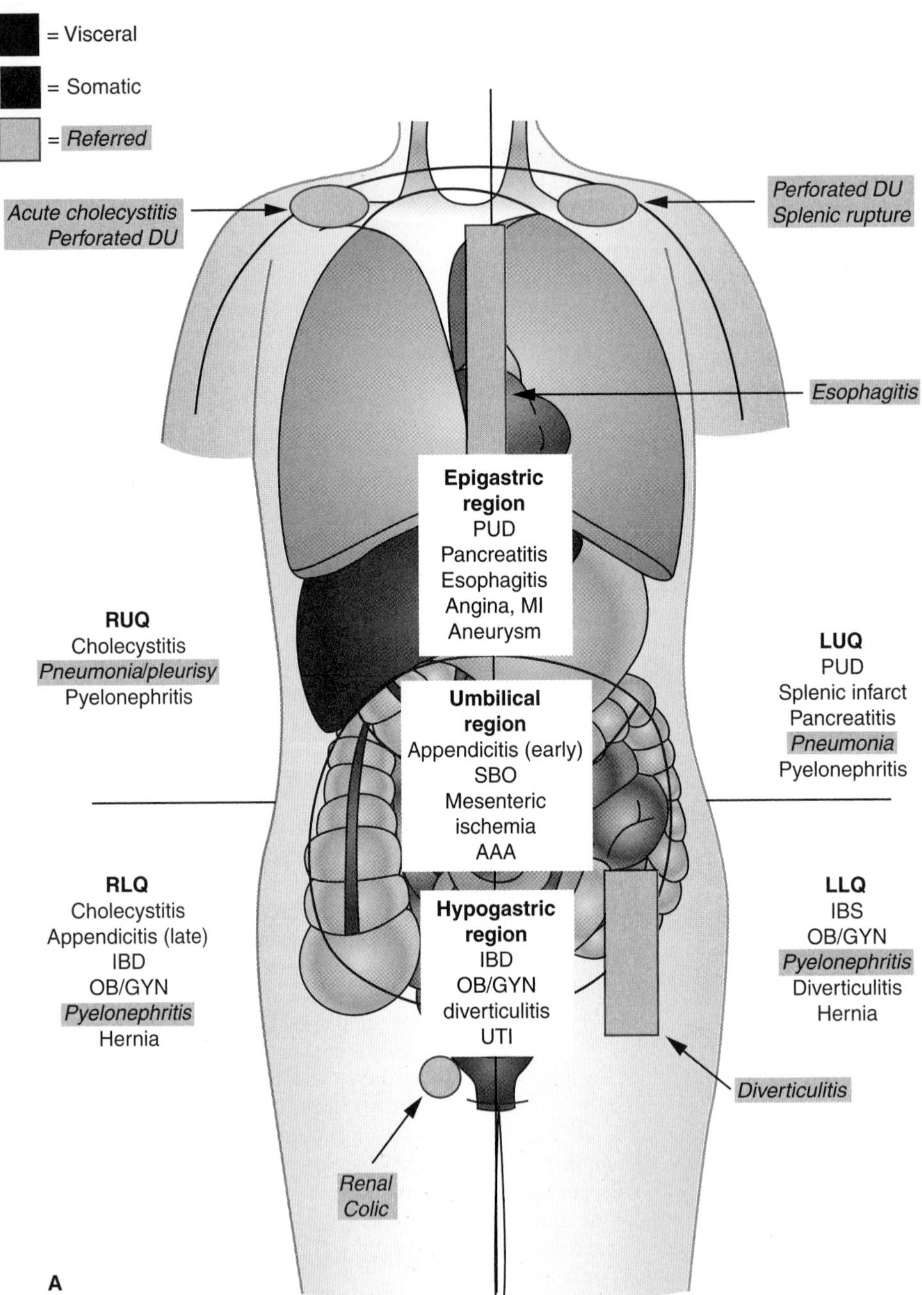

▲ **Figure 1–1.** Anatomy of abdominal pain: most frequent pain sites. **A.** Anterior view. **B.** Posterior view. AAA, abdominal aortic aneurysm; DU, duodenal ulcer; IBD, inflammatory bowel disease; IBS, irritable bowel syndrome; LLQ, left lower quadrant; LUQ, left upper quadrant; MI, myocardial infarction; OB/GYN, obstetric/gynecologic conditions; PUD, peptic ulcer disease; RLQ, right lower quadrant; RUQ, right upper quadrant; SBO, small bowel obstruction; UTI, urinary tract infection. (Used with permission from Frederick L. Makrauer, MD.)

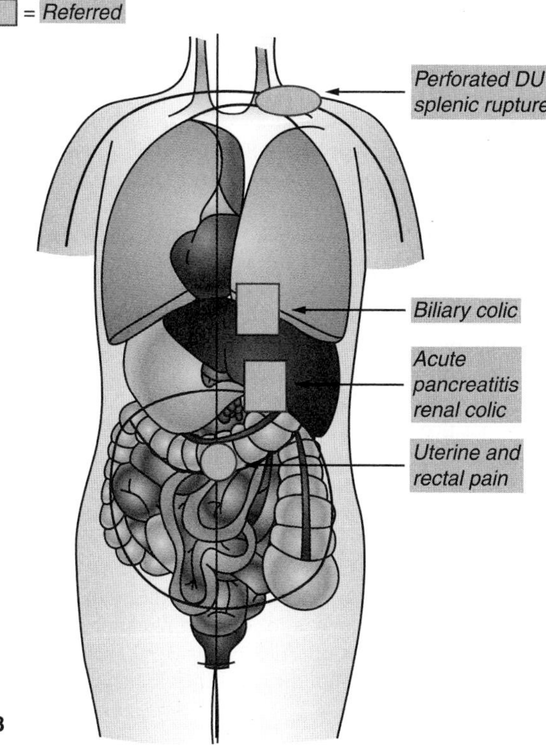

▲ **Figure 1–1.** (*Continued*)

pain, and the value of unexpected additional information that it yields. Ultrasound should always be the first consideration in the young, in women of childbearing age, and in the pursuit of biliary tract disease. MRI, also free of ionizing radiation, has particular value in the pursuit of biliary and pancreatic pathology. The most effective abdominal imaging methods currently available and their applications are discussed further in Chapters 9, 35, and 36. Detailed information about each imaging modality is provided in those chapters.

Cartwright SL, Knudson MP. Evaluation of acute abdominal pain in adults. *Am Fam Physician.* 2008;77:971–978. [PMID: 18441863]

Dixon AK, Watson CJ. Imaging in patients with acute abdominal pain. *BMJ.* 2009;338:b1678. [PMID: 19561055]

Karla MK, Francis IR. Personalized dose reduction for computed tomography scanning: size matters, so does prior radiation exposures. *Clin Gastroenterol Hepatol.* 2010;8:231–232. [PMID: 20005984]

Laméris W, van Randen A, van Es HW, et al. Imaging strategies for detection of urgent conditions in patients with acute abdominal pain: diagnostic accuracy study. *BMJ.* 2009;338:b2431. [PMID: 19561056]

Leschka S, Alkadhi H, Wildermuth S, et al. Multi-detector computed tomography of acute abdomen. *Euro Radiol.* 2005;15:2435–2447. [PMID: 16132914]

Pedrosa I, Rofsky NM. MR imaging in abdominal emergencies. *Radiol Clin North Am.* 2003;41:1243–1273. [PMID: 14661669]

ACUTE APPENDICITIS

General Considerations

Acute appendicitis is very common, with a lifetime risk of 7–8% that favors males slightly. Appendectomy is the most commonly performed emergency operation in the world. The reported incidence has dropped by more than 50% in the past three decades for unknown reasons. Over 250,000 patients per year are admitted for the management of appendicitis in the United States, with the highest incidence in the second and third decades of life. The rate of appendiceal perforation may be up to 80%. Mortality has dropped to less than 1% with more timely and accurate diagnosis in high-risk groups and advancements in imaging techniques. Delayed diagnosis in women, the elderly, and African Americans remains a concern.

The pathogenesis of acute appendicitis is bacterial proliferation secondary to luminal obstruction due to one of multiple disorders, including cytomegalovirus or adenovirus enteritis, Crohn disease, stone, foreign body, or tumor. The presentation of appendicitis depends on the patient's age, appendiceal length, body habitus, and trimester of pregnancy. The "classic" presentation (acute periumbilical pain migrating to McBurney point, followed by nausea and vomiting) occurs in only 30–60% of patients.

The perforation rate may reach 50–70% and is directly proportional to a delay in diagnosis of more than 24 hours. The elderly experience a mortality rate from appendicitis that is eightfold greater than that of the general population and accounts for 50% of all deaths from this disorder. Increased body mass index and smoking have also recently been implicated as risk factors for a complicated course.

Diagnosis is particularly challenging in the young and the elderly, as well as during pregnancy.

Grynspan D, Rabah R. Adenoviral appendicitis presenting clinically as acute appendicitis. *Pediatr Dev Pathol.* 2008;11:138–141. [PMID: 17990936]

Ingraham AM, Cohen ME, Bilimoria KY, et al. Effect of delay to operation on outcomes in adults with acute appendicitis. *Arch Surg.* 2010;145:886–892. [PMID: 20855760]

Papadopoulos AA, Polymeros D, Kateri M, et al. Dramatic decline of acute appendicitis in Greece over 30 years: index of improvement of socioeconomic conditions or diagnostic aids? *Dig Dis.* 2008;26:80–84. [PMID: 18277072]

Clinical Findings

A. Symptoms and Signs

The history and abdominal examination may vary depending on the location of the appendix. Diagnosis is delayed, and thus perforation occurs more commonly, in very young (<3 years), pregnant, and elderly (>64 years old) patients, the latter presenting atypically more than 70% of the time. Socioeconomic status, but not race, may also influence perforation rate.

The atypical location of the appendix in the third trimester of pregnancy represents a particular diagnostic challenge (see Figure 7–3). Fever may be low grade.

Pieracci FM, Eachempati SR, Barie PS, et al. Insurance status, but not race, predicts perforation in adult patients with acute appendicitis. *J Am Coll Surg.* 2007;205:445–452. [PMID: 17765161]

B. Laboratory Findings

Routine laboratory studies have limited value in the diagnosis of acute appendicitis. Leukocytosis may be modest or absent. Chemistry studies and urinalysis are usually normal. A pregnancy test must always be ordered in a woman of childbearing age.

C. Imaging Studies

1. Issues and controversies—The pathophysiology and imaging abnormalities of acute appendicitis are due to luminal obstruction, regardless of etiology. The advantage of preoperative imaging compared with clinical assessment alone continues to be challenged by some studies. Several centers have reported increased time to the operating room, operating time, length of stay, and cost without a reduction in negative appendectomy rate in patients whose surgery is postponed for the performance of CT (or ultrasound). On the other hand, even in patients with a high clinical probability of appendicitis, almost one third of those imaged will be found to have another diagnosis or a normal scan (Table 1–3). We believe the preceding discrepancies are largely due to variability in institutional experience and recommend that cross-sectional imaging (CT, MRI, or ultrasound) be performed in *all* patients suspected of having acute appendicitis, even those patients with high-probability clinical presentations (see Figure 9–17).

CT scan with an appendicitis protocol is appropriate in the majority of patients. The advantage of rectal contrast remains a matter of continued discussion.

2. Ultrasound—Ultrasound has a sensitivity and negative predictive value of nearly 98% and 100%, respectively, with a specificity of 70–100%. Results are highly operator dependent.

Findings suggestive of acute appendicitis include a thickened, blind-ended lumen (as opposed to an open-ended salpinx or gonadal vein) with a diameter greater than 6 mm that is noncompressible and fluid-filled and the presence of an appendicolith. There may be tenderness on compression. Ultrasound should be used as the sole imaging modality only for patients with a high probability of the disorder. False-positive findings occur commonly (33% of the time) in patients with inflammatory bowel disease, cecal diverticulitis, and pelvic inflammatory disease. The value of ultrasound is limited in morbidly obese patients, in the presence of perforation or a retrocecal position, and when there is inability to compress the right lower quadrant (RLQ).

Ultrasound should be considered as the study of choice in groups most vulnerable to ionizing radiation, especially children and women of childbearing age. The additional information gained about the female pelvic anatomy can also be clinically valuable.

3. CT scan—A contrast-enhanced helical CT scan performed for acute appendicitis is 96–98% sensitive and 83–89% specific, particularly with the demonstration of an appendicolith. MDCT may improve specificity even more. Positive findings include a diameter greater than 6 mm, thickened wall with enhancement, periappendiceal fat stranding, and appendicolith. An air-filled appendix on CT essentially excludes acute appendicitis.

Table 1–3. Value of preoperative imaging in acute appendicitis.

Final Operative Diagnosis	Clinical Presentation: Low Probability (n = 109)	Intermediate Probability (n = 97)	High Probability (n = 144)
Acute appendicitis	11 (10%)	23 (24%)	99 (65%)
Other	34 (31%)	37 (38%)	26 (18%)
Inflammatory bowel disease	7 (6%)	9 (9%)	6 (4%)
Enteritis	15 (14%)	8 (8%)	1 (<1%)
Right-sided diverticulitis	0 (0%)	1 (1%)	5 (3%)
Ovarian cyst	3 (3%)	3 (3%)	1 (<1%)
Normal findings	64 (59%)	37 (38%)	24 (17%)

Focal thickening of the terminal ileum or cecum may be confused with Crohn disease, and appendiceal dilation may be falsely attributed to an infected right fallopian tube. An ovoid fat-attenuation focus with hyperattenuating rim near the colonic serosa distinguishes epiploic appendagitis. Infectious enteritis should be easily differentiated by the diffuse nature of bowel thickening and enhancement in the presence of a normal appendix. Less common mimics include mucocele of the appendix, ovarian disorders, and endometriosis. An advantage of CT over ultrasound is its ability to visualize the entire abdomen, demonstrating an alternative diagnosis in 15% of cases. An additional 15% of patients will be found to be normal.

A high clinical index of suspicion for acute appendicitis mandates the use of a dedicated appendicitis protocol with intravenous and rectal contrast alone, reducing the time of study to only 15 minutes by eliminating the administration of oral contrast. CT scan during pregnancy must be used with great discretion; ultrasound or MRI is recommended. The lack of a reduction in the published rate of negative appendectomy since the introduction of CT most likely reflects inconsistent performance standards.

Rettenbacher T, Hollerweger A, Gritzmann N, et al. Appendicitis: should diagnostic imaging be performed if the clinical presentation is highly suggestive of the disease? *Gastroenterology.* 2002;123:992–998. [PMID: 12360459]

Differential Diagnosis

The differential diagnosis of acute appendicitis is broad, reflecting classic and atypical presentations of the disorder. It includes mesenteric lymphadenitis, bacterial enteritis, acute diverticulitis, ureteral calculus, Crohn disease, cholecystitis, appendagitis epiploica, Meckel diverticulitis, and several gynecologic disorders including acute salpingitis (pelvic inflammatory disease), ruptured ovarian follicle (mittelschmerz), and ruptured ectopic pregnancy. These disorders are reviewed in ensuing chapters, and only epiploic appendagitis will be discussed below in detail.

Treatment

A. Overview

Surgery has been recognized since 1886 as the definitive treatment for appendicitis. Active debate continues regarding the proper timing and choice of technique (ie, open appendectomy vs laparoscopic appendectomy) and what variables influence these decisions. The incidence of negative appendectomy remains as high as 20% in some patient groups, especially young women and patients with preexisting irritable bowel syndrome. Women aged 15–45 years have a 20% negative appendectomy rate, two to five times that of the general population, attributed to the multiple other causes for acute pelvic pain and the atypical location of the appendix in late pregnancy.

Clyde C, Bax T, Merg A, et al. Timing of intervention does not affect outcome in acute appendicitis in a large community practice. *Am J Surg.* 2008;195:590–593. [PMID: 18367138]

Ditillo MF, Dziura JD, Rabinovici R. Is it safe to delay appendectomy in adults with acute appendicitis? *Ann Surg.* 2006;244: 656–660. [PMID: 17060754]

Howell JM, Eddy OL, Lukens TW, et al. Clinical policy: critical issues in the evaluation and management of emergency department patients with suspected appendicitis. *Ann Emerg Med.* 2010;55:71–116. [PMID: 20116016]

Longstreth GF. Avoiding unnecessary surgery in irritable bowel syndrome. *Gut.* 2007;56:608–610. [PMID: 17440179]

B. Antibiotics

A third-generation intravenous cephalosporin may be initiated preoperatively in patients who are mildly ill. Sicker patients with signs of perforation and sepsis require broader coverage for anaerobes, including *Bacteroides.* Continuation of antibiotics postoperatively will depend on the surgical findings and the patient's clinical response. Antibiotic therapy as the sole treatment for acute appendicitis must be undertaken with great circumspection and extreme caution based on the current literature.

C. Interventional Radiology

Appendiceal rupture or abscess is found in 25% of patients at presentation. When an abscess is found on imaging, CT-guided drainage and dedicated parenteral antibiotic therapy should be considered the preferred alternative to immediate appendectomy. Interval appendectomy after resolution of the collection should then be performed at a later date. The final decision must be made by the surgeon after consultation with the gastroenterologist and radiologist.

D. Surgery

Surgery remains the treatment of choice for acute appendicitis. The timing and type of surgical approach for acute appendicitis is now the most debated aspect of management, with a balance sought between the desire for accurate diagnosis and stabilization of the patient versus prevention of perforation. Prevention of perforation remains a major goal, and the rate of perforation has become a quality-of-care indicator in some institutions. The identification of predictors more reliable than patient age and gender has been a challenge. A brief voluntary delay to perform diagnostic studies, begin antibiotics, or accommodate staffing needs has not been proven to increase the risk of complications, including perforation. A patient with a late or atypical presentation may actually benefit from a period of observation with the administration of antibiotics, while the gastroenterologist obtains additional history and reviews the imaging studies and the response to therapy with the surgeon or gynecologist/obstetrician. Primary therapy of acute appendicitis with antibiotics has been used when surgical intervention is not readily available or if antibiotics are deemed necessary by a surgeon prior to operation.

Laparoscopic appendectomy has gained increasing support as the operation of choice. Patients have fewer wound infections, less pain, and shorter hospital stays compared with those undergoing open cholecystectomy. The surgeon must first consider the degree of diagnostic certainty, imaging evidence for complicating disease, stage of appendicitis, and experience with the technique. Recent retrospective data suggest that race and insurance status may affect the decision. Debate continues over which procedure is medically appropriate, but in women, particularly during pregnancy, there appears to be a clear advantage to laparoscopic appendectomy associated with the ability to identify other gynecologic pathology and reduce the rate of negative appendectomy. Negative appendectomy rate, in women inversely proportional to fetal health, is becoming another benchmark for determining the proper procedure in any given institution. In men, the benefit of laparoscopic appendectomy is less well established. As noted earlier, the surgical experience in an institution must always be considered before a final choice of laparoscopic versus open cholecystectomy is made.

The resected appendix may reveal unexpected and clinically useful data in 2% of cases and, therefore, should always be submitted for histologic analysis. Surgeons should continue to submit the resected appendix for histologic analysis.

Jones AE, Phillips AW, Jarvis JR, et al. The value of routine histopathological examination of appendectomy specimens. *BMC Surg.* 2007;7:17. [PMID: 17692116]

Paterson HM, Qadan M, de Luca SM, et al. Changing trends in surgery for acute appendicitis. *Br J Surg.* 2008;95:363–368. [PMID: 17939131]

UNIQUE PRESENTATIONS OF APPENDICITIS

1. Appendicitis in Pregnancy (see Chapter 7)

Appendicitis occurs in approximately 1 in 800–1500 pregnancies, and appendectomy is the most common nonobstetric operation performed during pregnancy. The presence of the fetus and altered appendiceal location provide a major clinical challenge. Preoperative diagnosis is inaccurate 25–50% of the time. Maternal death is now virtually zero, but fetal loss is 2–3% without and 20% with appendiceal perforation. Appendiceal rupture is reported in 12–55% of pregnant women.

The proper choice of imaging in women with appendicitis has been discussed earlier. The risk of fetal harm from exposure to ionizing radiation of CT must be compared with the relatively reduced accuracy of ultrasound, especially in the third trimester. The imaging expertise in one's own institution, particularly in view of the increasing role of MRI, remains very important and should factor into the clinician's final choice of study.

Negative appendectomy is higher in pregnant (23%) than nonpregnant (18%) women and carries a 2.69 increased odds ratio for fetal loss. The goal of eliminating negative appendectomy during pregnancy with improvement in preoperative assessment must be balanced with the delay in surgical therapy and expected increase in complicated appendicitis and perforation. Laparoscopic appendectomy for the experienced surgeon appears safe and effective.

McGory ML, Zingmond DS, Tillou A, et al. Negative appendectomy in pregnant women is associated with a substantial risk of fetal loss. *J Am Coll Surg.* 2007;205:534–540. [PMID: 17903726]

2. Atypical Appendicitis

Retrocecal (ileal) appendicitis presents with less pain and rigidity due to shielding from the abdominal wall. In addition, localization of discomfort may be ill defined due to the lack of appendix contact with the peritoneum, and it is less common in the RLQ.

Pelvic appendicitis is characterized by severe, constant pain usually in the LLQ, with fecal and urinary urgency. Abdominal tenderness is variable, but severe tenderness on pelvic and rectal examination may be present. Atypical appendicitis is more common in the elderly but is considered less frequently as a cause for acute abdominal pain. Pain is vague and is present in the RLQ in only 20% of patients. There may be no fever. The abdominal examination may yield only a nontender mass. The white blood cell count can be lower than expected.

Proper management relies on a high index of suspicion, careful patient assessment, and CT findings.

3. Late ("Delayed") Appendicitis

Late appendicitis is defined as presentation following more than 72 hours of symptoms. It occurs most often in the young, the elderly, and women of childbearing age because accurate diagnosis is most difficult in these groups. A phlegmon may be palpable in the RLQ or be seen on CT, usually with an abscess component. Accurate diagnosis is difficult due to the surrounding inflammatory response. Crohn disease, infection, and neoplasm are part of the differential diagnosis. Malignancy (carcinoid, colonic adenocarcinoma, lymphoma, and ovarian cancer) may be present in 1% of cases. Studies of late appendicitis are retrospective, occurring before advanced CT imaging was widely available. Thirty percent of patients required a drainage procedure as their initial surgery, and appendectomy was usually postponed until abdominal sepsis could be controlled.

Patients should be kept NPO (nothing by mouth) with intravenous fluids and antibiotics. A nontoxic patient (without tachycardia, abdominal rigidity, or oliguria) should avoid immediate surgical intervention, if possible, to improve diagnostic accuracy and prevent recurrent episodes. The indications for percutaneous drainage of an abscess depend on the collection, size, consistency, and accessibility as well as the patient's stability. Percutaneous drainage as the sole treatment for delayed appendicitis is not recommended because the recurrence rate for abscess without appendectomy is 5–20%. Colonoscopy has a role in the preoperative and postoperative management of patients who are stable and have both clinical and radiographic features of ileocolonic Crohn disease. Note that the appendix can be involved in ileocolonic Crohn disease and obfuscate the diagnosis in patients with acute RLQ abdominal pain.

No clinical criteria have been developed to predict the clinical outcome of delayed appendectomy or the ideal timing of appendectomy. Curative surgery, ideally by laparoscopy, is usually performed within 2–3 months.

4. Chronic ("Recurrent," "Subacute") Appendicitis

Five to ten percent of patients with a surgical diagnosis of acute appendicitis may have had a previous attack, and 1.5% will have had symptoms for more than 3 weeks. Such observations have led to the description of a subset of patients with so-called chronic appendicitis. The literature is entirely retrospective, and no clinical distinction has been drawn between patients found to have a normal appendix at appendectomy and those with an inflamed appendix. Fibrosis with luminal obliteration has been described but not fistula or abscess. The role of appendectomy for such patients is controversial because they appear to represent a distinct clinical group without the poor prognosis associated with "late" or "delayed" appendicitis.

5. Epiploic Appendagitis

Epiploic appendagitis is very uncommon. In 70% of patients, illness is triggered by torsion with ischemia and pain in one or more of the approximately 100 epiploic (or omental) appendages that arise from the serosal surface of the colon. These appendages are oriented in two rows and are composed of adipose tissue and a vascular stalk, 0.5–5 cm in length. Less common manifestations are incarceration (20%) and obstruction (10%). The condition occurs more often in men, primarily in the fourth to fifth decades; and mimics acute appendicitis, diverticulitis, mesenteritis, and omental infraction with the acute onset of RLQ or LLQ pain often after eating or exercise in a previously healthy person. Risk factors are obesity, hernia, and physical inactivity. Fever and obstructive symptoms are uncommon. The white blood cell count is normal. Preoperative diagnosis is uncommon even with the availability of sensitive ultrasound and CT technology. CT findings, when present, consist of 2- to 4-cm, oval, fat-density lesions with surrounding inflammation and central attenuation. Unlike diverticulitis, colon wall thickness and diameter are normal. It is important to make the diagnosis so as to avoid unnecessary surgery. The prognosis is considered benign, but one study reported a 40% recurrence rate. Surgery, when performed for recurrent symptoms, involves resection of the inflamed appendages.

Sand M, Gelos M, Bechara FG, et al. Epiploic appendicitis—clinical characteristics of an uncommon surgical diagnosis. *BMC Surg.* 2007;7:11. [PMID: 17603914]

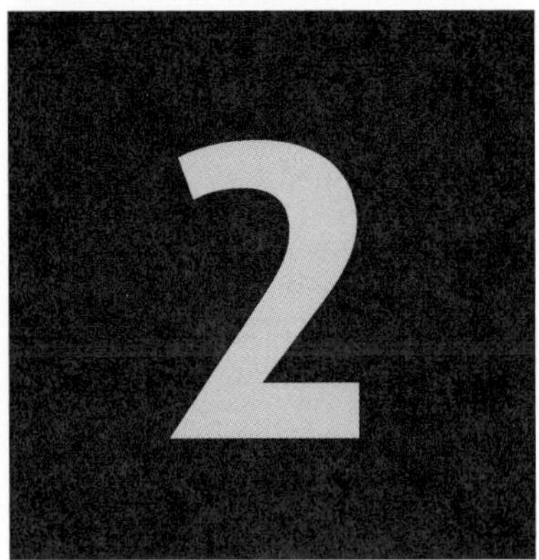

Inflammatory Bowel Disease: Immunologic Considerations & Therapeutic Implications

Richard S. Blumberg, MD
Scott B. Snapper, MD, PhD

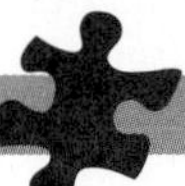

ESSENTIAL CONCEPTS

- Gut-associated lymphoid tissues (GALT) are characterized by a unique structure, physiologic inflammation, a tendency to suppress immune responses (oral tolerance), and production of secretory immunoglobulins.
- The immune response has two major arms: innate (rapid, hard-wired) and adaptive (delayed in onset with memory).
- Inflammatory bowel disease (IBD) offers a paradigm for understanding and treating intestinal inflammatory diseases.
- IBD is a dysregulated immune response of GALT to normal commensal microbes within the intestines of a genetically susceptible host; this response is modified by specific environmental factors (eg, tobacco).
- Numerous genetic loci defined as risk factors for IBD regulate innate immunity, adaptive immunity, the epithelial barrier, and the relationships of each of these with normal commensal microbiota (bacterial and nonbacterial).
- IBD is ultimately caused by overproduction of proinflammatory mediators relative to anti-inflammatory mediators, both of which are derived from cells associated with adaptive immunity (T helper [Th] cells) and innate immunity (macrophages and dendritic cells).
- Crohn disease (CD) preferentially exhibits overactivity of Th1 and Th17 cells, and ulcerative colitis (UC) may exhibit overactivity of Th2 cells.
- Excess production of cytokines derived from innate immune pathways (tumor necrosis factor [TNF] and interleukin-6 [IL-6]) occurs in both CD and UC.
- T regulatory cells secrete anti-inflammatory cytokines (eg, IL-10, transforming growth factor-β [TGFβ], and IL-35) that inhibit proinflammatory cytokine responses from innate and adaptive immune cells.
- Increased understanding of IBD immunopathogenesis has led to development of anti-inflammatory therapeutic agents that are increasingly being administered in a logical, mechanism-based manner.

General Considerations

Clinically, inflammatory bowel disease (IBD) is a chronic inflammatory condition of the intestines that is marked by remission and relapses and distills clinically into one of two major subtypes of disease: ulcerative colitis (UC) and Crohn disease (CD). Both diseases have a general commonality in their pathogenesis and are derived from a dysregulated mucosal immune response to antigenic components of the normal commensal microbiota that reside within the intestine in a genetically susceptible host (Figure 2–1).

This tripartite interaction between the genetic composition of the host, the mucosal immune response (including that associated with the epithelial barrier), and its relationship to the commensal microbiota is likely further modified by specific environmental factors that affect the lifetime risk of developing this disorder. *Although the influence of specific gene variations, as endogenous risk factors that clearly define susceptibility to this disease, is well accepted, only a limited number of environmental factors have clearly been proven to either modify these diseases or regulate the lifetime risk of developing them. These include tobacco use, enteropathogenic exposures, appendectomy, antibiotic use, and oral contraceptive pills. These do not, in and of themselves, cause the disease but likely modify the genetically defined or undefined aspects of the most critical components that underlie the immunopathogenesis of this disease: intestinal bacteria, epithelial barrier, and mucosal immune response.* Of the latter three factors, the best understood influence—which has, to date, generated the most information, resulting in novel and exciting new forms of therapy—involves the mucosal

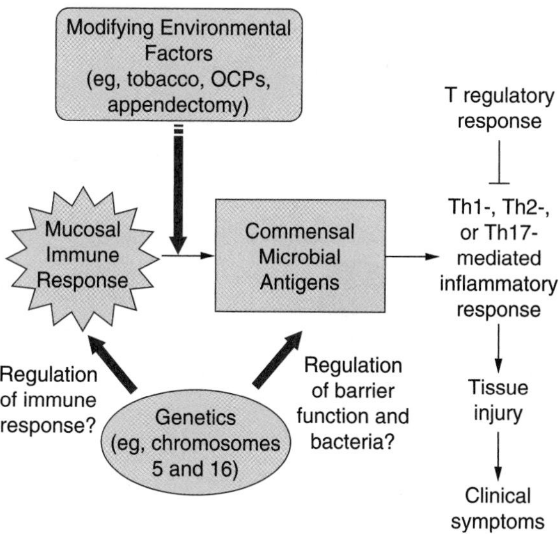

▲ **Figure 2–1.** Pathophysiologic mechanism of inflammatory bowel disease (IBD). IBD represents the dysregulated mucosal immune response to commensal microbial antigens in a genetically susceptible host that is modified by environmental factors. An exaggerated T-cell response of polarized T cells that secrete T helper (Th) 1, 2, or 17 cytokines causes tissue injury and clinical symptoms. An inadequate T regulatory cell response is likely to be a significant contributor to IBD pathogenesis. OCPs, oral contraceptive pills.

immune response associated with these disorders. *For this reason, a discussion of the immunopathogenesis of IBD not only is important for understanding the pathophysiology of these diseases but also provides a basis for understanding both the mechanisms and the rationale for using the wide variety of therapeutic approaches that have recently been developed or are soon to be developed for the treatment of these diseases.*

Friedman S, Blumberg RS. Inflammatory bowel diseases. In: Braunwald E, Fauci AS, Kasper DL, et al (editors). *Harrison's Principles of Internal Medicine,* 17th ed. McGraw-Hill, 2008: 1886–1899.

Kaser AK, Zeissig S, Blumberg RS. Inflammatory bowel disease. *Annu Rev Immunol.* 2010;28:573–621. [PMID: 20192811]

Loftus EV Jr. Clinical epidemiology of inflammatory bowel disease: incidence, prevalence and environmental influences. *Gastroenterology.* 2004;126:1504–1517. [PMID: 15168363]

Strober W, Fuss IJ, Blumberg RS. The immunology of mucosal models of inflammation. *Annu Rev Immunol.* 2002;20:495–549. [PMID: 11861611]

Tuvlin JA, Raza SS, Bracamonte S, et al. Smoking and inflammatory bowel disease: trends in familial and sporadic cohorts. *Inflamm Bowel Dis.* 2007;13:573–579. [PMID: 17345609]

GENERAL PRINCIPLES OF THE GUT-ASSOCIATED LYMPHOID TISSUES

The normal intestine has an enormous surface area that is exposed to a wide variety of exogenous, especially bacterial, antigens (Figure 2–2). Consequently, the mucosal immune system has had to develop a wide variety of very specific modifications and developmental structures to deal with and respond to these challenges. Importantly, the overwhelming majority of initial antigen encounters for the host occur at the mucosal surface, which is bathed by a heterogeneous population of microorganisms, most of which are congregated within the colon and distal small intestine where IBD most commonly occurs (see Figure 2–1). Thus, the intestines are confronted by a large number of antigenic stimuli that must be deciphered for pathologic potential.

Unique Characteristics of the Immune Response in the Gut

For the majority of antigenic challenges, a response that is characterized by either ignorance or active suppression would seem to be the most appropriate in the intestine to avoid a nonspecific inflammatory response. Obviously, for a few exposures such as to pathogens, a robust immune response is appropriate. The mucosal-associated lymphoid tissues associated with the gut, or so called gut-associated lymphoid tissues (GALT), are characterized by a unique organization and regulated state of physiologic (or controlled) inflammation. Thus, the gut is poised for, but actively restrained from, full action and notable for a tendency to suppress responses, a characteristic referred to as oral tolerance. Oral tolerance and physiologic inflammation are unique hallmarks of the GALT and are both manifestations of the tendency of mucosal-associated lymphoid tissues to tightly regulate immune responses (Table 2–1).

These two functional hallmarks of the GALT are representative of the fact that the GALT is a very large immunologic organ in addition to its obvious other functions associated with digestion and endocrine secretion. Its functions are organized anatomically and include two components. The first component is the so-called organized GALT, which includes the Peyer patches, isolated lymphoid follicles, and lymphocyte-filled villi. The second component, the so-called diffuse GALT, comprises anatomic structures that are diffusely contained within the lamina propria.

Organized GALT

The organized GALT structures are often characterized by specialized types of epithelium such as the so-called microfold cell (M cell). M cells are contained within the epithelium that overlies the Peyer patches, with its rich content of associated lymphocytes and dendritic cells that allows for selective uptake of and response to distinct types of antigens. The Peyer patches and other organized lymphoid structures

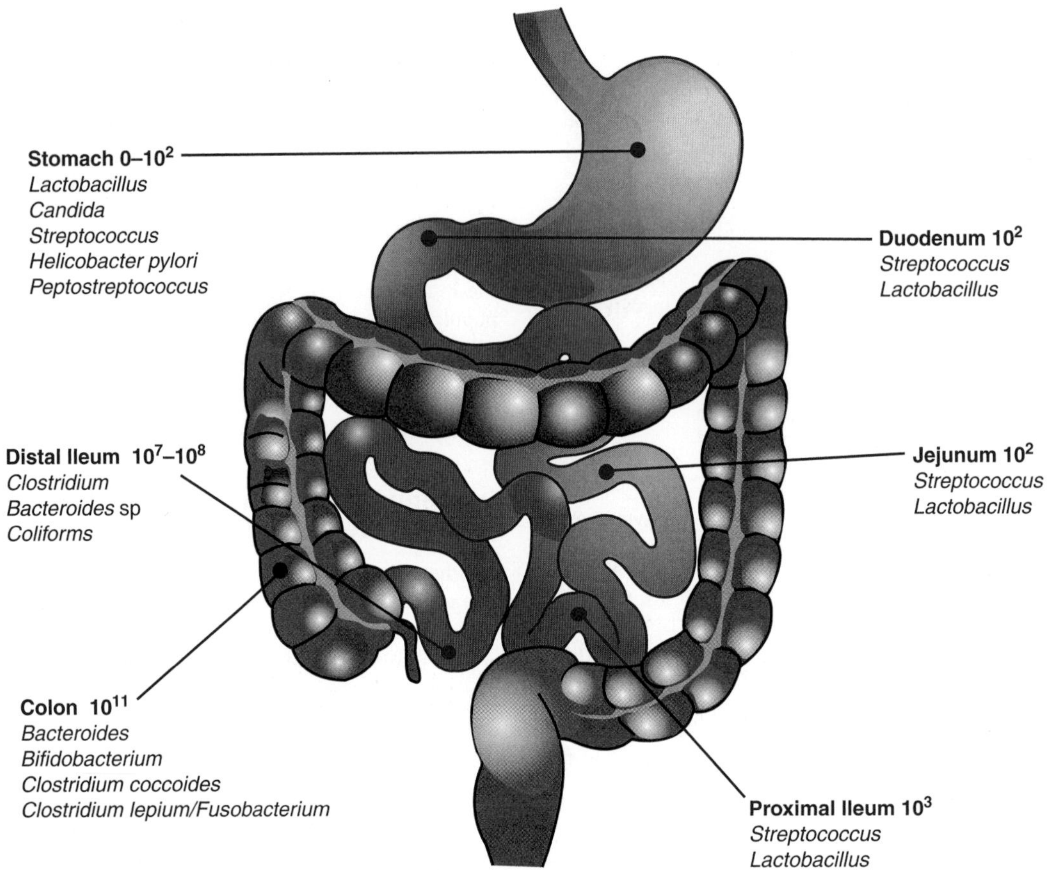

▲ **Figure 2–2.** The microbiologic composition of the gastrointestinal tract. (Adapted, with permission, from Sartor RB, Blumberg RS, Braun J, et al. CCFA microbial-host interactions workshop: highlights and key observations. *Inflamm Bowel Dis.* 2007;13:600–619.)

Table 2–1. Unique characteristics of gut-associated lymphoid tissue.

1. Physiologic inflammation
2. Special types of organized lymphoepithelial structures (eg, Peyer patches)
3. Oral tolerance
4. Immunoglobulin A production and secretion

are distributed throughout the gastrointestinal tract but are especially congregated in the distal ileum. They are mainly inductive sites where antigens, including bacterial antigens, are taken up, processed, and presented by dendritic cells for the education of the GALT-associated lymphocytes.

Diffuse GALT

The diffuse GALT constitutes the majority of the small and large intestine and is characterized by a single layer of simple epithelial cells that separates the lumen of the intestines from the lamina propria. This epithelium and its associated intraepithelial lymphocytes and dendritic cells are a major effector site for protecting the large surface of intestines that must be defended from epithelial exposures to pathogens. In addition, this epithelial surface is highly responsible for participating in the maintenance of a regulated immune response to the wide variety of microbes associated with the normal commensal microbiota.

Innate & Adaptive Immune Responses

Both the epithelial compartment above the epithelial basement membrane and the subepithelial compartment below the epithelial basement membrane that is contained within the lamina propria participate in the two major arms of the immune system. These are the innate and adaptive (or specific) immune systems (Table 2–2).

The innate immune system contains a pattern recognition system that provides a hard-wired and rapid response system for responding to microbial structures. A classic

Table 2–2. Innate and adaptive immunity.

Type of Immunity	Receptor	Ligand	Cell Type
Innate immunity (rapid, hard wired)	TLR2	Peptidoglycan	Macrophages
	TLR4	LPS	Macrophages/IEC
	TLR5	Flagellin	Macrophages/IEC
	TLR9	Bacterial DNA	Dendritic cells
	CRP	Bacterial carbohydrate	Serum
	NOD2	Muramyl dipeptide	Dendritic cells/IEC
Adaptive or specific immunity (delayed with memory)	TCR	HLA plus peptide	T cell
	BCR	Immunoglobulin	B cell
	IL-23R	IL-23	T cell

BCR, B-cell receptor; CRP, C-reactive protein; HLA, human leukocyte antigen; IEC, intestinal epithelial cell; IL-23R, interleukin-23 receptor; LPS, lipopolysaccharide; NOD2, nucleotide oligomerization domain–containing protein 2; TCR, T-cell receptor; TLR, toll-like receptor.

group of structures that are used by a wide variety of cell types in an innate immune response is the so-called toll-like receptors (TLRs), which respond to microbial structures as diverse as lipopolysaccharide or DNA of microbes. Another major class of pattern recognition receptors associated with innate immunity is the nucleotide oligomerization domain (NOD)-like receptors (NLRs), which recognize microbial structures such as muramyl dipeptide from the peptidoglycans of gram-negative and gram-positive bacteria. Innate, pattern-recognition receptors are distributed on virtually all cell types but are especially congregated on professional (dendritic cells, macrophages, and B cells) and nonprofessional (intestinal epithelial cells) antigen-presenting cells (APCs).

Adaptive or specific immunity has a delayed response and is characterized by memory. This type of immunity is characteristic of the immune response derived from T cells and B cells and requires the uptake, processing, and presentation of antigens by APCs to the lymphoid cell types (T and B cells) associated with the adaptive immune response. Moreover, innate and adaptive immunity interact with each other such that they both promote and regulate each other in the generation of a balanced and effective immune response.

Brandtzaeg P, Kiyono H, Pabst R, et al. Terminology: nomenclature of mucosa-associated lymphoid tissue. *Mucosal Immunol.* 2008;1:31–37.

Kaparakis M, Philpott DJ, Ferrero RL. Mammalian NLR proteins: discriminating foe from friend. *Immunol Cell Biol.* 2007;85: 495–502. [PMID: 17680011]

Sansonetti PJ. To be or not to be a pathogen: that is the mucosally relevant question. *Mucosal Immunol.* 2011;4:8–14. [PMID: 21150896]

PATHOGENESIS OF INFLAMMATORY BOWEL DISEASE

General Principles

The major operating paradigm of our current understanding of IBD is that this disease represents hyperreactivity or loss of (oral) tolerance of the mucosal immune system to one's own mucosal microbiota. This is consistent with the general localization of the disease, both UC and CD, to the regions of the intestine where microbes are most present. This concept is mainly derived from observations with numerous animal models of IBD, as well as a lesser number of human clinical studies. The latter have revealed some response to antibiotics, especially in CD, and the lack of any identifiable pathogens in both clinical subtypes of IBD. Thus, IBD likely represents a dysregulated mucosal immune response in a genetically susceptible host to commensal microbial antigens.

Genetic Basis

It has been known for almost 50 years that IBD in humans has a strong genetic basis. Specifically, 10–30% of patients will have a positive family history. There is also an extremely strong concordance of CD and, to a lesser extent (but which is still significant), of UC in monozygotic twins. The risk that both monozygotic twins will develop CD is approximately 60% (or 800-fold increased risk). Both CD and UC have been revealed as complex, polygenic disorders as opposed to simple mendelian disorders (ie, a disease caused by a single gene defect). That said, IBD is associated with several simple mendelian disorders such as Wiskott-Aldrich syndrome and glycogen storage diseases. However, it is clear

Table 2–3. Immunogenetic pathways to inflammatory bowel disease.

- Innate immunity and autophagy (eg, *NOD2, ATG16L1, IRGM*): inappropriate bacterial sensing and clearance by innate immune cells
- Adaptive immunity (eg, *IL23R, JAK2, STAT3, PTPN2, IL10*): imbalance between effector and regulatory pathways
- Inflammation pathways (eg, *MST1, CCR6*): dysfunction in leukocyte recruitment and inflammatory mediator production and response
- ER stress pathways & epithelium (eg, *XBP1*): abnormal intestinal epithelial cell regulation and sensing of bacteria
- Metabolic pathways (eg, *SLC22A5*): inappropriate energy metabolism in hypermetabolic cells

Human genes are listed in italics. ER, endoplasmic reticulum. Data from Kaser AK, Zeissig S, Blumberg RS. Inflammatory bowel disease. *Annu Rev Immunol.* 2010;28:573–621.

from genome-wide analyses that numerous loci on multiple chromosomes are involved in the development of these diseases. A genetic basis for IBD is further supported by observations in animal models.

Genome-wide association studies and candidate gene studies with DNA sequencing have identified nearly 100 genetic susceptibility loci throughout the human genome (Table 2–3). Genetic risk is an important, if not essential, variable in driving the causation of IBD. It should be noted, however, that the mechanism by which genetic risk factors impose risk for the development of IBD remains largely unknown. It can be surmised but not proven that any one of these genes alone cannot cause IBD, as is strongly supported by the well-known observation that deletion of *NOD2/CARD15*, the strongest genetic risk factor for CD in mice, does not result in spontaneous inflammation.

Several interesting observations have been derived from the susceptibility loci identified to date. First, as predicted by a wide variety of immunologic studies, the genetic evaluation of humans shows very clearly that components of the immune system associated with innate immunity (eg, *NOD2*) and adaptive immunity (eg, interleukin [IL]-23 receptor [*IL23R*]) and their relationships with the microbiota are clearly involved in the pathogenesis of these diseases. Moreover, the genetic studies show that alterations of intestinal epithelial cell function and especially that of Paneth cells, which secrete antimicrobial peptides into the lumen, contribute to the pathogenesis of these diseases. This occurs through genes such as *ATG16L1* (which regulates autophagy), *XBP1* (which regulates the unfolded protein response), and *NOD2* (which regulates intracellular bacterial sensing). In addition, the genes identified to date seem to associate with specific functional pathways that may be shared by CD and UC, as well as other immune-mediated diseases such as multiple sclerosis, type 1 diabetes mellitus, asthma, and others.

Abraham C, Cho JH. Inflammatory bowel disease. *N Engl J Med.* 2009;361:2066–2078. [PMID: 19923578]

Kobayashi KS, Chamaillard M, Ogura Y, et al. Nod2-dependent regulation of innate and adaptive immunity in the intestinal tract. *Science.* 2005;307:371–374. [PMID: 15692051]

Van Limbergen J, Russell RK, Nimmo ER, et al. Genetics of the innate immune response in inflammatory bowel disease. *Inflamm Bowel Dis.* 2007;13:338–355. [PMID: 17206667]

Immunologic Factors

It remains incompletely understood how the previously noted genetically imposed risk factors result in the development of IBD. However, it can be reasonably predicted that these genetic factors modify the intestinal epithelial cell barrier and have major effects on the function of innate and adaptive immune systems. They likely also regulate the composition of the microbiota itself. Furthermore, these genetic risk factors resolve into a final common pathway characterized by highly polarized T-cell responses associated with excess cytokine production derived from differentiated CD4-positive T helper cells and aggressive APCs (dendritic cells and macrophages). Animal models have shown the essential importance of the microbiota in these responses, as no disease is observed under germ-free conditions (ie, in the absence of intestinal bacteria). Finally, animal models have also revealed the importance of regulatory (anti-inflammatory) pathways and T regulatory cells, in particular, in both the prevention and resolution of IBD.

Given the importance of CD4-positive T helper (Th) cell polarization in IBD pathogenesis, some discussion of this topic is appropriate (Figure 2–3). T cells leave the thymus and migrate into peripheral tissues, such as the intestines, as naïve (antigen-inexperienced) cells. As such, they are considered to be Th0 cells without a bias for cytokine production other than the ability to secrete IL-2 upon stimulation through their antigen-specific receptor, the T-cell receptor (TCR), together with a co-stimulatory signal (so-called signal 2) that is classically delivered by cell surface molecules, such as CD80 or CD86 on APCs, to CD28 on the T cell (see Figure 2–3). When T cells are presented the antigen for which they are specific through their TCR (signal 1) by professional APCs (eg, dendritic cells in peripheral tissues such as the intestines) together with signal 2, they are induced to deviate to one of several polarized fates under the control of cytokines produced by the APC (dendritic cell) itself or other surrounding cells, or both. Importantly, these immune-deviating cytokines or other factors are typically produced by innate immune factors and cells (see Table 2–2 and Figure 2–3). Thus, cytokines associated with innate immune responses (eg, IL-12, IL-23) guide the adaptive immune response to one of several outcomes characterized by the development of T cells that are polarized to secrete a specific signature of cytokines, as shown in Figure 2–3 (eg, Th1, Th2, Th17, or T regulatory), through the actions of specific transcription factors (eg, T-bet in the case of Th1 cells).

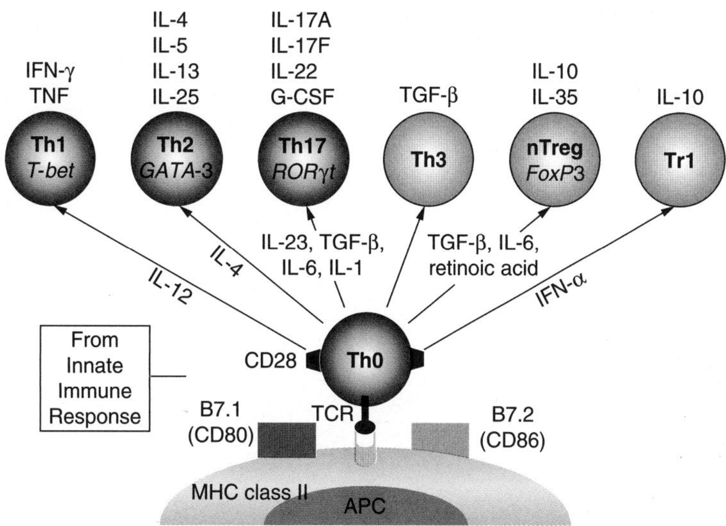

▲ **Figure 2–3.** Differentiation of T cells. Naïve CD4-positive T cells that have never experienced an antigen (Th0) are stimulated by an antigen-presenting cell (APC) such as a dendritic cell. The APC presents the antigen on a major histocompatibility complex (MHC) class II molecule to the T-cell receptor (TCR) on a T cell (signal 1). In the presence of co-stimulatory signals (so-called signal 2) provided by CD80 (B7.1) and CD86 (B7.2) on the APC to CD28 on the Th0 cell, the T cell is properly activated. The activated T cell is induced then to differentiate into one or more different fates that depend on the local cytokine milieu. This cytokine milieu is mainly derived from the APC itself and thus the innate immune response (boxed area in figure). In this manner, interleukin-12 (IL-12) induces Th1 cells; IL-4 induces Th2 cells; IL-23 induces transforming growth factor β (TGFβ), IL-6 and IL-1 induce Th17 cells; TGFβ, IL-6, and retinoic acid induce natural (n) T regulatory (Treg) cells; and interferon-α (IFNα) induces T regulatory 1 cells (Tr1). Each T cell is maintained in its differentiated state by intracellular transcription factors. These include T-bet (Th1), GATA-3 (Th2), RORt (Th17), and FoxP3 (nTreg). The differentiated T cells secrete a characteristic profile of cytokines (shown above the T cells). Cells in red are effector cells, and cells in gray are regulatory cells that inhibit inflammation. nTreg, natural T regulatory cell (see Figure 2–6).

Kim SC, Tonkonogy SL, Albright CA, et al. Variable phenotypes of enterocolitis interleukin 10-deficient mice monoassociated with two different commensal bacteria. *Gastroenterology.* 2005; 129:891–906. [PMID: 15825073]

Zhu J, Yamane H, Paul WE. Differentiation of effector CD4 T cell populations. *Annu Rev Immunol.* 2010;28:445–489. [PMID: 20192806]

PATHOGENESIS OF CROHN DISEASE: UNDERLYING MECHANISMS OF IMMUNE DYSREGULATION

A wide variety of animal studies of mucosal inflammation that model CD, as well as human CD itself, strongly support an excess of Th1 and Th17 cells and their respective cytokines as important in the development of this form of IBD. Thus, in human CD, increased IL-12, IL-23, interferon-γ, IL-17, and tumor necrosis factor (TNF) are present at high levels (Figure 2–4). This is consistent with the presence of granulomas in a subset of individuals with CD that is a well-known phenotypic consequence of Th1-related immune responses. Animal models and humans exhibit increased activity of transcription factors in T cells that are essential to development of these cytokine responses (eg, increased expression of T-bet, which is associated with Th1 cells). *The most definitive evidence to date that human CD is a Th1- or Th17-mediated disorder in subsets of patients is the efficacy, albeit limited, of biologic therapies directed at interferon-γ, IL-12, and IL-23 in the treatment of these diseases in human clinical studies.* IL-6 is another very significant proinflammatory cytokine that is also secreted by Th17 cells and activated macrophages and is highly present in human CD tissues. As will be discussed later, IL-6 is an important cytokine in UC, but in that case, it is mainly derived from innate immune cells. Human clinical trials have also investigated the efficacy of neutralization of IL-6 by blocking the IL-6 receptor in patients with CD. However, IL-6 can have both proinflammatory activities and beneficial properties for the intestinal epithelium.

When an activated Th1 or Th17 cell interacts with a professional APC such as a macrophage or dendritic cell, a wide variety of cell surface interactions between these cell types

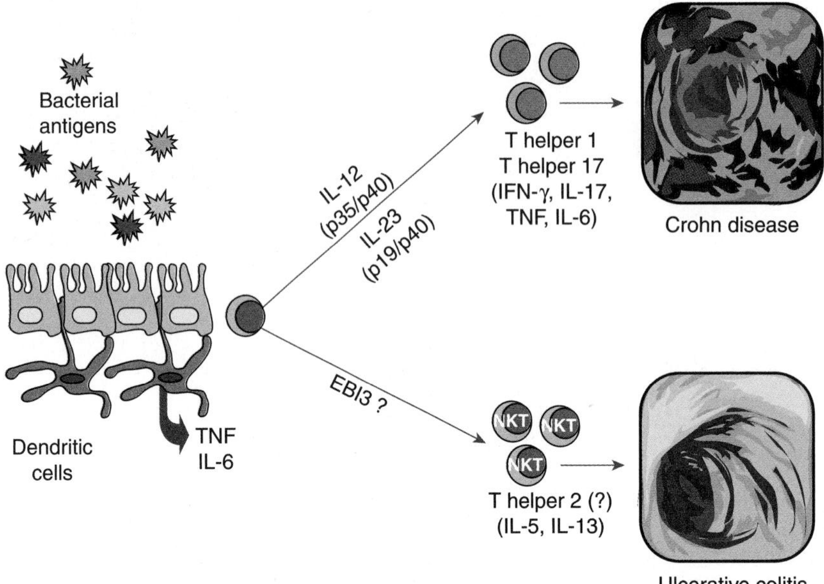

▲ **Figure 2–4.** Role of the dendritic cell in inflammatory bowel disease (IBD). Dendritic cells are always sensing the antigens within the bacterial milieu of the intestines. Through their innate immune function, dendritic cells then secrete cytokines that are proinflammatory (eg, tumor necrosis factor [TNF] and interleukin-6 [IL-6]) and others such as IL-12, IL-23, and Epstein-Barr virus—induced gene 3 (EBI3; IL-12-like protein) that promote the development of Th1 or Th17 cells in the case of Crohn disease or Th2-like cells in ulcerative colitis. These Th1, Th17, and Th2-like (or natural killer T [NKT] cells) cells secrete a variety of proinflammatory cytokines that are shown below the relevant cells. (Data from Neurath MF, Finotto S, Glimcher LH. The role of Th1/Th2 polarization in mucosal immunity. *Nat Med.* 2002;8:567–573.)

is induced to occur that are often called co-stimulatory and activate both cell types. These include the interaction between CD40 on the dendritic cell and CD40-ligand (CD40L) on the activated T cell, which leads to very high levels of secretion of TNF from the APC as well as from the activated Th1 T cell. This interaction makes TNF a very important cytokine in CD, although it is not strictly a Th1 cytokine because it is also secreted by other cell types, such as the APC. *Nonetheless, it is clear that TNF is a central mediator of CD that is derived from Th1 and innate immune cells, and is an important therapeutic target. Not surprisingly, a wide variety of therapies have been developed that have shown significant efficacy in the treatment of IBD through targeting of TNF. These include infliximab, adalimumab, and certolizumab pegol.* The mechanism by which the anti-TNF agents induce remission is not clear but may be a combination of neutralization of TNF itself and reverse signaling through membrane-bound TNF.

Hommes DW, Mikhajlova TL, Stoinov S, et al. Fontolizumab, a humanized anti-interferon gamma antibody, demonstrates safety and clinical activity in patients with moderate to severe Crohn's disease. *Gut.* 2006;55:1131–1137. [PMID: 16507585]

Ito H, Takazoe M, Fukuda Y, et al. A pilot randomized trial of a human anti-interleukin-6 receptor monoclonal antibody in active Crohn's disease. *Gastroenterology.* 2004;126:989–996. [PMID: 15057738]

Kasran A, Boon L, Wortel CH, et al. Safety and tolerability of antagonist anti-human CD40 Mab ch5D12 in patients with moderate to severe Crohn's disease. *Aliment Pharmacol Ther.* 2005;22:111–122. [PMID: 16011669]

Mannon PJ, Fuss IJ, Mayer L, et al; Anti-IL-12 Crohn's Disease Study Group. Anti-interleukin-12 antibody for active Crohn's disease. *N Engl J Med.* 2004;351:2069–2079. [PMID: 15537905]

Schreiber S, Khaliq-Kareemi M, Lawrance IC, et al; PRECISE 2 Study Investigators. Maintenance therapy with certolizumab pegol for Crohn's disease. *N Engl J Med.* 2007;357:239–250. [PMID: 17634459]

Strober W, Zhang F, Kitani A, et al. Proinflammatory cytokines underlying the inflammation of Crohn's disease. *Curr Opin Gastroenterol.* 2010;26:310–317. [PMID: 20473158]

Targan SR, Feagan BG, Fedorak RN, et al; International Efficacy of Natalizumab in Crohn's Disease Response and Remission (ENCORE) Trial Group. Natalizumab for the treatment of active Crohn's disease: results of the ENCORE trial. *Nat Clin Pract Gastroenterol Hepatol.* 2007;132:1672–1683. [PMID: 17484865]

Targan SR, Hanauer SB, van Deventer SJ, et al. A short-term study of chimeric monoclonal antibody cA2 to tumor necrosis factor alpha for Crohn's disease. Crohn's Disease cA2 Study Group. *N Engl J Med.* 1997;337:1029–1035. [PMID: 9321530]

PATHOGENESIS OF ULCERATIVE COLITIS: IMMUNOLOGIC FACTORS

UC is a diffuse superficial disease that is confined to the mucosa and is more commonly characterized by the presence of epithelial apoptosis and superficial ulcerations than is observed in CD. The immunologic profile in UC is also quite different from CD. It is characterized by cytokines that are more commonly associated with T cells that have been immune deviated or differentiated into so-called Th2 cells (which secrete IL-5 and IL-13) and cytokines derived from the activation of professional APCs that occur in response to these activated T-cell subsets (TNF and IL-6) (see Figure 2–4).

There is strong evidence that the origin of these Th2 cytokines in UC may be due to the activity of a unique subset of T cells. Specifically, animal models of UC and studies in humans show that IL-13 may be primarily derived from a unique subset of T cells that carries on its cell surface markers of both natural killer and T cells. These so-called NKT cells recognize a major histocompatibility complex (MHC) class I-like molecule, CD1d, which is structurally similar to human leukocyte antigen (HLA)-A, -B, and -C. In the presence of CD1d on an APC, these NKT cells, which represent approximately 1–2% of peripheral blood lymphocytes and a similarly small set of T cells in the intestines, respond to glycolipid antigens presented by the CD1d molecule on APC. This is in marked contrast to the presentation of peptide antigens in the case of classical MHC class I (HLA-A, -B, and -C) and class II (HLA-DR, -DP, and -DQ) molecules. *These studies in humans and animal models of IBD support the hypothesis that CD1d-restricted NKT cells are responsible for the elevated IL-13 observed in UC.* IL-13 is a highly inflammatory cytokine that has a strong tendency to disrupt the intestinal epithelial cell barrier, as do TNF and IL-6, which are also increased in UC due to the activity of inflamed macrophages and dendritic cells in this disease. *Disruption of the epithelial barrier in UC may be due to collateral damage from the deleterious effects of these cytokines (TNF and IL-13). These studies also suggest that therapies that target CD1d, the NKT cell, IL-13, TNF, and IL-6 may be important future therapies in the treatment of UC.* Studies in humans have indeed shown the efficacy of TNF-directed therapies in the treatment of UC.

Thus, the immune pathogenesis of IBD may be derived from a decision-making process initiated by dendritic cells and other innate immune cell types that take up and respond to microbial antigens derived from the normal commensal microbiota. *In the context of signals derived from innate immune responses by receptors (eg, TLRs) on the cell surface of these professional APCs, cytokines and other factors are secreted that drive the activity and differentiation of T cells within the mucosal tissues and lamina propria and damage the epithelium. In the case of CD, dendritic cells or macrophages, or both, respond to bacterial antigens with excess IL-12 and IL-23 secretion, leading to excessive differentiation and activation of Th1 and Th17 cells (see Figure 2–4).* Moreover, in the case of CD, this tendency to secrete IL-12 and IL-23 in response to commensal bacteria is likely under the control of innate immune receptors associated with risk for the development of IBD. For example, genetic polymorphisms in the *NOD2* gene may increase the risk of developing exaggerated secretion of cytokines that promote Th1 and Th17 cells. Similarly, T cells in CD may be more sensitive to cytokines secreted by dendritic cells (such as IL-12 and IL-23) given the detection of polymorphisms of the IL-23 receptor expressed on T cells that determine the responsiveness of this receptor. In a similar manner, dendritic cells in UC likely sample and respond to bacterial antigens in a manner that leads to the excess secretion of other cytokines that would tend to promote a Th2-like response derived from the activity of a unique subset of T cells, the NKT cells.

Fuss IJ, Strober W. The role of IL-13 and NK T cells in experimental and human ulcerative colitis. *Mucosal Immunol.* 2008;1(Suppl 1):S31–S33. [PMID: 19079225]

Zeissig S, Kaser A, Dougan S, et al. Role of NKT cells in intestinal immunity. *Am J Physiol Gastrointest Liver Physiol.* 2007;293:G1101–G1105. [PMID: 17717040]

REGULATORY PATHWAYS IN THE MAINTENANCE OF INTESTINAL TOLERANCE

As noted earlier, an important attribute of intestinal tissues is the tendency to suppress immune responses (see Table 2–1). This has been associated with the phenomenon of oral tolerance. Oral tolerance is thus a functional manifestation of a more general phenomenon of suppression of immune responses in the intestinal tissues. This tendency of the intestines to suppress is due to the presence of very strong regulatory pathways and high concentrations of regulatory molecules derived from these cells within the intestines. Regulatory cells that have been shown to be present in normal intestine and highly relevant to the development of IBD include natural T regulatory cells (CD4-positive, CD25-positive T cells), induced T regulatory cells, T regulatory 1 cells, Th3 cells, B cells, and possibly NKT cells and CD8-positive T cells. These cell types, either through cell surface-dependent interactions or the secretion of soluble mediators, are able to both maintain normal homeostasis in the baseline state and promote the inhibition of inflammation through the secretion of a variety of regulatory (anti-inflammatory) cytokines such as IL-10, TGFβ, and a recently identified IL-12 family member, IL-35. Although multiple different types of regulatory cells exist and may be operative in the intestines, the most important, thoroughly investigated cells likely to be involved in the regulation of IBD are the so-called natural and induced T regulatory cells; therefore, this discussion focuses mainly on these cells.

Natural T regulatory cells are CD4-positive, CD25 (IL-2 receptor α chain)-positive cells that are differentiated within the thymus and are dependent on the expression of a unique transcription factor called FoxP3 (see Figure 2–3). FoxP3 is a transcription factor that is homologous to the forked winged transcription family and induces T regulatory cell development. In the absence of FoxP3 expression, neither humans nor mice develop natural T regulatory cells. The human disorder IPEX (immune dysregulation, polyendocrinopathy, enteropathy, X-linked) is caused by FoxP3 deficiency. IPEX is characterized by autoimmune enteropathy, protein-losing enteropathy, insulin-dependent diabetes mellitus, dermatitis, and protracted diarrhea that is unresponsive to gluten withdrawal. Once educated in the thymus, FoxP3-positive T cells are exported into the bloodstream where they suppress the activity of effector (proinflammatory) T cells that have been differentiated to secrete Th1, Th2, or Th17 cytokines as well as innate immune cells (Figure 2–5). Thus, FoxP3-positive T regulatory cells are important in preventing autoimmunity (including IBD) and also play a role in allergy, tumor immunity, organ transplantation, and microbial infection.

FoxP3-positive natural T regulatory cells can be detected in human and mouse intestines and have been strongly linked to the regulation of inflammation that is driven by both innate and adaptive immune pathways. In the absence of an adequate natural T regulatory response, spontaneous inflammation of the intestines will develop, as shown in patients with IPEX. It is important to note that FoxP3-negative T cells can also be induced within the intestines to become FoxP3-positive cells when T cells are exposed to high concentrations of TGF-β and retinoic acid, which is a metabolic product derived from vitamin A. Thus, T regulatory cells can be induced and recruited into action for the amelioration of inflammation from FoxP3-negative T cells. Although T regulatory cells have been shown in murine models to be extremely important in the prevention of IBD, there is to date no guaranteed means to influence these important regulatory cells in a therapeutic manner. Nonetheless, this is an important goal of modern immunotherapy in these diseases. Studies of these very important cells show that IBD can evolve from either an overly exuberant, innate, T effector cell response and B-cell response through secretion of immunoglobulin G (IgG) with antibacterial specificities or a relatively inadequate T regulatory cell response, or both. *Thus, it is the balance between these various effector and regulatory pathways that leads to either the tendency to develop or the inability to prevent and thus regulate the inflammation that occurs in IBD.*

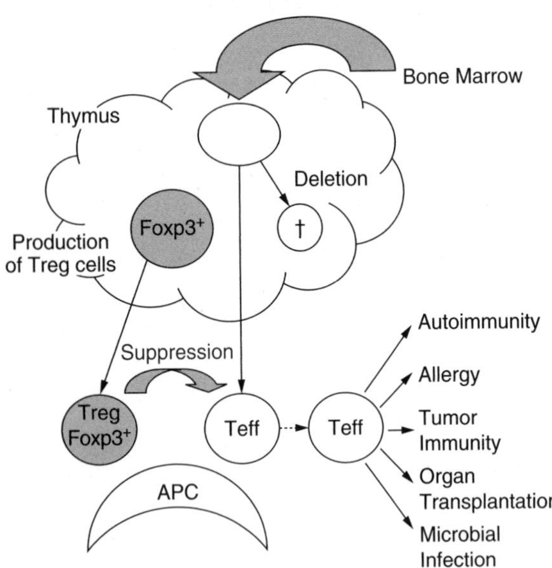

▲ **Figure 2–5.** Development of natural T regulatory (nTreg) cells. nTreg cells develop within the thymus and are induced to express the transcription factor (Foxp3) that results in their characteristic phenotypic and functional characteristics. They are important suppressors of effector T (Teff) cells, which play an important role in many immune-mediated pathways, including IBD. APC, antigen-presenting cell. (Adapted, with permission, from Sakaguchi S. Naturally arising Foxp3-expressing CD25$^+$CD4$^+$ regulatory T cells in immunological tolerance to self and non-self. *Nat Immunol.* 2005;6:345–352.)

Although it is important to discuss regulatory pathways in the pathogenesis of IBD, it should be recognized that a wide variety of other regulatory pathways are normally operative in the intestines under homeostatic conditions and presumably are of significance to the dampening or prevention of inflammation. Arguably, virtually every process in the immunologic cascade that leads to inflammation is regulated. A wide variety of molecules with natural regulatory properties have been described within intestinal tissues, including endogenous anti-inflammatory or proresolution mediators (eg, peroxisome proliferator-activated receptor γ [PPARγ], lipoxins, resolvins, opioids, cannabinoids), anti-adhesion factors (eg, apoAIV), inhibitory cytokines and suppressors (eg, TGF-β and suppressor of cytokine signaling), and finally an emerging group of co-inhibiting receptors on T cells and APCs (eg, CTLA-4, PD-1, and CEACAM1). Mesalamine has been proposed to work through PPARγ-mediated inhibition of the translocation of a potent proinflammatory transcription factor, nuclear factor-κB, into the nucleus. Therefore, the range of targets that might be useful for achieving regulation and thus remission of human IBD is enormous and represents a great therapeutic opportunity.

Boden EK, Snapper SB. Regulatory T cells in inflammatory bowel disease. *Curr Opin Gastroenterol.* 2008;24:733–741. [PMID: 19125486]

Coombes JL, Robinson NJ, Maloy KJ, et al. Regulatory T cells and intestinal homeostasis. *Immunol Rev.* 2005;204:184–194. [PMID: 15790359]

Kunos G, Pacher P. Cannabinoids cool the intestine. *Nat Med.* 2004;10:678–679. [PMID: 15229512]

Mucida D, Park Y, Kim G, et al. Reciprocal TH17 and regulatory T cell differentiation mediated by retinoic acid. *Science.* 2007;317:256–260. [PMID: 17569825]

Sakaguchi S. Naturally arising Foxp3-expressing CD25$^+$CD4$^+$ regulatory T cells in immunological tolerance to self and non-self. *Nat Immunol.* 2005;6:345–352. [PMID: 17659825]

Weaver CT, Hatton RD, Mangan PR, et al. IL-17 family cytokines and the expanding diversity of effector T cell lineages. *Annu Rev Immunol.* 2007;25:821–852. [PMID: 17201677]

THERAPEUTIC IMPLICATIONS OF THE IMMUNOBIOLOGY OF INFLAMMATORY BOWEL DISEASE

This discussion has shown that IBD emerges from a very specific immunologic cascade of events. The initial event is the interaction between a T cell, an APC, and an antigen (Figure 2–6). In this interaction, an APC responds to and takes up an antigen that is primarily derived from the commensal luminal microbiota, leading to innate receptor signaling of the APC followed by processing and presentation of nominal portions of this antigen to lymphocytes via the MHC-related molecules. Innate immune abnormalities alone associated with the epithelium or hematopoietic system (eg, macrophages) may also be the earliest origins of disease.

As a consequence of the cellular dialogue that occurs between T cells and APCs, both of these cells are activated to produce the cytokines that are characteristic of their stage of differentiation and are stimulated to display on their cell surface a wide variety of new receptors that may either promote or downregulate their activity. In turn, the cytokines and other soluble mediators that the activated T cell and APC are induced to express or secrete lead to the further activation of the endothelium.

The activated endothelium is induced to become very sticky for other leukocytes and thus encourages the so-called homing of T cells, monocytes, B cells, and polymorphonuclear leukocytes to the intestines by inducing adherence of these leukocytes to the endothelium and their diapedesis into the lamina propria. It should be noted that the adherence of T cells to the endothelium occurs through specific molecules on their cell surface (eg, an integrin called α4β7 and a chemokine called CCR9) and corresponding molecules on the endothelium (eg, MadCAM1), all of which are potential therapeutic targets.

In the context of an already inflammatory milieu, these recruited leukocytes find themselves within a highly inflammatory matrix that is replete with inflammatory cytokines. This leads to a further activation of the newly recruited leukocytes and their production of inflammatory mediators that further aggravate the tissue destruction through production of metalloproteinases and other proteases, leading to degradation of the matrix and tissue destruction. Most deleterious perhaps are the ultimate effects of these inflammatory cytokines and mediators, including proteases and reactive oxygen metabolites, which lead to disruption and degradation of the epithelial barrier, resulting in more promiscuous uptake of inflammatory antigens in the context of a highly active innate and adaptive immune system.

Given this scenario, one can understand both the mechanism of action of the therapeutic agents developed to date and the rationale for the development of new generations of agents to treat IBD (Table 2–4). Thus, one can understand the rationale for using probiotics to challenge the "pathogenic" commensal bacteria and their antigens that are driving the disease in the first instance, although this is an area of therapy that requires significantly more study before definitive therapeutic recommendations can be made. Similarly, it is logical to block so-called co-stimulatory molecules that are central to the initial interactions between a T cell and an APC, such as CD28 on the T cell, through the use of abatacept, for example. Abatacept (CTLA4-Ig), which is currently approved for the treatment of rheumatoid arthritis, binds to CD80 and CD86 on antigen-presenting cells, blocking the engagement of CD28 on T cells. However, blocking

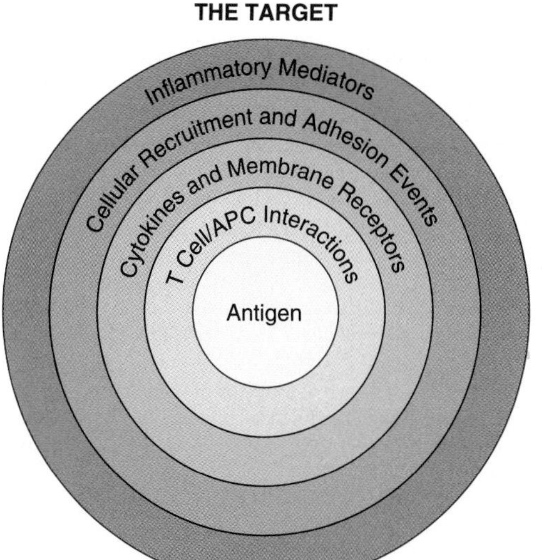

▲ **Figure 2–6.** The immunotherapeutic target in inflammatory bowel disease (IBD). IBD is initiated by a unique group of bacterial antigens that possess special qualities that allow them to interact with innate and adaptive immune pathways. These antigens are taken up by antigen-presenting cells (APCs) that both respond to the antigens (via innate immune pathways) and present the antigens (via adaptive immune pathways) to T cells. This leads to secretion of cytokines and upregulation of membrane receptors, activation of the endothelium and recruitment of inflammatory cells, and release of inflammatory mediators. Each level of this target is amenable to therapy, as described in the text and Table 2–4.

Table 2–4. Inflammatory bowel disease—therapeutic implications.

Target	Mechanism	Therapeutic
Antigen	Eliminate pathogenic bacterial strain	Antibiotic/probiotic (VSL#3)
T cell/APC interactions	Manipulate T cell activation	Anti-CD3 (visilizumab), CTLA4-Ig (abatacept), azathioprine/6-MP
Cytokines and membrane receptors	↓ Proinflammatory or ↑ anti-inflammatory cytokines	Anti-TNF (infliximab, adalimumab, certolizumab pegol), anti-IL-12, anti-IL-23, anti-IFNγ, anti-IL-6R, IL-10
Cellular recruitment	Block T-cell homing or endothelial cell addressin	Anti-α4β7 (natalizumab), Anti-MadCAM1
Inflammatory mediators	Block inflammatory signaling	Protease inhibitors, mesalamines, JAK-3 inhibitor
Barrier function and repair	↑ Epithelial barrier and restitution	Epidermal growth factor

APC, antigen-presenting cell; IFNγ, interferon-γ; IL, interleukin; MP, mercaptopurine; TNF, tumor necrosis factor.

CD28 signaling with CTLA4-Ig may also block the development and activity of T regulatory cells, emphasizing the challenges in translating insights from the immunobiology of IBD into therapeutics. Blockade of CD28 signaling may also be the mechanism by which azathioprine/6-mercaptopurine induces remission in IBD (see Table 2–4). It is obvious why anticytokine therapies that direct themselves at blocking proinflammatory cytokines (eg, anti-TNF and potentially anti-IL-6, anti-IL-12, anti-IL-23, and anti-IL-13) or promotion of anti-inflammatory cytokines (eg, IL-35 or IL-10) are of great significance. Moreover, it is clearly beneficial to disrupt leukocyte homing (eg, targeting molecules on the surface of the sticky endothelial cells such as MAdCAM1, or homing molecules on the leukocytes such as α4β7 on T lymphocytes) to treat these diseases. Finally, blocking proinflammatory signaling and the production of inflammatory mediators by inhibition of the transcription factor, nuclear factor-κB (NF-κB), through administration of mesalamines has been shown to be highly effective, especially in UC. However, even NF-κB has important protective effects on the intestinal epithelium, further demonstrating the challenges in effective translation of fundamental immunogenetic principles into human therapeutics. In conclusion, it is instructive to consider the immunobiology of IBD as a means to understand the rationale for the mechanism of action and utility of the current and emerging biologic therapies in IBD.

Feagan BG, Greenberg GR, Wild G, et al. Treatment of ulcerative colitis with a humanized antibody to the α4β7 integrin. *N Engl J Med.* 2005;352:2499–2507. [PMID: 15958805]

Gionchetti P, Rizzello F, Helwig U, et al. Prophylaxis of pouchitis onset with probiotic therapy: a double-blind, placebo-controlled trial. *Gastroenterology.* 2003;124:1202–1209. [PMID: 12730861]

Sandborn WJ, Colombel J, Enns R, et al. International Efficacy of Natalizumab as Active Crohn's Therapy (ENACT-1) Trial Group; Evaluation of Natalizumab as Continuous Therapy (ENACT-2) Trial Group. Natalizumab induction and maintenance therapy for Crohn's disease. *N Engl J Med.* 2005;353:1912–1925. [PMID: 16267322]

Tilg H, Moschen A, Kaser A. Mode of function of biological anti-TNF agents in the treatment of inflammatory bowel diseases. *Expert Opin Biol Ther.* 2007;7:1051–1059. [PMID: 17665993]

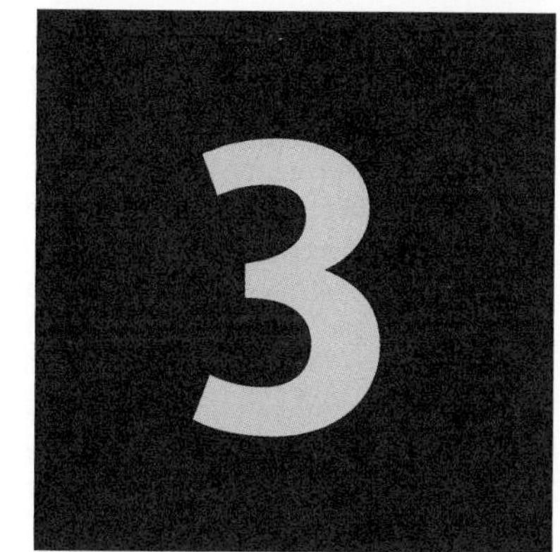

Inflammatory Bowel Disease: Medical Considerations

Jonathan S. Levine, MD
Robert Burakoff, MD, MPH

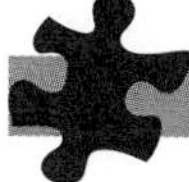

ESSENTIAL CONCEPTS

- Crohn disease and ulcerative colitis are chronic inflammatory diseases with well-described epidemiologic and clinical features.
- Genetic factors, immune dysregulation, and microbial gut flora all influence disease susceptibility.
- No single symptom, physical finding, or test result can diagnose inflammatory bowel disease (IBD); the diagnosis is a clinical one based on consistent findings obtained from the history, physical examination, and laboratory, endoscopic, histologic, and radiologic studies.
- Multiple conditions can mimic IBD; infectious pathogens are a particular concern.
- Intestinal complications commonly occur in IBD, many of which are predictable on the basis of disease type, location, severity, or duration; extraintestinal complications also occur, typically in association with active disease.
- Patients with long-standing colitis are at increased risk of developing colorectal cancer (CRC) and should be evaluated for dysplastic changes predictive of subsequent or synchronous malignancy.
- 5-Aminosalicylates, steroids, antibiotics, and immunomodulators have been mainstays of therapy; the choice of appropriate medication is based on multiple variables, including disease type, location, and severity.
- Biologic medications offer multiple powerful therapeutic options; the optimal time to apply these medications remains to be clarified.

General Considerations

The inflammatory bowel diseases, Crohn disease and ulcerative colitis, are chronic inflammatory illnesses of the gastrointestinal tract. Although significant advancements have been made in our understanding of the pathogenesis of these conditions, their ultimate cause remains idiopathic. The immunologic basis of IBD is discussed in Chapter 2. This chapter addresses the diagnosis and medical treatment of IBD. Surgical considerations are discussed in detail in Chapter 4.

A. Epidemiology

Crohn disease and ulcerative colitis have low incidences of new diagnosis; however, as a chronic condition typically diagnosed in the young, IBD has a relatively high prevalence. Estimates of incidence and prevalence vary among studies, with significant geographic and socioeconomic variations. The incidence of ulcerative colitis in North America is estimated to be 8–15 per 100,000 persons, with a prevalence of 170–230 per 100,000. Crohn disease has an estimated incidence of 5–15 per 100,000 and prevalence of 140–200 per 100,000. An increased incidence and prevalence of both forms of IBD is found in developed nations, northern locale (at least within the northern hemisphere), and urban environments; among Caucasians; and among persons of Jewish ethnicity. In industrialized countries, the incidence of Crohn disease has risen significantly over the past half century, whereas that of ulcerative colitis has remained relatively steady. In developing countries, the incidence of both forms of IBD has dramatically risen.

IBD typically presents at a relatively young age, often in adolescence. The median age of diagnosis for Crohn disease and ulcerative colitis is the third and fourth decades of life, respectively. Studies have suggested a second, smaller peak in incidence of IBD in the sixth and seventh decades, although this association is clearer for ulcerative colitis than for Crohn disease.

Sandler RS, Loftus EV. Epidemiology of inflammatory bowel disease. In: Sartor RB, Sandborn WJ (editors). *Inflammatory Bowel Diseases.* Saunders, 2004:245–262.

B. Etiology

The cause of IBD remains elusive, although interplay of genetic, microbial, and immunologic factors clearly exists. Twin and familial studies demonstrate a component of genetic susceptibility. However, the concordance rates among monozygotic twins for ulcerative colitis (6–18%) and Crohn disease (~50%) indicate that genetics play a relatively minor role in disease manifestation. Presumably, specific mutations confer susceptibility to IBD but are not sufficient per se. Various susceptibility genes have been identified, including *NOD2/CARD15* on chromosome 16 and *IL23R* on chromosome 1, in Crohn disease. Both play integral roles in immune regulation within the gut. At the same time, mutations in these genes are present in only a minority of Crohn disease cases. Clearly, other less well-described dysregulations in the gut immune defense systems exist. A more complete discussion of the immunopathology of IBD can be found in Chapter 2.

Animal studies have demonstrated that the presence of commensal gut bacteria is necessary for IBD to occur. In theory, the subsequent enteritis or colitis results from a dysregulated or inappropriate immune response to flora tolerated by healthy individuals. Other environmental factors appear important as well. Cigarette smoking increases the risk for Crohn disease but is protective for ulcerative colitis. Both oral contraceptive and nonsteroidal anti-inflammatory medications have been implicated as risk factors for IBD, although the association remains controversial. Various diets have been proposed as causes or remedies for IBD, but no rigorous scientific evidence supports their use.

Duerr RH, Taylor KD, Brant SR, et al. A genome-wide association study identifies IL23R as an inflammatory bowel disease gene. *Science.* 2006;314:1461–1463. [PMID: 17068223]

Podolsky DK. Inflammatory bowel disease. *N Engl J Med.* 2002;347: 417–429. [PMID: 12167685]

Clinical Findings

A. Crohn Disease

The inflammation in Crohn disease is typically transmural. This frequently leads to complications from perforating disease or from progressive fibrosis and stricturing. Crohn disease can thus be thought of as fitting one of three phenotypes: inflammatory, stricturing, or perforating disease (the latter including abscesses and fistulae). Disease behavior is not necessarily constant in an individual patient. Indeed, inflammatory disease frequently progresses to penetrating disease, and then to fibrosis and stricturing.

Unlike ulcerative colitis, Crohn disease may affect any part of the alimentary canal, and may do so in a nonconfluent (so-called skip lesion) pattern. Nearly half of all patients with Crohn disease have inflammation localized to the terminal ileum and cecum (Table 3–1). Isolated small bowel or colonic involvement is also common. Crohn disease of the esophagus, stomach, or duodenum is rare, and virtually unheard of in the absence of small bowel or colonic disease. Perianal disease, including abscesses and fistulae, is commonly encountered, particularly in conjunction with terminal ileal disease.

Table 3–1. Localization of Crohn disease within the gastrointestinal tract.

Location	Frequency (%)
Ileocolonic	35 (26–48)
Small bowel only	28 (11–48)
Colon only	32 (19–51)
Gastroduodenal[a]	1–4
Perianal[a]	18 (14–20)

[a]Typically in conjunction with disease elsewhere.

1. Symptoms and signs—The onset of symptoms in Crohn disease is typically insidious, and the subsequent clinical course highly variable. For the majority of patients, the clinical course is characterized by recurring episodes of symptomatic disease interspersed with periods of remission. Abdominal pain and diarrhea are the most typical symptoms. Unlike ulcerative colitis, the diarrhea in Crohn disease is often nonbloody. Fever and weight loss are common. As a general rule, the location and phenotype of disease (inflammatory, stricturing, or perforating), along with the severity of inflammation, dictate a patient's symptoms and signs.

Complications from fistulizing disease are common. Pain and drainage of purulent or fecal material are characteristic of perianal fistulae. Fistulae from the gut may cause a variety of symptoms, depending on the sites of origin and other organ(s) involved: gut—diarrhea, weight loss; skin—drainage; vagina—drainage; bladder—pneumaturia. Stricturing disease causes obstructive symptoms of pain, abdominal distention, nausea, and vomiting. Extraintestinal manifestations are frequently encountered with Crohn disease (as with ulcerative colitis) and are discussed in more detail below.

Signs of Crohn disease include abdominal tenderness, most classically in the right lower quadrant. An abdominal mass may be palpable. Temporal wasting and cachexia indicate significant malnutrition. Typical symptoms of small bowel obstruction (distention, tympany, high-pitched bowel sounds) may be present in stenosing disease. Perianal and cutaneous fistulae are readily identified on a careful perineal and skin examination.

2. Laboratory findings—No single laboratory test is diagnostic or specific for Crohn disease. Patients are typically at least mildly anemic, often with iron deficiency. Leukocytosis and thrombocytosis are common and typically reflect systemic inflammation. Serum albumin may be low in the case of protein-losing enterocolitis or in malnutrition. Malabsorption due to inflammation, bacterial overgrowth, or surgical resection may lead to diminished levels of various minerals (serum calcium and magnesium) and vitamins (B12, D, and folate). C-reactive protein (CRP)—and, to a lesser extent, erythrocyte sedimentation rate (ESR)—are nonspecific markers of inflammation that are frequently elevated in Crohn disease.

Stool studies may reveal excess fat, indicative of malabsorption, or fecal leukocytes, indicative of gut inflammation. Stool studies should be negative for infectious pathogens, including standard bacterial pathogens, *Clostridium difficile*, and ova and parasites.

Various serologic markers have been linked with Crohn disease, including antibodies to the yeast *Saccharomyces cerevisiae* (ASCA), to bacterial proteins Omp-C and I2, and to clostridial flagellin, CBir-1. Several antibodies to bacterial carbohydrates, including ALCA, ACCA, and AMCA, have been studied but are not yet commercially available. Antineutrophil cytoplasmic antibodies (ANCA, P-subtype) are associated with both ulcerative colitis and Crohn colitis. As individual tests, these markers have limited diagnostic accuracy, but in select situations may be helpful in distinguishing Crohn disease from other inflammatory conditions.

New stool tests, fecal lactoferrin and calprotectin, are available that can help distinguish IBD from irritable bowel syndrome (IBS) (conditions that often have overlapping symptoms), potentially gauge disease activity, predict flare, and monitor and/or assess response to treatment. Lactoferrin is the major component of secondary granules in neutrophils and inhibits bacterial proliferation by iron binding. It is stable in the stool for 7 days. Calprotectin is present in neutrophils, monocytes, and macrophages. It comprises 60% of the cytosolic protein in neutrophils and is stable in the stool for 7 days. Both appear to be promising markers for monitoring therapy as well as surrogates for mucosal healing. Insurance coverage for these tests, unfortunately, remains a major barrier. Future drug trials are incorporating these markers and will hopefully lead to improved coverage.

Greater than 60 distinct susceptibility loci for IBD have been identified, and advances in the technology for analyzing genetic information have improved dramatically. These have allowed for the identification of over 40 genes associated with IBD including multiple genes that regulate the innate immune response. Five genes, including *NOD2*, have been identified as regulating innate immune function in the pathogenesis of Crohn disease. Nine genes involved in Crohn disease have been implicated in dysregulation of adaptive immunity. Thirteen genes have been associated with ulcerative colitis by gene array studies. The *NOD2* (formerly *CARD15*) gene was the first to be well characterized, and its presence can predict the development of penetrating and fistulizing Crohn disease. *IL-23R* has been associated with both Crohn disease and ulcerative colitis and recently has been demonstrated to predict response to infliximab in ulcerative colitis patients. Recent studies have shown that using whole-blood gene array is a promising technology for distinguishing Crohn disease from ulcerative colitis and may have potential use in differentiating severity of disease and response to therapy.

Burakoff R, Chao S, Perencevich M, et al. Blood based biomarkers can differentiate ulcerative colitis from Crohn disease and non-IBD diarrhea. *Inflamm Bowel Dis.* January 6, 2011 [Epub ahead of print]. [PMID: 21213290]

Kane, SV, Sandborn WJ, Rufo PA, et al. Fecal lactoferrin is a sensitive and specific marker in identifying intestinal inflammation. *Am J Gastroenterol.* 2003;98:1309–1314. [PMID: 12818275]

Targan SR, Karp LC. Serology and laboratory markers of disease activity. In: Sartor RB, Sandborn WJ (editors). *Inflammatory Bowel Diseases.* Saunders, 2004:442–450.

3. Imaging studies—Standard abdominal plain films are useful for detecting obstructive disease and megacolon, but otherwise have a limited role in imaging Crohn disease. Small bowel series are useful for imaging small bowel mucosal disease, including strictures, ulcerations, and fistulae. Enteroclysis, although more sensitive, is limited by patient discomfort, increased radiation exposure, and its technically demanding nature. Barium enema remains an option for imaging colonic disease, especially to help delineate obstructive or fistulizing disease.

Computed tomography (CT) of the abdomen and pelvis has revolutionized the imaging of Crohn disease by allowing imaging of the bowel wall itself, as well as extraluminal disease such as abscesses or inflammatory masses. Common abnormalities of the gut include thickening and excessive mesenteric fat proliferation (so-called creeping fat). CT enterography, which uses a special low-density oral contrast, combines the advantages of CT and small bowel series by allowing detailed pictures of the small bowel mucosa, while at the same time imaging the extraintestinal abdomen. Three-dimensional CT reconstruction allows imaging of complicated transmural disease (see Figure 9–10). CT colonography has developed as a technology, but its role in Crohn disease remains limited in comparison to colonoscopy.

Magnetic resonance enterography (MRE) has been increasingly used. Studies have shown MRE to have better detection of mild disease than CT enterography (CTE) and slightly improved detection of wall thickening and enhancement. No significant difference was seen for moderate to severe disease. Other significant advantages include lack of ionizing radiation and, importantly, comprehensive evaluation of the perianal region. Disadvantages include higher cost compared to CTE and additional time needed to perform the study. Although not yet widely available, positron emission tomography (PET)/CT enterography in which glucose transporters are overexpressed in inflamed segments may show improved detection of lesions, better severity stratification, and improved monitoring of therapy.

Colonoscopy remains a mainstay in the assessment of Crohn disease, as it allows direct visualization of the bowel mucosa and sampling of tissue. Hallmark findings include ulcerations, erythema, granularity, and strictures. Pseudopolyps may be present. Ileal ulceration and skip lesions help distinguish Crohn disease from ulcerative colitis. The rectum is often spared. Fistulae are often difficult to locate endoscopically, and are best seen by contrast studies or magnetic resonance imaging (MRI). Endoscopic ultrasound, as previously mentioned, is useful in delineating perianal disease. Enteroscopy occasionally allows visualization of proximal small bowel lesions.

Capsule ("pill") endoscopy has been revolutionary in terms of allowing direct visualization of the small bowel in Crohn disease. The most common finding is ulceration, ranging from shallow aphthous-type to deep "punched-out" lesions. Strictures may also be encountered, occasionally causing pill retention and subsequent obstruction.

B. Ulcerative Colitis

Unlike Crohn disease, inflammation in ulcerative colitis is limited to the mucosal layer of the colon. The rectum is virtually always involved, with inflammation extending proximally in a confluent fashion. The extent of proximal involvement is variable. A significant proportion of patients have disease confined to the rectum (ulcerative proctitis). Roughly one third of patients have proctosigmoiditis, and the majority of patients have gross colitis only distal to the splenic flexure. Approximately one third of patients have disease that extends proximal to the splenic flexure (extensive colitis), often involving the entire colon (pancolitis or universal colitis).

On occasion, a so-called cecal patch of periappendiceal inflammation is encountered. This does not represent a true skip lesion suggestive of Crohn disease. Similarly, limited ileal involvement (backwash ileitis) can be seen in patients with ulcerative colitis who have pancolonic disease. Deep ileal ulcers, long segments of ileal involvement, or stricturing disease are consistent with Crohn disease and not ulcerative colitis. Although confluent disease involving the rectum is the rule in ulcerative colitis, patients on medical therapy, particularly topical therapy, may have apparent skip lesions or rectal sparing. This should be recognized as a treatment effect and not a manifestation of Crohn disease.

Unlike Crohn disease, ulcerative colitis is frequently acute or subacute in onset. Like Crohn disease, the subsequent clinical course is one of recurring episodes of symptomatic disease interspersed with episodes of relative (or complete) quiescence.

1. Symptoms and signs—As with Crohn disease, the symptoms of ulcerative colitis depend on the extent and severity of inflammation. Overt rectal bleeding and tenesmus are virtually universally present and may be the only symptoms in patients with proctitis alone. When the proximal colon is involved, diarrhea and abdominal pain are more frequent complaints. Nausea and weight loss portend more severe disease. Severe abdominal pain or fever suggests fulminant colitis or toxic megacolon.

Signs of ulcerative colitis include mild abdominal tenderness, often most localized in the hypogastrium or left lower quadrant. Digital rectal examination may disclose visible red blood. As with Crohn disease, signs of malnutrition may be evident. Severe tenderness, fever, or tachycardia heralds fulminant disease.

2. Laboratory findings—Patients with active disease are generally anemic and often iron deficient. Hypoalbuminemia suggests extensive disease with subsequent colonic protein losses. Leukocytosis, thrombocytosis, ESR, and CRP are nonspecific markers of systemic inflammation. Elevations in ESR and CRP are less common in ulcerative colitis than in Crohn disease.

Stool studies should be sent and found negative for typical bacterial pathogens, *C difficile*, and ova and parasites. Common positive findings in ulcerative colitis include fecal leukocytes and fecal lactoferrin.

Serologic markers have also been studied for ulcerative colitis. P-ANCA is the most commonly associated marker. However, as previously mentioned, it is also present in Crohn colitis, which limits its ability to distinguish the two conditions. As with markers in Crohn disease, P-ANCA may be helpful in predicting disease activity. Studies have suggested that P-ANCA-associated ulcerative colitis is more likely to be medically refractory, require early surgery, and result in chronic pouchitis in patients who have undergone ileal pouch anal anastomosis (IPAA).

Targan SR, Karp LC. Serology and laboratory markers of disease activity. In: Sartor RB, Sandborn WJ (editors). *Inflammatory Bowel Diseases.* Saunders, 2004:442–450.

3. Imaging studies—Plain films of the abdomen are useful predominantly in patients with symptoms of severe or fulminant colitis. So-called thumbprinting or thickening of the colon wall indicates severe colitis with bowel wall edema. With toxic megacolon, the bowel is dilated with loss of haustral markings. Intestinal pneumatosis is a late finding and signals bowel ischemia and infarction. Obstructive findings are less common in ulcerative colitis than in Crohn disease and usually suggest malignancy. Barium enema is less commonly used since the advent of flexible sigmoidoscopy and colonoscopy. Nonetheless, it can be useful for detecting active ulcerative disease, polyps, or masses. In ulcerative colitis, the colon typically appears granular and shortened, perhaps as a consequence of chronic inflammation or fibrosis. Pouchography (contrast study of the pouch) in patients who have undergone IPAA permits assessment of diseases related to this operation, including leaks, pouchitis, fistulae, or strictures.

CT of the abdomen typically reveals colonic wall thickening, as with other forms of colitis (see Figure 9–21). Small bowel disease is not present, other than perhaps mild ileal inflammatory changes. Once a diagnosis of ulcerative colitis has been made, CT has only a limited role as an imaging modality, because endoscopic examination is typically the preferred modality for disease assessment.

Colonoscopy allows assessment of the extent of disease and severity of involvement. Classic findings include confluent inflammation extending proximally from the anal verge, with mucosal erythema, edema, and granularity and loss of normal vasculature. With more severe disease, the mucosa becomes overtly hemorrhagic, with ulcerations and a purulent exudate. So-called backwash ileitis, characterized by mild terminal ileal erythema, is seen in patients who have pancolitis. Pseudopolyps are commonly encountered in patients with long-standing disease. These are polypoid nondysplastic colonic lesions of hypertrophied tissue, often with surrounding atrophic mucosa. They are thought to represent the sequelae of chronic recurrent inflammation and healing, and harbor no malignant potential. Dysplastic or frankly malignant polyps or mass lesions are also encountered at higher rates in patients with ulcerative colitis. These lesions are discussed in more detail under Complications, below. Both pseudopolyps and colitis-associated neoplastic lesions are also seen in patients with Crohn disease.

Flexible sigmoidoscopy is a useful tool for disease assessment in the setting of flares of colitis. In this setting, a full colonoscopy is typically overly cumbersome for the patient and may carry an undue risk of perforation in patients with severe colitis. Flexible colonoscopy can assist with assessment of disease severity and help to exclude alternative diagnoses, such as infectious or ischemic colitis.

C. Diagnostic Considerations

No single symptom, physical finding, or test result can diagnose IBD. The diagnosis of both Crohn disease and ulcerative colitis is a clinical one, based on compatible patient history; physical examination; and laboratory, radiographic, endoscopic, and histologic findings. Diagnostic tools have been discussed at length in the preceding sections. A detailed discussion of the histologic findings of IBD is beyond the scope of this chapter. Noncaseating granulomas and transmural disease both are highly specific to Crohn disease. Colonic biopsies in both ulcerative colitis and Crohn colitis demonstrate evidence of acute inflammation, characterized by neutrophilic cryptitis, and chronic inflammation, such as crypt distortion and a plasmacytic infiltration of the lamina propria. A skilled pathologist is indispensable in helping to characterize the histologic findings and make the diagnosis of IBD.

For both the initial diagnosis and subsequent flares, other conditions that mimic IBD should be excluded (see next section). Of particular importance is the exclusion of infectious pathogens, as the treatment of active IBD frequently involves immunosuppressive medications. For patients who do not respond to medical therapy (or worsen despite it), the diagnosis of IBD should be rechallenged.

Abreu MT, Harpaz N. Diagnosis of colitis: making the initial diagnosis. *Clin Gastroenterol Hepatol.* 2007;5:295–301. [PMID: 17368227]

Differential Diagnosis

Many medical conditions can mimic IBD clinically, radiographically, or endoscopically. Infectious diseases of the gastrointestinal tract are of particular concern (Table 3–2). First, they are common; second, many of the immunosuppressive therapies directed toward IBD are potentially deleterious if given to a patient with an infectious illness. Common enteric bacterial pathogens, such as *Campylobacter, Salmonella, Shigella,* and *Escherichia coli,* can cause an infectious colitis characterized by abdominal pain, diarrhea, and hematochezia. The onset is usually acute with a self-limited course. Colitis, suggestive of ulcerative colitis or Crohn colitis, is often apparent by CT and colonoscopy. The *E coli* serotype O157:H7 is of particular note due to its propensity to produce a hemorrhagic colitis that may closely mimic fulminant ulcerative colitis. *Campylobacter, Salmonella, Shigella,* and *Yersinia* can cause an ileitis, which may mimic the radiographic appearance of Crohn disease. *Yersinia* is particularly notable for its predilection for the terminal ileum and cecum. Gram stains and cultures of stool are helpful for establishing the diagnosis of bacterial colitis. However, stool cultures have limited sensitivity, and a negative Gram stain and culture does not rule out a bacterial infection, particularly in the setting of a suggestive clinical history.

Clostridium difficile infection is common in IBD patients, even among those who have not been hospitalized or recently received antibiotics. The symptoms of *C difficile* infection may be the frequent, watery stools seen in non-IBD patients. Alternatively, infection may trigger an IBD flare, with a patient's typical symptoms of pain and bloody diarrhea. Thus, any patient presenting with symptoms suggestive of an IBD flare should be tested carefully for *C difficile,* and if ill, treated empirically for this until infection is satisfactorily excluded.

Mycobacterial infections of the gastrointestinal tract, including *Mycobacterium tuberculosis,* have a predilection for the terminal ileum and cecum, and thus may mimic Crohn disease. Active pulmonary disease may or may not be present. A patient's history usually includes travel to or immigration from endemic areas, exposure to infected patients, or immunosuppression. The diagnosis may be difficult to make, as histologic stains and cultures have limited sensitivity. Polymerase chain reaction amplification of biopsied tissue increases the yield and should be ordered when the clinical suspicion is high. A missed mycobacterial infection can have severe consequences, as the therapies frequently used for Crohn disease (ie, steroids, anti-tumor necrosis factor [anti-TNF] agents) suppress the immune response to mycobacterial infection.

Appendicitis and diverticulitis are commonly encountered abdominal infections, and are typically readily distinguished from IBD by their acute nature. However, occasionally they have subacute presentations, in which case they may closely resemble Crohn disease both clinically and radiographically.

Noninfectious colitides may also mimic ulcerative colitis or Crohn colitis. Ischemic colitis may cause pain and bloody

Table 3–2. Infectious illness mimicking inflammatory bowel disease.

Infectious Agent	Site of Pathology	Risk Factors
Bacterial		
Salmonella (nontyphoid spp)	Ileum, colon	Foodborne and waterborne
Campylobacter jejuni	Ileum, colon	Foodborne and waterborne
Shigella sonnei	Ileum, colon	Foodborne and waterborne
Escherichia coli	Colon	Foodborne and waterborne
Yersinia enterocolitica	Ileum, colon	Foodborne and waterborne
Clostridium difficile	Colon	Antibiotic exposure, hospitalization
Plesiomonas shigelloides	Colon	Waterborne
Aeromonas spp	Colon	Waterborne
Mycobacteria (*tuberculosis* and atypical spp)	Ileum, colon	Endemic area, foodborne and waterborne; immunosuppression
Actinomyces israelii	Ileum, colon	Recent surgery or trauma
Treponema pallidum	Proctitis	Sexual exposure
Chlamydia trachomatis	Proctitis	Sexual exposure
Neisseria gonorrhoeae	Proctitis	Sexual exposure
Viral		
Cytomegalovirus	Entire GI tract	Immunosuppression
Herpes simplex	Entire GI tract	Immunosuppression
Protozoan		
Entamoeba histolytica	Ileum, colon	Endemic areas, foodborne and waterborne
Isospora, Cyclospora, Cryptosporidium, Giardia	Small bowel	Foodborne and waterborne, immunosuppression
Fungal		
Histoplasma capsulatum	Ileum, colon	Endemic areas, immunosuppression
Helminthic		
Strongyloides stercoralis	Small bowel	Endemic areas

GI, gastrointestinal.

diarrhea. However, it is typically acute in onset, self-limited, and localized to a specific segment of the colon. Biopsies readily identify acute ischemic injury. Radiation can cause proctitis, colitis, or enteritis. The injury can be chronic or acute, with symptoms similar to IBD. The diagnosis can usually be made on the basis of history, focal area of involvement, and characteristic biopsy findings. Diversion colitis is usually obvious by history, although distinguishing it from IBD can be a challenge when a patient with preexisting IBD (typically Crohn disease) undergoes a diversion. Segmental colitis is an idiopathic, recently appreciated entity characterized by focal colitis surrounding diverticula. Cardinal symptoms include rectal bleeding, abdominal pain, and diarrhea.

Gastrointestinal malignancies can manifest with symptoms similar to those of IBD. Adenocarcinoma of the colon or rectum may present with rectal bleeding, altered bowel habits, pain, and anemia. Lymphoma frequently involves the terminal ileum and cecum, creating a clinical picture similar to Crohn disease.

Irritable bowel syndrome is very common, and—like IBD—typically presents in younger patients. Hallmark symptoms include abdominal pain and diarrhea, which may make distinguishing irritable bowel syndrome from IBD challenging on a historical basis alone. Objective findings such as anemia, rectal bleeding, weight loss, or fever all point to IBD. A colonoscopy or small bowel study is helpful in documenting organic disease.

Lastly, Crohn disease and ulcerative colitis can have sufficient clinical overlap to make a definitive diagnosis difficult. The distinguishing features have already been discussed at length. Sometimes, however, a clear diagnosis of Crohn colitis versus ulcerative colitis cannot be made despite colonoscopy, biopsies, and other appropriate studies. In this circumstance, the term *indeterminate colitis* is used.

Forcione DG, Sands BE. Differential diagnosis of inflammatory bowel disease. In: Sartor RB, Sandborn WJ (editors). *Inflammatory Bowel Diseases.* Saunders, 2004:359–379.

Complications

As previously discussed, Crohn disease frequently causes complications from penetrating and stenosing disease, including perforation, abscess, fistulae, and obstruction. Active small bowel disease or extensive small bowel resection may lead to complications from malabsorption, the severity of which depends on the location and extent of nonfunctioning (or surgically excised) bowel. Deficiencies in iron, folate, vitamin B_{12}, and fat-soluble vitamins (A, D, E, and K) are common, with resulting complications including anemia and osteoporosis. Because Crohn disease has a predilection for the ileum, bile salt reabsorption is frequently compromised. Resection of 50–100 cm of ileum typically causes bile salts to spill into the colon, resulting in a bile-salt-induced diarrhea (responsive to bile-acid sequestrants). If more than 100 cm of ileum is resected or diseased, reabsorption of bile salts may be so impaired that the total pool is depleted, causing fat maldigestion and steatorrhea. Extensive small bowel disease or resection can also lead to short gut syndrome, with protein-calorie and micronutrient deficiency and dependence on parenteral nutrition. Small bowel bacterial overgrowth frequently complicates Crohn disease, particularly in the setting of stricturing disease or after resection of the ileocecal valve.

Malabsorption of fatty acids predisposes patients with Crohn disease to renal calculi. Calcium readily binds unabsorbed fatty acids, allowing oxalate to be taken up by the bowel in greater quantity. Subsequent renal excretion of this excess oxalate promotes the precipitation of calcium oxalate calculi.

The acute complications of ulcerative colitis (and Crohn colitis) are similar to that seen with other severe colitides. Severe, life-threatening hemorrhage occurs rarely. Toxic megacolon with subsequent infarction and perforation is also uncommon but requires a higher degree of clinical suspicion to diagnose. Colonic perforation bears a high mortality rate. Hence early diagnosis and treatment are critical.

Colorectal cancer (CRC) is the most feared long-term complication for ulcerative colitis. Risk factors include duration and extent of disease, severity of inflammation, family history of CRC, and concomitant primary sclerosing cholangitis (PSC). Early age of onset has been suggested to be a risk factor. The excess risk of CRC appears after 8–10 years of disease. Hence, a screening colonoscopy is recommended after 8 years for patients with extensive colitis, with surveillance examinations every 1–2 years. Unlike sporadic CRC, colitis-associated CRC does not typically arise from adenomatous polyps. Premalignant dysplastic epithelium may be flat and less readily recognized. For this reason, guidelines suggest random four-quadrant biopsies every 10 cm throughout the colon. Polyps should be resected and the flat mucosa at their base biopsied. Atypical polypoid lesions should also be biopsied. The presence of low-grade dysplasia in flat mucosa or any mass lesion other than a typical sporadic adenoma portends a high risk for synchronous or future CRC. In this situation, colectomy is advised, although in certain scenarios, intensive surveillance may be justified.

Although less well appreciated, Crohn colitis confers a risk of CRC comparable to that of ulcerative colitis. As with ulcerative colitis, the risk is proportional to the extent of colonic involvement. Surveillance guidelines are less well defined, but should roughly follow those for ulcerative colitis.

Other gastrointestinal malignancies occur with increased frequency in Crohn disease. Adenocarcinoma of the small bowel, although rare, is significantly more common among patients with small bowel Crohn disease than in the general population. Crohn patients also appear to have an excess risk of lymphoma, although the precise reason for this is unclear. Medications for treating Crohn disease have been implicated (see later discussion).

Pouchitis is a condition unique to patients who have undergone an IPAA. The etiology is unknown. Bacterial flora play a role, as evidenced by the effectiveness of antibiotic therapy. However, pouchitis is rare among non-IBD patients who have undergone IPAA, suggesting that other variables specific to IBD are at play. Typical symptoms include diarrhea, bleeding, urgency, incontinence, fever, and general malaise. Antibiotics (metronidazole and ciprofloxacin, among others), budesonide, and probiotics all have demonstrated efficacy.

Immunosuppressive therapy is a mainstay of treatment, and an increased risk of unique malignancies and infections has been documented. Thiopurine use has been proven to have a small increased risk of lymphoma, but it is concentrated in two populations: patients over the age of 65 and patients susceptible to mononucleosis infection. As a result, it is reasonable to check Ebstein-Barr virus (EBV) titers prior to instituting therapy in patients in their teens and twenties. Likewise, caution must be used in instituting therapy in the elderly. Initial reports linked the use of TNF-α agents with a rare type of lymphoma, hepatosplenic T-cell lymphoma (HSTCL). A review of cases shows numbers much smaller than initially reported and that most patients had received thiopurines either as monotherapy or in conjunction with TNF-α therapy. This issue may get more attention as further studies look at the use of combination therapy. Of note, most patients were men and less than 40 years old.

IBD may also cause extraintestinal complications (Table 3–3). PSC is linked to both ulcerative colitis and Crohn disease. The diagnosis of PSC may precede or follow that of IBD;

Table 3–3. Common extraintestinal manifestations of inflammatory bowel disease.

System or Site	Manifestation
Hepatobiliary	Primary sclerosing cholangitis Cholangiocarcinoma Gallstones
Dermatologic	Erythema nodosum Pyoderma gangrenosum Sweet syndrome
Oral	Aphthous ulceration
Ocular	Episcleritis Uveitis/iritis
Musculoskeletal	Enteropathic arthropathy Sacroiliitis Ankylosing spondylitis Osteopenia/osteoporosis
Hematologic	Thromboembolic disease

symptoms and signs may arise years after colectomy. In addition to being at increased risk for CRC, these patients carry a high risk for cholangiocarcinoma. Of the dermatologic considerations, erythema nodosum is most common and typically responds to therapy directed toward active bowel disease. Pyoderma gangrenosum is rarer and more worrisome. It may occur even when IBD is quiescent and often does not respond to front-line IBD therapies. Dapsone, thalidomide, calcineurin inhibitors, mycophenolate, and high-dose corticosteroids have been used. Dermatologic referral is suggested. Uveitis is of special concern, as it can lead to blindness if untreated. Patients with eye pain, redness, and visual disturbance require urgent ophthalmologic evaluation.

Itzkowitz SH, Present DH; Crohn's and Colitis Foundation of America Colon Cancer in IBD Study Group. Consensus conference: colorectal cancer screening and surveillance in inflammatory bowel disease. *Inflamm Bowel Dis.* 2005;11:314–321. [PMID: 15735438]

Vaccinations

Vaccination guidelines in IBD have been published in both the United States and Europe. IBD patients should receive the same vaccinations as patients in the general population with the exception of live vaccines. It is imperative that vaccines be brought up to date immediately upon diagnosis of IBD, with the presumption that patients will be receiving immunosuppressive therapy. Immunosuppressive medications should be held, if possible, to allow vaccines ample time to take effect. The recent European guidelines recommended adding prophylaxis against *Pneumocystis* if three immunomodulators are used concurrently (Table 3–4).

Table 3–4. ECCO consensus guidelines for vaccination of patients with IBD.

Item	Comment
General	Vaccinate as for general population
At diagnosis of IBD	Varicella vaccine (if no history of chickenpox and negative serology) Hepatitis B vaccine (if negative serology) Pneumococcal vaccine Influenza vaccine (inactivated) Human papilloma virus (in young women)
Annually	Influenza vaccine (inactivated)
Booster	Pneumococcal polysaccharide vaccine (3–5 years)
Discretionary	Travel vaccines: take advice from appropriate specialist Chest x-ray, tuberculin skin test, hepatitis B surface antibody/antigen prior to initiating anti-TNF therapy

ECCO, European Crohn's and Colitis Organization; IBD, inflammatory bowel disease; TNF, tumor necrosis factor.

Treatment

The primary goal of medical therapy for IBD is directed toward the relief of clinical symptoms. For both Crohn disease and ulcerative colitis, medical therapy is generally considered as a two-step approach: (1) achieving remission from symptoms of active disease, and (2) maintaining remission. To a large extent, the clinical presentation dictates the choice of pharmaceutical agent. Patients with severe disease generally require more aggressive therapy, whereas patients with milder disease may do well with less potent medications or no therapy at all. All medical therapeutic options carry risks of toxicity, and this risk must be considered carefully against the potential benefit.

The secondary goal of preventing IBD-related complications has only recently become a serious consideration. Recent studies have suggested that medical therapy may help prevent postoperative recurrence of Crohn disease, or reduce the risk of CRC in ulcerative colitis. Preventing complications may also mean avoiding medical therapies. The goal of achieving steroid-free remission is now well recognized in IBD care.

Sands BE. Therapy of inflammatory bowel disease: past, present, and future. *J Gastroenterol.* 2007;42:16–25. [PMID: 17322989]

A. Crohn Disease

1. 5-Aminosalicylates—The pharmacology of 5-aminosalicylate (5-ASA) medications is discussed in detail under ulcerative colitis, for which their therapeutic benefit is better established. Studies have indicated a modest benefit of sulfasalazine for achieving remission in patients with colonic Crohn disease. Other 5-ASA drugs that lack the sulfa moiety of sulfasalazine have yielded more equivocal results, with some studies suggesting a modest clinical benefit. Neither sulfasalazine nor other 5-ASA agents have been shown to be effective in maintaining clinical remission in Crohn disease. Certain mesalamine preparations allow release of the drug in the small bowel, theoretically allowing therapy to be directed there rather than the colon. Unfortunately, evidence that such treatment alters disease course is lacking. Despite the limited evidence supporting their use, the favorable safety profile of 5-ASA medications has made them a popular choice for the treatment of patients with mild to moderate disease.

2. Antibiotics—Both ciprofloxacin (500 mg twice daily) and metronidazole (1–1.5 g/day) are widely used in the treatment of mild to moderate Crohn disease. As with 5-ASA agents, studies regarding the utility of antibiotics have shown conflicting results. Uncontrolled trials have suggested a clinical benefit for these two antibiotics in colonic and perianal Crohn disease, but convincing randomized placebo-controlled evidence is lacking.

3. Corticosteroids—Oral and intravenous corticosteroids are effective in inducing clinical remission in Crohn disease. Oral prednisone (40–60 mg/day) is a common option for patients with moderate disease. For patients with severe disease or in whom enteric absorption is a concern, intravenous methylprednisolone (40–60 mg/day) or hydrocortisone (200–300 mg/day) is an option. Larger dosages of steroids have a higher risk of side effects but offer no additional clinical benefit. It should be noted that even though 75–80% of patients respond to initial therapy with corticosteroids, only 25% of patients after 1 year are well without steroids. Seventy-five percent become either steroid refractory or steroid dependent. Steroids do not help to heal fistulae.

Although useful in achieving remission, steroids are not effective in maintaining it. Therefore, once a satisfactory clinical response has been achieved (usually within 2 weeks), steroids should be tapered gradually but steadily. A common approach is to reduce the daily dose of prednisone by 5 mg every week. The risks of chronic steroid exposure have been well described (Table 3–5).

Budesonide is an oral corticosteroid with significant first-pass hepatic metabolism. As such, it offers therapy to the gut (typical dose 9 mg/day) with reduced systemic effect. Its predominant region of effect is the ileum and right colon; it is generally not recommended for left-sided colonic disease. Its role is typically reserved for patients with mild to moderate ileocecal disease. As with other steroids, budesonide has not been shown to be useful as a maintenance medication. Furthermore, common corticosteroid side effects may occur (eg, osteopenia and osteoporosis) but significantly less frequently than with prednisone.

Table 3–5. Corticosteroid toxicities.

Skin/soft tissue
Cushingoid appearance: moon facies, "buffalo hump"
Abdominal striae
Acne
Hirsutism
Edema
Easy bruisability
Psychiatric
Sleep disturbance/activation
Mood disturbance
Psychosis
Neurologic
Neuropathy
Pseudotumor cerebri
Musculoskeletal
Osteoporosis
Aseptic necrosis of bone
Myopathy
Endocrine
Diabetes mellitus
Adrenal cortex suppression → potential for adrenal crisis
Hypokalemia
Weight gain
Immunologic
Lymphocytopenia
Immunosuppression (opportunistic infection)
False-negative skin test
Cardiovascular
Hypertension
Ophthalmologic
Cataract
Narrow-angle glaucoma
Developmental
Growth retardation

Lichtenstein GR, Abreu MT, Cohen R, et al. American Gastroenterological Association Institute medical position statement and technical review on corticosteroids, immunomodulators, and infliximab in inflammatory bowel disease. *Gastroenterology.* 2006;130:940–987. [PMID: 16530532]

4. Thiopurines (azathioprine and 6-mercaptopurine)—Azathioprine and 6-mercaptopurine (6-MP) are purine analogs that function as immunosuppressive agents. Azathioprine is converted to 6-MP nonenzymatically. 6-MP is then converted via three distinct metabolic pathways to various metabolites, including the therapeutic metabolite, 6-thioguanine nucleotides. Both medications have been demonstrated to be effective for achieving and maintaining remission in Crohn disease. Moreover, they can help to heal fistulae and minimize steroid use. They are typically reserved for use in patients with moderate to severe disease due to their increased toxicity profile, which includes hepatitis, nausea, and pancreatitis. Perhaps the most serious common side effect is leukopenia, which can be life threatening. Several studies have suggested an increased risk of lymphoma, although the absolute risk appears to be well below 1%.

Standard therapeutic dosages for azathioprine and 6-MP are 2–2.5 mg/kg/day and 1–1.5 mg/kg/day, respectively. Over the past several years, studies have shown that 80% of patients will have an appropriate response to azathioprine/6-mercaptopurine (AZA/6-MP) if a serum level of the active metabolite (6-thioguanine, 6TGN) of the drug achieves a therapeutic range (235–450 pg/mL). Therefore, dosage adjustment is no longer based solely on weight. Because another metabolite of AZA/6-MP, 6-methylmercaptopurine (6-MMP), is associated with abnormal liver tests, it has become routine to check the metabolite levels of AZA/6-MP after 3–4 weeks to be sure the dose is appropriate in regard to a therapeutic level as well as risk for liver disease.

A minority of patients carry one or more mutant alleles in one of the genes that regulate thiopurine metabolism—thiopurine methyltransferase (*TPMT*). Patients carrying this mutation are highly susceptible to leukopenia, even with lower doses of drug. Therefore, it is common practice to test for this mutation prior to starting therapy with these medications. Patients homozygous for *TPMT* mutations (1%) should not be treated with azathioprine or 6-MP. Regular laboratory testing for leukopenia (every 1–2 weeks for first 3 months, then every 2–3 months indefinitely) is important for all patients (including those homozygous wild-type for *TPMT*), as leukopenia can occur late in the course of medical therapy.

5. Methotrexate—Methotrexate is a folate antimetabolite that has been shown to be effective for achieving remission when delivered intramuscularly or subcutaneously (25 mg/week). The drug is also effective at maintaining remission at lower doses (15 mg/week). Oral therapy has not been shown to be effective, possibly due to decreased absorption. Common toxicities include nausea, pancytopenia, pneumonitis, hepatitis, and hepatic fibrosis. Methotrexate is an abortifacient, and should be used only with extreme caution in women of childbearing age.

6. Anti-TNF agents (infliximab, adalimumab, certolizumab pegol)—The introduction of infliximab, a chimeric immunoglobulin G monoclonal antibody directed against TNF, revolutionized the medical therapy of moderate to severe Crohn disease. The importance of TNF as a proinflammatory cytokine in IBD has long been appreciated (see Chapter 2). Administered intravenously (starting dose 5 mg/kg) at weeks 0, 2, and 6, it is effective for achieving and maintaining remission in Crohn disease, including disease refractory to the standard medications discussed previously. Like 6-MP, it is steroid sparing and effective in healing fistulae. Infliximab also can maintain remission in Crohn disease (dosed every 8 weeks). However, despite an initial response rate of 80%, by the end of 1 year, only 25% of patients remain in a complete clinical remission. For patients who are losing response to infliximab, the dose may be increased to 10 mg/kg with no change in the infusion interval or, alternately, the interval to next infusion may be shortened to every 6 weeks. A recent trial comparing steroid-free remission in immunomodulator-naïve patients treated with combination of azathioprine and infliximab therapy showed statistically significant improvement in combination therapy over infliximab or azathioprine monotherapy up to 26 weeks (Table 3–6). Previous studies have not shown clinical benefit for patients who failed azathioprine and then started infliximab.

More recently, other anti-TNF biologic agents have been introduced (adalimumab, certolizumab pegol). All share the same putative mechanism of action and appear comparably effective. Both adalimumab (induction dose of 160 mg subcutaneously [SQ], followed by 80 mg SQ at week 2, then 40 mg SQ every 2 weeks) and certolizumab pegol (400 mg SQ at weeks 0, 2, and 4, followed by 400 mg SQ every 4 weeks) provide a similar response and remission rates as infliximab. Recent multicenter trials have demonstrated that both adalimumab (Table 3–7) and certolizumab pegol (Table 3–8) are effective in maintaining a clinical response in 50–60% of patients at either 6 months or 1 year and remission in 40–50% of patients. Additionally, among patients who have lost their response to infliximab, approximately 35% of patients will regain response with adalimumab or certolizumab therapy over 12 weeks. Patients who failed infliximab, including primary nonresponders, have been shown to have a clinical remission rate of approximately 45% after 2 years of adalimumab therapy. Adalimumab can heal

Table 3–6. Patients with corticosteroid-free remission and mucosal healing at 26 weeks after treatment with azathioprine and infliximab.

	Azathioprine	Infliximab	Infliximab + Azathioprine
Remission	51/170 (30%)	75/169 (44.4%)	96/169 (56.8%)
Mucosal healing	18/109 (16.5%)	28/93 (30.1%)	47/107 (43.9%)

Data from Colombel JF, Sandborn WJ, Reinisch W, et al. Infliximab, azathioprine, or combination therapy for Crohn's disease. *N Engl J Med.* 2010;362:1383–1395.

Table 3–7. Response to adalimumab (ADL) for maintenance of clinical response and remission in patients with Crohn disease.

Results	Placebo (n = 170)	ADL	
		40 mg/wk (n = 157)	40 mg every other week (n = 172)
Remission week 26	29 (17%)	74 (47%)	69 (40%)
Remission week 56	20 (12%)	64 (41%)	62 (36%)
Responsive CDAI↓ >100			
Week 26	45 (26.5%)	82 (52.2%)	89 (51.7%)
Week 56	28 (16.5%)	75 (47.8%)	71 (41.3%)
Responsive CDAI↓ >100			
Week 26	48 (28.2%)	93 (54.1%)	88 (56.1%)
Week 56	30 (17.6%)	74 (43%)	77 (49%)
Corticosteroid discontinuation			
Week 26	3%	30%	35%
Week 56	6%	23%	29%

CDAI, Crohn Disease Activity Index.
Data from Colombel JF, Sandbom WJ, Rutgeerts P, et al. Adalimumab for maintenance of clinical response and remission in patients with Crohn's disease: the CHARM trial. *Gastroenterology.* 2007;132:52–65.

fistulae in 40% of patients, and this outcome is maintained in 90% of patients over 2 years. As foreign proteins, these agents can generate an immune response in terms of antibody formation against the drug itself, particularly if administered intermittently. For this reason, continuous therapy is the current standard of care. Loss of response to one medication does not necessarily mean a loss of response to the class.

Infection is the most serious complication with anti-TNF biologic agents. Patients are particularly vulnerable to tuberculosis and should be screened carefully for this prior to initial administration. Patients with latent hepatitis B are vulnerable to reactivation. Anti-TNF therapy should be held in the setting of pyogenic infections. Concern has been raised about possible increased risk of lymphoma, although this remains controversial. Less serious adverse effects include infusion or injection reactions, lupus-like reaction, and serum sickness.

Colombel JF, Sandborn WJ, Reinisch W, et al. Infliximab, azathioprine or combination therapy for Crohn's disease. *N Engl J Med.* 2010;362:1383–1395. [PMID: 20393175]

Hanauer SB, Sandborn WJ, Rutgeerts P, et al. Human anti-necrosis factor monoclonal antibody (adalimumab) in Crohn's disease: the CLASSIC-I trial. *Gastroenterology.* 2006;130:323–333. [PMID: 16472588]

Sandborn WJ, Feagan BG, Stoinov S, et al. PRECISE 1 Study Investigators. Certolizumab pegol for the treatment of Crohn's disease. *N Engl J Med.* 2007;357:228–238. [PMID: 17634458]

Table 3–8. Response of patients to maintenance therapy with certolizumab pegol (CTZP) for Crohn disease.

Results at Week 26	Placebo (n = 210)	CTZP (n = 215)
Clinical response	36%	63%
Clinical remission	29%	48%
Fistula closure	13/30 (43%)	15/28 (43%)
Important adverse events	1%	3%

Data from Schreiber S, Khaliq-Kareemi M, Lawrence IC, et al; PRECISE 2 Study Investigators. Maintenance therapy with certolizumab pegol for Crohn's disease. *N Engl J Med.* 2007;357:239–250.

7. Other agents—The calcineurin inhibitor tacrolimus has demonstrated efficacy in fistulizing disease but is rarely used in adults due to its long-term risk of renal disease and opportunistic infections. Thalidomide appears effective, in part through anti-TNF effects, but is similarly limited by its known toxicities. Natalizumab is an antibody directed against α4 integrin, designed to inhibit trafficking of leukocytes. Although effective for Crohn disease, initial enthusiasm for natalizumab has been tempered by an apparent associated risk for developing progressive multifocal leukoencephalopathy. The drug is available in a strictly monitored setting for select patients. MLN-02, directed against α4β7 integrin, has shown early promise. Antibodies against interleukin (IL)-12,

IL-23, and IL-17, implicated in the pathogenesis or Crohn disease, are currently being studied as potential therapeutic agents.

8. Surgery—Surgery in Crohn disease is frequently required to address complications of stricturing, penetrating, or fistulizing disease. Because recurrence at anastomotic sites is common, surgery is not recommended as a primary treatment strategy. Refer to Chapter 4 for detailed discussion of surgical considerations in the treatment of Crohn disease.

Achkar JP, Hanauer SB. Medical therapy to reduce postoperative Crohn's disease recurrence. *Am J Gastroenterol.* 2000;95:1139–1146. [PMID: 10811318]

Panaccione R, Colombel JF, Sandborn WJ, et al. Adalimumab sustains clinical remission and overall clinical benefit after 2 years of therapy for Crohn's disease. *Aliment Pharmacol Ther.* 2010;31:1296–1309. [PMID: 20298694]

B. Ulcerative Colitis

1. 5-Aminosalicytes—5-ASA medications are the mainstay of therapy for mild to moderate ulcerative colitis. Sulfasalazine, the original drug in this class, consists of sulfapyridine attached to the 5-ASA moiety. The sulfa component causes the majority of side effects from sulfasalazine (nausea, vomiting, dyspepsia, headache, malaise). Hence, formulations consisting solely of the therapeutic 5-ASA compound have been developed, including both orally and rectally administered preparations. These formulations have used different mechanisms to control the site of drug delivery (Table 3–9). Medications that release 5-ASA at more than pH 7 selectively target the terminal ileum and colon. Those that require cleavage of an azo-bond by bacteria release 5-ASA only in the colon.

5-ASA medications have demonstrated efficacy in both the induction and maintenance of remission for ulcerative colitis. In the majority of patients, they are well tolerated. Interstitial nephritis, pulmonitis, pericarditis, rash, pancreatitis, or worsening of colitis occurs rarely. Patient adherence is a concern, as many formulations require three- to four-times-daily dosage. Rectally administered topical therapy is highly effective for distal ulcerative colitis but has similar problems with patient adherence.

Recent evidence has suggested that 5-ASA medications may decrease the risk for CRC. The mechanism is unclear but may involve decreased colonic inflammation. This apparent protective effect suggests that chronic 5-ASA therapy may be warranted not just as a maintenance drug, but as a chemopreventative agent.

Levine J, Burakoff R. Chemoprophylaxis of colorectal cancer in inflammatory bowel disease: current concepts. *Inflamm Bowel Dis.* 2007;13:1293–1298. [PMID: 17567870]

2. Corticosteroids—Much as with Crohn disease, corticosteroids are useful for the acute treatment of moderate to severe ulcerative colitis. Typical starting doses of prednisone are 40–60 mg, with methylprednisolone (40–60 mg/day) or hydrocortisone (200–300 mg/day) reserved for hospitalized patients. Approximately one third of patients with ulcerative colitis require steroids. Only about 50% of patients will achieve a remission and about 30% will have a response. However, after 1 year, about 20% of patients are steroid dependent and about 30% require surgery. As with Crohn disease, steroids are ineffective as maintenance medications. Therefore, they should be tapered off once a satisfactory maintenance medication has been started. Rectally administered steroid enemas offer the benefits of steroid therapy for flares of distal ulcerative colitis, and some may have less systemic side effects.

3. Thiopurines—The efficacy of 6-MP and azathioprine for ulcerative colitis has not been extensively studied. They are effective medications for the maintenance of remission in ulcerative colitis, although anecdotal experience suggests that they are less so than when used in Crohn disease.

Table 3–9. 5-Aminosalicylate (ASA) preparations.

Generic Name	Proprietary Name	Delivery Mechanism	Location of Release	Typical Dosage
Sulfasalazine	Azulfidine	5-ASA azo bond to sulfapyridine	Colon	1-4 g/day divided twice daily
Mesalamine	Asacol	pH > 7	Ileum, colon	2.4-4.8 g/day divided three times daily
	Pentasa	Timed release	Small bowel, colon	2-4 g/day divided four times daily
	Lialda	pH > 7	Colon	2.4-4.8 g/day once daily
	Rowasa	Enema	Rectum, sigmoid colon	1-4 g/day
	Canasa	Suppository	Rectum	1 g/day
Balsalazide	Colazal	5-ASA azo bond to inert carrier	Colon	6.75 g/day divided three times daily
Olsalazine	Dipentum	5-ASA azo bond to 5-ASA	Colon	1-3 g/day divided twice daily

Due to their slow onset of action, they are not appropriate as solo induction agents for patients with severe disease, especially in light of other available medical or surgical options. Dosing and adverse effects are as discussed earlier for Crohn disease.

4. Infliximab—Several years after infliximab had been in wide use for Crohn disease, it was demonstrated to be effective both for the induction and maintenance of remission in ulcerative colitis. It offers a valuable and less toxic alternative to cyclosporine for patients with severe disease who otherwise would be facing surgery. The appropriate time to initiate infliximab vis-a-vis steroid and thiopurine therapy remains controversial. However, infliximab may be considered in patients who are steroid refractory or steroid dependent and definitely for patients who are failing AZA/6-MP. Dosing and toxicity have previously been discussed. A recent study has identified several surrogate markers that predict a strong response to infliximab, including a high colitis activity index (CAI), ANCA seronegativity, and a genetic polymorphism called the *IL-23R* variant.

5. Cyclosporine—Cyclosporine is a calcineurin inhibitor used as last-line medical therapy to treat hospitalized patients with severe ulcerative colitis. Given as a continuous infusion (2–4 mg/kg/day), cyclosporine can induce a short-term response in 50–80% of patients. It is best begun in a hospitalized patient who has failed intravenous corticosteroids in hospital within 7 days. Toxicities limit its long-term use. Nephrotoxicity and opportunistic infections are prime concerns. Seizures are also possible; for this reason, cyclosporine should be avoided in patients with low cholesterol (<100 mg/dL) or hypomagnesemia. Moreover, long-term data suggest that half of patients treated with cyclosporine ultimately require colectomy within 1 year. Therefore, the risks of toxicity must be weighed carefully against the limited long-term benefit of even short-term cyclosporine use. Cyclosporine is not appropriate as a long-term maintenance medication.

6. Probiotics—Several recent studies have looked at the use of probiotics, specifically VSL #3, in both inducing and maintaining remission in mild to moderate ulcerative colitis as monotherapy or as an adjunct to 5-ASA and/or immunomodulator therapy. Limitations to the data include, varying dosages used in different studies and the fact that most probiotics are not currently covered by insurance and are costly.

7. Surgery—Unlike with Crohn disease, surgery offers a therapeutic option in ulcerative colitis. Total proctocolectomy removes the diseased tissue and eliminates the need for further medical therapy directed toward colitis. It is indicated in fulminant disease, severe disease refractory to maximal medical therapy, and when colitis-associated dysplasia or malignancy is detected. As discussed previously, colectomy does not preclude other complications, such as PSC or pouchitis. IPAA is the current surgery of choice in the elective setting. Total proctocolectomy with end ileostomy is also a reasonable choice, and may be more appropriate given the clinical setting. Surgical considerations in the treatment of ulcerative colitis are discussed in detail in Chapter 4.

Jurgens M, Laubender RP, Hartl F, et al. Disease activity, ANCA and IL23R genotype status determine early response to infliximab in patients with ulcerative colitis. *Am J Gastroenterol.* 2010;105: 1811–1819. [PMID: 21097757]

Sood A, Midha V, Makharia GK, et al. The probiotic preparation, VSL #3 induces remission in patients with mild-to-moderately active ulcerative colitis. *Clin Gastroenterol Hepatol.* 2009;7: 1202–1209. [PMID: 19631292]

Tursi A, Brandimarte G, Papa A, et al. Treatment of relapsing mild-to-moderate ulcerative colitis with the probiotic VSL #3 as adjunctive to a standard pharmaceutical treatment: a double-blind, randomized, placebo-controlled study. *Am J Gastroenterol.* 2010;105:2218–2227. [PMID: 20517305]

Prognosis

Ulcerative colitis and Crohn diseases are chronic, relapsing illnesses that can be managed for the most part with medical therapy. However, 75% of patients with Crohn disease can expect to have surgery over the course of the illness; this figure may be somewhat less with the introduction of biologic therapies. The majority of patients with ulcerative colitis can be managed using medical therapy with the prospect of surgery reaching 25%. It is important to remember that patients with ulcerative colitis and extensive Crohn colitis are at increased risk for CRC when the disease has been present for more than 8–10 years, and patients must be screened by colonoscopy every 1–2 years, depending on the extent of disease.

This chapter is a revised version of the chapter by Dr. Robert Burakoff and Dr. Scott Hande that was in the previous edition of Current Diagnosis & Treatment: Gastroenterology, Hepatology, & Endoscopy.

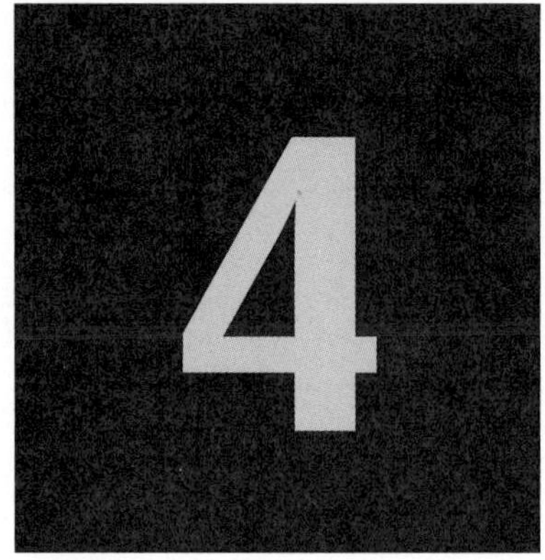

Inflammatory Bowel Disease: Surgical Considerations

Jennifer L. Irani, MD
Anthony Ramsanahie, MD
Ronald Bleday, MD

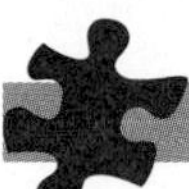

ESSENTIAL CONCEPTS

Ulcerative Colitis

- Surgery is indicated when (1) chronic intractable disease is not controlled with medication, or drug side effects are too severe; (2) patients with severe colitis require an urgent procedure; or (3) dysplasia or cancer is present.
- Most patients needing surgery are candidates for an ileoanal pouch anastomosis (IPAA); the main considerations are age, gender, type of job, and lifestyle.
- In most patients undergoing IPAA, a temporary diverting loop ileostomy is constructed to decrease the likelihood of pelvic sepsis.
- Laparoscopic-assisted and open IPAA give equivalent results.

Crohn Disease

- In general, surgery is indicated for complications (ie, abscess, fistula, perforation, obstruction); considerations include symptom severity, medical treatment failure or side effects, and operative risk.
- Most patients found to have Crohn disease at laparotomy for suspected appendicitis require early ileocolic resection.
- Perianal Crohn disease activity can be assessed using the Perianal Crohn Disease Activity Index.
- Surgical procedures for treatment of fistula-in-ano include fistulotomy, long-term draining setons, and endoanal flap closure, if the rectal mucosa is normal.
- Recent innovative therapy for anal fistula involves adhesive products, fibrin glue, and bioprosthetic plugs of porcine collagen.

General Considerations

The term *inflammatory bowel disease* (IBD) encompasses a collection of gastrointestinal diseases that medical and surgical specialists treat in a collaborative fashion. Chapter 2 discusses genetic and immunologic factors influencing the development of IBD. Chapter 3 describes medical therapy for IBD. This chapter discusses the indications and types of surgery used for ulcerative colitis and Crohn disease.

In general, these diseases are first treated with medications, and surgery is recommended after medical therapy has been exhausted. However, with certain presentations (eg, anal abscess, toxic colitis), surgery is the first line of therapy, with medication often given after a procedure. Our purpose in this chapter is to survey the surgical procedures used in the treatment of IBD, and to discuss indications and timings relating to their use.

Armuzzi A, Ahmad T, Ling KL, et al. Genotype-phenotype analysis of the Crohn's disease susceptibility haplotype on chromosome 5q31. *Gut.* 2003;52:1133–1139. [PMID: 12864271]

ULCERATIVE COLITIS

Ulcerative colitis is usually successfully treated medically; however, it is estimated that between 25% and 45% of patients with ulcerative colitis will ultimately require surgery. Surgical therapy is indicated in the following three cases: (1) in patients in whom medication is not controlling the disease, or side effects of the medication are too severe to be endured; (2) in patients with severe acute colitis requiring an urgent procedure; and (3) in patients with either cancer or dysplasia of the colorectal mucosa. Given that ulcerative colitis is a disease limited to the colon and rectum, one needs to remember that it is possible to "cure" this disease with surgical intervention. Further, in most patients, success rates of surgical therapy are high, and sphincter-sparing options exist. Despite the use of new therapies such as infliximab, the incidence of surgery has not significantly changed in the past few years.

Before discussing the specific indications for surgery, several general issues relating to the patient with colitis need to be reviewed.

1. IPAA or ileostomy?—When surgery is recommended for a patient with colitis, the surgeon needs to assess whether the patient is ultimately a candidate for a sphincter-sparing surgery that avoids a permanent ileostomy. Most patients are candidates for an ileoanal procedure (see later discussion), but some are not. The main considerations in determining whether a patient should have an ileostomy or a sphincter-sparing procedure include age, gender, type of job, and lifestyle. For example, an older woman who has had several children may at presentation to the surgeon already have some fecal incontinence issues. As difficult as it may be for the patient's body image, recommending an ileoanal procedure in this patient would do her a disservice because it is highly likely that there would be significant fecal leakage and hygiene issues. Further, if a patient has a job or hobby that does not allow for access to a bathroom, an ileostomy may provide for a better quality of life than an ileoanal procedure.

2. Emotional support and education—When surgery is recommended, the patient—and on occasion the medical team—may feel a sense of failure. In addition, the patient often has a significant fear of the procedure and the possible need for a permanent ostomy. The medical team, surgeon, and support staff need to be cognizant of this perception. Reassurance and education about the upcoming process is the best approach to the patient at this time. Availability of support staff, such as an ostomy nurse, and discussions with previous patients who have undergone the procedure are extremely helpful in improving the patient's outlook on the surgery.

3. Immunosuppression—The ill colitis patient is often referred to the surgeon after all immunosuppressive options have been exhausted. Surgical outcomes in avoiding infection and with wound healing can be significantly affected by immunosuppressive medications. The gastroenterologist, surgeon, and patient should discuss whether any medications can be stopped before the procedure without risk of a significant disease flare. It is not realistic to wean a patient off all immunosuppressive medications prior to surgery. In particular, many patients require and should remain on corticosteroids if these medications are necessary to avoid a significant exacerbation of a flare. Although patients undergoing surgery for inflammatory bowel disease are at increased risk of developing surgical site infections, recent studies have shown that the addition of biologics to the treatment of ulcerative colitis has not increased the risks of postoperative complications.

4. Nutrition—IBD and especially severe colitis can lead to weight loss, protein loss, and malnutrition. Intravenous nutrition preoperatively and perioperatively is essential in the most severe cases. Choice of operation is also affected by the nutritional status of the patient.

5. Medical comorbidities—Although colitis usually affects younger patients, the medical comorbidities of the patient need to be reviewed because they may affect the type of procedure recommended. In particular, patients with colitis seem to have an increased incidence of thrombotic complications in the postoperative period; therefore, a low threshold should be set for investigating any preoperative risk for venous thrombosis either of the extremities or the intestinal venous system.

6. Bowel preparation—Bowel preparation is recommended in any patient undergoing a colon resection. Recent studies have shown that mechanical preparation is not necessarily associated with a decreased risk of infectious complications. These studies, however, have been performed on the "average" colon patient and not on the subset of colitis patients with the issues already noted. We therefore recommend, when possible, that colitis patients undergo mechanical bowel preparation followed by administration of perioperative antibiotics to cover aerobic and anaerobic bacteria.

Indications for Surgery

A. Acute Colitis

Ideally operations for ulcerative colitis should be performed in a staged and deliberate manner. However, some patients develop severe acute colitis, requiring emergent surgical intervention.

Acute colitis is a term used to describe a series of signs and symptoms that include rapid onset of abdominal pain, bloody diarrhea, abdominal distention and tenderness, anorexia, fever, tachycardia, leukocytosis, and low urine output. It is important to remember that most of these patients use corticosteroids and other immunosuppressive agents that may mask the severity of many clinical symptoms. Severe colonic dilation or toxic megacolon is a feared complication of therapy that can lead to perforation, stool spillage, sepsis, and even death. Although acute colitis may occur in patients with known ulcerative colitis, it can also present as the heralding sign of colonic pathology in a patient not previously diagnosed with ulcerative colitis. Surgery is indicated for patients who exhibit signs of visceral perforation, generalized peritonitis, sepsis, or massive gastrointestinal bleeding. In addition, patients who do not improve despite maximized medical therapy after approximately 72 hours often require emergent operation. Other patients who improve with medical treatment while NPO but who then deteriorate once an oral diet is resumed often require surgery. The differential diagnosis of acute colitis includes *Clostridium difficile* infection, infectious diarrhea, and cytomegalovirus colitis. These conditions can coexist with and complicate ulcerative colitis. It is important to rule out these diseases, when possible, because their successful medical treatment can avoid an urgent or emergent surgical procedure. At times, however, the combination of baseline colitis and these secondary colitides necessitates an emergency procedure.

The choice of operation for an emergent procedure is discussed later in this chapter. In most cases, the goal of the surgeon is to "get in and get out." Typically, a total colectomy with ileostomy and Hartmann pouch (the oversewn rectum) is performed. This procedure can be completed quickly, removes about 90% of the large intestine, and avoids a complex pelvic dissection and anastomosis. The procedure also does not eliminate further treatment options for the patient; for instance, a sphincter-sparing ileoanal anastomosis can still be performed at a later date.

B. "Subacute" Colitis: Failure of Medical Therapy

Subacute colitis describes a disease pattern in which the patient is neither acutely ill with an unmistakable indication for resection, nor in remission and symptom free. Patients who experience symptoms of chronic intractable disease such as recurring acute colitis, steroid dependence, chronic fecal urgency, growth retardation, persistent active disease, or complications of medical therapy (eg, diabetes, hypertension, peptic ulcer disease, psychosis, myopathy, osteonecrosis, and cataracts) often benefit from surgical intervention. The long-term side effects of some of the new biologic medications have not yet been determined, and the patient, gastroenterologist, and surgeon need to balance the risks of long-term medical therapy against those of surgery. Again, it should be emphasized that one can "cure" ulcerative colitis with surgery, and most patients have an excellent quality of life without the need for medications. However, a small percentage of patients fail surgical therapy with a sphincter-sparing procedure and require an ileostomy, and some develop pouchitis, a postoperative condition that is rarely debilitating but can require chronic treatment.

C. Dysplasia or Cancer

In addition to failure of medical management, dysplasia or cancer is an indication for surgery in patients with ulcerative colitis. Patients with IBD are at increased risk of colorectal cancer (CRC). The risk of CRC in ulcerative colitis depends on the duration and extent of disease. A population-based study in the United States estimated the risk was significantly increased in those with extensive disease or pancolitis (standardized incidence ratio [SIR] 2.4, 95% CI 0.6–6.0). In addition, patients with ulcerative colitis complicating primary sclerosing cholangitis (PSC) may be at increased risk for CRC compared with those without PSC. A case-control study in which cases and controls were matched for the extent and duration of disease found that the risk of CRC was reduced with use of anti-inflammatory agents (including aspirin, nonsteroidal anti-inflammatory drugs, and 5-aminosalicylic acid [5-ASA] agents) and by surveillance colonoscopy, while it was increased in patients with a history of postinflammatory pseudopolyps.

Patients with disease extending to the hepatic flexure or more proximally have the greatest risk of CRC. Compared with an age-matched population, the risk begins to increase 8–10 years after the onset of symptoms. The approximate cumulative incidence of CRC is 5–10% after 20 years and 12–20% after 30 years of disease. Lower rates of CRC have also been found. In a population-based study from Copenhagen, the risk of CRC was not different from the general population, a finding that the authors hypothesize may have been due to an active surgical approach in medical treatment failures and long-term use of 5-ASA drugs. The highest cancer risks have been reported by medical centers that predominantly receive referral patients who may have more severe or long-standing disease.

In one series, the absolute risk of CRC in patients with pancolitis was 30% after 35 years of disease. The risk was increased in those with the onset of symptoms prior to age 15. However, in other reports, the age of onset of colitis did not increase the risk of CRC after adjusting for the longer period of time that young patients were at risk and the extent of the disease.

Most studies have found that the risk of CRC increases after 15–20 years (approximately one decade later than in pancolitis) in patients with colitis confined to the left colon (ie, distal to the splenic flexure). However, rates of CRC and dysplasia similar to those seen in patients with pancolitis have been described. Patients with ulcerative proctitis and proctosigmoiditis are probably not at increased risk for CRC. Although optimal surveillance strategies for colon cancer in patients with IBD have not been established, the following recommendations for patients with ulcerative colitis have been issued by major national medical societies in the United States.

1. American Gastroenterological Association (AGA)—The AGA recommends that colonoscopic surveillance begin after 8 years in patients with pancolitis, and after 15 years in patients with colitis involving the left colon. Colonoscopy should be repeated every 1–2 years.

2. American College of Gastroenterology (ACG)—The ACG recommends annual surveillance colonoscopy beginning after 8–10 years of disease in patients who are surgical candidates. Multiple biopsies should be performed at regular intervals. The finding of definite dysplasia (of any grade) should be confirmed by an expert pathologist and is an indication for colectomy. Patients whose biopsy specimens are indefinite for dysplasia after review by an expert pathologist should undergo repeat surveillance colonoscopy at a shorter interval. The ACG recommendations do not specify whether surveillance can begin later in patients with disease limited to the left colon.

Velayos FS, Loftus EV Jr, Jess T, et al. Predictive and protective factors associated with colorectal cancer in ulcerative colitis: a case-control study. *Gastroenterology.* 2006;130:1941–1949. [PMID: 16762617]

Surgical Options

The choice of operation(s) for a patient with ulcerative colitis is dependent on the presenting condition (emergent vs urgent vs elective), general issues previously discussed, and the experience of the surgeon. There are three eventual choices for the patient: (1) proctocolectomy and creation of an ileoanal anastomosis with a pouch (IPAA), (2) proctocolectomy with end ileostomy, and (3) continent ileostomy (Koch pouch or variation).

Another surgical issue is how to stage these procedures. Can the procedure be completed in one operation, or does it require a two-stage or three-stage approach? Finally, in patients undergoing IPAA, should the anorectal mucosa that lines the sphincter complex and distal rectal wall just proximal to the dentate line be "stripped," or should 0–3 cm of this mucosa be left intact and the pouch stapled to this anorectal cuff?

Many factors are taken into account when the surgeon and patient choose an operation, including age, comorbidities, patient size, extent of disease, and patient preference. Ultimately, however, surgery results in complete removal of the colon and rectum, and near complete removal of the proximal anal mucosa, which effectively eliminates the disease.

A. Emergency Surgery

When an emergency operation is indicated, the best surgical option consists of total colectomy, end ileostomy, and the Hartmann pouch (stapling or sewing off the stump of the rectum). As mentioned, this procedure avoids a pelvic dissection, removes most of the large intestine, avoids an anastomosis, and does not eliminate any future options. The procedure also is used in patients in whom the diagnosis of ulcerative colitis is not clear. If the differential diagnosis includes Crohn disease, indeterminate colitis, or *C difficile* or other infectious colitis, this procedure should be performed; the eventual surgical choice can then be discussed after the pathologist has been able to examine the whole specimen. On extremely rare occasions, the surgeon's only option is a diverting ileostomy. The only indication for this procedure is a patient who is hemodynamically unstable on the operating room table.

B. Ileoanal J Pouch Procedure

In the ileoanal J pouch procedure, the colon and rectum are removed in either one or two stages, and a reservoir is created using the distal ileum. This reservoir or pouch is then anastomosed to the anus in one of two ways: either with a hand-sewn anastomosis combined with stripping of the distal rectal mucosa down to the dentate line, or with a specialized stapling device that leaves 0–3 cm of distal rectum. The pouch procedure (IPAA) is a very attractive option because it not only removes the diseased areas, but it also allows the patient to remain continent and with normal anal defecation. It is usually performed as a two-stage operation: the first stage involves a complete proctocolectomy with ileoanal J pouch anastomosis and temporary diverting ileostomy, and the second (final) stage involves removal of the diverting ileostomy and restoration of intestinal continuity. The IPAA can also be performed after a patient has had emergency surgery (see later discussion). Once a patient has recovered sufficiently, both medically and psychologically, from an emergency total colectomy, the surgeon can proceed to removal of the remaining rectum and creation of the pouch.

The purpose of the pouch in the IPAA is to provide a reservoir for stool as a means of decreasing the frequency of bowel movements. When the ileoanal procedure was first performed, creation of the pouch was not part of the procedure. Instead, the patient would have a "straight" ileoanal anastomosis. However, stool frequency during the first year following surgery was extremely high—as many as 20 times per day. Although the frequency diminished after 1 year, the pouch procedure was added to the ileoanal anastomosis to correct this functional problem.

There are several different configurations for an ileoanal pouch. The most common shape is the J pouch, so named because it resembles the letter "J." The J pouch is created by folding the end of the oversewn ileum back on itself by 12–15 cm and then creating a common channel between the limbs via the apex of the J. The procedure can be performed with a surgical stapling device, which is quick and reliable. The pouch has an increased capacity, which then allows for a decreased frequency of bowel movements. The J pouch is anastomosed to the anus or very distal rectum through the opening at the apex that had been used to create the reservoir.

Several other pouch configurations (S, W, Q, etc) exist; however, one pouch shape rarely has an advantage over another. The S pouch is the only other configuration that is commonly used. To create an S pouch, the distal ileum is folded on itself three times for 8–10 cm, with the most distal limb having a short "spout." The spout is anastomosed to the anus. The key technical issue with the S pouch is to make sure the spout is not too long, since this can lead to difficulties in emptying of the pouch. Typically the spout is no longer than 2 cm.

In most patients, after creation of the pouch and the ileoanal anastomosis, a temporary diverting loop ileostomy is constructed. The goal is to decrease the pelvic sepsis rate from a suture line leak either at the ileoanal anastomosis or along the suture or staple lines of the pouch. Pelvic sepsis rates are decreased significantly when a temporary diverting ileostomy is used. Because pelvic sepsis can lead to poor pouch function and, in women, can lead to significant rates of infertility, the diversion is nearly always performed (ie, in >95% of all patients undergoing IPAA). In carefully selected patients, however, this temporary diversion can be eliminated. These patients tend to be thin and well nourished, tend to undergo a stapled anastomosis, and are not receiving immunosuppressive medications.

C. Total Proctocolectomy and End Ileostomy

The IPAA is not suitable for all patients. For example, in patients who do not have sufficient anal sphincter function, an ileoanal J pouch may lead to involuntary soilage and leakage of stool. In these patients, the best surgical option is proctocolectomy with end ileostomy. This procedure removes all of the large bowel, including the colon, rectum, and anal glands, which are lined with columnar mucosa, thereby removing any subsequent risk of inflammation or carcinoma. It is usually performed as a one-stage procedure and, because there are no suture or staple lines, is often performed without major septic complications.

The disadvantage of the procedure is that it obligates the patient to a permanent ileostomy. Any stoma can have an effect on the patient's body image; however, this decrease in quality of life is counterbalanced by the overall increase in well-being that results from elimination of the disease. Additionally, for patients who have had problems with fecal incontinence, an ostomy can bring a significant improvement in quality of life.

Total proctocolectomy and end ileostomy are indicated in the following cases: poor anal sphincter control, those who need postoperative chemoradiation for cancer treatment, body habitus (ie, obese patients) that precludes an IPAA, prior small bowel resection, severe dysplasia in the distal rectal mucosa, and patient preference.

D. Continent Ileostomy

Another surgical option for patients with ulcerative colitis is total proctocolectomy and continent ileostomy. This procedure combines a total proctocolectomy with complex pouch and nipple configuration of the distal ileum. The nipple valve is sutured flush with the abdominal skin, and the pouch is then emptied using a catheter at regular intervals. Although ideal in theory, the continent ileostomy is associated with many complications, including fistulization, valve necrosis, prolapse of the valve, extrusion of the valve, dessusception, and incontinence. Additionally, the continent pouch uses significant amounts of distal ileum and if revised or removed, can result in significant loss of small bowel. This procedure is usually performed only at specialized centers, and its complexity and complication rate make it the third choice for patients who need surgery for colitis.

E. Laparoscopic Approach

As with all colonic surgery, laparoscopic techniques can be applied to surgery for ulcerative colitis. The use of laparoscopic instruments does not, however, lead to a significant difference in hospitalization. Although the time to discharge may be decreased in patients undergoing a segmental colon resection, in those undergoing total colectomy or total proctocolectomy, the length of stay is often the same for both laparoscopic and open surgery. The laparoscopic procedure does have some advantage in cosmesis. The overall length of the small incisions is less than the incision length for open surgery, and sometimes the main laparoscopic incision can be placed low on the abdomen in a transverse manner so it can be hidden below a belt or panty line. The laparoscopic procedure is best reserved for thin patients who are undergoing an elective procedure. Larson and colleagues studied the functional outcome of laparoscopic-assisted versus open IPAA and found equivalent results for frequency and consistency of stool, medication usage, daytime and nocturnal incontinence, and quality of life in regard to social life, home life, family, travel, sports, recreation, and sex life.

Larson DW, Dozois EJ, Piotrowicz K, et al. Laparoscopic-assisted vs. open ileal pouch-anal anastomosis: functional outcome in a case-matched series. *Dis Colon Rectum.* 2005;48:1845–1857. [PMID: 16175324]

F. Fertility Considerations in Female Patients

Female patients requiring restorative proctocolectomy are usually in their reproductive years at the time of surgery. Cornish and colleagues reviewed the effect of restorative proctocolectomy on sexual function, urinary function, fertility, pregnancy, and delivery. They found that the incidence of dyspareunia increases after restorative proctocolectomy. There was a decrease in fertility, although pregnancy was not associated with an increase in complications. Vaginal delivery is safe after restorative proctocolectomy, and pouch function after delivery returns to pregestational function within 6 months.

Cornish JA, Tan E, Teare J, et al. The effect of restorative proctocolectomy on sexual function, urinary function, fertility, pregnancy and delivery: a systematic review. *Dis Colon Rectum.* 2007;50:1128–1138. [PMID: 17588223]

CROHN DISEASE

Crohn disease can affect the entire gastrointestinal tract, from mouth to anus. It may be confined to the colon alone or involve only the anal canal. Segmental involvement, rectal sparing, fistulas, perianal disease, strictures, and abscess formation are all characteristic of granulomatous colitis. Characteristic "fat creeping" (subserosal extension of fat around the surface of the bowel) and prominent vascularity in the serosa are characteristics of the disease seen on gross inspection. The disease usually affects the bowel in a segmental fashion, leaving so-called skip lesions. Ulcerations and bowel wall thickening occur with areas of sparing in between pathologic areas. Fistulas often form in Crohn disease and may involve small or large bowel, bladder, vagina, uterus, ureter, or skin, most commonly originating from the mesocolic (rather than antimesocolic) border of the bowel. Histologically, the three primary findings in Crohn colitis are transmural inflammation and fibrosis, granulomas, and narrow, deeply penetrating ulcers or fissures.

Although the majority of patients with Crohn disease require surgery during the course of their disease, the indications for surgery are not completely clear-cut. In general, surgery is indicated primarily for complications of the disease, including abscess, fistula, perforation, and obstruction. The decision to operate involves consideration of symptom severity, medical treatment failure or side effects, and operative risks.

Ileocolic Disease

Ileocecal Crohn disease may masquerade as appendicitis. Traditionally, patients found to have terminal ileitis at laparotomy for presumed appendicitis, and who have a normal cecum, undergo appendectomy, leaving the diseased ileum in place. However, recent studies demonstrate that the majority of patients found to have Crohn disease at laparotomy for appendicitis required early ileocolic resection; therefore, the traditional advice to leave the diseased bowel in place may be reconsidered.

The ileocecal region is the most common site of Crohn disease. The diagnosis of ileocolic Crohn disease may be delayed up to 1 year. The second surgery rate for ileocolic disease is 44% over 10 years, but this rate may change with the introduction of biologics and other therapies given postoperatively as "maintenance" therapy.

Strictures & Fistulas

The rectum and anal region can be involved in this chronic inflammatory bowel disease (Figure 4–1), either together (as rectal and perianal Crohn disease) or as separate entities, and the perianal disease often heralds the onset of intestinal symptoms of Crohn disease (see Figure 9–23). Perianal disease on its own has a better prognosis than disease associated with rectal involvement. However, it is important that definitive diagnosis be confirmed by histologic examination, as ulcerative colitis and Crohn disease share similar features. Perianal involvement is present in 3.8–80% of patients, as seen in literature reviews (refer to Armuzzi and colleagues; McClane and Rombeau, listed later), and it recently has been cited as a distinct phenotype of Crohn disease by identification of a susceptibility locus on chromosome 5.

There is a wide spectrum of presentation of perianal disease, with the perianal skin appearing bluish in active disease.

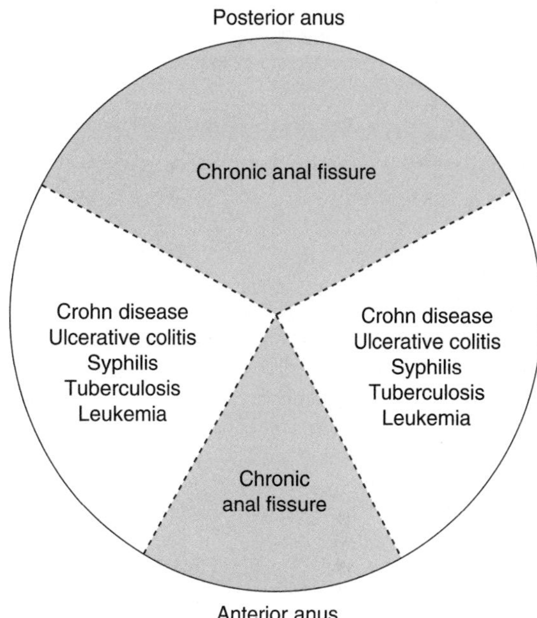

▲ **Figure 4–1.** Common locations of chronic anal fissures and other anal conditions.

Superficial ulcers may extend into the anal canal or be present on edematous fleshy tags protruding from the anal verge. These ulcers may be painless, whereas deep cavitating ones in the upper anal canal can be painful, causing abscesses and fistulas. The anus can be distorted with fistulating disease and is sometimes described as a "watering can anus." Pain and swelling are common findings, and individuals with fistulas have persistent purulent discharge, pain, and possibly bleeding as well as fever and a preceding history of abscess development. The external opening on the skin is evident, and on digital rectal examination, anoscopy, or proctoscopy, an indurated area in the anal canal corresponding to the internal opening may be obvious. The involved rectal mucosa has a characteristic thickened, nodular feel and a congested and granular appearance.

Perianal lesions are classified as primary or secondary. Primary lesions comprise anal fissure, ulcerated edematous pile, cogitating ulcer, and aggressive ulceration. Secondary lesions consist of skin tags, anal or rectal stricture, perianal abscess or fistula, fistulas of the vagina or bladder, and carcinoma.

An assessment of perianal Crohn disease activity can be made using the Perianal Crohn Disease Activity Index (Table 4–1), which looks at discharge, pain, restriction of sexual activity, type of perianal disease, and degree of induration. Other scoring systems also are available that require additional evaluation. A thorough assessment of intestinal pathology should be undertaken to determine the extent

Table 4–1. Perianal Crohn Disease Activity Index.

Categories Affected by Fistulas	Score
Discharge	
None	0
Minimal mucous discharge	1
Moderate mucous or purulent discharge	2
Substantial discharge	3
Gross fecal soiling	4
Pain and Restriction of Activities	
No activity restriction	0
Mild discomfort, no restriction	1
Moderate discomfort, some limitation of activities	2
Marked discomfort, marked limitation of activities	3
Severe pain, severe limitation of activities	4
Restriction of Sexual Activity	
No restriction	0
Slight restriction	1
Moderate limitation	2
Marked limitation	3
Unable to engage in sexual activity	4
Type of Perianal Disease	
None or skin tags	0
Anal fissure or mucosal tear	1
<3 perianal fistulas	2
≥3 perianal fistulas	3
Anal sphincter ulceration or fistulas with substantial undermining skin	4
Decree of Induration	
None	0
Minimal	1
Moderate	2
Substantial	3
Gross fluctuance or abscess	4

and severity of the disease, because terminal ileal disease sometimes manifests as a perianal fistula, and at other times, medical treatment of intestinal disease improves the outcome or healing of local surgery of perianal disease.

Armuzzi A, Ahmad T, Ling KL, et al. Genotype-phenotype analysis of the Crohn's disease susceptibility haplotype on chromosome 5q31. *Gut.* 2003;52:1133–1139. [PMID: 12865271]

Basu A, Wexner SD. Perianal Crohn's disease. *Curr Treat Options Gastroenterol.* 2002;5:197–206. [PMID: 12003714]

McClane SJ, Rombeau JL. Anorectal Crohn's disease. *Surg Clin North Am.* 2001;81:169–183. [PMID: 11218163]

Pikarsky AJ, Gervaz P, Wexner SD. Perianal Crohn disease: a new scoring system to evaluate and predict outcome of surgical intervention. *Arch Surg.* 2002;137:774–777. [PMID: 12093328]

Indications for Surgery

Traditionally, owing to poor or delayed healing, a conservative approach to the management of perianal Crohn disease has been followed. Surgical procedures range from simple suppurative drainage to proctocolectomy and ileostomy, the latter reserved for intractable disease or complications associated with intestinal disease.

Indications for local surgery in perianal Crohn disease are limited to the drainage of pus in abscesses, bothersome fistulas-in-ano that are refractory to medical or nonsurgical management, rectovaginal fistulas, and, in severe proctitis, anal stenosis, or severe recurrent abscesses, proctectomy.

It is important to note that medical therapy alone or surgical therapy alone does not have as high a success rate in the treatment of anal fistulae in Crohn disease as does a combined approach. Surgery, antibiotics, and medical therapy, especially the use of infliximab, used in sequence or combination have shown the best results.

Sciaudone G, Di Stazio C, Limongelli P, et al. Treatment of complex perianal fistulas in Crohn disease: infliximab, surgery or combined approach. *Can J Surg.* 2010;53:299–304. [PMID: 20858373]

Surgical Options

A. Incision & Drainage of Abscesses

A common emergency presentation of perianal Crohn disease is abscess formation requiring incision and drainage to allow maximum drainage of sepsis (Figure 4–2). Appropriate antimicrobial cover is needed when significant cellulitis surrounds the abscess, or the patient is immunocompromised or has cardiac valvular pathology. A cruciate incision or an elliptical excision of skin overlying the area of maximum fluctuance is undertaken under general anesthesia if the abscess cavity is large. Any loculations are then gently broken up with a digit, and the wound is loosely packed (Figure 4–2A). This approach should suffice for superficial abscesses. For deep or high abscesses, placement of a mushroom or Malecot catheter allows adequate drainage and thus prevents premature closure of the surgical incision (Figure 4–2B).

At this time an examination to find any fistulas is undertaken under anesthesia. Usually a probe is inserted through the external opening to delineate the fistulous tract. If any resistance to the passage of the probe is encountered, care is

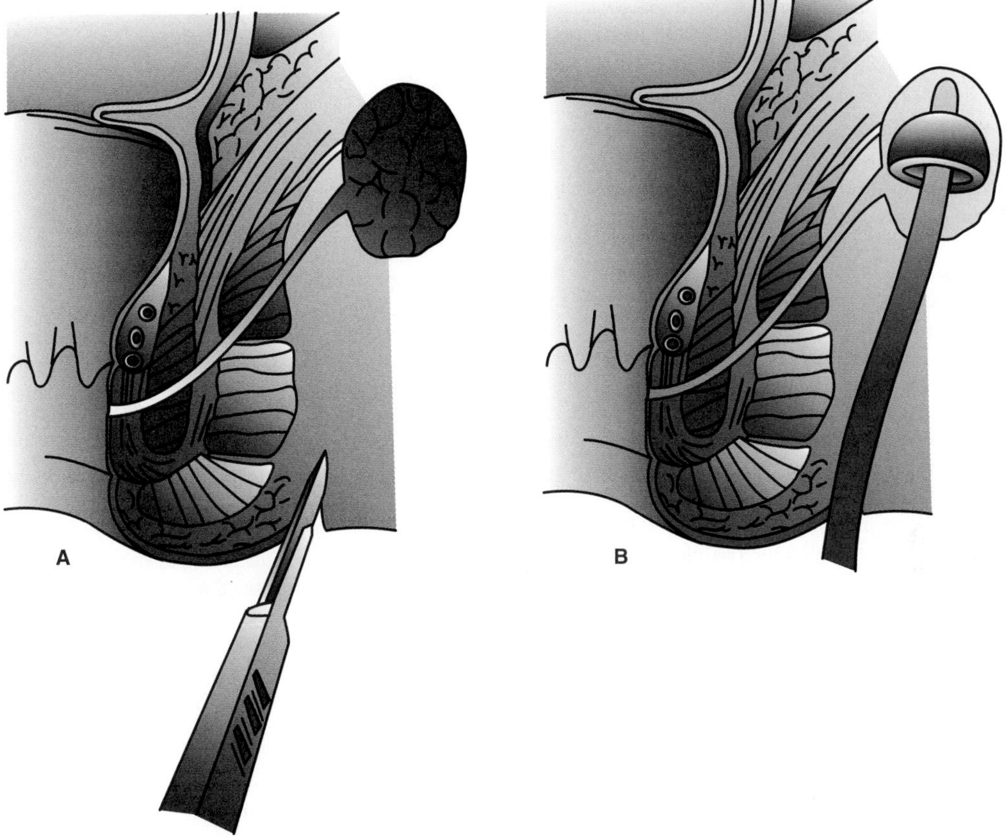

▲ **Figure 4–2.** Surgical approach to perianal abscess drainage. **A:** Simple incision and drainage procedure for an abscess. **B:** Incision and drainage followed by placement of a mushroom drainage catheter for an abscess. (Reproduced, with permission, from Schwartz DA, Pemberton JH, Sandborn WJ. Diagnosis and treatment of perianal fistulas in Crohn disease. *Ann Intern Med*. 2001;135:906–918.)

taken to avoid creating false passages. If the internal opening is not evident, injection of dilute methylene blue dye or hydrogen peroxide into the external opening with an angiocatheter may facilitate visualization. The track, if found, is curetted, and a loose seton is inserted to allow drainage. The seton is a thread of foreign material that is passed through a fistula tract and tied into a loop. (Silastic tubing or a vessel loop is preferred because they are soft and can remain in place for prolonged periods.) Drainage of sepsis decreases the risk of further abscess formation and avoids iatrogenic incontinence due to division of any sphincteric muscle, particularly in high anal fistula.

These simple procedures alleviate pain and improve the quality of life in most patients. They also permit magnetic resonance imaging or endoanal ultrasonographic imaging of the anus to delineate more complex fistula tracks or distorted anorectal anatomy. Later, as the sepsis resolves, a more definitive surgical procedure can be undertaken.

Some patients require long-term seton drainage because of the risk of complications that may occur with surgery (eg, delayed wound healing and incontinence). However, healing of the perianal pathology occurs with removal of the seton in some patients.

B. Surgical Management of Fistulas

Surgical procedures for treating fistula-in-ano in patients with Crohn disease vary, depending on the severity of symptomatology and the complexity of the fistulous track. The following guidelines are suggested: (1) Asymptomatic fistulas need not be treated immediately. However, they often reclose at the level of the skin, and placement of a draining seton is often required to keep the tract open. (2) Simple, low fistulas may be treated by fistulotomy. (3) Complex fistulas may be well palliated with long-term draining setons. (4) Complex fistulas may be treated with advancement flap closure if the rectal mucosa is grossly normal or with placement of a porcine plug, and on rare occasions, a Crohn fistula can be treated with a LIFT (ligation of intersphincteric fistula tract) procedure.

1. Fistulotomy—Fistulotomy involves laying open the fistula tract and merging it with the anal canal. This allows the tissues to heal from the inside out. Primary fistulotomy in Crohn disease patients with low, simple fistulas demonstrates excellent healing rates, particularly in the absence of rectal disease. The procedure is contraindicated for complex and high fistulas where division of a large proportion of the anorectal sphincter would be necessary.

When a fistula occurs anterior to the anal canal in a woman, primary fistulotomy almost invariably causes some degree of fecal incontinence. Wound healing occurs in 3–6 months, and complications of fecal incontinence and anal stenosis have been reported. In complex cases, a more conservative surgical approach is taken to minimize the risk of incontinence, by using a noncutting or draining seton. Medical therapy can also be instituted, thus reducing the risk of recurrence. One report found that 85% of patients treated with noncutting setons experienced fistula closure; however, rates of fistula recurrence may be as high as 39% after removal of noncutting setons, highlighting the need for concomitant medical therapy with antibiotics, azathioprine, or 6-mercaptopurine and infliximab. More than one seton may be placed if multiple tracts are present, although fecal seepage and drainage along the seton can be problematic.

In patients with rectal-sparing disease, endoanal or rectal flaps are advocated. These flaps are advantageous because they avoid the risk of incontinence, problems of open wounds, and possibly poor healing that may occur in the presence of sepsis. Apart from flap failure, few complications are seen. Thus, fistulotomy can be performed as a primary procedure or following seton drainage with the use of flaps or interposition grafts.

For longer, more complex fistulae with no evidence of anal sepsis, a porcine plug can be placed in the tract. The tract is usually curetted of all granulation tissue, and the plug is sutured to the anorectal wall with the rectal mucosa covering the plug (see below). A new procedure called a LIFT technique can also be used. The surgeon divides the fistula tract in the intersphincteric groove. All of these techniques for complex fistulae have a lower success rate with Crohn disease. Success is improved when there is no evidence of anorectal sepsis and with quiescent rectal disease.

Bahadursingh AM, Longo WE. Colovaginal fistulas. Etiology and management. *J Reprod Med.* 2003;48:489–495. [PMID: 12953321]

Person B, Wexner SD. Management of perianal Crohn's disease. *Curr Treat Options Gastroenterol.* 2005;8:197–209. [PMID: 15913509]

Rojanasakul A, Pattanaarun J, Sahakitrungruang C, et al. Total anal sphincter saving technique for fistula-in-ano; the ligation of intersphincteric fistula tract. *J Med Assoc Thai.* 2007;90:581–586. [PMID: 17427539]

Rutgeerts P. Review article: treatment of perianal fistulizing Crohn's disease. *Aliment Pharmacol Ther.* 2004;20(Suppl 4):106–110. [PMID: 15352905]

Schwartz DA, Pemberton JH, Sandborn WJ. Diagnosis and treatment of perianal fistulas in Crohn disease. *Ann Intern Med.* 2001:135:906–918. [PMID: 11712881]

Singh B, McMortenson NJ, Jewell DD, et al. Perianal Crohn's disease. *Br J Surg.* 2004;91:801–814. [PMID: 15227686]

2. Endoanal advancement flap—An endoanal advancement flap consists of anal mucosa, submucosa, and usually part of the underlying circular muscle. The base of the flap should be twice the width of its apex to ensure adequate blood supply for healing. The optimal depth of the flap is controversial; some surgeons believe that the flap should entail the full thickness of the rectal wall to reduce the chance of flap failure. The fistula tract is cored out or curetted before mobilization, and suturing of the flap distal to the internal opening of the fistula is carried out. Any secondary tracts can be treated by curetting or laying open the tract.

A curvilinear mucosal flap is most commonly used. It involves a semicircular incision starting at the dentate line and continuing proximally for 4–5 cm. The fistula tract is cored out, and the fistula is closed in layers, with mobilization of the flap. The diseased distal portion of the flap is trimmed before the flap is sutured to the mucosal edge of the anus.

If the location of the fistula is high, or there is too much tension on the flap, a linear mucosal flap is used. In this repair, the fistula tract is excised in a linear fashion perpendicular to the dentate line. The defect is closed in layers. The mucosa and submucosa are mobilized on each side and sutured together.

An anocutaneous flap is another option for closing the internal opening. It has the theoretical advantage of not involving any sphincter and can be a more feasible option than an endoanal flap if the internal opening is located distally or if the anal canal is changed by stenosis or scarring after previous surgery or inflammation. The sleeve advancement flap originally described by Berman has also been used to treat anal stricture and a combination of rectal and perianal fistulas.

Using these variations of flaps, healing rates of 68% have been achieved for a curvilinear rectal flap in scenarios of minimal rectal-sparing disease and for rectal ulceration, a sleeve flap and a linear flap for high rectovaginal fistula. Based on a literature review, Sher and colleagues advised using a transvaginal approach to develop a vaginal flap with a protective defunctioning ileostomy for the management of rectovaginal fistula in patients with Crohn colitis. They achieved a success rate of 93% in their series of patients. In cases of high rectovaginal or colovaginal fistula, an approach via the abdomen would be preferable. However, in intractable disease, some women may choose to accept residual fistula drainage over proctectomy or stoma formation.

Bahadursingh AM, Longo WE. Colovaginal fistulas. Etiology and management. *J Reprod Med.* 2003;48:489–495. [PMID: 12953321]

Hull TL, Fazio VW. Surgical approaches to low anovaginal fistula in Crohn's disease. *Am J Surg.* 1997;173:95–98.[PMID: 9074371]

Sher ME, Bauer JJ, Gelernt I. Surgical repair of rectovaginal fistulas in patients with Crohn's disease: transvaginal approach. *Dis Colon Rectum.* 1991;34:641–648. [PMID: 1855419]

Singh VV, Draganov P, Valentine J. Efficacy and safety of endo scopic balloon dilation of symptomatic upper and lower gastro-intestinal Crohn's disease strictures. *J Clin Gastroenterol.* 2005; 39:284–290. [PMID: 15758621]

3. Fecal diversion—Diversion of the fecal stream by the creation of an ileostomy or a colostomy has been employed to manage anal fistulas in Crohn disease, an approach first reported by Truelove. A loop defunctioning stoma, which should be easy to reverse, is constructed either laparoscopically or by open surgery. The decrease in fecal flow through the rectum and across the fistula tract allows the rectal mucosa to heal and the fistula to close. Creation of the stoma may improve the results of subsequent anal procedures, and also allows the patient to adjust to the prospect that life with a stoma is feasible. Symptomatic improvement after diversion is not predictable, and new manifestations of perianal Crohn disease can develop. Approximately 50% of patients with symptomatic perianal Crohn disease require permanent fecal diversion.

There are limited indications for fecal diversion in Crohn disease. These include severe perianal sepsis, deep persistent anal ulceration, and complex anorectal or rectovaginal fistula, as well as complications refractory to medical and local surgical measures. In some patients, fecal diversion can be considered before commencement of combination medical therapy. Initially there is a high rate of perianal healing with reversal of the stoma in patient with rectal-sparing disease. However, in individuals with rectal or colonic Crohn involvement, restoration of bowel continuity almost invariably leads to recurrence of perianal symptoms, eventually necessitating proctectomy.

Galandiuk S, Kimberling J, Al-Mishlab TG, et al. Perianal Crohn disease: predictors of need for permanent diversion. *Ann Surg.* 2005;241:796–801. [PMID: 15849515]

Yamamoto T, Allan RN, Keighley MR. Effect of fecal diversion alone on perianal Crohn's disease. *World J Surg.* 2000;24: 1258–1262. [PMID: 11071572]

C. Proctectomy

Patients with active anorectal disease that fails to respond to medical and previous surgical therapy may require proctectomy with end colostomy. Rates of 10–18% have been reported. Patients who also have colonic involvement require proctocolectomy with permanent end ileostomy. In ill or high-risk patients, this may be performed in two stages, with colectomy and end ileostomy comprising the first procedure, followed by completion proctectomy. In contrast to an abdominoperineal resection for rectal cancer, an intersphincteric dissection may be considered for the perineal component, as this leaves a smaller, more vascularized wound that heals with less morbidity. However, deep fistulating disease or sepsis may make this impossible. When a tension-free closure is not possible, the use of rectus abdominis, gluteal myocutaneous, and gracilis transposition flaps promote healing.

A recognized complication of proctectomy is a persistent perineal sinus. In such cases, it is important to rule out pelvic sepsis or an enteroperineal fistula, which would require resection of the affected bowel. Some patients experience phantom sensations after proctectomy that are analogous to those occurring after limb amputation. Explanation and reassurance is usually sufficient to allay patients' concerns. Persistent perineal pain after proctectomy can be troublesome and may be caused by a neuroma.

Patients with long-standing Crohn disease, like those with ulcerative colitis, are at increased risk (3.7%) of developing adenocarcinoma as well as squamous cell carcinomas. This increased risk has been attributed to an early onset and prolonged duration of disease. The incidence of carcinoma is 0.7% in patients with perineal Crohn disease. Patients with adenocarcinoma require proctectomy. Those with squamous cell carcinoma may be considered for chemoradiotherapy; however, the functional outcome may be unsatisfactory. Therefore, proctectomy may be the preferred option. The diagnosis is usually made based on examination of biopsy specimens and brushings of the curetted fistulous tract.

Rius J, Nessim A, Noguerasa JJ, et al. Gracilis transposition in complicated perianal fistula and unhealed perineal wounds in Crohn's disease. *Eur J Surg.* 2000;166:218–222. [PMID: 10755336]

D. Other Techniques

Recent innovative therapy involves the use of adhesive products. Several studies have reported on fibrin glue treatment of anal fistula using both autologous fibrin tissue adhesives and commercially available fibrin glue. The adhesive is instilled in the fistula tract after curetting, and sometimes irrigation of the tract, to allow glue adhesion to the tissue. Insertion of the fibrin glue is continued until glue appears at the internal opening of the fistula. The sealant not only acts as a closing plug for the fistula, but also as the substrate for the in-growth of fibroblasts. The technique is not suitable for fistulas with extensions.

The reported success rates in patients have varied from 40% to 85%, with a mean of 67% for the various materials. Buchanan and colleagues reported long-term healing of only 14%, whereas Sentovich showed a healing rate of 60%

when all patients had a draining seton preoperatively and the internal opening was closed with a suture at the time of glue instillation. In a later review by Swinscoe and colleagues of 12 studies, the overall healing rate was 53%. However, in patients with Crohn disease, fistula results have been considerably lower. Recent data have shown no value in using fibrin glue over fistula surgery without glue. Currently, we do not recommend or use fibrin glue for the treatment of fistulae. The use of human granulocyte colony-stimulating factor instead of fibrin glue has been shown to heal perianal Crohn-associated fistula in some patients.

Johnson and colleagues introduced a new method of closure for anal fistula with a bioprosthetic plug. The conically shaped plug, made of porcine collagen, is pulled into the primary tract through the internal opening until it fills out the whole length of the tract. Both ends of the plug are secured with sutures, and at the internal opening, the end of the plug is covered with mucosa and also preferably with internal sphincter. The remaining external opening is left open for drainage. Champagne and colleagues reported a success rate of 83% with a median follow-up of 12 months for high cryptoglandular anal fistulas, and the method has also been used in a smaller group of patients with Crohn fistulas reported by O'Connor and colleagues. However the exact place that these modalities have in the management of Crohn fistula remains unclear, but their use does not preclude other surgical procedures should the treatment fail.

Asymptomatic fissures, hemorrhoids, and skin tags in Crohn patients should be left alone, and if surgery is requested, the patient should be informed of complications such as poor healing, stenosis, incontinence, and ulcer formation. Anal ulcers are likely to be worsened by surgery, and a trial with medical therapy should be instituted to promote healing. In refractory symptomatic anal fissures without proctitis, lateral sphincterotomy is indicated. Symptomatic strictures should be cautiously dilated with Hegar dilators or an endoscopic balloon, as perforation is a risk. The stricture may be primary or occur as a complication of anorectal or ileal pouch surgery performed on the basis of an incorrect preoperative diagnosis of ulcerative colitis or indeterminate colitis. Severe strictures that do not respond to dilation may require an advancement flap (in low anal strictures) or ultimately fecal diversion or proctectomy (in anorectal stenosis).

Given the unpredictable disease process of perianal Crohn fistulas and the variety of surgical options, management should be individually tailored, using combined medical and surgical approaches to offer the patient an improved quality of life.

Buchanan GN, Bartram CI, Phillips RK, et al. Efficacy of fibrin sealant in the management of complex anal fistula: a prospective trial. *Dis Colon Rectum.* 2003;46:1167–1174. [PMID: 12972959]

Champagne BJ, O'Connor LM, Ferguson M, et al. Efficacy of anal fistula plug in closure of cryptoglandular fistulas: long term follow-up. *Dis Colon Rectum.* 2006;49:1817–1821. [PMID: 17082891]

Cintron JR, Park JJ, Orsay CP, et al. Repair of fistulas-in-ano using fibrin adhesive: long-term follow-up. *Dis Colon Rectum.* 2000;43:944–949. [PMID: 10910240]

Johnson EK, Gaw JU, Armstrong DN. Efficacy of anal fistula plug vs. fibrin glue in closure of anorectal fistulas. *Dis Colon Rectum.* 2006;49:371–376. [PMID: 16421664]

Lindsey I, Smilgin-Humphreys MM, Cunningham C, et al. A randomized, controlled trial of fibrin glue vs. conventional treatment for anal fistula. *Dis Colon Rectum.* 2002;45:1608–1615. [PMID: 12473883]

Loungnarath R, Dietz DW, Mutch MG, et al. Fibrin glue treatment of complex anal fistulas has low success rate. *Dis Colon Rectum.* 2004;47:432–436. [PMID: 14978618]

O'Connor L, Champagne BJ, Ferguson MA, et al. Efficacy of anal fistula plug in closure of Crohn's anorectal fistulas. *Dis Colon Rectum.* 2006;49:1569–1573. [PMID: 16998638]

Sentovich SM. Fibrin glue for anal fistulas: long-term results. *Dis Colon Rectum.* 2003;46:498–502. [PMID: 12682544]

Swinscoe MT, Ventakasubramaniam AK, Jayne DG. Fibrin glue for fistula-in-ano: the evidence reviewed. *Tech Coloproctol.* 2005;9:89–94. [PMID: 16007368]

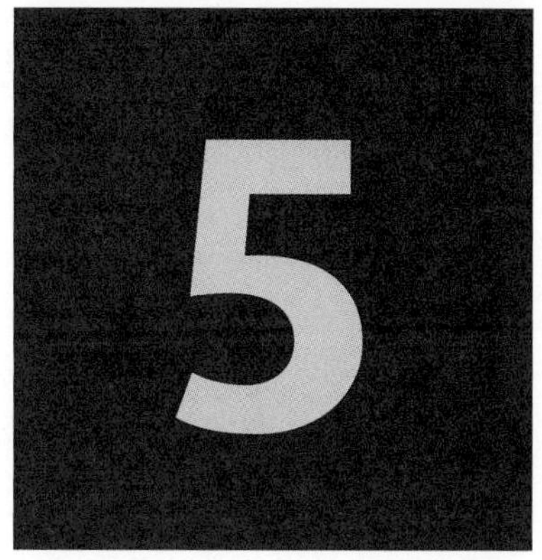

Acute Diarrheal Disorders

Jerry S. Trier, MD

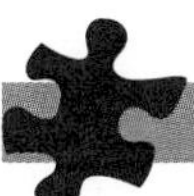

ESSENTIALS OF DIAGNOSIS

- High fever, frequent bloody stools, severe abdominal pain, dehydration, and no improvement after 3–4 days of initial supportive treatment are worrisome features.
- Sigmoidoscopy and biopsy are indicated in patients with bloody dysenteric stools and tenesmus lasting more than 3–4 days.
- Upper endoscopy and biopsy are indicated in patients with persistent diarrhea and evidence of malabsorption.
- Routine stool cultures aid in identifying *Salmonella, Shigella,* and *Campylobacter* but rarely provide useful information if diarrhea develops 2–3 days after hospitalization.
- Clinical features of shigellosis, salmonellosis, and *Campylobacter* colitis (diarrhea, tenesmus, fever, abdominal cramps) often overlap.
- Consider *Clostridium difficile* infection after both recent and remote (within 3 months) use of antibiotics and if diarrhea develops during hospitalization.
- Risk factors for severe *C difficile* infection include age >65, renal failure, immunosuppression, and white blood cell count >20,000/μL.
- Consider enterohemorrhagic *Escherichia coli* (*E coli* O157:H7) in patients with bloody diarrhea, abdominal pain, leukocytosis, and little or no fever, especially if uremia or microangiopathic anemia develops; if suspected, avoid antibiotics.
- Giardiasis is best diagnosed using stool enzyme-linked immunosorbent assay (ELISA) directed against *Giardia* antigens as an adjunct to microscopic stool exam.
- Up to 10% of patients who have had infectious diarrhea may develop a postinfectious irritable bowel syndrome.

ACUTE DIARRHEA

General Considerations

Acute diarrheal diseases remain a major global public health problem, responsible for an estimated two million or more deaths annually. Most deaths occur in developing countries and many occur in infants and young children. The majority of acute diarrheal episodes reflect gastrointestinal infections, but medications, food intolerances, or the abrupt onset of chronic disease may be causative (Table 5–1). In the United States, acute diarrheal diseases are a major health and economic problem resulting in between 200 million and 400 million total episodes, 900,000 hospitalizations, and approximately 6000 deaths per year.

Acute diarrheal diseases are second only to respiratory infections as a cause of time lost from work in the United States. As a symptom, diarrhea can be defined as an increase in frequency, volume, and often urgency of the passage of stool and as a decrease in stool consistency. More objectively as a sign, diarrhea is an increase in stool mass to greater than 200 g/24 h, the upper limit of normal stool weight. Acute diarrheal disease is generally defined as having begun within 2 weeks of presentation; diarrhea that persists for more than 3 weeks is considered subacute or chronic.

Thielman NM, Guerrant RL. Clinical practice. Acute infectious diarrhea. *N Engl J Med.* 2004;350:38–47. [PMID: 14702526]

Pathogenesis

A. Normal Absorption and Secretion

Under normal circumstances, adults ingest approximately 2 L of fluid per day. An additional 7 L of endogenous secretions from salivary, gastric, pancreatic, biliary, and enteric sources enter the intestine for an approximate 24-hour load of 9 L.

Table 5–1. Major causes of acute diarrhea.

Viral infections
Bacterial infections
Parasitic infections
Medication related
Laxatives
Antibiotics
Antacids
Nonsteroidal anti-inflammatory agents
Nutritional supplements
Others (colchicine, gold, and many more)
Food related
Allergies (shellfish)
Additives (sulfites)
Sorbitol
Carbohydrate intolerances
Abrupt onset of chronic disease
Inflammatory bowel disease
Celiac disease
Irritable bowel syndrome

Ingested nutrients are dissolved or suspended in this 9-L fluid load. The healthy small intestine will absorb about 7.5 L, largely in the duodenum and jejunum. Of the 1.5 L that traverse the ileocecal valve, the colon absorbs approximately 1.3 L, resulting in a stool mass of no more than 200 g/24 h. The maximum absorptive capacity of the small intestine is about 12 L and that of the colon, 4–6 L, for a total of 18 L; roughly double the normal daily fluid load.

B. Major Mechanisms of Diarrhea (Table 5–2)

An increased fluid load sufficient to overwhelm the intestinal and colonic absorptive capacity of about 12 L usually results in diarrhea. Excessive endogenous fluid secretion is the usual culprit, but excessive fluid intake may contribute. Examples of diseases that cause diarrhea by excessive secretion include cholera, toxigenic *E coli* infection, or, rarely, a vasoactive intestinal peptide-secreting tumor.

Epithelial cell absorptive and digestive function in the small and large intestine is impaired and permeability of the epithelial barrier is increased by the mucosal damage caused by a variety of gastrointestinal viral, bacterial, and protozoal infections and protozoal infestations. In addition, the available absorptive surface may be reduced as in, for example, rotavirus and norovirus enteritis and in giardiasis. Increased intraluminal osmolality is a cause of acute diarrhea. Ingestion of poorly absorbed or nonabsorbable laxatives such as magnesium citrate or magnesium hydroxide or polyethylene glycol 3350 are the classic examples, but impaired nutrient absorption in some intestinal infections contributes to diarrhea by increasing intraluminal osmolality. All of the mechanisms detailed above may be causative in acute diarrheal diseases in which there is substantial mucosal inflammation as occurs in most invasive and some toxigenic bacterial enterocolitides. If mucosal inflammation is mild or absent, as in cholera, enhanced fluid secretion, altered permeability, enhanced motility, or, in the case of laxative ingestion, increased intraluminal osmolality are the major mechanisms.

Table 5–2. Major mechanisms of diarrhea.

Enhanced mucosal secretion
Impaired epithelial absorptive and digestive activity
Increased permeability of the epithelial barrier
Decreased absorptive surface
Altered motility
Increased intraluminal osmolality

Clinical Findings

A. Symptoms and Signs

A careful history and physical examination are crucial in the evaluation of patients presenting with acute diarrhea and should provide information as to the possible nature, underlying cause, and severity of the diarrhea. Historical points that should be explored include (1) any recent travels; (2) the nature of recent food ingestion, including type, preparation (fully cooked, rare, or raw), and location (home, restaurant, or street vendor); (3) occurrence of a similar illness among recent contacts; (4) medication history, especially new medications or past or current use of antibiotics; (5) sexual history; and (6) predisposing conditions, such as compromised immune status.

The character of the diarrhea also provides clues as to the site of involvement by the process causing the diarrhea. A large stool volume with little urgency, no tenesmus, and only a moderate increase in stool number suggests involvement primarily of the small intestine and more proximal colon, whereas frequent, low-volume dysenteric stools containing blood and mucus associated with urgency and tenesmus suggest disease involving the rectum and distal colon. Although a patient's subjective description of the nature of the diarrhea is helpful, examination of the stool by the clinician is most useful.

On physical examination, the presence or absence of fever should be determined. Hypotension, orthostasis, tachycardia, poor skin turgor, and dry mucous membranes indicate dehydration, a major cause of morbidity and mortality in acute diarrheal diseases, especially in the young and the elderly. A careful abdominal examination is essential to assess for evidence of localized abdominal infections (eg, appendicitis or diverticulitis) that may be associated with diarrhea. The abdomen should also be assessed for distention, which might suggest megacolon, and for the presence of peritoneal signs.

Centers for Disease Control and Prevention. Diagnosis and management of foodborne illness: a primer for physicians. *MMWR Recomm Rep*. 2004;53:1–40. [PMID: 15123984]

B. Laboratory Findings

The majority of patients with acute diarrhea in developed countries have relatively mild, self-limited illness, which resolves in a day or two and requires no specific diagnostic studies. A major goal of the initial assessment, including the history and physical examination, is to identify patients who have more serious disease meriting prompt and specific diagnostic studies and aggressive treatment (Figure 5–1).

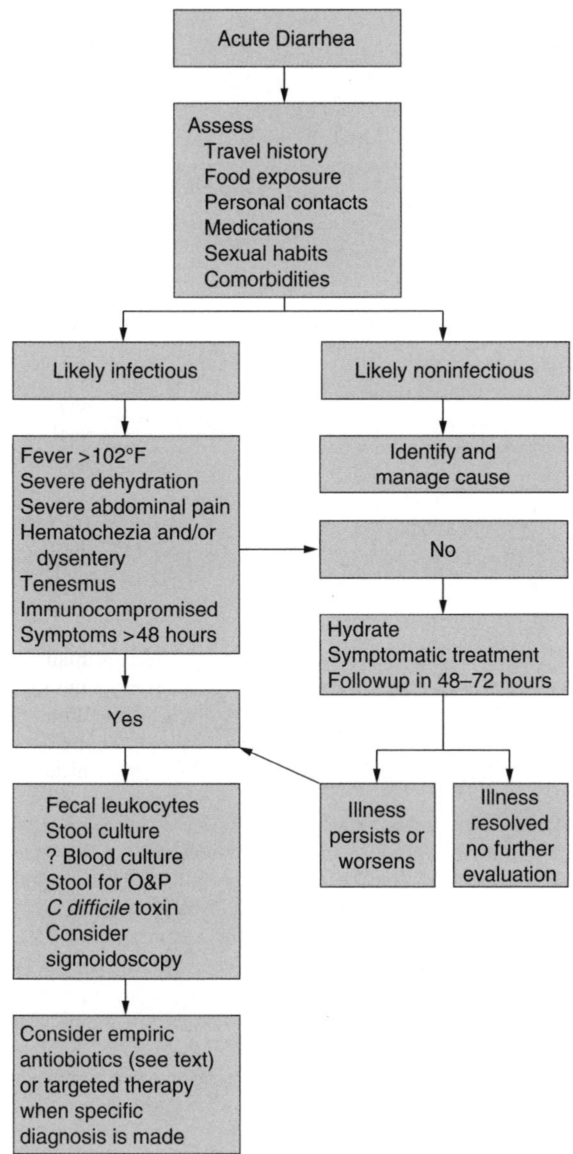

▲ **Figure 5–1.** Algorithm showing the approach to the patient with acute diarrhea. O&P, ova and parasites.

Worrisome features include high fever, dehydration, frequent bloody stools with tenesmus (dysentery), severe abdominal pain, an immunosuppressed host, and no improvement in or progression of symptoms after 3–4 days of supportive treatment (see Figure 5–1). Useful tests for further evaluation include assessment of stool for fecal leukocytes, stool culture, blood culture, stool examination for ova and parasites, stool testing for *C difficile* toxin, endoscopy and mucosal biopsy, and, in selected cases, abdominal imaging studies.

1. Fecal leukocytes and stool lactoferrin—Examination of stool suspensions stained with methylene blue for the presence of fecal leukocytes is a time-honored test for evaluation of patients with acute diarrhea. Neutrophils are usually present in patients with dysenteric stools (containing blood and mucus) caused by infection with invasive bacteria (Table 5–3) and colitides unassociated with infection, as can occur in acute onset or during acute exacerbations of inflammatory bowel disease (IBD). In other words, the presence of neutrophils indicates the presence of an inflammatory colitis or enterocolitis but not its cause. Thus, the test lacks specificity for infectious colitis, and its reported sensitivities for invasive bacterial infections are only in the range of 60–70%, in part because the presence of neutrophils in stools is variable in patients with diarrhea caused by *Salmonella* or *Yersinia* infection. Fecal leukocytes are usually absent from the watery stools caused by viral infections and toxin-producing bacteria with exceptions being *C difficile*- and cytomegalovirus-induced enterocolitis, in which fecal neutrophils may be present (see Table 5–3).

Despite its limitations, fecal leukocyte testing remains worthwhile and, if positive, helps select patients who merit more extensive diagnostic evaluation and possibly empiric antibiotic therapy. Fecal lactoferrin, a surrogate marker for fecal neutrophils, can be measured using a latex agglutination assay. The test has been used most widely in assessing patients with IBD. It appears to be more sensitive, less observer dependent, but more costly than the conventional fecal leukocyte assay. Falsely positive results may occur in breast-fed infants.

2. Stool culture—The indications for and cost-effectiveness of obtaining stool cultures from patients with acute diarrhea are still being debated. However, there is general consensus that too many are obtained. Most surveys report an incidence of positive stool cultures in only 1.5–3% of submitted stools with an estimated cost of more than $1000 per positive culture. As indicated earlier, most episodes of acute diarrhea are self-limited and resolve within 48–72 hours, often before the results of a stool culture are available. Stool cultures are rarely informative in nonimmunosuppressed patients who develop diarrhea 3 or more days after hospitalization.

Stool cultures should be obtained from patients with severe dehydration, fever exceeding 102°F (38.9°C), dysenteric stools, and stools that contain neutrophils, and from those in whom the culture may ultimately guide therapy. Stool cultures should also be obtained from all immunosuppressed patients who

Table 5–3. Fecal leukocytes in infectious diarrhea.[a]

Usually Present	Usually Absent	Variable
Shigellosis *Campylobacter* Invasive *Escherichia coli*	Noroviruses Rotavirus *Vibrio cholerae* Enterotoxic *E coli* Enterohemorrhagic *E coli* *Staphylococcus* or *Bacillus cereus* food poisoning Giardiasis	Salmonellosis Noncholera vibrios *Clostridium difficile* *Yersinia* Amoebiasis Cytomegalovirus

[a]Fecal leukocytes are also present in noninfectious colitides such as active ulcerative colitis.

develop diarrhea or patients with other severe comorbidities, including idiopathic IBD. Stool cultures should be obtained for epidemiologic purposes if an outbreak of diarrheal disease is suspected.

Once obtained, the stool specimen should be sent to the laboratory as soon as possible to minimize false-negative results. The clinician should also be cognizant of which organisms are identified by the particular laboratory performing the culture. In some laboratories, only *Salmonella, Shigella,* and *Campylobacter* are identified during routine processing. Hence, the clinician should specify other organisms if suspected, such as *Yersinia,* enterohemorrhagic *E coli* (EHEC), *Aeromonas,* or noncholera *Vibrio,* so that proper media and culture conditions are used.

3. Blood culture—Blood cultures should be obtained from patients with high fever, those with shaking chills, and those who are immunosuppressed.

4. Stool examination for ova and parasites—The yield of positive examinations for ova and parasites is low among patients with acute diarrhea as most parasitic infestations that cause diarrhea cause symptoms lasting several weeks or more. Indications for assessment include diarrhea that persists for more than 2 weeks, a history of travel to areas endemic for parasitic disease, exposure to children in day care centers or summer camps, a concomitant history of immunosuppression (HIV, chemotherapy, immunosuppressive drugs), known idiopathic IBD, homosexuals, and unexplained peripheral eosinophilia. As ova and parasites can be passed intermittently, optimal testing requires prompt examination of each of three specimens collected on separate days. If giardiasis or cryptosporidiosis is suspected, enzyme-linked immunosorbent assays (ELISAs) or immunochromatographic assays that detect *Giardia* and/or *Cryptosporidium* antigens are useful adjuncts to microscopic examination of the stool, with sensitivities of 80–90%.

5. *Clostridium difficile* toxin—The recently reported rising incidence and increased morbidity and mortality of *C difficile* colitis (see later discussion) underscores the importance of *C difficile* toxin testing of the stool for timely diagnosis and implementation of therapy for this important disease. Groups at risk and, hence, indications for the test include patients who have received recent or even distant antibiotic therapy, patients who develop diarrhea in a hospital or other institutional setting, immunosuppressed patients, and patients with idiopathic IBD. Community-acquired cases in the absence of known recent antibiotic use are being increasingly recognized.

The cytotoxicity assay using cultured fibroblasts has been the gold standard for testing for *C difficile* toxin, with sensitivity of approximately 70–90% and almost absolute specificity. However, the test is costly and requires 2–3 days for completion. Also available are several less expensive ELISAs for stool *C difficile* toxin, which are somewhat less sensitive but provide a result within 1 day. A new commercial quantitative polymerase chain reaction (PCR) test that provides results in hours has recently been approved for use in the United States. Sensitivity and specificity documented with this PCR are comparable to or greater than those of the time-consuming cytotoxicity assay.

Peterson LR, Robicsek A. Does my patient have *Clostridium difficile* infection? *Ann Intern Med.* 2009;151:176–179. [PMID 19652187]

C. Endoscopy and Biopsy

Sigmoidoscopy and biopsy can be very useful in selected patients with acute diarrhea. Sigmoidoscopy is indicated in patients with bloody, dysenteric stools and tenesmus lasting more than 3–4 days. The endoscopic appearance of the mucosa is often indistinguishable in patients with acute infectious diarrhea caused by invasive organisms compared with patients with idiopathic IBD, but in such patients, it provides some information as to extent and severity of disease. Additionally, rectosigmoid biopsies may help distinguish acute infectious diarrhea from diarrhea caused by an acute flare of IBD (Plates 1 and 2). Sigmoidoscopy can also help to exclude ischemic colitis, which may present with abdominal pain and bloody diarrhea. Sigmoidoscopy can provide a rapid, tentative diagnosis of *C difficile* colitis if the characteristic pseudomembranous lesions are present.

Additionally, sigmoidoscopy can provide rapid diagnosis of amoebiasis if secretions from the edge of ulcers are examined microscopically and the organism is seen. Mucosal biopsy from immunosuppressed patients may detect cytomegalovirus or herpetic proctocolitis. Upper endoscopy is indicated in patients with persistent diarrhea and malabsorption and, through examination of duodenal aspirates and mucosal biopsies, may detect parasitic infections including giardiasis, cryptosporidiosis, *Isospora* infection, and occasionally strongyloidiasis.

Shen B, Kahn K, Ikenberry SO, et al. ASGE Guidelines. The role of endoscopy in management of patients with diarrhea. *Gastrointest Endosc.* 2010;71:887–892. [PMID: 20346452]

D. Imaging Studies

Imaging studies are usually not required in patients with uncomplicated acute diarrhea. An abdominal flat and upright film may be useful if there is worrisome abdominal distention in order to screen for toxic megacolon, which can occur in *C difficile* colitis and colonic amoebiasis. On occasion, computed tomography (CT) or ultrasound scan of the abdomen and pelvis may be indicated, if there is associated severe abdominal pain, tenderness, or evidence of peritoneal irritation, to exclude a focal intra-abdominal or pelvic process.

Treatment

A. General Principles

Some general principles of treatment of acute diarrhea are summarized next. When specific therapy of a defined cause of acute diarrhea is indicated as, for example, for *C difficile* colitis, such treatment is described later, in the section entitled "Acute Diarrheal Disease Caused by Specific Infections."

B. Treatment of Dehydration

Oral rehydration therapy will suffice in most patients who develop acute diarrhea. In milder cases, juices, broth, and water along with salted crackers usually suffice. If dehydration is more severe, oral rehydration fluids should be utilized. The World Health Organization (WHO) recommends the following formula per liter of water:

2.6 g sodium chloride

2.5 g sodium bicarbonate or 2.9 g trisodium citrate

1.5 g potassium chloride

13.5 g glucose or 27 g sucrose

Several oral rehydration solutions in addition to that recommended by the WHO are commercially available. Rehydrate closely mimics WHO oral rehydration solutions, whereas others (Pedialyte, Enfalyte) contain less sodium and may require intake of a larger volume. Maintaining a 1:1 molar ratio of sodium to carbohydrate facilitates sodium transport in diarrheal diseases in which the enteric sodium–glucose co-transport mechanism remains intact as, for example, in cholera or enterotoxigenic *E coli* (ETEC) infection. Some clinicians favor preparations formulated with complex carbohydrates such as rice-based solutions (CeraLyte). The WHO recommends zinc supplementation of oral rehydration solutions for children (10 mg/day for infants <6 months old; 20 mg/day for children >6 months old), but there are no recommendations for adults due to lack of data.

Intravenous hydration is often overutilized in developed countries such as the United States. However, if diarrhea is massive and dehydration severe, especially in infants and young children, the elderly, and patients unable to rehydrate orally due to nausea, vomiting, or other comorbidities, intravenous rehydration is indicated. Serum electrolyte levels should be closely monitored and imbalances corrected.

Atia A, Buchman AI. Oral rehydration solutions in non-cholera diarrhea: a review. *Am J Gastroenterol.* 2009;104:2596–2604. [PMID: 19550407]

Sentongo TA. The use of oral rehydration solutions in children and adults. *Curr Gastroenterol Rep.* 2004;6:307–313. [PMID: 15245700]

C. Antidiarrheal Drugs

The antimotility agent loperamide can be used with caution to provide symptomatic relief in patients without high fever, colonic distention, or dysenteric stools. The usual dose is 4 mg initially followed by 2 mg every 4–6 hours, as required for persistent diarrhea, not to exceed 10 mg/24 h. Absorption may be increased by prolonging contact time of luminal contents with mucosa, although oral fluid intake should be continued. Fluid may pool in the gut lumen as antimotility agents do not decrease intestinal secretion. Diphenoxylate has also been used but is less desirable as it crosses the blood-brain barrier and has central opiate actions. Antimotility drugs should generally be avoided in patients with dysentery, and no antimotility drug should ever be used if the possibility of toxic megacolon is a concern. Moreover, there is some evidence that suggests that the use of antimotility agents, while reducing the number of stools, may prolong the course of some enteric infections, including those caused by *Shigella* and ETEC, perhaps by prolonging the time required for clearance of causative organisms and toxins from the gut. Bismuth subsalicylate reduces stool number, but there is no evidence that fecal fluid losses are decreased significantly.

D. Empiric Antibiotic Therapy

Although a controversial topic, antibiotics are overutilized in acute infectious diarrhea. Most episodes are self-limited and clear within 2–4 days or less without specific therapy; hence, most patients would derive little or no benefit and risk potential harm if antibiotics were indiscriminately prescribed. Their use predisposes to the development of resistant organisms. They provide no benefit in viral diarrhea caused by rotaviruses or noroviruses and may be harmful in EHEC infections, prolong fecal excretion of nontyphoidal *Salmonella*, and precipitate *C difficile* colitis. Their benefit in *Yersinia*, *Campylobacter*, and *Aeromonas* infections is controversial.

Generally accepted indications for the use of an empiric antibiotic (at this writing usually a quinolone) include fever greater than 102°F (38.9°C) and chills, severe dysentery, traveler's diarrhea that is severe or affects an individual in whom a shortened duration of illness is critical, individuals with severe dehydration and prolonged, severe diarrhea (1 week or more), and the immunocompromised host.

Antibiotics should be avoided in patients with bloody stools, abdominal pain, but little or no fever until EHEC has been excluded from consideration.

E. Specific Antibiotic Therapy

Recommendations regarding antibiotic therapy for specific pathogens that cause acute infections are discussed in the next section.

Pawlowski SW, Warren CA, Guerrant R. Diagnosis and treatment of acute or persistent diarrhea. *Gastroenterology.* 2009;136:1874–1886. [PMID: 19457416]

ACUTE DIARRHEAL DISEASE CAUSED BY SPECIFIC INFECTIONS

As indicated previously, most acute diarrheal disease is caused by transmissible infectious viruses, bacteria, or parasites. Infectious organisms cause disease by a number of mechanisms (Table 5–4). Some actually invade and proliferate in the intestinal epithelium, underlying mucosa, and lymphoid follicles. Others produce tissue-damaging cytotoxins while in the lumen and in contact with the epithelium. Still others elaborate enterotoxins that produce profound functional alterations but no detectable histologic lesion. Some adhere to the epithelial surface and induce epithelial damage and mucosal inflammation without invasion. Finally, still others produce toxins in vitro that, when ingested, induce symptomatic gastrointestinal illness.

Table 5–4. Mechanisms of intestinal infections and infestations.

Mechanisms	Examples
Invasive	Rotavirus *Campylobacter* *Salmonella* *Shigella*
Cytotoxic	*Clostridium difficile* Enterohemorrhagic *Escherichia coli*
Enterotoxic	*Vibrio cholerae* Enterotoxigenic *E coli*
Enteroadherent	Enteropathogenic *E coli* Giardiasis
Toxin produced in vitro	*Bacillus cereus* *Staphylococcus aureus*

The human host has defenses that resist enteric infections. Gastric acid secretion reduces bacterial colonization of the proximal small intestine, and there is evidence that individuals who have had acid-reducing gastric surgery are more susceptible to nontyphoidal salmonellosis and selected other enteric infections. Normal gastric motility is a defense factor; stasis predisposes to intestinal intraluminal bacterial proliferation, and there is evidence that the use of antimotility agents prolongs diarrhea caused by some enteric pathogens. The normal intestinal flora itself is protective. Its alteration by antibiotic therapy predisposes to *C difficile* colitis and reduces the number of organisms required to produce nontyphoidal salmonellosis. Antibodies secreted into the intestinal lumen by the intestine and via the biliary tract appear to play a protective role in reducing colonization of pathogens in the gut.

Musher DM, Musher BL. Contagious acute gastrointestinal infections. *N Engl J Med.* 2004;351:2417–2427. [PMID: 15575058]

1. Viral Infections

A. Noroviruses

Noroviruses, which include Norwalk agent, Hawaii agent, and Snow Mountain agent, are caliciviruses—small, single-stranded RNA viruses that, despite extensive efforts, have not been cultured (Table 5–5). It is estimated that these viruses produce approximately 25 million episodes of illness annually worldwide and are responsible for over 90% of outbreaks of viral gastroenteritis in the United States. Epidemic outbreaks in hospitals, nursing homes, in schools from catered food, in restaurants, and on cruise ships have been widely publicized, but endemic cases also occur. Transmission is via the fecal-oral route through contaminated food and water, from virus-contaminated environmental surfaces, and direct person-to-person contact. Histologic studies of volunteers have shown that after ingestion, noroviruses induce a mild to moderate mucosal enteritis that peaks in severity approximately 48 hours after viral ingestion and resolves completely within 4–6 weeks or earlier. Lesions of the gastric mucosa were not detected after ingestion of Norwalk agent.

The incubation period is usually 12–48 hours, and clinical symptoms may include nausea, vomiting, watery diarrhea, and abdominal cramps. Fever, if present, is usually mild

Table 5–5. Viral gastroenteritis.

Feature	Noroviruses	Rotavirus
Size	27 nm	70 nm
Nucleic acid	SS RNA	DS RNA
Age	>2 years	Infants, young children
Transmission	Fecal-oral: food, water	Fecal-oral
Pathologic findings	Mild enteritis	Mild to severe enteritis
Incubation	1–2 days	1–3 days
Duration	1–3 days	5–7 days
Diagnostics	RT-PCR and immunoassays are available; used largely to identify outbreaks	Commercial ELISA, latex agglutination, and RT-PCR assays useful for diagnosis
Treatment	Rehydration as needed	Vigorous rehydration
Vaccine	None	RotaTeq, Rotarix

ELISA, enzyme-linked immunosorbent assay; RT-PCR, reverse transcriptase polymerase chain reaction.

(<101.5°F [38.6°C]). The duration of clinical symptoms is short, usually ranging from a few hours to 3 days. The characteristic histologic lesion has been observed in asymptomatic volunteers after norovirus ingestion, providing evidence that some infections are subclinical. Routine laboratory studies remain normal unless severe dehydration develops, in which case elevations of blood urea nitrogen and creatinine and leukocytosis may be seen.

The diagnosis depends on the epidemiology and clinical features. A reverse transcription PCR assay and diagnostic immunoassays are available and are used largely to identify outbreaks but are not generally used to diagnose individual patients.

Treatment is supportive and consists of oral rehydration with carbohydrate–electrolyte solutions (see earlier discussion) and, in a small minority of patients with severe dehydration, by intravenous hydration. Symptomatic treatments such as bismuth subsalicylate and loperamide can be used but are usually not needed, and there is little evidence that they significantly influence fecal fluid losses. There is no effective antiviral agent and no available vaccine.

The prognosis is excellent for this generally self-limited disease, although deaths may occur in association with norovirus gastroenteritis, largely in debilitated, elderly patients with significant comorbidities.

Blanton LH, Adams SM, Beard RS, et al. Molecular and epidemiologic trends of caliciviruses associated with outbreaks of acute gastroenteritis in the United States, 2000–2004. *J Infect Dis.* 2006;193:413–421. [PMID: 16388489]

Glass RI, Parashar UD, Estes MK. Norovirus gastroenteritis. *N Engl J Med.* 2009;361:1776–1185. [PMID: 19864676]

B. Rotaviruses

Rotaviruses are a major cause of infectious diarrhea worldwide, accounting for an estimated 500,000 or more deaths each year. In the United States, prior to the widespread use of rotavirus vaccines, approximately 2.7 million children developed rotavirus gastroenteritis yearly, resulting in over 50,000 hospitalizations and an estimated 30 deaths. However, there is increasing evidence that with the introduction of effective vaccines, those numbers have decreased substantially.

Rotaviruses are double-stranded RNA viruses (see Table 5–5) whose classification is complex. There are several groups, which, in turn, may contain subgroups and multiple serotypes. Most but not all disease in humans is caused by group A. The virus invades, proliferates in, and destroys enterocytes, resulting in the passage of abundant virions in the stool of infected individuals for 7–10 days; however, virions can be shed for up to 3–4 weeks. Significant enteritis develops, with patchy shortening or even complete loss of villi, crypt hyperplasia, and inflammation of the lamina propria.

Symptomatic illness is more common in winter and occurs largely in infants and young children. Watery diarrhea, which can be profuse, and vomiting are the major symptoms, accompanied by fever in 50% or more of cases. Reinfections in older children and adults are usually asymptomatic or mild but can occasionally cause severe symptoms. Dehydration is a hazard—especially in infants, if diarrhea is accompanied by vomiting that precludes adequate oral fluid intake—and is the major cause of morbidity and death. The illness generally lasts from 4–7 days, but more protracted diarrhea has been reported. The diagnosis can be confirmed by demonstrating rotavirus antigen in the stool by specific ELISA, latex agglutination, or PCR assays.

Hydration is the cornerstone of therapy and can often be achieved with oral rehydration regimens containing sugar, salt, and water or commercial oral rehydration formulations unless diarrhea is profuse and accompanied by vomiting, in which case intravenous rehydration may be lifesaving. The American Academy of Pediatrics does not recommend symptomatic therapy, including antimotility drugs, bismuth subsalicylate, and probiotics, for children younger than age 5 years.

The overall prognosis is excellent, with the vast majority of patients recovering completely within 7–10 days, except as noted earlier.

A pentavalent human-bovine reassortant rotavirus vaccine (RotaTeq) and a monovalent attenuated human rotavirus vaccine (Rotarix) are licensed in the United States. Vaccination is recommended for all infants who have no contraindications.

Kahn MA, Bass DM. Viral infections: new and emerging. *Curr Opin Gastroenterol.* 2010;26:26–30. [PMID: 19907323]

Widdowson MA, Bresee JS, Gentsch JR, et al. Rotavirus disease and its prevention. *Curr Opin Gastroenterol.* 2005;21:26–31. [PMID: 15687881]

C. Other Viruses

Enteric adenovirus causes a rotavirus-like endemic gastroenteritis primarily in children younger than 2 years of age. Its incubation period is longer than that of rotavirus, but it appears to be less contagious. Astrovirus also causes endemic gastroenteritis primarily in children but also among elderly and immunocompromised adults; occasional multicase outbreaks have been described. Clinically, gastroenteritis caused by adenovirus and astrovirus resembles that caused by rotavirus and norovirus, and the principles of therapy are the same. Diarrhea may also accompany enterovirus and coxsackievirus infections, although manifestations involving other systems often overshadow any accompanying diarrhea.

Whereas cytomegalovirus infections of the gastrointestinal tract notoriously affect immunocompromised patients, as discussed in Chapter 10, occasional cases of cytomegalovirus colitis have been described in apparently immunocompetent adults. In one review, 15 cases over a wide age range were described. Presenting features included diarrhea, hematochezia, fever, and abdominal pain. Endoscopy generally revealed colitis with frank ulcers, and mortality (27%) was high. When diagnosed, antiviral therapy with agents such as ganciclovir or foscarnet is indicated.

Galiatsatos P, Shrier I, Lamoureux E, et al. Meta-analysis of outcome of cytomegalovirus colitis in immunocompetent hosts. *Dig Dis Sci.* 2005;50:609–616. [PMID: 15844689]

2. Bacterial Infections

Although specific bacterial infections are discussed on the following pages, the presentation of patients with shigelloses, invasive *E coli* and EHEC, *Campylobacter,* and nontyphoidal *Salmonella* enterocolitis may be clinically indistinguishable. As a result, the decision about whether or not to begin empiric antibiotic treatment can be difficult. Although antibiotics may be of benefit in a few infections (shigelloses, invasive *E coli*), they may have undesirable effects in others (EHEC, uncomplicated nontyphoidal *Salmonella* enterocolitis) and predispose to *C difficile* colitis. Hence, potential benefits versus risks must be weighed carefully.

A. Shigelloses

Shigella species are a major cause of dysenteric infectious colitis, with an estimated annual incidence of 450,000 in the United States. Four pathogenic species have been identified (*Shigella dysenteriae, Shigella flexneri, Shigella sonnei,* and *Shigella boydii*). Disease is caused by ingestion of contaminated food, water, or direct person-to-person fecal-oral spread. The *Shigella* species are acid-resistant; hence, a very small inoculum (≤100 bacteria) can produce disease. The bacteria invade and spread through the epithelium, produce several enterotoxins, including Shiga toxin, and induce severe, acute inflammation of the mucosa (see Plates 1 and 2) probably by causing the release of proinflammatory cytokines. There is no available vaccine.

After an average 3-day incubation period, patients usually develop watery diarrhea, which rapidly progresses to dysenteric stools with mucus and blood, tenesmus, and, usually, fever. Some patients also develop nausea and vomiting. The severity varies and ranges from watery stools without dysentery or significant fever to severe dysentery with more than 20 low-volume stools per day, abdominal cramps, tenesmus, and high fever. Sigmoidoscopy in patients with dysentery caused by shigellosis is usually grossly indistinguishable from that observed with other dysenteric infections (*Campylobacter,* nontyphoidal *Salmonella*) or a flare of idiopathic IBD. Biopsy can be useful in distinguishing infectious proctocolitis from a flare of idiopathic proctocolitis in that chronic changes such as crypt distortion and dropout are absent despite the presence of substantial inflammation, most prominently in the upper half of the mucosa (compare Plate 1 with Plate 2). Stools from the majority of patients contain neutrophils, and the diagnosis is established by stool culture.

In previously healthy individuals who are not immunosuppressed, shigellosis is usually self-limited and clears within about 1 week without treatment. Antibiotic therapy shortens the duration of symptoms and the fecal shedding of *Shigella* organisms by about 50% and should be considered if fever is high and dysentery is severe or the stool cultures are positive, especially in infants and young children but also in adults. Antibiotic therapy is clearly indicated in patients with bacteremia (<10%), food handlers, elderly or malnourished patients with comorbidities, and the immunosuppressed. If possible, it should be guided by the antibiotic sensitivity of the *Shigella* species isolated from stool or blood culture. If antibiotic susceptibility is unknown, the current treatment of choice is a fluoroquinolone in adults, although reports of resistance to quinolones are appearing especially in Asia, and azithromycin in children younger than 18 years of age. In all patients, supportive measures such as hydration are important, but antimotility agents are not recommended as they may prolong symptoms and fecal shedding of *Shigella.*

Gastrointestinal complications are uncommon, but rectal prolapse, toxic megacolon, and even intestinal perforation have been reported. The most common gastrointestinal complication of this and other intestinal bacterial infections appears to be postinfectious irritable bowel syndrome, which occurs in as many as 10% of patients (see Chapter 24). Systemic complications include a sterile reactive arthritis occurring usually 1–2 weeks after the onset of gastrointestinal symptoms and, in rare instances, the hemolytic uremic syndrome with microangiopathic anemia, thrombocytopenia, and acute renal failure. In addition, seizures associated with high fever may occur, especially in infants and young children.

Kosek M, Yori PP, Olortegui MP. Shigellosis update: advancing antibiotic resistance, investment empowered vaccine development, and green bananas. *Curr Opin Infect Dis.* 2010;23:475–480. [PMID: 20689423]

Sivapalasingam S, Nelson JM, Joyce K, et al. High prevalence of antimicrobial resistance among *Shigella* isolates in the United States tested by the National Antimicrobial Resistance Monitoring System from 1999 to 2002. *Antimicrob Agents Chemother.* 2006;50:49–54. [PMID: 16377666]

B. Nontyphoidal Salmonellosis

Salmonella organisms that cause disease in humans are a zoonosis widely distributed throughout the animal kingdom. Salmonellosis is the most common cause of foodborne enterocolitis in the United States. Most of the estimated one and a half to two million annual cases that occur in the United States result from ingestion of fecally contaminated, incompletely cooked food such as meat (especially poultry and ground beef), eggs, milk and other dairy products, contaminated vegetables, and even processed foods such as peanut butter. Direct person-to-person spread and spread from common and exotic pets, especially reptiles, occur. Outbreaks from contaminated water have been described.

Salmonella typhimurium and *Salmonella enteritidis* are the most common causes in the United States, but other serotypes may be isolated. Unlike *Shigella* organisms, salmonellae are acid-sensitive; hence, a larger inoculum is required for induction of clinical illness. Reduction of gastric acid secretion through surgery, disease, or pharmacotherapy and prior antibiotic treatment that disrupts the normal intestinal flora reduce the number of organisms required to produce infection. The extremes of age, immunosuppression, and malignancy also predispose to infection. *Salmonellae* adhere to and invade the intestinal epithelium. They enter macrophages, in which virulent forms can survive and then may disseminate to distant sites.

The clinical features of *Salmonella* gastroenteritis are not distinctive and vary from case to case. Nausea, vomiting, and fever are common early in the course followed by abdominal cramps and diarrhea, which may be voluminous. Dysentery may occur but is less common than in shigellosis or *Campylobacter* enterocolitis. In most healthy adults, the disease is self-limited, with fever abating within 2–3 days and diarrhea lasting no more than 10 days. Clinical features are often more severe in those with predisposing factors such as immunosuppression, in neonates and the elderly, and in those with other comorbidities. As there are no available tests for rapid diagnosis, confirmation awaits a positive stool culture, which requires 2–3 days. Blood cultures should be obtained in those with severe symptoms and those with conditions predisposing to disseminated or recurrent disease.

There is general agreement that antibiotics are not indicated for individuals in good general health with mild to moderate illness who are not at the extremes of age. There is no convincing evidence that such treatment significantly alters the clinical course, and several studies indicate that antibiotic treatment prolongs fecal shedding of nontyphoidal *Salmonellae.* Thus, supportive care with rehydration forms the basis of treatment. Whether immunocompetent patients with more severe and prolonged illness should be treated is somewhat controversial. Some authorities favor a short course of antibiotics, such as 4–7 days of a fluoroquinolone in that setting. Also controversial is whether infected food handlers and health care workers should be routinely treated.

More definite indications for antibiotic treatment include the immunosuppressed host; those with sickle cell disease or known atherosclerotic disease, in whom dissemination may cause osteomyelitis or infection of an atherosclerotic plaque; those with vascular grafts or orthopedic prostheses; and the elderly, especially those with additional comorbidities. Most authorities would recommend at least 2 weeks of treatment for these high-risk patients, with a choice of antibiotics guided by the antibiotic resistance pattern of the infecting organism and the patient's comorbidities.

Hohmann EL. Nontyphoidal salmonellosis. *Clin Infect Dis.* 2001; 15:263–269. [PMID: 11170916]

Patrick ME, Adcock PM, Gomez TM, et al. *Salmonella enteritidis* infections, United States, 1985–1999. *Emerg Infect Dis.* 2004;10: 1–7. [PMID: 15078589]

C. *Campylobacter*

Like nontyphoidal *Salmonella* infections, *Campylobacter* species that infect humans, notably *Campylobacter jejuni* and *Campylobacter coli,* are carried by a wide array of domestic and wild species. Hence, human *Campylobacter* infections are second only to *Salmonella* as a cause of foodborne enterocolitis in the United States, with contaminated poultry responsible for approximately 50% of infections. However, beef, lamb, and pork, as well as contaminated water or improperly pasteurized milk, have caused major outbreaks. Like *Salmonella* and *Shigella, Campylobacter* adhere to and then invade the intestinal epithelium of the small intestine and colon, although the exact mechanisms of adhesion and invasion differ. Like *Salmonella, Campylobacter* species are acid-sensitive; as a result, conditions that reduce gastric acid secretion predispose to infection by reducing the number of ingested bacteria required to produce symptomatic disease. The immunosuppressed, especially AIDS patients, and the elderly with comorbid conditions are at risk of more severe *Campylobacter*-induced illness.

The clinical features are not distinctive and often closely resemble those seen with shigellosis or nontyphoidal salmonellosis. After an average 3-day incubation period, a brief prodromal phase with fever and malaise in some patients is rapidly followed by crampy periumbilical abdominal pain and diarrhea. Hematochezia occurs in 30–50% of patients, and the abdominal cramps and diarrhea are often severe. Fever occurs in 70–90% of patients. The disease is usually self-limited, with recovery in 5–9 days, although a minority (~10%) of patients suffer a relapse, usually within a few days following apparent resolution. The abdominal pain in patients with *Campylobacter* infection may be severe and lead to consideration of other diagnoses, such as acute appendicitis, especially in children. As with *Salmonella* and *Shigella* infections, the clinical presentation and gross endoscopic appearance of the colonic mucosa in *Campylobacter* enterocolitis can be indistinguishable from the acute onset or an acute relapse of colitis caused by IBD, especially ulcerative colitis.

Definitive diagnosis requires identification of *Campylobacter* in stool culture. A tentative diagnosis can be made more rapidly by microscopic examination of a stool suspension using phase-contrast or darkfield optics in those instances in which large numbers of *Campylobacter* organisms are excreted in diarrheal stool. The rapidly motile spiral-shaped organisms are characteristic.

Antibiotics may shorten the duration of symptoms if given within 1–2 days of onset. However, as the diagnosis is rarely established that rapidly, and the disease is self-limited in otherwise healthy individuals, routine treatment is not recommended, although this may change as some data now indicate that antibiotic treatment may reduce the incidence of postinfectious irritable bowel syndrome. Supportive therapy with rehydration is recommended. Antibiotic treatment is indicated for patients with prolonged or relapsing illness, the immunosuppressed, those with serious comorbidities, and the elderly. A 3–5-day course of a macrolide such as erythromycin or azithromycin is recommended. Fluoroquinolones are an alternative, although resistance to this group of antibiotics is high, especially in parts of Asia.

Rarely, reactive arthritis or Guillain-Barré syndrome may complicate *C jejuni* infection, with a range of onset of 1 week to 2 months after the presentation with gastrointestinal symptoms.

Kirkpatric BD, Tribble DR. Update on human *Campylobacter jejuni* infections. *Curr Opin Gastroenterol.* 2011;27:1–7. [PMID: 21124212]

Ternhag A, Askikainen T, Giesecke J, et al. A meta-analysis on the effects of antibiotic treatment on duration of symptoms caused by infection with *Campylobacter species. Clin Infect Dis.* 2007;44:696–700. [PMID: 17278062]

D. *Yersinia*

Yersinia enterocolitica and *Yersinia pseudotuberculosis* produce enterocolitis with diarrhea in humans. Although *Yersinia* species are widespread throughout the animal kingdom, the strains pathogenic to humans do not produce disease in animals but may be carried by them, especially pigs. Ingestion of contaminated food—especially undercooked pork, but also vegetables grown in contaminated soil, dairy products, and contaminated water—transmits the infection to humans. Both outbreaks and sporadic infections occur in the United States and, more commonly, in Europe. Individuals with diseases that result in increased iron stores, such as hemochromatosis and thalassemia, appear to be more susceptible to infection. *Yersinia* organisms invade via the epithelium overlying lymphoid follicles, which are most abundant as aggregates in the ileum and cecum (Peyer patches) but are present along the length of the alimentary tract. The organisms then proliferate in the lymphoid tissues and can spread to regional mesenteric lymph nodes.

After an incubation period of 1–10 days (median, 4 days), two major patterns of clinical symptoms develop. A typical acute enterocolitis with fever, abdominal cramps, diarrhea (which may be bloody), and, in the minority of patients, nausea and vomiting occurs. This presentation is nonspecific and indistinguishable from that observed with *Salmonella, Shigella,* or *Campylobacter* enteritis. However, the duration of symptoms among patients with *Yersinia* enterocolitis tends to be longer, averaging 2 weeks in several reported outbreaks. Also, in contrast to gastroenteritis caused by other invasive bacteria, pharyngitis involving the lymphoid-rich tonsils may accompany *Yersinia* enterocolitis. In the other pattern of illness seen most often in adolescents and young adults, diarrhea may be mild or absent, whereas severe right lower quadrant abdominal pain, fever, and leukocytosis predominate, often mimicking acute appendicitis. If such patients undergo surgery, an acute ileitis and mesenteric adenitis is usually observed.

Diagnosis is best established by culture of *Yersinia* from stool, body fluids, or tissue, if surgical specimens are available. Throat culture may be positive, especially if pharyngitis is present. The laboratory should be alerted when *Yersinia* infection is suspected as screening for *Yersinia* is usually not routine. Serologic tests can be helpful; the presence of immunoglobulin M antibodies to *Yersinia* and a significant rise in antibody titers between acute and convalescent sera support the diagnosis of recent infections, although the latter is of little help during acute illness. In patients in whom symptoms mimic appendicitis, imaging of the right lower quadrant via CT or ultrasound is important; ileitis and mesenteric adenitis are usually present, but the appendix generally appears normal.

Supportive therapy with hydration is the mainstay of treatment. There is no convincing evidence that antibiotic treatment alters the clinical course of uncomplicated *Yersinia* enterocolitis. Indications for treatment are the immunosuppressed host, complications such as invasive infections and septicemia, and, perhaps, patients with conditions associated with increased iron stores. If oral therapy suffices, in adults a fluoroquinolone and in children trimethoprim–sulfamethoxazole are recommended for 5–7 days. If intravenous administration is required, a third-generation cephalosporin is recommended for 2–3 weeks. Complications include reactive arthritis, erythema nodosum, and, rarely, other conditions with autoimmune overtones, including myocarditis, glomerulonephritis, thyroiditis, and hepatitis.

Black RE, Slome S. *Yersinia enterocolitica. Infect Dis Clin North Am.* 1988;2:625–641. [PMID: 3074119]

E. Listeriosis

Listeria monocytogenes is an invasive, gram-positive, rod-shaped organism resembling diphtheroids in appearance. *Listeria monocytogenes* is widely found in soil, many animal species, and foodstuffs, most notably cheese, sausage, and other processed delicatessen meats. *L monocytogenes* can proliferate in refrigerated foods. Most infections occur sporadically, but foodborne outbreaks have also been well documented.

In otherwise healthy immunocompetent individuals, the organism invades the intestinal mucosa and causes a self-limited febrile gastroenteritis of relatively short duration, usually 2 days or less. Symptoms are nonspecific and include fever, malaise, muscle aches, nausea, vomiting, and diarrhea. Pregnant patients commonly present with a flulike illness with or without gastrointestinal symptoms. There is a predilection for invasion of placental tissue, especially during the last trimester, with spread of the organism to the fetus and fetal death or birth of an infected neonate. In immunosuppressed hosts and the elderly, there is a predilection for central nervous system invasion with resulting meningitis, meningoencephalitis, and, rarely, brain abscess.

The diagnosis is usually made by culture of *L monocytogenes* from the blood and cerebrospinal fluid. The significance of isolation of the organism from the stool is unclear as it can be isolated occasionally from asymptomatic individuals. Isolation from stool requires the use of selective media not generally used for routine stool culture. Blood cultures should be obtained from pregnant and immunocompromised patients with febrile gastroenteritis.

There is no evidence that antibiotic therapy influences the course of uncomplicated, febrile *Listeria* gastroenteritis in otherwise healthy patients; in many instances, the diagnosis is not established by bacterial isolation and, if it is, symptoms will have resolved. On the other hand, infection in pregnant, elderly, or immunosuppressed patients or in any individual with evidence of spread to other tissues should be treated. Ampicillin, penicillin G, and trimethoprim–sulfamethoxazole have been effective.

Ooi ST, Lorber B. Gastroenteritis due to *Listeria monocytogenes*. *Clin Infect Dis*. 2005;40:1327–1332. [PMID: 15825036]

F. Noncholera *Vibrio*

Several *Vibrio* species distinct from *Vibrio cholerae*, including *Vibrio parahaemolyticus*, can cause diarrheal disease in humans. These organisms thrive in high salt concentrations and are found in saltwater estuaries, especially in the summer and fall, although they also can contaminate fresh water. Most outbreaks and sporadic cases of diarrheal disease result from ingestion of contaminated raw or improperly cooked seafood, especially mollusks (eg, oysters, mussels, or clams) and crustaceans, including crab and shrimp. Most noncholera *Vibrio* species induce diarrhea by producing enterotoxins similar to the heat-labile toxin produced by *V cholerae* or a heat-stable toxin similar to that produced by ETEC. *V parahaemolyticus* produces hemolysins, which appear to correlate with virulence.

The clinical features of noncholera *Vibrio*–induced gastroenteritis are nonspecific and include diarrhea, which may be grossly bloody in 25–30% of patients, abdominal cramps, fever, and, less commonly, nausea and vomiting. The duration of illness ranges from an average of 3 days for *V parahaemolyticus* to 6 days for the other noncholera *Vibrio* species. Most species may also cause wound infections and, especially in patients who are immunosuppressed or have liver disease, septicemia, the latter with mortality as high as 20%.

Isolation from stool samples requires use of selective media; hence, the laboratory should be alerted that infection with noncholera *Vibrio* is suspected.

Supportive therapy and hydration are the mainstays of treatment. Although controlled trials are lacking and diarrhea is self-limited in immunocompetent individuals, doxycycline or quinolones have been reported to reduce the duration of diarrhea and shedding of *Vibrio* organisms in the stool.

Daniels NA, MacKinnon L, Bishop R, et al. *Vibrio parahaemolyticus* infections in the United States, 1973–1998. *J Infect Dis*. 2000;981:1661–1666. [PMID: 10823766]

G. *Vibrio cholerae*

Cholera is endemic in developing countries in Asia, Africa, and Central and South America and also causes epidemic outbreaks in these continents largely through contamination of water supplies and, less often, foodstuffs. In North America, a few sporadic cases have occurred in recent years, probably though ingestion of contaminated food, largely shellfish. There are more imported infections among travelers than sporadic indigenous infections in the United States. The recent major cholera epidemic in Haiti raises the possibility that an increase in imported infections may become evident in neighboring Caribbean islands and throughout the Western hemisphere including the United States. *Vibrio cholerae* is acid-sensitive; hence, a large inoculum is required to cause infection in individuals with normal gastric acid secretion. Surviving organisms colonize the small intestine by attaching to the epithelial surface via pili and subsequently elaborate toxins that induce electrolyte and water secretion and alter epithelial permeability in the absence of mucosal inflammation.

Infections range from asymptomatic colonization to devastating, watery diarrhea with fluid losses that can approach 1 L/h. Vomiting may accompany the diarrhea, but a significant fever is uncommon. Massive fecal fluid losses, if not replaced, can rapidly lead to severe dehydration and profound electrolyte disturbances, including hypokalemia and metabolic acidosis, with associated renal failure. The epidemiologic history and clinical picture facilitate diagnosis. *Vibrio* can often be seen in stool examined by phase-contrast or darkfield microscopy and on Gram stain. *V cholerae* is cultured on selective media.

Prompt rehydration is imperative. Oral rehydration solution (see "General Principles of Treatment," earlier) is sufficient for most infections and has saved hundreds of thousands of lives and reduced mortality from cholera to less than 1% in adults and older children. Ongoing stool fluid losses should be measured to help guide the volume of oral fluid administration. If dehydration is severe or nausea and vomiting preclude adequate oral intake, intravenous hydration is indicated. If facilities or supplies needed for intravenous hydration are unavailable, oral solutions should be administered via nasogastric tube, although aspiration is a hazard. Antibiotics (tetracycline, doxycycline, or azithromycin, depending on susceptibility) reduce fluid losses and shorten the duration of diarrhea. The rBS-WC vaccine, an oral, killed, whole cell vaccine containing the nontoxic cholera toxin B subunit, has recently been approved for use for prophylaxis of traveler's diarrhea (see later) and provides significant protection against *V cholerae* and ETEC infections.

Seas C, Gotuzzo E. *Vibrio cholerae.* In: Mandell GL, Bennett JE, Dolin R (editors). *Principles and Practice of Infectious Diseases,* 6th ed. Churchill Livingston, 2005:2536.

Tobin-D-Angelo M, Smith AR, Bulens SN, et al. Severe diarrhea caused by cholera toxin-producing *Vibrio cholera* serogroup O75 infections acquired in the southeastern United States. *Clin Infect Dis.* 2008;47:1035–1040. [PMID: 18781876]

H. *Aeromonas*

Aeromonas species, like noncholera vibrios, thrive in brackish and freshwater environments but also cause disease in fish as well as many land animals. They produce several toxins, adhesins, hemolysins, and proteases, but the exact role of these putative virulence factors in the pathogenesis of disease in humans remains uncertain.

The role of *Aeromonas* species in human diarrheal disease is somewhat controversial. Although small outbreaks among travelers are described and the organisms are sporadically cultured from patients with diarrheal disease, *Aeromonas* have been isolated from 5–15% of asymptomatic individuals in developing countries. An effort to induce disease in normal volunteers by oral challenge was inconclusive. However, there is general consensus that some *Aeromonas* species can cause diarrheal disease in some individuals.

Symptoms range from watery to dysenteric diarrhea and may be accompanied by nausea and vomiting and, in the minority of patients, fever. Although most cases are self-limited, more protracted diarrhea lasting several weeks has been observed. *Aeromonas,* like noncholera vibrios, can also cause wound infections. Gram-negative sepsis may occur in immunosuppressed patients or patients with liver disease. The diagnosis is made by stool culture, but the laboratory should be alerted that *Aeromonas* species are being sought. Although *Aeromonas* grows readily on conventional media, identifying these organisms is not generally routine.

The disease is self-limited in most patients with *Aeromonas*-associated diarrhea. Anecdotal reports suggest that patients with protracted diarrhea merit antibiotic treatment with trimethoprim–sulfamethoxazole or a fluoroquinolone, depending on the results of susceptibility testing. Controlled trials showing the benefit of antibiotic treatment are not available.

I. *Plesiomonas*

Plesiomonas shigelloides, like *Aeromonas* species, is widely distributed in aquatic environments and among a broad range of sea and land animals. Rare or undercooked shellfish, notably oysters, as well as contaminated water have been incriminated in outbreaks of human diarrheal disease. Unlike *Aeromonas,* the carriage rate among asymptomatic individuals is very low. However, like *Aeromonas,* an attempt to induce disease in volunteers was inconclusive.

The pathogenesis of *Plesiomonas*-induced gastroenteritis is poorly understood, and specific disease-producing virulence factors have not been identified. The clinical features closely resemble those of *Aeromonas*-induced gastroenteritis and range from watery to, in the minority of patients, dysenteric diarrhea. Nausea and vomiting are common, and abdominal cramps may be present. Fever is uncommon. Although most cases are self-limited with only a few days of symptoms, prolonged diarrhea has been reported. Diagnosis is generally made by culture of *P shigelloides* from the stool, but again, the bacteriology laboratory should be notified that the organism is being sought.

There are no available controlled trials defining efficacy of treatment with antibiotics. Most cases require no more than supportive treatment. Patients who are immunocompromised and those who have chronic liver disease, bacteremia, extraintestinal infections, or prolonged diarrhea should be treated. Trimethoprim–sulfamethoxazole, quinolones, and cephalosporins are usually effective, but the choice of antibiotic should be guided by sensitivity testing.

J. Enterotoxigenic *E coli* (ETEC)

ETEC have been recognized for years as a major cause of diarrheal disease in infants and children younger than 2 years of age in the developing world and, in some series, as the most common cause of traveler's diarrhea at any age. In recent years, large outbreaks in the United States and Europe have also been reported. Transmission generally is via contaminated food or water, and a large inoculum is required. Important virulence factors characterizing ETEC are heat-labile toxin (LT) and a heat-stable toxin (STa). LT closely resembles cholera toxin, stimulating cyclic adenosine monophosphate production, resulting in intestinal crypt chloride and water secretion and reduced sodium chloride absorption by enterocytes. STa stimulates cyclic guanosine monophosphate production, which, much like LT, causes enhanced chloride and water secretion and impaired sodium chloride absorption by the small intestine.

The major clinical manifestation is diarrhea, which ranges from just a few loose stools lasting less than a day to severe, watery diarrhea that may persist for several days to a week and result in significant dehydration. Fever is uncommon and, when present, low grade. Nausea and abdominal cramps may accompany the diarrhea, but vomiting is uncommon.

As in cholera, the involved mucosa is not inflamed; hence, fecal leukocytes are absent. ETEC require research techniques (serotyping or bioassay) for identification; they cannot be differentiated from nonpathogenic *E coli* by routine stool culture. In the absence of research facilities, the diagnosis is a clinical one.

Rehydration, again, is the cornerstone of therapy; short courses of antibiotics, including fluoroquinolones and rifaximin, shorten the duration of illness by a day or so. Lack of a definitive diagnosis in most instances and the self-limited nature of the illness limit their therapeutic use. Prophylaxis is discussed later in the section on traveler's diarrhea.

Beatty ME, Adcock PM, Smith SW, et al. Epidemic diarrhea due to enterotoxigenic *Escherichia coli*. *Clin Infect Dis*. 2006;42: 329–334. [PMID: 16392076]

K. Enteropathogenic *E coli* (EPEC)

EPEC primarily cause disease in infants and children younger than 2 years of age. Older children and adults may harbor the causative organism, but overt illness is uncommon. Both outbreaks and sporadic episodes are most common in developing countries. EPEC attaches to the brush-border surface of enterocytes, activating signal transduction pathways. These activated pathways in turn alter cytoskeletal components, resulting in the effacement of the absorptive surface as well as increased epithelial permeability and altered epithelial barrier function. The resulting diarrhea in neonates and young children can be severe, may be associated with vomiting, and can cause severe dehydration. Most cases are self-limited.

Some commercial laboratories offer a Hep-2 cell adherence assay, but definitive diagnosis usually requires the resources of reference or research laboratories. Rehydration therapy is critical. Antibiotics appear effective; trimethoprim–sulfamethoxazole and colistin have been used.

L. Enteroaggregative *E coli* (EAEC)

EAEC are a relatively recently recognized diarrhea-causing phenotype of *E coli*. EAEC cause disease in all ages and have been identified in both developing and fully industrialized countries. In one recent study, EAEC was detected in 4.5% of patients presenting with diarrhea to emergency rooms of two academic centers in Baltimore and New Haven. There is evidence that transmission by contaminated food is a major source of infection. EAEC adhere to cultured Hep-2 cells in a characteristic "stacked brick" fashion; hence, the term *aggregative* has been included in their name. Cytotoxin and enterotoxin secretion and specific adherence factors together with still other virulence factors have been incriminated, but the pathogenesis of diarrhea caused by EAEC is incompletely understood.

Watery diarrhea is a prominent clinical feature and may be accompanied by low-grade fever and abdominal pain. Bloody diarrhea has been reported. Although many episodes of diarrhea are self-limited, EAEC has been identified in stools of children in developing countries and in adults with AIDS in the United States and Europe with chronic diarrhea.

Identification of EAEC in stools requires use of the Hep-2 adherence assay, which is not performed in conventional clinical laboratories. Ciprofloxacin, rifaximin, and azithromycin have been reported to be effective therapy, shortening the duration of diarrhea caused by EAEC.

Huang DB, Nataro JP, DuPont HL, et al. Enteroaggregative *Escherichia coli* is a cause of acute diarrheal illness: a meta-analysis. *Clin Infect Dis*. 2006;43:556–563. [PMID: 16886146]

Nataro JP, Mai V, Johnson J, et al. Diarrheagenic *Escherichia coli* infection in Baltimore, Maryland and New Haven, Connecticut. *Clin Infect Dis*. 2006;43:402–407. [PMID: 16838226]

M. Enteroinvasive *E coli* (EIEC)

EIEC is a relatively uncommon cause of diarrhea found largely in developing nations and, occasionally, among travelers returning to industrialized nations. It shares virulence factors with *Shigella* strains and invades intestinal epithelial cells, causing mucosal inflammation. The clinical picture is identical to that observed in shigellosis (see earlier discussion), with watery diarrhea often progressing to dysentery accompanied by fever and, in some patients, nausea and vomiting. Diagnosis requires DNA-probe testing by reference or research laboratories. Treatment guidelines follow those for shigellosis; severe cases, especially in children or immunocompromised adults, should be treated with fluoroquinolone (adults) or azithromycin (children) along with vigorous rehydration as needed.

N. Enterohemorrhagic *E coli* (EHEC)

Since its description 25 years ago, EHEC has become recognized as a major health problem. Over 50% of outbreaks are foodborne. EHEC inhabit the intestinal tract of cattle, deer, sheep, and goats, and outbreaks have been traced to undercooked meat, especially ground beef, contaminated vegetables, fruit, and fruit products. Contaminated recreational water sites and direct animal contact, especially at petting zoos, have also been incriminated in outbreaks. Person-to-person contact in venues such as day care centers or nursing homes may also cause outbreaks as only a small inoculum (<100 organisms) can induce disease.

Following ingestion, EHEC adhere to gut epithelial cells and cause epithelial apical surface effacement by mechanisms similar to EPEC. All EHEC strains produce one or more Shiga toxins, which, on entering the systemic circulation, damage endothelial cells, producing vascular damage that may contribute to bloody diarrhea and predispose to hemolytic uremic syndrome, thrombotic thrombocytopenic purpura, and microangiopathic hemolytic anemia. *E coli* O157:H7 is the most common EHEC serotype isolated in the United States, but other Shiga toxin-producing serotypes are being increasingly isolated from outbreaks in the United States and other countries.

After an average incubation period of 3–5 days, the illness often begins with watery diarrhea for 2–5 days, progressing to bloody diarrhea in up to 90% of patients. Severe cramps and abdominal pain are common, with right lower quadrant tenderness prominent in some patients. Notably, fever is absent in most patients and, when present, is low grade. Peripheral leukocytosis of 10,000–20,000/μL is common. The duration of gastrointestinal symptoms can be only a few days to as long as 2 weeks or more. In some outbreaks, *E coli* O157:H7 has been isolated from patients with much milder or no symptoms, further suggesting a broad range of severity of clinical manifestations.

Endoscopy, if performed, shows a friable, edematous, erythematous colonic mucosa with superficial ulceration. Imaging studies show colonic wall thickening, thumbprinting, and, if contrast is used, mucosal hyperemia, which is often most severe in the right colon. Fecal leukocytes may or may not be present.

The diagnosis can often be suspected from the clinical presentation (bloody stools, abdominal pain, leukocytosis, but little or no fever) and is confirmed by stool cultures using sorbitol-MacConkey agar. An ELISA that detects Shiga toxins in the stool is also available, but occasional false-positive results have been reported.

Treatment is supportive. Rehydration is important. Antimotility agents should be avoided. There is no evidence that antibiotic treatment provides any benefit in EHEC colitis. Indeed, some series indicate that in children, antibiotic treatment increases the risk of associated hemolytic uremic syndrome. A trial of administration of a Shiga toxin-binding agent to children with diarrhea and hemolytic uremic syndrome showed no benefit when compared with placebo.

Hemolytic uremic syndrome, thrombotic thrombocytopenic purpura, and microangiopathic anemia are the dreaded complications of EHEC infection and occur most often in children younger than 10 years, although older children and adults are not always spared. Details of treatment for these conditions are beyond the scope of this chapter, but treatment is largely supportive, often requiring dialysis for renal disease and, less often, plasma exchange for thrombotic thrombocytopenic purpura.

Wong CS, Jelacic S, Habeeb RL, et al. The risk of the hemolytic uremic syndrome after antibiotic treatment of *Escherichia coli* O157:H7 infections. *N Engl J Med.* 2000;342:1930–1936. [PMID: 10874060]

Pennington H. *Escherichia coli* O157. *Lancet.* 2010;376:1428–1435. [PMID: 20971366]

O. *Staphylococcus aureus*

Staphylococcus aureus gastroenteritis is a common cause of food poisoning. The causative food is often contaminated by a food handler. Foods rich in sugar and cream, such as custards, cakes with creamy frostings, salty meat such as ham, and mayonnaise- and cream-containing salads favor *Staphylococcus* growth and enterotoxin production at room temperature. Within 6 hours of ingestion of foodstuffs containing sufficient toxin, patients develop nausea and vomiting, which may be severe; abdominal cramps; and subsequently, in some, diarrhea. Fever is uncommon. Duration of symptoms rarely exceeds 24 hours, and rapid recovery is the rule.

The diagnosis can best be established by isolating *S aureus* or enterotoxin from the suspected food if an outbreak is suspected. Additionally, vomitus or diarrheal stool can be tested for enterotoxin, but this in not routinely done. Treatment is supportive, with hydration and correction of metabolic alkalosis, if present, due to severe vomiting.

P. *Bacillus cereus*

Bacillus cereus, a gram-positive, spore-forming bacillus, can produce two distinct types of food poisoning. Some strains produce a heat-stable toxin in vitro that induces vomiting; other strains produce a heat-labile enterotoxin that causes diarrhea.

The organisms that produce the vomiting syndrome have largely been associated with ingestion of rice, notably fried rice. The vegetative forms are destroyed when rice is boiled, but the spores survive. If the rice is not refrigerated, the spores germinate and toxin is produced that may not be inactivated by flash frying as the fried rice is prepared. A short 2–3-hour incubation period follows toxin ingestion. Then vomiting associated with abdominal cramping develops, which may be associated with mild diarrhea. The illness is self-limited, averaging about 8 hours, and can be treated with antiemetics and, if needed, rehydration. The organisms that produce the diarrheal syndrome have been associated with contaminated meats, sauces, and dairy products. Their longer incubation following ingestion of contaminated food (6–18 hours) suggests that the enterotoxin is produced in vivo. Major symptoms include diarrhea and abdominal cramps; vomiting occurs in less than 25% of cases. Symptoms usually clear within 24 hours and should be treated supportively with rehydration, if needed.

Q. *Clostridium perfringens*

Clostridium perfringens is a gram-positive, anaerobic, spore-forming bacillus widely found in nature in the intestinal flora of many animals and in soil. Type A strains produce a heat-labile enterotoxin that causes intestinal fluid secretion and is also cytotoxic to intestinal epithelium. Disease is caused almost exclusively by ingested meat that is inadequately refrigerated after cooking. After a 12–24-hour incubation, patients develop watery diarrhea and abdominal crampy pain that may be severe, usually in the absence of nausea, vomiting, or fever. Symptoms generally last less than a day and treatment is supportive; oral rehydration is usually sufficient. Type C strains can produce a much more severe illness, which has been termed enteritis necroticans or pigbel. It is characterized by intestinal necrosis that may produce perforation requiring surgery. Mortality rates as high as 40% have been reported. This disease has been described largely in South Pacific islands after festive consumption of large amounts of improperly cooked pork.

R. *Clostridium difficile*

Clostridium difficile, a gram-positive, spore-forming bacillus, is the major cause of hospital-acquired infectious diarrhea but can also cause community-acquired diarrhea albeit less frequently. *C difficile* spores are heat and alcohol resistant and can remain infectious in vitro. They may colonize up to 40% of hospitalized patients and 3% of healthy individuals.

Alteration of the normal enterocolonic bacterial flora by prior antibiotic administration is required for the development of *C difficile* colitis in the large majority of those who develop the disease. Antibiotics most often associated with *C difficile*-induced disease include aminopenicillins, fluoroquinolones, cephalosporins, and clindamycin, but virtually all antibiotics, even metronidazole, have been incriminated. Occasionally, cancer chemotherapy or preexisting IBD, especially with colonic involvement, appears to trigger *C difficile* colitis. Increasingly, the disease appears to develop in the absence of antecedent antibiotic administration even in otherwise healthy individuals. Other risk factors for development of *C difficile* infection include prolonged exposure in any health care facility, debilitating comorbidities, gastrointestinal surgery, and old age. Although still controversial, there is increasing evidence that chronic acid suppression with proton pump inhibitors and, to a lesser degree, H_2-receptor antagonists increase the risk for developing *C difficile* colitis or its recurrence after seemingly effective treatment.

Upon colonizing the intestine, most virulent *C difficile* strains produce toxin A and toxin B. These induce colonic epithelial cytoskeletal damage, mucosal inflammation, and mucosal fluid secretion, resulting in the clinical features described below. The toxin-induced mucosal lesion is characterized by damaged epithelium, mucosal inflammation, and the exudative pseudomembrane, which consists of necrotic debris, inflammatory cells, and mucus adherent to the mucosal surface. Strains that produce only toxin B have been isolated from patients with clinically manifest *C difficile* colitis.

Recently, the highly virulent strain of *C difficile* (BI/NAP1/027 or PCR ribotype 027) has been identified in North American and European outbreaks. This toxinotype III strain has been shown to produce up to 16- and 23-fold greater amounts of toxin A and B, respectively. This has been ascribed to a partial deletion of the *tcdC* gene that normally downregulates toxin A and toxin B production. This highly virulent strain has emerged in concert with the wide use of fluoroquinolones, is frequently resistant to fluoroquinolones, and has been implicated in the increasing frequency and morbidity of *C difficile* enterocolitis in North America and in Europe. Another high toxin-producing hypervirulent strain (PCR ribotype 078, toxinotype V) has been isolated more recently with increasing frequency in Europe and North America.

The clinical features of *C difficile* colonization may range, at the one extreme, from total lack of symptoms in carriers to, at the other extreme, fulminant diarrhea and toxic megacolon requiring emergency surgery. Symptoms usually begin a few days to 2 weeks after initiation of antibiotic treatment, although the latency period may be as long as several months. Malaise, watery diarrhea, lower abdominal pain and tenderness, and low-grade fever are characteristic features. Frank hematochezia is rare, although occult blood loss is common. Mild peripheral leukocytosis is common, and fecal leukocytes are often present, especially in patients with more than mild colitis.

It should be stressed that many of the milder episodes of diarrhea that occur in concert with antibiotic treatment are not infectious in nature. Rather, alterations in the balance of the colonic flora impair salvage carbohydrate digestion and absorption. As a result, the amount of unabsorbed carbohydrates in the colonic lumen is increased, resulting in an osmotic diarrhea.

Demonstration of *C difficile* diarrhea cytotoxin in stool samples is the gold standard for establishing the diagnosis of *C difficile* colitis. This test is performed by culturing fibroblasts in the presence of stool supernate. If toxin is present, the fibroblasts show evidence of cytotoxicity. Sensitivity and specificity of this test range from 95–99%, but the assay requires 2–3 days. Available enzyme immunoassays (EIAs) are more rapid and less costly, but less sensitive, and may miss 10–20% or more of stool samples that are positive when tested using the cytotoxicity assay. Some laboratories employ a two-step algorithm, initially utilizing an EIA for glutamate dehydrogenase (GDH), an enzyme produced by *C difficile* whether or not it is a toxigenic strain, followed by an EIA for toxin in GDH-positive stools. A recently approved rapid direct stool PCR assay is a promising diagnostic tool with reported high sensitivity and specificity.

In some patients, an immediate, albeit only provisional, diagnosis can be made at anoscopy or sigmoidoscopy if the characteristic pseudomembrane is observed. However, the absence of the pseudomembrane does not exclude *C difficile* colitis as the disease may be confined to the more proximal colon and the rectum and distal colon may be spared. Moreover, not all patients with *C difficile* colitis develop the characteristic pseudomembrane. Imaging studies including abdominal flat films or abdominal CT are nonspecific and may show colonic wall thickening and mucosal contrast enhancement. In patients with fulminant colitis, ileus or toxic megacolon may be evident.

Worrisome signs suggesting fulminant, potentially life-threatening colitis include florid diarrhea in excess of 10 stools per day; abrupt reduction of diarrhea in the absence of other signs of clinical improvement, which may signal the development of toxic megacolon; increasing abdominal pain and distention; high fever; hypotension, especially if pressors are required; hypoalbuminemia; a rising serum creatinine; and colonic dilation on imaging. Patients showing such symptoms and signs must be monitored closely in conjunction with a surgeon and may require vigorous therapeutic intervention (see below).

Treatment recommendations depend on the severity of clinical illness and host of risk factors. Hospitalized patients should be isolated, and in all cases, caregivers should wash their hands with soap and water after patient contact. Purell and other alcohol-based hand cleaners do not destroy *C difficile* spores.

Recently, treatment guidelines have been published by the Society for Healthcare Epidemiology of America and the Infectious Diseases Society of America. Whenever possible, causative antibiotics should be discontinued and antimotility agents should be avoided. For patients with mild to moderate disease, metronidazole (500 mg three times daily for 10–14 days) should be begun as the initial treatment. In patients with severe disease, oral vancomycin (125 mg every 6 hours for 10–14 days) should be started. A limitation of these guidelines is that clear-cut definitions or firm consensus on what constitutes mild, moderate, and severe disease are lacking in the literature. Clearly, diarrhea in excess of 8–10 stools/24 h, leukocytosis >15,000/μL, fever >101°F, hypoalbuminemia, and a rising creatinine point to severe disease. For patients with disease characterized by fulminant diarrhea (>10 stools/24 h), fever greater than 102°F, leukocytosis >25,000/μL, marked abdominal pain or tenesmus, colonic dilation, or hemodynamic instability, both vancomycin orally or via nasogastric tube (500 mg every 6 hours) and intravenous metronidazole (500 mg every 8 hours) should be begun. In addition, if ileus is present, intracolonic administration of vancomycin (500 mg four to six times daily) should be considered. These very ill patients should be closely monitored with frequent abdominal examinations and daily abdominal flat films to assess for developing megacolon along with serial surgical assessment for the possible need for colectomy. Metronidazole or vancomycin, or both, should be continued for at least 14 days or for 10 days after symptoms have disappeared. Emergency colectomy may be lifesaving in those few patients who develop progressive fulminant diarrhea, severe ileus, and megacolon with impending perforation or generalized sepsis.

Management of patients with *C difficile* infection complicating IBD can be challenging as the clinical presentations of *C difficile* colitis and a flare of IBD can be quite similar. If such a patient fails to improve promptly with treatment for *C difficile* colitis, appropriate concurrent treatment of the coexistent IBD should be implemented.

Relapses after apparent complete resolution occur in approximately 10–25% of treated patients, most likely caused by reinfection or germination of residual spores remaining in the colon. Retreatment should follow the guidelines outlined above for initial therapy as there is no evidence that antibiotic resistance plays a role. If there are multiple relapses, tapering doses of vancomycin can be tried, starting with 125 mg four times daily and then reducing the dose frequency by 50% every week until 125 mg of vancomycin every 3 days has been administered for 2 weeks. If that fails, other antibiotics, including nitazoxanide, bacitracin, rifampin, or rifaximin, can be tried. The role, if any, of probiotics in the prevention or treatment of *C difficile* colitis remains unclear. As a last resort, intravenous immunoglobulin G can be tried, as some responses of refractory *C difficile* colitis to this treatment have been reported. In a recently published promising study, neutralizing human monoclonal antibodies against *C difficile* toxins A and B were administered intravenously to patients simultaneously being treated for *C difficile* colitis with metronidazole or vancomycin. The incidence of recurrent *C difficile* colitis was reduced approximately fourfold in recipients of the antibodies compared to randomized placebo recipients. Recently the macrocyclic antibiotic, fidaxomicin, which appears to have therapeutic equivalence to vancomycin with a lower incidence of post-treatment recurrence has been approved for treatment of *C. difficile* colitis.

Cohen SH, Gerding DN, Johnson S, et al. Clinical practice guidelines for *Clostridium difficile* infection in adults: 2010 update by the Society for Healthcare and Epidemiology of America (SHEA) and the Infectious Diseases Society of America (IDSA). *Infect Control Hosp Epidemiol.* 2010;31:431–455. [PMID: 20307191]

McDonald LC, Killgore GE, Thompson A, et al. An epidemic, toxin gene-variant strain of *Clostridium difficile. N Engl J Med.* 2005;353:2433–2441. [PMID: 16322603]

O'Connor JR, Johnson S, Gerding DN. *Clostridium difficile* infection caused by epidemic BI/NAP1/027 strain. *Gastroenterology.* 2009;136:1913–1924. [PMID: 19457419]

O'Donoghue C, Kyne L. Update on *Clostridium difficile* infection. *Curr Opin Gastroenterology.* 2011;27:38–47. [PMID: 21099432]

S. *Klebsiella oxytoca*

Klebsiella oxytoca causes a relatively uncommon but distinctive antibiotic-associated hemorrhagic colitis. *K oxytoca* has been shown to produce a cytotoxin that has been implicated in the pathogenesis of colitis. Colitis generally occurs during the first week after the introduction of antibiotic therapy, usually with a penicillin, although cases that occurred in concert with administration of other antibiotics, including cephalosporins and quinolones have been described. Most reported patients have been relatively young to middle aged. Bloody diarrhea (uncommon in *C difficile* colitis), abdominal cramps, low-grade fever, and mild to moderate leukocytosis are clinical features. The rectum is often spared, and a patchy hemorrhagic colitis with superficial ulcers but without a pseudomembrane is observed in colonic segments. Mucosal biopsies show an ulcerated mucosa that resembles the lesion observed in patients with EHEC with both inflammatory and ischemic features. The condition is generally self-limited, resolving promptly after the discontinuation of the causative antibiotic and requires only supportive treatment.

Högenauer C, Langner C, Beubler E, et al. *Klebsiella oxytoca* as a causative organism of antibiotic-associated hemorrhagic colitis. *N Engl J Med.* 2006;355:2418–2426. [PMID: 17151365]

3. Protozoal Infections

A. *Giardia lamblia*

Giardia lamblia is the most common protozoal infestation in the United States, where it occurs both endemically and in epidemic outbreaks. It is a common cause of illness worldwide, especially in the developing world where sanitation is suboptimal and, hence, is a common cause of traveler's diarrhea. *G lamblia* infects other mammals, including beavers, dogs, and cattle. The cyst form of *Giardia* can survive for prolonged periods in most environments. Once cysts are ingested, the distinctive trophozoites are released in the upper small intestine where they multiply by binary fission and colonize the host. The trophozoites attach to the intestinal epithelium but do not invade the mucosa; however, they can produce significant enteritis with mucosal inflammation and architectural changes. Hence, biopsy specimens can range from those revealing normal mucosal structure to an almost flat mucosa architecturally reminiscent of a lesion of severe celiac sprue.

Several factors increase the risk of contracting *G lamblia* infection. These include travel to areas where the water supply may be contaminated, drinking mountain and forest stream or lake water that has not been filtered or boiled, attendance at day care or preschool, and swimming in pools with improperly treated water or in contaminated lakes. The risk of developing giardiasis is higher in patients with immunoglobulin deficiencies and in homosexuals, although, interestingly, HIV infection by itself is not a risk factor.

Approximately 50% of individuals infested with *G lamblia* have no symptoms and can be asymptomatic carriers of the parasite for many months. Those that develop symptoms commonly experience diarrhea, flatulence, abdominal cramps, and epigastric pain and nausea. Approximately one third of symptomatic patients experience vomiting. Significant malabsorption with steatorrhea and weight loss may develop. If left untreated, most symptomatic patients recover spontaneously and eliminate the parasite within 3–4 weeks. However, up to a quarter develop chronic infection if untreated, which may result in significant signs and symptoms of intestinal malabsorption (see Chapter 20).

Stool examination for ova and parasites has been used for years to establish the diagnosis, but a single specimen has a yield of only approximately 50%, whereas examination of three separate stool samples increases the yield of positive examinations to 80–90%. The cysts and trophozoites may be seen in diarrheal stools, but only cysts are usually observed in formed stools. Several stool immunoassays, including an ELISA with reported sensitivities and specificities approaching 100%, are now being widely used by clinical laboratories. Though rarely needed now, sensitivity and specificity of examining duodenal aspirates and mucosal biopsies for trophozoites also approach 100%. It is wise to exclude the diagnosis among household members of symptomatic patients.

Metronidazole (250 mg three times daily for 5–7 days) is the most commonly used treatment. Although the drug is not approved by the U.S. Food and Drug Administration (FDA) for treatment of giardiasis, reported efficacy rates from a single course of therapy are in the 85–95% range. A single 2-g dose of tinidazole has been reported to be 90% effective. The effectiveness of albendazole is similar to that of nitroimidazoles. Nitazoxanide (500 mg twice daily for 3 days) is 85% effective and also treats other protozoa such as *Entamoeba* and *Cryptosporidium*. Paromomycin is recommended for the treatment of pregnant patients.

Rossingnol JF, Ayoub A, Ayers MS. Treatment of diarrhea caused by *Giardia intestinalis* and *Entamoeba histolytica* or *E. dispar*: a randomized, double-blind, placebo-controlled study of nitazoxanide. *J Infect Dis.* 2001;184:381–384. [PMID: 11443569]

B. Cryptosporidiosis

Cryptosporidia are widely found in the animal kingdom. Two coccidial species, *Cryptosporidium hominis* and *Cryptosporidium parvum,* are responsible for most human infections. Cryptosporidiosis is transmitted via contaminated food or water, human-to-human contact, and, occasionally, animal-to-human contact. Major waterborne outbreaks have been well documented. Ingestion of a small number of oocysts can produce colonization and disease. The oocysts release sporozoites, which attach to and invade endodermal epithelia. Ultimately, newly formed oocysts are excreted in large numbers in stools of infected individuals. Both cellular and humoral immune defects predispose to symptomatic disease; indeed, many of the earlier recognized cases of cryptosporidial infection coincided with the recognition of HIV infection.

Although *Cryptosporidium* can cause biliary tract, pancreatic, and respiratory tract disease (see Chapter 10), intestinal infection is the most common manifestation. Infected persons may remain asymptomatic or develop an enteritis characterized by watery diarrhea, abdominal cramps, nausea, and malaise, which usually resolves spontaneously in 2–3 weeks in immunocompetent hosts. The diarrhea can be voluminous, especially in immunosuppressed patients in whom chronic infections with debilitating secretory diarrhea and weight loss may develop.

The diagnosis rests upon identification of cryptosporidia organisms in stool, bile, or tissue samples. A modified acid-fast stain of stool has high specificity but mediocre sensitivity and requires the examination of at least three stool specimens if initial specimens are negative. Fluorescent ELISA tests for stool examination have high specificity and sensitivity, as does a PCR-ELISA assay that is now commercially available. Intestinal mucosal biopsy samples often reveal cryptosporidia within the extreme apical cytoplasm of the enterocytes.

If treatment is required for immunocompetent patients, nitazoxanide is the drug of choice, although spontaneous resolution of symptoms is the rule. Immunosuppressed patients can also be treated with nitazoxanide, although only some respond. An attempt to restore immunologic competence with highly active antiretroviral therapy (HAART) in HIV-infected patients is crucial. Other agents that have been tried, with generally disappointing results, include paromomycin, metronidazole, clarithromycin, and other antibiotics. Supportive treatment with hydration and antidiarrheal agents is important in the immunosuppressed, and parenteral nutrition may be required. Octreotide has been tried, but few patients respond.

Smith HV, Corcoran, GD. New drugs for the treatment for cryptosporidiosis. *Curr Opin Infest Dis.* 2004;17:557–564.

C. *Cyclospora cayetanensis*

Cyclospora cayetanensis, like *Cryptosporidium* and *Isospora*, is a coccidian that is widely distributed geographically and, hence, a cause of traveler's diarrhea. In immunosuppressed patients, it is a cause of protracted diarrheal illness. The major recognized vectors for human infection in the United States have been contaminated fruits and vegetables, although contaminated water is also likely in developing countries.

After a relatively prolonged 1-week incubation period, patients develop watery diarrhea, flatulence, abdominal cramps, and malaise. The illness even in immunocompetent hosts may range from minimal to no symptoms to prolonged illness lasting several weeks and even months if left untreated. In immunosuppressed hosts, especially AIDS patients, prolonged, debilitating illness virtually identical to that caused by other coccidia (*Cryptosporidium* or *Isospora*) may develop. Diagnosis is established by demonstrating oocysts in the stool. The oocysts are autofluorescent; hence, fluorescence microscopy is useful. Alternatively, modified acid-fast staining is used. Biopsies of the intestinal mucosa reveal mucosal inflammation and protozoal epithelial invasion.

Trimethoprim–sulfamethoxazole (160 mg/800 mg twice daily for 1 week) is effective treatment for otherwise healthy hosts; larger doses and more prolonged treatment are indicated for immunosuppressed patients. Ciprofloxacin or nitazoxanide can be used for patients intolerant of trimethoprim–sulfamethoxazole.

Herwaldt BL. *Cyclospora cayetanensis*: a review, focusing on the outbreaks of cyclosporiasis in the 1990s. *Clin Infect Dis.* 2000;31:1040–1057. [PMID: 11049789]

D. *Isospora belli*

Isospora belli, like the other coccidial pathogens, is widely distributed geographically. Ingestion of contaminated food or water and person-to-person contact are probably important in transmission. Travelers and immunosuppressed patients are most likely to be infected, but sporadic illness in otherwise healthy hosts occurs in the United States and other developed countries.

Clinical features are not specific and include diarrhea, abdominal discomfort, steatorrhea, weight loss, nausea, vomiting, and malaise. Symptoms are generally self-limited in immunocompetent patients but may wax and wane for months without specific treatment. Among AIDS and other severely immunosuppressed patients, protracted illness with severe diarrhea, malabsorption, and weight loss is the rule without specific therapy.

The diagnosis is established by identifying oocysts in the stool using autofluorescence or modified acid-fast staining. Oocysts can also be identified in duodenal aspirates, and examination of mucosal biopsy specimens reveals invasive protozoal forms in the epithelium as well as mild to severe enteritis with mild to marked architectural changes and a mixed inflammatory infiltrate containing many eosinophils. Peripheral eosinophilia may also be present.

Treatment with trimethoprim–sulfamethoxazole for 3–4 weeks is effective in most patients, but more prolonged and even indefinite treatment may be required in AIDS and other immunosuppressed patients to prevent frequent relapses. Quinolones have been used successfully in those intolerant of trimethoprim–sulfamethoxazole. Where possible, immune reconstitution with HAART treatment is important for AIDS patients.

E. *Entamoeba histolytica*

Entamoeba histolytica infection occurs throughout the world, but the highest prevalence rates are found in developing countries in Asia, Africa, and Central and South America, where sanitation is suboptimal. Simply finding amoeba by microscopic examination in stool in the course of epidemiologic studies and clinical evaluation is compromised by the fact that only 10% of *E histolytica* infections are symptomatic and that two noninvasive, nonpathogenic species, *Entamoeba dispar* and *Entamoeba moshkovskii*, colonize humans with far greater frequency than does *E histolytica*.

E histolytica cysts are ingested by consuming contaminated food or water or via fecal-oral contact, often during sexual activity; hence, there is a higher prevalence among homosexuals. Following excystation, trophozoites bind to the colonic epithelial glycocalyx sugars via a trophozoite surface lectin and subsequently invade the colonic mucosa, causing inflammation and ulceration. Systemic dissemination may occur, most often to the liver, resulting in abscess formation.

Clinically, colonic colonization by *E histolytica* produces a wide spectrum of symptoms ranging from no symptoms in the majority of patients to devastating pancolitis with toxic megacolon, requiring emergency colectomy and carrying a mortality rate as high as 50%. In most symptomatic individuals, mild initial diarrhea progresses to dysentery with blood and mucus in the stool and crampy abdominal pain, often with tenesmus. Low-grade fever may be present in the minority of amoebic colitis patients. Anemia and hypoalbuminemia may be present depending on the severity and duration of the colitis. The clinical features can closely mimic ulcerative colitis or Crohn colitis. Indeed, it is crucial to exclude amoebiasis before administering corticosteroids or other immunosuppressive drugs to presumed ulcerative colitis patients to avoid precipitating fulminant amoebic colitis with toxic megacolon or perforation. Localized infections may produce mass lesions (amoebomas), mimicking colonic malignancy.

Testing for *E histolytica*-specific antigen in the stool is now available and has the advantage of selective identification of *E histolytica* and not morphologically identical nonpathogenic strains. Sensitivities and specificities in the range of 90% have been reported. Stool microscopy is less sensitive and less specific. Using stool concentration techniques and special stains, examination of three specimens results in a sensitivity of approximately 85%. Sigmoidoscopy with collection of mucus from ulcers for microscopy and biopsy samples from the edge of ulcers may supplement antigen testing and stool microscopy. Blood serologic testing is also useful in that absence of antibodies in someone with 7–10 days of symptoms makes the diagnosis less likely. Because antibody levels may persist for prolonged periods after exposure, a positive serologic test does not necessarily indicate acute amoebiasis.

Patients with *E histolytica* colonization should be treated whether symptomatic or not with metronidazole (750 mg three times daily for 10 days) or, alternatively, with tinidazole (2 g daily for 3 days), which has fewer side effects. To eliminate residual cysts, treatment with a nitroimidazole should be followed by an intraluminally active drug such as iodoquinol (650 mg three times daily for 20 days) or paromomycin (10 mg three times daily for 7 days). Patients with severe colitis must be observed very closely for the development of surgically emergent toxic megacolon or perforation until a response to metronidazole treatment is evident.

Gonzales ML, Dans LF, Martinez EG. Antiamoebic drugs for treating amoebic colitis. *Cochrane Database Syst Rev.* 2009; 15:CD006085. [PMID: 19370624]

Haque R, Huston CD, Hughes M, et al. Amebiasis. *N Engl J Med.* 2003;348:1565–1573. [PMID: 12700377]

4. Fungal Infections: Microsporidia

Previously considered to be protozoa, microsporidia are now classified as fungi. Numerous species infect many life forms, and over 10 species are known to cause disease in humans, with *Enterocytozoon bieneusi* the most common. Involvement of many organs in addition to the intestine has been reported and will not be described here. The majority of clinically significant infections occur in AIDS and other immunosuppressed patients, although infections in travelers and otherwise healthy individuals have been documented.

Ingestion of spores via person-to-person, animal-to-person, foodborne, or waterborne routes has been incriminated as sources of transmission. Microsporidia spores have been isolated from the stools of asymptomatic, healthy, immunocompetent individuals raising questions as to whether the organisms are always the cause of gastrointestinal symptoms ascribed to them. Nevertheless, both self-limited diarrhea and occasionally chronic diarrhea have been reported, especially in travelers and in the elderly.

In immunosuppressed AIDS patients and some immunosuppressed transplant patients, dehydration and malabsorption clinically indistinguishable from that associated with coccidial infections such as cryptosporidiosis have been noted in association with microsporidial organisms invading intestinal mucosa and with identification of *E bieneusi* or *Enterocytozoon intestinalis* in stool specimens. As in cryptosporidiosis, biliary tract involvement can occur.

Diagnosis is established by stool examination, which is facilitated by using special stains such as a modified trichrome stain or identification of the organism in tissue samples such as intestinal mucosal biopsies by light or electron microscopy.

Albendazole (400 mg twice daily for 2–4 weeks) is the treatment of choice for microsporidiosis but is of limited efficacy in the treatment of *E bieneusi* infections, the most common form associated with diarrheal disease. Hence, restoration of immunocompetence with HAART in AIDS patients and reduced immunosuppression in transplant patients is desirable if possible. Numerous other antibiotic, antiparasitic, and antifungal agents have been tried without much benefit in immunosuppressed patients with chronic diarrhea who harbor these organisms. Treatment with the antibiotic fumagillin at 60 mg daily for 2 weeks showed promising results in one small placebo-controlled trial and in several uncontrolled reports, although worrisome bone marrow depression was noted in some drug recipients.

Didier ES, Weiss LM. Microsporidiosis: current status. *Curr Opin Infect Dis.* 2006;19:485–492. [PMID: 16940873]

5. Traveler's Diarrhea

With increasing economic globalization and the increased popularity of tourism to developing nations, traveler's diarrhea affects literally millions of travelers each year. A generally accepted definition for traveler's diarrhea is the passage of three or more loose to diarrheal stools in 24 hours often but not invariably associated with other symptoms, including abdominal discomfort, nausea, vomiting, hematochezia, and fever, depending on the cause. Symptoms most often develop 2–10 days after arrival of the traveler but may occur at any time during foreign exposure.

The incidence of traveler's diarrhea varies greatly with geographic region and correlates with the level of sanitation at the travelers' destination. Incidence rates as high as 50% have been noted for selected Asian, Central African, and Latin American countries, whereas estimated rates are 10–20% in Southern European countries, the Caribbean Islands, and Northern African countries. Estimated rates among travelers to and in Northern Europe, the United States and Canada, Australia, and New Zealand are well under 10%. Risk factors for the individual traveler other than destination are conditions that interfere with host defenses against enteric infections, as discussed earlier in this chapter. In particular, immunosuppressed patients and patients with hypochlorhydria caused by pharmacologic agents or gastric surgery may be especially vulnerable to developing traveler's diarrhea.

Virtually any of the specific organisms discussed individually in this chapter may be the causative agent for any given case of traveler's diarrhea. Pathogenic bacteria have been estimated to cause up to 90% of traveler's diarrhea in some studies in which an etiologic agent was identified. ETEC and EAEC appear as the most common causes, but invasive bacteria including *Campylobacter*, *Salmonella*, *Shigella* species, and invasive *E coli* predominate among those with dysentery. Both rotaviruses and noroviruses are established causes, the latter being increasingly recognized in outbreaks among cruise passengers. Protozoa such as *Giardia* and cryptosporidia, while less common, have been isolated from a substantial number of travelers with more protracted diarrhea, especially among those who develop malabsorption.

The clinical features will not be belabored here, and the reader is referred to the descriptions of specific infections earlier in the chapter. By far the most common presentation is that associated with ETEC or EAEC infection, with abrupt onset of watery diarrhea lasting a few hours to as long as 5 days. However, the entire spectrum of the clinical features of gastrointestinal infections may be seen, ranging from a few loose stools to severe dysentery with fever or protracted diarrhea with malabsorption, depending on the cause of the infection and the host's immune response capacity.

Because a specific diagnosis is rarely established during travels, treatment is largely empiric. If diarrhea is severe, rehydration is crucial, preferably using an oral rehydration solution with a formula similar to that recommended by the WHO or, if necessary, intravenous hydration. Loperamide (2 mg up to four times daily) can provide symptomatic relief but should not be used in patients with dysentery of unknown cause and should be avoided in patients with possible *C difficile* (those taking prophylactic antibiotics) given the risk of development of toxic megacolon. There is also some evidence, though not conclusive, that antimotility agents can prolong the duration of some enteric infections such as shigellosis. Effective antibiotic therapy reduces the duration of ETEC and EAEC, the most common causes of traveler's diarrhea. Development of antibiotic resistance is a major problem and has reduced the efficacy of trimethoprim–sulfamethoxazole, aminopenicillins, and tetracyclines. Instead, ciprofloxacin or azithromycin are now recommended. The nonabsorbed antibiotic rifaximin is effective against ETEC and, although expensive, may ultimately become the empiric antibiotic treatment of choice for nondysenteric traveler's diarrhea.

Prevention is the most effective approach to reducing the burden of traveler's diarrhea. Patient education is a crucial component of this strategy. Travelers should be instructed not to consume water that has not been thoroughly boiled, filtered with iodine-containing filters, or chemically treated with bleach or tincture of iodine. Drinks, especially those with ice, should be avoided. Teeth should be brushed with bottled or treated water, and ingestion of water while showering should be avoided. Only thoroughly cooked vegetables, fish, shellfish, and meat should be eaten. Sauces and dips such as guacamole are a frequent source of infection. Fruits, unless freshly peeled, should not be eaten. Fruit-, vegetable-, and meat-containing salads should be avoided.

Bismuth subsalicylate (two tablets or 30 mL of the liquid preparation four times daily) can be taken as prophylaxis. However, compliance is generally poor due to the inconvenience, and salicylate toxicity is a small risk especially if intake is prolonged. Antibiotic prophylaxis for the casual, healthy tourist, although often used, is not generally recommended in view of cost and the risk of inducing antibiotic resistance among pathogens. Rather, providing a prescription for ciprofloxacin or azithromycin for use should the traveler develop diarrhea is more appropriate. Undesirable side effects of antibiotic prophylaxis may include allergic reactions, antibiotic-induced diarrhea, *C difficile* colitis, and yeast infections. Antibiotic prophylaxis can be justified for individuals who are immunocompromised, who have IBD or other significant comorbidities, or for those travelers whose responsibilities and schedule are such that severe traveler's diarrhea would be more than an inconvenience and would potentially negate the purpose of their journey. Quinolones such as ciprofloxacin (500 mg daily) are most widely used, although resistance to these agents is increasing. Rifaximin (200 mg twice daily) is promising, reducing diarrhea more than threefold among travelers to Mexico in one study with little apparent alteration of the colonic flora. The orally administered whole cell vaccine with the nontoxic cholera toxin B subunit (Dukoral) is effective against ETEC. It is FDA approved in the United States for prophylaxis of traveler's diarrhea, but as recommended by the Infectious Diseases Society of America, casual use must be weighed against cost, potential side effects, and the fact that only some of the episodes of traveler's diarrhea caused by ETEC will be prevented by the vaccine.

Goodgame R. Emerging causes of traveler's diarrhea: *Cryptosporidium, Cyclospora, Isospora* and *Microsporidia. Curr Infect Dis Rep.* 2003; 5:66–73. [PMID: 12525293]

Hill DR, Ericsson CD, Pearson RD, et al. The practice of travel medicine: guidelines by the Infectious Diseases Society of America. *Clin Infect Dis.* 2006;43:1499–1539. [PMID: 17109284]

Koo HL, DuPont HL. Rifaximin: a unique gastrointestinal-selective antibiotic for enteric diseases. *Curr Opin Gastroenterol.* 2010;26: 17–25. [PMID: 19881343]

6. Medication-Related Diarrhea

Literally hundreds of medications can produce diarrhea. One only has to peruse the adverse reaction sections related to individual medications in the current *Physician's Desk Reference* to appreciate the scope of the problem. Only a few of the major causes are listed in Table 5–1. To that list could be added antiarrhythmics, cholinergic agents, prokinetics, prostaglandins, and many more. A careful history of all medications, both prescription and nonprescription, as well as herbal remedies and nutritional supplements—*including when they were begun*—must be obtained if unnecessary and costly evaluation seeking the cause of the diarrhea is to be avoided. In the vast majority of cases, though not all, medication-related diarrhea begins within a few days of the initiation of treatment with or a change in dosage of the offending agent.

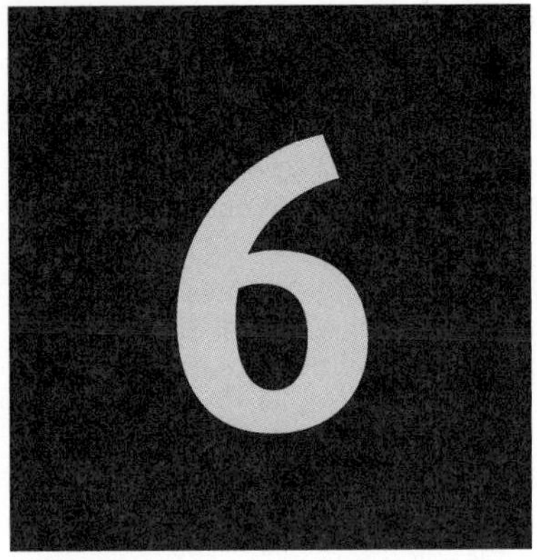

Mesenteric Vascular Disease

Elena M. Stoffel, MD, MPH
Norton J. Greenberger, MD

MESENTERIC ISCHEMIA

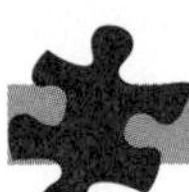

ESSENTIAL CONCEPTS

- Acute mesenteric ischemia (AMI) is a medical and surgical emergency. Delay in diagnosis is associated with high mortality.
- Patients often present with abdominal pain out of proportion to physical examination findings.
- Clinical suspicion of AMI necessitates early radiologic evaluation (computed tomographic [CT] angiography, conventional angiography) or exploratory surgery in patients with peritoneal signs.
- Chronic intestinal ischemia is a clinical diagnosis; patients report classic symptoms (eg, abdominal angina) and have radiographic findings showing severe stenoses or occlusion of two or more mesenteric arteries.
- Colonic ischemia is rarely life threatening and usually resolves with supportive care.

1. Etiology & Pathogenesis

Intestinal ischemia is caused by a reduction in intestinal blood flow, most commonly as a result of occlusion, vasospasm, or hypoperfusion of the mesenteric circulation. It is categorized as acute or chronic, depending on the rapidity and the extent to which blood flow is compromised and whether it is episodic or constant, as might occur in chronic mesenteric ischemia. Ischemia can involve the small intestine or colon. Acute small intestinal ischemia is a medical and surgical emergency that requires prompt diagnosis and a coordinated, interdisciplinary approach. By contrast, acute colonic ischemia (ie, ischemic colitis) is rarely an emergent condition. Acute intestinal ischemia can be further categorized as arterial versus venous, embolic versus thrombotic, and occlusive versus nonocclusive. Other causes of bowel ischemia include strangulating obstructions (adhesions, hernias, metastatic malignancy, intussusceptions) and vasculitis (systemic lupus erythematosus, polyarteritis nodosa).

2. Splanchnic Circulation: Anatomy & Physiology

The vascular supply to the intestines includes the celiac artery, the superior mesenteric artery (SMA), and the inferior mesenteric artery (IMA) (Figure 6–1). The celiac axis supplies blood to the stomach and duodenum. The SMA supplies the small bowel from the distal duodenum to the mid-transverse colon. The inferior mesenteric artery supplies the transverse colon to the rectum. Anastomoses exist between branches of the major vessels, and if one artery is occluded, some flow may be maintained via a patent collateral vessel.

When a major vessel is occluded, collateral pathways open immediately in response to a fall in arterial pressure distal to the obstruction. The superior and inferior pancreaticoduodenal vessels are collaterals that connect the celiac axis to the SMA. The phrenic artery connects the aorta to the celiac axis. The marginal artery of Drummond and the arc of Riolan are collaterals that connect the SMA and the IMA. The internal iliac arteries provide collaterals to the rectum. Griffith point in the splenic flexure and Sudeck point in the rectosigmoid area are watershed areas within the colonic blood supply and common locations for ischemia.

The splanchnic circulation receives 25% of the cardiac output under basal conditions and 35% or more postprandially. Approximately 70% of splanchnic inflow goes to the mucosa, which is the most metabolically active area of the gut. The villus tips are the most vulnerable to ischemic injury. Intestinal blood flow is under complex regulation controlled primarily by resistance arterioles and precapillary sphincters. Several vasoactive substances influence intestinal perfusion. Catecholamines, angiotensin II, and vasopressin all can cause vasoconstriction, whereas vasoactive intestinal peptide causes vasodilation. Products of ischemia such as acidosis, hypoxemia, and hyperkalemia have been shown to cause vasodilation. Ischemic damage is caused by both hypoxia and reperfusion injury.

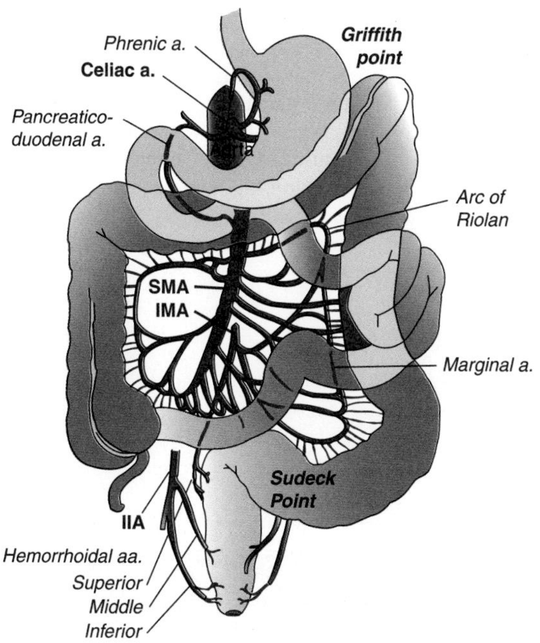

▲ **Figure 6–1.** Distribution of blood supply to the small intestine and colon from the celiac artery, superior mesenteric artery (SMA), inferior mesenteric artery (IMA), and internal iliac artery (IIA). (Reproduced, with permission, from Kasper DL, Braunwald E, Fauci AS, et al [editors]. *Harrison's Principles of Internal Medicine,* 17th ed. McGraw-Hill, 2008.)

Brandt LJ, Boley SJ. AGA technical review on intestinal ischemia. American Gastrointestinal Association. *Gastroenterology.* 2000;118:954–968. [PMID: 10784596]

Kirkpatrick ID, Kroeker MA, Greenberg HM. Biphasic CT with mesenteric CT angiography in the evaluation of acute mesenteric ischemia: initial experience. *Radiology.* 2003;229:91–98. [PMID: 12944600]

ACUTE MESENTERIC ISCHEMIA

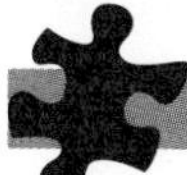

ESSENTIALS OF DIAGNOSIS

- Maintain a high index of clinical suspicion.
- Consider in patients >50 years who present with sudden onset of severe abdominal pain lasting >2 hours, especially if a history of cardiovascular disease (congestive heart failure, myocardial infarction, arrhythmia) is present.
- Consider in patients with abdominal pain out of proportion to physical findings.
- Angiography is the diagnostic procedure of choice and is potentially therapeutic.

General Considerations

Acute mesenteric ischemia (AMI) remains a challenging diagnosis, with a mortality rate exceeding 50%. The incidence of AMI has increased over the past 20 years due to longer life expectancies, increased awareness of ischemic syndromes, and enhanced diagnostic and therapeutic techniques. The various causes of AMI include SMA embolism (50%), SMA thrombosis (15–20%), nonocclusive mesenteric ischemia (NOMI; 20–25%), and mesenteric venous thrombosis (5–10%).

1. Mesenteric Artery Embolism & Thrombosis

Embolism to the SMA is most frequently due to a dislodged thrombus originating from the left atrium, left ventricle, or cardiac valves. One third of patients have a history of a prior embolic event, and 20% have synchronous emboli. The onset of symptoms is abrupt and dramatic. SMA thrombosis usually occurs at the origin of the vessel, which is frequently an area of severe atherosclerotic narrowing. Acute thrombosis usually occurs in a patient with underlying chronic intestinal ischemia. This process is analogous to plaque rupture in acute coronary syndromes. Approximately 50% of patients have a history of chronic mesenteric ischemia, and the acute event occurs after closure of a collateral vessel.

Clinical Findings

A. Symptoms & Signs

Patients with AMI present with severe, acute, unremitting abdominal pain strikingly out of proportion to the initial physical findings. On examination, the abdomen may be soft and either nontender or minimally tender. Distention is often the first sign. Later findings may include signs of peritonitis, especially if infarction or gangrene has occurred. Associated symptoms may include nausea, emesis, and transient diarrhea due to urgent bowel evacuation. Occult blood is found in the stool in 50–75% of cases.

B. Laboratory Findings

Leukocytosis with a white blood cell count greater than 15,000/μL is found in 75% of patients. However, most patients with early intestinal ischemia do not have abnormal laboratory findings. Lactic acidosis, hemoconcentration, and raised serum aminotransferase levels are usually late findings indicative of intestinal infarction.

C. Imaging Studies

Historically, standard radiologic imaging has not been useful in diagnosing AMI, because most of the reported "classic" findings (eg, bowel edema, pneumatosis intestinalis, portal venous gas) are not seen until late in the course of the illness. Plain films of the abdomen are usually normal, and the utility of these studies is to exclude other acute abdominal processes such as perforation or obstruction. Mesenteric angiography has been the gold standard for making the diagnosis of AMI; however, recent studies have demonstrated that CT scans may have an overall sensitivity of 80% for AMI, thanks to technical advances, including spiral CT, rapid intravenous bolus injection of contrast, and multidetector-row CT (MDCT) with three-dimensional reconstruction. CT findings may be either more specific or nonspecific. More specific findings include thromboembolism in mesenteric vessels, portal venous gas, bowel wall intramural gas or pneumatosis, lack of bowel wall enhancement, and signs of ischemia in other organs. Less specific signs include diffuse bowel wall thickening, striking vascular engorgement, dilated fluid-filled loops of bowel, and mesenteric edema (Figure 6–2). Magnetic resonance angiography (MRA) can produce similar images; however, image acquisition takes longer than for MDCT, which limits its use in the setting of an acutely ill patient.

Initial evaluation should include radiographic imaging to exclude other causes of acute abdominal pain such as perforation or obstruction. MDCT can provide detailed information about the mesenteric vessels and small bowel and is particularly sensitive in the diagnosis of mesenteric venous thrombosis.

D. Angiography

Angiography is important in both diagnosis and management of AMI and remains the gold standard for evaluation of patients with suspected AMI and no peritoneal signs.

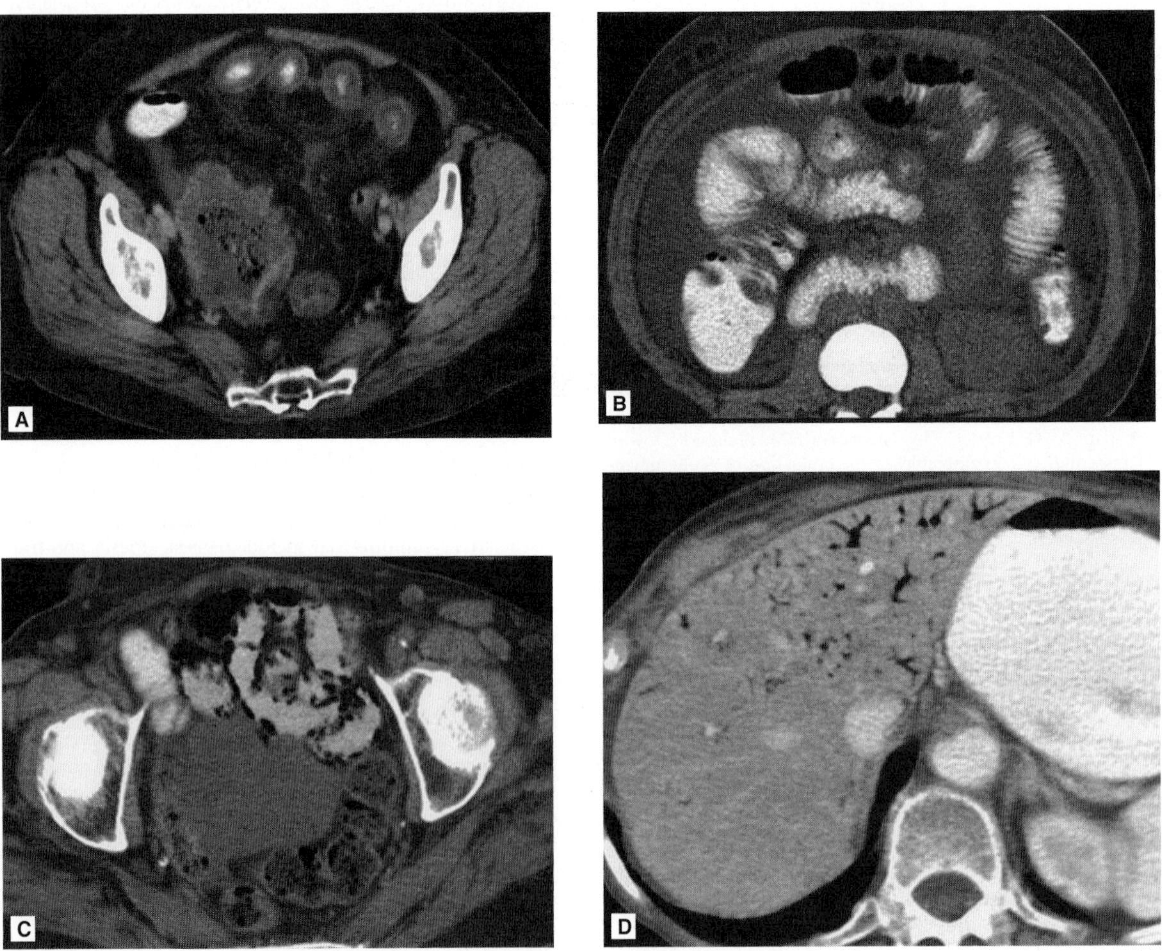

▲ **Figure 6–2.** CT scan findings of intestinal ischemia. **A** and **B:** Small bowel thickening. **C:** Small intestinal pneumatosis. **D:** Portal venous gas. (Used with permission from Koenraad Mortele, MD.)

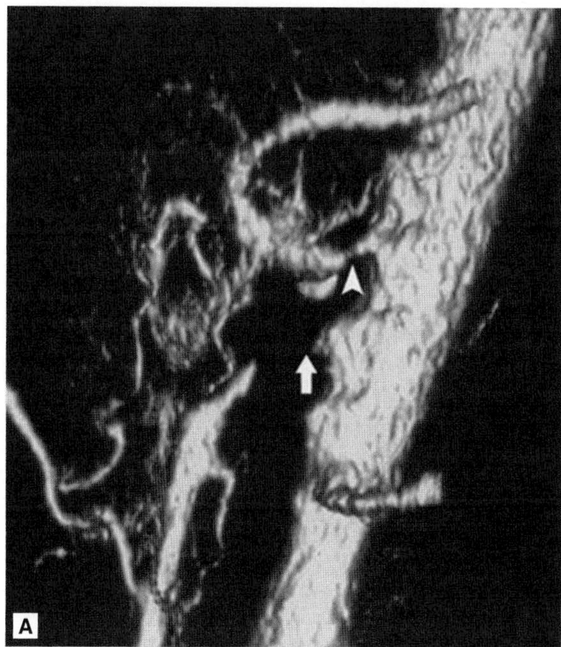

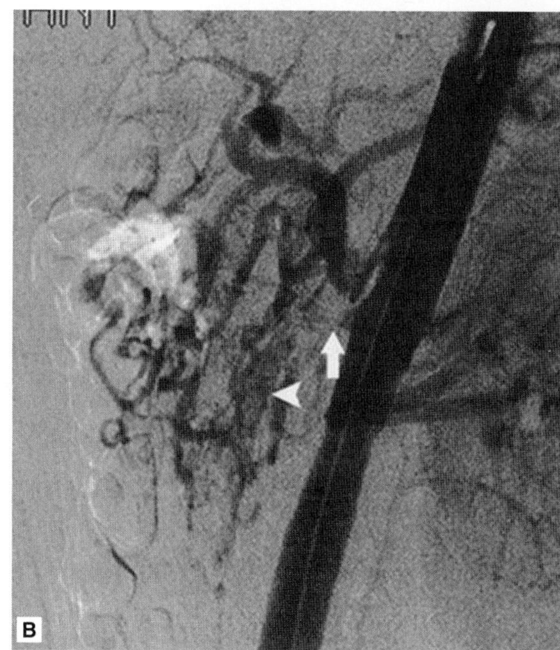

▲ **Figure 6–3. A:** Volume-rendered three-dimensional CT scan showing narrowing of the celiac trunk (*arrowhead*) and occlusion of the proximal SMA (*arrow*). **B:** Conventional angiogram showing SMA occlusion (*arrow*). (Reproduced, with permission, from Kirkpatrick Kroeker MA, Greenberg HM. Biphasic CT with mesenteric CT angiography is the evaluation of acute mesenteric ischemia: initial experience. *Radiology*. 2003;229:94.)

It is the mainstay of diagnosis and treatment for both occlusive mesenteric ischemia and NOMI. It can be both diagnostic and therapeutic. Placement of a catheter into the SMA allows visualization of obstructing lesions and facilitates interventions such as infusion of vasodilators into the SMA, angioplasty, stenting, or infusion of thrombolytics (Figure 6–3).

Treatment

The goal of treatment in AMI is to restore intestinal blood flow as rapidly as possible. However, initial management must include hemodynamic resuscitation and correction of precipitating causes of AMI such as arrhythmias, congestive heart failure, or volume depletion. Patients require aggressive hemodynamic monitoring and support, correction of fluid and electrolyte abnormalities, and treatment with broad-spectrum antibiotics.

Patients with peritoneal signs or clinical suspicion of perforation or gangrene require emergent laparotomy, after hemodynamic stabilization, to immediately restore mesenteric blood flow and resect nonviable bowel. Patients who are hemodynamically stable with no peritoneal signs should undergo angiography to diagnose obstructive lesions and begin treatment with vasodilators, such as papaverine, which when infused directly into mesenteric vessels can help increase blood flow by reversing vasospasm. Once an obstructing lesion is confirmed with angiography, patients can undergo either surgical revascularization (through aortomesenteric bypass grafting, embolectomy, or thromboendarterectomy) or endovascular revascularization (using techniques such as balloon dilation and angioplasty with or without stenting, or catheter-directed thrombolytic therapy, in selected cases). The American Gastroenterological Association algorithm for diagnosis and management of acute intestinal ischemia is presented in Figure 6–4.

Oldenburg WA, Lau LL, Rodenberg TJ, et al. Acute mesenteric ischemia: a clinical review. *Arch Intern Med.* 2004;164:1054–1062. [PMID: 15159262]

Segatto E, Mortelé K, Ji H, et al. Acute small bowel ischemia: CT imaging findings. *Semin Ultrasound CT MR.* 2003;24:364–376. [PMID: 14620718]

Wiesner W, Khurana B, Ji H, et al. CT of acute bowel ischemia. *Radiology.* 2003;226:635–650. [PMID: 12601205]

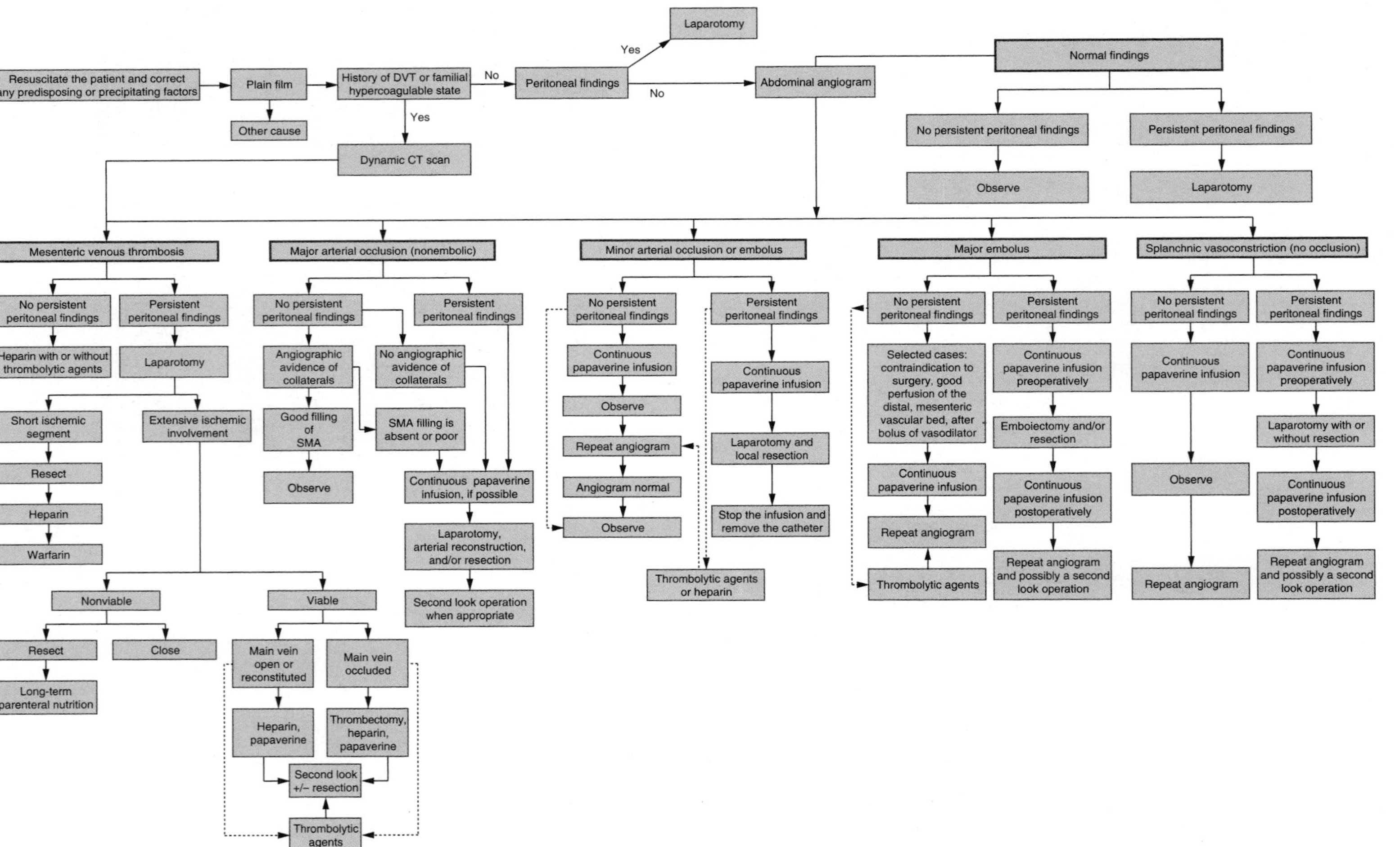

▲ **Figure 6–4.** Algorithm for diagnosis and management of acute intestinal ischemia. DVT, deep venous thrombosis; SMA, superior mesenteric artery. (Reproduced, with permission, from American Gastroenterological Association Medical Position Statement: guidelines on intestinal ischemia. *Gastroenterology*. 2000;118:951.)

2. Mesenteric Venous Thrombosis

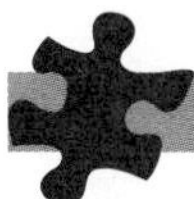

ESSENTIALS OF DIAGNOSIS

- Acute form—maintain a high index of suspicion in patients with recent onset of acute abdominal pain associated with a predisposing condition (ie, heritable or acquired hypercoagulable states).
- Diagnosed with 90% sensitivity by contrast CT, MDCT, or vascular angiography.

General Considerations

Mesenteric venous thrombosis (MVT) accounts for 5–10% of all cases of AMI. The conditions responsible for the development of MVT can be identified in over 80% of cases, and risk factors are summarized in Table 6–1. The clinical presentation of MVT can be acute, characterized by the sudden onset of symptoms; subacute, in which symptoms occur for days or weeks without bowel infarction; or chronic, involving portal or splenic vein thrombosis and stigmata of portal hypertension with or without variceal bleeding.

Pathogenesis

MVT leads to resistance to mesenteric venous blood flow and intestinal ischemia, with resultant bowel wall edema, fluid efflux into the bowel lumen, and systemic hypotension. As a consequence of venous congestion, arterial inflow is diminished, which can lead to bowel ischemia and, ultimately, infarction. The extent of the venous collateral circulation is a key variable influencing whether submucosal hemorrhage or bowel infarction will develop following MVT.

Table 6–1. Causes of mesenteric venous thrombosis.

1. **Hypercoagulable states**
   a. Heritable disorder of coagulation
      (1) Factor V Leiden-resistance to activated protein C
      (2) Prothrombin gene mutation—*A20210*
   b. Acquired hypercoagulable states
      (1) Paroxysmal nocturnal hemoglobinuria
      (2) Myeloproliferative disorders
   c. Deficiencies of anticoagulant proteins
      (1) Protein C and protein S
      (2) Antithrombin
   d. Acquired hypercoagulable states
      (1) Neoplasms
      (2) Oral contraceptives
      (3) Pregnancy
2. **Inflammatory disorders**
   a. Pancreatitis
   b. Intra-abdominal sepsis
3. **Cirrhosis and portal hypertension**

Clinical Findings

A. Symptoms and Signs

As noted, the presentation of MVT can be acute, subacute, or chronic. Symptoms of acute MVT usually begin a few days to a few weeks (mean, 7 days) before presentation and, in 25% of patients, have been present for 30 days before admission. Nausea, vomiting, and diarrhea are common, and over 50% of patients have occult blood in the stool. Examination findings include fever (50%), abdominal distention with mild to moderate tenderness and signs of dehydration, and hypotension (25%). Hematochezia, found in 15% of patients, usually signifies severe ischemia or bowel infarction. Fever, guarding, rebound tenderness, lactic acidosis, and increased transaminases are late findings that may be associated with bowel infarction.

In the subacute form of MVT, symptoms such as abdominal pain can be present for several weeks along with an unremarkable physical examination. Patients with chronic MVT may not have experienced abdominal pain and often present with stigmata of portal hypertension, varices (esophageal, gastric, intestinal), and splenomegaly or bleeding from varices. The latter can be manifested by hematemesis or fecal blood loss.

Over 50% of patients with MVT have a personal or family history of deep venous thrombosis or pulmonary embolism. MVT should be suspected in patients with pain out of proportion to physical findings, especially if there is a personal or family history of such coagulation abnormalities.

B. Imaging Studies

The gold standard for the diagnosis of MVT is CT scan with intravenous contrast. Classical findings with a sensitivity of greater than 90% include a dilated superior mesenteric vein with a clot or filling defect in the lumen (Figure 6–5).

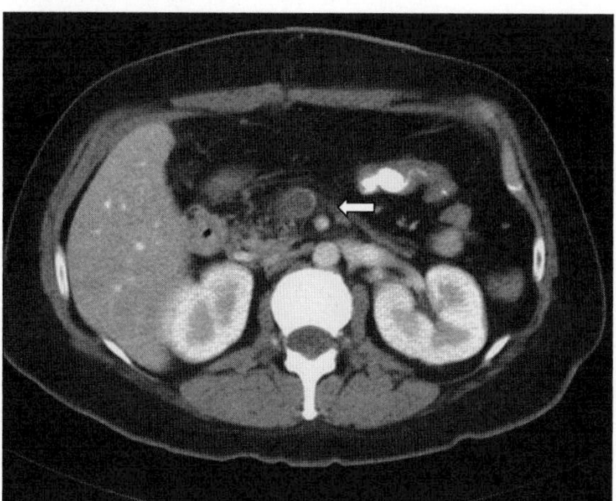

▲ **Figure 6–5.** Acute superior mesenteric vein thrombosis; arrow points to a large thrombus in the proximal superior mesenteric vein. (Used with permission from David Stockwell, MD.)

It should be noted, however, that CT may be less reliable in early thrombosis if small vessels are involved. Portal venous gas, air in the small bowel, or free intraperitoneal air usually indicates intestinal infarction.

Treatment

The treatment of acute MVT depends on whether intestinal infarction has occurred or is strongly suspected. For example, persistent peritoneal findings such as guarding or rebound tenderness should raise suspicion for gut infarction and warrant laparotomy (see Figure 6–4). By contrast, in patients with clinical and radiologic evidence of MVT, but no infarction, and with good mesenteric blood flow demonstrated by angiography, conservative management can be attempted using anticoagulation therapy (ie, heparin). Anticoagulation is usually continued for 6 months or longer if coagulation abnormalities preceded MVT. Few data are available regarding long-term follow-up or the need for treatment after 6 months. Use of thrombolytics such as streptokinase, urokinase, and tissue plasminogen activator has not been studied in a large group of patients; however, catheter-directed thrombolysis has been performed in some cases.

When there is suspicion of bowel infarction, laparotomy is required to restore mesenteric blood flow and resect gangrenous bowel segment(s). In cases in which there is extensive ischemic damage, massive intestinal resection followed by long-term parenteral nutrition may be required.

Amitrano L, Brancaccio V, Guardascione MA, et al. High prevalence of thrombophilic genotypes in patients with acute mesenteric vein thrombosis. *Am J Gastroenterol.* 2001;96:146–149. [PMID: 11197244]

Harnik IG, Brandt LJ. Mesenteric venous thrombosis. *Vasc Med.* 2010;15:407–418. [PMID: 20926500]

3. Nonocclusive Mesenteric Ischemia

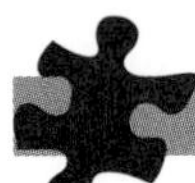

ESSENTIALS OF DIAGNOSIS

- Accounts for ~20% of cases of AMI and results from intense mesenteric vasoconstriction, leading to splanchnic hypoperfusion.
- Maintain a high index of clinical suspicion.
- Suspect in patients with diffuse atherosclerotic disease under conditions of hemodynamic stress (hypotension), in the setting of vasoconstrictive agents (vasopressin, cocaine), and in patients with vasculitis (eg, systemic lupus erythematosus, polyarteritis nodosa).
- Angiography may be both diagnostic and therapeutic.

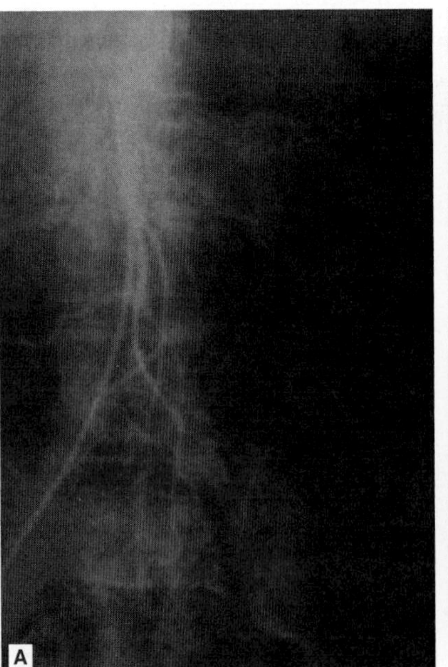

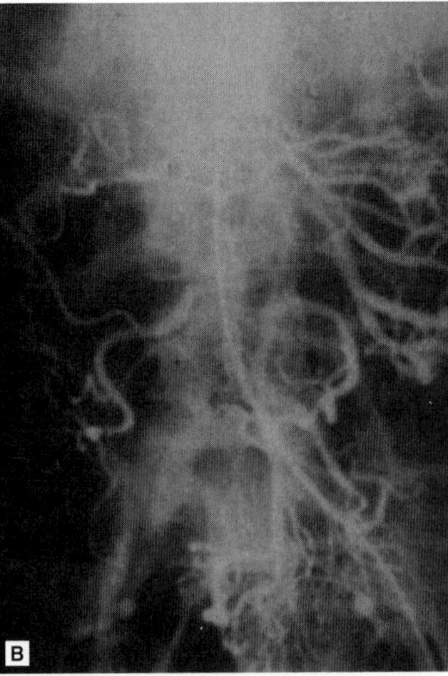

▲ **Figure 6–6.** Angiogram of the superior mesenteric artery in a patient with nonocclusive mesenteric ischemia (NOMI). **A:** Initial angiogram demonstrating diffuse vasoconstriction in setting of hypotensive shock. **B:** Angiogram after 48 hours of papaverine infusion, showing dilation. (Reproduced, with permission, from Boley SJ, Brandt LJ. Mesenteric ischemia. In: Baum S [editor]. *Abram's Angiography*, 4th ed. Little, Brown, 1997:1627.)

Clinical Findings

Signs and symptoms of NOMI may be similar to those of AMI. Patients who develop NOMI are typically elderly with diffuse vascular disease, but NOMI can also be seen in patients with vasculitis or who are on vasoconstricting medications. Predisposing factors include conditions such as myocardial infarction with decreased cardiac output, congestive heart failure, cardiac arrhythmias, sepsis, dehydration, and shock; medications such as diuretics, digoxin, and adrenergic agonists; and therapies such as dialysis. Vasopressin and angiotensin are the most likely mediators of the marked vasoconstriction. NOMI has also been reported after cocaine use.

The mortality rate from NOMI is high for several reasons, including advanced patient age, comorbidities, and difficulty in making the diagnosis and reversing ischemia once it has started. When NOMI is suspected, angiography is the gold standard for diagnosis and management (Figure 6–6).

Treatment

Treatment of NOMI includes hemodynamic resuscitation, antibiotics, and intra-arterial infusion of papaverine, a smooth muscle dilator, which reverses vasoconstriction and restores mesenteric blood flow.

Bassiouny HS. Nonocclusive mesenteric ischemia. *Surg Clin North Am.* 1997;97:319–326. [PMID: 9146715]

Brandt LJ, Boley SJ. AGA technical review on intestinal ischemia. American Gastrointestinal Association. *Gastroenterology.* 2000;118:954–968. [PMID: 10784596]

Prognosis in Patients with AMI

Survival of patients with AMI depends on early diagnosis and treatment. Mortality rates from AMI have been reported at 70–90% if diagnosis is delayed and intestinal gangrene develops. However, patients with angiographically proven AMI who do not have peritonitis can have improved survival rates, approaching 90%. Early diagnosis and prompt intervention with angiography, or surgery, or both, are of critical importance for improving outcomes for patients with AMI.

Schoots IG, Koffeman GI, Legemate DA, et al. Systemic review of survival after acute mesenteric ischaemia according to disease aetiology. *Br J Surg.* 2004;91:17–27. [PMID: 14716789]

CHRONIC MESENTERIC ISCHEMIA

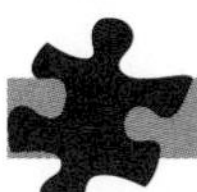

ESSENTIALS OF DIAGNOSIS

- Postprandial abdominal pain, avoidance of eating (which triggers pain), weight loss, abdominal bruit (50% of patients).
- Angiography shows involvement of at least two of three major splanchnic blood vessels.

General Considerations

Chronic mesenteric ischemia (CMI) is the result of reduced blood flow due to atherosclerotic narrowing of at least two of three major vessels (ie, celiac axis, SMA, or IMA). Usually, an adequate collateral circulation has developed that prevents intestinal infarction. However, acute or chronic mesenteric ischemia and infarction can develop suddenly if thrombosis or embolism occurs in a severely narrowed artery.

Clinical Findings

A. Symptoms and Signs

The classic diagnostic triad for CMI consists of postprandial abdominal pain, weight loss, and an abdominal bruit. Pain from abdominal angina is typically recurrent, dull, crampy, epigastric, and periumbilical, occurring 10–30 minutes after meals and lasting 1–3 hours. Because eating consistently triggers pain, food fear causes patients to eat progressively less, resulting in weight loss and often cachexia. Most patients have a history of peripheral vascular disease (PVD). It is important to note that some patients with PVD develop abdominal angina after undergoing surgical repair of peripheral vascular lesions because of so-called steal syndrome (ie, increased blood flow to the extremities and away from the mesenteric circulation).

Physical examination of CMI patients usually reveals a soft abdomen without tenderness during episodes of pain, hence the classic description of pain disproportionate to physical findings. As many as 50% of CMI patients have an epigastric bruit, especially postprandially, and nausea, emesis, and early satiety are common associated symptoms. The average duration of symptoms prior to diagnosis is 1 year. Diagnosis is often difficult because of the vague nature of complaints, absence of physical findings, and lack of an accurate noninvasive test.

B. Imaging Studies

Angiography is the diagnostic test of choice for CMI; however, the diagnosis of CMI remains a clinical rather than an anatomic one. Angiograms in patients with CMI typically demonstrate high-grade stenosis in at least two vessels. CT angiography, magnetic resonance angiography (MRA), and Doppler ultrasound measuring mesenteric blood flow are noninvasive imaging modalities. However, it is important to correlate angiographic findings with symptoms, because some individuals who have complete occlusion of all three major mesenteric arteries may remain asymptomatic because of collateral blood flow. Although there have been preliminary reports of "stress tests" for abdominal angina, at present there is no functional test with high sensitivity or specificity for confirming a clinical diagnosis of CMI.

Treatment

Once the diagnosis of CMI is made based on symptoms and high-grade stenosis or occlusion of two or more mesenteric arteries, the goal is to restore mesenteric arterial flow. Although open surgical revascularization using aortomesenteric grafting is the gold standard, studies suggest that endovascular therapy using percutaneous angioplasty with or without stenting may be effective in treating CMI, albeit with a higher risk of symptom recurrence.

Gupta PK, Horan SM, Turaga KK, et al. Chronic mesenteric ischemia: endovascular versus open revascularization. *J Endovasc Ther.* 2010;17:540–549. [PMID: 20681773]

COLONIC ISCHEMIA

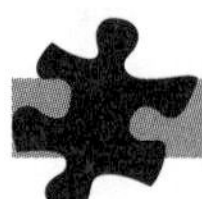

ESSENTIALS OF DIAGNOSIS

- Typically, sudden onset of left lower quadrant pain followed by hematochezia within 24 hours.
- Diagnosed by colonoscopy or imaging studies (CT, barium enema).
- Bleeding is not massive and transfusion only rarely required.

General Considerations

Colonic ischemia, also referred to as ischemic colitis, is the most frequent form of mesenteric ischemia, accounting for 75% of all intestinal ischemia and affecting primarily the elderly. It is estimated that colonic ischemia may account for as many as 3 per 1000 hospital admissions. Findings of colonic ischemia are seen in 1 of every 100 colonoscopies and may be misdiagnosed as inflammatory bowel disease or infectious colitis (Plate 3). Colonic ischemia has been described in several clinical settings (Table 6–2), although in many instances, no specific cause can be identified. Many cases are initially misdiagnosed as inflammatory bowel disease or infectious colitis, especially in individuals younger than age 50 years. The risk of colonic ischemia appears to be highest for patients who have recently undergone cardiovascular surgery, and these patients may experience more severe episodes.

Pathogenesis

Ischemic injury to the colon usually occurs as a consequence of a sudden and transient reduction in blood flow, resulting in a low-flow state. In the majority of cases, a specific occluding anatomic lesion cannot be identified. Although it may occur anywhere, colonic ischemia most commonly affects the so-called watershed areas with a limited collateral blood supply, such as the splenic flexure and left colon (Figure 6–7). Ischemia is usually mucosal and rarely transmural; consequently, gangrenous colitis and colonic strictures are infrequent. Eighty-five percent of cases of colonic ischemia resolve spontaneously within 2 weeks.

Table 6–2. Risk factors for colonic ischemia.

Precipitants of colonic ischemia
Hypotension
Congestive heart failure
Cardiopulmonary bypass
Dialysis
Aortoiliac surgery
Cholesterol emboli
Dehydration
Precipitants in patients <50 years
Vasculitis (eg, systemic lupus erythematosus)
Hypercoagulable states (factor V Leiden), phospholipid antibody syndrome
Sickle cell crisis
Long-distance running
Medications (estrogens, danazol, vasoconstrictors [pseudoephedrine, sumatriptan], gold, psychotropic drugs, alosetron, antihypertensives, diuretics)
Cocaine
Infections resulting in hemorrhagic colitis (*Shigella, Escherichia coli* 0157:H7, *Campylobacter, Klebsiella oxytoca* [especially with use of penicillin derivative], *Clostridium difficile* [10% hemorrhagic colitis])

Clinical Findings

A. Symptoms and Signs

Patients with colonic ischemia usually present with abrupt onset of crampy left lower quadrant abdominal pain, and mild to moderate rectal bleeding or bloody diarrhea within the first 24 hours. Over 90% of patients are older than 60 years. Cardiovascular disease is common, and frequent precipitating factors include hypotension, cardiovascular surgery (coronary artery bypass grafting, aortic aneurism repair), dialysis, and dehydration. Physical examination reveals mild to moderate abdominal tenderness over the affected bowel, most often left-sided.

In contrast to patients with AMI, those with colonic ischemia do not usually appear acutely ill. Bleeding is usually mild, and patients rarely require blood transfusion. Peritoneal signs, if present, would suggest perforation or peritonitis. Ischemic colitis is usually a singular event, and only 5% of patients develop a recurrence.

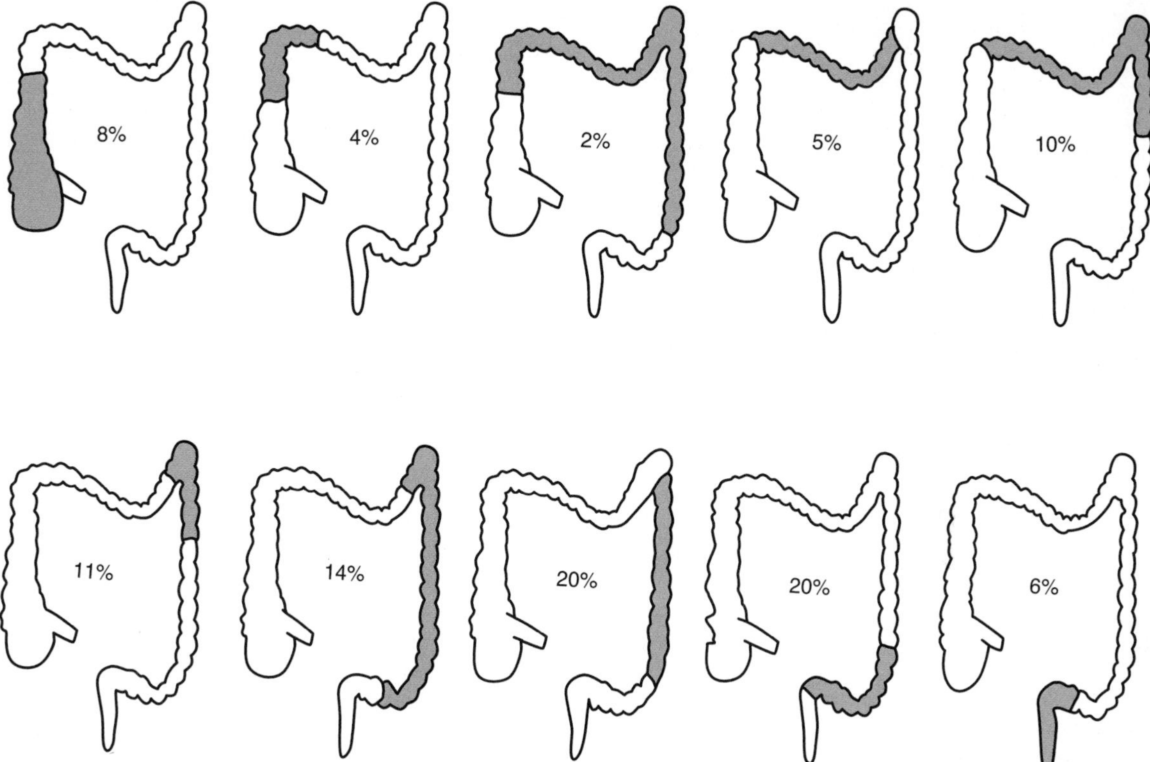

▲ **Figure 6–7.** Distribution of colonic ischemia in 250 cases. (Reproduced, with permission, from Brandt L, Boley SJ. Colonic ischemia. *Surg Clin North Am*. 1992;72:212. Copyright Elsevier.)

The diagnosis is usually established on the basis of clinical history, physical examination, and endoscopic or radiologic studies. Although most patients who develop colonic ischemia are elderly, the condition can also occur in younger patients. For patients who are younger than age 50, several precipitants of colonic ischemia should be considered (see Table 6–2). In young women, the triad of smoking, use of oral contraceptives, and carriage of the factor V Leiden mutation may be associated with increased risk of colonic ischemia. Recent reports indicate that giving penicillin derivatives to patients who harbor *Klebsiella oxytoca* may precipitate hemorrhagic colitis.

B. Diagnostic Tests

Diagnostic modalities include flexible sigmoidoscopy or colonoscopy, plain films of the abdomen, and CT scan. Colonoscopy with biopsies makes the definitive diagnosis; however, endoscopy should be avoided in patients with significant abdominal pain or distention because air insufflation may precipitate perforation in cases of severe ischemia. Endoscopic findings frequently include petechial bleeding, pale mucosa, and, in more severe cases, hemorrhagic ulceration (see Plate 3), and biopsy specimens show characteristic findings. Plain films of the abdomen are usually nondiagnostic, but thumbprinting representing submucosal hemorrhage and edema may be seen in 20–25% of cases. The use of plain films has been largely superseded by the ready availability and accuracy of CT scans. CT scans can demonstrate wall thickening, mucosal and submucosal hemorrhage, and pericolic fat stranding, and occasionally bowel wall pneumatosis (Figure 6–8).

Angiography is usually not necessary in the evaluation of colonic ischemia; however, it should be considered if the clinical findings raise concern for concomitant small bowel ischemia or infarction.

Stool studies should be performed to exclude infections such as *Escherichia coli* O157:H7, *Campylobacter* enteritis, *Klebsiella oxytoca, Shigella,* or *Clostridium difficile,* which can be associated with hemorrhagic colitis.

▶ Treatment

Patients with colonic ischemia are usually placed on bowel rest. Patients should be followed with serial abdominal examinations and monitored for bleeding, fever, leukocytosis, and electrolyte abnormalities. Although there are no controlled

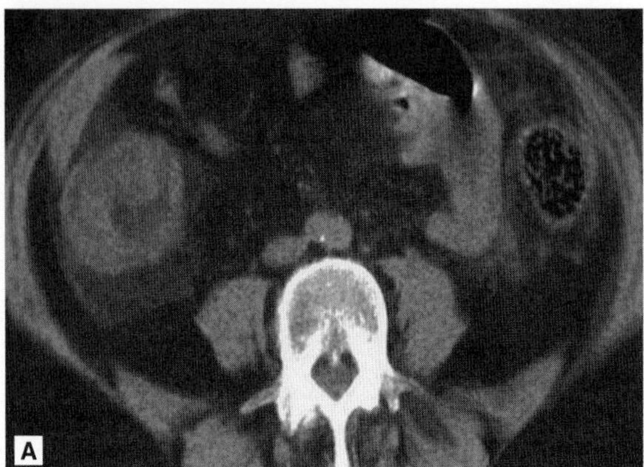

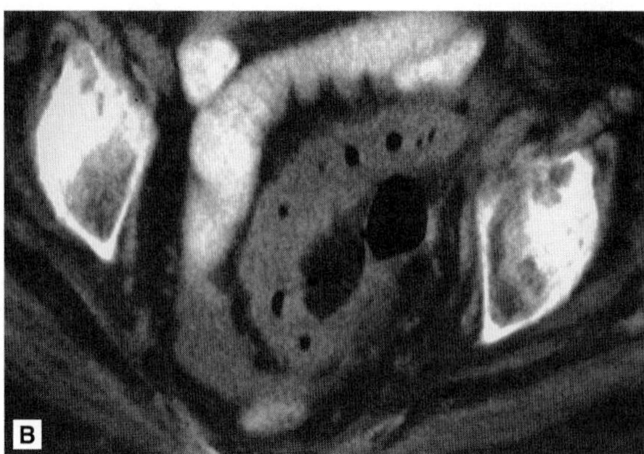

▲ **Figure 6–8.** CT scans demonstrating findings in colonic ischemia. **A:** Colonic thickening. **B:** Pneumatosis. (Used with permission from Koenraad Mortele, MD.)

randomized trials proving the effectiveness of antibiotics in reducing morbidity and mortality, broad-spectrum intravenous antibiotics are recommended. Any medications that can cause vasoconstriction and promote ischemia should be withdrawn (ie, digitalis, glycosides, vasopressin, and diuretics). Marked colonic distention is treated with rectal tubes and nasogastric decompression if necessary. There is no role for anticoagulation or corticosteroids. Prognosis is favorable, and most patients improve within a few days and demonstrate clinical and radiologic resolution within 2 weeks.

Indications for surgery include peritoneal signs suggesting perforation, gangrenous colitis, massive bleeding, toxic megacolon, and recurrent sepsis. Long-term complications, including persistent recurrent colitis and colonic structures, are infrequent but may require resection of the affected colonic segment.

In contrast to small bowel ischemia, colonic ischemia is rarely life threatening. However, some reports suggest that ischemia of the right colon may have a worse prognosis compared with ischemia of other parts of the colon. Furthermore, the development of colonic ischemia in the setting of recent cardiovascular surgery also deserves special mention, as the natural history of colonic ischemia in these patients may be more severe. Prolonged colonic ischemia, such as can occur in patients with ruptured abdominal aortic aneurysms or prolonged aortic cross-clamp time, can lead to acute gangrenous colitis and transmural infarction of the colon. Although emergent operative intervention may be necessary in the setting of sepsis and peritoneal signs, most cases of colonic ischemia resolve with conservative management.

Brandt LJ, Feuerstadt P, Blaszka MC. Anatomic patterns, patient characteristics, and clinical outcomes in ischemic colitis: a study of 313 cases supported by histology. *Am J Gastroenterol.* 2010;105:2245–2252. [PMID: 20531399]

Hogenauer C, Langner C, Beubler E, et al. Klebsiella oxytoca as a causative organism of antibiotic-associated hemorrhagic colitis. *N Engl J Med.* 2006;355:2418–2426. [PMID: 17151365]

Gastrointestinal & Biliary Complications of Pregnancy

7

Sonia Friedman, MD
Jaya R. Agrawal, MD, MPH

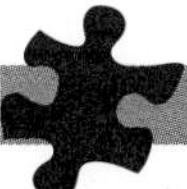

ESSENTIAL CONCEPTS

- Pregnancy can exacerbate many chronic gastrointestinal disorders; the central goal of evaluation is to control symptoms and rule out an urgent need for surgery while minimizing exposure to excessive tests and medications.
- Inflammatory bowel disease (IBD) patients should be in remission while trying to conceive, and most IBD medications are safe in pregnancy.
- Appendicitis is the most common indication for surgery during pregnancy.
- Indications for urgent surgery are the same in pregnant as in nonpregnant patients.
- Incidence of gallstone-related disease is increased in pregnancy.
- Efforts should be made to minimize risk to mother and fetus when performing diagnostic endoscopic and radiologic tests.

General Considerations

The management of gastrointestinal disease during pregnancy poses multiple challenges. First, gastrointestinal diseases are common during pregnancy, and many predisposing gastrointestinal disorders are aggravated by pregnancy. Second, diagnostic options are often limited in pregnancy as there is a need to minimize testing out of concern for both maternal and fetal exposure. Finally, the management of these diseases is more complex due to the need to consider additional risks to both the pregnant mother and the fetus incurred by medications, endoscopic procedures, and surgeries. Data on safety and efficacy of both medications and procedures during pregnancy are often scarce or inadequate; few controlled trials have included pregnant women, and fewer still were designed specifically to study gastrointestinal disease in this population. Table 7–1 summarizes the U.S. Food and Drug Administration (FDA) categories for medication use in pregnancy.

Biertho L, Sebajang H, Bamehriz F, et al. Effect of pregnancy on effectiveness of laparoscopic Nissen fundoplication. *Surg Endosc.* 2006;20: 385–388. [PMID: 16391963]
Cohen-Kerem R, Railton C, Oren D, et al. Pregnancy outcome following non-obstetric surgical intervention. *Am J Surg.* 2005; 190:467–473. [PMID: 16105538]
Malangoni MA. Gastrointestinal surgery and pregnancy. *Gastroenterol Clin North Am.* 2003;32:181–200. [PMID: 12635416]

GASTROESOPHAGEAL REFLUX DISEASE

Heartburn symptoms attributed to gastroesophageal reflux occur in nearly two thirds of pregnancies and in women with no preexisting gastroesophageal reflux disease (GERD), often resolve following delivery. Symptoms are more common and more severe during the third trimester. Risk factors for heartburn during pregnancy include a history of heartburn before pregnancy or during previous pregnancies, multiparity, and younger maternal age. Reduced lower esophageal sphincter (LES) pressure and decreased gastric and small bowel motility, possibly mediated by progesterone and to a lesser extent by estrogen, and increased abdominal pressure secondary to the gravid uterus are all implicated in the pathogenesis.

Clinical Findings

Heartburn is the predominant symptom of GERD, and regurgitation may accompany it. Symptoms are exacerbated by reclining and eating, and patients may also report hoarseness, cough, and asthma-like symptoms. Diagnosis is based on symptoms. Esophageal manometry and pH studies are rarely needed, and barium studies should be avoided in pregnancy. If required for severe symptoms,

Table 7–1. FDA categories for the use of medications in pregnancy.

FDA Pregnancy Category	Interpretation
A	Controlled studies in animals and women have shown no risk in the first trimester, and possible fetal harm is remote
B	Either animal studies have not demonstrated a fetal risk but there are no controlled studies in pregnant women, or animal studies have shown an adverse effect that was not confirmed in controlled studies in women in the first trimester
C	No controlled studies in humans have been performed, and animal studies have shown adverse events, or studies in humans and animals are not available; give if potential benefit outweighs the risk
D	Positive evidence of fetal risk is available, but the benefits may outweigh the risk if life-threatening or serious disease
X	Studies in animals or humans show fetal abnormalities; drug contraindicated

Reproduced, with permission, from Mahadevan U, Kane S. American Gastroenterological Association Institute technical review on the use of gastrointestinal medications in pregnancy. *Gastroenterology*. 2006;131:283–311.

esophagogastroduodenoscopy (EGD) can be performed during pregnancy with careful monitoring (see later discussion on endoscopy during pregnancy).

Treatment

Lifestyle modification should be the first line of therapy. This includes avoidance of alcohol, caffeine, mint, chocolate, tobacco, and fatty and spicy foods. Avoiding late night meals and raising the head of the bed can also prevent nighttime symptoms.

Medications used in the treatment of GERD during pregnancy are listed in Table 7–2. Limited data are available about either the efficacy or the safety of antacids; however, aluminum- and calcium-containing antacids are considered acceptable in normal therapeutic doses during pregnancy, and limited studies have not shown evidence of teratogenicity in animals. Calcium-based antacids are considered the first line of pharmacologic therapy. All magnesium-containing compounds should be avoided during the last few weeks of pregnancy, as magnesium can slow or arrest labor and may cause convulsions. Antacids containing alginic acid or magnesium trisilicate should be avoided, as these chemicals have been associated with nephrolithiasis, hypotonia, respiratory distress, and cardiovascular impairment. Antacids containing sodium bicarbonate should not be used because they can cause maternal or fetal metabolic acidosis and fluid overload. Finally, antacids should be taken separately from iron preparations as they can interfere with absorption of iron.

Overall, sucralfate, histamine-2 blockers (H_2-blockers), and the majority of proton pump inhibitors (PPIs) have been found to be safe in pregnancy even when used in the first trimester. Sucralfate, like antacids, is a nonabsorbable medication and has been studied in a randomized controlled trial in pregnancy and found to be effective in the treatment of heartburn and regurgitation without presenting any risk to the fetus of pregnant women with normal renal function. H_2-receptor blockers are commonly used and considered safe in pregnancy. Ranitidine has demonstrated safety and efficacy and is probably the H_2-blocker of choice. Cimetidine is also considered safe; however, some authorities recommend avoiding its use in pregnancy because of feminization seen in some animal and human studies. Fewer data are available for famotidine and nizatidine.

Although PPIs are more effective than H_2-blockers for controlling symptoms of GERD and healing esophagitis, they are not as well studied in pregnancy. Some investigators suggest documenting failure with H_2-blockers and considering upper endoscopy before empiric trial. Observational studies suggest omeprazole can be used safely during pregnancy; however, increased fetal toxicity in animal studies and some evidence of cardiac malformations in human studies have led to class C categorization by the FDA. Animal studies support the safety of lansoprazole and rabeprazole; pantoprazole and esomeprazole also appear to be safe based on animal data, although studies in humans are limited.

Antireflux surgery during pregnancy should be avoided and is often not necessary as symptoms resolve or improve with delivery. Metoclopramide can be used in very refractory cases and may help treat pregnancy-related bowel hypomotility, which is hypothesized to contribute to pregnancy-related reflux. It is used to treat pregnancy-associated nausea and vomiting, and one study shows no association with fetal malformations. For patients who have already undergone antireflux surgery prior to pregnancy, these methods appear to be effective in controlling GERD symptoms during and after pregnancy, and pregnancy does not appear to affect long-term outcomes and failure rates of antireflux surgery.

For patients experiencing symptoms in the postpartum period, antacids and sucralfate are considered safe because of limited maternal absorption. All H_2-blockers are excreted in breast milk; however, cimetidine, ranitidine, and famotidine are felt to be safe during breast-feeding. Nizatidine has been associated with growth retardation in one animal study.

Gonzalez R, Bowers SP, Swafford V, et al. Pregnancy and delivery after antireflux surgery. *Am J Surg.* 2004;188:34–38. [PMID: 15219482]

Richter JE. Gastroesophageal reflux disease during pregnancy. *Gastroenterol Clin North Am.* 2003;32:235–261. [PMID: 12635418]

Table 7–2. Medications used in the treatment of gastroesophageal reflux and peptic ulcer disease.

Drug	FDA Pregnancy Category	Recommendations for Pregnancy	Recommendations for Breast-Feeding
Antacids			
Aluminum containing	None	Most low risk: minimal absorption	Low risk
Calcium containing	None	Most low risk: minimal absorption	Low risk
Magnesium containing	None	Most low risk: minimal absorption	Low risk
Magnesium trisilicates	None	Avoid long-term or high doses	Low risk
Sodium bicarbonate	None	Not safe: alkalosis	Low risk
Mucosal Protectants			
Sucralfate	B	Low risk	No human data: probably compatible
H_2 Receptor Antagonists			
Cimetidine	B	Controlled data: low risk	Compatible
Famotidine	B	Paucity of safety data	Limited human data: probably compatible
Nizatidine	B	Limited human data: low risk in animals	Limited human data: probably compatible
Ranitidine	B	Low risk	Limited human data: probably compatible
Proton Pump Inhibitors			
Esomeprazole	B	Limited data: low risk	No human data: potential toxicity
Lansoprazole	B	Limited data: low risk	No human data: potential toxicity
Omeprazole	C	Embryonic and fetal toxicity reported, but large data sets suggest low risk	Limited human data: potential toxicity
Pantoprazole	B	Limited data: low risk	No human data: potential toxicity
Rabeprazole	B	Limited data: low risk	No human data: potential toxicity
Promotility Agents			
Cisapride	C	Controlled study: low risk, limited availability	Limited human data: probably compatible
Metoclopramide	B	Low risk	Limited human data: potential toxicity
Treatment of *Helicobacter pylori* Infection			
Amoxicillin	B	Low risk	Compatible
Bismuth	C	Not safe: teratogenicity	No human data: potential toxicity
Clarithromycin	C	Avoid in first trimester	No human data: probably compatible
Metronidazole	B	Low risk: avoid in first trimester	Limited human data: potential toxicity
Tetracycline	D	Not safe: teratogenicity	Compatible

Reproduced, with permission, from Mahadevan U, Kane S. American Gastroenterological Association Institute technical review on the use of gastrointestinal medications in pregnancy. *Gastroenterology*. 2006;131:283–311.

NAUSEA & VOMITING

Almost 50% of women experience nausea and vomiting during early pregnancy and an additional 25% have nausea alone. In a prospective study of 160 pregnant women, 80% of the women reporting nausea stated that it lasted all day, suggesting that "morning sickness" may be a misnomer. The onset of nausea is within 4 weeks after the last menstrual period in most patients and typically peaks at 9 weeks of gestation. Sixty percent of cases resolve by the end of the first trimester, and 91% resolve by 20 weeks of gestation. The stimulus for nausea and vomiting is likely produced by the placenta. Nausea and vomiting are less common in older women, multiparous women, and smokers probably due to smaller placental volumes in these women. Nausea and vomiting during pregnancy are associated with a decreased risk of miscarriage.

The clinical course of nausea and vomiting during pregnancy correlates closely with the level of human chorionic gonadotropin (hCG). It is theorized that hCG may stimulate estrogen production from the ovary; estrogen is known to increase nausea and vomiting. Women with twins or hydatidiform moles, who have higher hCG levels than do other pregnant women, are at a higher risk for these symptoms. Vitamin B deficiency may also contribute since the use of multivitamins containing vitamin B reduces the incidence of nausea and vomiting.

Clinical Findings

A. Symptoms and Signs

A careful evaluation to exclude other disorders and contributing factors is important (Figure 7–1). The presence of heartburn suggests the coexistence of GERD and should prompt treatment with antacid medications (see the earlier discussion of GERD). Although patients can experience soreness of the abdominal muscles and ribs in the setting of recurrent vomiting and retching, abdominal pain is not typically associated with nausea and vomiting during pregnancy.

Epigastric, periumbilical, or right-sided pain can suggest gallstone disease, peptic ulcer disease (PUD), pancreatitis, or appendicitis, and an appropriate workup should be performed to exclude these disorders. Vomitus typically contains recently ingested food or yellow juice. Bilious vomitus or severe periumbilical pain can suggest bowel obstruction.

The patient with uncomplicated pregnancy-associated nausea and vomiting should have normal findings on physical examination. The presence of dehydration or orthostatic hypotension can suggest hyperemesis gravidarum (see later discussion). The presence of abdominal tenderness, rebound, palpable masses, abdominal distention, or a succussion splash should prompt laboratory evaluation and imaging to rule out other causes.

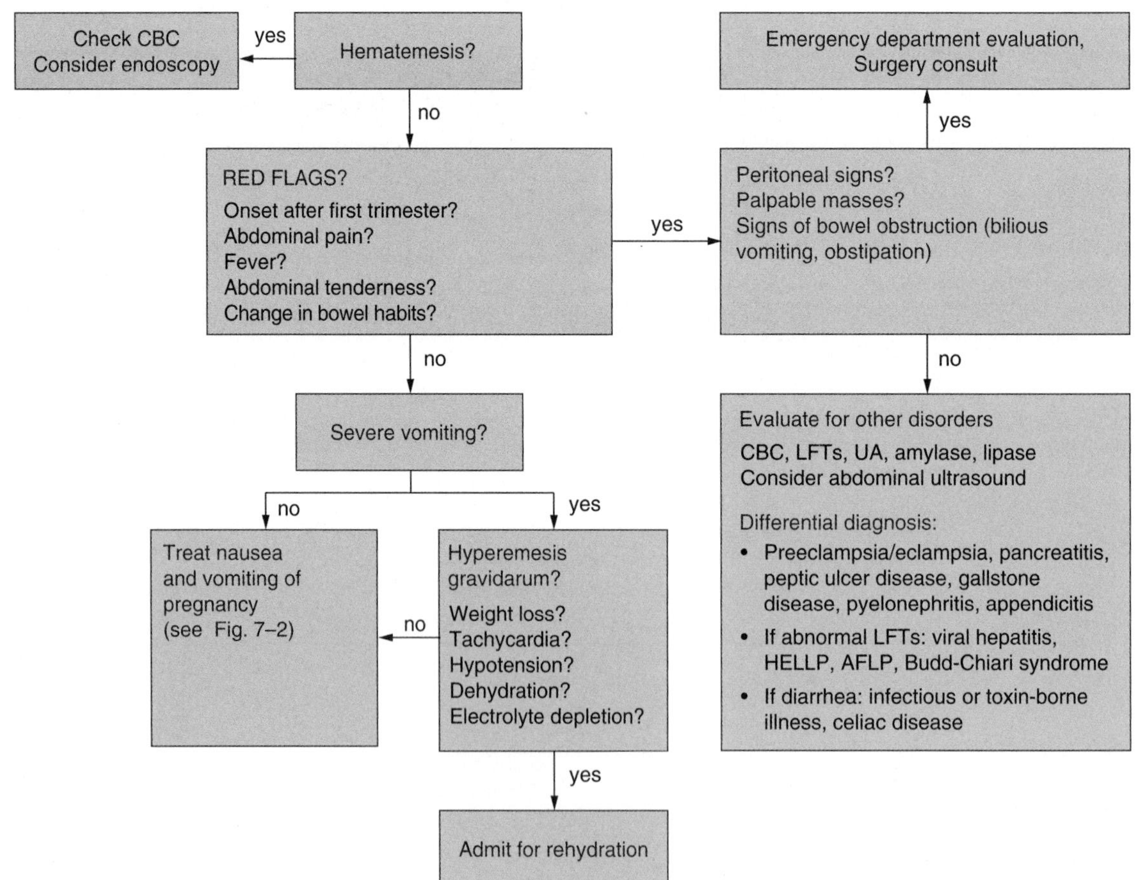

▲ **Figure 7–1.** Evaluation of nausea and vomiting during pregnancy. AFLP, acute fatty liver of pregnancy; CBC, complete blood count; LFT, liver function tests; HELLP, syndrome of hemolysis, elevated liver enzymes, and low platelets; UA, urinalysis.

B. Laboratory Findings

An elevated white blood cell count (beyond physiologic leukocytosis of pregnancy or accompanied by a neutrophilia) can suggest the presence of cholecystitis, pancreatitis, appendicitis, or pyelonephritis. A urine specimen for urinalysis and urine culture to exclude urinary tract infection should be obtained. Other relevant testing includes thyroid function testing, liver blood tests (chronic hepatitis C infection can be associated with a high incidence of nausea), hepatitis serologies, and fasting glucose level. Severely abnormal serum electrolytes resulting from vomiting suggest the diagnosis of hyperemesis gravidarum.

Treatment

The medical and nonmedical literature is replete with dietary suggestions for women suffering from this problem. Medical treatment is directed toward control of symptoms (Figure 7–2).

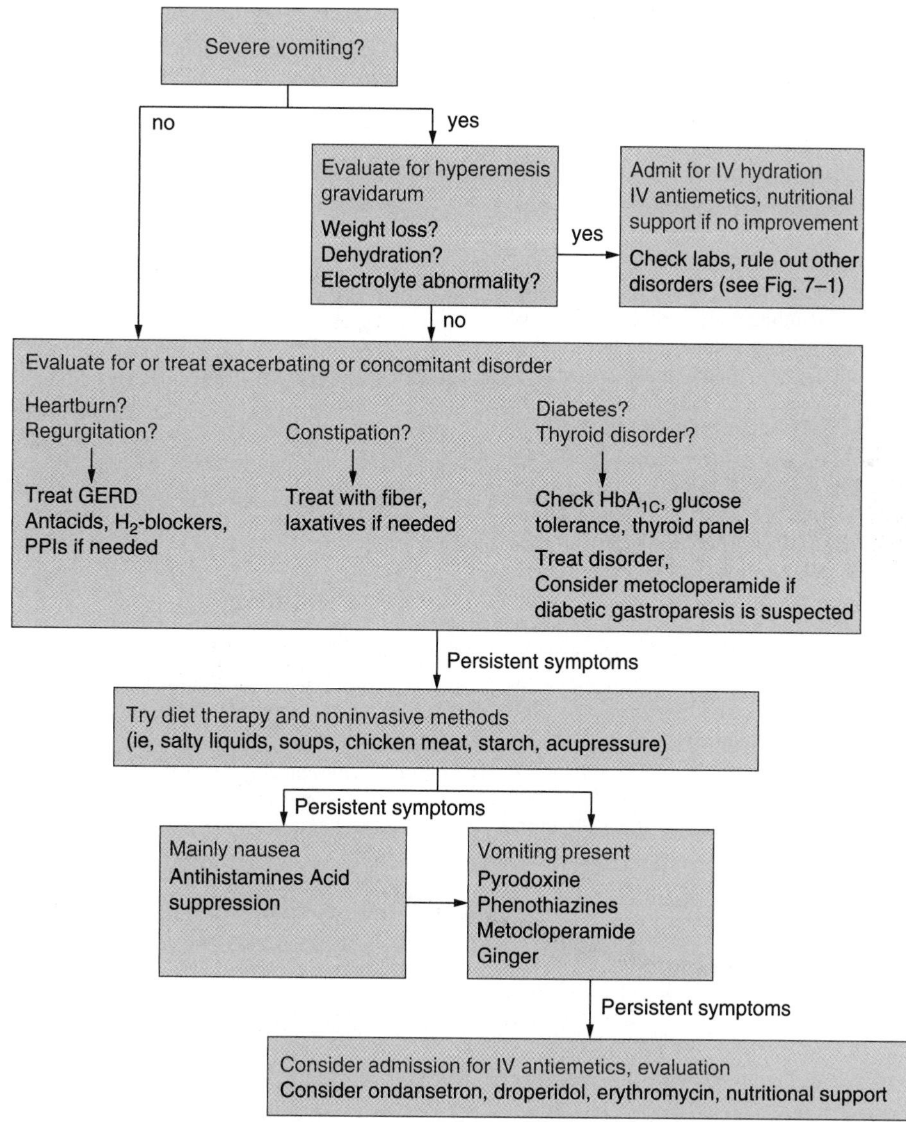

▲ **Figure 7–2.** Management of nausea and vomiting in pregnancy. GERD, gastroesophageal reflux disease; IV, intravenous; PPI, proton pump inhibitor.

Women should avoid exposure to odors, foods, or supplements that appear to trigger nausea. Typically, fatty foods are avoided because these can delay gastric emptying. Small, frequent meals of bland carbohydrates (starches such as noodles, potatoes, and rice), chicken, and fish are recommended. For patients with severe nausea and vomiting, small sips of salty liquids such as sports beverages or broth are recommended. Juices and creamy or dairy beverages are not advised as these can exacerbate symptoms. Some authors also recommend avoidance of vegetables or high-fiber foods, which can form bezoars. Acupressure is often performed with the use of wrist bands (Seabands) worn continuously for a period of a few days, followed by a hiatus of few days; it is noninvasive, and many women report a reduction in the number of episodes of nausea, although data are equivocal about whether this benefit is actual or partially a placebo effect. Most studies did not show a significant benefit in the treatment of severe vomiting. A recent Cochran review supports the use of pyridoxine (B_6) for control of nausea symptoms, and another small trial comparing 1.05 g of ginger daily for 3 weeks with 75 mg of pyridoxine found a similar modest benefit in reducing symptoms of nausea.

Women who have persistent nausea and vomiting and high concentrations of ketones require intravenous hydration with multivitamins, including thiamine, with follow-up measurement of levels of urinary ketones and electrolytes. Antiemetic agents should be prescribed in these patients.

Antihistamines such as meclizine have been used with no reports of teratogenicity. Studies of dimenhydrinate and diphenhydramine during pregnancy have shown conflicting results on safety and efficacy. Phenothiazines such as promethazine, prochlorperazine, and trimethobenzamide are considered low-risk drugs based on studies in pregnant women and also have clinical efficacy in this setting. Metoclopramide is used frequently in Europe for this indication, and one study shows no association with fetal malformations. In a recent randomized trial, intravenous metoclopramide and intravenous promethazine had similar efficacy in the treatment of hyperemesis, but metoclopramide caused less drowsiness and dizziness. An Israeli cohort study involving 3458 women who were exposed to metoclopramide in the first trimester (in most cases for 1–2 weeks) showed no significant association between exposure and the risk of congenital malformations, low birth weight, preterm delivery, or perinatal death.

Other prokinetics such as domperidone (used in Canada), bethanechol, and erythromycin have not been studied. Ondansetron is considered low risk in pregnancy, although its use is typically limited to cases of hyperemesis gravidarum. Granisetron and dolasetron have not been studied in human pregnancies.

Jewell D, Young G. Interventions for nausea and vomiting in early pregnancy. *Cochrane Database Syst Rev.* 2003;(4):CD000145. [PMID: 14583914]

Koch KL, Frissora CL. Nausea and vomiting during pregnancy. *Gastroenterol Clin North Am.* 2003;32:201–234. [PMID: 12635417]

Matok I, Gorodischer R, Koren G, et al. The safety of metoclopramide use in the first trimester of pregnancy. *N Engl J Med.* 2009;360:2528–2535. [PMID: 19516033]

Smith C, Crowther C, Willson K, et al. A randomized controlled trial of ginger to treat nausea and vomiting in pregnancy. *Obstet Gynecol.* 2004;103:639–645. [PMID: 15051552]

Tan PC, Khine PP, Vallikkannu N, et al. Promethazine compared with metoclopramide for hyperemesis gravidarum: a randomized controlled trial. *Obstet Gynecol.* 2010;115:975–981. [PMID: 20410771]

HYPEREMESIS GRAVIDARUM

This condition is characterized by severe vomiting with concurrent dehydration, electrolyte abnormalities, or weight loss. The reported incidence is 0.3–1% of pregnancies, and symptoms nearly always begin in the first trimester, although hyperemesis can sometimes be indicated by vomiting that persists after the first trimester. This condition is characterized by persistent vomiting, weight loss of more than 5%, ketonuria, electrolyte abnormalities (hypokalemia), and dehydration (high urine specific gravity). Hyperemesis gravidarum is associated with high estrogen levels and is more likely to occur with multiple gestations, gestational trophoblastic disease, and fetal abnormalities such as triploidy, trisomy 21, and hydrops fetalis. It has also been associated with hyperthyroidism, preeclampsia, eclampsia, HELLP syndrome (hemolysis, elevated liver enzymes, and low platelets), and acute fatty liver of pregnancy (AFLP). Although overall, patients with hyperemesis have good fetal outcomes, one study found that patients who experience a loss of 5% or more of body weight have a greater risk of growth retardation or fetal anomalies.

Clinical Findings

A. Symptoms and Signs

Patients may report dry mouth, sialorrhea, hyperolfaction, dysgeusia (altered or metallic taste), and decreased taste sensation. Physical examination may reveal signs of dehydration, including dry mucous membranes and poor skin turgor. The presence of epigastric or right upper quadrant pain, headache, and diplopia can suggest preeclampsia or eclampsia. Blood pressure should be measured and urinalysis performed; hypertension and proteinuria support the diagnosis of preeclampsia. Hyperreflexia and edema may also be present in preeclampsia, and the development of seizures defines eclampsia.

B. Laboratory Findings

Blood chemistries should be evaluated as hypochloremic metabolic alkalosis, hypokalemia, hypomagnesemia, and hyponatremia are common. Complete blood count and liver blood tests should also be checked to evaluate for HELLP syndrome (elevated transaminases without significant elevation of alkaline phosphatase or bilirubin, often with low platelets). AFLP can present with fulminant hepatic failure (elevated prothrombin time, jaundice, and elevated transaminases) and sometimes concurrent renal failure and hypoglycemia. These patients must be transferred to an intensive care unit, and a hepatologist should be consulted immediately. HELLP syndrome and AFLP typically occur late in pregnancy, usually in the third trimester. Other diseases associated with severe vomiting include hepatic vein thrombosis or Budd-Chiari syndrome, which can be diagnosed with a Doppler ultrasound. Celiac sprue can be diagnosed by tissue transglutaminase immunoglobulin A (IgA) and antiendomysial IgA or endoscopy, or both. *Helicobacter pylori* can be diagnosed by serology, endoscopy, or hydrogen breath test. Hyperemesis does not typically cause elevation in liver blood tests or renal failure unless severe dehydration is present.

Complications

Pregnancies of women with hyperemesis gravidarum can be complicated by low birth weight if the mother has experienced weight loss; however, fetal fatality is rare. Severe vomiting can rarely cause Mallory-Weiss tears or esophageal rupture. Rarely, women can develop peripheral neuropathies due to vitamin B_6 and B_{12} deficiencies. The most serious complication is Wernicke encephalopathy resulting from thiamine deficiency. Poor dietary intake can also result in deficiency of other vitamins and nutrients such as iron, calcium, and folate. Infants of mothers who have lost weight in early pregnancy, as compared with infants of women whose weight increased or stayed the same, have lower mean birth weights and lower percentile weights for gestational age.

Treatment

Oral and intravenous hydration and repletion of electrolytes is the primary treatment. Thiamine should be administered prior to dextrose to avoid Wernicke encephalopathy. After 24 hours of aggressive intravenous hydration, the infusion should be adjusted to maintain urine output. Once oral hydration is tolerated, broth or salty liquids should be started, followed by small carbohydrate meals such as crackers and noodles. In some cases, nasogastric or nasojejunal feeding may be required. In rare cases, parenteral nutrition has been used, but this should be avoided if possible due to risks of infection, diabetes, cholelithiasis, and risks associated with central line placement. Four cases have been reported of placement of percutaneous endoscopic gastrostomy tubes with jejunal extensions for this indication, during which fetal monitoring and anesthesia support were provided. Although procedure-related adverse fetal outcomes were not reported, this procedure should be reserved for patients at high nutritional risk, after nasoenteric feeding has failed and parenteral nutrition is contraindicated (hyperglycemia, hypercoagulability, or inadequate venous access). Medications used to control nausea and vomiting are often effective for hyperemesis. One study demonstrated some benefit of powdered root of ginger (20 mg orally, four times daily) in controlling symptoms. A few case reports describe benefits of erythromycin in controlling hyperemesis. Another study showed some efficacy of methylprednisolone, but steroids can be associated with adverse fetal outcomes.

Irving PM, Howell RJS, Shidrawi RG. Percutaneous endoscopic gastrostomy with a jejunal port for severe hyperemesis gravidarum. *Eur J Gastroenterol Hepatol.* 2004;16:937–939. [PMID: 15316422]

CONSTIPATION

New-onset constipation and exacerbation of chronic constipation are common complaints during pregnancy. Several physiologic changes are believed to contribute to this problem, including poor fluid intake in the setting of nausea and vomiting, iron supplementation, bed rest or decreased exercise, and hormonal changes such as increased progesterone and estrogen, which is thought to depress the migrating motor complex and slow orocecal transit time.

Clinical Findings

A. Symptoms and Signs

In uncomplicated constipation, the physical examination should be normal. Fever, abdominal pain, tenderness, distention, nausea or vomiting, or obstipation should prompt evaluation for other causes such as bowel obstruction or volvulus.

Treatment

The treatment of constipation during pregnancy is similar to its treatment in nonpregnant patients. First-line therapy consists of dietary fiber, which is the safest and most physiologic way to treat constipation; however, many patients will not respond to dietary fiber alone.

Psyllium, calcium polycarbophil, and methylcellulose are bulk laxatives that can be used as an alternative or adjunct to dietary fiber. These agents should be diluted and taken with food during meals. Fiber increases fecal water content, increases stool weight, decreases colonic transit time, and improves stool consistency. The laxative effect may be delayed for days. Pregnant patients should be warned that fiber can cause bloating and flatulence and instructed to consume sufficient fluids with it. Docusate, a stool softener, can be used alongside fiber supplements and is used routinely in pregnancy; however, there is one case report of neonatal hypomagnesemia associated with maternal oral administration of sodium docusate.

Osmotic laxatives can be used if fiber supplementation fails. Sorbitol and lactulose are poorly absorbed sugars that stimulate fluid accumulation in the colon by an osmotic effect. Lactulose is more expensive and should not be used in diabetic patients because it contains galactose. In addition, it can exacerbate nausea in pregnant patients with this symptom. Polyethylene glycol has been used to treat chronic constipation during pregnancy and causes less abdominal bloating and flatulence than other osmotic laxatives. It is now available over-the-counter and is recommended by many obstetric societies.

Stimulant laxatives are generally reserved for patients who do not respond to fiber or osmotic laxatives. If used chronically, electrolytes should be monitored as hypokalemia, hypomagnesemia, hyponatremia, and dehydration can result. Senna is generally safe in pregnancy and can be used in combination with bulk laxatives. It can be used at bedtime with fluids up to three times per week. Cascara is milder and is less often associated with abdominal discomfort. Bisacodyl is also safe in pregnancy as tablets or suppository, but can produce some abdominal discomfort when administered orally.

Fecal impaction should be treated with digital disimpaction. Mineral oil, tap water, or retention enemas can be used to soften stool. Bisacodyl suppository can then be used along with oral agents to treat constipation.

Agents to avoid during pregnancy include castor oil, which can initiate premature uterine contractions; aloe, which has been associated with congenital malformations; and saline hyperosmotic agents such as magnesium laxatives and phosphosoda, which can promote sodium and water retention. Orally administered mineral oil should also be avoided because it prevents absorption of fat-soluble vitamins. Tegaserod is no longer available for use in either pregnant or nonpregnant patients. Lubiprostone is class C and should not be used during pregnancy.

Wald A. Constipation, diarrhea, and symptomatic hemorrhoids during pregnancy. *Gastroenterol Clin North Am.* 2003;32:309–322. [PMID: 12635420]

DIARRHEA

Acute or chronic diarrhea can occur in pregnant women, and it is believed that pathogenesis and differential diagnosis are similar in pregnant and nonpregnant patients. Most cases of acute diarrhea are caused by viral infections such as rotavirus and Norwalk virus and are associated with large-volume, watery diarrhea that is self-limited. Bacterial illness often produces more frequent stools of small volume, abdominal pain, occasional fever, and blood and leukocytes in the stool.

Clinical Findings

A. Symptoms and Signs

Evaluation of diarrhea is typically warranted only if diarrhea is profuse, leads to dehydration, is bloody, is associated with high fevers, or if the illness persists for 48 hours without improvement or becomes chronic. Noninfectious causes of acute and chronic diarrhea include functional diarrhea, food intolerance, use of sugar substitutes such as sorbitol and mannitol, and IBD. A careful dietary and family history should be obtained.

B. Laboratory and Imaging Studies

Stool cultures for bacterial pathogens, ova, and parasites, and toxin or enzyme-linked immunosorbent assay (ELISA) for *Clostridium difficile* are the next step in evaluation. Flexible sigmoidoscopy with biopsy is considered safe in pregnancy and can be performed if needed to evaluate bloody or persistent diarrhea.

Treatment

Uncomplicated diarrhea should be treated with oral rehydration using juices, noncaffeinated beverages, and broth. Orange juice and bananas provide potassium, and salted crackers and broth can provide sodium. Small, frequent meals and avoidance of high-fat food, caffeine, dairy, and artificial sweeteners are recommended.

Antibiotics should be used only in the setting of documented infection with bacterial or parasitic microbes. Albendazole is teratogenic in animals, but in the setting of helminthic infections during pregnancy, the benefit is felt to be greater than the theoretical risk. Metronidazole can be used for *C difficile, Giardia lamblia,* and *Entamoeba histolytica,* but should be avoided during the first trimester and should not be administered long term because there are no data supporting its use for more than 2–3 weeks at a time. Ampicillin and erythromycin stearate have been used for bacterial causes of diarrhea, the latter specifically for *Campylobacter jejuni* infection. Less data are available on vancomycin, but it is also considered a low-risk drug. Azithromycin is not associated with congenital defects but may cause maternal gastrointestinal discomfort during pregnancy. Second-generation cephalosporins such as cefuroxime and cefixime can be used for acute shigellosis. Fluoroquinolones, tetracycline, doxycycline, erythromycin estolate, and trimethoprim–sulfamethoxazole should not be used based on current data available. Rifaximin is a nonabsorbable antibiotic with a wide spectrum of gram-negative and anaerobic coverage that is currently FDA approved for traveler's diarrhea. Although it should eventually be useful during pregnancy, no data are currently available regarding its use in pregnant women.

Antidiarrheal agents can be used to control symptoms in severe or persistent disease once active infection has been excluded. Kaolin and pectin are not absorbed and are probably safe although impairment of iron absorption is a possibility. Loperamide in small doses has been used in and is rated category B during pregnancy. Codeine can also be used in small amounts. Agents to avoid include bismuth subsalicylate (contained in Kaopectate), mainly because of the teratogenicity of salicylates. Diphenoxylate with atropine has also been found to be teratogenic. Alosetron should be avoided as well, because there are few data on its use during pregnancy. Cholestyramine has been used to treat cholestasis of pregnancy safely; however, its use can result in fat-soluble vitamin deficiencies including coagulopathy, which can lead to neonatal intracerebral hemorrhage.

HEMORRHOIDS

Hemorrhoids are common in the U.S. adult population and often become symptomatic or worsen during pregnancy. Pregnancy-associated constipation, poor venous return, increase in circulating blood volume, and extended time in the sitting position are all believed to contribute to this problem.

Clinical Findings

A. Symptoms and Signs

The perianal area should be inspected to rule out other contributions to pain and pruritus such as pinworms, fissures, fistulas, or ulcers. Other causes of rectal bleeding should be evaluated for, and a flexible sigmoidoscopy performed if needed. Internal hemorrhoids should be graded: first-degree hemorrhoids bleed but do not prolapse and can be visualized by anoscopy; second-degree hemorrhoids protrude during defecation or with straining but revert when straining stops; third-degree hemorrhoids are continuously prolapsed but easily reduced; fourth-degree hemorrhoids cannot be reduced.

Treatment

External hemorrhoids require treatment if they become thrombosed, which often results in pain or discomfort with sitting. If conservative measures such as stool softeners, daily warm sitz baths, and mild analgesics are not effective, surgical excision under local anesthesia is safe during pregnancy and does not affect the fetus. Clot incision and removal is generally only a temporizing measure as thrombosis usually recurs.

Internal hemorrhoids can cause bleeding, pain, or pruritus that may require treatment. Treatment of constipation is essential. Topical therapies such as witch hazel, hydrocortisone cream, and topical anesthetics (eg, benzocaine, dibucaine, or pramoxine) can help treat pruritus. Products containing epinephrine or phenylephrine should be avoided, especially in women with hypertension, diabetes, or fluid overload. If topical measures fail, band ligation for first-, second-, or third-degree internal hemorrhoids or injection sclerotherapy for first- or second-degree hemorrhoids is safe in pregnancy. Band ligation carries the associated risk of acute necrotizing perianal sepsis; however, this complication is rare.

Infrared photocoagulation or laser coagulation of first- and second-degree hemorrhoids is also minimally invasive, although safety in pregnancy has not been demonstrated. For patients who fail office-based procedures or those with fourth-degree lesions, closed excisional hemorrhoidectomy using local anesthesia has been reported to be safe and effective in pregnancy.

Wald A. Constipation, diarrhea, and symptomatic hemorrhoids during pregnancy. *Gastroenterol Clin North Am.* 2003;32: 309–322. [PMID: 12635420]

IRRITABLE BOWEL SYNDROME

The symptom complex and defining criteria of irritable bowel syndrome is described in Chapter 24. Irritable bowel syndrome is common in pregnancy, partly because it is a common syndrome in women of childbearing age and partly because pregnancy seems to exacerbate gastrointestinal symptoms associated with the syndrome. Many women experience an increase in constipation, or conversely, an increase in stool frequency. Abdominal pain, bloating, flatulence and nausea are also exacerbated by pregnancy, it is thought because of the impact of female hormones on gastrointestinal motility.

Clinical Findings

A. Symptoms and Signs

In patients with preexisting irritable bowel syndrome, evaluation mainly consists of ruling out other causes of constipation, irregular stools, and abdominal discomfort. Failure to respond to medical management or alarm symptoms such as bleeding, weight loss, or fever should prompt a search for other causes. In patients who present with irritable bowel syndrome during pregnancy, the diagnosis of irritable bowel syndrome is suggested by the combination of pain, flatulence, irregular defecation, and mucus in stools, and the exacerbation of symptoms by eating and relief by defecation. (See Chapter 24.)

Treatment

Dietary measures are the safest way to treat irritable bowel syndrome in pregnancy. Fiber supplementation can be implemented for constipation-predominant, diarrhea-predominant, and alternating irritable bowel syndrome. Patients can add bran to each meal or purchase supplements such as psyllium. Patients should be warned that an increase in bloating and flatulence occurs initially with fiber but may improve with time.

Medications used in the treatment of irritable bowel syndrome are outlined in Table 7–3. For patients with constipation-predominant symptoms who do not respond

Table 7–3. Medications used in the treatment of irritable bowel syndrome.

Drug	FDA Pregnancy Category	Recommendations for Pregnancy	Recommendations for Breast-Feeding
Alosetron	B	Avoid: restricted access	No human data: potential toxicity
Amitriptyline	C	Avoid: no malformations, but worse outcomes	Limited human data: potential toxicity
Bisacodyl	C	Low risk in short-term use	Safety unknown
Bismuth subsalicylate	C	Not safe: teratogenicity	No human data: potential toxicity
Castor oil	X	Uterine contraction and rupture	Possibly unsafe
Cholestyramine	C	Low risk, but can lead to infant coagulopathy	Compatible
Desipramine	C	Avoid: no malformations, but worse outcomes	Limited human data: potential toxicity
Dicyclomine	B	Avoid: possible congenital anomalies	Limited human data: potential toxicity
Diphenoxylate/atropine	C	Teratogenic in animals: no human data	Limited human data: potential toxicity
Docusate	C	Low risk	Compatible
Hyoscyamine	C	No available data	No human data: probably compatible
Imipramine	D	Avoid: no malformations, but worse outcomes	Limited human data: potential toxicity
Kaopectate	C	Unsafe because now contains bismuth	No human data: probably compatible
Lactulose	B	No human studies	No human data: probably compatible
Loperamide	B	Low risk: possible increased cardiovascular defects	Limited human data: probably compatible
Lubiprostone	C	No human studies but pregnancy loss in guinea pigs	Avoid use
Magnesium citrate	B	Avoid long-term use: hypermagnesemia, hyperphosphatemia, dehydration	Compatible
Mineral oil	C	Avoid: neonatal coagulopathy and hemorrhage	Possibly unsafe
Nortriptyline	D	Avoid: no malformations, but worse outcomes	Limited human data: potential toxicity
Paroxetine	D	Avoid: twice as many birth defects as other antidepressants	Potential toxicity
PEG	C	First-choice laxative in pregnancy	Low risk
Senna	C	Low risk in short-term use	Compatible
SSRIs (except paroxetine)	C	Avoid: no malformations, but increased adverse events in fetus	Limited human data: potential toxicity
Simethicone	C	No available data: low risk	No human data: probably compatible
Sodium phosphate		Avoid long-term: hypermagnesemia, hyperphosphatemia, dehydration	Safety unknown
Tegaserod	B	Low risk: human data negative for malformations	Safety unknown

PEG, polyethylene glycol; SSRI, selective serotonin reuptake inhibitor.
Reproduced, with permission, from Mahadevan U, Kane S. American Gastroenterological Association Institute technical review on the use of gastrointestinal medications in pregnancy. *Gastroenterology*. 2006;131:283–311.

to bulk laxatives, osmotic laxatives such as polyethylene glycol, sorbitol, or lactulose can be used and are considered low risk in pregnancy. Tap-water enemas can be used to treat fecal impaction. Magnesium citrate and sodium phosphate should be avoided. For a full discussion of laxatives that can be used in pregnancy, see the earlier discussion of constipation. For patients with diarrhea-predominant symptoms, a low-fat, nondairy diet should be tried first. After this, loperamide or codeine can be used in small doses after infection is ruled out. For information about antidiarrheal agents for use during pregnancy, see the earlier section on treatment of diarrhea in pregnancy.

Antispasmodic agents such as anticholinergics, calcium channel blockers, and direct gut smooth muscle relaxants are used in patients whose irritable bowel syndrome is associated with severe pain, but these agents have not been well studied in pregnancy, and there is a lack of efficacy data to support use. Dicyclomine has been associated with phocomelia in animals and is a category B drug in pregnancy. Most other anticholinergics, such as hyoscyamine, and calcium channel blockers, such as nifedipine, are category C drugs and are not well studied in pregnancy. Antidepressant drugs have been used during pregnancy for treatment of depression, but have not been studied for the treatment of irritable bowel syndrome in pregnancy. Tricyclic antidepressants and selective serotonin reuptake inhibitors (SSRIs) have been associated with short-term neonatal withdrawal symptoms, and cases of neonatal heart failure and electrocardiographic abnormalities have been reported with tricyclic antidepressants. SSRIs such as fluoxetine, paroxetine, sertraline, and citalopram are FDA category C. Paroxetine is associated with increased congenital malformation. The tricyclic agents nortriptyline and imipramine are category D drugs, but desipramine and amitriptyline are category C. Narcotics should be avoided because of the risk of tolerance, and benzodiazepines are category D in pregnancy.

Hasler WL. The irritable bowel syndrome during pregnancy. *Gastroenterology Clin North Am.* 2003;32:385–406. [PMID: 12635423]

FECAL INCONTINENCE

Fecal incontinence following vaginal delivery can be caused by anal sphincter tears, denervation injury, or rectovaginal fistulas. Risk factors for anal sphincter tears after vaginal delivery include third- or fourth-degree perineal lacerations (those that extend into the muscular layers of the anal sphincter), incomplete repairs of these lacerations, nerve injury or partial dehiscence following laceration repair, episiotomies (particularly midline episiotomies), a history of anal tears from previous deliveries, and forceps or vacuum delivery. The incidence of anal sphincter tears is lower in elective caesarean deliveries, but fecal incontinence is still common following emergency caesarean deliveries, presumably because some injury to the pelvic floor has already occurred. Anovaginal and rectovaginal fistulas are more common in pregnant women in underdeveloped countries and are felt to be partly due to prolonged labor leading to pressure necrosis. Fistulas can also be seen after laceration repair or in infected episiotomy sites. Nerve injury, particularly pudendal nerve injury during delivery, has also been implicated in fecal incontinence, but this has not been demonstrated conclusively.

Clinical Findings

A. Symptoms and Signs

Patients can present with pregnancy-related fecal incontinence immediately after or many years following delivery. In most patients, the rectal examination will be normal and rectal tone will be grossly normal; in some cases, it is possible to palpate a defect in the anterior wall.

B. Imaging Studies

The mainstay of evaluation is the endoanal ultrasound (EAUS). Defects in either the external or internal anal sphincter are seen as asymmetries in concentric rings of tissues that surround the anal canal. The internal anal sphincter appears hypoechoic, and defects in this layer appear hyperechoic. The external anal sphincter appears hyperechoic, and defects appear hypoechoic. Typically, pregnancy-related trauma from tears or episiotomies is located anteriorly. Fistulas appear as hypoechoic tracts; air within these tracts appears as focal hyperechoic areas. Findings on EAUS have been validated by anorectal manometry and correlate with anal squeeze pressure and surgical findings and histology. Other studies of EAUS performed before and after surgical repair of sphincter defect show that EAUS documentation of closure of the sphincter defect predicts improvement in fecal incontinence. Anorectal manometry can demonstrate changes in resting and squeeze pressure due to sphincter trauma but is less sensitive in being able to detect tears than anorectal manometry. Pelvic magnetic resonance imaging (MRI) may be a useful and noninvasive modality but is currently not widely available and has not been well studied for this indication. Pudendal nerve injury can be documented by pudendal nerve terminal motor latency measurements, but the role of pudendal nerve injury in fecal continence is controversial.

Treatment

The treatment of sphincter tears and rectovaginal fistulas is surgical. Sphincteroplasty, when closure of the defect is successful, often leads to improvement in symptoms.

Chong AK, Hoffman B. Fecal incontinence related to pregnancy. *Gastrointest Endosc Clin N Am.* 2006;16:71–81. [PMID: 16546024]

Mimura T, Kaminishi M, Kamm MA. Diagnostic evaluation of patients with faecal incontinence at a specialist institution. *Dig Surg*. 2004;21:235–241. [PMID: 15237257]

INFLAMMATORY BOWEL DISEASE

Clinical Findings

A. Impact of Pregnancy on Disease Activity

For a patient with ulcerative colitis (UC) in remission at the time of conception, there is about a one-third chance that she will flare during the 12 months of gestation and the puerperium. This is similar to the relapse rate of nonpregnant patients with colitis followed for a year. In UC patients with active disease at the time of conception, roughly 45% will get worse, whereas 25% will improve and 25% will remain unchanged. Thus, virtually three out of four patients will have active disease during the course of their pregnancy with a subsequent ill effect on the fetus. For patients with Crohn disease (CD) in remission at conception, approximately 25% will relapse in the following 12 months, which is the same rate as for nonpregnant CD patients. For patients with active disease at the time of conception, one third will improve and one third will worsen. Thus, two thirds will have to contend with active disease during pregnancy.

It is common for disease activity to vary from pregnancy to pregnancy in a particular individual, despite the fact that disease may be inactive at conception. The only study examining this question investigates the effect of human leukocyte antigen (HLA) mismatch on disease activity. The authors study 50 pregnancies in 38 women with CD or UC. Both mother and child were HLA tested. Thirty of the 50 pregnancies were disparate at both the DRB1 and the DQ loci. Twelve pregnancies were mismatched at the DRB1 locus and four at the DQ locus. Four were disparate at neither. When comparing the calculated average disease score for pregnancies disparate at one versus both loci, an odds ratio of 22 was seen. By logistic regression analysis, HLA disparity at both DRB1 and DQ predicted a lower postpartum disease activity score. Thus, maternal immune response to paternal HLA antigens may play a role in pregnancy-induced remission of IBD.

B. Effect of Disease Activity on Pregnancy

Perhaps the most important thing doctors should remember when counseling an IBD patient about a potential pregnancy is that the patient should be in remission at the time of conception. This remission should be durable, for at least 3–6 months on stable medications, prior to conception. Most IBD medications are safe during pregnancy, and the biggest problem most patients have is stopping their long-term medications prior to conception. A frank discussion about pregnancy, reinforced at each office visit, for both women and men with IBD helps both doctor and patient anticipate any potential problems. Since something can always go wrong with a pregnancy (eg, there is a 14% rate of miscarriage in the United States), it is always best to give the patient and her or his partner all of the facts and not decide for them about stopping certain medications such as azathioprine or 6-mercaptopurine.

It is fairly well documented that babies born to women with CD and UC are at greater risk for adverse pregnancy outcomes including premature birth and low birth weight when compared to controls in the general population. Women with IBD, and probably CD in particular, are at greater risk for having a cesarean section. A meta-analysis of 12 prior studies encompassing 3907 patients with IBD and 320,531 controls was published in 2006. Overall, there was a 1.87-fold increase in the incidence of prematurity (<37 weeks of gestation), compared with controls. The incidence of low birth weight (<2500 g) was over twice that of normal controls. Women with IBD were 1.5 times more likely to undergo cesarean section, and the risk of congenital anomalies was found to be 2.37-fold increased. The greater risk of low birth weight and cesarean section was significant only in patients with CD. The greater risk of congenital anomalies was found only in women with UC in a single study. All types of congenital anomalies, including ones of minor significance, were included in this particular study, and the authors did not take disease activity or medications into consideration. When just the higher quality studies were analyzed, there was no greater risk of congenital anomalies. Neither disease activity nor medication use was used as a confounder in this meta-analysis.

There is even newer and more specific information about the impact of CD activity per se on pregnancy outcomes. A recent paper examined all births by women with CD in North Jutland County, Denmark from January 1977 to December 2005. All individual medical records were reviewed. The authors found 71 pregnancies in women with low to moderate-high disease activity and 86 pregnancies in women with inactive disease. There was no increased incidence of low birth weight, low birth weight at term, or congenital abnormalities among the two groups of women. However, there was a 3.4-fold increased risk of preterm birth in women with moderate to high disease activity. The authors controlled for the influence of drug therapy, particularly immunomodulator use, as a confounder.

Another recent, even more comprehensive paper looked at pregnancy outcomes in women with IBD in a large health maintenance organization (HMO) in Northern California. This was a cohort study of 461 pregnant women with IBD matched to 493 pregnant women without IBD. All medical records were reviewed, and data were gathered on many factors, including disease activity and IBD medications during pregnancy. Very few patients were on biologics or immunomodulators (4%) during pregnancy and conception, whereas 21% had some corticosteroid exposure and 51% had some aminosalicylate exposure. Pregnant women with IBD were less likely to have a live birth (60% vs 68%, $P = .01$) and more likely to have a cesarean section (13.8% vs 9.5%, $P = .05$) than women without IBD. The rates of therapeutic abortion and congenital anomalies were similar between the two groups. There was no difference in the rate of congenital anomalies between children born to mothers with UC or CD ($P = .45$). Women with IBD were also more likely to have an adverse conception outcome (eg, spontaneous abortion, abortion for unknown reason) (23% vs 17%, $P = .03$), an adverse pregnancy outcome (eg, preterm birth, small for gestation age, still birth) (25% vs 19%, $P = .058$), or a complication of pregnancy (25% vs 16%, $P < .01$) compared with women without IBD. There was no statistically significant difference in newborn outcomes between the two groups (10% vs 7%, $P = .18$). Low birth weight was also more common among IBD patients than among patients without IBD (7.4% vs 3.6%, $P = .04$).

Among all patients, predictors of an adverse conception outcome in a multivariate model included the presence of IBD, non-Caucasian ethnicity, a history of IBD surgery, and increasing maternal age (odds ratio per year of age, 1.10; 95% confidence interval [CI], 1.05–1.14). Predictors of an adverse pregnancy outcome were non-Caucasian ethnicity and the presence of IBD. Predictors of a pregnancy complication were a diagnosis of IBD, CD, and a history of IBD surgery. The only predictor of a newborn adverse outcome was a diagnosis of CD.

Among patients with IBD, maternal age was a predictor of an adverse outcome. IBD surgery was a predictor of adverse outcome when IBD patients with surgery were compared with controls, but not when IBD patients with surgery were compared with IBD patients without surgery.

Disease activity, IBD medication use, and moderate to severe disease activity were not associated with adverse outcomes. The majority of patients (about 80%) with both CD and UC had inactive or mild disease throughout pregnancy. Although limited by its homogeneous study population, this study should reassure us that women in remission should have healthy pregnancies. Because only 4% of patients were on immunomodulators or biologics, we need to look elsewhere for the safety of these specific medications during pregnancy.

C. Management of IBD During Pregnancy

Patients with active disease should be considered as having high-risk pregnancies and should be followed by the appropriate obstetric service. Unlike many other diseases in pregnancy, delivery will rarely cure an IBD flare, although early delivery in some situations may protect the fetus and allow for more aggressive treatment of the mother. Disease activity should be monitored carefully prior to conception and throughout the pregnancy. Patients should be encouraged to be compliant with treatment if needed for flares or for maintenance, as active disease is the greatest threat to normal pregnancy, not the medications used to treat it. As patients with IBD can develop other gastrointestinal complications during pregnancy, an evaluation for infection, ulcer disease, nausea and vomiting associated with pregnancy, and biliary disease should be undertaken before starting treatment for a flare.

Disease assessment during pregnancy in IBD patients should rely heavily on clinical features, and patients should be questioned about abdominal pain, stool frequency, nocturnal stools, and blood and mucous in the stool. Laboratory parameters will often not be accurate because, during gestation, hemoglobin and albumin levels will fall as a result of hemodilution and erythrocyte sedimentation rate (ESR) will rise. During pregnancy, the C-reactive protein level is a more accurate measure of IBD activity than ESR. The pulse rate and temperature should be recorded, and stool cultures and stool *C difficile* toxin should be performed in the event of diarrhea. Maintaining adequate nutrition, hydration, and electrolyte balance is critical for the patient and fetus. Antidiarrheal therapy can be used as an adjunct to IBD treatment to help avoid hospitalization in refractory diarrhea.

D. Imaging and Endoscopic Studies

1. Diagnostic radiology during pregnancy—Various imaging modalities are available for diagnostic use in IBD patients during pregnancy. These include x-ray, ultrasonography, MRI in the second and third trimesters, and computed tomography (CT) after 25 weeks of gestation. In humans, growth retardation, microcephaly, and mental retardation are the most common adverse effects from high-dose radiation. Based on data from atomic bomb survivors, it appears that the risk of central nervous system effects is greatest with exposure at 8–15 weeks of gestation, with no proven risk at less than 8 weeks of gestation or greater than 25 weeks of gestation. Thus, at 8–15 weeks of gestation, the fetus is at greatest risk for radiation-induced mental retardation, and the risk appears to be at doses of at least 20 rad. For example, the risk of severe mental retardation in fetuses exposed to ionizing radiation is approximately 40% at 100 rad of exposure and as high as 60% at 150 rad of exposure. Even multiple diagnostic x-ray procedures rarely result in ionizing radiation exposure to this degree. Fetal risks of anomalies, growth restriction, or abortions are not increased with radiation exposure of less than 5 rad, a level above the range of exposure of most diagnostic procedures. The risk of carcinogenesis as a result of in utero exposure to ionizing radiation is unclear but is probably very small. It is estimated that a 1–2 rad fetal exposure may increase the risk of leukemia by a factor of 1.2–2.0 over natural incidence and that an estimated 1 in 2000 children exposed to ionizing radiation in utero will develop childhood leukemia. This is increased from a background rate of 1 in 3000.

With MRI, magnets that alter the energy state of hydrogen protons are used instead of ionizing radiation. MRI is somewhat useful in establishing the diagnosis or evaluating the activity of CD in the second and third trimesters. Ultrasonography involves the use of sound waves and is not a form of ionizing radiation. It is less useful than MRI in evaluating IBD activity.

Most intravenous contrast agents used with CT contain derivatives of iodine and have not been studied in humans; however, many have been studied in animals and do not appear to be teratogenic. Neonatal hypothyroidism has been associated with some iodinated contrast agents taken during pregnancy, and for this reason, these compounds are avoided unless essential for the correct diagnosis. Neonatal thyroid function should be checked during the first week if iodinated contrast media have been given during pregnancy. Paramagnetic contrast agents used during MRI have not been studied in pregnant women. Animal studies have demonstrated increased rates of spontaneous abortion, skeletal abnormalities, and visceral abnormalities when given at two to seven times the recommended human dose. The agents should be used if the potential benefit justifies the potential risk. Only a tiny amount of iodinated or gadolinium-based contrast medium given to the lactating mother reaches the milk and only a minute proportion is absorbed.

2. Endoscopy during pregnancy—Flexible sigmoidoscopy is generally safe during pregnancy and can be performed if needed to evaluate the severity of a flare or to rule out hematochezia or diarrhea from another source. Colonoscopy is generally avoided in pregnancy (see later discussion of endoscopy during pregnancy). The indications for performing sigmoidoscopy in pregnant patients are similar to indications in nonpregnant patients and include evaluation of diarrhea, hematochezia, and abdominal pain or mass. In one study, 15 of 17 patients with IBD who underwent sigmoidoscopy during pregnancy had a change in management based on findings. When lower endoscopy is required, flexible sigmoidoscopy is much lower risk than colonoscopy and should be considered first, particularly in patients with left-sided disease.

Treatment

Treatment of IBD during pregnancy is similar to that of nonpregnant patients.

A. Pharmacotherapy

Tables 7–4 and 7–5 outline considerations relating to medication use in pregnant and breast-feeding women.

1. Sulfasalazine—Sulfasalazine is useful for colonic CD and UC, particularly in the treatment of mild disease and maintenance of remission. It is category B in pregnancy but has a high rate of side effects in both pregnant and nonpregnant patients (nausea, vomiting, rash, fever, anorexia, heartburn, epigastric pain, diarrhea, pancreatitis, interstitial nephritis, hepatotoxicity). For patients starting this medication, a low dose of 500 mg/day should be prescribed initially due to high rate of side effects; if tolerated, this can be increased to the goal of 4–6 g/day over several days. Patients taking sulfasalazine should take higher amounts of folic acid than normally recommended (2 g/day).

2. 5-Acetylsalicylic acid—5-Acetylsalicylic acid (5-ASA) compounds are more expensive than sulfasalazine, but have minimal side effects, and mesalamine may be effective in treating small bowel CD. Side effects reported are the same in pregnant as in nonpregnant patients and include renal toxicity, headache, abdominal pain, nausea, fever, IBD flare, pancreatitis, leukopenia, and hepatocellular toxicity. Asacol (mesalamine) releases 5-ASA in the distal ileum and colon and can be used in doses of 4.8 g/day orally or as enemas or suppositories in patients with distal disease. Pentasa (mesalamine), used in oral doses of 4 g/day, is a formulation that contains coated micro-granules that release 5-ASA

Table 7–4. Inflammatory bowel disease medications and pregnancy.

Category B	Category C	Category D	Category X
Balsalazide Adalimumab Certolizumab pegol Infliximab Loperamide Mesalamine (except Asacol and Asacol HD) Metronidazole[a] Prednisone/prednisolone Sulfasalazine	Budesonide Ciprofloxacin Codeine Cyclosporine Diphenoxylate Olsalazine Asacol Asacol HD Tacrolimus Rifaximin	Azathioprine[b] 6-Mercaptopurine[b]	Methotrexate Thalidomide

[a]Safe during the second and third trimester.
[b]Studies in women with IBD and renal transplants have shown that these medications are relatively safe during pregnancy (see text discussion).

Table 7–5. Inflammatory bowel disease medications and breast-feeding.

Safe to Use When Needed	Limited Data Available	Should Be Avoided
Balsalazide Oral mesalamine Prednisone/prednisolone Sulfasalazine Topical mesalamine	Azathioprine Infliximab/Adalimumab/Certolizumab pegol 6-Mercaptopurine Tacrolimus	Ciprofloxacin Cyclosporine Methotrexate Metronidazole

throughout the gastrointestinal tract; it is effective in gastric and small bowel CD. Balsalazide releases 5-ASA into the colon and is also safe in pregnancy. Few data are available on slow-release Lialda (MMX mesalamine) and olsalazine sodium. The FDA classification has recently changed to class C for Asacol and Asacol HD because of the dibutyl phthalate (DBP) that is present in the Eudragit-S delayed-release coating of Asacol and Asacol HD tablets.

3. Antibiotics—There are no studies of long-term antibiotic use during pregnancy. The safest antibiotics to use for CD in pregnancy for short periods of time (weeks, not months) are ampicillin and cephalosporins. These are category B drugs, and human studies have not shown increased teratogenic risk. They are compatible with breast-feeding and may provide an alternative to ciprofloxacin or metronidazole. Metronidazole is a pregnancy category B drug, and multiple studies have suggested that it is not associated with birth defects. These include two meta-analyses, two retrospective cohort studies, and a prospective controlled study of 228 women exposed to metronidazole during pregnancy. It can be used in the second or third trimester. There is toxicity associated with long-term use of metronidazole, and therefore, it is not recommended for breast-feeding.

Ciprofloxacin causes cartilage lesions in immature animals and should be avoided because of the absence of data on its effects on growth and development in humans. Although a prospective study did not find any increased congenital anomalies, the effects on bone and cartilage may take years to develop, and therefore, it is not recommended during pregnancy. It should also be held during breast-feeding due to lack of data.

Rifaximin is pregnancy category C. It should be useful in pregnancy because there is very little systemic absorption (<0.4%). It has not been shown to affect fertility or pregnancy outcome in rats but can cause teratogenic complications in rats and rabbits. Safety in breast-feeding is unknown.

4. Azathioprine and 6-mercaptopurine—Azathioprine and 6-mercaptopurine (6-MP) are FDA pregnancy category D. However, decades of experience in IBD, transplantation, and other immune diseases do not show a clear association with congenital anomalies. The oral bioavailability of these agents is low in humans, and the fetal liver in the first trimester lacks inosinate pyrophosphorylase, the enzyme needed to metabolize the agent. Both of these are factors that may be protective to the fetus during organogenesis. There are only two retrospective IBD studies of the use of 6-MP in pregnancy that control for disease activity. One looked at the effect of 6-MP at conception and during pregnancy and found no statistical difference in conception failures (defined as a spontaneous abortion), abortion secondary to a birth defect, major congenital malformations, neoplasia, or increased infections among female or male patients taking 6-MP compared with controls (relative risk, 0.85; 95% CI, 0.47–1.55; $P = .59$). There were 155 patients (79 females) and 325 pregnancies. This paper did not look at prematurity or low birth weight. All patients were in clinical remission at the time of conception with no patient being moderately or severely ill during pregnancy.

Another paper by this same group looked at 6-MP and azathioprine in addition to other IBD medications taken during pregnancy. These other medications used sometime during pregnancy included 5-ASA (100 of 207 conceptions), prednisone (49 conceptions), 6-MP or azathioprine (101 conceptions), metronidazole (27 conceptions), ciprofloxacin (18 conceptions), and cyclosporine (2 conceptions). Eighty-five of the conceptions were free of any medication. The authors reported that the "great majority of patients were in remission at the time of conception." In multivariate analyses controlling for the age of the mother, there was no evidence that any type of drug therapy influenced pregnancy outcomes. Outcomes measured were spontaneous or therapeutic abortion, maternal or fetal illness resulting in abortion, premature birth, healthy full-term birth, multiple births, ectopic pregnancy, congenital abnormalities, birth weight, and type of delivery.

A more recent study found that among 20 women with IBD exposed to azathioprine/6-MP during pregnancy, the risks of preterm birth and congenital abnormalities was 4.2 (95% CI, 1.4–12.5) and 2.9 (95% CI, 0.9–8.9), respectively. However, the authors did not adequately control for disease activity. It is generally agreed that for women who need azathioprine/6-MP, it is safer to stay on these drugs during pregnancy than to risk a flare and a potential pregnancy complication.

Breast-feeding has traditionally been discouraged, but recent data showing zero to minimal levels in breast milk and no detectable levels in the breast-feeding infant suggest that it may be safe, but more studies are needed.

5. Glucocorticoids—Glucocorticoids are generally reserved for acute flares of disease often presenting as diarrhea, hematochezia, and abdominal pain. They are believed to be safe during pregnancy and nursing, although one uncontrolled human study did demonstrate a possible increased risk of cleft palate (and there is also the risk of premature rupture of membranes). Patients with left-sided colitis or proctosigmoiditis may benefit from once- or twice-daily steroid enemas (hydrocortisone enemas, 100 mg/60 mL), foam (10% hydrocortisone acetate), or suppositories (hydrocortisone acetate, 30 mg). For those who require systemic steroids the standard dose for acute flares is 40 mg/day of oral prednisone. For those with severe flares or who fail a trial of oral steroids, the next step is intravenous hydrocortisone, 300 mg/day in divided doses, or the equivalent dose of methylprednisolone for 7–10 days or until there is improvement in symptoms (solid stool, absence of blood or abdominal pain). Patients are then transitioned to oral prednisone. Side effects are the same in pregnant as in nonpregnant patients (weight gain, fluid retention, hypertension, avascular necrosis, mood swings, psychosis, PUD, diabetes, obesity, myopathy, immunosuppression, metabolic bone disease); however, electrolyte abnormalities such as hypernatremia, volume overload, and hypokalemia are more common in pregnancy and can produce preeclampsia. Careful monitoring of electrolytes is required, and dietary salt restriction may be needed. Budesonide is an orally administered synthetic steroid with limited systemic absorption that is particularly effective in right-sided CD, but data in pregnancy are currently lacking.

6. Immunosuppressants—Cyclosporine is a category C drug during pregnancy. A meta-analysis of 15 studies of pregnancy outcomes after cyclosporine therapy reported a total of 410 patients with data on major malformations. The calculated odds ratio of 3.83 for malformations did not achieve statistical significance (95% CI, 0.75–19.6). In IBD, case reports have noted the successful use of intravenous cyclosporine during pregnancy. In the setting of severe steroid-refractory UC, cyclosporine is a better option than colectomy, which is associated with a 50–60% fetal mortality. Cyclosporine is excreted in the breast milk in high concentrations and is contraindicated during nursing.

Tacrolimus is also category C. There is an increased incidence of perinatal hyperkalemia and prematurity. The reported malformation rate is 5.6% with no persistent anomalies seen. There is a single case report of the successful use of tacrolimus in a pregnant patient with UC.

The anti-tumor necrosis factor (TNF) α agents infliximab and adalimumab are immunoglobulin G1 (IgG1) antibodies and are FDA category B. IgG1 does not cross the placenta in the first trimester during organogenesis. However, they do cross highly efficiently in the third trimester. One paper reported on 133 infliximab exposures in women with CD or rheumatoid arthritis, and data were available on 96 pregnancies. Fetal adverse outcomes in women exposed to infliximab were no different than those outcomes in women who had not been exposed. Another retrospective analysis of 10 women with CD treated intentionally with infliximab during pregnancy did not show any congenital anomalies, intrauterine growth retardation, or small for gestational age parameters.

Infliximab has been detected in cord blood, and levels are detectable in the infant up to 6 months after birth. The effects of infliximab on the developing infant immune system and response to vaccines are not known, although limited data do not show harm. The recent recommendation for the live rotavirus vaccine in the second month of life may need to be avoided if the infant has detectable infliximab levels. Common practice in the United States is to give the last dose of infliximab at the beginning of the third trimester and the next dose after birth if the mother is in remission. If the mother flares during the third trimester, she is given her usual dose of infliximab. The infant should be monitored until infliximab levels are undetectable, especially before the live vaccines varicella and MMR (measles, mumps, rubella) are given at 1 year of life. Limited data have shown that infliximab is not detectable in breast milk and mothers can probably safely nurse their infants.

Adalimumab is listed as a category B drug and has recently been approved by the FDA for treatment of CD. Animal data have shown no evidence of harm to the fetus. There are several case reports of successful use of adalimumab during pregnancy in CD patients.

Certolizumab is also listed as a category B drug and crosses the placenta by passive diffusion. There are very low levels in cord blood and no levels in breast milk. A handful of case reports have shown it to be safe in pregnancy.

B. Adjunctive Measures

Maintaining adequate nutrition, hydration, and electrolyte balance is critical for the patient and the fetus. Antidiarrheal therapy can be used as an adjunct in the treatment of IBD to help avoid hospitalization in refractory diarrhea. The safest agent is loperamide, but codeine has also been used (see the earlier discussion of antidiarrheal agents). Parenteral nutrition is safe in pregnancy and should be used in patients requiring bowel rest.

C. Surgery

Indications for surgery during pregnancy include uncontrollable bleeding, obstruction, perforation, fulminant disease refractory to medical management, or intra-abdominal abscess that cannot be drained by other methods. Surgery during the second trimester carries a lower rate of miscarriage than during the first trimester and is technically less complicated than during the third trimester. Total colectomy for fulminant UC has a 50–60% fetal mortality rate, and if possible, intravenous cyclosporine, possibly infliximab, or early delivery is preferable.

D. Delivery

In general, the method of the delivery should be dictated by obstetric indication. Vaginal delivery and cesarean delivery are safe for patients with an ileal pouch–anal anastomosis, and episiotomy is not contraindicated in IBD. Many patients with active perianal disease report worsening of their disease after vaginal delivery; therefore, it is generally recommended that these patients undergo cesarean deliveries. Patients with fulminant UC should also undergo cesarean delivery. Women in remission or with mild disease without perianal activity generally deliver vaginally unless the circumstances of pregnancy dictate otherwise.

ACOG Committee on Obstetric Practice. ACOG Committee Opinion. Guidelines for diagnostic imaging during pregnancy. *Obstet Gynecol.* 2004;104:647–651. [PMID: 15339791]

Bertoli D, Borelli G. Fertility study of rifaximin (L/105) in rats. *Chemioterapia.* 1986;5:204–207. [PMID: 3719854]

Christensen LA, Dahlerup JF, Nielsen MJ, et al. Azathioprine treatment during lactation. *Aliment Pharmacol Ther.* 2008;28: 1209–1213. [PMID: 18761704]

Cornish JA, Tan EKW, Teare J, et al. A meta-analysis on the influence of inflammatory bowel disease on pregnancy. *Gut* 2007;56: 830–837. [PMID: 17185356]

Diav-Citron O, Shechtman S, Gotteiner T, et al. Pregnancy outcome after gestational exposure to metronidazole: a prospective controlled cohort study. *Teratology.* 2001;63:186–192. [PMID: 11320529]

Francella A, Dyan A, Bodian C, et al. The safety of 6-mercaptopurine for childbearing patients with inflammatory bowel disease: a retrospective cohort study. *Gastroenterology.* 2003;124:9–17. [PMID: 12512024]

Kane S, Kisiel J, Shih L, et al. HLA disparity determines disease activity through pregnancy in women with inflammatory bowel disease. *Am J Gastroenterol.* 2004;99:1523–1526. [PMID: 15307871]

Katz JA, Antonini C, Keenen GF, et al. Outcome of pregnancy in women receiving infliximab for the treatment of Crohn's disease and rheumatoid arthritis. *Am J Gastroenterol.* 2004;99: 2385–2392. [PMID: 15571587]

Larsen H, Nielsen GL, Schonheyder HC, et al. Birth outcomes following maternal use of fluoroquinolones. *J Antimicrob Agents.* 2001;18:259–262. [PMID: 11673039]

Mahadevan U, Kane S. American Gastroenterological Association Institute position statement on the use of gastrointestinal medications in pregnancy. *Gastroenterology.* 2006;131:278–282. [PMID: 16831610]

Mahadevan U, Kane S. American Gastroenterological Association Institute technical review on the use of gastrointestinal medications in pregnancy. *Gastroenterology.* 2006;131:283–311. [PMID: 16831611]

Mahadevan U, Sandborn WJ, Li DK, et al. Pregnancy outcomes in women with inflammatory bowel disease: a large community-based study from northern California. *Gastroenterology.* 2007;133:1106–1112. [PMID: 17764676]

Malangoni MA. Gastrointestinal surgery and pregnancy. *Gastroenterol Clin North Am.* 2003;32:181–200. [PMID: 12635416]

Norgard B, Fonager K, Pedersen L, et al. Birth outcome in women exposed to 5-aminosalicylic acid during pregnancy: a Danish cohort study. *Gut.* 2003;52:243–247. [PMID: 12524407]

Norgard B, Hundborg HH, Jacobsen BA, et al. Disease activity in pregnant women with Crohn's disease and birth outcomes: a regional Danish cohort study. *Am J Gastroenterol.* 2007;102: 1947–1954. [PMID: 17573787]

Qureshi WA, Rajan E, Adler DG, et al. ASGE guideline: guidelines for endoscopy in pregnant and lactating women. *Gastrointest Endosc.* 2005;61:357–362. [PMID: 17212888]

Sau A, Clarke S, Bass J, et al. Azathioprine and breastfeeding: is it safe? *BJOG.* 2007;114:498–501. [PMID: 17261122]

Siddiqui U, Proctor DD. Flexible sigmoidoscopy and colonoscopy during pregnancy. *Gastrointest Endosc Clin North Am.* 2006;16: 59–69. [PMID: 16546023]

ABDOMINAL PAIN

The differential diagnosis of abdominal pain in pregnant patients, just as in nonpregnant patients, is extensive and deserves careful evaluation. Because imaging tests are often avoided during pregnancy, there is often heavy reliance on the history, physical examination, and laboratory testing. Location and severity of pain are critical to evaluation. Diffuse pain can suggest intestinal obstruction; peritoneal inflammation from pancreatitis, appendicitis, or intra-abdominal abscess; or metabolic abnormalities such as uremia, porphyria, and diabetes. Upper abdominal pain can suggest biliary disease, PUD, or mediastinal pathology such as esophageal rupture, pneumonia, rib fracture, pulmonary embolism, Mallory-Weiss tear, esophageal stricture, and myocardial infarction. In addition, some diseases may present with epigastric pain or localize to the left side, such as PUD, splenic infarcts or abscess, splenic artery aneurysm (more common in pregnancy), gastric volvulus, and incarcerated paraesophageal hernia. Right upper quadrant pain can suggest hepatitis, hepatic vascular engorgement, hepatic hematoma, hepatic malignancy, preeclampsia, or HELLP syndrome. Biliary diseases such as biliary colic, choledocholithiasis, cholangitis, and cholecystitis may also present with epigastric discomfort or localize to the right side. Right lower quadrant pain can indicate appendicitis, ruptured Meckel diverticulum, CD, intussusception, bowel infection or perforation, or colon cancer. Left lower quadrant pain can indicate diverticulitis, sigmoid volvulus, colon cancer, bowel infection or perforation, IBD, and irritable bowel syndrome. Any lower abdominal discomfort can suggest gynecologic or obstetric causes such as ruptured ectopic pregnancy (severe pain), ovarian cyst rupture, pelvic inflammatory disease, tubo-ovarian abscess, uterine fibroids, impending abortion, adnexal mass, salpingitis, endometriosis, ruptured corpus luteum, or cervical or ovarian cancer. Nephrolithiasis and pyelonephritis can manifest right- or left-sided, upper or lower abdominal pain.

Vascular causes such as mesenteric ischemia and abdominal aortic aneurysm can cause diffuse or localized pain and should always be considered in the differential as they may present as medical or surgical emergencies. Spontaneous hepatic rupture is an abdominal emergency unique to pregnancy. It typically occurs late in pregnancy; is associated with subcapsular hematoma, preeclampsia, and HELLP syndrome; and presents with severe right-sided or epigastric pain, sometimes radiating to the right shoulder. It can be diagnosed with ultrasound, and when signs of rupture or expanding subcapsular hematoma are seen, the patient should undergo immediate cesarean delivery; intraoperative packing, hepatic resection, or hepatic artery ligation are often needed to control bleeding.

Clinical Findings

A. Symptoms and Signs

A careful history of pain onset, character, severity, and location is critical. Important signs on physical examination include the presence of fever, hypotension, and tachycardia; these findings should prompt a search for causes of abdominal infection or acute abdomen. Classic physical examination findings of peritonitis may be absent due to abdominal wall laxity in pregnancy; however, the presence of a rigid abdomen is a likely indicator of peritonitis.

B. Laboratory and Imaging Studies

Any patient presenting with significant abdominal pain should undergo laboratory tests, including complete blood count and differential, serum electrolytes, liver function tests, coagulation profile, and amylase and lipase levels. Physiologic changes in these values that occur normally during pregnancy, such as elevation in white blood cell count, anemia, elevated alkaline phosphate, elevated erythrocyte sedimentation rate, and mild hyponatremia, all should be kept in mind during evaluation.

Ultrasound is considered low risk and should be the imaging study of choice if needed. Abdominal radiographs are avoided if possible due to radiation exposure to the fetus, but may be indicated when bowel perforation or obstruction is suspected. MRI is preferable to CT scanning to avoid ionizing radiation, but gadolinium should be avoided during the first trimester if possible. Any radiologic testing should be preceded by counseling of the patient.

Treatment

Treatment is based on the disorder. Evaluation and treatment of common biliary and gastrointestinal problems in pregnancy are discussed in later sections of this chapter. Liver diseases of pregnancy are discussed in Chapter 8.

Capell MS, Friedel D. Abdominal pain during pregnancy. *Gastroenterol Clin North Am.* 2003;32:1–58. [PMID: 12635413]

PEPTIC ULCER DISEASE

There is no evidence to support an increased incidence of PUD during pregnancy, and in fact, many studies suggest a decreased incidence. Nevertheless, both gastric and duodenal ulcers do occur and detection is difficult, as avoidance of invasive testing is desirable during pregnancy.

Clinical Findings

A. Symptoms and Signs

The symptoms of PUD are the same in pregnant as in nonpregnant patients and include epigastric pain, abdominal distention, eructation, postprandial nausea and vomiting, anorexia, and rarely, hematemesis, melena, hematochezia, or peritonitis. Differentiating ulcer disease from other conditions that present with similar symptoms is an important part of evaluation. Nausea and vomiting associated with pregnancy are often most pronounced in the first trimester, whereas PUD worsens during the third trimester. The physical examination may reveal signs of complications from PUD; heme-positive stool or visible blood on rectal examination may suggest bleeding from an ulcer. Peritoneal signs should prompt surgical consultation for possible perforated ulcer.

B. Laboratory, Imaging, and Endoscopic Studies

Liver blood tests and an ultrasound scan should be obtained to evaluate for cholelithiasis, choledocholithiasis, viral hepatitis, AFLP, and HELLP syndrome. Right upper quadrant tenderness, a history of fatty food intolerance, fever, and leukocytosis can suggest cholecystitis, which can also be diagnosed by ultrasound. Pancreatitis can be suggested by pain that is exacerbated with eating, pain radiating to the back, a history of alcoholism, gallstones, prior pancreatitis, leukocytosis, and fever; amylase and lipase levels should be checked. An electrocardiogram should be obtained to exclude myocardial ischemia. Urinalysis and urine culture should also be obtained to exclude urinary tract infection.

Abdominal radiographs are avoided in pregnancy but should be obtained in suspected perforation. Barium studies are also avoided, but upper endoscopy should be performed when symptoms are severe and refractory to intensive medical therapy, when complications including hemorrhage and gastric outlet obstruction occur, or when gastric adenocarcinoma or lymphoma is suspected. The safety of endoscopy in pregnancy is discussed separately, later in this chapter.

Treatment

The symptoms of PUD are difficult to distinguish from GERD; however, the medical treatment for both is identical and should be attempted first unless indications for endoscopy, discussed earlier, are present. Medical treatment for suspected PUD and GERD includes antacids, sucralfate,

H_2-blockers, and if needed PPIs (see earlier discussion of treatment of GERD in pregnancy). Misoprostol is contraindicated in pregnancy. Triple-drug therapy for treatment of *H pylori* should be deferred if possible until after delivery due to the low risk of complications from PUD and possible fetal risk from antibiotics. Treatment of *H pylori* associated with mucosa-associated lymphoid tissue tumor is indicated, however, and should not be deferred. Amoxicillin (class B), metronidazole (class B), and clarithromycin (class C), can be used, although treatment during the first trimester should be avoided if possible. Both tetracycline and bismuth subsalicylate are relatively contraindicated during pregnancy.

Endoscopy is indicated in patients with gastrointestinal bleeding suspected to be from PUD. Very little is known about the risks of therapeutic endoscopic therapy for PUD or hemostasis for other disorders such as variceal bleeding or Mallory-Weiss tear. Therapeutic endoscopy is currently an experimental procedure during pregnancy but is justifiable when the only alternative is surgery. The indications for surgery for PUD are the same in pregnant as in nonpregnant patients and include uncontrollable hemorrhage, perforation, and gastric outlet obstruction.

Capell MS. Gastric and duodenal ulcers during pregnancy. *Gastroenterol Clin North Am.* 2003;32:263–308. [PMID: 12635419]

BILIARY DISEASE

Pregnancy predisposes to gallstone formation; increased bile lithogenicity mediated by estrogen and decreased gallbladder contractility mediated by progesterone are implicated in the causality. The incidence of cholelithiasis in pregnancy has been reported to be between 2.5% and 12.5%, but most patients with gallstones remain asymptomatic. Obesity, prepregnancy weight gain, Hispanic ethnicity, and maternal age are risk factors for gallstone disease during pregnancy.

Clinical Findings

A. Symptoms and Signs

Symptomatic patients may present with anorexia, nausea, vomiting, right upper quadrant or epigastric pain, and a history of symptoms exacerbated by fatty foods. The pain can radiate to the back or right shoulder. Although termed "biliary colic," severe pain from gallstones can last several hours. The presence of fever, tachycardia, leukocytosis, elevated neutrophil count, right upper quadrant tenderness, and Murphy sign may indicate the presence of cholecystitis.

B. Laboratory and Imaging Studies

Abnormal liver blood tests may indicate the presence of choledocholithiasis (keeping in mind physiologic elevation of alkaline phosphatase in pregnancy). Elevated amylase and lipase can indicate pancreatitis. A right upper quadrant ultrasound is safe in pregnancy and has a high degree of accuracy in detecting gallstones. The presence of sonographic Murphy sign, gallbladder wall thickening, pericholecystic fluid, or stranding can suggest cholecystitis. Common bile duct or intrahepatic duct dilation can suggest choledocholithiasis. The ultrasonographer should evaluate for liver and pancreatic disease as well.

Treatment

The management of gallstones in the absence of cholecystitis or choledocholithiasis is medical, including avoidance of fatty foods and a brief period of bowel rest and pain control if needed. For patients who do not respond to medical therapy or who develop recurrent symptoms, early operative management is advocated as there is a high rate of recurrence and risk of complications during pregnancy.

When cholecystitis is present, intravenous antibiotics should be started. Intravenous cefazolin and extended-spectrum penicillin are effective and generally considered safe in pregnancy. Because of the risk of fetal loss, teratogenesis, and preterm labor during the first trimester, and the risk of preterm labor, premature delivery, and technical difficulties due to the gravid uterus during the third trimester, surgery is often delayed until the second trimester or after delivery if possible. Recent improvements in less-invasive surgical techniques may lead to improved surgical outcomes. One study showed an overall benefit of medical versus surgical management of cholelithiasis during pregnancy, and another showed no significant increase in major birth defects in patients who underwent surgery during the first trimester.

Gallstone pancreatitis, choledocholithiasis, or acute cholecystitis that fails to resolve is an indication for early surgery. Typically, laparoscopic surgery is performed during the first two trimesters, but open procedures are often required in the third trimester.

Routine intraoperative cholangiography is not recommended during pregnancy; however, bile duct exploration and intraoperative ultrasound are alternatives. Successful laparoscopic common bile duct exploration during acute gallstone pancreatitis has been reported in a patient who was 14 weeks pregnant. If needed, cholangiography can be done with a fetal shield to minimize radiation.

Choledocholithiasis is rare in pregnancy, but endoscopic retrograde cholangiopancreatography (ERCP) with stone extraction, sphincterotomy, or stent insertion can all be performed and is indicated for common bile duct stones and cholangitis.

Bagci S, Tuzun A, Erdil A, et al. Treatment of choledocholithiasis in pregnancy: a case report. *Arch Gynecol Obstet.* 2003;267: 239–241. [PMID: 12592428]

Ko CW. Risk factors for gallstone-related hospitalization during pregnancy and the postpartum. *Am J Gastroenterol.* 2006;101:2263–2268. [PMID: 17032191]

Ko CW, Beresford SA, Schulte SJ, et al. Incidence, natural history, and risk factors for biliary sludge and stones during pregnancy. *Hepatology.* 2005;41:359–365. [PMID: 15660385]

Lu EJ, Curet MJ, El-Sayed YY, et al. Medical versus surgical management of biliary tract disease in pregnancy. *Am J Surg.* 2004;188:755–759. [PMID: 15619495]

Tarnasky PR, Simmons DC, Schwartz AG, et al. Safe delivery of bile duct stones during pregnancy. *Am J Gastroenterol.* 2003;98:2100–2101. [PMID: 14499796]

PANCREATITIS

Acute pancreatitis can complicate up to 1% of pregnancies and is most common during the third trimester and postpartum. Gallstones are the cause in the vast majority of pregnant patients with pancreatitis; however, the typical differential diagnosis of pregnancy still applies, and alcoholism, hypercalcemia, hypertriglyceridemia, infections, trauma, and medication-induced causes should be ruled out.

Clinical Findings

Clinical presentation and elevated amylase and lipase levels are typically diagnostic, as pancreatic enzyme levels are not affected by pregnancy. Ultrasound can diagnose gallstones and choledocholithiasis (bile duct dilation) and can also sometimes visualize pancreatic inflammation. CT scan is reserved for severe, refractory pancreatitis to evaluate for areas of pancreatitis necrosis, and MRI may be a safer alternative during pregnancy.

Treatment

Medical management includes stopping oral intake, aggressive intravenous fluids, histamine blockers, and PPI. Laboratory values such as calcium, blood urea nitrogen, creatinine, white blood cell count, and hematocrit should be monitored carefully (see Chapter 25). Meperidine is typically chosen for pain control and is a category B drug; it appears to be safe for use in pregnancy. For severe pancreatitis, surgical debridement or endoscopic or percutaneous drainage of abscesses or pseudocysts should not be delayed. Severe pancreatitis may in rare cases require antibiotics and parenteral nutrition. Although endoscopic procedures and tests involving radiation are generally avoided during pregnancy, one study noted a significant relapse rate in patients with gallstone pancreatitis. These findings argue for ERCP, cholecystectomy, or both. Currently, acute gallstone pancreatitis complicated by evidence of persistent biliary obstruction is one of the indications for ERCP with sphincterotomy during all stages of pregnancy. Cholecystectomy is often deferred until the second trimester or postpartum period. Pancreatitis is associated with fetal wastage in the first trimester and premature labor in the third trimester. Maternal mortality can be as high as 10% in severe, complicated pancreatitis but is low if pancreatitis improves quickly with medical management.

Kim YW, Zagorski SM, Chung MH. Laparoscopic common bile duct exploration in pregnancy with acute gallstone pancreatitis. *JSLS.* 2006;10:78–82. [PMID: 16709365]

APPENDICITIS

Acute appendicitis is the most common gastrointestinal disorder requiring surgery during pregnancy. The key to management is prompt diagnosis.

Clinical Findings

A. Symptoms and Signs

Patients typically present with anorexia, nausea, vomiting, and abdominal pain; however, in pregnancy, this presentation needs to be distinguished from conditions such as nausea and vomiting of pregnancy, particularly in the first trimester. Abdominal pain associated with appendicitis can be located in nontraditional places. During the first trimester, the appendix has the usual right lower quadrant location, and patients typically present with periumbilical pain that migrates to the right lower quadrant. During the second and third trimesters, however, the appendix gradually moves upward and laterally until by the third trimester, it is located in the right upper quadrant (Figure 7–3). This changes the presentation of appendicitis and can delay diagnosis and management. Fever, tachycardia, abdominal tenderness, and peritoneal signs can be clues to an inflamed appendix, but their absence does not rule out appendicitis.

B. Laboratory and Imaging Studies

Although pregnancy can elevate the white blood cell count, a finding of more than 80% neutrophils on the differential is suggestive of an acute disorder. Abdominal ultrasound can be diagnostic during the first trimester but less helpful when the appendix migrates. Abdominal CT scan can be used to diagnose appendicitis; however, this exposes the fetus to radiation teratogenicity. Diagnostic laparoscopy can also be performed if there is diagnostic uncertainty. If there is any suspicion of appendicitis, surgical consultation should be obtained immediately.

Treatment

Once appendicitis is diagnosed, either clinically or by imaging, immediate surgery is indicated, as appendiceal perforation can increase maternal mortality to as high as 4% and

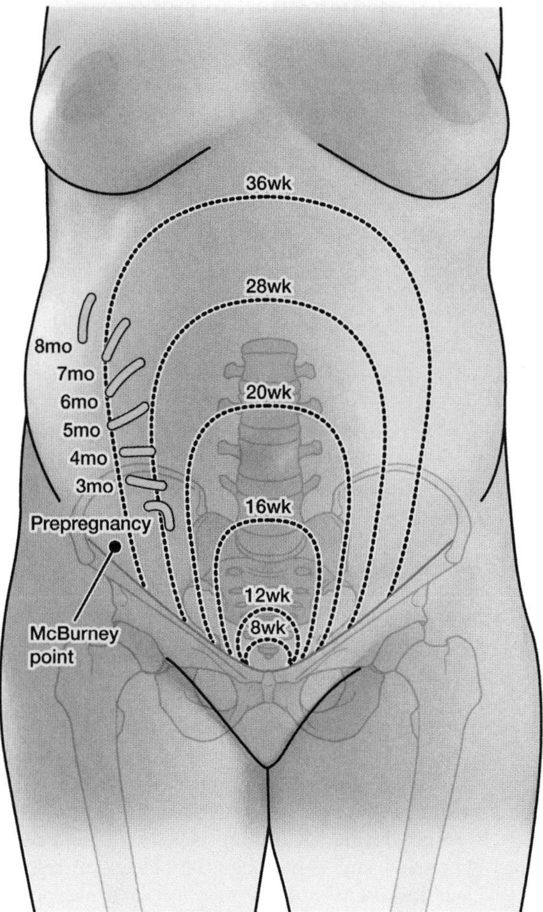

▲ **Figure 7–3.** Changes in location and direction of the appendix during pregnancy in relationship to the McBurney point and the height of the fundus at various weeks of gestation.

fetal mortality to as high as 20%. The only exception to this is in the setting of active labor, in which case it is undertaken after vaginal or cesarean delivery if labor is prolonged. In the first two trimesters, laparoscopic appendectomy can be done safely; however, in the third trimester or in the setting of diffuse peritonitis, laparotomy is generally indicated. Fetal complications are similar between laparoscopic and open approaches.

Carver TW, Antevil J, Egan JC, et al. Appendectomy during early pregnancy: what is the preferred surgical approach? *Am Surg.* 2005;71:809–812. [PMID: 16468524]

Palanivelu C, Rangarajan M, Parthasarathi R. Laparoscopic appendectomy in pregnancy: a case series of seven patients. *JSLS.* 2006;10:321–325. [PMID: 17212888]

INTESTINAL OBSTRUCTION, PSEUDO-OBSTRUCTION, & GASTROINTESTINAL CANCER

Although the most common cause of intestinal obstruction in pregnancy is adhesions, another important cause is volvulus, which accounts for more than 20% of cases. Most cases of volvulus during pregnancy occur near term, presumably because the gravid uterus can push a redundant colon out of the pelvis to twist around a point of fixation. Other causes of intestinal obstruction include intussusception, hernia, acute appendicitis, and gastric and colorectal cancer. Incarcerated diaphragmatic hernias are rare but more common during pregnancy and have a high rate of complications.

Clinical Findings

Prompt recognition and treatment of obstruction and pseudo-obstruction are critical. Sigmoid volvulus during pregnancy is associated with high maternal and fetal mortality even with appropriate intervention. Patients present with constipation, progressive abdominal pain, and abdominal distention. Later on, bilious vomiting and obstipation can be present. Abdominal radiographs and CT scans may be required for evaluation and are typically diagnostic of this condition. Flexible sigmoidoscopy or colonoscopy may be required for diagnosis or decompression. Pseudo-obstruction or colonic distention without obstruction can occur following delivery; symptoms are similar to those of intestinal obstruction. Pseudo-obstruction is typically diagnosed with abdominal radiographs. Colon and gastric cancer are the most common gastrointestinal malignancies during pregnancy and can cause bleeding, anemia, abdominal pain, or obstruction.

Treatment

Conservative management includes nasogastric decompression, fluid resuscitation, monitoring of electrolytes, bowel rest, and careful use of analgesia. Prophylactic antibiotics should be considered. Pseudo-obstruction and some cases of volvulus or adhesion-induced small bowel obstruction will resolve with conservative management. Suspected intestinal ischemia, perforation, persistent tachycardia, fever, abdominal tenderness, and failure to resolve with conservative management are indications for surgery.

Patients with postpartum pseudo-obstruction should be followed radiographically if required. A colonic diameter greater than 10–12 cm increases the risk of colonic perforation. Neostigmine or colonic decompression can be performed for pseudo-obstruction if required to avoid surgery.

Volvulus during pregnancy may be treated by decompression with colonoscopy, flexible sigmoidoscopy, or rectal tube; however, surgery may be required if the condition is recurrent or persistent. Hernias frequently require surgical repair, and an incidental incarcerated diaphragmatic hernia should be repaired during surgery due to risk of strangulation.

Mortality can be high for volvulus or intestinal ischemia, and preterm delivery is common in patients who require surgery.

Patients with gastrointestinal cancer diagnosed during pregnancy should undergo colonoscopy for biopsy and for evaluation of synchronous lesions. Resections can be performed during the first half of pregnancy but are often deferred until after delivery. There is no contraindication to vaginal delivery as long as the birth canal is not obstructed. All options should be discussed with the patient. Chemotherapy is typically delayed until the second trimester, and pelvic radiation is often delayed until after delivery to protect the fetus. Maternal outcome in colorectal cancer diagnosed during pregnancy is similar to that of the general population; however, pregnant women with gastric cancer often present with advanced disease and have a worse survival rate than nonpregnant women.

Lal SK, Morgenstern R, Vinjirayer EP, et al. Sigmoid volvulus an update. *Gastrointest Endoscopy Clin N Am.* 2006;16:175–187. [PMID: 16546032]

ENDOSCOPY IN PREGNANCY

Although endoscopy is routine in the evaluation of many gastrointestinal disorders, it is typically only performed when absolutely needed in pregnancy due to the risk to the fetus of sedative medications, particularly in the first trimester, and technical complexity during the third trimester. The risks of sedative medications include overdosage, allergic reaction, teratogenesis, and hemodynamic instability of the mother leading to hypoxia and hypotension of the fetus.

In general, maternal hypotension should be avoided as much as possible; patients with gastrointestinal bleeding should be resuscitated with packed erythrocytes and fluid as needed before the procedure. Antihypertensives prior to the procedure and colonic overdistention during the procedure should be avoided. Patients should not be placed or moved to the supine position (because the gravid uterus compresses the vena cava and can lead to hypotension), and sedative medications should be used judiciously but sparingly. If hypotension occurs during the procedure, intravenous fluids should be used and the patient's position should be changed to drain blood from the lower extremities to the vital organs. Consideration should be given to terminating the procedure.

Premature uterine contractions during endoscopy may require tocolytics such as magnesium sulfate or terbutaline. Consultation with an obstetrician is important, and anesthesiologic assistance with the procedure should always be considered, particularly in the first trimester, during a high-risk pregnancy, in the presence of maternal or fetal instability, or for a prolonged procedure such as ERCP. The risks of medications used during endoscopy and considerations relating to specific procedures are outlined below.

1. Medications Used During Endoscopy (Table 7–6)

A. Meperidine

Meperidine is generally a category B drug in pregnancy; it has a rating of D when used in high doses and for a prolonged period of time at term. Although it is rapidly transferred across the placenta, it has been used extensively in pregnancy and, with the exception of one study that noted a higher rate of congenital inguinal hernias, teratogenicity has not been observed even with exposure during the first trimester. The drug can cause diminished fetal beat-to-beat cardiac variability that can last 1 hour after administration; however, this is generally transient and not considered a poor prognostic sign. It is preferred over benzodiazepines for endoscopic procedures and is approved by the American Academy of Pediatrics in single dose administration for breast-feeding women. Dosage should be restricted to 50 or 75 mg intravenously during routine endoscopy.

B. Diazepam and Midazolam

Diazepam is categorized as a class D drug during pregnancy due to earlier studies suggesting an association between use during pregnancy and cleft palates in animals and humans, as well as other congenital malformations and neonatal neurobehavioral abnormalities. Recent data suggest, however, that it may be safer than previously appreciated when administered at low doses for a brief period of time.

Less is known about the effects of midazolam exposure in utero. Exposure during parturition suggests transient respiratory depression and abnormal neurobehavioral responsiveness, but little is known about the effects of fetal exposure during the first or second trimester. Because of its similarity to diazepam, midazolam is classified as category D during pregnancy; in general, however, it is preferable to diazepam if one of these agents is required during endoscopy.

C. Propofol

Propofol is used by anesthesiologists and some gastroenterologists for sedation during endoscopy. The advantages include a greater depth of sedation, quicker onset, and shorter duration of action than the benzodiazepines. Propofol is also a pregnancy category B drug; it is considered safe for use during parturition, but at this time, there is inadequate experience to recommend its use during the first trimester.

D. Fentanyl

Fentanyl is a pregnancy category C drug. Studies in rats showed injury to embryos, but some human studies of use during labor found no evidence of neonatal toxicity. It is used in low doses for endoscopy during pregnancy despite some case reports describing respiratory depression and muscle rigidity in neonates. Frequent use has been associated with neonatal withdrawal in a mother with opiate addiction.

Table 7–6. Medications used for endoscopy.

Drug	FDA Pregnancy Category	Recommendations for Pregnancy	Recommendations for Breast-Feeding
Ampicillin	B	Low risk to use when prophylaxis required	Compatible
Diatrizoate	D	Minimal use for therapeutic ERCP	Limited human data: probably compatible
Diazepam	D	Midazolam preferred benzodiazepine	Limited human data: potential toxicity
Electricity	—	Use for therapeutic ERCP	No human data
Epinephrine	C	Avoid unless for hemostasis	No human data: potential toxicity
Fentanyl	C	Use in low doses	Compatible
Flumazenil	C	Only for significant benzodiazepine overdose	No human data: probably compatible
Gentamicin	C	Short courses low risk, check serum levels if used for >48 h	Compatible
Glucagon	B	Avoid except for ERCP	No human data
Lidocaine	B	Gargle and spit	Limited human data: probably compatible
Meperidine	B	Use in low doses	Compatible
Midazolam	D	Use in low doses	Limited human data: potential toxicity
Naloxone	B	Only for severe narcotic overdoses	No human data: probably compatible
PEG electrolyte	C	No human studies available	Probably low risk
Propofol	B	Avoid in first trimester	Limited human data: probably compatible
Simethicone	C	Can be avoided, but low risk	No human data: probably compatible
Sodium glycol electrolyte	C	Low risk one-time use	No human data

ERCP, endoscopic retrograde cholangiopancreatography; PEG, polyethylene glycol.
Reproduced, with permission, from Mahadevan U, Kane S. American Gastroenterological Association Institute technical review on the use of gastrointestinal medications in pregnancy. *Gastroenterology*. 2006;131:283–311.

E. Ketamine

Ketamine is used by anesthesiologists during endoscopy because of its rapid action of onset, short duration of effects, and ability to sedate people who experience insufficient sedation from propofol. Ketamine has been used during labor and delivery, and although some neonatal respiratory depression may occur, it is often less than that of other sedatives. It has not been associated with teratogenicity and is classified as pregnancy category B; however, it is relatively unstudied during the first trimester.

F. Reversal Agents

Naloxone is an opioid reversal agent with a pregnancy category B designation. It is appropriate for administration in pregnant patients with signs of narcotic toxicity from sedation, such as respiratory depression, hypotension, or unresponsiveness. It should not be used in patients who are opiate dependent, however, due to the risk of maternal and fetal withdrawal. Naloxone should be used only when necessary and carefully; overdose can cause maternal myocardial infarction, pulmonary edema, or severe hypertension.

Flumazenil is a benzodiazepine reversal agent and a pregnancy category C drug because little is known about fetal risk. Overdose can cause maternal seizures and maternal and neonatal withdrawal, especially in patients who chronically use benzodiazepines. It should be used only if absolutely needed for benzodiazepine toxicity. There are no data regarding either reversal agent during breast-feeding.

G. Lidocaine

Lidocaine is classed as a pregnancy category B drug based on studies showing no harm in rats and safety during parturition and appears safe for use as a numbing agent for the oropharynx during upper endoscopy. It is recommended that the patient gargle and spit it out rather than swallow it to minimize systemic absorption.

H. Simethicone

Simethicone is used to coalesce gastric bubbles during endoscopy and is a pregnancy category C drug. When used during endoscopy, however, it is unlikely to be absorbed and therefore unlikely to be a risk during either pregnancy or breast-feeding.

I. Glucagon

Glucagon is a pregnancy category B drug. Although there is no evidence of harm in rats, it is uncharacterized in pregnant humans. The American Gastroenterological Association supports its use in decreasing motility in endoscopy with the goal of decreasing procedure time, particularly during therapeutic ERCP.

J. Contrast Agents

Diatrizoate contrast is used during ERCP and is classified as pregnancy category D because of the risk to fetal thyroid function during amniography. However, it has been used in diagnostic and therapeutic endoscopy without fetal harm and in the setting of maternal cholangitis, the benefits likely outweigh the risks.

Briggs GG, Freeman RY, Yaffe SJ. *Drugs in Pregnancy and Lactation: A Reference Guide to Fetal and Neonatal Risk,* 7th ed. Lippincott Williams & Wilkins, 2005.

Cappell MS. Sedation and analgesia for gastrointestinal endoscopy during pregnancy. *Gastrointest Endosc Clin N Am.* 2006;16:1–31. [PMID: 16546020]

Hawkins JL. Obstetric anesthesia and analgesia. In: Scott JR, Gibbs RS, Karlan BY, et al (editors). *Danforth's Obstetrics and Gynecology,* 9th ed. Lippincott Williams & Wilkins, 2003:57–73.

Mahadevan U, Kane S. American Gastroenterological Association Institute position statement on the use of gastrointestinal medications in pregnancy. *Gastroenterology.* 2006;131:278–282. [PMID: 17261292]

Mahadevan U, Kane S. American Gastroenterological Association Institute technical review on the use of gastrointestinal medications in pregnancy. *Gastroenterology.* 2006;131:283–311. [PMID: 16831610]

2. Endoscopic Retrograde Cholangiopancreatography (ERCP)

Choledocholithiasis occurs in one out of every 1200 deliveries and is the most common indication for ERCP during pregnancy. Other indications for ERCP include severe acute gallstone pancreatitis, cholangitis, bile duct injury, and pancreatic duct disruption. To minimize risk in pregnancy, less-invasive testing should be considered to confirm the presence of gallstones in the bile duct in the setting of choledocholithiasis, cholangitis, and gallstone pancreatitis. Endoscopic ultrasound has been used with high diagnostic accuracy to confirm or exclude choledocholithiasis. There are a few reports of the use of ultrasound-guided or endoscopic needle-knife papillotomy for choledocholithiasis without exposure to fluoroscopy. One group has described the use of magnetic resonance cholangiopancreatography (MRCP) in a pregnant patient to demonstrate a stone in a dilated common bile duct. There were no adverse outcomes; however, the safety of MRI, especially in the first trimester, has not been rigorously tested.

The predominant concern with ERCP is the effect of radiation, a known teratogen, on the health of the fetus. Nineteen case and clinical series have been published on use of ERCP during pregnancy. Fetal and maternal outcome data were available for a total of 164 ERCP procedures, and the overall complication rate of 8.5% mainly involved pancreatitis and postsphincterotomy bleeding. Most cases involved sphincterotomy or stent placement, or both, to prevent future recurrence. Eighty-nine percent of these pregnancies resulted in the birth of healthy term infants. Six percent of births were premature, and there were three spontaneous abortions. Two infants had intrauterine growth restriction.

The second trimester is felt to be the safest time to perform ERCP; however, often the need arises during the first or third trimester. Although a growing body of data supports the safety of ERCP during pregnancy, precautions to minimize radiation risk to the fetus should be taken, particularly during the first trimester. One group has reported a case series of six pregnant patients who underwent ERCP and bile duct cannulation without fluoroscopy. The common bile duct was cannulated and a guidewire advanced approximately 10–15 cm into the bile duct under endoscopic view. The catheter was then advanced over the wire and bile aspirated to confirm placement, after which sphincterotomy with balloon stone extraction was performed. This method, if technically possible, minimizes exposure to radiation. Some authors also advocate using a lead apron to protect the entire abdomen from radiation until cannulation, during which time the apron can be repositioned to expose the necessary area. The patient should be in the left lateral recumbent position, facilitating both the procedure and blood flow to the fetus. The grounding pad should be placed so that the uterus is not between the pad and the sphincterotome. If antibiotics are required, penicillins or cephalosporins are preferred. Clindamycin is generally safe in patients with allergies to penicillin. Tetracycline, quinolones, and streptomycin should be avoided. Metronidazole should be avoided during the first trimester, and sulfonamides and nitrofurantoin should be avoided in the third trimester.

There are a few case reports of endoscopic cystogastrostomy for pseudocysts; if drainage is required, endoscopic methods may be safer than the alternative surgical or percutaneous techniques that expose the patient to risks of surgery and radiation from imaging studies, respectively.

Kahaleh M, Hartwell GD, Arseneau KO, et al. Safety and efficacy of ERCP in pregnancy. *Gastrointest Endosc.* 2004;60:287–292. [PMID: 15278066]

Menees S, Elta G. Endoscopic retrograde cholangiopancreatography during pregnancy. *Gastrointest Endosc Clin N Am.* 2006;16:41–57. [PMID: 16546022]

Simmons DC, Tarnasky PR, Rivera-Alsina ME, et al. Endoscopic retrograde cholangiopancreatography in pregnancy without the use of radiation. *Am J Obstet Gynecol.* 2004;190:1467–1469. [PMID: 15167871]

Tham TC, Vandervoort J, Wong RC, et al. Safety of ERCP during pregnancy. *Am J Gastroenterol.* 2003;98:308–311. [PMID: 12591046]

3. Esophagogastroduodenoscopy (EGD)

The most common indications for upper endoscopy during pregnancy include upper gastrointestinal bleeding, particularly to rule out variceal bleeding or PUD, and severe dyspepsia or epigastric comfort to rule out PUD. Severe hyperemesis that is unresponsive to management and odynophagia or dysphagia are other possible indications. Recent studies have not demonstrated an increase in complications in pregnant patients who have undergone EGD. Informed consent should still involve a discussion of possible fetal risks related to sedation and the procedure. An obstetrician should be involved to determine if fetal monitoring is needed. The American Society for Gastrointestinal Endoscopy (ASGE) also recommends that patients not lie in the supine position during recovery due to the risk of inferior vena cava compression. During the procedure the patient should be placed in the left lateral position with the head elevated due to an increased risk of regurgitation of gastric contents in pregnant patients. Aspiration should be avoided by aggressive perioral suctioning, elevation of the head of the patient, nasogastric aspiration in patients with upper gastrointestinal bleeding before EGD, and aspiration of the gastric lake during the procedure. For patients with gastrointestinal bleeding, resuscitation should be performed before the procedure to the extent possible.

Bruno JM, Kroser J. Efficacy and safety of upper endoscopy procedures during pregnancy. *Gastrointest Endosc Clin N Am.* 2006;16:33–40. [PMID: 16546021]

Qureshi WA, Rajan E, Adler DG, et al. ASGE guideline: guidelines for endoscopy in pregnant and lactating women. *Gastrointest Endosc.* 2005;61:357–362. [PMID: 17212888]

4. Flexible Sigmoidoscopy & Colonoscopy

The most common symptom leading to the use of lower endoscopy during pregnancy is hematochezia. Severe diarrhea, abdominal pain, colonoscopic decompression of volvulus, and evaluation of a mass lesion are other possible indications. Another indication for lower endoscopy during pregnancy is incarceration of the gravid uterus; in this condition, the uterus becomes lodged beneath the inferior margin of the sacral promontory. One report has described five patients who underwent successful colonoscopic release by intubating the sigmoid colon to apply pressure to the anterior wall of the rectum after manual reduction had failed. No adverse fetal outcomes were observed, and the alternative would have been surgery, which carries a much higher risk.

The safety of flexible sigmoidoscopy has been demonstrated in multiple case reports and studies. Flexible sigmoidoscopy has been performed without adverse outcome in all three trimesters of pregnancy. Most procedures are done with minimal bowel preparation (tap-water enemas) and without sedation to minimize adverse effects. Although hemodynamic monitoring of the mother should always be a part of the procedure, most reported cases did not involve any fetal monitoring, though this may be considered, especially in cases of maternal hemodynamic instability.

Colonoscopy is rarely indicated during pregnancy and less is known about the safety of this procedure. If required, the second trimester is generally considered the safest time to perform colonoscopy during pregnancy. The theoretical risks of colonoscopy include premature labor, uterine rupture, placental abruption, and fetal compression. Most data come from case reports, case series, and retrospective studies, which have not shown adverse fetal effects from the procedure performed during any trimester. The use of colonoscopy should be restricted to strong indications or life-threatening emergencies. Patients should be placed in the left or right lateral decubitus position, minimal external compression away from the uterus should be used, and maternal and fetal monitoring should be utilized. Trauma to the uterus from compression or colonoscope looping should be avoided.

In regard to bowel preparation, the risk of polyethylene glycol, a category C drug in pregnancy, is not known, although one study indicated safety when used to treat constipation. There is one report of repeated use of phosphate enemas in combination with phosphate solution leading to neonatal bone demineralization. One-time use of sodium phosphate enemas has been done safely in pregnancy, although this has not been studied. In general, phosphate solutions are associated with electrolyte shifts, and the effect of these shifts on the fetus is unknown.

Siddiqui U, Proctor DD. Flexible sigmoidoscopy and colonoscopy during pregnancy. *Gastrointest Endosc Clin N Am.* 2006;16: 59–69. [PMID: 16546023]

5. Gastrointestinal Bleeding & Endoscopic Therapy

There are very few data on the risks related to endoscopic therapy in pregnancy. Because endoscopy is often performed for the indication of gastrointestinal bleeding, endoscopic hemostasis may be required to maintain hemodynamic stability of the mother and fetus and to avoid the greater risks of persistent bleeding or surgery. No adverse events related to the use of thermocoagulation in pregnancy have been reported in case reports and small studies; however, electric current can cross the amniotic fluid, and the risk of fetal exposure remains. The ASGE recommends that bipolar cautery should be used rather than monopolar to reduce the risk of fetal exposure to stray current. The patient should be positioned so that the uterus is not between the electrical catheter and the grounding pad.

Epinephrine is a category C drug during pregnancy because of the theoretical risk of decreasing placental perfusion. Although no adverse outcomes have been reported in pregnancy when used during endoscopy, the drug should be used sparingly, to avoid systemic effects on both the mother and the fetus. Hemoclips have not been studied but may be safer than methods that involve injection of substances or electric current.

In the case of lower endoscopy, lesions such as polyps may be identified. If there is no urgent need to remove or biopsy the lesion, many endoscopists will defer intervention until after delivery to avoid exposure to bleeding risks or risks of electrocautery. In these situations, tattooing the lesion can be considered; India ink is generally felt to be safe in nonpregnant patients, although there are no existing studies examining its use in pregnant patients. Methylene blue is labeled as a teratogen and should be avoided during pregnancy.

Patients with cirrhosis and portal hypertension are at increased risk for variceal bleeding during pregnancy due to physiologic rises in portal pressure and increased volume in the splanchnic vessels during pregnancy. Variceal bleeding is associated with poor fetal outcomes, and effective hemostasis is critical. Case reports of esophageal banding and sclerotherapy have shown effectiveness in controlling variceal hemorrhage without any reports of fetal harm. Because there is a theoretical risk of the sclerosant entering the fetal circulation, many authors recommend banding as the preferred method, and some suggest that it may be more effective. Somatostatin and octreotide have not been studied in pregnancy but are thought to be relatively safe. Vasopressin is not recommended due to the risk of placental ischemia. Additionally, a reported series of cases has described the control of gastric varices with cyanoacrylate glue during pregnancy.

6. Alternatives to Diagnostic Endoscopic Procedures

Upper gastrointestinal series, barium enemas, abdominal radiographs, angiography, and CT are generally avoided in pregnancy due to radiation teratogenicity. Bleeding scans are also contraindicated due to ionizing radiation. MRI, on the other hand, is believed to be safer in pregnancy than CT scans; short-term exposure to electromagnetic radiation from MRI does not appear to produce harmful fetal effects. MRCP may be an alternative to diagnostic ERCP during pregnancy.

Video capsule endoscopy may be a useful alternative or adjunct to endoscopy during pregnancy as it does not require sedation and does not exert mechanical pressure on the uterus. Theoretically the gravid uterus and effect of pregnancy on motility may retard the passage of the capsule, but these factors should not predispose to retention in the absence of strictures or bowel obstruction. On the other hand, radiographs to confirm passage, and surgery in the event of retention, would involve risks to the mother and the fetus. The safety of this method has not been evaluated in pregnancy, but it is theoretically promising as a less-invasive diagnostic approach to luminal disease.

Kanal E, Borgstede JP, Barkovich AJ, et al. American College of Radiology white paper on MR safety. *AJR*. 2002;178:1135–1147. [PMID: 15100103]

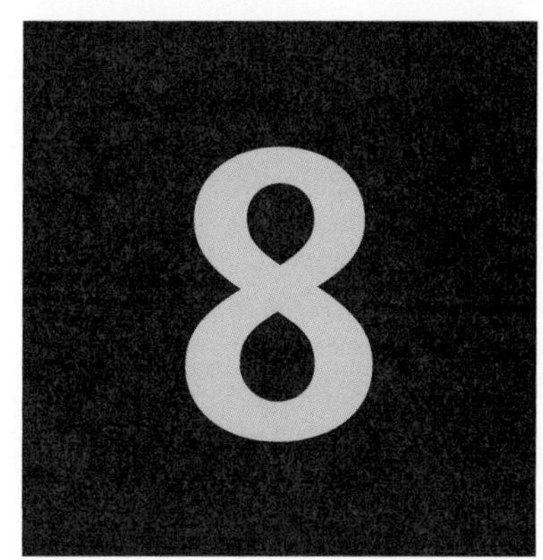

Hepatic Complications of Pregnancy

Chinweike Ukomadu, MD, PhD

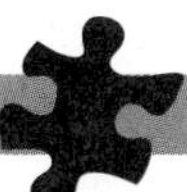

ESSENTIAL CONCEPTS

- Most liver biochemical tests are unchanged during pregnancy.
- Exceptions are albumin, total protein, and bilirubin (decreased) and alkaline phosphatase and cholesterol (increased).
- Several conditions unique to pregnancy may lead to hepatic impairment:
  - Hyperemesis gravidarum, often in the first trimester, invariably before the 20th week of pregnancy.
  - Intrahepatic cholestasis of pregnancy (IHCP), often in the third trimester (pruritus and mild liver tests abnormalities).
  - Acute fatty liver disease of pregnancy (AFLP) in the third trimester (nausea and vomiting, jaundice, and oliguria; typically mild increase in transaminases, hyperbilirubinemia, coagulopathy, thrombocytopenia, and hypoglycemia).
  - Preeclampsia (classic triad of hypertension, proteinuria, and edema) and eclampsia (preeclamptic triad plus seizures and coma) in the second or third trimester.
  - HELLP syndrome (hemolysis, elevated liver enzymes, and low platelets), between the start of the third trimester and the immediate postpartum period, often manifesting with right upper quadrant pain, edema, and hypertension.

General Considerations

Various hepatic conditions may occur in pregnancy, and the interpretation of common liver biochemical tests in women who are pregnant can sometimes be challenging. Among the specific conditions unique to pregnancy that may manifest with altered liver tests are hyperemesis gravidarum, IHCP, AFLP, preeclampsia/eclampsia, and HELLP syndrome. Other common hepatic conditions, such as viral hepatitis and cirrhosis, are not unique to but can manifest during pregnancy.

Guntupalli SR, Steingrub J. Hepatic disease and pregnancy: an overview of diagnosis and management. *Crit Care Med.* 2005; 33:S332–S339. [PMID: 16215356]

Hay JE. Liver disease in pregnancy. *Hepatology.* 2008;47:1067–1076. [PMID: 18265410]

INTERPRETATION OF LIVER BIOCHEMICAL TESTS DURING PREGNANCY (TABLE 8–1)

The pregnant state is accompanied by a 30–50% increase in blood volume. As a result, several biochemical tests have reduced values during pregnancy. These include albumin, total protein, and bilirubin.

The most significant change is noted during the second trimester. The alkaline phosphatase level is elevated because of the presence of placental-derived alkaline phosphatase. The biliary-derived alkaline phosphatase stays within the normal range as illustrated by normal levels of γ-glutamyl transpeptidase (GGT) and 5′-nucleotidase (5′ NT). Cholesterol also increases to approximately twice its prepregnancy level. Lastly, the hepatic markers of inflammation, alanine aminotransferase (ALT) and aspartate aminotransferase (AST), are unchanged.

Pathologic conditions that result in abnormal biochemical tests during pregnancy tend to be divided into three broad categories: (1) those that lead to a mild increase in transaminases, (2) those that lead to marked increase in transaminases, and (3) those that result in predominantly cholestatic biochemical abnormalities. Conditions that lead to mild increase in transaminases include AFLP, preeclampsia, eclampsia, HELLP syndrome, Budd-Chiari syndrome, IHCP, drug-induced hepatitis, and chronic liver diseases. Those that result in

Table 8–1. Liver biochemical test findings in pregnancy.

Biochemical Test	Value During Pregnancy
Albumin	Decreased
Total protein	Decreased
Bilirubin	Decreased
Alkaline phosphatase	Increased
ALT	Normal
AST	Normal
GGT	Normal
5′ NT	Normal
Cholesterol	Increased

ALT, alanine aminotransferase; AST, aspartate aminotransferase; GGT, γ-glutamyl transpeptidase; 5′ NT, 5′-nucleotidase.

marked increase in ALT and AST also include preeclampsia and eclampsia, especially in the setting of hepatic infarct, Budd-Chiari syndrome with portal vein thrombosis, hepatic rupture, acute viral hepatitis, drug-induced hepatitis, and hepatic shock. Lastly, conditions that result predominantly in cholestasis include IHCP, choledocholithiasis, or drug-induced cholestatic conditions.

HEPATIC CONDITIONS UNIQUE TO PREGNANCY (TABLE 8–2)

1. Hyperemesis Gravidarum

This disorder produces occasional severe and intractable nausea and vomiting. It begins characteristically in the first trimester but can last late into pregnancy. Liver biochemical abnormalities, specifically elevations in aminotransferases and bilirubin, are seen in more than 50% of patients hospitalized as a result of hyperemesis gravidarum. The level of aminotransferase elevation is on average two to three times the upper limit of normal, but occasional reports of transaminase elevations of greater than 1000 IU exist in the literature.

The cause of hepatic dysfunction in hyperemesis gravidarum is unknown, and in the few well-documented instances, results of liver biopsies have been normal. Regardless, the consequences of hypovolemia, ketosis, and malnutrition likely contribute to observed biochemical abnormalities.

Treatment is symptom management-based with intravenous hydration and antiemetic therapy. In the most severe cases, parenteral feeding may be necessary.

2. Intrahepatic Cholestasis of Pregnancy

IHCP is a rare disease in the United States, occurring in less than 0.1% of all pregnancies. The highest incidence is in Chile, where approximately 12–22% of all pregnancies are affected. The disease is very rare among African Americans. The major risk factors for IHCP include multiparity, advanced maternal age, family history of IHCP, and pruritus while on oral contraceptive medicines.

The molecular basis of IHCP remains unclear, but a mutation in the gene for multidrug resistance protein 3 (*MDR3*) has been implicated as a potential cause in two families. However, a study of Finnish patients with IHCP did not reveal linkage with *MDR3* or for other cholestatic genes, specifically the bile salt export pump (*BSEP*) and familial intrahepatic cholestasis type 1 (*FIC1*).

Patients with IHCP present with cholestasis in the third trimester of pregnancy. Pruritus occurs in 80% of patients; it usually begins peripherally and then progresses centrally. In approximately 20% of patients with pruritus, jaundice may occur. The diagnosis is often made by clinical history, although laboratory abnormalities, especially mild ALT, AST, and alkaline phosphate elevations, may occur. Serum levels of bile acids are elevated 30–100 times the upper limit of normal.

Control of pruritus is important for maternal comfort, and ursodiol and cholestyramine are the first agents of choice. Studies have demonstrated the efficacy of ursodiol in control of pruritus, improvement of biochemical parameters, and increasing the likelihood of a term birth. Finally, there have been reports that dexamethasone can be used to good effect in controlling pruritus and also in enhancing fetal lung maturity.

There are usually no postpregnancy sequelae for the mother, and pruritus usually resolves postpartum. Fetal complications include prematurity (38%), meconium staining, fetal distress, and intrauterine fetal demise.

Dixon PH, Weerasekera N, Linton KJ, et al. Heterozygous *MDR3* missense mutation associated with intrahepatic cholestasis of pregnancy: evidence for a defect in protein trafficking. *Hum Mol Gen.* 2000;9:1209–1217. [PMID: 10767346]

Savander M, Ropponen A, Avela K, et al. Genetic evidence of heterogeneity in intrahepatic cholestasis of pregnancy. *Gut.* 2003;52:1025–1029. [PMID: 12801961]

Zapata R, Sandoval L, Palma J, et al. Ursodeoxycholic acid in the treatment of intrahepatic cholestasis of pregnancy. A 12-year experience. *Liver Int.* 2005;25:548–554. [PMID: 15910492]

3. Acute Fatty Liver of Pregnancy

AFLP is a potentially fatal disease that occurs most often in the third trimester and is reported in 1 in 13,000 pregnancies. Complications include preeclampsia (see later discussion) in 20–40% of cases. Maternal mortality is estimated at around 18%.

The medical basis of the disease has been identified as a defect in β-oxidation of long chain fatty acids in the fetus. The most commonly invoked molecular defect is a mutation in the long chain-3 hydroxyacyl CoA dehydrogenase (*LCHAD*). Mothers who are heterozygotes for *LCHAD* are at risk. The disorder arises from excess unmetabolized long chain fatty acids,

Table 8–2. Clinical features of liver disorders unique to pregnancy.

Disorder	Onset	Symptoms and Signs	Laboratory and Imaging Findings
Hyperemesis gravidarum	Mostly first trimester (unusual after 20 weeks)	Nausea and vomiting	ALT/AST 1–2× Bilirubin <5 mg/dL Positive urinary ketone
IHCP	Second and third trimesters	Pruritus and jaundice	ALT/AST 1–4× Bilirubin <5 mg/dL Bile acids 30–100×
AFLP	Third trimester	RUQ pain, jaundice, nonspecific symptoms	ALT/AST 1–5× Bilirubin >10× Hypoglycemia PT/PTT increased Platelets decreased CT/US—fatty infiltration Liver biopsy—microvesicular steatosis
Preeclampsia/eclampsia	Second and third trimesters (20 weeks prior to delivery)	Hypertension, edema	ALT/AST 1–10× Bilirubin <5 PT/PTT increased Proteinuria Platelets decreased
HELLP syndrome	Third trimester	Nonspecific RUQ pain ± hypertension	ALT/AST 1–10× Bilirubin <5 mg/dL PT/PTT increased Platelets decreased Hemolysis
Hepatic rupture	Late second to third trimester	Acute abdominal pain Hypotension Nausea Vomiting	ALT/AST 2–100× PT/PTT increased Platelets decreased CT/US—hematoma, hemoperitoneum

AFLP, acute fatty liver disease of pregnancy; ALT, alanine aminotransferase; AST, aspartate aminotransferase; CT, computed tomography; HELLP, hemolysis, elevated liver enzymes, and low platelets; IHCP, intrahepatic cholestasis of pregnancy; PT, prothrombin time; PTT, partial thromboplastin time; RUQ, right upper quadrant; US, ultrasound.
Adapted, with permission, from Wolf JL. Liver disease in pregnancy. *Med Clin North Am.* 1996;80:1167–1187.

generated by a fetus homozygously defective for *LCHAD*. This results in elevated levels of long chain fatty acids in the serum of the mother heterozygously defective for *LCHAD*, leading to subsequent hepatotoxicity. Indeed, mutations in the gene for *LCHAD* have been identified in affected women; specifically, the *G1528C* a cytosine for guanine mutation that results in a missense substitution is the most common. Although *LCHAD* is implicated in the disease, other disorders of β-oxidation of long chain fatty acid may produce a similar disease syndrome. There is at least one case report of a deficiency in palmitoyl transferase that led to AFLP.

The clinical presentation may be nonspecific, with nausea and vomiting present in 70% of patients. However, jaundice encephalopathy and oliguria often follow. Laboratory evaluation may show mild serum transaminase elevation, hyperbilirubinemia, coagulopathy, thrombocytopenia, and hypoglycemia. Ultrasound and computed tomography (CT) scans often show fatty infiltration of the liver. Liver biopsy examination shows microvesicular steatosis, easily discernible on oil red O staining.

Early delivery is the recommended therapeutic intervention, although some clinicians argue that mild cases should be managed expectantly. Regardless, management decisions should consider the rapidity in which complications develop and the significant mortality rate in patients with AFLP. There are no long-term sequelae for the mother as most recover; however, at least one case report exists of liver transplantation in AFLP. For the child, mortality is estimated at 13–18%, and developmental delay, hypoglycemia, and striated muscle dysfunction are all potential complications. Therapy with medium chain fatty acids is often necessary for infants with homozygous *LCHAD* deficiency.

Ibdah JA. Acute fatty liver of pregnancy: an update on pathogenesis and clinical implications. *World J Gastroenterol.* 2006; 12:7397–7404. [PMID: 17167825]

Innes AM, Seargeant LE, Balachandra K, et al. Hepatic carnitine palmitoyltransferase I deficiency presenting as maternal illness in pregnancy. *Pediatr Res.* 2000;47:43–45. [PMID: 10625081]

4. Preeclampsia & Eclampsia

This complication of pregnancy, which occurs during the second or third trimester, is characterized by hypertension (defined as an elevation of at least 30 mm Hg systolic, 15 mm Hg diastolic, or a blood pressure >140/90) and proteinuria. Edema, a former component of the definition, is no longer required due to its commonality in all pregnancies. Preeclampsia or eclampsia occurs in 5–10% of all pregnancies. Eclampsia includes the above triad plus seizures and coma. The risk factors include preexisting hypertension, family history of preeclampsia, primigravida, multiple gestations, and early and late ages at the time of childbearing.

Clinical presentation may include headache or visual changes, right upper quadrant pain with or without signs of liver failure, pulmonary edema, oliguria, hemolysis with or without thrombocytopenia, and grand mal seizures. The ALT level is abnormal in approximately 20% of patients with preeclampsia and in 90% of those with full-blown eclampsia. The diagnosis is often made on clinical grounds with elimination of other potential causes of late pregnancy liver abnormalities. Hypoglycemia as seen in AFLP is unusual.

Endothelial dysfunction due to placental function is felt to be the major culprit in preeclampsia. Supporting evidence for this includes the occurrence of preeclampsia in women with hydatiform mole pregnancies even in the absence of a fetus. In these cases, the removal of the mole leads to resolution of preeclampsia. In addition, postpartum retention of the placenta leads to preeclampsia with resolution often after the delivery of the placenta. Scientific evidence shows that transformation of small but high-resistance uterine spiral arteries to high-capacitance vessels mediated by invasion of fetal cytotrophoblasts is incomplete in persons with preeclampsia. This abnormality in placentation ultimately leads to a systemic vascular dysfunction characterized by leaky capillaries and vasospasm.

Management of preeclampsia relies on the delivery of the (abnormal) placenta. At experienced institutions, the mortality rate is less than 1%. Complications include seizure, coma, hepatic rupture, and fulminant hepatic failure.

Hay JE. Liver disease in pregnancy. *Hepatology.* 2008;47:1067–1076. [PMID: 18265410]

Young BC, Levine RJ, Karumanchi SA. Pathogenesis of preeclampsia. *Ann Rev Pathol.* 2010;5:173–192. [PMID: 20078220]

5. HELLP Syndrome (Hemolysis, Elevated Liver Enzymes, & Low Platelets)

This syndrome is a potential complication of preeclampsia, occurring in 0.1–0.6% of all pregnancies and in 4–12% of all preeclamptic patients. Seventy percent of patients with HELLP syndrome develop this problem between the 27th week of pregnancy and the time of delivery. However, approximately 30% develop the problem postpartum.

Signs and symptoms are right upper quadrant pain, occurring in 65–90% of patients; jaundice, in around 5%; edema, in 60%; and hypertension, in 80%. Laboratory abnormalities include a mean ALT level of around 150 IU/L; serum bilirubin is often normal or minimally elevated. Hypoglycemia as seen in AFLP is unusual.

Delivery remains the mainstay of management, and it is recommended that if the pregnancy has progressed beyond 34 weeks, the infant should be delivered. Observation for 24–48 hours is recommended, but only if hypertension and central nervous system abnormalities are not present.

Complications of HELLP include a mortality rate of 1–3%, disseminated intravascular coagulation (DIC) in 20% of patients, placenta abruptio in 16%, acute renal failure in 7%, and pulmonary edema in 6%. Perinatal mortality is approximately 35%.

Barton JR, Sibai BM. Diagnosis and management of hemolysis, elevated liver enzymes, and low platelets syndrome. *Clin Perinatol.* 2004;31:807–833. [PMID: 15519429]

6. Liver Hematoma & Rupture

This is a severe and devastating complication of pregnancy, which often occurs in the third trimester and almost always in the setting of HELLP, preeclampsia, AFLP, cocaine abuse, neoplasms, sickle cell disease, polyarteritis nodosa, and rupture of hepatic adenoma during pregnancy. Intraparenchymal hemorrhage always precedes the rupture. This diagnosis should be suspected in any pregnant woman with right upper quadrant pain, preeclampsia, and shock. Maternal mortality is estimated at 57–75%, and fetal mortality of approximately 62–77% is seen.

CONDITIONS NOT UNIQUE TO PREGNANCY

1. Viral Hepatitis

Acute viral hepatitides from hepatitis A, B, C, D, and E can occur in pregnant women as in nonpregnant patients. Nonhepatotropic viruses such as cytomegalovirus, Epstein-Barr virus, and herpes simplex virus (HSV) can also cause hepatic injury in pregnant women. Considerations in managing pregnant patients with some of these hepatitides are presented here. For additional information about acute and chronic hepatitis, see Chapters 39 and 40.

A. Hepatitis A

The incidence and management of hepatitis A are the same in pregnant as in nonpregnant individuals (see Chapter 39). The management of hepatitis A is conservative. Perinatal transmission is rare, but there may be horizontal transmission at the time of delivery. Hepatitis A vaccine and immunoglobulin are safe during pregnancy.

B. Hepatitis B

The risk of vertical transmission to the fetus of acute infections in the second and third trimesters is 10% and 90%, respectively. Intrauterine infections are rare. Most infections occur in intrapartum. In women who are positive for hepatitis B e antigen (HBeAg), there is a 70–90% chance of vertical transmission. Hepatitis B vaccine is safe during pregnancy, and once infants are administered protective immunoglobulins (hepatitis B immunoglobulin [HBIG]) at the time of birth, there is no additional risk from breast-feeding. All children born to hepatitis B surface antigen-positive mothers should receive HBIG at the time of birth and the first of their hepatitis B vaccines before discharge from the hospital.

It is known that the combination of HBIG and vaccination decreases the vertical transmission rate from around 90% to between 3% and 7%. The residual failure rate appears to occur in children born to mothers with very high viral loads often greater than 1×10^8 IU/mL. While there is no consensus on whether pregnant women with high hepatitis viral loads should be treated with antiretroviral agents, many cite experiences with therapy against human immunodeficiency virus (HIV) and herpes simplex as examples where treatment in late pregnancy reduces the risk of maternal to fetal transmission. In support, data on mothers with high viral load who were treated with or without antiretroviral agents (lamivudine and telbivudine in separate studies) show that treatment during the third trimester decreased vertical transmission rates in this group of patients.

C. Hepatitis C

Hepatitis C virus (HCV) infection is not a contraindication to pregnancy, but perinatal transmission is around 5% in mothers who are positive for HCV RNA. If patients are coinfected with HIV, the risk of infection increases to 19%. Amniocentesis and fetal blood monitoring are contraindicated in HCV-positive mothers because of worries regarding percutaneous exposure. Breast-feeding is permitted.

D. Hepatitis E

The hepatitis E virus causes a fulminant hepatitis resembling hepatitis A. The mortality rate in pregnant mothers is around 30%.

E. Herpes Simplex Virus Hepatitis

HSV hepatitis is a rare disorder seen in immunocompromised and in pregnant patients. There is usually a short prodrome of between 2 days and 2 weeks. Symptoms are mostly nonspecific, although fever and abdominal pain can occur. Oropharyngeal or genital lesions, or both, are seen in roughly 50% of infected persons; thus, their absence does not eliminate this as a possible etiology.

Factors associated with possible diagnosis include low bilirubin in the presence of elevated transaminases (anicteric hepatitis), AST greater than ALT, third trimester of pregnancy, and immunocompromised state. Diagnosis can be made through HSV-1 and HSV-2 serologies, viral cultures, or liver biopsy, which is the gold standard. The biopsy sample often shows minimal inflammatory infiltrate and is characterized by zonal necrosis of hepatocytes.

In untreated patients, the mortality rate exceeds 80%. In one study of 14 pregnant patients who received acyclovir, 10 patients survived. Because the results of serologic tests, viral cultures, and biopsy examination often are not available for several days, clinical decision making in the absence of these findings is important. If suspicion is high, therapy should be begun immediately while awaiting diagnostic results.

Bzowej NH. Hepatitis B therapy in pregnancy. *Curr Hepat Rep.* 2010;9:197–204. [PMID: 20949113]

Kang AH, Graves CR. Herpes simplex hepatitis in pregnancy: a case report and review of the literature. *Obstet Gynecol Surv.* 1999;54:463–468. [PMID: 10394584]

Shi Z, Yang Y, Ma L, et al. Lamivudine in late pregnancy to interrupt in utero transmission of hepatitis B virus: a systematic review and meta-analysis. *Obstet Gynecol.* 2010;116:147–159. [PMID: 20567182]

Valladares G, Chacaltana A, Sjogren MH. The management of HCV-infected pregnant women. *Ann Hepatol.* 2010;9:S92–S97. [PMID: 20714003]

2. Budd-Chiari Syndrome

This syndrome results from an obstruction of the hepatic vein or the suprahepatic portion of the vena cava. The most common reason is thrombosis. Because of increased risk of thrombotic events in pregnancy, this disorder should be considered in any pregnant with right upper quadrant pain, rapid weight gain, and ascites.

Evaluation relies heavily on ultrasonographic Doppler examination. Occasionally CT or venography may be necessary.

If the patient is stable, heparin is the therapy of choice. If unstable, transjugular intrahepatic portosystemic shunts should be performed if feasible. Warfarin cannot be used during pregnancy.

Horton JD, San Miguel FL, Ortiz JA. Budd-Chiari syndrome: illustrated review of current management. *Liver Int.* 2008;28:455–466. [PMID: 18339072]

3. Wilson Disease

Wilson disease is a disorder of copper metabolism that results in systemic manifestations, with hepatic and neurologic symptoms as the most prominent components (see Chapter 40). Many patients are diagnosed in their teenage years; thus issues related to disease management become a concern during their childbearing years.

In general, patients whose disease is well controlled during pregnancy do well. Therapy should continue throughout pregnancy as fulminant liver failure has been reported in patients who discontinue therapy. Penicillamine, trientine, and zinc have been used with success during pregnancy. Many practitioners decrease the dose of penicillamine to between 25% and 50% during pregnancy.

Roberts EA, Schilsky ML. Diagnosis and Treatment of Wilson's disease: an update. *Hepatology.* 2008;47:2089–2111. [PMID: 18506894]

Sternlieb I. Wilson's disease and pregnancy. *Hepatology.* 2000;31: 531–532. [PMID: 10655282]

4. Autoimmune Hepatitis

Autoimmune hepatitis (AIH) is a chronic heterogeneous hepatic disorder characterized by the presence of autoantibodies and elevated γ-globulins (see Chapter 40). It is more common in women than in men and can lead to cirrhosis, and therapy often involves the use of azathioprine, a medicine with suspected teratogenicity. Thus, issues related to maternal and fetal welfare may surface in the management of women of childbearing age.

AIH frequently improves during pregnancy, although there is a tendency toward postpartum flare and disease reactivation. Because of concerns regarding the use of azathioprine in pregnancy, some practitioners withdraw azathioprine during early pregnancy and reinstate it late in the third trimester. Although azathioprine is a pregnancy class D agent based on congenital malformation in rodents, there has been no evidence of increased teratogenicity among children born to mothers receiving azathioprine or any adverse effects of breast-feeding in this population. Regardless, counseling is recommended prior to conception in women actively treated with azathioprine. Overall pregnancy is well tolerated, and pregnancy outcomes in patients with AIH, with regard to fetal loss, cesarean sectioning, and still births, are similar to that of the general population.

Heneghan MA, Norris SM, O'Grady JG, et al. Management and outcome of pregnancy in autoimmune hepatitis. *Gut.* 2001;48;97–102. [PMID: 11115829]

Schramm C, Herkel J, Beuers U, et al. Pregnancy in autoimmune hepatitis: outcome and risk factors. *Am J Gastroeneterol.* 2006;101:555–560. [PMID: 16464221]

5. Cirrhosis

Although infertility is common in persons with advanced liver disease, pregnancy does occur in cirrhotic patients. Maternal mortality in pregnant patients with cirrhosis is estimated at 10–18%. In a large case series of 117 pregnant women with cirrhosis, portal hypertension, or both, 50% had uncomplicated term pregnancies, but variceal bleeding occurred in 24 women and was responsible for death in 4% of the patients. The few case reports available indeed confirm that variceal bleeding is by far the most common complication of cirrhosis in pregnancy. This is not surprising given the 30–50% increase in plasma volume that accompanies the pregnant state.

Although no uniformed consensus exists on management in these cases, most agree that endoscopic evaluation for esophageal varices should be performed and patients with high-grade varices treated either by nonselective β-blockade or by esophageal variceal band ligation if β-blockers are contraindicated. There are no reliable data to show superiority of cesarean delivery over vaginal delivery; thus, decisions should be made based on the individual clinical information.

Cerqui AJ, Haran M, Brodribb R. Implications of liver cirrhosis in pregnancy. *Aust N Z J Obstet Gynaecol.* 1998;38:93–95. [PMID: 9521402]

Shaheen AA, Myers RP. The outcomes of pregnancy in patients with cirrhosis: a population-based study. *Liver Int.* 2010;30: 275–283. [PMID: 19874491]

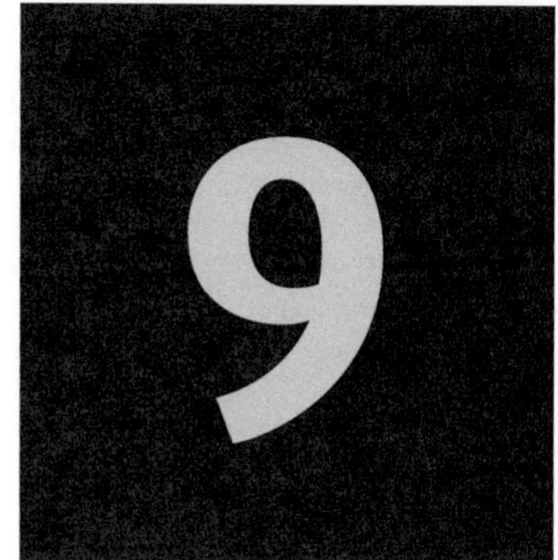

State-of-the-Art Imaging of the Gastrointestinal System

Koenraad J. Mortele, MD

General Considerations

During the last decade, many new tools became part of the radiologist's armamentarium to image the gastrointestinal (GI) system. Developments in computerized tomography (CT), magnetic resonance (MR) technology, and positron emission tomography (PET) made GI radiologists essential physicians in the diagnosis and evaluation of a vast array of diseases involving the abdomen and pelvis. Moreover, these major innovations mandated the replacement of some classic invasive diagnostic methods with noninvasive and efficient ones.

Multidetector-row CT (MDCT), initially introduced in 1998, has diffused into clinical imaging practice in a short time. Rapid volume coverage speed combined with thin image thickness allows creation of a volume data set. In addition to technical advances, such as shorter scanning times, multiplanar imaging, and improved ability to perform true multiphasic contrast-enhanced studies, advances in postacquisition data-processing techniques have made MDCT a powerful imaging tool in abdominal visceral imaging.

Compared with CT, magnetic resonance imaging (MRI) still plays a relatively minor role in the diagnosis and imaging workup of patients with abdominal diseases. However, technical improvements, such as the development of phased array multicoils and faster sequences, allow excellent contrast resolution images of the liver, pancreas, biliary tree, and even GI tract with an acceptable spatial and temporal resolution. Published results of MRI compared with CT and sonography have allowed, in a vast array of abdominal diseases, not only a more accurate delineation of the extent of disease, but also improvements in disease characterization. Furthermore, the evaluation of abdominal organs by means of contrast-enhanced dynamic MRI can be optimized with the use of MR angiography, which visualizes the vessels, and MR cholangiopancreatography (MRCP), which depicts the biliopancreatic ductal system. At present, this "all-in-one" approach is presumably the most cost-effective imaging technique in the evaluation of a vast array of liver function abnormalities, exocrine pancreatic diseases, and biliary disorders. Currently, the indications for MRI of the GI tract are limited to staging of rectal cancer and assessing the extent of perianal fistulae and anal sphincter tears. However, the value of MR colonography, MR enterography, and MRI of appendicitis is rapidly emerging.

PET-CT is another rapidly evolving technique with increasing applications in GI diseases. The majority of investigations allow staging of cancer and monitoring therapy, using the glucose analog 2-deoxy [18F] fluoro-D-glucose (FDG). Because tumor cells preferentially utilize glucose as a metabolic substrate, FDG-PET depicts areas of increased metabolism as "hot spots"; a CT scan performed in the same session allows linking these areas to morphologic abnormalities.

Coupled with these recent innovations in cross-sectional imaging, there has been a serious decline in the utilization of more routine diagnostic imaging methods used in the past to evaluate the GI system. Nowadays, fluoroscopic examinations of the small bowel and colon have very specific but limited indications. Nevertheless, some contrast examinations, such as barium swallow and upper GI studies, remain cost-effective investigations and continue to play an important role in the evaluation of the upper GI tract.

This chapter details the current imaging algorithms and key imaging features of various diseases involving the GI system, with special emphasis on new imaging techniques currently available in clinical practice.

GASTROINTESTINAL TRACT IMAGING

1. Esophagus

A. Imaging Algorithm

Although endoscopy may comprise the initial examination to evaluate the esophagus in many centers, fluoroscopic examination of the esophagus after contrast administration still has a high yield to detect clinically significant pathology and can complement endoscopy in several ways. Using a biphasic technique (single and double contrast), the esophagogram has proven invaluable in the evaluation of dysphagia, odynophagia, gastroesophageal reflux disease, and especially motility disorders; assessment of the integrity of the esophagus following local surgery or invasive procedures is another useful and common indication. Nowadays, CT and especially PET-CT are used increasingly in the evaluation of patients with esophageal neoplasms in order to stage the cancer locally and more distantly.

Levine MS, Rubesin SE, Laufer I. Barium esophagography: a study for all seasons. *Clin Gastroenterol Hepatol.* 2008;6:11–25. [PMID: 18083069]

B. Morphologic Abnormalities

Esophageal carcinoma. Double-contrast esophagography has a sensitivity of greater than 95% in the detection of esophageal cancer. Approximately 70% of esophageal neoplasms are squamous cell carcinomas, and the remaining 30% are adenocarcinomas arising in Barrett esophagus. The appearance of esophageal cancers on barium studies is variable and has been described as infiltrating, polypoid, ulcerative, or varicoid (Figure 9–1). Fistula formation is seen in approximately 5–10% of cases. Nowadays, PET-CT imaging is increasingly used to detect nonregional lymphadenopathy or distant metastases (Plate 4).

Zenker diverticulum (see Chapter 13) is an acquired mucosal herniation between the horizontal and oblique fibers of the cricopharyngeus muscle; it is more common in men and probably associated with GI reflux disease. On barium studies, a contrast-filled midline sac is seen posterior to the pharyngoesophageal junction (Figure 9–2). Below the opening of the sac, a prominent cricopharyngeal muscle is commonly identified. It is important for a Zenker diverticulum to be diagnosed on barium swallow because of an increased risk of perforation at endoscopy.

Gastroesophageal reflux disease (GERD). (See Chapter 11.) Barium studies have proved invaluable in patients with GERD to document the presence of a hiatal hernia, gastroesophageal reflux, and reflux esophagitis, and to detect complications, such as ulcerations, strictures, Barrett esophagus, and neoplasms. Early esophagitis in patients with GERD is manifested by a fine nodular or granular appearance with small well-defined radiolucencies caused by mucosal edema. In more advanced disease, contrast-filled ulcers may be present near the gastroesophageal junction on the posterior esophageal wall and peptic strictures may be detected in the distal esophagus above a hiatal hernia (Figure 9–3). The classic signs of Barrett esophagus include a high, midesophageal stricture, ulcer, or reticular pattern (see Chapter 12).

Infectious esophagitis is most frequently encountered in patients who are immunocompromised; among the possible infectious agents are *Candida albicans*, herpes simplex virus, cytomegalovirus (CMV), and HIV. *Candida* esophagitis (moniliasis) is typically manifested on barium studies as discrete, linear, plaque-like lesions separated by normal intervening mucosa, with a predilection for the upper and midesophagus. Herpes esophagitis shows the presence of small barium-filled ulcers on a normal background mucosa, while CMV and HIV esophagitis is manifested by giant, flat ulcerations that are typically several centimeters in length.

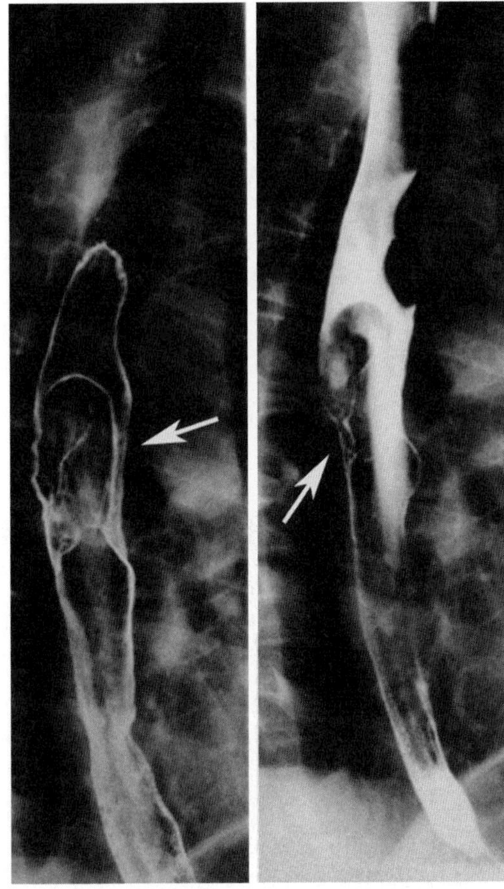

▲ **Figure 9–1.** Polypoid esophageal carcinoma. Upright double-contrast esophagogram shows a thick, polypoid, and irregular tumor (*arrows*) in the midesophagus.

C. Motility Disorders (See Chapter 13)

Achalasia can be categorized as primary when it is idiopathic and as secondary when it is caused by other conditions, such as tumors or Chagas disease. Patients with idiopathic achalasia are typically young and demonstrate lack of esophageal peristalsis and incomplete relaxation of the lower esophageal sphincter. On barium studies, the esophagus appears dilated, flaccid, and obstructed by a tapered, bird beak-like narrowing

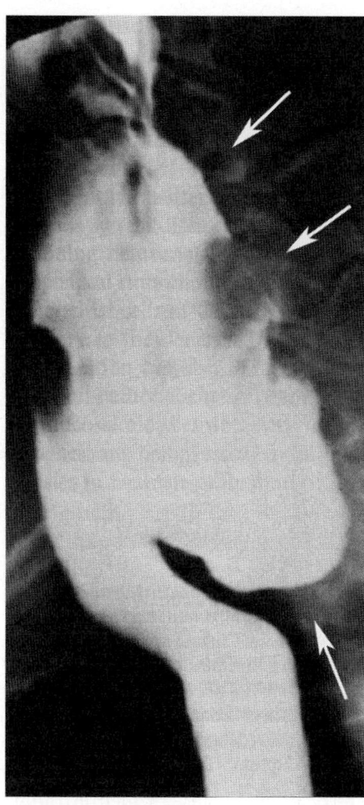

▲ **Figure 9–2.** Zenker diverticulum. Lateral view from a single-contrast esophagogram shows a barium-filled diverticulum (*arrows*) posterior to the cervical esophagus.

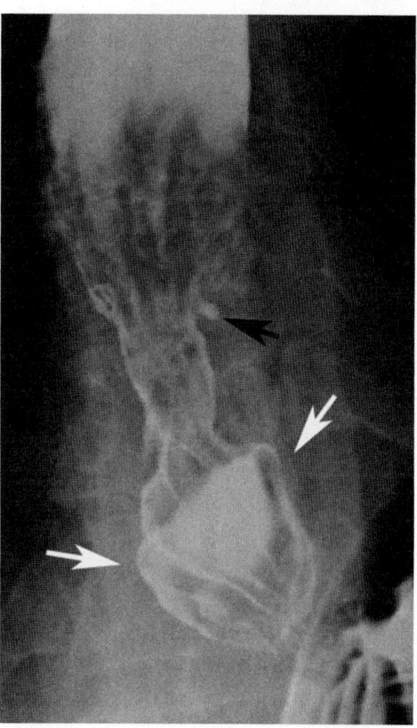

▲ **Figure 9–3.** Peptic stricture and ulceration. Upright double-contrast esophagogram shows a smooth, tapered stricture in the distal esophagus above a hiatal hernia (*white arrows*). Also note a small barium-filled ulceration (*black arrow*) on the left lateral wall.

at the gastroesophageal junction. In patients with secondary achalasia, due to destruction of ganglion cells caused by miscellaneous processes, the length of the narrowed segment is often greater and may appear nodular or ulcerated.

Diffuse esophageal spasm (DES) is characterized by intermittent, abnormal esophageal peristalsis with presence of multiple, simultaneous nonperistaltic contractions. In approximately 15% of patients with DES, lumen-obliterating nonperistaltic contractions can be seen that compartmentalize the esophagus, producing the classic "corkscrew" esophagus on barium studies.

2. Stomach

A. Imaging Algorithm

Upper endoscopy has largely replaced fluoroscopic studies as the primary investigation in patients with suspected gastric or duodenal pathology. Nevertheless, if endoscopy is contraindicated or unsuccessful, a well-performed upper GI study is the next sensitive diagnostic test. In addition to displaying the morphology of the stomach in patients following bariatric surgery, with suspected gastric volvulus, or gastric outlet obstruction, upper GI studies also readily detect mucosal and submucosal abnormalities that distort the gastric wall with high sensitivity. More recently, MDCT with neutral contrast material has been proposed as an excellent imaging test to evaluate the gastric wall, especially in the evaluation of gastric neoplasms. Other diagnostic methods utilized to diagnose and stage gastric neoplasms include ultrasonography, endoscopic ultrasound (EUS), MRI, and PET (CT) scan.

Rubesin SE, Levine MS, Laufer I. Double-contrast upper gastrointestinal radiography: a pattern approach for diseases of the stomach. *Radiology*. 2008;246:33–48. [PMID: 18096527]

B. Neoplasms

Adenocarcinoma is by far the most common gastric malignancy and represents approximately 90% of all gastric malignancies. CT is currently the staging modality of choice because it can identify the primary tumor, assess for local

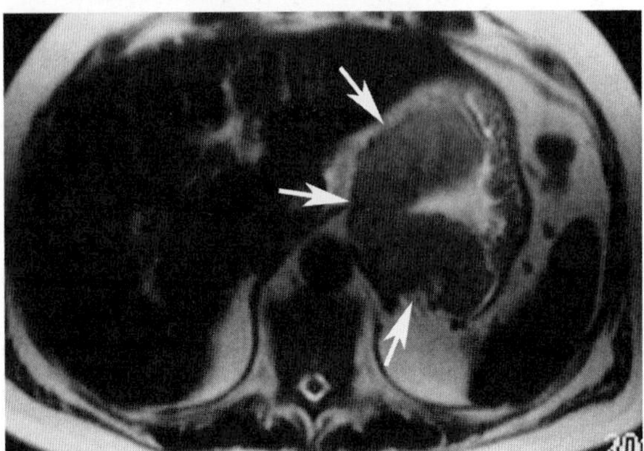

▲ **Figure 9–4.** Gastric adenocarcinoma. Axial T2-weighted MR image shows a thick hyperintense mass (*arrows*) arising from the gastric cardia.

spread, and detect nodal involvement and distant metastases. On CT, if larger than 5 mm, gastric cancer may present as a focal enhancing soft tissue mass or as diffuse thickening of the gastric wall (Figure 9–4). Both CT and PET-CT have a reported sensitivity of 90% in detecting distant metastases. Classic features of gastric cancer include the presence of a lobulated or nodular mass with associated irregular ulceration (Figure 9–5). In scirrhous adenocarcinoma, the stomach demonstrates a long segment of circumferential narrowing and focal areas of mucosal nodularity.

Other gastric malignancies occur much less frequently and include lymphoma (<5%), GI stromal tumors (<2%), and malignant carcinoid (<1%). Gastric lymphoma typically appears as segmental or diffuse gastric wall thickening.

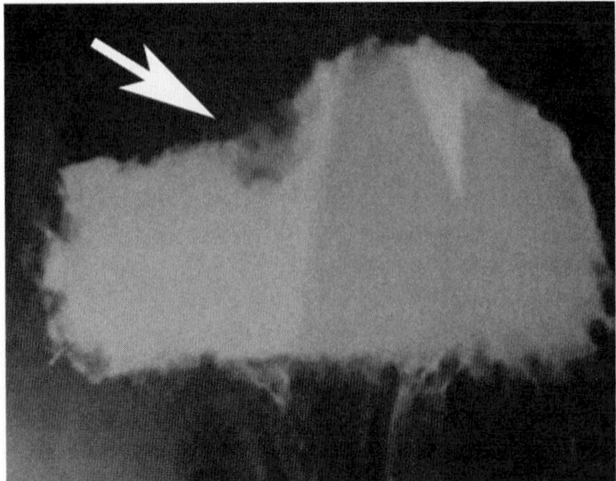

▲ **Figure 9–5.** Gastric adenocarcinoma. Upright double-contrast upper GI image shows a large irregular mass (*arrow*) arising from the fundus.

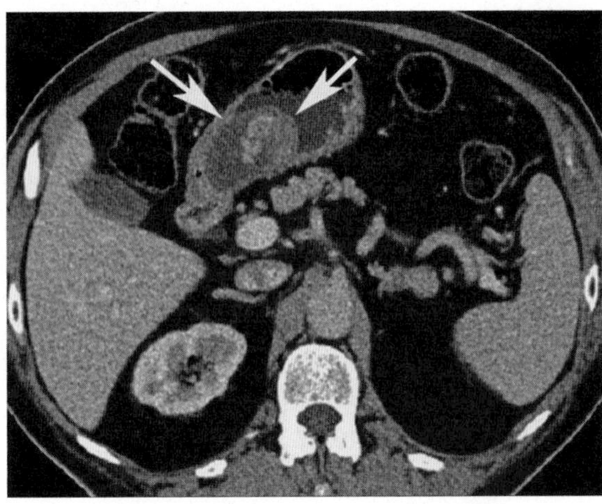

▲ **Figure 9–6.** Gastrointestinal stromal tumor. Axial MDCT image shows a well-defined hypervascular mass (*arrows*) in the gastric body.

In contrast to gastric cancer, lymphoma typically involves more than one region of the stomach, is unlikely to cause gastric outlet obstruction, and may be associated with lymphadenopathy below the renal hila. Gastric stromal tumors can be benign or malignant, and 90% of them originate in the gastric fundus or body. Because of their extramucosal origin, upper GI series may be negative. Small masses appear as intramural hypervascular lesions on CT. Larger stromal tumors tend to necrose, hemorrhage, or ulcerate (Figure 9–6). They typically are partially exophytic in location. Associated lymphadenopathy is uncommon, in contrast with gastric adenocarcinoma or lymphoma.

C. Infectious and Inflammatory Conditions

Peptic ulcer disease (see Chapter 15) is most commonly caused by infection by *Helicobacter pylori* or by nonsteroidal anti-inflammatory drugs (NSAIDs). Most duodenal ulcers are caused by *H pylori,* while most gastric ulcers are caused by NSAIDs. Erosion is an area of focal necrosis confined to the epithelium or lamina propria, whereas a true ulcer extends through the muscularis mucosa into the deeper layers of the gastric wall. On upper GI studies, a depressed lesion greater than several millimeters in depth is called an ulcer. When viewed en face, most peptic ulcers are manifested as round or ovoid collections of barium filling the ulcer crater with smooth, straight folds radiating to the ulcer's edge (Figure 9–7). The presence of a Hampton line (a thin radiolucent line traversing the base of the crater due to undermining of the submucosa) is diagnostic of a benign gastric ulcer. CT does not detect most peptic ulcers because they affect only the superficial layers of the gastric wall. However, deep or perforated ulcers manifest as focal wall thickening with associated inflammatory changes in the adjacent soft tissues.

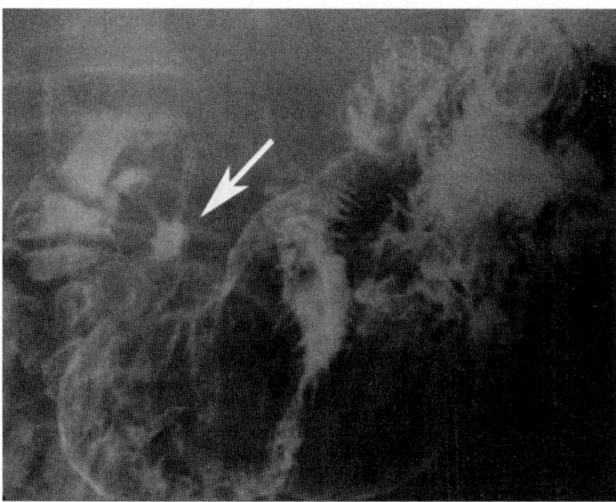

▲ **Figure 9–7.** Gastric benign ulcer. Double-contrast upper GI study shows a small ulcer (*arrow*) with radiating folds surrounding it.

Gastritis, due to *H pylori* or other causes, typically appears on barium studies as thickened, scalloped folds that have a longitudinal or transverse orientation. Similarly, the most common CT finding in patients with gastritis is thickening of the gastric folds (Figure 9–8). In severe cases, the gastric wall appears stratified due to extensive submucosal edema and mucosal hyperenhancement. This striated appearance helps to distinguish gastritis from gastric cancers. *H pylori* gastritis, the most common infection in humans, is by far the most likely cause of focally or diffusely thickened folds, especially involving the antrum. Gastritis by a gas-producing organism (eg, *Escherichia coli*) may cause the classic appearance of emphysematous gastritis, a condition with a high mortality rate. Ménétrier disease typically causes massive enlargement of the rugal folds predominantly involving the gastric fundus and body with sparing of the antrum.

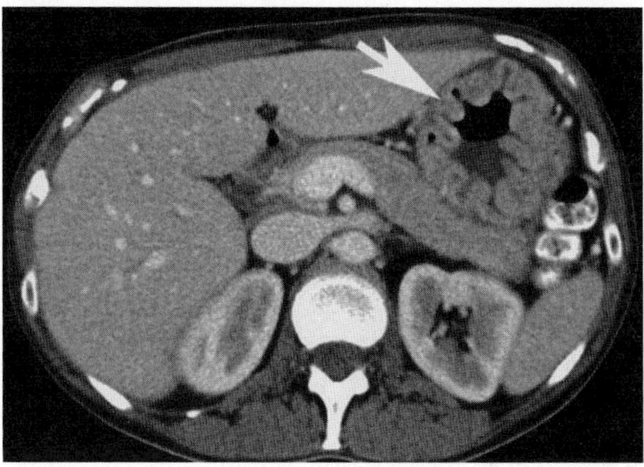

▲ **Figure 9–8.** Gastritis. Axial MDCT image shows severe thickening of the gastric folds (*arrow*).

3. Small Bowel

A. Imaging Algorithm

Traditionally, the small bowel has been studied noninvasively with fluoroscopic imaging techniques, such as small bowel follow-through (SBFT) or enteroclysis. The accuracy of SBFT and enteroclysis for detecting and characterizing small bowel abnormalities, however, varies widely among radiologists and institutions. Moreover, the inherent disadvantage of studying only the mucosa represents another limitation of enteroclysis and SBFT. CT enteroclysis is a successful alternative imaging method for a more detailed evaluation of bowel wall disease and for accurate diagnosis of extraluminal pathologies. With this technique, a nasogastric tube is fluoroscopically placed and oral contrast agent is infused subsequently; for most patients, however, the intubation remains a traumatizing experience. Today, imaging of the small bowel with noninvasive adequate distention of bowel loops is possible without fluoroscopically guided intubation. Recent studies have demonstrated that noninvasive, peroral CT enterography is an accurate and feasible technique for detecting active small bowel inflammation in patients with Crohn disease. The use of a neutral oral contrast agent provides a better evaluation of the bowel wall due to the inherent contrast between the neutral bowel content and the enhancing bowel wall.

MR enteroclysis or enterography is performed with increasing frequency due to the lack of ionizing radiation, which allows it to be used in young patients with Crohn disease who need repeated evaluation. MR enterography is also performed using oral and intravenous contrast material.

Remaining indications for plain film of the abdomen, SBFT, and enteroclysis in the evaluation of the small bowel include the detection and evaluation of adynamic ileus, small bowel perforation, small bowel obstruction, correct placement of jejunostomy tubes, and functional small bowel abnormalities.

B. CT Enterography Technique

CT enterography is preferably performed using an MDCT scanner after the oral administration of barium sulfate 0.1% w/v suspension. Patients drink 1350 mL of VoLumen (low-density barium sulphate preparation) prior to the scan. For specific indications, such as obscure GI bleeding, small bowel neoplasms, and chronic ischemia, a biphasic contrast-enhanced MDCT study is performed: images are acquired during the late arterial phase (40 seconds) and parenchymal phase (70 seconds) following intravenous administration of nonionic contrast material.

Patak MA, Mortele KJ, Ros PR. Multidetector row CT of the small bowel. *Radiol Clin North Am.* 2005;43:1063–1077. [PMID: 16253662]

C. Crohn Disease

In many institutions, SBFT is still the most common imaging technique used in the evaluation of suspected small bowel Crohn disease. Nevertheless, although SBFT can demonstrate early active mucosal disease, such as ulcers, it has limitations; most importantly, the radiologist must rely on secondary signs to evaluate the complete small bowel wall and mesentery.

Although CT has traditionally been used to assess extra-enteric complications of Crohn disease, including abscesses, fistulas, or obstruction, it has been shown that CT features of the small bowel wall itself, such as mural stratification, mucosal and mural hyperenhancement, edema in the mesenteric fat, and engorged ileal vasa recta, correlate with active inflammation (Figure 9–9). Furthermore, submucosal fat deposition and mural thickening without hyperenhancement or mural stratification typically correlate with fibrotic or quiescent disease. Large studies have evaluated the sensitivity and specificity of MDCT for detection of Crohn disease using SBFT as the gold standard; the sensitivity and specificity of MDCT for advanced disease were reported as 95% and 98%, respectively. In particular, adding multiplanar reconstructions to the axial data significantly improves the diagnostic confidence.

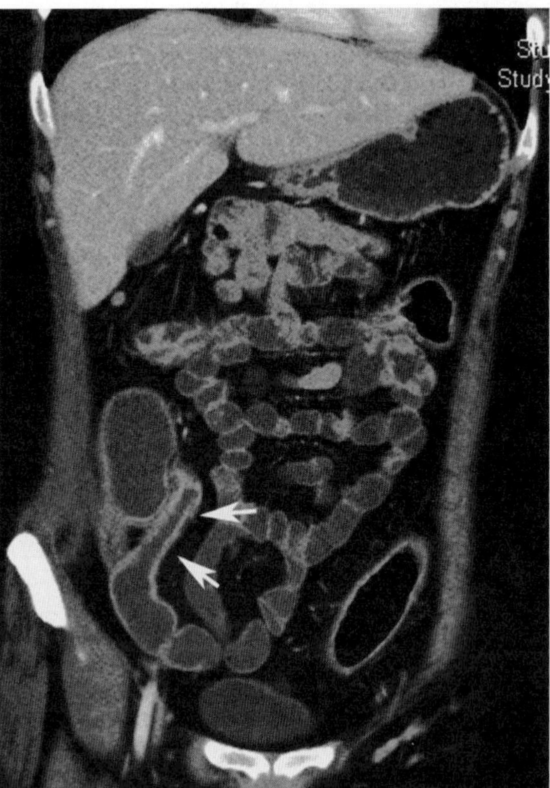

▲ **Figure 9–9.** Crohn disease. Coronal CT enterography image shows mucosal hyperenhancement of the wall of the terminal ileum (*arrows*).

D. Small Bowel Obstruction

The early diagnosis of bowel obstruction is critical in preventing complications, particularly perforation and ischemia. The accuracy of conventional radiography in determining the presence of obstruction is 46–80% (Figure 9–10). Today, while abdominal radiography is often still the preferred initial radiologic examination, CT has gained favor because it can be effectively used to reveal the site, level, and cause of obstruction and it displays the signs of threatened bowel viability with high accuracy.

Adhesions are responsible for more than half of all small bowel obstructions, followed by hernias and extrinsic compression from neoplasms. Improvements in MDCT technology allow the transition point to be viewed from a variety of perspectives, increasing the diagnostic confidence once other causes have been appropriately excluded. Recently, Jaffe and colleagues reported a specificity of 87% and a sensitivity of 90% for diagnosing small bowel obstruction. MDCT is also excellent for detecting external hernias and for characterizing the bowel and mesentery in the hernia sac in patients with internal herniation.

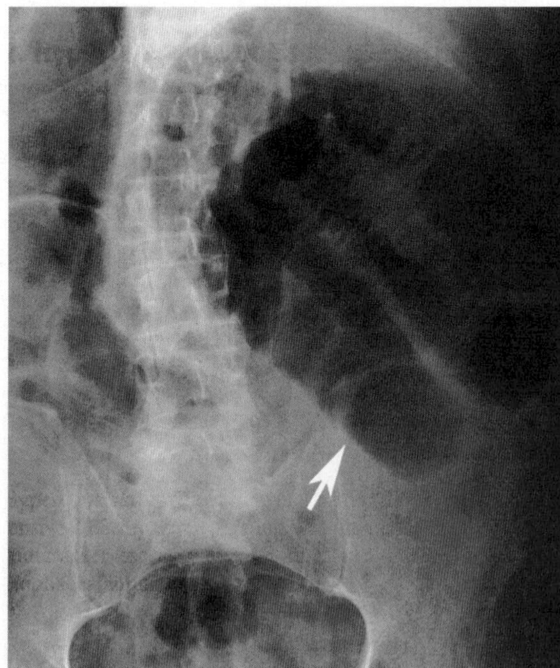

▲ **Figure 9–10.** Small bowel obstruction. Abdominal radiograph image shows severe dilation of jejunal small bowel loops with acute transition (*arrow*).

Jaffe TA, Martin LC, Thomas J, et al. Small-bowel obstruction: coronal reformations from isotropic voxels at 16-section multidetector row CT. *Radiology*. 2006;238:135–142. [PMID: 16293807]

E. Mesenteric Ischemia (See Chapter 6)

Dual-phase MDCT can demonstrate changes in ischemic bowel segments accurately, is often helpful in determining the primary cause of ischemia, and can demonstrate important concomitant findings or complications. CT findings in acute bowel ischemia may consist of various morphologic changes, including homogeneous or heterogeneous hypoattenuating or hyperattenuating wall thickening, dilation, abnormal or absent wall enhancement, mesenteric stranding, vascular engorgement, ascites, pneumatosis, and portal venous gas (Figure 9–11). Dual-phase imaging of the abdomen is necessary during the arterial and the portal phases of enhancement to adequately opacify both the mesenteric arteries and veins. Three-dimensional (3D) imaging is crucial to visualize even the more distal branches of mesenteric arteries, which sometimes are not easily visualized on axial images. MDCT 3D imaging also can be used in the follow-up of patients after surgery, which typically includes bypass with grafts, whose patency is well documented by 3D imaging.

F. Neoplasms

Diagnosis of small bowel tumors is still challenging because they are uncommon, usually produce nonspecific symptoms, and often are small. Therefore, MDCT, because of the thinner collimation, is achieving an even more important role in the detection and staging of small bowel tumors.

Benign small bowel tumors are uncommon and are typically detected on SBFT and CT as incidental findings. The most common of these tumors are lipomas and leiomyomas. Lipomas are easily recognized by their fat attenuation values (–90 to –120 Hounsfield units [HU]). Leiomyomas are typically smooth, homogenous submucosal masses that enhance up to 1.5 times baseline following injection of intravenous contrast material.

The most common primary malignant tumor of the small intestine is adenocarcinoma; it accounts for approximately 40% of all small bowel neoplasms. Most adenocarcinomas are located in the duodenum (Figure 9–12). On MDCT images, adenocarcinoma is typically visualized as a focal area of wall thickening that encases the lumen. The second most common primary small bowel neoplasm is carcinoid, representing approximately 25% of all primary small bowel tumors. Carcinoid tumors usually present as small enhancing nodules, which when bigger, may cause metastatic infiltration of the mesentery (Figure 9–13). On CT, this appears as an infiltrating mesenteric mass that contains calcifications in up to 70% of cases. Non-Hodgkin lymphoma represents approximately 10–15% of all small bowel neoplasms. The primary tumor often can be detected with small bowel contrast studies and CT; however, CT offers the advantage of simultaneously detecting adenopathy and the extraluminal extent of disease. Primary small bowel lymphomas often appear as a focally thickened, aneurysmally dilated loop. Celiac disease is a predisposing factor for small bowel lymphoma (Figure 9–14). Gastrointestinal stromal tumors

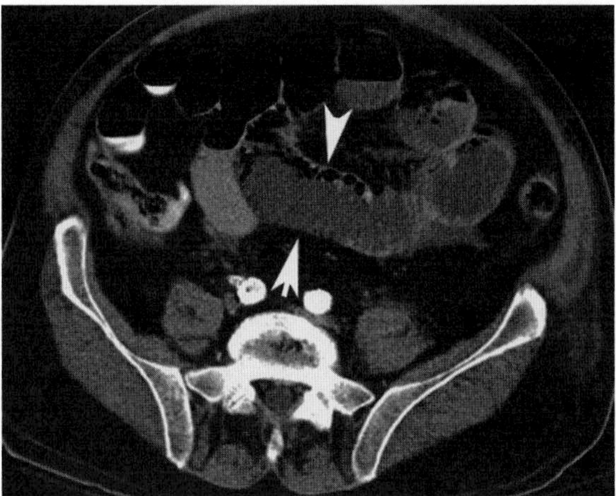

▲ **Figure 9–11.** Mesenteric ischemia. Axial MDCT image shows lack of enhancement of the small bowel wall (*arrow*) and presence of pneumatosis (*arrowhead*).

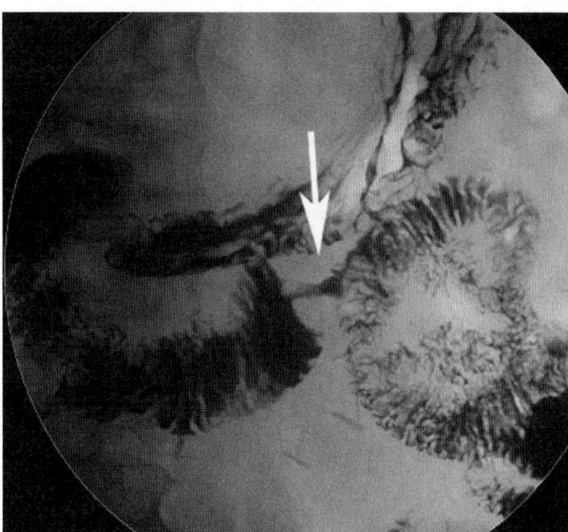

▲ **Figure 9–12.** Duodenal adenocarcinoma. Upright double-contrast upper GI image shows an apple-core lesion (*arrow*) at the level of the third portion of the duodenum.

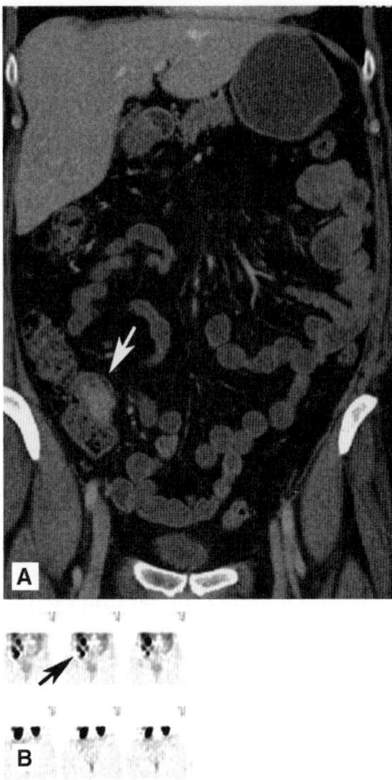

▲ **Figure 9–13.** Ileal carcinoid. **A:** Coronal CT enterography image shows a hypervascular mass (*arrow*) in the wall of the terminal ileum. **B:** Selected images from an octreotide nuclear medicine study show increased uptake of the tracer in the terminal ileum (*arrow*).

(GISTs) are estimated to comprise 9% of all small bowel neoplasms. They typically appear as large, bulky masses. Central necrosis and ulceration are common. MDCT imaging may be especially helpful in defining the exact site of origin and helping the surgeon plan for resection and, more importantly, may improve the capability of CT to detect small lesions.

Sailer J, Zacherl J, Schima W. MDCT of small bowel tumours. *Cancer Imaging.* 2007;17:224–233. [PMID: 18083648]

G. Miscellaneous Conditions

Several uncommon small bowel abnormalities, such as graft versus host disease, diverticulitis, radiation enteritis, intussusception, hernia, and volvulus, may be better visualized using multiplanar MDCT images than SBFT. On CT, the key to the diagnosis of radiation enteritis is the presence of abnormal findings only in the bowel loops localized to the area corresponding to the radiation port. Inguinal hernias can be either direct or indirect. Indirect hernias are the most common and occur predominantly in males. The peritoneal sac enters the inguinal canal and exits at the external ring. Because of their long course, indirect hernias can become incarcerated, leading to bowel obstruction and infarction. Direct hernias are less common and occur when the hernia enters the inguinal canal medial to the inferior epigastric vessels. On CT, finding of abdominal contents (small bowel, sigmoid, rectum, mesenteric fat) in the inguinal canal anterior to the femoral vessels is virtually diagnostic of an inguinal hernia (Figure 9–15).

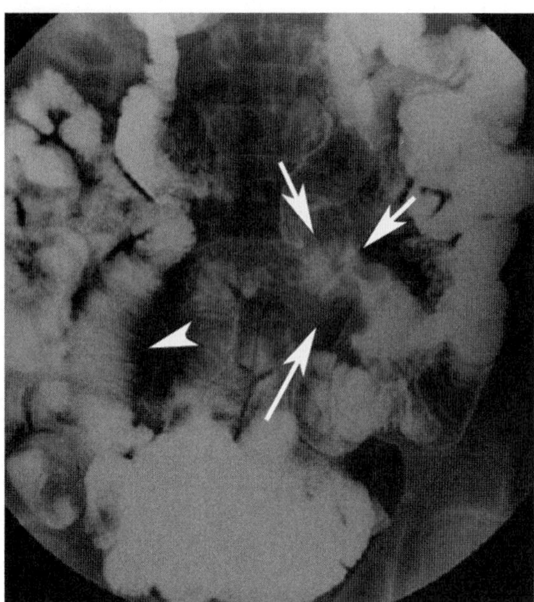

▲ **Figure 9–14.** Small bowel lymphoma in celiac sprue. SBFT image shows an irregular mass in the distal jejunum (*arrows*), mild dilation of small bowel loops, and jejunization of the ileum (*arrowhead*).

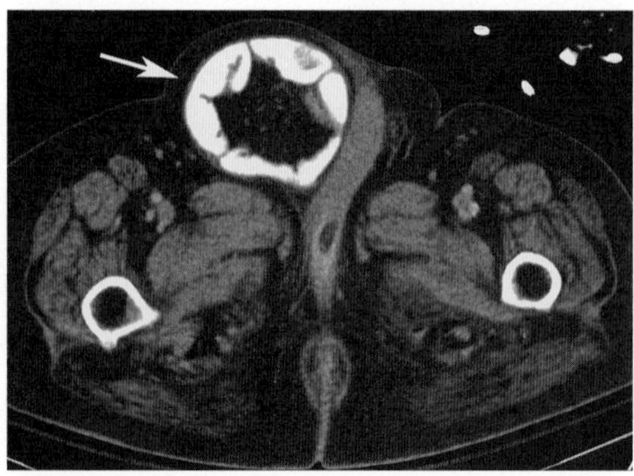

▲ **Figure 9–15.** Inguinal hernia. Axial MDCT image shows the presence of nonobstructed small bowel loops (*arrow*) in a right-sided inguinal hernia.

4. Appendix

A. Imaging Algorithm

Although sonography has proven to be a reliable technique to diagnose acute appendicitis in children and slim patients, it may be significantly limited in obese patients. Moreover, mild inflammatory changes of the appendix as well as retrocecal appendicitis may be missed if the cecum is air filled. In contrast, CT has an accuracy of up to 98% in diagnosing appendicitis and allows for diagnosis of even very mild and early stages of the disease. Furthermore, CT can often diagnose other pathologies that may clinically mimic appendicitis; CT is, therefore, able to decrease significantly the rate of negative appendectomies. Currently, MRI of appendicitis is increasingly used, with excellent accuracy, in pregnant patients presenting with right lower quadrant pain and leukocytosis.

B. Appendicitis

Typical CT findings of appendicitis are a thickened appendix with a diameter of more than 6 mm, an edematous or hyperemic wall of the appendix, infiltration of the surrounding mesenteric fat, and, sometimes, inflammatory changes in the adjacent cecum (Figure 9–16). If an appendolith is present, along with pericecal inflammation, the scan is virtually diagnostic for appendicitis. The presence of inflammation in the surrounding mesenteric fat is reported to have a sensitivity of 100% and a specificity of 80%. Perforation is one of the serious complications that may occur in acute appendicitis, and CT can confirm this diagnosis. In cases with pronounced surrounding fluid collections, perforation should be considered. If extraluminal air can be identified in the peritoneal cavity or in the retroperitoneum or if the fluid collections have already taken on the appearance of a phlegmon or an abscess, perforation can be diagnosed with certainty. Lastly, in complicated cases, CT can be also used to diagnose pylephlebitis or pylephlebitic liver abscesses and for CT-guided abscess drainage in cases in which surgeons prefer to operate electively.

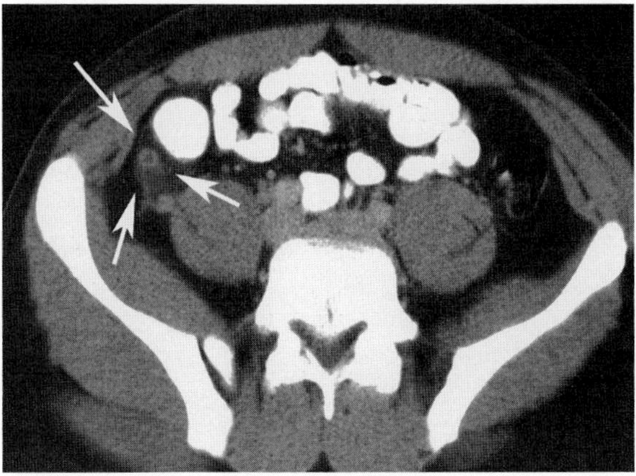

▲ **Figure 9–16.** Appendicitis. Axial MDCT image shows hyperenhancement of the wall of the appendix and periappendiceal fat stranding (*arrows*).

Nitta N, Takahashi M, Furukawa A, et al. MR imaging of the normal appendix and acute appendicitis. *J Magn Reson Imaging.* 2005;21:156–165. [PMID: 15666398]

5. Large Bowel

A. Imaging Algorithm

CT is almost universally accepted as the primary screening modality for the evaluation of patients suspected of having colonic disease. Key advantages of CT over other imaging modalities include the fact that CT not only allows accurate demonstration of the colonic wall but also outlines the pericolonic tissues and adjacent structures. CT can help assess infectious and inflammatory conditions, as well as facilitate diagnosis and staging of colonic neoplasms. The latter is typically performed using a dedicated CT method, known as CT colonography or virtual colonoscopy.

CT colonography has several advantages over optical colonoscopy: no sedation is needed, it is only minimally invasive, and the examination is less time consuming. However, there is still a need for bowel cleansing and insufflation of gas to expand the colon. Moreover, exposure to radiation is inherent to CT, and there is no possibility of biopsy or polypectomy or treatment. Failed optical colonoscopy or a medical contraindication for endoscopy is a good indication for CT colonography. There is still substantial debate about the usefulness of CT colonography as a general screening tool for colonic polyps and colorectal cancer.

MR colonography is performed using contrast within the colonic lumen, resulting in increased and decreased signal intensity accordingly to the contrast used.

Remaining indications for single- and double-contrast barium enema are rapidly declining and are typically reserved for the postoperative patient, to detect strictures, fistula formation, or anastomotic leaks.

Ajaj W, Goyen W. MR imaging of the colon: "technique, indications, results and limitations." *Eur J Radiol.* 2007;61:415–423. [PMID: 17145153]

B. CT Colonography Technique

Optimal CT colonography technique requires careful cleansing and distention of the colon. Residual stool causes problems similar to those encountered with barium enema as it simulates polyps or masses. In theory, any preparation that results in a clean colon will suffice. Stool markers (mostly barium, eg, Tagitol) or iodine can be administered orally 24–48 hours before CT to improve differentiation of soft tissue intraluminal lesions and retained stool. This technique is called fecal tagging.

Three-dimensional endoluminal images are useful to confirm the presence of a lesion and to improve diagnostic confidence. Most investigators use a primary two-dimensional (2D) interpretation with so-called lumen tracking, starting from the rectum and following the course of the bowel from slice to slice to the cecum. Primary 3D endoluminal assessment of the colon (endoluminal "fly-through") is less often performed as it is more time consuming and more susceptible to pitfalls. It is imperative that the 2D images be reviewed by using colon window settings (approximately W: 1600, C: –400). In addition, soft tissue windows must be used for further characterization of suspected lesions and when searching for extracolonic abnormalities.

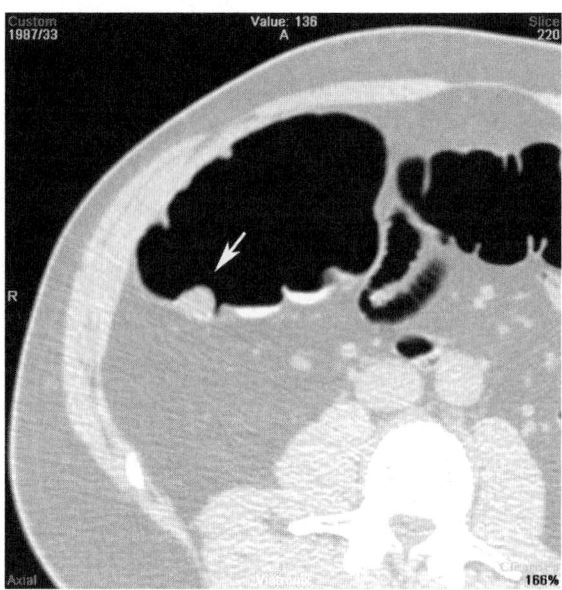

▲ **Figure 9–17.** Colonic polyp. Axial MDCT image displayed in a "colon" window shows a 1.2-cm polyp (*arrow*) in the ascending colon. (For corresponding 3D endoluminal reconstructed image, see Plate 5.)

C. Polyps and Malignancies

The majority of colorectal cancers are believed to arise within benign adenomatous polyps and follow the adenoma-carcinoma sequence. The duration of this sequence is very long (±10 years) and the removal of these precursor adenomatous polyps decreases the risk for lethal colorectal cancer significantly.

The aim of colorectal imaging and screening is to detect early malignancies or premalignant lesions (see Chapter 22). Colorectal polyps appear as round, oval, or lobulated intraluminal projections and are homogeneous in attenuation (Figure 9–17 and Plate 5). Most large colorectal carcinomas appear as fungating masses, often causing luminal narrowing (Figure 9–18). Flat colorectal adenomas and carcinomas are difficult to identify, not only on 3D endoluminal images, but also on thin 2D images. It is important to remember that the adenomatous polyp (particularly advanced lesions) is the primary target of screening. Because the prevalence of malignancy is extremely low in lesions smaller than 10 mm (only 1%), this could be a good target. Patients with polyps larger than 10 mm should undergo immediate colonoscopy for excision of the lesion. Diminutive filling defects (<5 mm) can represent normal mucosal protrusion, adherent fecal material, hyperplastic polyps, or small adenomatous polyps. The clinical significance of missing a diminutive adenoma is probably minimal, and the question can be asked whether these very small polyps (<5 mm) should be reported at all. What about lesions between 5 and 9 mm? This remains a dilemma. Most gastroenterologists remove these lesions when endoscopically visualized.

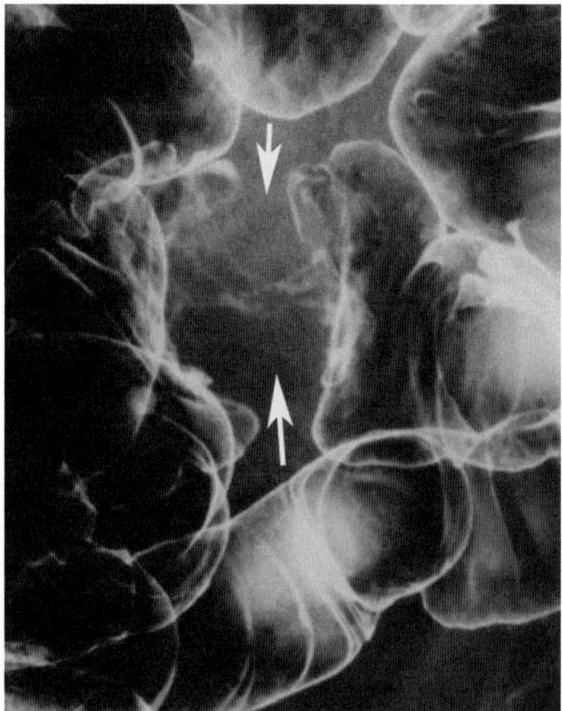

▲ **Figure 9–18.** Colon cancer. Double-contrast barium enema image shows an apple-core lesion in the sigmoid colon with irregularity of the mucosal lining (*arrows*).

D. Inflammatory Bowel Disease

Both patients with Crohn disease and those with ulcerative colitis may have isolated colonic disease. Many of the imaging features used to diagnose inflammatory bowel disease on

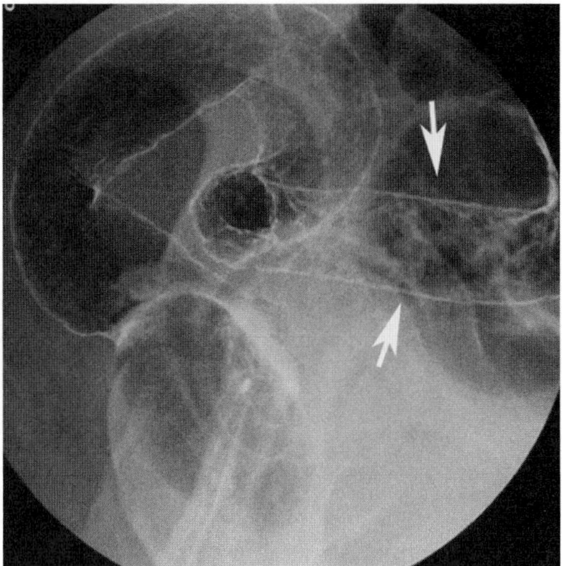

▲ **Figure 9–19.** Ulcerative colitis. Double-contrast barium enema image shows numerous contrast-filled superficial ulcerations (*arrows*) with loss of normal colonic haustrations.

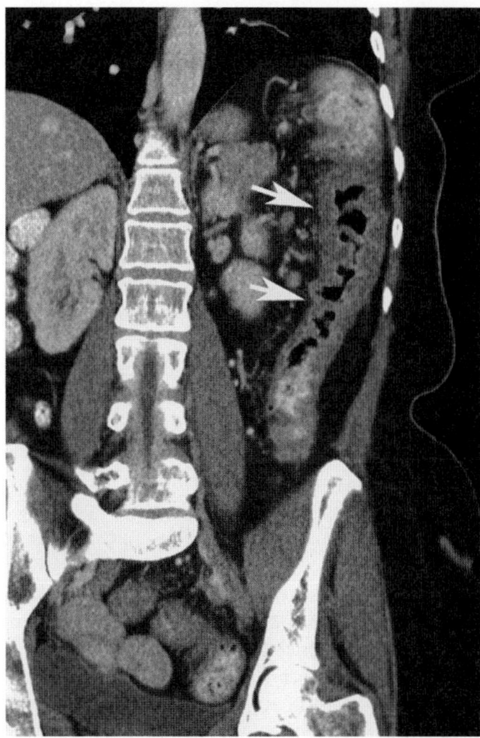

▲ **Figure 9–20.** Ulcerative colitis. Coronal MDCT image shows mild symmetric wall thickening (*arrows*) of the left colon with associated lymphadenopathy in the mesocolon.

CT are derived from the appearance of the colon at barium enema examinations. Double-contrast enemas and optical colonoscopy are superior to CT for demonstrating superficial changes in the mucosa (Figure 9–19). Despite considerable overlap between the CT features seen in Crohn disease and ulcerative colitis, some differentiating findings can be detected. In Crohn disease, the wall thickening is eccentric or asymmetric, typically along the mesenteric border; the rectum is typically spared; the distribution of disease is typically discontinuous and involves mainly the right-sided colon; the wall thickening is usually greater than 10 mm; and pericolonic phlegmon formation and presence of sinus tracts and fistulas are common. In ulcerative colitis, the wall is typically symmetrically thickened; the wall measures less than 10 mm; the rectum is always involved; the distribution of disease is continuous and mainly involves the left colon; and pericolonic abnormalities are rare (Figure 9–20).

E. Infectious Conditions

Pseudomembranous colitis is a toxin-mediated disease without evidence of microbial invasion into the bowel wall. The causative organism is *Clostridium difficile*, and disease occurs typically after antibiotic use. On CT, pseudomembranous colitis usually manifests as marked bowel wall thickening (average, 15 mm). The thickening is homogeneously low in attenuation due to edema. Contrast material insinuating between the large pseudomembranes of pseudomembranous colitis, also known as the "accordion" sign, is considered relatively specific.

Typhlitis classically occurs in neutropenic patients receiving chemotherapy to treat leukemia. Mechanisms probably related to its occurrence include infection with CMV, neoplastic infiltration, ischemia, and mucosal hemorrhage. The disease usually presents acutely with abdominal right lower quadrant pain, fever, and bloody diarrhea. Pathologically, typhlitis is characterized by cecal wall edema and inflammation, frequently also involving the ascending colon and terminal ileum. In more advanced disease, bowel wall necrosis and perforation may be present. Because barium enema or colonoscopy carries a high risk for bowel perforation in these patients, CT is the imaging modality of choice for the diagnosis of neutropenic colitis. Typically, a circumferential thickening of the cecum is detected along with inflammatory changes in the adjacent mesenteric fat. Due to extensive edema, the affected bowel wall is hypoattenuating. Complications important to recognize include intramural perforation with pneumatosis, transmural necrosis with pneumoperitoneum, and pericolic abscesses because they indicate a need for urgent surgical intervention.

Thoeni RF, Cello JP. CT imaging of colitis. *Radiology*. 2006;250: 623–638. [PMID: 16926320]

F. Ischemic Colitis (See Chapter 6)

The spectrum of ischemic lesions in the colon ranges from mild, superficial necrosis and mucosal hemorrhage to total transmural infarction, with or without perforation. Acute occlusion of mesenteric vessels due to thromboembolism, dissection, or arteriosclerosis is a well-known cause that may lead to severe ischemic damage or even infarction of the large bowel. Although all these conditions are due to partial or total extrinsic or intrinsic vascular occlusion, ischemic colitis is most commonly caused by nonocclusive reduction of the blood supply. If blood pressure falls in hypovolemic, cardiogenic, or septic shock, systemic and local regulatory mechanisms try to preserve blood supply to the brain, heart, and muscles by, among other means, reducing intestinal perfusion dramatically. As a result, intestinal ischemia may develop, especially around the watershed areas at the splenic flexure or in the rectosigmoid. Rarely and especially in younger patients, such nonocclusive ischemic colitis may also appear in the cecum and ascending colon.

On CT, colonic ischemia may be diffuse or localized, segmental, or even focal. Imaging findings may include wall thickening, fold enlargement, or loss of haustra in the affected bowel segments (due to the submucosal edema, hemorrhage, or both). If edema is dominating, the affected segment will present with a more hypodense wall thickening and a shaggy inner layer. In contrast, the wall thickening will appear hyperdense if mucosal and submucosal hemorrhage or reactive hyperperfusion are dominating. Following the administration of iodinated contrast material, the ischemic bowel wall may show heterogeneous or even absent wall enhancement with zones of low attenuation. Sometimes, discrete findings such as pericolic streakiness may be found in the surrounding mesenteric fat. Although wall thickening is the most common finding, it seems that decreased or even absent wall enhancement is the most specific CT finding for bowel ischemia (Figure 9–21).

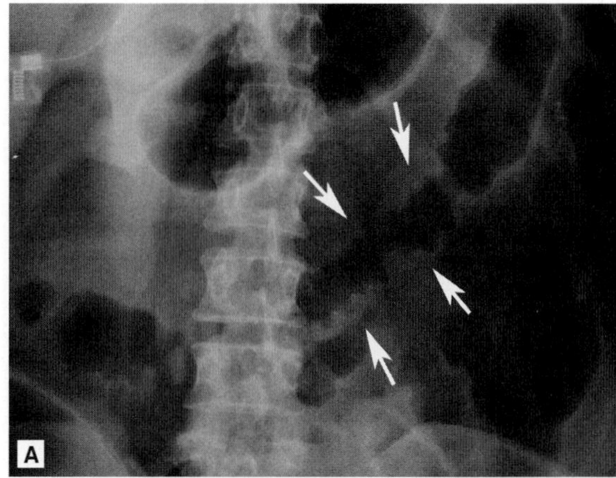

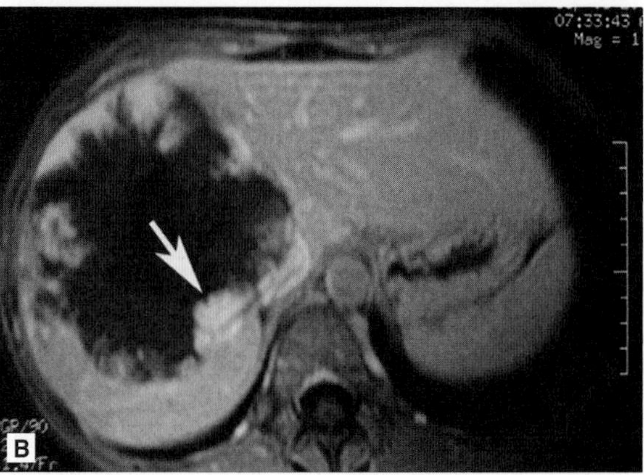

▲ **Figure 9–21.** Ischemic colitis. **A:** KUB (kidney, ureter, bladder) image shows wall thickening (*arrows*) of the transverse colon with thumbprinting. **B:** Axial MDCT image shows thickening of the wall of the left colon (*arrow*) with lack of wall enhancement.

6. Anorectum

A. Imaging Algorithm

Clinical history and physical examination under anesthesia often are sufficient for the diagnosis of perianal fistula. The major role of imaging is in establishing the relation of the fistula to the anal sphincter and related structures. MRI assessment of perianal fistula provides important anatomic and pathologic information required to guide surgical management. MRI is the investigation of choice in accurately classifying perianal fistulas.

MRI was first introduced for staging of anorectal cancer in 1986. MRI has been used increasingly because it gives more information for preoperative staging than any other diagnostic method. It can show a clear relationship between the rectal cancer and the rectal wall and any adjacent pelvic organ. It can also show the status of the lateral pelvic lymph nodes and any involvement of pelvic floor muscles beyond the reach of transrectal ultrasonography. MRI is also valuable as it is able to provide surgeons with information regarding the presence of sphincter invasion and the surrounding structures in patients with distal rectal cancer, which is important for making a decision on whether to perform sphincter preservation surgery or not.

MRI of the anal sphincter muscles using an endoanal coil has been applied to study the integrity of the anal sphincters in patients with fecal incontinence. The external anal sphincter muscle and pelvic floor muscles are clearly visualized, and muscle atrophy and tears may be detected accurately.

Pelvic floor weakness is characterized by abnormal symptomatic displacement of pelvic organs. It represents a complex clinical problem most commonly seen in middle-aged and elderly parous women. Fluoroscopic colpocystodefecography has been proven to surpass physical examination in the detection and characterization of functional abnormalities of the anorectum and surrounding pelvic structures. Similarly, MR defecography appears to be an accurate imaging technique to assess clinically relevant pelvic floor abnormalities. Moreover, MR defecography negates the need to expose the patient to harmful ionizing radiation and allows excellent depiction of the surrounding soft tissues of the pelvis.

B. Perianal Fistula

Perianal disease encompasses a wide range of conditions including skin tags, ulceration, fissures, abscesses, and fistulas. Fistulas associated with Crohn disease tend to be complex, with secondary extensions and abscesses; as a result, their diagnosis and treatment can be particularly challenging. Accurate anatomic mapping and the identification of abscesses are imperative as this determines the outcome of both medical and surgical treatment. The preferred investigation for perianal disease depends in part on local expertise, facilities available, and patient tolerance. High soft tissue contrast resolution, multiplanar capability, and lack of ionizing radiation all make MRI a well-suited examination for the diagnosis of perianal Crohn disease. Imaging can be supplemented with dynamic intravenous gadolinium-enhanced sequences and by MR fistulography. T1-weighted images provide anatomic information of the sphincter complex and demonstrate active fistulas as low signal with enhancement post-gadolinium administration. The active fistula track is of high signal on T2-weighting (Figure 9–22).

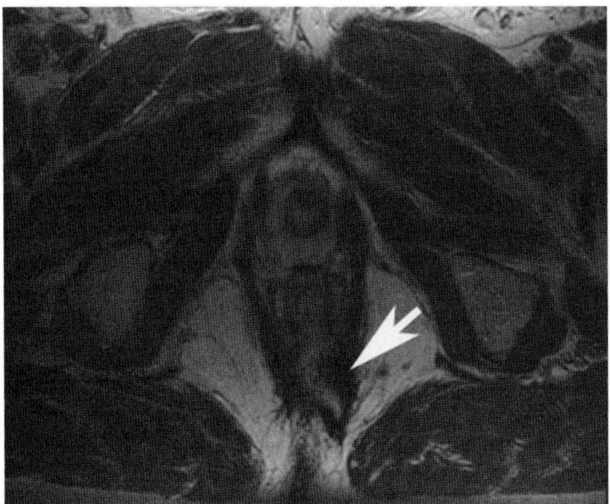

▲ **Figure 9–22.** Anal fistula. Axial T2-weighted MR image shows the presence of a fluid-filled hyperintense fistula (*arrow*) that transgresses the external anal sphincter.

Fistula appearance is accentuated by using fat suppression techniques, which eliminate the high signal from fat in the pelvis thus maximizing tissue contrast. Inactive fistulas have low signal on T2-weighted images. Fistulas can be classified according to the Parks classification, a surgically based classification, to provide the surgeon with a road map, which should minimize both operative trauma to the anal sphincters and subsequent recurrence. Fistulas can also be classified according to the St James's University Hospital classification, which is an MRI-based classification.

Recently, there has been a shift in emphasis in the use of radiology in perianal Crohn disease. Traditionally, its indication was confined to the diagnosis and mapping of disease preoperatively. However, the development of the drug infliximab has resulted in a role for radiology in monitoring response to therapy.

Sahni VA, Ahmad R, Burling D. Which method is best for imaging of perianal fistula? *Abdom Imaging.* 2008;33:26–30. [PMID: 17805919]

C. Neoplasms

Transrectal ultrasound (TRUS) has been applied to the staging of rectal cancer for many years. Its ability to visualize the different layers of the rectal wall was its main strength. The main problem with TRUS is the overstaging of T2 tumors due to the extensive peritumoral tissue reaction surrounding the growing tumor. TRUS has some other limitations, such as operator dependency, limitation to tumors located 8–10 cm from the anal verge when a rigid probe is used, and inability to assess stenotic tumors or the mesorectal fascia. This may explain the more recent widespread use of MRI as these limitations do not apply to MRI.

The optimal imaging sequences for endoluminal MRI are multiplanar T2-weighted and axial T1-weighted sequences. The T2-weighted images clearly demonstrate normal anorectal anatomy and allow differentiation of the rectal wall layers. T1-weighted imaging is particularly helpful to determine the extent of the lesion in the mesorectal fat. The use of intravenously administered gadolinium may be helpful to determine tumor extent, especially to differentiate T2 from T3 tumors. A drawback of the endorectal MRI technique is that coil insertion can be difficult or impossible in patients with stenosing rectal tumors. The major limitation of endoluminal MRI, however, is its limited ability to detect lymph node metastases. Pelvic MRI for rectal carcinoma uses a phased array coil. These high-resolution images demonstrate local tumor stage (Figure 9–23), and scanning the entire pelvis may be of further help in detecting distant lymphadenopathy.

The preoperative evaluation of a patient with rectal cancer determines the type of surgical approach and the need for chemotherapy and radiotherapy. Tumor size,

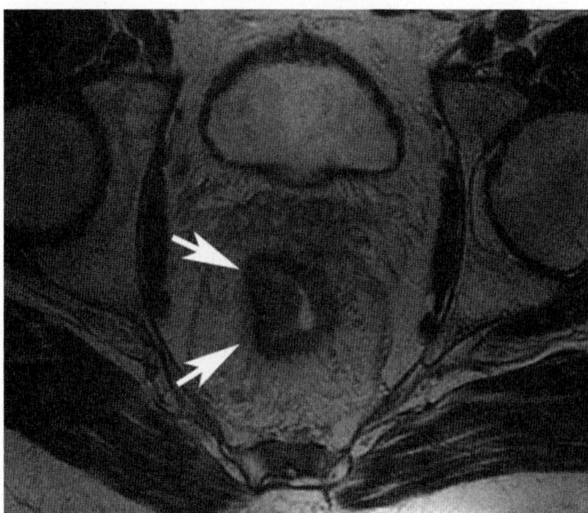

▲ **Figure 9–23.** Rectal cancer. Axial T2-weighted MR image shows a T2 rectal cancer arising from the right lateral wall of the rectum with involvement of the muscularis propria (*arrows*).

local stage, presence of distant metastases, and proximity to the anal sphincter decide which individuals are eligible for local excision and which require either transanal resection or abdominoperineal or low anterior resection. Furthermore, an accurate preoperative assessment and staging of the patient is valuable for the centers administrating neoadjuvant chemoradiotherapy prior to the surgery.

Bipat S, Glas AS, Slors FJ, et al. Rectal cancer: local staging and assessment of lymph node involvement with endoluminal US, CT, and MR imaging—a meta-analysis. *Radiology.* 2004;232: 773–783. [PMID: 15273331]

D. Functional Abnormalities: Pelvic Floor Abnormalities

At present, functional pelvic floor abnormalities represent a common health care problem. These abnormalities result in more than 300,000 surgeries in the United States annually, and it is estimated that approximately 15% of older multiparous women suffer from some sort of pelvic support defect. These conditions often have a significant impact on quality of life and result in a variety of symptoms, including chronic pelvic pain, urinary or fecal incontinence, and constipation. Because physical examination is not a reliable method for evaluating these symptoms, an objective assessment of rectal evacuation that is reproducible and allows quantification is extremely valuable. Fluoroscopic defecography is conventionally used to evaluate functional and anatomic anorectal disorders (Figure 9–24). The development of fast MRI sequences provides a new and better alternative to study all pelvic visceral movements in a dynamic fashion. MR defecography has several important advantages over conventional defecography. First, it avoids exposure of the patient to harmful ionizing radiation. Second, it provides excellent soft tissue resolution of all pelvic floor compartments and supporting structures, including pelvic floor muscles and fascial planes. Therefore, MR defecography is a much more comprehensive examination that allows assessment of coexisting bladder and uterocervical prolapse, which is vital when planning surgical treatment.

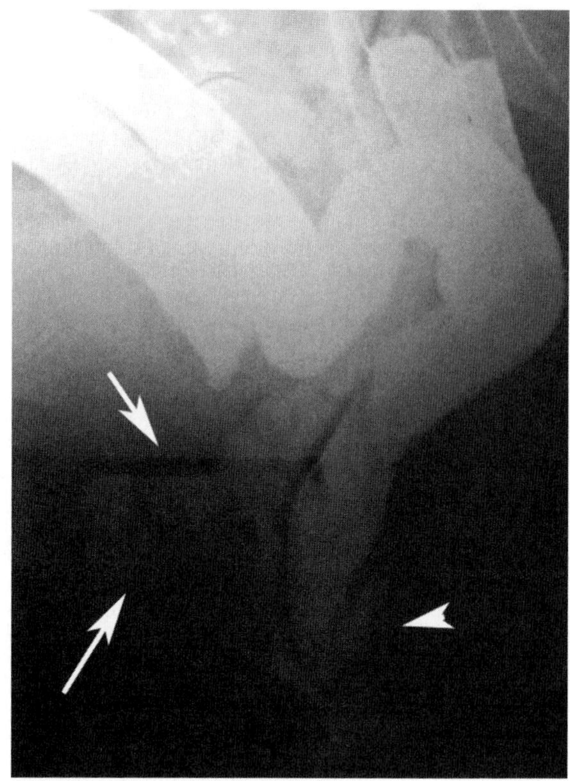

▲ **Figure 9–24.** Rectal intussusception and enterocele. Sagittal image from a fluoroscopic defecography study shows intra-anal rectal intussusception (*arrowhead*) and the presence of a large enterocele (*arrows*).

Mortele KJ, Fairhurst J. Dynamic MR defecography of the posterior compartment: indications, techniques, and MRI features. *Eur J Radiol.* 2007;61:462–472. [PMID: 17145152]

LIVER IMAGING

1. Focal Liver Lesions

A. Imaging Algorithm

Because the clinical implications and therapeutic strategies of focal liver lesions vary tremendously depending on their causes, the ability to differentiate focal hepatic lesions is extremely important. The development of both dynamic multiphasic CT and fast MRI and the ability to use tailored MR techniques (such as fat-suppression sequences and in/out phase imaging) have facilitated assessment of the morphologic and hemodynamic features of liver tumors. In the majority of cases, familiarity with the most relevant CT and MRI features, in combination with additional clinical information, provides enough information for adequate lesion characterization. MRI is typically used as a problem-solving tool in cases where CT remains inconclusive.

B. Benign Liver Lesions (See Chapter 49)

Hepatic cysts are developmental anomalies present in 2.5% of the population. They can be either solitary or multiple as part of hepatorenal polycystic disease. Hepatic cysts are well defined and anechoic on ultrasound, homogeneously hypodense on nonenhanced CT scans, and show no enhancement following administration of contrast. On MRI, hepatic cysts reveal very low signal intensity on T1-weighted and very high signal intensity on T2-weighted images, especially heavily T2-weighted images. They are typically round or ovoid shaped, well delineated, without a capsule, and lack enhancement following gadolinium administration.

Hemangioma is the most common benign hepatic tumor. Hemangiomas are usually solitary (80%), measure less than 4 cm in diameter, and are most often peripherally located. A giant hemangioma is larger than 10 cm in diameter and often contains a central cleft-like area of fibrosis or cystic degeneration. Typical hemangiomas appear homogeneously hyperechoic on ultrasound with acoustic enhancement. The classic appearance on CT is that of a well-defined hypodense lesion showing foci of peripheral globular enhancement during early phase imaging after contrast administration. On delayed images, the mass usually shows a centripetal fill-in with persistent delayed enhancement. MRI findings in hemangiomas reflect their vascular nature. On T1- and T2-weighted images, the lesions show decreased and markedly increased signal intensity, respectively. Dynamic T1-weighted imaging obtained following administration of gadolinium also shows a peripheral nodular centripetal enhancement pattern progressing to homogeneity. In 94% of the large hemangiomas, however, a persistent hypointense center is present on the delayed images due to variable degree of fibrosis and cystic degeneration (Figure 9–25).

Focal nodular hyperplasia (FNH) is a rare (3%) benign tumor predominantly diagnosed in asymptomatic women during the third to fifth decades of life. The size of FNH ranges between 0.5 and 15 cm with an average of 5 cm in greatest dimension. On CT, FNH is classically seen as a solitary hypodense area with immediate intense enhancement (96%) and homogeneity (85%) after contrast material injection. The presence of an enhancing central scar has been reported to occur in 14–43% of cases (Figure 9–26A). Typical MRI features of FNH are isodensity on T1- and T2-weighted images, homogeneity (96%), hypervascularity, and the presence of a central scar, which is hyperintense on T2-weighted images due to its vascular and biliary components and presence of myxoid stroma (Figure 9–26B).

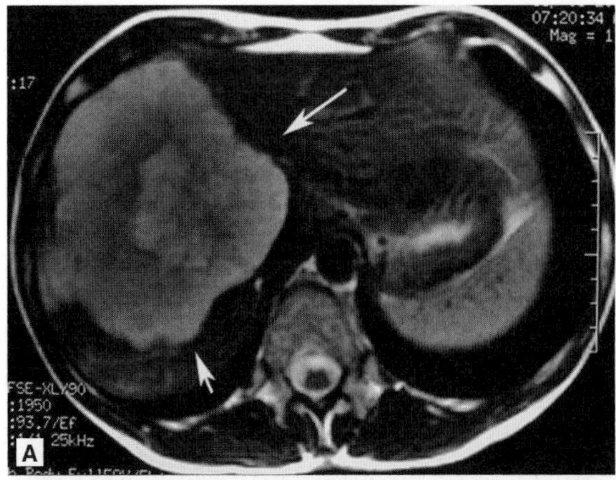

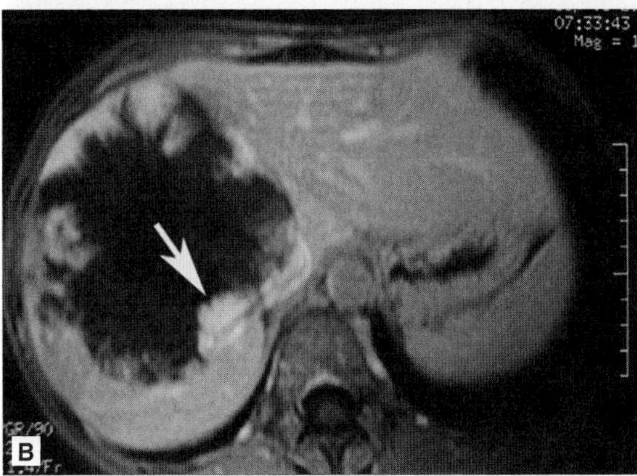

▲ **Figure 9–25.** Hepatic hemangioma. **A:** T2-weighted axial MR image shows a well-defined hyperintense mass (*arrows*) in the right lobe of the liver. **B:** Contrast-enhanced T1-weighted axial MR image shows peripheral nodular incomplete enhancement (*arrow*) of the lesion.

Hepatic adenoma is a rare benign neoplasm associated with oral contraceptive use and most commonly seen in women of childbearing age. Adenomas are usually solitary, and the presence of intratumoral fatty infiltration, necrosis, hemorrhage, peliotic changes, a capsule, and central scar are common pathologic features. Unenhanced CT usually reveals

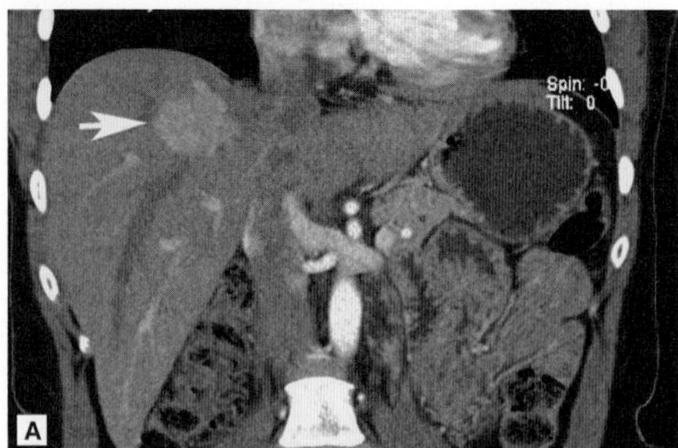

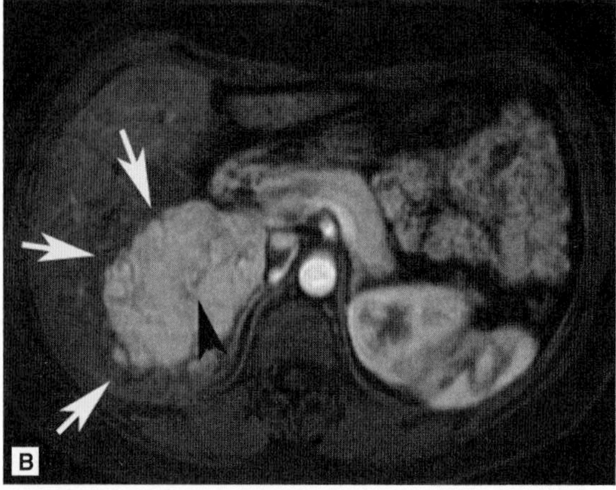

▲ **Figure 9–26.** Focal nodular hyperplasia. **A:** Coronal MDCT image shows a homogeneous, lobulated, hypervascular mass in the liver (*arrow*). **B:** Contrast-enhanced T1-weighted axial MR image shows a homogeneous hypervascular mass (*arrows*) with the presence of a central scar (*black arrowhead*).

a neoplasm that is slightly more hypodense than surrounding liver. Hyperdense foci represent intratumoral hemorrhage. Following contrast administration, they usually enhance early and appear heterogeneous and strong due to their hypervascular nature (Figure 9–27). MRI classically shows a heterogeneous (93%) mass, with predominantly hyperintense signal intensity on T2-weighted images (47–75%), and variable signal intensity on T1-weighted images, according to fatty changes (25%), hemorrhage (38%), and necrosis (16%). On dynamic gadolinium-enhanced T1-weighted images, 86% of adenomas show early arterial enhancement. Small lesions tend to enhance homogeneously during the arterial phase with early washout of contrast material.

Mortele KJ, Ros PR. Benign liver neoplasms. *Clin Liver Dis.* 2002;6:119–145. [PMID: 11933585]

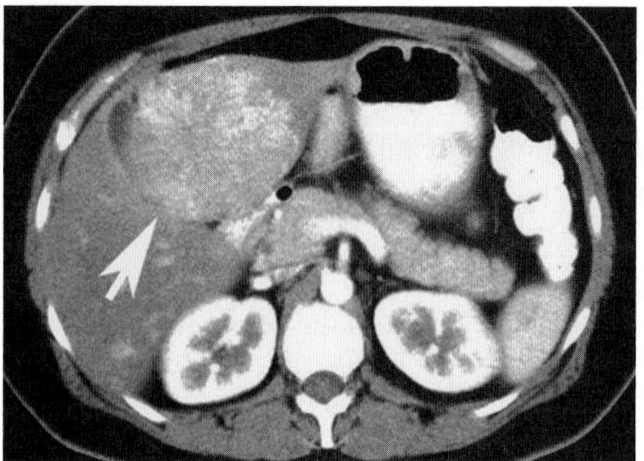

▲ **Figure 9–27.** Hepatic adenoma. Axial MDCT image shows a large heterogeneously hyperenhancing mass (*arrow*) in segment IV of the liver.

C. Malignant Liver Lesions (See Chapter 49)

Hepatocellular carcinoma is the most common primary epithelial neoplasm of the liver. In classical cases, it presents on unenhanced CT, in a patient with underlying cirrhosis, as a hypodense mass. Following the administration of contrast material, smaller lesions tend to be hypervascular (with early hyperdense enhancement) and larger lesions more hypovascular (revealing a mosaic-like enhancement pattern) (Figure 9–28). Signs of vascular invasion and arterial-portal shunting are frequently present. On T2-weighted MRI

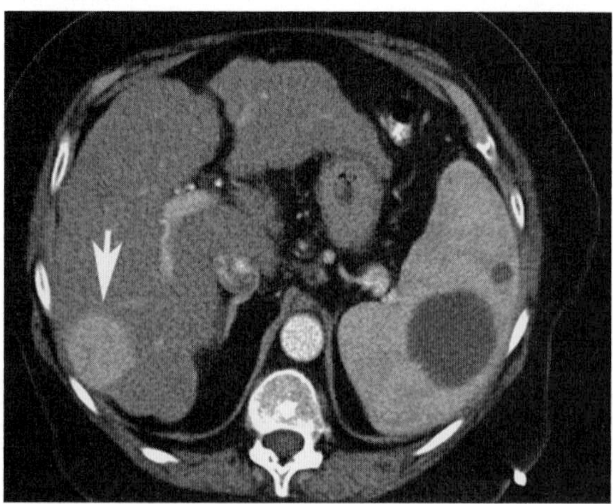

▲ **Figure 9–28.** Hepatocellular carcinoma. Axial MDCT image shows a round homogeneous and hypervascular mass in the right lobe of the liver (*arrow*) in a patient with underlying cirrhosis.

images, typical cases of hepatocellular carcinoma demonstrate a mild hyperintensity relative to normal liver. The variable signal intensity seen on T1-weighted images depends on the presence or absence of glycogen, steatosis, or hemorrhage. High signal intensity on T2-weighted images is especially meaningful in the setting of underlying cirrhosis for the differential diagnosis with dysplastic nodules. The latter typically have a low intensity on T2-weighted images due to accumulation of iron. Following intravenous administration of gadolinium, enhancement patterns similar to those seen on CT are described (Figure 9–29).

Intrahepatic cholangiocarcinoma (I-CAC) is relatively uncommon, although it is the second most common primary hepatic malignant neoplasm. Some underlying liver diseases, such as Caroli disease, primary sclerosing cholangitis, and clonorchiasis, may favor the development of I-CAC. The average age of the patients with I-CAC ranges from 50 to 60 years. Because of the peripheral localization relative to the bile ducts, jaundice is seldom present at presentation. On CT, I-CAC usually presents as a large hypoattenuating mass (6–10 cm), irregularly delineated, with satellite nodules (62%), and sometimes a central scar. Other MRI features of I-CAC are encasement of the portal vein, usually without evidence of thrombus (25–75%), focal liver atrophy (43%), dilation of peripheral intrahepatic bile ducts (29%), capsular retraction (21%), and small calcifications.

Metastases. Neoplastic infiltration due to metastatic disease can occur with many primary tumors. CT appearances of hepatic metastases depend on the vascularity of the lesions compared with the normal liver parenchyma. Hypovascular lesions, such as metastases of colorectal adenocarcinoma, show a lower attenuation compared with normal liver and are best detected on portal venous phase contrast-enhanced images (Figure 9–30). Hypervascular metastases, including

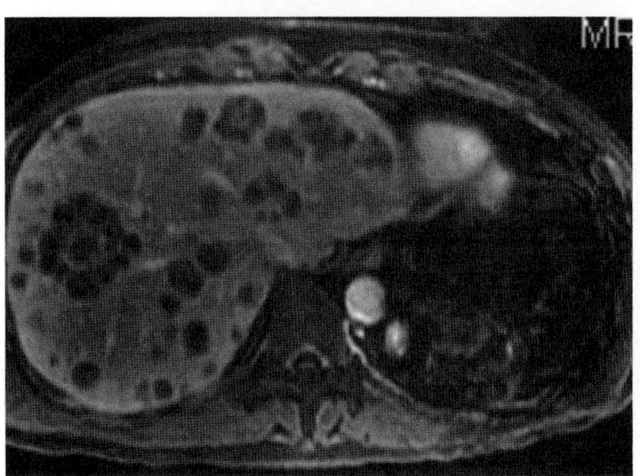

▲ **Figure 9–30.** Colorectal cancer metastases. Contrast-enhanced T1-weighted axial MR image shows numerous hypovascular masses scattered throughout the liver.

those from endocrine tumors, melanoma, sarcoma, renal cell carcinoma, and certain subtypes of breast and lung carcinoma, enhance more rapidly than normal liver and require arterial phase imaging for accurate depiction. Infrequently, metastatic involvement is very discrete and only detectable through indirect features, such as diffuse parenchymal heterogeneity, vascular and architectural distortion, or alterations of the liver contour. The latter, especially seen in breast cancer patients, has been reported as the so-called "pseudocirrhosis sign." Other suggestive features that may be seen with both small and large metastases include central amorphous calcifications in mucinous primary malignancies, "peripheral washout" sign during the delayed phase, capsular retraction, and presence of biliary or vascular invasion. On MRI, hepatic metastases are typically moderately hyperintense on T2-weighted images, are hypointense on T1-weighted images, and appear hypointense or hyperintense following gadolinium administration, depending on their vascularity. Hepatospecific contrast agents, such as iron oxide particles, may be useful in the detection of hepatic metastatic disease; because Kupffer cells are not present in metastases, they do not show uptake of contrast medium and hence appear significantly more conspicuous.

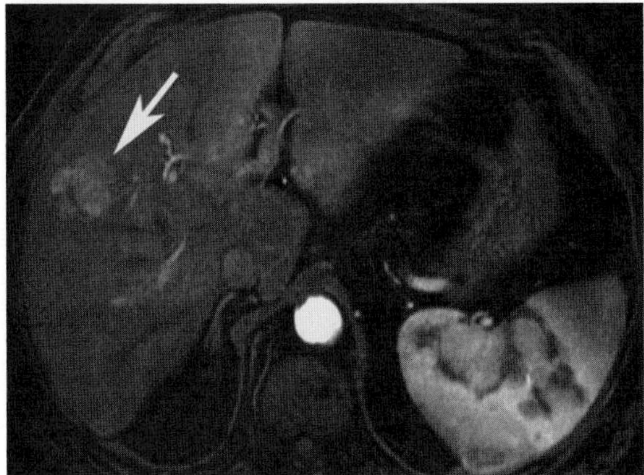

▲ **Figure 9–29.** Hepatocellular carcinoma. Contrast-enhanced T1-weighted axial MR image shows a homogeneous hypervascular mass (*arrow*).

2. Diffuse Liver Diseases

A. Imaging Algorithm

During the last decade, the role of the radiologist in evaluating patients with diffuse liver diseases has increasingly expanded. In some cases, such as fatty liver and iron overload, imaging (especially MRI) may point directly to the diagnosis; in many others, such as hepatitis and cirrhosis, imaging helps in narrowing the differential diagnosis substantially or is crucial in the follow-up of patients.

Mortele KJ, Ros PR. Imaging of diffuse liver disease. *Semin Liver Dis.* 2001;21:195–212. [PMID: 11436572]

B. Cirrhosis

Cirrhosis is a diffuse, progressive process of liver fibrosis, pathologically characterized by architectural distortion and nodular regenerative change. The presence of intrahepatic and extrahepatic imaging findings of cirrhosis (eg, surface nodularity, hepatic morphologic changes, splenomegaly, ascites, portosystemic collaterals) depends on the severity of the cirrhosis (Figure 9–31). Enlargement of the hilar periportal space, in the absence of other conventional signs, has been described as a helpful sign in the diagnosis of early cirrhosis. More pronounced lobar or segmental changes of hepatic morphology such as atrophy of the right hepatic lobe and left medial segment, enlargement of the caudate lobe and left lateral segment, and the expanded gallbladder fossa sign are seen in advanced cirrhosis.

Accurate identification of different types of hepatocellular nodules arising in the cirrhotic liver is crucial. Nowadays, MRI is by far the most specific imaging technique for differentiating those nodules based on characteristic features, such as signal intensity and enhancement pattern. *Regenerative nodules*, like normal liver, invariably have a portal venous blood supply with minimal contribution from the hepatic artery. As a consequence, they are usually isointense with background liver on both T1- and T2-weighted images, and they show no predominant enhancement following gadolinium administration. *Dysplastic nodules* are neoplastic premalignant nodules found in approximately 25% of cirrhotic livers. Similar to regenerative nodules, the main blood supply to dysplastic nodules is from the portal venous system. A dysplastic nodule is typically homogeneously hyperintense on T1-weighted images, hypointense on T2-weighted images, shows a portal-venous phase enhancement, is smaller than 3 cm, and has no capsule. In cases of dysplastic nodules with foci of hepatocellular carcinoma, the classic appearance is that of a "nodule within a nodule," consisting of a high signal intensity focus of hepatocellular carcinoma within a low signal intensity dysplastic nodule on T2-weighted images.

Extrahepatic associated signs of cirrhosis include features of portal hypertension, such as splenomegaly and the formation of portosystemic collateral vessels, and findings related to hepatocellular dysfunction (ascites, bowel wall edema, gallbladder wall thickening). MR angiography provides useful information regarding the presence, location, and flow pattern in portosystemic shunts. These findings are useful both for diagnostic purposes (eg, detection of bleeding varices) and for treatment planning (eg, prior to transjugular intrahepatic portosystemic shunt placement or shunt surgery).

C. Storage Diseases

Hepatic steatosis results from a variety of abnormal metabolic processes. The distribution of steatosis can be variable, ranging from focal, to regional, to diffuse (Figure 9–32). Undoubtedly the most sensitive technique to detect microscopic fatty change of the liver is the use of gradient echo MR pulse sequences. With those, by varying the echo time to image water and fat in and out phase, chemical shift between water and lipid protons can be demonstrated. On out-of-phase images, areas with a significant amount of intracellular fat will show lower signal intensity than on the corresponding in-phase images, and this loss of signal intensity between the

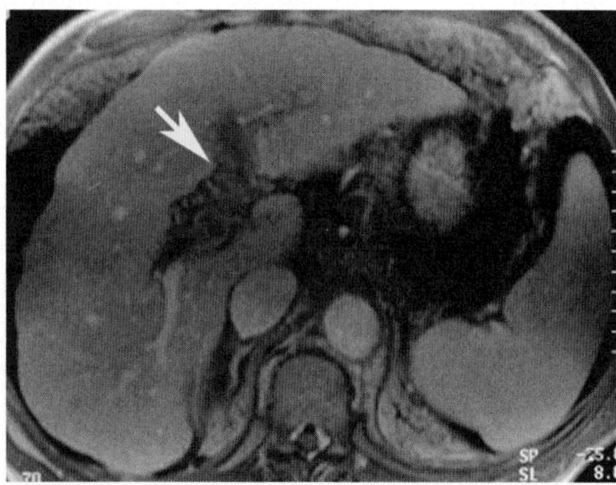

▲ **Figure 9–31.** Cirrhosis. Contrast-enhanced T1-weighted axial MR image shows a nodular contour of the liver, splenomegaly, and ascites. Note portal vein thrombosis (*arrow*).

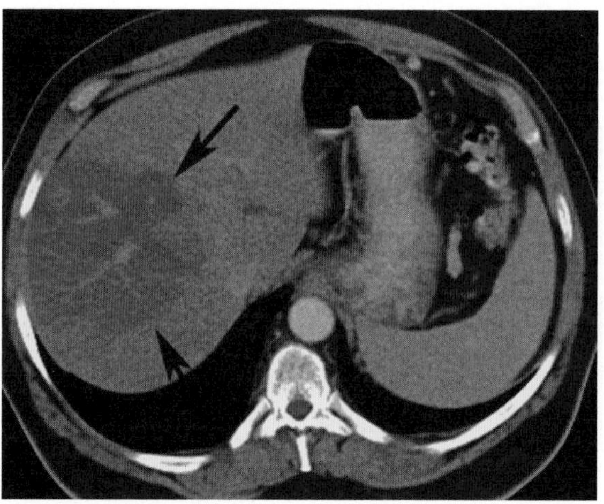

▲ **Figure 9–32.** Steatosis. Axial MDCT image shows a wedge-shaped area of low attenuation (*arrows*) in the right lobe of the liver with vessels coursing through it.

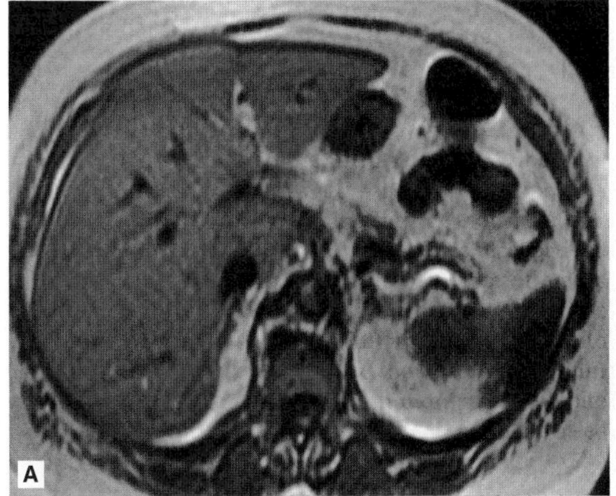

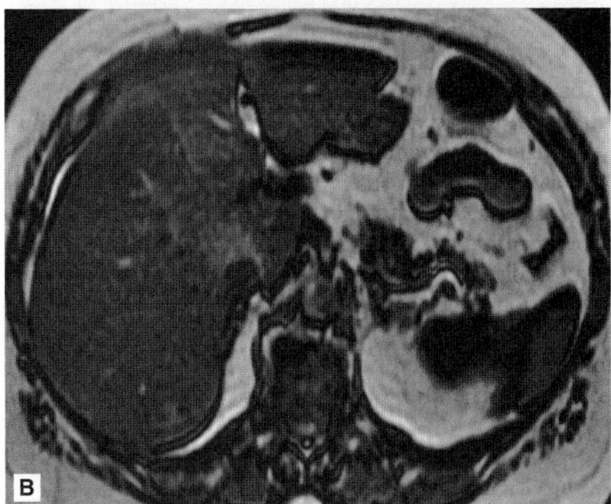

▲ **Figure 9–33.** Steatosis. **A:** Axial in-phase unenhanced T1-weighted MR image shows a normal hyperintense appearance of the liver parenchyma. **B:** Axial out-off-phase unenhanced T1-weighted MR image shows a significant drop in signal of the liver compatible with steatosis.

two types of images allows the radiologist to establish the diagnosis of fatty change of the liver (Figure 9–33). On imaging, several features enable correct identification of focal fatty change or focal spared areas: the typical periligamentous and periportal location, lack of mass effect, sharply angulated boundaries of the area, nonspherical shape, absence of vascular displacement or distortion, and lobar or segmental distribution.

Hereditary or primary hemochromatosis is characterized by excessive deposition of iron into the hepatocytes, pancreatic acinar cells, myocardium, joints, endocrine glands, and skin. MRI is far more specific than any other imaging modality for the characterization of iron overload due to the unique magnetic susceptibility effect of iron. The superparamagnetic effect of accumulated iron in the hepatocytes results in significant reduction of signal intensity of the liver parenchyma on T2-weighted images, particularly T2*-weighted gradient-echo sequences. Comparison of the signal intensity of liver with that of paraspinal muscles, which are normally less intense than liver and not prone to excessive iron accumulation, provides a useful internal control.

In patients with *hemosiderosis or siderosis*, either due to transfusional iron overload states or dyserythropoiesis, the excessive iron is processed and accumulates in organs containing reticuloendothelial cells, including liver, spleen, and bone marrow. As a result, although the distribution of iron in patients with siderosis is demonstrated in the liver as diffuse low signal intensity changes similar to those seen in primary hemochromatosis, extrahepatic signal intensity changes in the spleen and bone marrow enable MRI to distinguish primary hemochromatosis from hemosiderosis.

D. Diffuse Vascular Disorders

Budd-Chiari syndrome is defined as obstruction of the large hepatic venous outflow pathways, typically at the level of the hepatic veins or inferior vena cava (IVC). Imaging findings associated with Budd-Chiari syndrome include direct findings of hepatic venous obstruction, secondary morphologic changes of the liver, and extrahepatic features. Direct diagnostic features are the visualization of intraluminal echogenic or hyperdense material (web, tumor, thrombus) within the hepatic veins or IVC. The absence of hepatic vein flow or presence of flow disturbances on Doppler ultrasound is also diagnostic. Additional features supporting the diagnosis include presence of intrahepatic venous collaterals, nonvisualization of the hepatic veins or IVC, and dilation of the azygos venous system. Indirect morphologic changes in the liver result from the tremendous venous congestion produced by the outflow obstruction. In the acute setting, the peripheral portion of the liver becomes congested and swollen and appears hypoechoic on sonography, hypodense on CT, and hyperintense on T2-weighted images. In contrast, the central portions of the liver, because of the direct drainage into the IVC, show increased enhancement on contrast-enhanced imaging studies. Over time, in the chronic phase, these central portions of the liver become hypertrophic while the periphery of the liver becomes atrophic (Figure 9–34).

Veno-occlusive disease is another cause of hepatic outflow obstruction but differs from Budd-Chiari syndrome in that veno-occlusive disease involves inflammation and obstruction of the postsinusoidal venules. Hepatic veno-occlusive disease is usually associated with prior full-body chemoradiation in leukemia patients or certain herbal medications and tea ("bush tea" disease). On imaging, the liver appears congested and enhances heterogeneously (mosaic-like). The hepatic veins and IVC, although narrowed due to the hepatic edema, are patent, and no morphologic hepatic changes are identified.

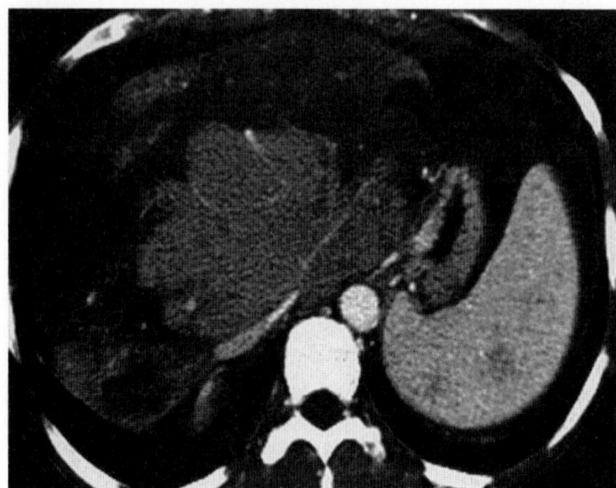

▲ **Figure 9–34.** Budd-Chiari syndrome. Axial MDCT image shows enlargement and hyperenhancement of the caudate lobe with congestion and atrophy of the periphery of the liver. Note the presence of ascites.

Passive hepatic congestion is typically caused by right-sided heart failure. Although the liver also shows a heterogeneous mosaic-like enhancement in patients with passive congestion, it can be easily differentiated from Budd-Chiari syndrome and veno-occlusive disease, because in passive hepatic congestion, the IVC and hepatic veins are abnormally dilated due to reflux of blood from the heart.

BILIARY IMAGING

1. Stone Disease (See Chapter 53)

A. Imaging Algorithm

Ultrasound is still the modality of choice for the evaluation of the gallbladder and biliary ductal system. Ultrasound is fast, readily available, and noninvasive, and does not use ionizing radiation. However, ultrasound also has some inherent limitations; these include the dependence of diagnostic accuracy on the skill of the operator, body habitus, bowel gas interference, and patient cooperation. Because many biliary stones do not contain a sufficient amount of calcium, CT performs very poorly in the detection of gallstones and choledocholithiasis. However, thin-section unenhanced CT imaging may be useful in detecting partially calcified ductal stones. CT cholangiography is a relatively novel technique that provides high-resolution images of the biliary tree based on thin-section MDCT after the intravenous administration of a biliary contrast agent.

MRI has an increasing role in the routine workup of patients with suspected choledocholithiasis when compared with ultrasound or CT. Today, in the initial diagnostic workup of choledocholithiasis, especially in patients with low and intermediate probability of having common bile duct stones, MRCP has replaced the use of diagnostic endoscopic retrograde cholangiopancreatography (ERCP) in many institutions. Compared with ERCP, MRCP offers several advantages, such as noninvasiveness and short examination times. It avoids a variety of possible complications, including pancreatitis and hemorrhage, which occur in 5% of ERCP attempts. Unlike ERCP, MRCP does not expose patients to ionizing radiation or iodinated contrast material. It can be performed in patients in whom it is almost impossible to perform ERCP due to anatomic alterations from previous surgery. Nevertheless, the major strength of ERCP is the access it offers for therapeutic interventions; unlike ERCP, MRCP is a purely diagnostic technique.

Bennett GL, Balthazar EJ. Ultrasound and CT evaluation of emergent gallbladder pathology. *Radiol Clin North Am.* 2003;41:1203–1216. [PMID: 14661666]

Levy AD, Murakata LA, Abbott RM, et al. From the archives of the AFIP. Benign tumors and tumorlike lesions of the gallbladder and extrahepatic bile ducts: radiologic-pathologic correlation. Armed Forces Institute of Pathology. *Radiographics.* 2002;22:387–413. [PMID: 11896229]

Mortele KJ, Wiesner W, Cantisani V, et al. Usual and unusual causes of extrahepatic cholestasis: assessment with magnetic resonance cholangiography and fast MRI. *Abdom Imaging.* 2004;29:87–99. [PMID: 15160760]

B. Cholelithiasis and Choledocholithiasis (See Chapter 53)

Gallstones. In approximately 80% of gallstones, the main component is cholesterol, and 10% of these are pure cholesterol stones. The term *pigment stone* is used for gallstones that contain calcium bilirubinate as the major component and less than 25% cholesterol. The other constituent, calcium carbonate, is relatively less common. Only approximately 15–20% of gallstones contain enough calcium to be demonstrable on plain radiographs. Ultrasound has 95% sensitivity for the detection of cholelithiasis. A gallstone can be diagnosed with certainty when a mobile hyperechoic intraluminal filling defect is identified along with acoustic shadowing (Figure 9–35). CT detects only approximately 80% of gallstones seen via sonography. In depicting cholelithiasis, MRCP with conventional MRI has sensitivity comparable to sonography (90–95%). It is especially useful when sonography results are equivocal or there is a clinical suspicion of diseases of adjacent organs, such as pancreatitis. Furthermore, common bile duct stones can be detected with much greater sensitivity with MRCP than with ultrasonography.

Choledocholithiasis is the most common cause of biliary obstruction. Ultrasound is less capable of detecting common bile duct (CBD) stones than gallstones, with reported sensitivities ranging from 13 to 75%. The major difficulty lies in

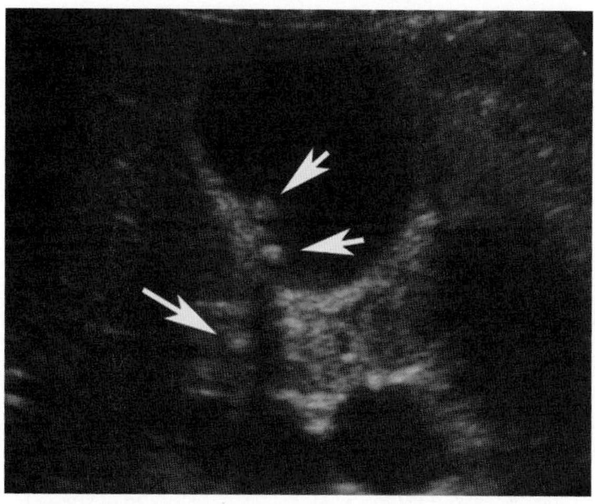

▲ **Figure 9–35.** Gallstones. Sagittal ultrasound image shows hyperechoic stones in the gallbladder along with shadowing (*short arrows*). Also note a nonshadowing stone in the cystic duct (*long arrow*).

detecting distal CBD stones, especially when there is no associated acoustic shadowing or ductal dilation (30% of cases). MRI is highly accurate in the detection and characterization of CBD stones. CBD stones are usually hypointense on both T1- and T2-weighted images and are typically surrounded by bile (Figure 9–36). On axial images, the stone typically reveals a dependent position in the duct, thus differentiating it from pneumobilia (air is located in the nondependent position) and bile flow artifacts (typically central in location).

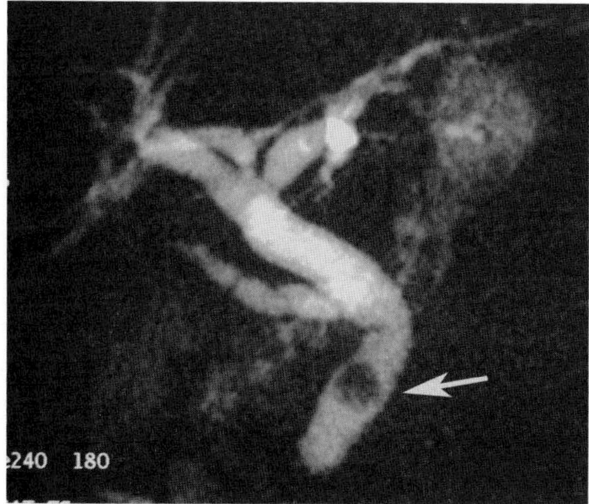

▲ **Figure 9–36.** Choledocholithiasis. Coronal oblique thick-slab MRCP image shows a round filling defect (*arrow*) in the distal common bile duct.

2. Inflammatory Conditions

A. Imaging Algorithm

Ultrasound is the initial imaging modality of choice in cases of suspected cholecystitis. Hepatobiliary scintigraphy has a similar diagnostic sensitivity to ultrasound for acalculous cholecystitis. CT and MRI, imaging modalities with excellent sensitivity and specificity, are typically reserved for cases in which ultrasound shows equivocal results. Cross-sectional imaging techniques, especially MRI with MRCP, have proven to be as sensitive as the more invasive test ERCP in the detection of cholangitis.

B. Acute Cholecystitis (See Chapter 53)

Sonographic findings supportive of the diagnosis of acute cholecystitis include the presence of gallstones, gallbladder wall thickening greater than 3 mm, pericholecystic fluid, and the detection of tenderness directly over the gallbladder (sonographic Murphy sign). When all these findings are present, the sensitivity for the diagnosis of acute cholecystitis with ultrasound is more than 90%. CT features of acute cholecystitis include the presence of gallstones, gallbladder wall thickening greater than 3 mm, pericholecystic fluid and fat stranding, hydrops, and hyperenhancement of segment IV of the liver due to hyperemia (Figure 9–37). On T2-weighted unenhanced MR images, inflammatory pericholecystic changes are visualized as linear and strand-like structures of high signal intensity around the gallbladder. MRI shows the thickened gallbladder wall, which has increased signal intensity on T2-weighted images. Gadolinium-enhanced T1-weighted images are useful in depicting inflammatory changes of the gallbladder wall, pericholecystic fat, and intrahepatic periportal tissues. Contrast enhancement of the gallbladder wall is increased, and on dynamic imaging, there is a transient enhancement of liver segments adjacent to the gallbladder on early images. The role of MRCP in the diagnostic workup of acute cholecystitis is mainly to detect small cystic duct and gallbladder neck calculi. Impacted cystic duct or gallbladder neck calculi can be demonstrated with MRCP accurately to a resolution as low as 2 mm.

C. Chronic Cholecystitis (See Chapter 53)

Chronic cholecystitis may be asymptomatic or may present as acute cholecystitis on a background of chronic disease. Other manifestations of this entity may be biliary colic, fistula formation, and hydrops of the gallbladder or perforation. Deposition of calcium within the gallbladder wall, a condition termed porcelain gallbladder, is an uncommon manifestation of chronic cholecystitis and is associated with an increased prevalence of gallbladder carcinoma (Figure 9–38).

On imaging studies, chronic cholecystitis may have findings similar to those of acute cholecystitis, such as wall thickening and stones. However the gallbladder is typically contracted around the stones rather than distended.

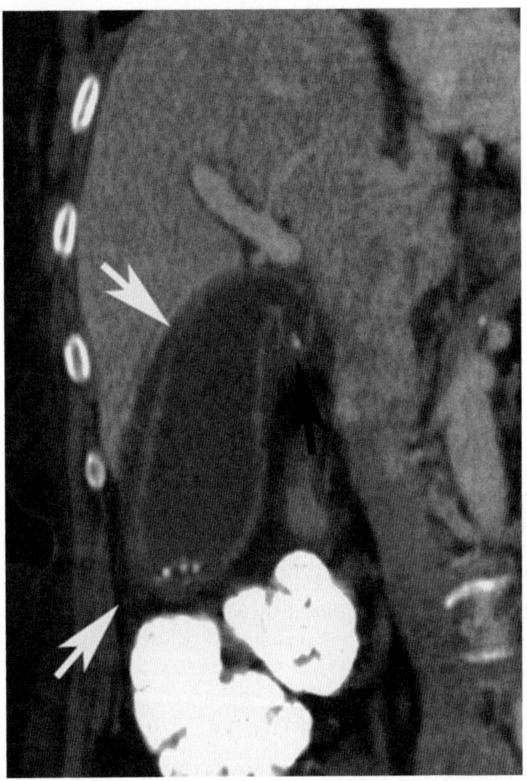

▲ **Figure 9–37.** Acute cholecystitis. Coronal MDCT image shows hydrops of the gallbladder (*white arrows*), pericholecystic fluid, and gallstones. Note a stone in the neck of the gallbladder (*black arrow*).

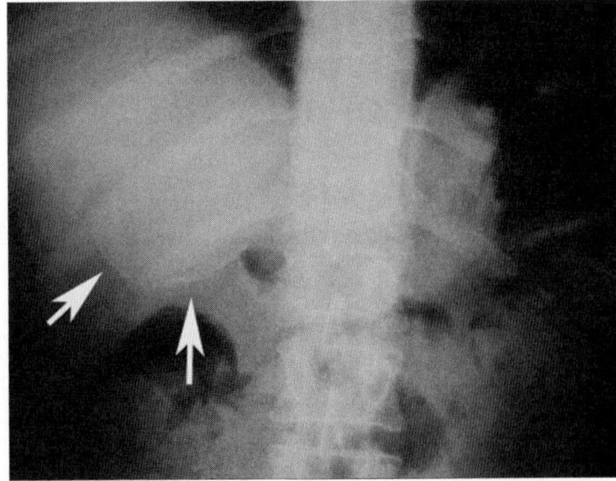

▲ **Figure 9–38.** Porcelain gallbladder. KUB (kidney, ureter, bladder) image shows linear calcifications in the wall of the gallbladder (*arrows*).

Furthermore, on contrast-enhanced images, the degree of contrast enhancement of the gallbladder wall is significantly lower in comparison with acute cholecystitis. The transient pericholecystic liver enhancement on early postcontrast images, which is described with acute cholecystitis, is also not evident in chronic cholecystitis. Secondary signs of malignancy, such as local invasion, distant metastases, and bile duct dilation, are helpful in distinguishing chronic cholecystitis from gallbladder carcinoma.

D. Cholangitis (See Chapter 52)

Cholangitis can be categorized as bacterial cholangitis, primary sclerosing cholangitis, and secondary sclerosing cholangitis or chronic pyogenic (obstructive) cholangitis. Primary sclerosing cholangitis is an autoimmune disorder characterized by obliterative fibrotic inflammation of the bile ducts and, typically, both intrahepatic and extrahepatic bile ducts are involved simultaneously. On MRI, the characteristic appearance is marked by the presence of multiple stenoses, minor dilation of the proximal segments (due to periductal fibrosis), a beaded appearance of intrahepatic bile ducts, presence of sacculations resembling diverticula, enhancing bile duct wall, and intrahepatic lithiasis.

3. Neoplastic Processes

A. Imaging Algorithm

Ultrasound is very valuable in the evaluation of the patient with jaundice caused by malignant biliary obstruction. The accuracy of MRCP in assessing the level and the morphology of the malignant obstruction is comparable to that of ERCP or percutaneous transhepatic cholangiography. However, compared with ERCP, MRCP may more accurately depict the suprahilar tumor extension in cases of severe stenosis of the confluence (because in such cases the accuracy of ERCP will be impaired due to insufficient contrast filling). Another advantage of MRCP is its ability to visualize an undrained bile duct without injection of contrast material, thus avoiding secondary cholangitis. In addition, portal venous invasion and hepatic metastases in patients can be detected accurately with dynamic contrast-enhanced MR sequences coupled to the MRCP protocol. It offers significant advantages in the preoperative staging of hilar cholangiocarcinoma, because it becomes possible to simultaneously assess the bile duct, the vascular structures, and the liver parenchyma. For all these reasons, ERCP should not be performed for diagnostic purposes but be reserved for therapeutic interventions.

B. Gallbladder Carcinoma

Gallbladder carcinoma is the most common malignancy of the biliary tree and the fifth most common GI malignancy. More than 90% of gallbladder cancers are adenocarcinomas, but other cell types such as squamous cell carcinoma, anaplastic carcinoma, and sarcomas also have been reported.

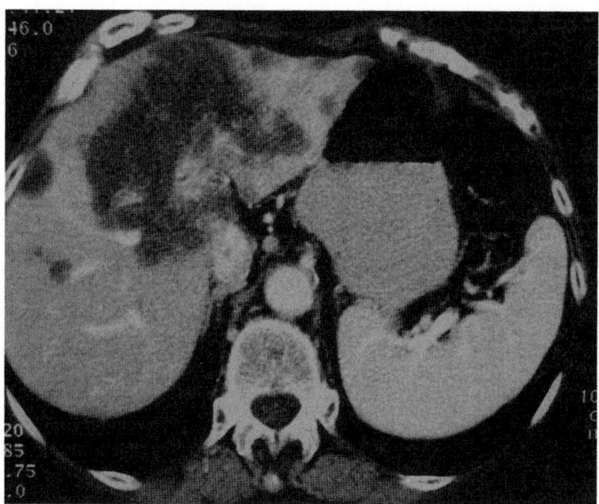

▲ **Figure 9–39.** Gallbladder carcinoma. Axial MDCT image shows large mass replacing the gallbladder fossa with presence of intrahepatic metastases.

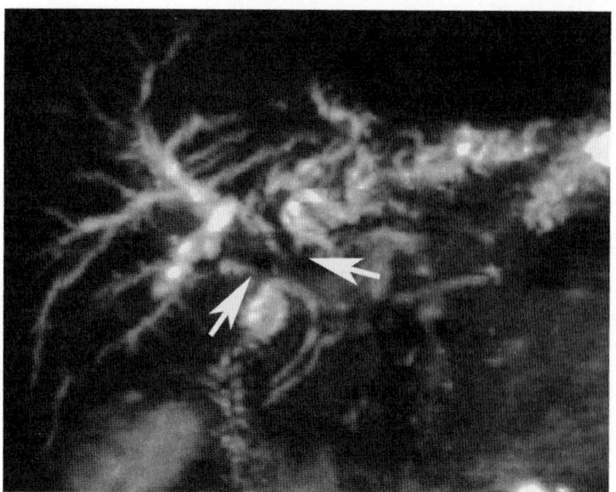

▲ **Figure 9–40.** Klatskin tumor. Maximum intensity projection (MIP) image of a multislice MRCP data set shows intrahepatic biliary ductal dilation with the presence of an obstructing mass (*arrows*) at the level of the porta hepatis.

Gallstones are detected in more than 70% of the cases. There are three common radiologic appearances for gallbladder carcinoma. The most common appearance is that of a mass replacing the gallbladder fossa (55%) (Figure 9–39). The second most common appearance is that of either focal or diffuse gallbladder wall thickening (25%); this pattern is the most difficult to diagnose because of the small size of early masses. In addition, diffuse wall thickening is also caused by a wide variety of other pathologic conditions, such as acute and chronic cholecystitis, adenomyomatosis, and low protein states. The third presentation is an intraluminal polypoid mass. Metastases are present at the time of diagnosis in approximately 75% of cases.

C. Extrahepatic Cholangiocarcinoma

Extrahepatic cholangiocarcinomas include biliary adenocarcinomas located at the bifurcation or proximal hepatic duct (Klatskin tumors) and the distal duct types. They are usually seen in older patients presenting with painless jaundice, weight loss, and cholangitis. Once the diagnosis has been established, accurate local staging of the tumor is essential for the planning of patient management, because few patients are eligible for surgery at time of diagnosis. The staging system described by Bismuth and Corlette is widely accepted as a guide for the extension of surgery required.

On MRI, these tumors typically present as a mass located at the liver hilum and causing biliary dilation. They are usually hypointense on T1-weighted images and slightly hyperintense on T2-weighted images, with heterogeneous and variable enhancement following gadolinium administration. MRCP images typically reveal a stenotic lesion at the bifurcation, with proximal biliary dilation; nodular intraductal tumor components are occasionally seen (Figure 9–40). Hilar extrahepatic cholangiocarcinomas can involve the distal common hepatic duct alone (Bismuth type I), the confluence of the left and right hepatic duct (Bismuth type II), the confluence and either the right (Bismuth type IIIa) or the left (Bismuth type IIIb) hepatic duct, or both the left and right secondary confluence (Bismuth type IV).

4. Developmental Disorders

A. Imaging Algorithm

Congenital biliary anomalies are commonly encountered on imaging studies and can be accurately diagnosed, with increasing level of specificity, by ultrasound, CT, MRI with MRCP, and ERCP.

B. Choledochal Cysts

Choledochal cysts are rare congenital biliary tract anomalies characterized by biliary ductal dilation. The five subtypes, as described by Todani, have different pathophysiologies but are grouped together by the commonality of the cystic changes present.

The *type I choledochal cyst* (Figure 9–41) is a choledochal cyst confined to the extrahepatic bile duct. This cyst results from an anomalous pancreaticobiliary union characterized by formation of a long common channel, frequently ectatic.

The *type II choledochal cyst* represents a true diverticulum of the extrahepatic bile duct.

The *type III choledochal cyst* (Figure 9–42), also known as a choledochocele, is formed by ectasia of the intramural

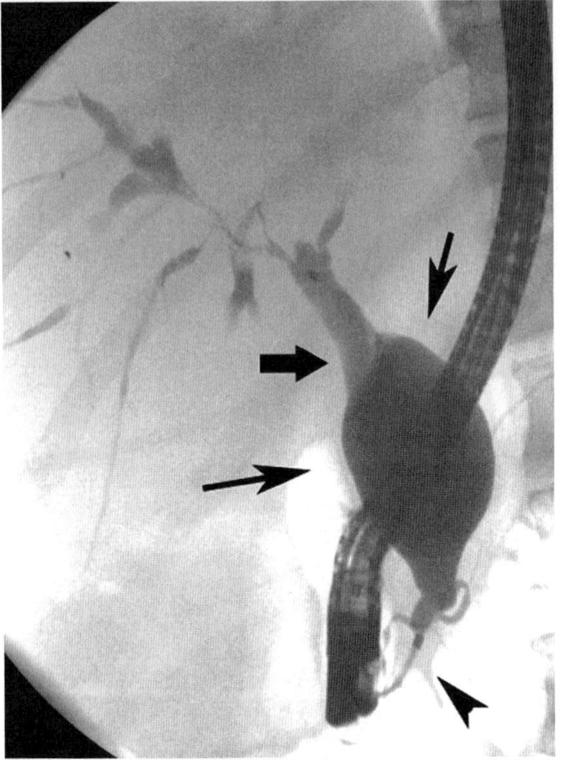

▲ **Figure 9–41.** Type I choledochal cyst. ERCP image shows saccular dilation of the extrahepatic bile duct (*arrows*) with presence of a long common channel (*arrowhead*) and mass cholangiocarcinoma (*thick arrow*) arising from the cranial aspect of the cyst.

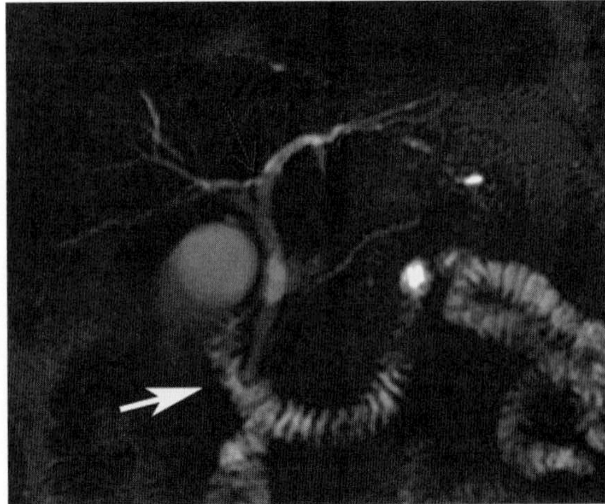

▲ **Figure 9–42.** Type III choledochal cyst. Oblique coronal MRCP image shows telescoping of the distal common bile duct (*arrow*) in the duodenum.

common bile duct segment. It is not embryologically related to the other cystic dilations of the choledochal cysts. This subtype occurs typically as focal dilation of the intraduodenal segment of the distal common bile duct.

The *type IV choledochal cysts* are, by definition, multiple and can have both intrahepatic and extrahepatic components.

Caroli disease (Todani type V choledochal cyst) is a rare congenital cystic dilation of the intrahepatic bile ducts. It is an autosomal-recessive disorder resulting from the arrest of or a derangement in the normal embryologic remodeling of ducts that, in turn, causes varying degrees of destructive inflammation and segmental dilation. If the large intrahepatic bile ducts are affected, the result is Caroli disease, whereas abnormal development of the small interlobular bile ducts results in congenital hepatic fibrosis. If all levels of the intrahepatic biliary tree are involved, features of both congenital hepatic fibrosis and Caroli disease are present; this condition has been termed Caroli syndrome. Imaging methods show intrahepatic saccular or fusiform dilated cystic structures of varying sizes that communicate with the biliary tree. The presence of tiny dots with contrast enhancement within the dilated intrahepatic bile duct ("central dot sign") is considered very suggestive of Caroli disease. The "central dot sign" represents the enhancing portal branches surrounded by cystic alterations of the intrahepatic biliary ducts.

PANCREATIC IMAGING

1. Pancreatic Neoplasms (See Chapter 28)

A. Imaging Algorithm

With the introduction of MDCT, the visualization of the pancreas has dramatically improved. Therefore, MDCT has become a superb tool for detection of solid neoplasms, with an increasing overall diagnostic accuracy (by means of better differentiating pancreatitis from neoplasm and characterizing the different neoplasms) and an able method to assess unresectability. Recent studies have compared the accuracy of MRI in staging pancreatic carcinoma with CT. With breath-hold imaging and the use of phased array coils, dynamic MRI was shown to be superior to CT in determining the degree of tumor extension, while both modalities performed equally well in establishing the degree of vascular involvement. Other studies indicate that the two modalities perform comparably in the global assessment of resectability. PET-CT may be helpful to stage pancreatic cancer accurately by detecting distant metastatic disease.

Because MRI is so sensitive to fluid, it is not surprising that this modality has great potential to accurately assess cystic pancreatic neoplasms. The cyst fluid improves contrast resolution within the mass, often rendering subtle irregularities of the cyst wall that aid in differential diagnosis between benign and malignant neoplasms. When combined with MR pancreatography, the duct system can be visualized and the relation of these lesions to the main and branch ducts may be predicted. MRCP has been shown to be more sensitive than CT and ERCP in the depiction of these lesions.

Mortele KJ, Ji H, Ros PR. CT and magnetic resonance imaging in pancreatic and biliary tract malignancies. *Gastrointest Endosc.* 2002;56(Suppl):S206–S212. [PMID: 12447269]

Shah S, Mortele KJ. Uncommon solid pancreatic neoplasms: ultrasound, computed tomography, and magnetic resonance imaging features. *Semin Ultrasound CT MR.* 2007;28:357–370. [PMID: 17970552]

B. Ductal Adenocarcinoma

Ductal pancreatic adenocarcinoma accounts for nearly 95% of all malignant pancreatic neoplasms and is the ninth most common malignancy. Prognosis is poor, with a 5-year survival rate ranging from 1 to 5%; at the time of clinical presentation, 66% of patients have an advanced tumor stage, with metastatic disease present in 85% of cases. The majority of tumors are located in the pancreatic head, and because of the involvement of the common bile duct, they present earlier than tumors arising in the body or tail of pancreas.

CT is the imaging modality of choice for the detection and preoperative staging of pancreatic cancer. The new MDCT scanners provide radiologists enormous capabilities for fast data acquisition and narrow collimation, resulting in accuracies of 96% for detecting pancreatic tumors. On contrast-enhanced MDCT images, adenocarcinomas present as hypoattenuating lesions with respect to the surrounding normal pancreatic parenchyma (Figure 9–43). There are also some indirect signs for the presence of a tumor on CT without identification of the tumor itself: dilation of the common bile and pancreatic duct without calculi, dilation of the pancreatic duct in the body and tail but not in the head, a homogenous zone within a heterogeneous atrophic gland, bulging of the uncinate process, and atrophy of the pancreatic tail. The detection of hepatic metastases is critical in the preoperative staging of the patients, because presence of metastatic foci within the liver makes the tumor unresectable. MDCT scanners have the ability to depict very small lesions (<5 mm). In the absence of obvious liver metastases, tumor resectability depends on the presence of local invasion or vascular involvement. In a recent prospective study comparing EUS, CT, MRI, and angiography in preoperative staging and tumor resectability assessment of pancreatic cancer, Soriano and colleagues reported that CT is the mainstay for pancreatic cancer staging, with the best figures in the evaluation of extent of primary tumor, locoregional extension, vascular invasion, and metastatic spread (with accuracies of 73%, 74%, 83%, and 88%, respectively). In this study, EUS was evaluated as essential in assessing tumor size and lymph node involvement. Nevertheless, it can be assumed that the initial enthusiasm for EUS staging of pancreatic cancer has today diminished as a result of studies reporting that EUS is not as accurate as it was earlier suggested in locoregional staging, especially in the diagnosis of vascular involvement. Furthermore, detection of distant metastases, including nonregional lymph node groups, is far beyond the capability of EUS, thus favoring MDCT as a single imaging technique for staging pancreatic cancer.

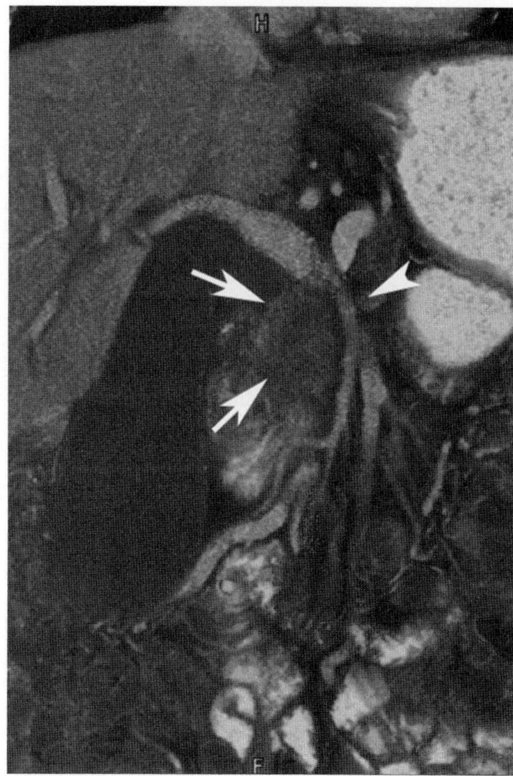

▲ **Figure 9–43.** Pancreatic adenocarcinoma. Curved, reformatted CT image shows a low-density pancreatic mass (*arrows*) with invasion of the superior mesenteric vein (*arrowhead*).

Detection of pancreatic adenocarcinoma is based on noncontrast T1-weighted fat-suppressed images and immediate postgadolinium T1-weighted images. On T1-weighted fat-suppressed images, pancreatic cancer appears as a low signal intensity mass and is clearly separated from normal pancreatic tissue, which is high in signal intensity (Figure 9–44). MRCP has proven an accurate means of evaluating the level and causes of pancreatic ductal obstruction. A major advantage of MRCP is that the visualization of the duct is based on the signal features in the pancreatic secretions. Thus, one can visualize the duct before and after an obstructing lesion.

PET with F-18 fluorodeoxyglucose (F-18 FDG PET) is a relatively novel modality in pancreatic imaging. In a comparison between CT and F-18 PET, F-18 PET was more sensitive than CT for detecting malignancy (92% vs 65%), as well as

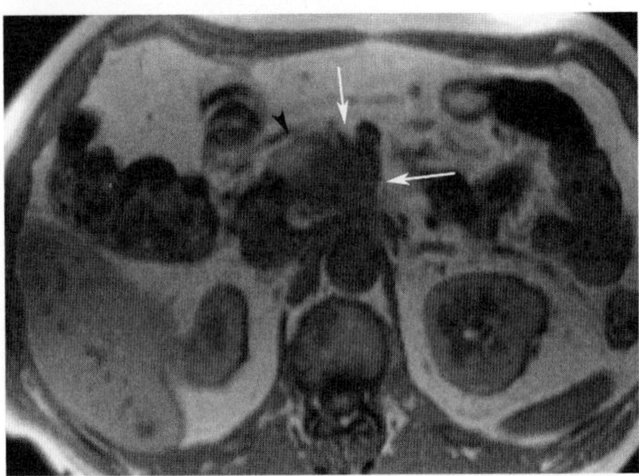

▲ **Figure 9–44.** Pancreatic adenocarcinoma. T1-weighted axial MR image shows a hypointense pancreatic mass (*arrows*). Note the normal hyperintense residual pancreas (*arrowhead*).

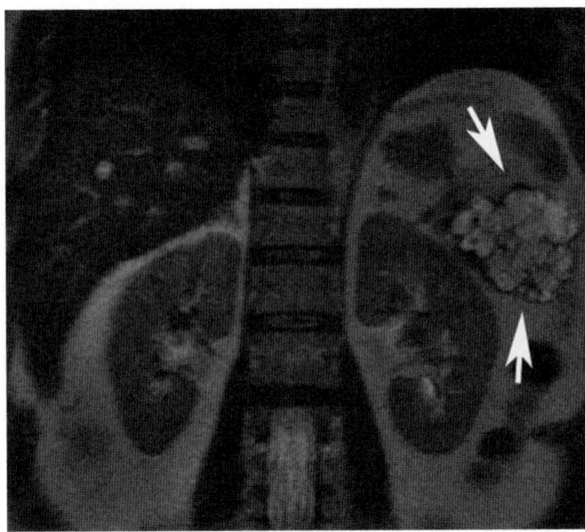

▲ **Figure 9–45.** Serous cystadenoma. Coronal T2-weighted image shows a lobulated cystic mass (*arrows*) composed of numerous small cysts.

more specific (85% vs 61%). Whereas for pancreatic tumors less than 2 cm in diameter, the sensitivity of F-18 FDG PET is markedly superior to that achieved with CT, CT is superior to F-18 FDG PET when pancreatic lesions are large (>4 cm in diameter).

Soriano A, Castells A, Ayuso C, et al. Preoperative staging and tumor resectability assessment of pancreatic cancer: prospective study comparing endoscopic ultrasonography, helical computed tomography, magnetic resonance imaging, and angiography. *Am J Gastroenterol.* 2004;99:492–501. [PMID: 15156091]

C. Cystic Pancreatic Tumors (See Chapter 28)

Serous cystadenoma is a benign neoplasm that occurs most frequently in the pancreatic head of elderly female patients. This well-circumscribed tumor is often lobulated and contains a central, stellate, calcified scar in addition to multiple small cysts divided by thin septations. Imaging studies may show this tumor as either homogeneously solid, or, more commonly, a predominantly cystic mass with multiple small cysts. It has been stated that the presence of six or more small cysts within the mass is suggestive of serous rather than mucinous cystic neoplasm. On unenhanced MDCT scans, serous cystic tumors are low-density, solid, or, more commonly, multiple cyst-containing lesions with Hounsfield values similar to water. If present, the characteristic central stellate scar with dystrophic calcifications is demonstrated. The amount of fibrous stroma determines the appearance of the tumor on contrast-enhanced CT images. An innumerable cyst-containing tumor appears as an irregular heterogeneously enhancing mass, whereas a tumor with microscopic cysts and a dominant fibrous stroma presents as a homogenous mass on postcontrast images. Serous cystic tumors are usually markedly hyperintense on T2-weighted MR images, although some central areas of low signal intensity may occasionally be seen related to the presence of a fibrous scar (Figure 9–45). On T1-weighted MR images, the tumor is of low signal intensity, except in cases in which hemorrhage is present. The tumor is hypervascular secondary to its rich subepithelial capillary network.

Mucinous cystic tumors range from tumors with malignant potential to frankly malignant mucinous cystadenocarcinomas. In 95% of cases, they occur in women during their fourth to sixth decades. Most tumors are located in the tail or body of the pancreas. These encapsulated hypovascular tumors are most frequently multilocular. They may contain internal septations, solid papillary excretions, and occasionally peripheral calcifications and septations. Unenhanced MDCT studies show a round mass, which is well delineated and has smooth external margins. Attenuation values are usually similar to that of water. MDCT scans obtained after the intravenous administration of contrast material may demonstrate enhancement of the wall and the presence of thin septations; on the internal surface of the tumor, nodularities representing papillary projections may be demonstrated. MRI studies show the unilocular or multilocular fluid nature of this mass. If a mucinous cystic neoplasm appears unilocular and without septations on imaging, differentiation from a pseudocyst may not be possible. MR is advantageous to show internal septations, mural nodules, and solid excrescences in the tumor wall.

Intraductal papillary mucinous neoplasm (IPMN) is a relatively new and increasingly reported entity typically presenting either as a dilated main pancreatic duct or a unilocular or multilocular cystic lesion. IPMNs are cystic pancreatic neoplasms characterized by proliferation of pancreatic ductal

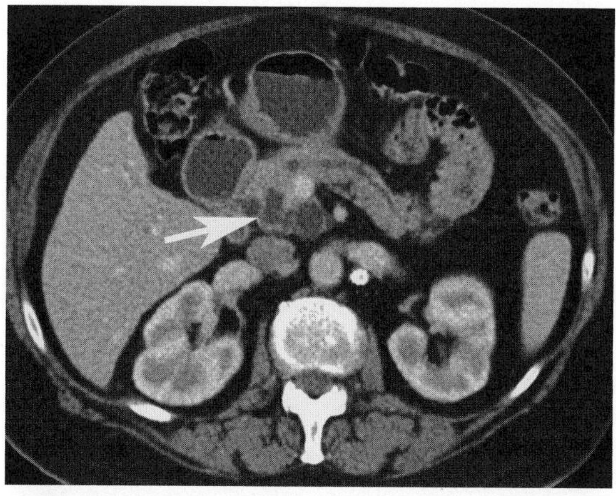

▲ **Figure 9–46.** Intraductal papillary mucinous neoplasm. Axial CT image shows a dilated pancreatic side-branch duct (*arrow*) in the uncinate process.

epithelium and excess mucin production. They are classified into main and branch duct types. The branch duct type mostly presents in the uncinate process or pancreatic head, but it can also involve the body or tail. On unenhanced MDCT, branch-duct tumor appears as clusters of multiple small cysts or as a single cystic lesion with irregular, lobulated margins and septations (Figure 9–46). Diffuse or segmental dilation of the main pancreatic duct is typical for main-duct type tumors. Contrast-enhanced thin section MDCT images may demonstrate communications between dilated cystic segments and the main pancreatic duct. MDCT may also depict the papilla bulging into the duodenal lumen and hyperdense filling defects secondary to mucin in the dilated duct. On MRI and MRCP, a dilated main pancreatic duct with a unilocular or multilocular cystic lesion is typical (Figure 9–47); communication between the main pancreatic duct and the cystic lesion may be depicted. Biliary obstruction, a bulging papilla, large size (>3 cm) of a side-branch lesion, and large caliber of the main pancreatic duct (>1 cm) are more common in patients with malignant IPMN.

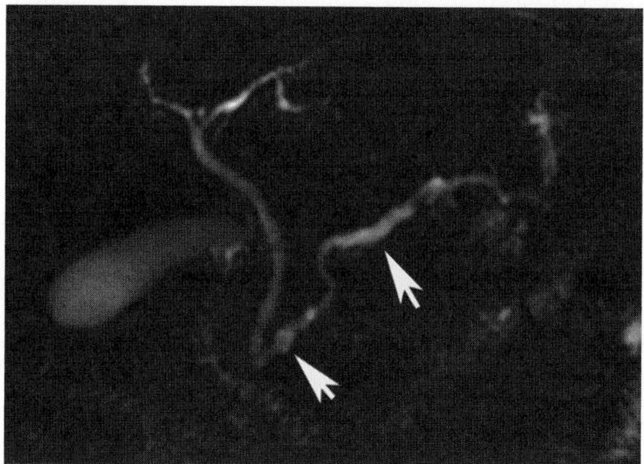

▲ **Figure 9–47.** Intraductal papillary mucinous neoplasm. Oblique coronal MRCP image shows irregular segmental dilation of the main pancreatic duct.

Sidden CR, Mortele KJ. Cystic tumors of the pancreas: ultrasound, computed tomography, and magnetic resonance imaging features. *Semin Ultrasound CT MR.* 2007;28:339–356. [PMID: 17970551]

D. Endocrine Tumors

Islet cell tumors are benign or malignant neoplasms with endocrine cell differentiation. *Insulinoma* is the most common and, at the time of diagnosis, is usually smaller than 1.5 cm; only 5–10% are malignant. *Gastrinoma* (see Chapter 16) is the second most common endocrine tumor of the pancreas. *Glucagonomas* and *vipomas* represent less than 10% of endocrine pancreatic tumors, and the majority of them are malignant. The tumors are found predominantly in the pancreatic body and tail and tend to be larger than insulinomas or gastrinomas. *Somatostatinoma* is the rarest endocrine pancreatic tumor (<1%), and at the time of diagnosis, the majority are malignant (75%).

On multiphasic contrast-enhanced MDCT, islet cell tumors present as hypervascular lesions, best seen in the early phases of pancreatic enhancement (Figure 9–48). Using optimized thin-slice CT scans, even small tumors can be visualized. The most striking evidence of malignancy is evidence of metastatic disease to the liver or local lymph nodes.

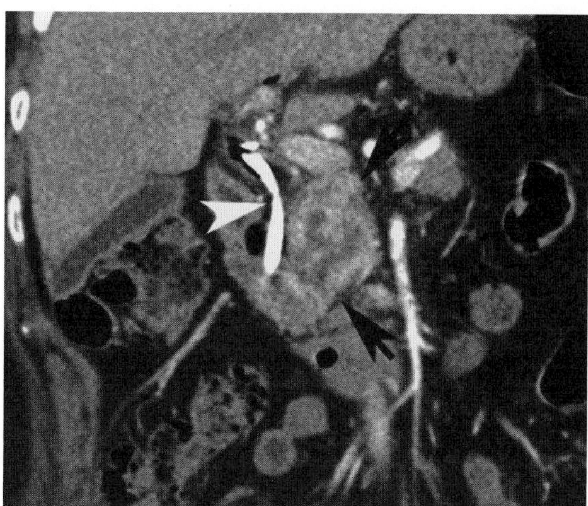

▲ **Figure 9–48.** Islet cell tumor. Coronal MDCT image shows a heterogeneously enhancing hypervascular mass in the pancreatic head (*arrows*). Note the presence of a biliary stent (*arrowhead*).

On MRI, insulinomas and gastrinomas appear as lesions with low signal intensity on T1-weighted and high signal intensity on T2-weighted imaging. The use of intravenous gadolinium is helpful as they are hypervascular. Ring-like enhancement in the periphery of the tumor is typically seen, while the center may remain hypointense secondary to fibrosis. The more uncommon but generally larger hyperfunctioning and nonhyperfunctioning tumors present with slightly low signal intensity on T1-weighted and bright signal intensity on T2-weighted MRI.

2. Pancreatic Inflammation

A. Imaging Algorithm

The role of radiologic imaging in patients with suspected pancreatitis is to help diagnose pancreatitis, try to establish the cause of the disease, assess disease severity, and detect complications. In assessment of acute pancreatitis, MRI, as well as CT, can depict the presence and extent of necrosis and peripancreatic fluid collections. MRI is used instead of routine CT in some cases because mild pancreatitis cannot be well visualized by CT, MRI is better in defining the internal composition of peripancreatic fluid collections, and MRI is capable of detecting underlying causes of pancreatitis (eg, pancreas divisum, choledocholithiasis).

B. Acute Pancreatitis (See Chapter 25)

Of all the imaging modalities, CT is the most commonly used to evaluate acute pancreatitis. Contrast-enhanced CT plays a critical role in establishing necrosis in acute pancreatitis. CT features in mild acute pancreatitis consist of normal findings or focal or diffuse enlargement of the pancreas, a normal pancreatic enhancement (50–60 HU above baseline) with or without peripancreatic fat stranding. In more severe cases, pancreatic parenchymal necrosis develops with acute fluid collections that occur mostly around the pancreas, in the anterior or posterior pararenal spaces and in the lesser sac (Figure 9–49). CT is also used for staging of severity; for diagnosis, follow-up, and monitoring of established local pancreatic complications; for demonstrating other nonpancreatic sequelae, such as renal, splenic, vascular, and GI complications; and for guidance of interventional procedures.

In assessment of acute pancreatitis, MRI can depict the presence and extent of necrosis and peripancreatic fluid collections. Gadolinium-enhanced MRI is particularly useful for the assessment of pancreatic parenchymal perfusion and presence of necrosis. T2-weighted sequences are the most sensitive in demonstrating fluid collections. Furthermore, by using additional MRCP or MR angiography sequences, MRI enables underlying etiologies, such as choledocholithiasis or pancreas divisum, or vascular complications to be accurately diagnosed.

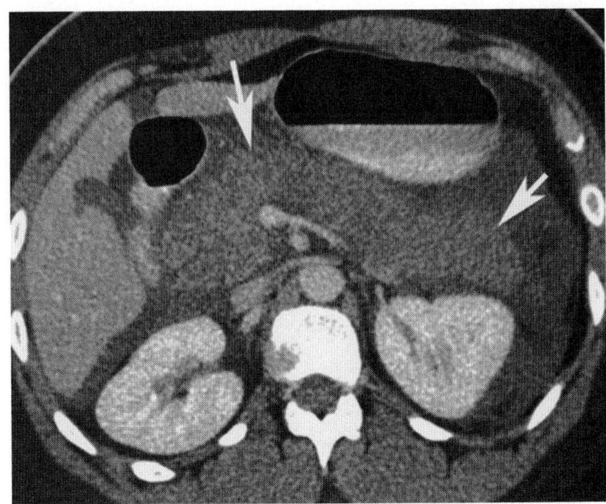

▲ **Figure 9–49.** Acute pancreatitis. Axial MDCT image shows a diffusely enlarged pancreatic gland (*arrows*). Note the lack of normal enhancement and presence of acute fluid collections in the retroperitoneum.

Mortele KJ, Wiesner W, Intriere L, et al. A modified CT severity index for evaluating acute pancreatitis: improved correlation with patient outcome. *AJR Am J Roentgenol.* 2004;183:1261–1265. [PMID: 15505289]

C. Chronic Pancreatitis (See Chapter 26)

Chronic pancreatitis is a progressive, irreversible inflammatory and fibrosing disease of the pancreas. CT findings of chronic pancreatitis include dilation of the main pancreatic duct, parenchymal atrophy, pancreatic calcifications, and pseudocysts (Figure 9–50). In chronic pancreatitis, optimal MRI examination should include T1- and T2-weighted images and MRCP sequences. The role of MRCP in chronic pancreatitis is still controversial but evolving. Comparisons between MRCP and ERCP in cases of chronic pancreatitis have revealed agreement of 83–100% for identification of ductal dilation, 70–92% for identification of narrowing, and 92–100% for identification of filling defects, respectively. Several centers have investigated functional MR pancreatic evaluation by obtaining MRCP images before and after intravenous secretin administration, and it showed improved visualization of the pancreatic duct and its side branches. Furthermore, the volume of effluent into the duodenal lumen can be graded, allowing a relative estimation of the exocrine function.

De Backer AI, Mortele KJ, Ros PR, et al. Chronic pancreatitis: diagnostic role of computed tomography and magnetic resonance imaging. *JBR-BTR.* 2002;85:304–310. [PMID: 12553661]

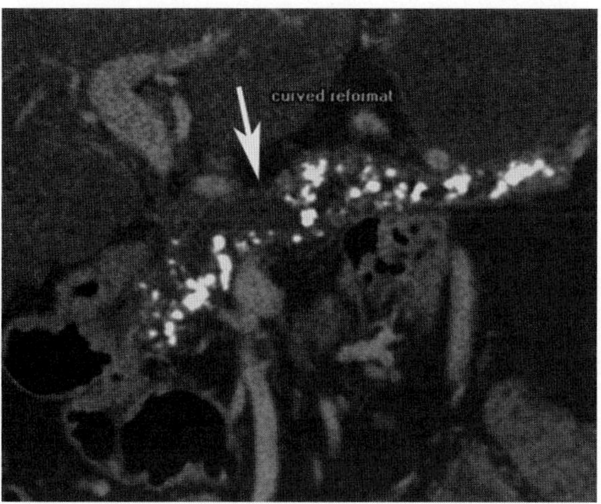

▲ **Figure 9–50.** Chronic pancreatitis. Curved, reformatted CT image shows an atrophic pancreas with numerous calcifications and irregular ductal dilation (*arrow*).

3. Developmental Disorders

A. Imaging Algorithm

The definitive diagnosis of the two most important pancreatic developmental disorders, pancreas divisum and annular pancreas, is made with ERCP. MDCT and MRI, however, may depict both pancreas divisum and annular pancreas. MR pancreatography has been shown to be highly sensitive and specific for depicting pancreas divisum.

B. Congenital Anomalies

Pancreas divisum is the most common congenital anomaly of the pancreatic ductal system, being reported in up to 10% of the population. The ventral duct (duct of Wirsung) drains only the ventral pancreatic anlage through the major papilla while the majority of the gland empties into the minor papilla through the dorsal duct or duct of Santorini. Pancreas divisum usually causes no symptoms but is found more frequently in patients with chronic abdominal pain, elevated pancreatic function tests, and idiopathic pancreatitis than in the general population. MRCP demonstrates the noncommunicating dorsal and ventral ducts with their independent drainage sites.

Annular pancreas is a rare congenital anomaly in which incomplete rotation of the ventral anlage leads to a segment of the pancreas encircling the second part of the duodenum. The incidence of annular pancreas is 1 in 2000. Annular pancreas can be diagnosed on the basis of CT, MRI, and ERCP findings that reveal pancreatic tissue and an annular duct encircling the descending duodenum.

Mortele KJ, Rocha TC, Streeter JL, et al. Multimodality imaging of pancreatic and biliary congenital anomalies. *Radiographics.* 2006;26:715–731. [PMID: 16702450]

Mortele KJ, Wiesner W, Zou K, et al. Asymptomatic nonspecific serum hyperamylasemia and hyperlipasemia: spectrum of MRCP findings and clinical implications. *Abdom Imaging.* 2004;29: 109–114. [PMID: 15160763]

SUMMARY OF CURRENT RECOMMENDATIONS

Developments in imaging technology in recent years have led to many improvements in the field of diagnostic GI radiology. Many semi-invasive diagnostic methods are being replaced by noninvasive imaging technologies. MRCP has widely replaced ERCP in the diagnosis and staging of pancreatobiliary disorders; virtual colonoscopy proved itself as an efficient screening method for colon cancer; and MDCT enterography is becoming the standard imaging technique for many small bowel disorders. As a result, there is a significant decline in the use of fluoroscopic imaging techniques. CT continues to be the most effective modality for the initial evaluation of patients with diseases involving the GI system. Additional imaging procedures, such as MRI and MRCP and PET-CT scanning are best reserved for patients who cannot undergo a contrast-enhanced CT, or for patients in whom ultrasound or CT show equivocal findings. Nevertheless, in many centers, MRI has been adopted as the primary imaging technique in the diagnosis and staging of a variety of hepatobiliary, pancreatic, and GI tract diseases.

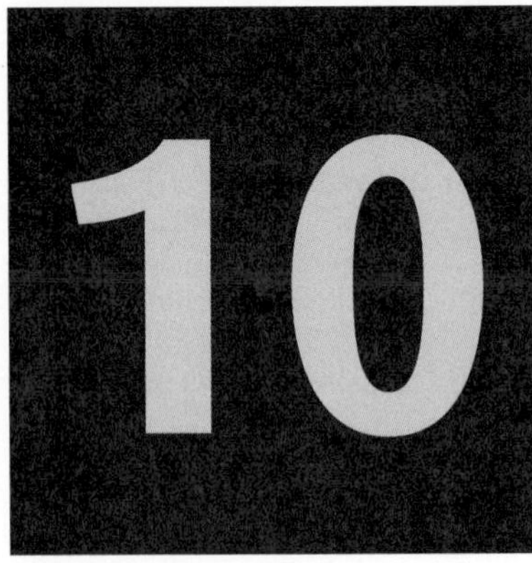

Gastrointestinal Manifestations of Immunodeficiency

Zhenglun Zhu, MD, PhD

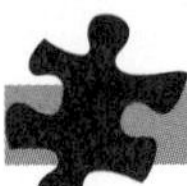

ESSENTIAL CONCEPTS

- Recurrent infections and diarrhea are the most common gastrointestinal manifestations of immunodeficiency.
- Some pathogens (eg, *Mycobacterium avium* complex), are unique to immunocompromised hosts; others (eg, *Cryptosporidium, Giardia lamblia*) cause self-limited diarrhea in healthy hosts but chronic diarrhea in immunosuppressed patients.
- In patients without a specific diagnosis after routine study, endoscopic evaluation with biopsy is important in establishing the diagnosis.
- *Candida* species, herpes simplex virus, cytomegalovirus, and *Mycobacterium* species are the most frequent causative agents of infectious esophagitis in an immunocompromised host.
- In immunocompromised patients, opportunistic infections are a major cause of abdominal pain and can evolve rapidly.
- The frequency of intestinal lymphomas is increased in patients with common variable immunodeficiency.

General Considerations

The gastrointestinal (GI) tract is the largest lymphoid organ and dysfunction of the GI tract is one of the most common manifestations of immunodeficiency. Some studies have suggested that 50–90% of patients with secondary (acquired) immunodeficiency syndromes, such as full-blown AIDS, develop significant GI symptoms. The most common GI manifestations of immunodeficiency are infection and malignancy, which correlate with the progressive deterioration of host defense systems. Patients often develop diarrhea, abdominal pain, dysphagia, and odynophagia, as well as nausea, vomiting, weight loss, and GI bleeding. The overall goal of evaluation is, therefore, to identify treatable causes of the symptoms and to preserve the function of the GI tract.

The impaired host immune system results from either primary inherited defects or secondary acquired deficiencies resulting from infectious agents (eg, HIV) or pathologic insults, including nutritional deficiencies or the iatrogenic effects of medical interventions (eg, immunosuppressive therapies). In addition, the chronic disease burden associated with advanced age and, to a lesser degree, the poorly understood physiologic decline of host defense systems associated with aging play an important role in the development of GI symptoms in geriatric populations. A detailed description of the nature and mechanisms of the GI manifestations of each individual primary and acquired (secondary) immunodeficiency is beyond the scope of this chapter. However, a comprehensive understanding of the composition and development of the immune defense systems of the GI tract and their alterations in pathologic conditions is essential for the clinical management of GI problems associated with immunodeficiency patients.

Castle SC, Uyemura K, Fulop T, et al. Host resistance and immune responses in advanced age. *Clin Geriatr Med.* 2007;23:463–479. [PMID: 17631228]

Pathogenesis

A. Pathophysiology of Gastrointestinal Defense Systems

The intestinal epithelium serves as the major frontier of self-protection from exogenous injurious events. To defend against the vast quantity of infectious agents and toxins and ensure homeostasis of the gut epithelium for nutritional absorption, the body relies on the proper development and maintenance of the immunologic defense systems associated with the intestinal epithelium, which employs both innate and adaptive immune systems. Abnormalities occurring during normal development of the GI defense systems or inability to maintain the function of these systems, stemming from congenital abnormalities, nutritional defects, or insults from toxins (eg, immunosuppressives) or infections, can lead to disturbances of mucosal homeostasis and defense. These disturbances, in turn, can produce a variety of GI symptoms, including chronic diarrhea, abdominal pain, and bleeding.

Innate immunity is characterized by a rapid response to specific general structures associated with microbes of all classes (bacteria, mycobacteria, viruses, and fungi). Innate immunity is initiated by specific so-called pattern recognition receptors such as toll-like receptors (TLRs). TLR4, for example, recognizes bacterial lipopolysaccharides. Pattern recognition receptors are expressed on a wide variety of cell types, including natural killer (NK) cells, a subclass of T cells called NK-T cells, and most importantly phagocytes, mast cells, dendritic cells, and epithelial cells. Innate immunity functions as part of a first line of defense to ward off pathogenic invasions and to recruit other components of the defense system to protect the host. For example, in response to pathogenic bacteria as induced by pattern recognition receptor interactions with microbes, phagocytes engulf microorganisms (by phagocytosis), NK cells remove damaged cells (from either pathogen or malignant transformation) by secretion of lytic enzymes such as granzymes and perforins, and NK and NK-T cells alarm other immune defense cells against the microbial invasion by secreting cytokines, such as interferon-γ.

The molecular mechanisms that underlie host interactions with microbes reflect the nature of the innate immune response, which is, as noted, mediated by specific pattern recognition receptors that recognize the commonly conserved features of microbes. These pathogen-associated molecular patterns, such as the lipopolysaccharides recognized by TLR4, peptidoglycans recognized by TLR2, and double-stranded RNA recognized by TLR3, are not expressed by host cells. Recognition of these microbial products by the host immune cell receptors triggers signal transduction pathways that initiate acute phase inflammatory reactions, which typically occur within a few hours of exposure. For example, the recognition of a common pathogen-associated molecule, lipopolysaccharide, by TLR4 leads to activation of nuclear factor-κB (by destroying the inhibitory factor IKKα), which initiates an acute phase inflammatory response. In addition to the cellular components of innate immunity, noncellular components of innate immunity—such as normal peristalsis, gastric acid, bile secretion, pancreatic enzymes, mucus, epithelial cellular tight junctions, and the indigenous microbial flora—also play an important role in protecting the host from adverse reactions associated with pathogenic infection.

In comparison to innate immunity, the adaptive (specific or acquired) immune response is characterized by the large number of clonally expanded and distinct B cells and T cells that have been selected to respond to specific foreign antigens and are, at the same time, trained by the host to be tolerant to self-antigens in order to avoid autoimmunity. The selective expansion of the B-cell or T-cell clones is a complex process that involves bone marrow (for B cells) and thymus (for T cells) and requires specific receptors on the lymphocyte cell surface. Moreover, peripheral tissues and organs, such as the intestine, are also involved in the development of adaptive immunity and lymphocyte maturation and, especially, the Peyer patches and mesenteric lymph nodes. The involvement of the intestine in the development and maturation of the immune system characterizes the GI tract as both a site of immune regulation (eg, for the induction of oral tolerance) and a target of immunologic alterations associated with dysregulated immune responses.

As a result of clonal selection, the selected B cells secrete specific classes of immunoglobulins, such as immunoglobulin (Ig) A, IgG, and IgM. Decreased or dysregulated production of immunoglobulins constitutes one of the most common symptomatic forms of immunodeficiency, termed common variable immunodeficiency (CVID). CVID frequently manifests during early adulthood with recurrent respiratory and GI infections, and lymphoid hyperplasia, which is presumably a compensatory response to the immunodeficiency associated with inadequate immunoglobulin production. Although there have been a number of genes that regulate B-cell function (including genes that are expressed by T cells) that have been associated with familial forms of CVID, most cases occur spontaneously, and the pathogenesis in these cases is unclear. However, given the reduction in immunoglobulin production in all forms of CVID, some of the symptoms associated with this syndrome, at least in part, are amenable to infusions with intravenous immunoglobulin (IVIG). Defects in immunoglobulin class switching or secretion (or transcytosis) can also be associated with immunodeficiency. One such example is selective IgA deficiency, which is the most common primary immune deficiency. Patients with selective IgA deficiency are often asymptomatic and require no treatment (partially due to compensation by secreted IgM and IgG). Recognition of selective IgA deficiency is important because it can obscure the diagnosis of celiac disease and may be associated with unusual chronic infections such as *Giardia lamblia*. There is an increased risk of lymphoma in CVID patients. Possible factors include genetics, immune dysregulation, radiosensitivity, and chronic infections such as *Helicobacter pylori*, human herpes virus type 8, and CMV.

The other major class of lymphocytes associated with adaptive immunity is the T cell. T cells originate in the bone marrow, like B cells, but receive their final maturation and education within the thymus before trafficking into the systemic circulation and mucosal tissues. Once these so-called naïve T cells leave the thymus, they are instructed by dendritic cells to specific differentiated fates that are either regulatory and inhibit immune responses (so-called T regulatory cells) or effector cells (such as T helper [Th] 1, Th2, or Th17 cells). T cells express an enormous array of specific receptors that are selected within the thymus for recognition of the multitude of antigens to which the host may be exposed within a lifetime. Many rare primary immunodeficiency syndromes are associated with defects in T-cell development that result in susceptibility to infection, malignancy, autoimmunity, or a combination of all three. For example, mutations of the transcription factor FoxP3 lead to a disease called immune-mediated polyendocrinopathy, eczema X-linked (IPEX), in which there is poor formation of T regulatory cells. In addition, mutations of the cell surface molecule CTLA4, which normally inhibits T cells, are associated with autoimmune diseases.

External factors also play an important role in maintaining the normal function of the GI immune system and may form the basis for the development of acquired (secondary) types of immunodeficiency. Nutritional defects, either from malnourishment or protein-loosing enteropathy, or selective nutrient deficiency (eg, vitamin A and zinc deficiency) often lead to impaired host responses to pathogens and the development of recurrent infections. Extensive use of cytotoxic agents in a variety of clinical settings often causes depletion of neutrophils, leading to acute infections that may be associated with inflammation, such as neutropenic enterocolitis or typhlitis. In comparison with the primary immunodeficiencies, the acquired immunodeficiencies are much more common and may be involved in diseases as diverse as severe trauma, burns, cancer, myeloproliferative diseases, and immune-depleting infections such as those associated with HIV and AIDS.

Chua I, Quinti I, Grimbacher B. Lymphoma in common variable immunodeficiency: interplay between immune dysregulation, infection and genetics. *Curr Opin Hematol.* 2008;15:368–374. [PMID: 18536576]

Geissmann F, Manz MG, Jung S, et al. Development of monocytes, macrophages, and dendritic cells. *Science.* 2010;327:656–661. [PMID: 20133564]

Medzhitov R, Janeway C Jr. Innate immunity. *N Engl J Med.* 2000;343:338–344. [PMID: 10922424]

Takahashi I, Kiyono H. Gut as the largest immunologic tissue. *JPEN J Parenter Enteral Nutr.* 1999;23(Suppl):S7–12. [PMID: 10483885]

Viswanathan VK, Hecht G. Innate immunity and the gut. *Curr Opin Gastroenterol.* 2000;16:546–551. [PMID: 17031136]

B. Gastrointestinal Immunodeficiency Syndromes

1. Primary GI immunodeficiency syndromes—These syndromes result from congenitally derived abnormalities in the structure or function of immune components within the GI immune system, as outlined earlier. This category therefore includes abnormalities of T cells, B cells, and other cellular components, such as macrophages. Primary GI immunodeficiencies are often characterized by abnormalities in antibody production (either synthesis or release). These diseases include X-linked hypogammaglobulinemia, selective IgA deficiency, CVID, and hyper IgM syndromes. In addition to abnormalities of B-cell development, primary GI immunodeficiency may be a consequence of T-cell developmental defects, such as congenital thymic aplasia (DiGeorge syndrome) or abnormalities of phagocyte dysfunction, such as chronic granulomatous disease. Some primary immunodeficiencies, which are commonly associated with GI manifestations, can affect both innate and adaptive immune cell function including the Wiskott-Aldrich syndrome and nuclear factor-κB essential modulator (NEMO) deficiency.

Table 10–1. Common causes of acquired immunodeficiency.

Patient Group	Cause
Organ transplantation (renal, liver, heart, lung, bone marrow, small intestine)	Immunosuppressive therapy with corticosteroids, cyclosporine, azathioprine, methotrexate
Cancer	Malignancy or chemotherapy
Autoimmune diseases and chronic obstructive pulmonary disease	Corticosteroid therapy
Viral infection	HIV, measles
Neutropenia	Drug induced
Splenectomy	Surgical or traumatic
Advanced age	Immunosenescence
Malnutrition	Famine, infections, protein-losing enteropathy, vitamin A or zinc deficiency

2. Acquired (secondary) GI immunodeficiency syndromes—These immunodeficiency syndromes may result from a variety of insults, such as physical (eg, radiation), chemical (eg, chemotherapeutic agents, steroids, immunosuppressive drugs such as methotrexate), or infectious agents (eg, HIV), as well as decreased immunity due to severe malnutrition, old age, protein-losing enteropathy, and selective nutrient deficiency (Table 10–1).

Clinical Findings

A detailed history and physical examination provide the initial clues to the possible presence of immunodeficiency. However, the establishment of a definitive diagnosis of immunodeficiency often requires laboratory tests that quantify specific elements of the immune system such as quantitative T-cell subset analysis (eg, CD4-positive T-cell numbers), immunoglobulin isotype evaluation, or both.

A. Symptoms and Signs

A history of prolonged and severe GI symptoms (diarrhea, dysphagia, odynophagia, nausea, vomiting, abdominal pain, anorectal disease, GI bleeding, or jaundice), relapse of symptoms after proper treatment, recurrent respiratory tract or GI tract infection since childhood, or being a recipient of immunosuppressive treatments are supportive of an underlying state of immunodeficiency.

On physical examination, patients may demonstrate facial abnormalities (DiGeorge syndrome), oral thrush, oral ulcers, a

Table 10–2. Gastrointestinal pathogens in immunocompromised hosts.

Site	Viral	Parasitic	Fungal	Bacterial
Oral cavity	HSV, Epstein-Barr virus		*Candida* spp	
Esophagus	HSV, CMV		*Candida* spp, *Histoplasma capsulatum*	*Mycobacterium*, *Pseudomonas*
Small intestine	CMV, rotavirus, adenovirus, coxsackievirus, astrovirus, calicivirus, picornavirus/parvovirus	*Giardia lamblia*, *Cryptosporidium*, *Strongyloides*, *Microsporidia*	*Aspergillus*, *Histoplasma*	*Salmonella*, *Campylobacter*, *Aeromonas*
Colon	CMV, HSV	*Entamoeba*	*Histoplasma*, *Aspergillus*	*Clostridium difficile*, *Campylobacter*, *Shigella sonnei*
Liver	CMV, HSV		*Candida*	*Mycobacterium*

CMV, cytomegalovirus; HSV, herpes simplex virus.
Adapted, with permission, from Yamada T (editor). *Textbook of Gastroenterology*, Vol 1, 4th ed. Lippincott Williams & Wilkins, 2003:1021.

paucity of lymphoid tissues (X-linked agammaglobulinemia), focal or diffused lymphadenopathy, edema (protein-losing enteropathy), or eczema (Wiskott-Aldrich syndrome, IgA deficiency, hyper IgE, or Job syndrome).

Unlike the GI symptoms observed in immunocompetent hosts (eg, diarrhea and abdominal pain), which are often a self-limited process, GI symptoms in immunocompromised patients are commonly associated with chronicity and significantly higher rates of morbidity and mortality. The impaired immune function of immunocompromised patients leads to both uncommon presentations of common infections and the development of uncommon opportunistic infections. For example, in immunocompromised hosts, cytomegalovirus (CMV) infection may lead to necrotizing colitis or perforation of the gut. Therefore, the prompt recognition and management of GI symptoms in an immunocompromised host are crucial for the rapid relief of symptoms and, consequently, reduction of morbidity and mortality.

B. Laboratory Findings

Routine laboratory evaluation may reveal neutropenia, lymphopenia, or altered albumin and globulin levels. These studies are often supplemented by microscopic examination of the stool. More specific laboratory tests of the cellular and humoral components of the immune system are often required to establish a definitive diagnosis of the specific cause of the immunodeficiency. Because the most common GI manifestations of immunodeficiency are recurrent infections and diarrhea, the discussion that follows focuses on the evaluation and management of these common symptoms.

Treatment

A. Diarrhea (See also Chapter 5)

Diarrhea is typically defined as the passage of three or more loose or watery stools per day for more than 2 days. Chronic diarrhea is defined as diarrhea lasting for more than 30 days in adults and 14 days in children. In immunocompetent hosts, chronic diarrhea is caused predominately by noninfectious conditions, such as inflammatory bowel disease, celiac sprue, endocrinopathies, eating disorders, laxative abuse, malignancies, short bowel syndrome, and bacterial overgrowth. In comparison, in immunocompromised hosts, infections resulting from a variety of pathogens are the most common causes of diarrheal disease (Table 10–2).

Some pathogens are unique to immunocompromised hosts; for example, *Mycobacterium avium* complex (MAC) infections are unique to HIV infection and AIDS, occurring when the CD4 T-cell count declines below 100/mm^3. Other pathogens, such as *Cryptosporidium*, cause self-limited diarrhea in healthy hosts but chronic diarrhea in immunosuppressed patients.

Small bowel bacterial overgrowth is defined as more than 10^4 bacteria per milliliter in the small intestine, comprising gram-negative anaerobes of colonic origin rather than gram-positive aerobes of the stomach and oral microflora. It occurs more often in immunocompromised hosts with both primary immunodeficiency (eg, hypogammaglobulinemia) and acquired immunodeficiency from HIV infection or aging.

To evaluate diarrhea in a patient with an immunocompromised condition, a detailed history is necessary to rule out the common causes of diarrhea, which include medications (use of multiple medications is common in immunocompromised patients), diet (lactose, food, or fatty acid intolerance), or inadvertent use of cathartics. Although symptoms alone are unlikely to identify the cause of the diarrhea, it may facilitate the evaluation. For example, diarrhea with cramps, bloating, and nausea suggests the involvement of the stomach and small bowel or both (eg, infection with *Cryptosporidium, Microsporidia, Isospora belli,* or *Giardia*). Diarrhea associated with hematochezia and tenesmus implies large bowel involvement (and therefore the possible involvement of CMV, *Shigella,* or *Campylobacter* infection).

Stool examination is very important for making the diagnosis of a pathogenic cause of diarrhea in immunocompromised patients. The stool examination should include stool culture for enteric bacteria, three samples for *Clostridium difficile* toxin analysis (when patients are on antibiotics), and at least three stool specimens for ova and parasite examination to increase the sensitivity of the examination.

In cases refractory to routine study, endoscopic evaluation with biopsy is of particular importance in helping to establish the diagnosis. Colonoscopy or sigmoidoscopy is helpful in identifying CMV infection, and upper endoscopic examination can help to uncover small bowel infection with *Cryptosporidium, Microsporidia,* or *M avium.*

Once the cause of diarrhea is identified, specific therapy should be administrated. Unlike patients with an intact immune system, in whom supportive care is usually sufficient for self-recovery, immunocompromised patients may require chronic administration of antibiotics for recurrent *Salmonella, Shigella, Campylobacter,* or *Isospora* infection. An empiric trial of oral antibiotics or antiparasite therapy for possible small bowel bacterial overgrowth or undetected infection should also be considered in the immunocompromised patient who has persistent symptoms and in whom a specific diagnosis is not made, even after extensive evaluation. Some of the reasonable regimens that might be considered are the use of sulfonamides, ciprofloxacin, tetracyclines, or metronidazole.

Symptom relief with antidiarrheal agents, such as loperamide (Imodium) and Lomotil (diphenoxylate with atropine), may also be considered, using careful clinical judgment. In patients with debilitating conditions, nutritional support may carry a direct benefit for patient well-being and contribute to the restoration of immune function. In some patients with chronic diarrhea, in whom the specific cause cannot be established, a trial of the somatostatin analog octreotide may be effective, presumably by inhibition of secretion of a broad array of GI hormones. However, this potential benefit must be counterbalanced by the possible risk of gallbladder ileus and gallstone formation.

Camilleri M. Chronic diarrhea: a review on pathophysiology and management for the clinical gastroenterologist. *Clin Gastroenterol Hepatol.* 2004;2:198–206. [PMID: 15017602]

Kearney DJ, Steuerwald M, Koch J, et al. A prospective study of endoscopy in HIV-associated diarrhea. *Am J Gastroenterol.* 1999;94:596–602. [PMID: 10086637]

B. Dysphagia and Odynophagia

As in the case of diarrhea, the symptoms of dysphagia and odynophagia in immunocompetent and immunocompromised patients usually have different causes. In immunocompetent patients, the most frequent causes of dysphagia and odynophagia are usually acid reflux damage, malignancy, or neuromuscular diseases. In immunocompromised patients, by comparison, infections are the most frequent cause for these symptoms. In fact, because symptomatic infectious esophagitis is extremely rare in the immunocompetent host, the development of infectious esophagitis serves as a strong clinical indicator in and of itself of an underlying state of immunodeficiency that requires further immunologic evaluation.

Candida species, herpes simplex virus (HSV), CMV, and *Mycobacterium* species are the most frequent causative agents of infectious esophagitis in an immunocompromised host (see Table 10–2). Although each pathogen is associated with characteristic clinical manifestations (eg, *Candida* infection with oral thrush, HSV with gingivostomatitis, CMV with abdominal pain and diarrhea, and *Mycobacterium* with fever, cough, and weight loss), it is impossible to identify the particular pathogen causing dysphagia or odynophagia, or both, on the basis of clinical symptoms alone. Endoscopic evaluation with biopsies is therefore extremely valuable in establishing the cause of the esophageal symptoms in order to commence specific treatment. It has been suggested that multiple biopsies (more than three) are necessary to establish the diagnosis of a single infection, and additional biopsies may be necessary to establish causative agents in complex infections, which may be polymicrobial.

One exception to this general approach to the evaluation of esophageal symptoms is that of immunocompromised patients who develop oral thrush. In these patients, empiric treatment of possible esophageal candidiasis is warranted. In a large clinical study of 110 HIV-infected patients, the presence of oral thrush had a positive predictive value of 77% for *Candida* esophagitis.

The most frequently used regimen for esophageal candidiasis is either fluconazole, 100–200 mg/day, or itraconazole, 200 mg/day orally. Amphotericin B can be effective in patients with refractory *Candida* esophagitis. Most HSV esophagitis responds well to acyclovir, 200 mg orally every 4 hours. In the rare case of acyclovir resistance, patients may require foscarnet, which is associated with possible adverse effects of nephrotoxicity and hypocalcemia. CMV esophagitis usually responds well to a 2- to 3-week course of ganciclovir. However, a maintenance regimen or an additional course of treatment is often required to suppress CMV infection.

C. Abdominal Pain (See also Chapter 1)

Unlike diarrhea and esophageal symptoms, the common causes of abdominal pain in immunocompetent persons are also the common causes of abdominal pain in immunocompromised patients (Table 10–3). Nevertheless, in immunocompromised patients, opportunistic infection presents a major cause of abdominal pain which, in the setting of immunodeficiency, can proceed more rapidly and lead to a medical catastrophe. Therefore, to evaluate abdominal pain in immunocompromised patients, the early use of computed tomographic scanning and abdominal sonography is warranted to identify the origin of abdominal pain and uncommon diseases that manifest by bowel wall thickening. In such

Table 10–3. Causes of abdominal pain in immunocompromised hosts.

Cytomegalovirus (CMV) infection
Colonic perforation caused by CMV, *Candida* species, *Histoplasma capsulatum*, lymphoma
Typhlitis
Cholecystitis caused by CMV, *Cryptosporidium parvum, Isospora belli, Microsporidia, Pneumocystis carinii*
Pancreatitis caused by CMV, immunosuppressive and antiviral drugs
Graft-versus-host disease
Hepatosplenic candidiasis
Veno-occlusive liver diseases
Tissue infiltration by tumor or lymphoma
Bleeding secondary to drug-induced thrombocytopenia

cases, patients should be further evaluated with endoscopic studies and biopsies, which often reveal CMV infection, lymphoma, and MAC infection.

CMV infection is a frequent cause of abdominal pain in immunocompromised patients, such as HIV-infected patients and transplant recipients. Different from biliary pain and intestinal obstruction, which often fluctuate in intensity, enteric pain caused by CMV often presents as constant cramping in the lower abdomen. CMV may also cause severe epigastric pain by inducing pancreatitis, cholecystitis, or cholangitis. Perforation should be considered in an immunocompromised patient with an acute exacerbation of abdominal pain.

The location of abdominal pain can be indicative of the underlying cause, although further imaging or invasive studies are usually required to establish the diagnosis. For example, in patients with severe neutropenia, right lower quadrant abdominal pain is suggestive of typhlitis or necrotizing enterocolitis, whereas right upper quadrant abdominal pain and tenderness associated with nausea and fever may be a typical presentation of hepatosplenic candidiasis encountered during the treatment of acute leukemia or lymphoma. Another common right upper quadrant pain syndrome is veno-occlusive disease of the liver in a recent bone marrow transplant recipient (within 20 days), which often manifests with right upper quadrant pain and tenderness, hepatomegaly, hyperbilirubinemia, and ascites.

Similar to the management of the general population, the initial question to be answered in immunocompromised patients with abdominal pain is whether or not surgical intervention is required. In general, intestinal perforation and obstruction almost always require surgical management. Once the cause of the pain has been identified, treatable infections should be managed promptly. Symptoms resulting from lymphoma or Kaposi sarcoma may require chemotherapy or radiation therapy.

D. Other Gastrointestinal Symptoms in Immunocompromised Patients

1. Gastrointestinal bleeding—GI bleeding is a rare presentation in patients with immunodeficiency. The evaluation and management of GI bleeding in these patients is the same as that in the immunocompetent population. The location and severity of the bleeding should be determined. Upper endoscopy is usually necessary to define the source of any severe upper GI bleeding, whereas nuclear red blood cell scan is more useful to define the approximate site of lower GI bleeding. During the acute phase, endoscopic mucosal biopsy is generally not advisable to avoid the risk of precipitating more severe bleeding. A follow-up examination with mucosal biopsy can be performed when the acute bleeding subsides.

In addition to the common causes of GI bleeding in the general population, immunocompromised patients may also exhibit bleeding as a result of infection. The most common infectious cause of esophageal bleeding in immunocompromised patients is HSV, which induces shallow ulcers in the esophagus. In the case of HSV, the bleeding is typically slow and self-limited. CMV is the more common cause of intestinal bleeding, which again tends to be slow and self-limited. Both HSV and CMV are, however, rare causes of bleeding among immunocompromised patients. The possibility that CMV infection is the cause of intestinal bleeding is increased with concurrent symptoms of fever, abdominal pain, and diarrhea.

2. Anorectal and perianal disease—Anorectal disease is one of the most important GI complications of immunodeficiency and occurs in 5–7% of neutropenic patients with leukemia or lymphoma. If not managed properly, devastating morbidity and high mortality are ensured. The various manifestations of anorectal disease in neutropenic patients include abscess formation, fissure, fistula, ulceration, and infected hemorrhoids. Extensive tissue necrosis and breakdown can occur. Surgical intervention with incision and drainage is usually needed to reduce the high recurrence (12%) and high mortality (18%) rate associated with nonoperative management in neutropenic patients. Early treatment with antibiotics, which should include aminoglycosides and agents with anaerobic coverage, is advisable. HSV infection, which often begins with perianal vesicular lesions, should be treated promptly with acyclovir to prevent the devastating progression to perianal ulcers.

3. Neutropenia—A decline in the absolute number of circulating neutrophils below $1000/mm^3$ is associated with an increased susceptibility to infections. When the number of neutrophils decreases below $500/mm^3$, the host's ability to manage the endogenous GI flora is also significantly impaired, and patients often develop fever and sepsis due to passage of commensal bacteria across the epithelial barrier into the circulation. It must also be remembered that in the context of an abnormal immune system, symptoms may be subtle due to the inability of the host to respond properly.

Three GI syndromes are often associated with neutropenia: oral infection (gingivitis, periodontitis, and oral ulcers), anorectal infection, and typhlitis (typically in the area of the cecum). Early recognition of these complications and commencement of medical and surgical treatment are mandatory to prevent severe morbidity and mortality, as previously discussed.

In neutropenic patients who present with fever, right lower quadrant abdominal pain, diarrhea (which may be bloody), or a combination of these findings, computed tomography scan is critical for establishing the diagnosis of typhlitis. For localized disease, bowel rest with broad-spectrum antibiotics can be effective in preventing disease progression. Diffuse disease or evidence of perforation warrants consideration of surgical intervention.

4. Transplant-associated GI illness—GI disease is an important cause of morbidity and mortality in bone marrow and solid organ transplant recipients. In general, bone marrow transplant recipients experience more frequent and severe GI disease. Acute graft-versus-host disease (GVHD) usually occurs during the first 3–4 weeks posttransplantation. Patients often present with diarrhea and a variety of other GI symptoms, including anorexia, nausea, vomiting, and abdominal pain. GVHD occurs in as many as 40% of bone marrow transplant recipients. Acute GVHD is often accompanied by symptoms of skin rash and jaundice. Establishment of the diagnosis, however, requires histologic examination demonstrating single-cell apoptosis of the epithelium, crypt distortion, abscesses, and periglandular infiltrates. CMV infection has been shown to be a significant cause of GI bleeding in patients with acute GVHD.

Chronic GVHD typically occurs between 3 and 12 months after bone marrow transplantation and presents as mucositis of the oral cavity, dysphagia, and small bowel dysmotility associated with bacterial overgrowth. GI symptoms in recipients of solid organ transplants usually are infectious in nature and less severe than those observed in bone marrow transplant recipients, due presumably to less severe immune suppression in the latter patient group.

Gastroesophageal Reflux Disease

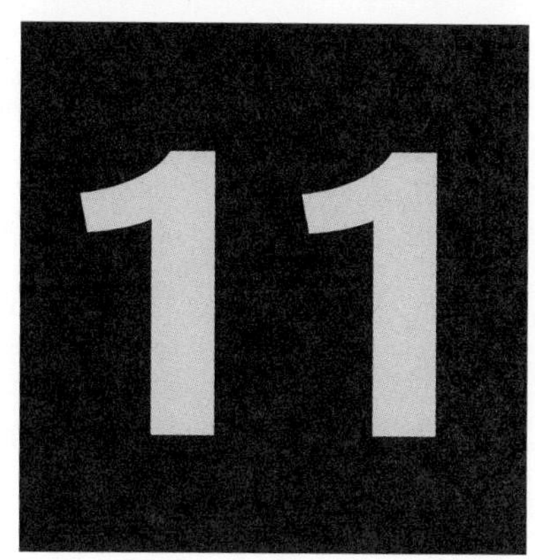

John R. Saltzman, MD

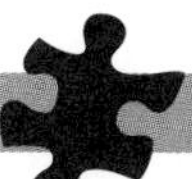

ESSENTIALS OF DIAGNOSIS

- ▶ Heartburn, regurgitation, and dysphagia.
- ▶ "Alarm signs"—dysphagia, odynophagia, weight loss, family history of upper gastrointestinal (GI) tract cancers, persistent nausea and emesis, long duration of symptoms (>10 years), and incomplete response to treatment.
- ▶ Atypical manifestations (eg, asthma) are common.

General Considerations

Gastroesophageal reflux disease (GERD) is the most common and costly digestive disease. It accounts for at least 9 million physician office visits in the United States each year, and annual direct costs for managing GERD are estimated to exceed 9 billion dollars. GERD is a chronic disorder resulting from the retrograde flow of gastroduodenal contents into the esophagus or adjacent organs, and producing a variable spectrum of symptoms, with or without tissue damage. Transient inappropriate relaxation of the lower esophageal sphincter (LES) is the predominant pathophysiologic mechanism in the majority of GERD patients. Gastroparesis and a reduced LES pressure play a significant role in patients with moderate to severe disease.

Sandler RS, Everhart JE, Donowitz M, et al. The burden of selected digestive diseases in the United States. *Gastroenterology.* 2002;122:1500–1511. [PMID: 1984534]

A. Epidemiology

The prevalence of GERD in the United States appears to be increasing. In Western populations, 25% of people report having heartburn at least once a month, 12% at least once per week, and 5% describe having symptoms on a daily basis. There appears to be no gender predominance of heartburn symptoms; men and women are affected equally. The relationship of age and reflux is unclear. One study has suggested an association between advancing age and fewer reflux symptoms but the presence of more severe esophagitis. There is an unequivocal positive association between body mass index and reflux symptoms. Inappropriate relaxation of the LES can be exacerbated by obesity. Even moderate weight gain among persons of normal weight is thought to cause or exacerbate reflux symptoms. These epidemiologic characteristics should be considered when evaluating a patient with typical and atypical GERD.

Johnson DA, Fennerty MB. Heartburn severity underestimates erosive esophagitis severity in elderly patients with gastroesophageal reflux disease. *Gastroenterology.* 2004;126:660–664. [PMID: 14988819]

Moayyedi P, Axon AT. Review article: gastroesophageal reflux disease: the extent of the problem. *Aliment Pharmacol Ther.* 2005;22(Suppl 1):11–19. [PMID: 16042655]

B. Pathogenesis

Pathologic reflux of gastric contents occurs when the refluxate overcomes the antireflux barriers of the gastroesophageal junction, typically in a postprandial state. The antireflux barrier of the gastroesophageal junction is anatomically and physiologically complex and vulnerable to a number of potential mechanisms of reflux. The primary antireflux mechanism is the LES, a segment of smooth muscle in the lower esophagus that is chronically contracted to maintain a pressure that is approximately 15 mm Hg above intragastric pressure. The two main patterns of LES dysfunction are (1) a hypotensive LES and (2) pathologic transient LES relaxations. Anatomic disruption of the gastroesophageal junction, commonly associated with a hiatal hernia, contributes to the pathogenesis of reflux disease by impairing LES function.

A large hiatal hernia predisposes to transient LES relaxations and increases the risk of developing esophagitis. Transient LES relaxations account for the majority of reflux events in individuals with normal LES pressure and clinically mild reflux disease. Chronically low LES pressure is the predominant GERD mechanism in patients with severe reflux disease, such as in patients with scleroderma.

Gastric factors can play a significant role in producing GERD. Gastric factors that promote GERD include increased gastric volume after meals, increased gastric pressure due to obesity, recumbency after meals, and delayed gastric emptying or gastroparesis, which can be idiopathic or drug induced. Increased gastric distention can cause an increase in transient LES relaxations and the volume of refluxate, particularly in GERD patients with large hiatal hernias. Delayed gastric emptying, or gastroparesis, may be present in approximately 15% of patients with GERD and is frequently underdiagnosed.

Other factors that decrease LES pressure and contribute to GERD are medications, lifestyle behaviors, and the ingestion of certain foods. Certain medicines can exacerbate GERD by lowering LES pressure; others can cause esophagitis by direct mucosal injury (Table 11–1). Certain foods, beverages, and behaviors will cause heartburn by reducing LES pressure (Table 11–2). Fatty foods, peppermint, chocolate, caffeinated beverages, alcohol, and smoking can all decrease LES pressure.

El-Serag HB, Ergun GA, Pandolfino J, et al. Obesity increases oesophageal acid exposure. *Gut.* 2007;56:749–755. [PMID: 17127706]

Horowitz M, Su YG, Rayner CK, et al. Gastroparesis: prevalence, clinical significance and treatment. *Can J Gastroenterol.* 2001;15:805–813. [PMID: 11773947]

Jacobson BC, Somers SC, Fuchs CS, et al. Body-mass index and symptoms of gastroesophageal reflux in women. *N Engl J Med.* 2006;354:2340–2348. [PMID: 16738270]

Table 11–1. Medications that can cause GERD or esophagitis.

Decrease LES Pressure	Cause Direct Mucosal Injury
β-Adrenergic agonists, including inhalers	Alendronate
α-Adrenergic antagonists	Aspirin
Anticholinergics	Iron salts
Calcium channel blockers	Nonsteroidal anti-inflammatory drugs
Diazepam	Potassium chloride tablets
Estrogens	Quinidine
Narcotics	Tetracycline
Progesterone	
Theophylline	
Tricyclic antidepressants	

LES, lower esophageal sphincter.

Table 11–2. Factors that can precipitate or exacerbate GERD symptoms.

Medications (see Table 11-1)
Foods
Caffeine
Chocolate
Peppermint
Alcohol (red wine pH = 3.25)
Carbonated beverages (cola pH = 2.75)
Citrus fruits (orange juice pH = 3.25)
Tomato-based products (tomato juice pH = 3.25)
Vinegar (pH = 3.00)
Lifestyle factors
Weight gain
Smoking
Eating prior to recumbency

Jones MP, Sloan SS, Rabine JC, et al. Hiatal hernia size is the dominant determinant of esophagitis presence and severity in gastroesophageal reflux disease. *Am J Gastroenterol.* 2001;96:1711–1717. [PMID: 11419819]

Kahrilas PJ. GERD pathogenesis, pathophysiology and clinical manifestations. *Cleve Clin J Med.* 2003;70(Suppl 5):S4–19. [PMID: 14705378]

Clinical Findings

A. Symptoms and Signs

GERD is defined in a guideline by the American College of Gastroenterology as symptoms or mucosal damage produced by the abnormal reflux of gastric contents into the esophagus. The typical manifestations of GERD are heartburn, regurgitation, and dysphagia. Other symptoms associated with GERD include water brash, a globus (lump in the throat) sensation, odynophagia, and nausea. Heartburn (pyrosis) is defined as a retrosternal burning discomfort located in the epigastric area that may radiate up toward the neck and typically occurs in the postprandial period, especially after a high-fat or a large-volume meal. Postural changes such as bending over often exacerbate patients' symptoms. Symptoms can also be aggravated by ingestion of certain foods or beverages, such as tomato sauce, peppermint, chocolate, coffee, tea, and alcohol. When assessing a patient with heartburn symptoms, the duration and severity of symptoms should be investigated. Patients who present with typical symptoms with a minimum frequency of twice a week for 4–8 weeks or more should be considered as having GERD. At initial presentation, it is important to consider a patient's age and the presence of "alarm signs" (Table 11–3). The presence of any alarm signs necessitates the evaluation of GERD symptoms with an upper endoscopy or imaging modality.

Atypical manifestations of GERD refer to symptoms that are extraesophageal, including pulmonary, ear, nose,

Table 11–3. "Alarm" signs that necessitate further evaluation of GERD.

Dysphagia
Odynophagia
Weight loss
Gastrointestinal (GI) bleeding
Family history of upper GI tract cancer
Anemia
Advanced age

and throat manifestations, as well as noncardiac chest pain (Table 11–4). According to published studies in the literature, pathologic GERD can be found in 30–80% of adults patients with asthma. Microaspiration of gastric acid and subsequent airway irritation are considered the possible triggers for asthma. Any adult with new-onset asthma should be evaluated for GERD as a possible etiology. A new, more frequently recognized atypical manifestation of GERD is otitis media in children. Otitis media with effusion is the most common cause of childhood hearing loss. High concentrations of pepsin/pepsinogen were found in greater than 90% of middle ear effusion samples from children with otitis media with effusion. Reflux of gastric juice into the middle ear may be the primary factor in precipitating this disease in children.

Patients with gastroparesis and GERD may present with concomitant nausea, vomiting, or early satiety. These patients may not respond to antisecretory agents alone, as the refluxate contains bile and digestive enzymes in addition to gastric acid. Gastroparesis should be suspected in patients with an acute or subacute onset of GERD, particularly after an episode of viral upper respiratory infection or gastroenteritis. The natural history of GERD with acute gastroparesis is that the majority of patients will achieve symptomatic resolution, although some will need treatment with prokinetic agents. Antisecretory agents may offer some symptomatic relief and reduce gastric volume. Dietary changes such as low-fat, frequent, small meals may also be helpful in controlling symptoms.

Table 11–4. Extraesophageal manifestations of GERD.

Otitis media	Frequent throat clearing
Asthma	Globus
Chronic sinusitis	Tracheobronchitis
Dental erosions	Chronic cough
Aphthous ulcers	Aspiration pneumonia
Halitosis	Pulmonary fibrosis
Pharyngitis	Chronic bronchitis
Laryngitis	Bronchiectasis
Laryngospasm	Noncardiac chest pain
Postnasal drip	Sleep apnea

American Lung Association Asthma Clinical Research Centers, Mastronarde JG, Anthonisen NR, et al. Efficacy of esomeprazole for treatment of poorly controlled asthma. *N Engl J Med.* 2009;360:1487–1499. [PMID: 19357404]

Horowitz M, Su YG, Rayner CK, et al. Gastroparesis: prevalence, clinical significance and treatment. *Can J Gastroenterol.* 2001;15:805–813. [PMID: 11773947]

Tasker A, Dettmar PW, Panetti M, et al. Is gastric reflux a cause of otitis media with effusion in children? *Laryngoscope.* 2002;112:1930–1934. [PMID: 12439157]

B. Laboratory, Imaging, and Endoscopic Studies

Classic GERD can be diagnosed by taking a thorough symptom history and confirmed by a complete response to medical therapy (a "PPI [proton pump inhibitor] test"). In general, diagnostic testing is reserved for patients who fail to respond to a trial of adequate medical therapy or for patients who have alarm symptoms with GERD (Figure 11–1). Available tests include upper GI series, upper endoscopy, 24-hour esophageal pH study, wireless capsule pH study, and esophageal impedance testing.

PPI therapy is very effective in healing esophagitis. Patients who have no symptom response to PPI therapy are unlikely to have GERD. A meta-analysis that assessed the accuracy of normal or high-dose PPI for 1–4 weeks in the diagnosis of GERD found a pooled sensitivity of 78% (95% confidence interval [CI] 66–86%) and a specificity of 54% (44–65%) when ambulatory pH was used as a gold standard. Diagnostic testing for GERD patients is indicated in those who fail a PPI test or have alarm signs.

Radiologic studies are of limited use in the management of GERD due to poor sensitivity in milder forms of GERD, but they can detect moderate to severe esophagitis, strictures, hiatal hernias, and tumors. The studies that are most commonly used are the barium swallow, which only examines the esophagus, and the upper GI series, which examines the esophagus, stomach, and upper small intestine. The primary utility of radiographic studies in GERD is to rule out other diseases in patients in whom there is a low clinical suspicion that significant disease is present. These studies can help exclude peptic ulcer disease and tumors as a cause of a patient's symptoms. In addition, radiographic studies can be helpful in the evaluation of a patient with dysphagia to rule out peptic rings, which can sometimes be difficult to visualize on upper endoscopy. Compared with endoscopy, radiologic studies are noninvasive, widely available, and relatively inexpensive. However, they are less sensitive and specific than upper endoscopy and require an operator skill that may be becoming scarcer in the era of cross-sectional imaging.

Upper endoscopy, in addition to excluding the presence of other diseases such as tumors and peptic ulcers, can detect and grade the severity of GERD-induced esophagitis (Plate 6). Upper endoscopy is highly specific (90–95%) for GERD but has limited sensitivity (~50%). The extent and severity of mucosal injury can be assessed endoscopically.

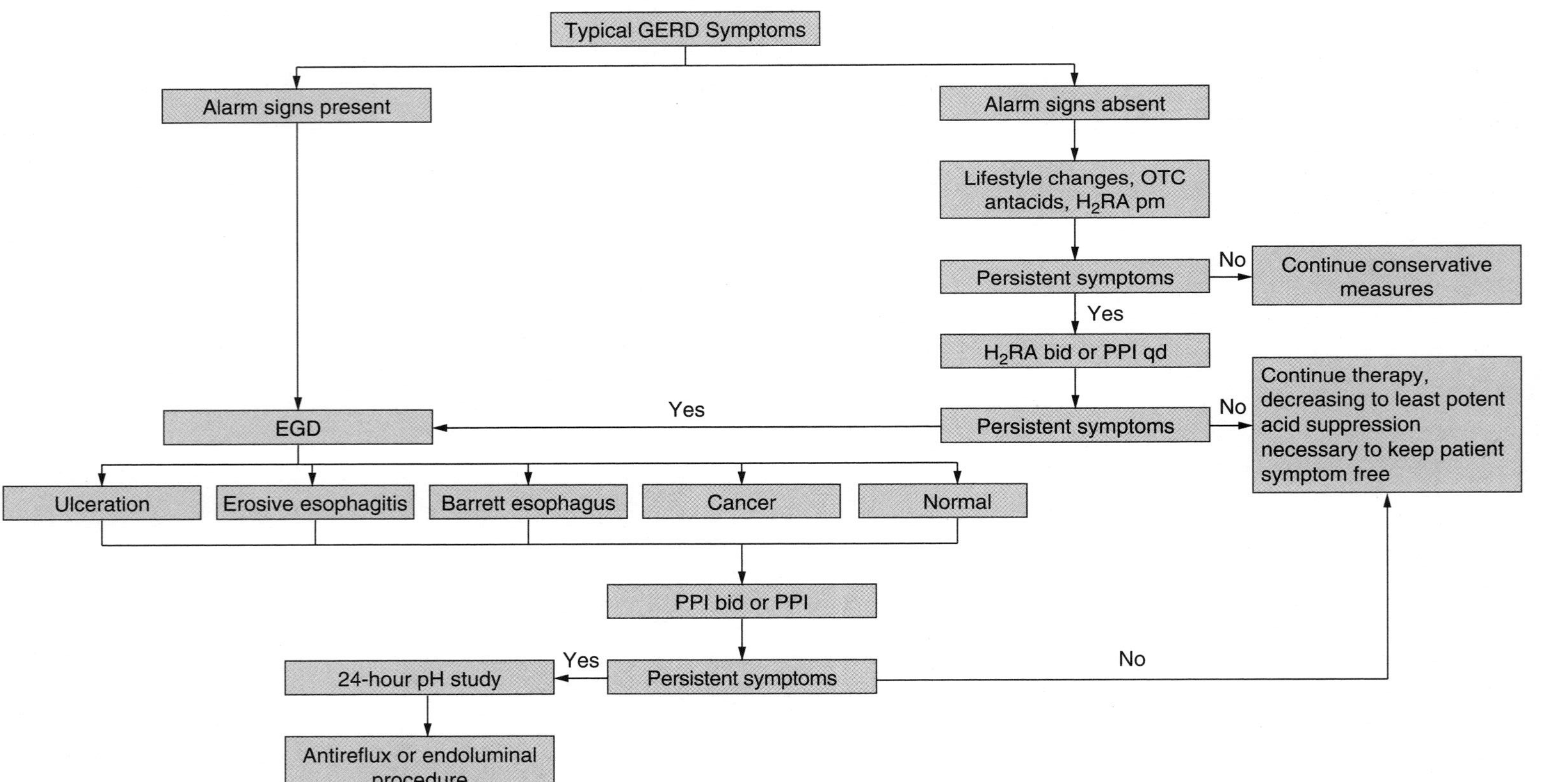

▲ **Figure 11–1.** Algorithm for the diagnosis and treatment of gastroesophageal reflux (GERD). bid, twice daily; EGD, esophagogastroduodenoscopy; H_2RA, H_2-receptor antagonist; OTC, over-the-counter; prn, as needed; qd, daily.

The Los Angeles classification of esophagitis quantifies the length and circumference of mucosal breaks. Upper endoscopy also allows the evaluation of any complications of the disease, such as strictures or Barrett esophagus. It is therefore the test of choice in patients with alarm signs. If a patient has dysphagia and a stricture is detected, dilation of the stricture can be performed during the same procedure. Esophageal biopsy is also the best test for patients in whom eosinophilic esophagitis is suspected, namely younger patients with a history of intermittent dysphagia and possibly atopy. Upper endoscopy is the test of choice in evaluating complicated GERD patients.

Intraesophageal ambulatory pH monitoring utilizes a probe that can record the distal esophageal pH continuously for 24 hours. The test is done with a pH probe that is passed transnasally to 5 cm above the manometrically determined LES. The data are collected by a battery-powered device carried by the patient, who also records when meals are eaten and symptoms experienced. This technique allows for correlation of symptoms with reflux episodes. Ambulatory esophageal pH monitoring records the timing, length, and number of reflux episodes. Acid reflux episodes are defined as an esophageal pH below 4. Normally the total amount of time during which the esophagus has a pH of 4 or less is 4% or less. Intraesophageal pH probe monitoring is a sensitive test to detect the presence of intraesophageal acid.

Despite its sensitivity, esophageal pH testing should only be used in a select minority of GERD patients. Twenty-four hour pH monitoring is useful in patients who have typical GERD symptoms but are unresponsive to therapy. When performed in this patient population, ambulatory pH monitoring can determine if the diagnosis of GERD is correct or if additional medical or surgical therapy is required. It is also helpful in patients with atypical GERD symptoms, such as asthma and chronic cough, when these symptoms are not responsive to acid suppression therapy. Ambulatory esophageal pH monitoring is also important in the postoperative evaluation of a patient who has had antireflux surgery, in order to determine whether GERD is still present.

Although extremely useful in selected patients, esophageal pH testing is not widely available, can be uncomfortable, and is expensive. The discomfort associated with nasal probe placement has prompted the development of a wireless pH monitoring system. The Bravo wireless capsule pH monitoring system (Medtronic, Inc) allows for a wireless, pill-sized capsule to be attached to the distal esophageal mucosa during an upper endoscopy. The pH monitoring lasts for 48 hours (vs 24 hours with a conventional pH probe). The capsule detaches and is spontaneously passed within 2 weeks. The main disadvantage of this system is that up to 10% of patients experience discomfort due to the presence of the pH capsule or may feel that the capsule is present (mild foreign body sensation). In some patients, the capsule may dislodge prematurely, not allowing for the full 48-hour period of pH monitoring. There have also been isolated reports of esophageal bleeding requiring transfusion and esophageal perforation.

Esophageal impedance testing detects changes in the resistance of electrical current on a catheter placed within the esophagus. In addition to recording esophageal pH, this catheter can differentiate both antegrade and retrograde transit of liquid and gas. Thus acid, weakly acid, and nonacid reflux can be detected, and this test has greater sensitivity than pH testing alone for the detection of GERD. This test is helpful in patients who have suspected GERD or extraesophageal symptom of GERD but negative esophageal pH tests (in patients with suspected nonacid GERD and in patients on PPI therapy with suspected symptoms related to GERD). This test is recommended after standard testing has not demonstrated significant GERD in patients with typical, atypical, or refractory symptoms of GERD. Although this test is not yet widely available, it has the potential to change patient management by directing further therapies.

DeVault KR, Castell DO. American College of Gastroenterology. Updated guidelines for the diagnosis and treatment of gastroesophageal reflux disease. *Am J Gastroenterol.* 2005;100:190–200. [PMID: 15654800]

Hirano I, Richter JE; Practice Parameters Committee of the American College of Gastroenterology. ACG practice guidelines: esophageal reflux testing. *Am J Gastroenterol.* 2007;102:668–685. [PMID: 17335450]

Numans ME, Lau J, de Wit NJ, et al. Short-term treatment with proton pump inhibitors as a test for gastroesophageal reflux disease: a meta-analysis of diagnostic test characteristics. *Ann Intern Med.* 2004;140:518–527. [PMID: 15068979]

Pritchett JM, Aslam M, Slaughter JC, et al. Efficacy of esophageal impedance/pH monitoring in patients with refractory gastroesophageal reflux disease, on and off therapy. *Clin Gastroenterol Hepatol.* 2009;7:743–748. [PMID: 19281866]

Standards of Practice Committee, Lichtenstein DR, Cash BD, et al. Role of endoscopy in the management of GERD. *Gastrointest Endosc.* 2007;66:219–224. [PMID: 17643692]

U.S. Food and Drug Administration. Center for Devices and Radiological Health. Available at: http://www.accessdata.fda.gov/scripts/cdrh/cfdocs/cfMAUDE/search.cfm.

Complications

Complications from chronic GERD include bleeding from esophageal erosions or ulceration, stricture formation, and Barrett esophagus.

A. Esophageal Ulcers

Although somewhat counterintuitive, the severity and duration of GERD symptoms poorly correlates with the presence or severity of esophagitis. Esophageal ulcers due to esophagitis account for approximately 2% of all upper GI bleeding. The vast majority of esophageal peptic ulcers heal completely with acid-suppression therapy using PPIs.

B. Peptic Esophageal Strictures

Peptic esophageal strictures have been described in 10% of patients who seek medical attention for GERD symptoms.

When questioned, most patients with esophageal strictures report dysphagia for an average of 4–6 years, and up to 25% deny any prior GERD. Weight loss, a cardinal symptom of esophageal cancer, is uncommon with peptic strictures because patients gradually learn to change their dietary habits to avoid foods that cause dysphagia.

C. Esophageal Carcinoma

Although the severity and duration of GERD symptoms appears to have little correlation with the presence of esophagitis, there is increasing evidence that frequent, severe GERD, particularly nocturnal, is a major risk factor for the development of esophageal adenocarcinoma. The incidence of esophageal adenocarcinoma is increasing in the United States and Europe at a very rapid rate. Esophageal adenocarcinoma and its predisposing risk factor, Barrett esophagus, are discussed in Chapter 12.

Treatment

The goals of treatment for GERD are to resolve symptoms, heal esophagitis, and prevent complications of GERD. Once a patient is in remission, the goal is to maintain remission from symptoms and prevent further tissue injury.

A. Lifestyle, Medical, and Mechanical Therapies

A cornerstone of the treatment of GERD is lifestyle modifications. Patients are instructed to avoid foods and acid-containing beverages that can exacerbate their symptoms of GERD (see Table 11–2). Patients should avoid lying down for 3 hours after eating as ingested food may remain in the stomach and contribute to reflux. This practice is a frequent trigger of GERD symptoms and one of the most effective lifestyle changes a patient can institute to control symptoms. Smaller and frequent meals are also recommended for GERD patients. Elevation of the head of the bed by 6 inches (by placing blocks underneath the feet at the head of the bed) can also reduce symptoms by using gravity to prevent reflux. It is recommended that patients avoid wearing tight-fitting clothing. Patients should be instructed to stop smoking and lose weight, which can be critical to reducing or eliminating symptoms. The current epidemic of obesity is a major contributing factor to increasing prevalence of GERD.

Medical treatment is characterized by antacid and antisecretory agents. Over-the-counter antacids are taken at least twice a month by more than one fourth of the U.S. population. Antacids provide symptom relief by neutralizing refluxed gastric acid thereby increasing esophageal pH and inactivating pepsin. Antacids are inexpensive, readily available, convenient, and effective. Short-term use of antacids for occasional symptoms is safe.

Histamine-2 (H_2)-receptor antagonists inhibit the secretion of gastric acid by competitively blocking the H_2-receptors located on gastric parietal cells. H_2-blockers have an excellent safety record and have been approved by the U.S. Food and Drug Administration (FDA) for over-the-counter sales. Low-dose H_2-receptor antagonists not only prevent heartburn symptoms when taken before meals but also relieve meal-induced heartburn symptoms in 15–40 minutes when taken after meals. H_2-receptor antagonists should be given twice daily to be most effective in patients with frequent GERD. These drugs are approximately 75% effective in patients with mild to moderate degrees of esophagitis; however, in patients with moderate to severe esophagitis, they are only 50% effective in healing esophagitis. H_2-receptor antagonists are appropriate for patients with mild to moderate GERD and remain a major treatment modality for GERD.

PPIs act by blocking the hydrogen–potassium ATPase on the apical surface of the parietal cell. PPIs are more effective than H_2-receptor antagonists because they act on the final common pathway of acid secretion rather than one of its three receptors (histamine, acetylcholine, and gastrin). The timing of PPI use is important as these drugs are most effective when taken in a fasting state 30 minutes before meals when parietal cells have large numbers of active proton pumps.

Side effects can occur in up to 3% of patients and can include headaches and diarrhea. Rare side effects include hepatitis and interstitial nephritis. PPIs induce the cytochrome P450 system, necessitating dosage adjustments of warfarin, phenytoin, and diazepam. There has been recent controversy about the effect of PPIs on clopidogrel as this medication is a prodrug that is converted to its active form via the cytochrome P450 system (CYP2C19). PPIs are both a substrate and an inhibitor of CYP2C19 and potentially reduce clopidogrel's inhibitory effect on platelet P2Y12. At this time, observational clinical studies on the influence of PPIs on the effectiveness of clopidogrel have shown conflicting results. Prospective clinical trials will be needed to definitively answer the question of whether the association between PPIs and clopidogrel has any clinically significant consequences. The only large randomized trial in clopidogrel users of omeprazole versus placebo showed no significant difference in cardiovascular events (hazard ratio with omeprazole 0.99, 95% CI 0.68–1.44, $P = .96$) along with a significant reduction in GI events (hazard ratio with omeprazole 0.34, 95% CI 0.18–0.63, $P < .001$). At the current time, the available evidence does not justify a conclusion that PPI use is associated with clinical cardiovascular events among clopidogrel users.

PPIs are indicated as initial therapy in patients with moderate to severe GERD and in patients with complications of GERD such as bleeding and strictures. A recent study reviewed 26 trials involving 4064 patients that compared PPIs with H_2-receptor antagonists. PPI therapy was significantly better than H_2-receptor antagonist therapy in treatment of esophagitis at 4–8 weeks.

Independent comparisons of the currently available PPIs have consistently shown first-generation PPIs (all except esomeprazole) to be essentially equal in esophagitis healing rates and intragastric profiles. There have been several reports that rabeprazole has a faster onset of action than the others; however, the clinical significance of this is debatable. A comparison of all five available PPIs in controlling 24-hour intragastric pH showed a statistically significant advantage for esomeprazole on day 5 of therapy (Table 11–5).

The safety of long-term PPI therapy has been demonstrated by the treatment of millions of patients over the past 20 years and the approval by the FDA for the over-the-counter availability of several of these drugs. During the initial testing of these medicines, gastric carcinoids were seen in animal models. This complication has not been demonstrated to occur in humans. There is also a theoretical concern about interference with nutrient absorption (especially magnesium, calcium, iron, and protein) due to a significant decrease in gastric acid production. However, there has only been a demonstrable reduction in absorption of magnesium. A modest reduction of vitamin B_{12} levels has been seen with long-term PPI use, which may be due to a decrease in protein-bound vitamin B_{12} absorption. Therefore, vitamin B_{12} levels should be periodically monitored in patients who are on continuous PPI therapy for more than 5 years. Clinically insignificant bacterial overgrowth of the small bowel has been noted to occur in patients on chronic PPIs. However, the bacterial overgrowth can become significant if there is an underlying motility disorder of the small intestine or surgically altered anatomy. Recently the use of PPIs has been associated with increased rates of community-acquired pneumonias, *Clostridium difficile* infection, and hip fractures.

Although most patients with GERD are successfully managed with lifestyle modifications and medical therapy, some patients may have persistent symptoms despite treatment. Mechanical antireflux therapies, either surgical or endoscopic, can be employed in patients with a good clinical response to medical treatments who wish to discontinue medications or in patients who have failed medical therapy.

B. Surgical Considerations

Gastroesophageal reflux surgery has been performed since the early 1950s. The goal of antireflux surgery is to narrow the lower esophageal luminal diameter to prevent the reflux of gastroduodenal contents. The most widely performed procedure is the Nissen fundoplication. Several studies have reported a symptomatic response of 80–90% in patients undergoing this fundoplication procedure. A review of six randomized controlled trials comparing open and laparoscopic fundoplications found no difference in the GERD recurrence rate between the two procedures but demonstrated a lower operative morbidity and shorter postoperative hospital stay with the laparoscopic approach. However, it has been noted that 62% of patients again require medications 10 years after antireflux surgery.

Complications of fundoplication include dysphagia, chest pain, gas-bloat syndrome, postoperative flatulence, and vagal nerve injuries leading to gastroparesis and diarrhea. The prevalence of these complications ranges between 5% and 20%. Postoperative dysphagia occurs in up to 18% of patients, with early dysphagia occurring in approximately 20% of patients and late dysphagia occurring in 6% of patients at 2 years. The benefit of antireflux surgery must also be balanced against the 0.5–1% risk of operative mortality. The risk of mortality is reduced by the laparoscopic approach and the experience of the surgeon.

C. Endoscopic Antireflux Procedures

Various endoscopic techniques have been developed for the treatment of GERD. Most studies of endoscopic therapy have reported limited follow-up information for a relatively small number of patients. Each endoscopic antireflux technique was designed to alter the anatomy of the gastroesophageal junction to prevent GERD.

Although some studies demonstrated an improvement in 24-hour intraesophageal acid exposure, normalization of

Table 11–5. Efficacy of proton pump inhibitors in decreasing intragastric pH.

Therapy	% Time pH > 4.0[a]	No. Hours pH > 4.0[b]	Mean pH
Esomeprazole, 40 mg	58.43	14.0	4.04
Rabeprazole, 20 mg	50.53	12.1	3.70
Omeprazole, 20 mg	49.16	11.8	3.54
Lansoprazole, 30 mg	47.98	11.5	3.56
Pantoprazole, 40 mg	41.94	10.1	3.33

[a]Percentage of time that intragastric pH was 4.0.
[b]Mean 24-h intragastric pH on day 5 by treatment group (n = 34).
Adapted, with permission, from Miner P Jr, Katz PO, Chen Y, et al. Gastric acid control with esomeprazole, lansoprazole, omeprazole, pantoprazole, and rabeprazole: a five-way crossover study. *Am J Gastroenterol.* 2003;98:2616–2620.

acid exposure was the exception rather than the rule for these techniques. Complications associated with these endoscopic antireflux procedures include bleeding, aspiration pneumonia, perforation, mediastinitis, and rarely, death. Future studies are needed to better understand the mechanism of these treatments and improve the efficacy and durability of these endoscopic procedures before they can be recommended.

D. Nonerosive Reflux Disease

Fewer than half of patients with typical reflux symptoms have evidence of esophagitis on upper endoscopy, giving rise to the term *nonerosive reflux disease* (NERD). NERD patients have typical GERD symptoms, but only half have evidence of abnormal acid exposure. The causes of symptoms in such patients include nonacid reflux, visceral hypersensitivity, and abnormal esophageal motor function. The treatment of NERD patients is similar to that of patients with erosive esophagitis; however, several studies have shown that these patients are less likely to respond to PPI therapy. Low-dose tricyclic antidepressants can be used in NERD patients who do not respond to conventional acid-reducing therapy.

Aseeri M, Schroeder T, Kramer J, et al. Gastric acid suppression by proton pump inhibitors as a risk factor for *Clostridium difficile*-associated diarrhea in hospitalized patients. *Am J Gastroenterol.* 2008;103:2308–2313. [PMID: 18702653]

Bhatt DL, Cryer BL, Contant CF, et al. COGENT Investigators. Clopidogrel with or without omeprazole in coronary artery disease. *N Engl J Med.* 2010;363:1909–1917. [PMID: 20925534]

Bytzer P, Morocutti A, Kennerly P, et al. ROSE Trial Investigators. Effect of rabeprazole and omeprazole on the onset of gastroesophageal reflux disease symptom relief during the first seven days of treatment. *Scand J Gastroenterol.* 2006;41:1132–1140. [PMID: 15990197]

Catarci M, Gentileschi P, Papi C, et al. Evidence-based appraisal of antireflux fundoplication. *Ann Surg.* 2004;239:325–337. [PMID: 15075649]

Corley DA, Kubo A, Zhao W, et al. Proton pump inhibitors and histamine-2 receptor antagonists are associated with hip fractures among at-risk patients. *Gastroenterology.* 2010;139: 93–101. [PMID: 20353792]

Cundy T, Mackay J. Proton pump inhibitors and severe hypomagnesemia. *Curr Opin Gastroenterol* 2011;27:180–185. [PMID: 20856115]

Dial S, Delaney JA, Barkun AN, et al. Use of gastric acid-suppressive agents and the risk of community-acquired *Clostridium difficile*-associated disease. *JAMA.* 2005;294:2989–2995. [PMID: 16414946]

Finlayson SR, Laycock WS, Birkmeyer JD. National trends in utilization and outcomes of antireflux surgery. *Surg Endosc.* 2003;17:864–867. [PMID: 12632134]

Flum DR, Koepsell T, Heagerty P, et al. The nationwide frequency of major adverse outcomes in antireflux surgery and the role of surgeon experience, 1992–1997. *J Am Coll Surg.* 2002;195: 611–618. [PMID: 12437246]

Kahrilas PJ, Shaheen NJ, Vaezi MF. American Gastroenterological Association Institute, Clinical Practice and Quality Management Committee. American Gastroenterological Association Institute technical review on the management of gastroesophageal reflux disease. *Gastroenterology.* 2008;135:1392–1413. [PMID: 18801365]

Kaltenbach T, Crockett S, Gerson LB. Are lifestyle measures effective in patients with gastroesophageal reflux disease? An evidence-based approach. *Arch Intern Med.* 2006;166:965–971. [PMID: 16682569]

Klinkenberg-Knol EC, Nelis F, Dent J. Long-term omeprazole treatment in resistant gastroesophageal reflux disease: efficacy, safety, and influence on gastric mucosa. *Gastroenterology.* 2000;118:661–669. [PMID: 10734017]

Klok RM, Postma MJ, van Hout BA, et al. Meta-analysis: comparing the efficacy of proton pump inhibitors in short-term use. *Aliment Pharmacol Therapeut.* 2003;17:1237–1245. [PMID: 12755827]

Laheij RJ, Sturkenboom MC, Hassing RJ, et al. Risk of community-acquired pneumonia and use of gastric acid-suppressive drugs. *JAMA.* 2004;292:1955–1960. [PMID: 15507580]

Laine L, Hennekens C. Proton pump inhibitor and clopidogrel interaction: fact or fiction? *Am J Gastroenterol.* 2010;105:34–41. [PMID: 19904241]

Liu JJ, Carr-Locke DL, Osterman MT, et al. Endoscopic treatment for atypical manifestations of gastroesophageal reflux disease. *Am J Gastroenterol.* 2006;101:440–445. [PMID: 16542278]

Moayyedi P, Soo S, Deeks J, et al. Pharmacologic interventions for non-ulcer dyspepsia. *Cochrane Database System Rev.* 2006;(4):CD001960. [PMID: 17054151]

Spechler SJ, Lee E, Ahnen D, et al. Long-term outcome of medical and surgical therapies for gastroesophageal reflux disease: follow-up of a randomized controlled trial. *JAMA.* 2001;285: 2331–2338. [PMID: 11343480]

Targownik LE, Lix LM, Leung S, et al. Proton-pump inhibitor use is not associated with osteoporosis or accelerated bone mineral density loss. *Gastroenterology.* 2010;138:896–904. [PMID: 19931262]

Yang YX, Lewis JD, Epstein S, et al. Long-term proton pump inhibitor therapy and risk of hip fracture. *JAMA.* 2006;296: 2947–2953. [PMID: 17190895]

Yang YX, Metz DC. Safety of proton pump inhibitor exposure. *Gastroenterology.* 2010;139:1115–1127. [PMID: 20727892]

E. Management of Peptic Esophageal Strictures

1. Esophageal dilation—Peptic strictures of the esophagus due to GERD account for nearly 80% of esophageal strictures, although this may be decreasing due to the use of PPIs. The primary indication for esophageal dilation is to relieve dysphagia; empiric dilatation with large-bore dilators cannot be recommended if no structural abnormalities are seen endoscopically.

Three general types of dilators are currently in use. These are (1) mercury or tungsten-filled bougies (Maloney or Hurst), (2) wire-guided polyvinyl dilators (Savary-Gilliard or American), and (3) TTS ("through the scope") balloon dilators. Maloney bougies have a tapered tip and can be passed blindly or under fluoroscopic control. Savary and American dilators are passed over a guidewire that has been positioned in the antrum, with or without fluoroscopic guidance. TTS dilating balloons are available in either single or multiple diameters that may be passed with or without wire guidance.

In preparation for endoscopic dilation, anticoagulants should be discontinued. Routine antibiotic coverage is not recommended; however, endocarditis prophylaxis should be followed. Patients should be informed of the risks associated with esophageal dilation; the principal complications are perforation, bleeding, and aspiration. The perforation rate for esophageal strictures after dilation has been reported to be 0.1–0.4%. Perforation is more common in radiation-induced strictures, malignant strictures, complex strictures due to lye ingestion, and in patients with achalasia.

The degree of dilation within an endoscopic session should be based on the severity of the luminal narrowing (Plates 7 and 8). A "rule of three" has been described for esophageal dilation using bougie dilators. After moderate resistance is encountered, no more than three consecutive dilators in increments of 1 mm should be passed in a single session. This rule does not appear to directly apply to balloon dilators in simple esophageal strictures, which may be incrementally dilated greater than 3 mm. No data exist on the optimal time the balloon should remain inflated. Dilation therapy for a symptomatic Schatzki ring should be directed toward achieving rupture of the ring.

No clear advantage has been demonstrated between bougie and TTS dilators. In patients with benign peptic strictures, the long-term benefits of dilation appear greatest when a luminal diameter of more than 12 mm is achieved. For peptic strictures, smaller lumen diameter, presence of a hiatal hernia greater than 5 cm, persistence of heartburn after dilation, and number of dilations needed for initial dysphagia relief were significant predictors of early symptomatic recurrence.

2. Proton pump inhibitors—Patients with peptic strictures should be treated with PPI therapy. Patients with peptic strictures complicated by food impactions should undergo treatment with PPIs prior to dilation of the peptic stricture. PPI use decreases stricture recurrence and the need for repeat stricture dilation.

Hernandez LV, Jacobson JW, Harris MS. Comparison among the perforation rates of Maloney, balloon and Savary dilation of esophageal strictures. *Gastrointest Endosc.* 2000;51:460–462. [PMID: 10744819]

Said A, Brust DJ, Gaumnitz EA, et al. Predictors of early recurrence of benign esophageal strictures. *Am J Gastroenterol.* 2003;98:1252–1256. [PMID: 12818265]

Standards of Practice Committee, Egan JV, Baron TH, Adler DG, et al. Esophageal dilatation. *Gastrointest Endosc.* 2006;63: 755–760. [PMID: 16650533]

Course & Prognosis

Once patients without esophagitis have responded to lifestyle changes and medical therapy and achieved remission from clinical symptoms, most should have a trial of medication withdrawal. Symptom relief should be sustained for 2–3 months before attempting to withdraw medications. PPI therapy can be tapered to an every-other-day regimen or to a reduced dose (if possible), or switched to a H_2-blocker. Most patients who are treated with H_2-blockers are on twice-daily medications, and the initial tapering should be to a once-a-day regimen. If a patient tolerates a taper for 2–4 weeks without an increase in symptoms, the dosage can be further decreased or the medication discontinued. The goal of long-term treatment is to step down management to the lowest level of medical therapy that controls symptoms, or consider surgery. However, if a patient experiences recurrent symptoms, the medication regimen should be increased until symptom resolution is achieved.

If GERD patients on long-term PPI therapy are abruptly withdrawn (not tapered) from their medicine, many will experience symptoms that are worse than their initial presenting complaints. This phenomenon of "rebound hypersecretion" occurs when parietal cells secrete elevated amounts of acid after a prolonged blockade. A prolonged tapering of PPI therapy helps improve these symptoms. *Helicobacter pylori* eradication has been found to worsen rebound gastric hypersecretion.

Therapy for GERD is frequently chronic and long-term in most patients as the underlying disorder is dysfunction of the LES, which is not directly affected by medical therapy. Among patients with erosive esophagitis, more than 80% will relapse if their therapy is stopped. The same medication that induces remission is usually required in the same dosage to maintain remission. In those with nonerosive GERD, on-demand therapy is a cost-effective alternative to maintenance treatment.

Long-term GERD treatment can be challenging, but empowering patients to recognize the dietary and lifestyle choices that produce symptoms enables the majority of motivated patients to wean themselves off medical therapy. For those patients who are unable to discontinue acid suppression therapy due to symptom recurrence, the medical therapies available are fortunately very effective and generally safe.

Inadomi JM, Jamal R, Murata GH, et al. Step-down management of gastroesophageal reflux disease. *Gastroenterology.* 2001;121:1095–1100. [PMID: 11677201]

Inadomi JM, McIntyre L, Bernard L, et al. Step-down from multiple-to single-dose proton pump inhibitors (PPIs): a prospective study of patients with heartburn or acid regurgitation completely relieved with PPIs. *Am J Gastroenterol.* 2003;98:1940–1944. [PMID: 14499769]

This chapter is a revised version of the chapter by Dr. John R. Saltzman and Dr. John M. Poneros that was in the previous edition of Current Diagnosis & Treatment: Gastroenterology, Hepatology, & Endoscopy.

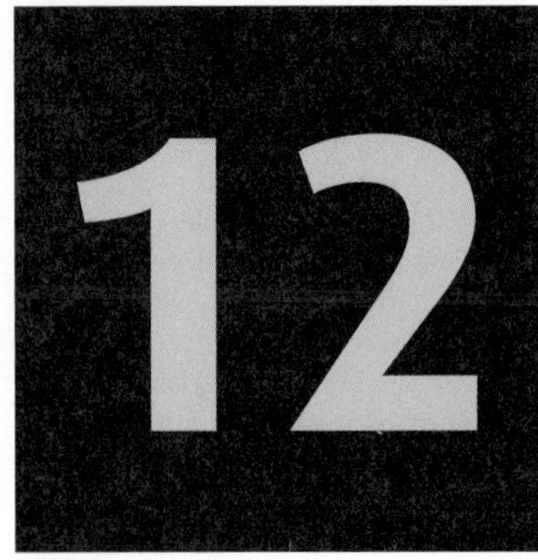

Barrett Esophagus

Kunal Jajoo, MD
John R. Saltzman, MD

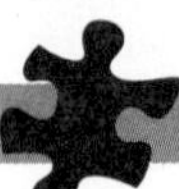

ESSENTIALS OF DIAGNOSIS

- ▶ Replacement of normal squamous epithelium of the distal esophagus with specialized intestinal metaplasia.
- ▶ Endoscopy and biopsy are essential for an accurate diagnosis.
- ▶ Presence of high-grade dysplasia should be confirmed by two expert gastrointestinal pathologists.
- ▶ Risk factors for progression to adenocarcinoma include a large hiatal hernia, long segment of Barrett esophagus, and mucosal abnormalities (nodules, ulcerations, or strictures).

General Considerations

Barrett esophagus is named after a London thoracic surgeon who published a paper in 1950 entitled "Chronic Peptic Ulcer of the Esophagus and 'Oesophagitis.'" In this article, Norman Barrett described cases of esophageal ulcers surrounded by columnar mucosa found at autopsy. Barrett esophagus is the replacement of the normal squamous epithelium of the distal esophagus with specialized intestinal metaplasia (SIM). It is thought to be caused by chronic gastroesophageal reflux disease (GERD), which leads to esophagitis and subsequent metaplastic change of the esophageal lining. SIM may be protective against further injury by gastric acid; however, this metaplastic epithelium is also associated with an increased risk for esophageal adenocarcinoma. There is considerable ongoing debate regarding various aspects of Barrett esophagus, such as the exact neoplastic risk it confers as well as its management if it has become dysplastic.

Barrett NR. Chronic peptic ulcer of the oesophagus and "oesophagitis." *Br J Surg.* 1950;38:175–182. [PMID: 14791960]

Sharma P. Clinical practice. Barrett's esophagus. *N Engl J Med.* 2009;361:2548–2556. [PMID: 20032324]

A. Epidemiology

The overall prevalence of Barrett esophagus in the general adult population is thought to be 1.6–1.7% (although estimates have varied widely from 0.9% to more than 20% depending on the population studied and the definition of Barrett esophagus). As of the 2010 Census, this would translate to nearly 4.0 million individuals with the condition in the United States. In patients with GERD, the prevalence of Barrett esophagus is higher, approximately 5–10%. In patients with severe GERD, such as those with erosive esophagitis, the prevalence is approximately 10%; in patients with peptic strictures of the esophagus, the prevalence is almost 30%. Barrett esophagus affects males more than females by a ratio of approximately 3:1. The typical patient is a Caucasian, middle-aged male. Although the prevalence of Barrett esophagus in Hispanics appears to be similar to that in Caucasians, Barrett esophagus is uncommon in blacks and Asians. In certain studies, alcohol and smoking have been found to be risk factors for the presence of Barrett esophagus. The conclusion that Barrett esophagus is an acquired complication of chronic GERD is supported by the fact that Barrett esophagus is exceedingly rare in children with competent lower esophageal sphincters (LES).

El-Serag HB, Gilger MA, Shub MD, et al. The prevalence of suspected Barrett's esophagus in children and adolescents: a multicenter endoscopic study. *Gastrointest Endosc.* 2006;64: 671–675. [PMID: 17055854]

Evans DE, Barron WG. *2000 Census of Population and Housing.* U.S. Department of Commerce Economics and Statistics, 2005.

Ronkainen J, Aro P, Storskrubb T, et al. Prevalence of Barrett's esophagus in the general population: an endoscopic study. *Gastroenterology.* 2005;129:1825–1831. [PMID: 16344051]

Spechler SJ, Fitzgerald RC, Prasad GA, et al. History, molecular mechanisms, and endoscopic treatment of Barrett's esophagus. *Gastroenterology.* 2010;138:854–869. [PMID: 20080098]

B. Pathogenesis

The components of the refluxate in GERD (both gastric acid and bile salts) are important etiologic factors in the development of Barrett esophagus. Esophageal pH monitoring studies have shown that patients with Barrett esophagus have more esophageal acid exposure than healthy controls or even patients with mild heartburn. The greater acid exposure in Barrett esophagus results from longer periods of acid reflux (ie, >5 minutes), rather than from a greater number of reflux episodes. Patients with Barrett esophagus may be predisposed to more severe acid reflux episodes due to mechanical dysfunction of the LES as well as the decreased amplitude of distal esophageal contractions.

Helicobacter pylori infection of the stomach causes chronic inflammation that can result in gastric intestinal metaplasia and cancer. However, there is no clear association between *H pylori* infection and GERD, and the organism does not infect the esophagus. In fact, *H pylori* infection of the stomach may actually protect the esophagus from GERD and Barrett esophagus.

The role of bile salts in refluxed gastric acid in the development of Barrett esophagus continues to be debated and investigated. Increased levels of refluxed bile acid concentrations have been found in patients with Barrett esophagus. Acid and bile have been shown to induce a class of homeobox genes (*Cdx*), which are regulators of cell differentiation, and this has been postulated to result in metaplasia. Some clinicians argue that the increased reflux of bile salts in these patients necessitates a mechanical treatment for their GERD, such as a fundoplication. Finally, the genetic and environmental factors that also play a role in the development of Barrett esophagus are only beginning to be understood.

Souza RF, Krishnan K, Spechler SJ. Acid, bile and CDX: the ABCs of making Barrett's metaplasia. *Am J Physiol Gastrointest Liver Physiol.* 2008;295:G211–G218. [PMID: 18556417]

Wang C, Yuan Y, Hunt RH. *Helicobacter pylori* infection and Barrett's esophagus: a systematic review and meta-analysis. *Am J Gastroenterol.* 2009;104:492–500. [PMID: 19174811]

Clinical Findings

Barrett esophagus cannot be detected on clinical grounds as there are no specific symptoms that distinguish this condition from GERD without Barrett esophagus. In addition, Barrett esophagus cannot be reliably detected radiologically. The gold standard for the diagnosis of Barrett esophagus is upper endoscopy with biopsy of the distal esophagus.

A. Endoscopic and Biopsy Findings

Barrett esophagus is diagnosed when mucosal biopsies confirm the presence of SIM in a columnar-lined distal esophagus. In normal individuals, the squamocolumnar junction (SCJ) coincides with the gastroesophageal junction (GEJ). The SCJ is the transition from the pale squamous mucosa of the esophagus to the salmon-colored gastric mucosa. Endoscopically, the GEJ is best defined as the top of the gastric folds. If there is proximal displacement of the SCJ above the top of the gastric folds into the tubular esophagus, a columnar-lined esophagus is present and biopsies should be taken (Plate 9).

Early studies defined the diagnosis of Barrett esophagus as the presence of 3 cm of columnar-lined distal esophagus with SIM (Plate 10). Subsequent work deemed the presence of less than 3 cm of SIM as "short-segment" Barrett esophagus. Finally, a study in which investigators biopsied the normal-appearing SCJ of consecutive patients undergoing upper endoscopy found a SIM prevalence of 18%. The significance of intestinal metaplasia at the SCJ is debatable, and at present, it is not recommended that a normal-appearing SCJ be biopsied.

It is important to note that intestinal metaplasia of the cardia cannot be distinguished from intestinal metaplasia of the esophagus. Therefore, the proximal displacement of the SCJ into the tubular esophagus must be documented endoscopically in order to diagnose a patient with Barrett esophagus.

The clinical significance of Barrett esophagus length is important as studies have confirmed that longer segments have higher risks of progression to adenocarcinoma. To maintain consistency across studies of Barrett esophagus, the Prague C and M criteria were established to determine the extent of disease. By these criteria, the extent of circumferential (C) and maximal (M) visualized Barrett esophagus is measured, and standard definitions of endoscopic landmarks are used. These criteria have good interobserver reliability for Barrett esophagus ≥1 cm in length. It remains to be determined whether these criteria will become adopted broadly.

Biopsy specimens of Barrett esophagus are classified as negative for dysplasia (or non-dysplastic), indefinite for dysplasia (or indefinite-grade dysplasia), low-grade dysplasia, or high-grade dysplasia. The diagnosis of dysplasia is typically reserved for lesions in which nuclear atypia is present on the mucosal surface.

Avidan B, Sonnenberg A, Schnell T, et al. Hiatal hernia size, Barrett's length and severity of acid reflux are all risk factors for esophageal adenocarcinoma. *Am J Gastroenterol.* 2002;97: 1930–1936. [PMID: 12190156]

Sharma P, Dent J, Armstrong D, et al. The development and validation of an endoscopic grading system for Barrett's esophagus: the Prague C & M criteria. *Gastroenterology.* 2006;131: 1392–1399. [PMID: 17101315]

Sharma P, McQuaid K, Dent J, et al. A critical review of the diagnosis and management of Barrett's esophagus: the AGA Chicago workshop. *Gastroenterology.* 2004;127:310–330. [PMID: 15236196]

Wang KE, Sampliner RE. Practice Parameters Committee of the American College of Gastroenterology. Updated guidelines for the diagnosis, surveillance and therapy of Barrett's esophagus. *Am J Gastroenterol.* 2008;103:788–797. [PMID: 18341497]

B. Screening

Screening refers to performing a test on a large asymptomatic sample of the population to identify a disease. The role of screening upper endoscopy for Barrett esophagus is unclear, and the major gastroenterologic societies are not unanimous in their recommendations. Patients with chronic GERD are at increased risk for Barrett esophagus, and the prevalence of Barrett esophagus is higher in middle-aged white males, suggesting that screening should be reserved for this higher risk subgroup. The recent American College of Gastroenterology guideline acknowledges the controversy in screening for Barrett esophagus and only states that the highest yield is achieved in screening patients with chronic GERD symptoms who are over age 50.

If the only criteria for Barrett esophagus screening were the presence of GERD symptoms, however, the population to be screened would be enormous as it is estimated that 20% of the U.S. adult population experiences weekly acid reflux. Conversely, a recent meta-analysis demonstrated that GERD symptoms are not associated with the presence of short-segment Barrett esophagus, but these symptoms do confer a five-fold increase in the risk of long-segment Barrett esophagus.

Decision analysis studies that have examined the cost-effectiveness of screening for Barrett esophagus have shown conflicting results. In addition, a significant proportion of patients with esophageal adenocarcinoma report no prior symptoms of reflux. What cannot be debated, however, is that the majority of patients newly diagnosed with esophageal cancer have not had a previous diagnosis of Barrett esophagus, emphasizing a need for more effective screening strategies. As the cost of esophageal visualization decreases with newer techniques such as transnasal and video capsule endoscopy, these issues will need to be readdressed.

Gerson LB, Groeneveld PW, Triadafilopoulos G. Cost-effectiveness of endoscopic screening and surveillance in patients with gastroesophageal reflux disease. *Clin Gastroenterol Hepatol.* 2004;2:868–879. [PMID: 15476150]

Inadomi JM, Sampliner R, Lagergren J, et al. Screening and surveillance for Barrett's esophagus in high-risk groups: a cost utility analysis. *Ann Intern Med.* 2003;138:176–186. [PMID: 12558356]

Sharma P, Falk GW, Weston AP, et al. Dysplasia and cancer in a large multicenter cohort of patients with Barrett's esophagus. *Clin Gastroenterol Hepatol.* 2006;4:566–572. [PMID: 16630761]

Taylor JB, Rubenstein JH. Meta-analyses of the effect of symptoms of gastroesophageal reflux on the risk of Barrett's esophagus. *Am J Gastroenterol.* 2010;105:1730–1737. [PMID: 20485283]

C. Surveillance

Surveillance in patients with Barrett esophagus refers to the performance of serial endoscopies at regular intervals with the goal of detecting dysplasia and early cancer at a curable stage. If the incidence of cancer in patients with Barrett esophagus were high, surveillance would be cost-effective; however, if the incidence were low, an extremely small proportion of the at-risk population would benefit. The overall risk of cancer in Barrett esophagus patients is estimated to be approximately 0.5% per year. Stated another way, the risk of any given patient with Barrett esophagus developing cancer is approximately 1 in 200 per year.

As with screening, the cost-effectiveness of surveillance in Barrett esophagus is debated. Retrospective data have shown that cancers detected during Barrett esophagus surveillance are more likely to be found at an early stage and are associated with better survival compared with those not detected during surveillance. Such retrospective studies are subject to both lead time and length of time bias. A few studies have demonstrated no difference in overall survival between patients with Barrett esophagus and the general population, calling into question the utility of Barrett esophagus endoscopic surveillance. Barrett esophagus patients more frequently die from causes other than esophageal adenocarcinoma, suggesting that surveillance is of no benefit to the vast majority of these patients. It is not clear which patients who are known to have Barrett esophagus benefit from surveillance.

At present, until better markers of risk stratification are found, the surveillance interval of upper endoscopy is determined by the degree of dysplasia found in a Barrett esophagus segment. Until better biomarkers are validated, dysplasia remains the best indicator of risk of cancer development. Barrett esophagus biomarkers are being actively investigated because the diagnosis and detection of dysplasia have significant limitations. There is a high interobserver variability in the reading of dysplasia, particularly among community pathologists. Many pathologists have difficulty distinguishing between inflammatory changes and dysplasia. In addition, random biopsy surveillance introduces the possibility of sampling error given that the distribution of dysplasia throughout a Barrett esophagus segment can be patchy. At present, the presence of dysplasia in a Barrett esophagus segment remains the best method of cancer risk stratification. It is strongly recommended that when a diagnosis of dysplastic Barrett esophagus is being considered, the histopathologic slides be reviewed by two senior pathologists with expertise in this area.

Currently upper endoscopy with four-quadrant "jumbo" biopsies at 2-cm intervals remains the best method for obtaining surveillance biopsies once esophageal inflammation related to GERD has been well controlled with antisecretory therapy. Biopsy specimens should be obtained in four quadrants at 2-cm intervals beginning at the end of the tubular esophagus (top of the gastric folds) and continuing proximally to the SCJ. Any mucosal abnormalities such as ulcerations, strictures, or nodules should be extensively sampled, ideally by endoscopic mucosal resection (EMR). At present, chromoendoscopy and other "optical biopsy" techniques have not been validated on a large scale and are not recommended for standard use.

Table 12–1. Summary of recommendations for surveillance endoscopies in Barrett esophagus.

	ASGE	ACG	AGA
Screening	Selected patients, no further screening if Barrett not present on initial EGD	Screening is controversial; highest yield is in patients with chronic GERD over age 50	Screening of white males over age 50 with GERD may be cost-effective
No dysplasia	Repeat at 1 y then every 3 y	Repeat EGD, then every 3 y	Repeat at 1 y then every 5 y
Low-grade dysplasia	Yearly EGD	Yearly EGD	If 2 pathologists agree, then yearly; if disagreement that dysplasia is present, then every 2 y
High-grade dysplasia	Confirm path; repeat EGD to exclude cancer; consider ablative therapy, surgery, or surveillance every 3 mo	Confirm path; repeat EGD to exclude cancer; if mucosal irregularity, then EMR; treat with ablative therapies or surgery depending on local expertise	Confirm path; repeat EGD to exclude cancer; consider patient, local expertise, focality of dysplasia; consider intensive surveillance, ablation, or surgery

ACG, American College of Gastroenterology; AGA, American Gastroenterological Association; ASGE, American Society for Gastrointestinal Endoscopy; EGD, esophagogastroduodenoscopy; EMR, endoscopic mucosal resection; GERD, gastroesophageal reflux disease.

The recommendations of the major gastroenterologic societies differ slightly regarding the time interval between surveillance endoscopies in Barrett esophagus (Table 12–1). If a patient is found to have Barrett esophagus without dysplasia on incident endoscopy, it is generally recommended that a repeat esophagogastroduodenoscopy (EGD) be performed in 1 year for repeat biopsies. If no dysplasia is found on the second surveillance endoscopy performed 1 year later, it is reasonable to repeat surveillance endoscopies every 2–3 years. Some investigators advocate that this interval be extended to every 3–5 years or longer given that Barrett esophagus surveillance has not been proven cost-effective. A large trial of over 1200 patients demonstrated that 98.6% of patients with nondysplastic Barrett esophagus were cancer free at the 5-year follow-up. It is important to note that in a recent retrospective study of patients with Barrett esophagus, 53% of patients who developed high-grade dysplasia or cancer had two consecutive initial endoscopies with biopsies that revealed nondysplastic mucosa.

Corley DA, Levin TR, Habel LA, et al. Surveillance and survival in Barrett's adenocarcinomas: a population-based study. *Gastroenterology*. 2002;122:633–640. [PMID: 11874995]

Wani S, Falk G, Hall M, et al. Patients with non-dysplastic Barrett's esophagus have low risks for developing dysplasia or esophageal adenocarcinoma. *Clin Gastroenterol Hepatol*. 2011;9:220–227. [PMID: 21115133]

D. Risk Factors for Progression to Adenocarcinoma

Many studies have assessed risk factors for the development of adenocarcinoma in patients with Barrett esophagus (Table 12–2). Dysplasia is a risk factor for progression to adenocarcinoma, as well as a risk for having an occult, coincident carcinoma present in the Barrett esophagus segment. Dysplastic transformation of Barrett esophagus epithelium is thought to precede the development of adenocarcinoma, although whether this progression occurs without interruption from nondysplastic Barrett esophagus to low-grade dysplasia to high-grade dysplasia is unclear. Patients with short-segment Barrett esophagus appear to have a lower incidence of dysplasia since less mucosa is involved (6–8% in short-segment Barrett esophagus vs 15–24% in long-segment Barrett esophagus).

Table 12–2. Risk factors for esophageal adenocarcinoma in patients with Barrett esophagus.

Clinical factors	Diet low in fruits and vegetables High body mass index Male gender Older age Tobacco smoking Heavy alcohol use Working in a stooped posture Less use of proton pump inhibitors Fewer heartburn symptoms Use of medicines that relax the lower esophageal sphincter
Endoscopic factors	Large hiatal hernia Long segment of Barrett esophagus Mucosal abnormalities Nodularity Ulceration Strictures
Histologic factors	High-grade dysplasia
Biomarkers	Aneuploidy p53 loss of heterozygosity

Furthermore, the risk of adenocarcinoma has been estimated to be 2–15 times higher with long-segment Barrett esophagus compared to short-segment Barrett esophagus. Biomarkers for the development of adenocarcinoma in Barrett esophagus patients, such as aneuploidy and p53 loss of heterozygosity as determined by flow cytometry, immunohistochemistry, and fluorescence in situ hybridization (FISH) to aid in the detection of dysplasia, are still experimental.

Cooper BT, Chapman W, Neumann CS, et al. Continuous treatment of Barrett's oesophagus patients with proton pump inhibitors up to 13 years: observations on regression and cancer incidence. *Aliment Pharm Ther.* 2006;23:727–733. [PMID: 16556174]

Hirota WK, Zuckerman MJ, Adler DG, et al. Standards of Practice Committee, American Society for Gastrointestinal Endoscopy. ASGE guideline: the role of endoscopy in the surveillance of premalignant conditions of the upper GI tract. *Gastrointest Endosc.* 2006;63:570–580. [PMID: 16564854]

Prasad GA, Bansal A, Sharma P, et al. Predictors of progression in Barrett's esophagus: current knowledge and future directions. *Am J Gastroenterol.* 2010;105:1490–1502. [PMID: 20104216]

Wang KK, Sampliner RE. Practice Parameters Committee of the American College of Gastroenterology. Updated guidelines 2008 for the diagnosis, surveillance and therapy of Barrett's esophagus. *Am J Gastroenterol.* 2008;103:788–797. [PMID: 18341497]

Wang KK, Wongkeesong M, Buttar NS. American Gastroenterological Association technical review on the role of the gastroenterologist in the management of esophageal carcinoma. *Gastroenterology.* 2005;128:1471–1505. [PMID: 15887129]

Wongsurawat VJ, Finley JC, Galipeau PC, et al. Genetic mechanisms of TP53 loss of heterozygosity in Barrett's esophagus: implications for biomarker validation. *Cancer Epidemiol Biomarkers Prev.* 2006;15:509–516. [PMID: 16537709]

Treatment

A. Nondysplastic Barrett Esophagus

It is our practice to put every patient with Barrett esophagus on proton pump inhibitor (PPI) therapy indefinitely. There are data demonstrating that patients on PPIs have a lower rate of progression to dysplasia and adenocarcinoma than patients not taking PPIs. In one study, the cumulative incidence of dysplasia was significantly lower among patients who received PPI after Barrett esophagus diagnosis than in those who received no therapy or histamine receptor antagonists. Furthermore, among those on PPIs, a longer duration of use was associated with a less frequent occurrence of dysplasia. Every patient diagnosed with Barrett esophagus should be treated with a PPI whether or not symptomatic GERD is present.

At present there are not enough data to support ablative therapies for nondysplastic Barrett esophagus. In the future, biomarkers may provide better risk stratification justifying endoscopic ablation of nondysplastic Barrett esophagus in high-risk patients. However, given that the vast majority of patients with Barrett esophagus do not progress to adenocarcinoma, the use of these methods for this indication cannot currently be recommended.

Data suggest that, despite long-term antisecretory therapy, long segments of Barrett esophagus do not regress. Normalization of SIM has been described in cases of "ultra-short" Barrett esophagus and short-segment Barrett esophagus. Patients with long segments of Barrett esophagus should be informed that their Barrett esophagus will not regress and that they should remain on PPI therapy indefinitely and undergo surveillance endoscopies.

Cyclooxygenase (COX)-2 inhibitors (both aspirin and nonsteroidal anti-inflammatory drugs [NSAIDs]) are being studied as chemoprevention of Barrett esophagus progression. A study of esophagectomy specimens correlating COX-2 immunopositivity and clinical course demonstrated that tumors expressing higher levels of COX-2 were more likely to be associated with distant metastases, local recurrence, and reduced survival. A recent meta-analysis of cohort studies estimated that aspirin use was inversely associated with esophageal adenocarcinoma (odds ratio [OR] 0.64, 95% confidence interval [CI] 0.52–0.79) with a similar reduction in risk observed for NSAIDs (OR 0.65, 95% CI 0.50–0.85). Statin medications have also been proposed as chemopreventive agents for esophageal carcinoma. A recent large case-control study demonstrated that patients with Barrett esophagus on antisecretory therapy who filled prescriptions for either NSAID medications or statin medications had a reduced risk of developing esophageal adenocarcinoma. In the future, chemoprevention of Barrett esophagus progression may become the standard of care if further human clinical studies can substantiate these findings.

Abnet CC, Freedman ND, Kamangar F, et al. Non-steroidal anti-inflammatory drugs and risk of gastric and oesophageal adenocarcinomas: results from a cohort study and a meta-analysis. *Br J Cancer.* 2009;100:551–557. [PMID: 19156150]

El-Serag HB, Aguirre TV, Davis S, et al. Proton pump inhibitors are associated with reduced incidence of dysplasia in Barrett's esophagus. *Am J Gastroenterol.* 2004;99:1877–1883. [PMID: 15447744]

Horwhat JD, Baroni D, Maydonovitch C, et al. Normalization of intestinal metaplasia in the esophagus and esophagogastric junction: incidence and clinical data. *Am J Gastroenterol.* 2007;102:497–506. [PMID: 17156135]

Nguyen DM, Richardson P, El-Serag HB. Medications (NSAIDs, statins, proton pump inhibitors) and the risk of esophageal adenocarcinoma in patients with Barrett's esophagus. *Gastroenterology.* 2010;138:2260–2266. [PMID: 20188100]

B. Indefinite-Grade Dysplasia

In indefinite-grade dysplasia, nuclear enlargement, crowding, hyperchromatism, prominence of the nucleoli, and mild stratification can be seen but are confined to the lower portion of the glands, whereas the upper portion of the glands and surface epithelium show less abnormality or are normal. The diagnosis of dysplasia should be made with caution when atypical changes do not involve the mucosal surface.

Active inflammation due to GERD may cause nuclear changes that mimic both low-grade and high-grade dysplasia. If a biopsy specimen is obtained adjacent to an ulcer and numerous neutrophils infiltrate the epithelium, the diagnosis of dysplasia may not be possible and the diagnosis of "indefinite for dysplasia" may be assigned.

If Barrett esophagus surveillance biopsy specimens are obtained and indefinite-grade dysplasia is the highest grade lesion found, aggressive antisecretory therapy should be instituted and repeat surveillance biopsies should be performed in 3 months.

C. Low-Grade Dysplasia

Low-grade dysplasia is characterized by mucosal cells with nuclei that are larger and hyperchromatic, with irregular contours that are basally located in the cell with minimal or no stratification (Plate 11). As with other grades of dysplasia, the interpretations of low-grade dysplasia biopsy specimens should be considered for review by experts in esophageal pathology. Extensive surveillance biopsies should be done to confirm that low-grade dysplasia is the highest grade lesion in a Barrett esophagus segment.

Several clinical studies have not demonstrated a significantly increased malignant potential of Barrett esophagus with low-grade dysplasia. In these studies, the risk of progression to esophageal adenocarcinoma was not significantly higher in patients with low-grade dysplasia than in those without dysplasia. In addition, some case series have demonstrated a transient nature to low-grade dysplasia, which can regress and revert to nondysplastic Barrett esophagus on subsequent biopsies. More recent data suggest that the extent of low-grade dysplasia measured as the mean proportion of low-grade dysplastic crypts may be a more significant predictor of esophageal adenocarcinoma outcome than the presence of low-grade dysplasia alone.

The natural history of low-grade dysplasia is variable; it can persist for long periods of time or even revert to nondysplastic Barrett esophagus. A repeat EGD with surveillance biopsies should be performed within 3–6 months after low-grade dysplasia is detected to confirm it is the highest grade lesion present and then annually as long as low-grade dysplasia persists. Given the emerging data regarding the implications of a large dysplastic burden, a shorter interval may be considered if multiple biopsies reveal a large number of low-grade crypts.

Sharma P. Low-grade dysplasia in Barrett's esophagus. *Gastroenterology.* 2004;127:1233–1238. [PMID: 15481000]

Srivastava A, Hornick JL, Li X, et al. Extent of low-grade dysplasia is a risk factor for the development of esophageal adenocarcinoma in Barrett's esophagus. *Am J Gastroenterol.* 2006;102:483–493. [PMID: 17338734]

D. High-Grade Dysplasia

The accurate pathologic diagnosis of high-grade dysplasia is critically important because therapeutic intervention may be initiated based on its diagnosis. Histopathologically, at low magnification power, distortion of the glandular architecture is usually present and may be marked. The glands are composed of branching and lateral budding of crypts and a villi-form configuration of the mucosal surface. Most importantly, the diagnosis of high-grade dysplasia requires that the dysplastic epithelium on the mucosal surface demonstrate loss of nuclear polarity and the absence of a consistent relationship of nuclei to each other (Plate 12).

The clinical implications of the presence of high-grade dysplasia in Barrett esophagus remain somewhat controversial. Owing to the risk of occult, coincident malignancy in a Barrett esophagus segment as well as the higher risk of progression to malignancy, the previous standard recommendation was that all patients diagnosed with high-grade dysplasia undergo esophagectomy once the diagnosis was confirmed by two experienced GI pathologists. Esophagectomy is a very invasive surgery and is associated with 3–10% mortality and up to 45% morbidity. Subsequent studies found that the rate of progression to esophageal adenocarcinoma in patients with high-grade dysplasia can vary widely from 15–60% and, in a subset of patients, may not occur at all. A recent retrospective review of patients referred for esophagectomy for Barrett esophagus with high-grade dysplasia or intramucosal carcinoma found that only 6.7% had submucosal invasion, suggesting that endoscopic therapies could have been considered. Therefore, the recommendations regarding the management of high-grade dysplasia have become more patient specific and tailored to each clinical scenario.

It is imperative that the diagnosis of high-grade dysplasia be confirmed by two expert GI pathologists prior to formulating a treatment plan. Extensive surveillance biopsies must be performed every 1 cm in all four quadrants of the Barrett esophagus segment in order to rule out the presence of any occult malignancy. Any suspicious nodules or ulcerations must be extensively sampled. An assessment of the patient's operative risk should be performed. After the preceding information has been obtained, a treatment plan can be formulated with the patient's input regarding the risks and benefits of each course of action.

The extent of high-grade dysplasia present in a patient's Barrett esophagus segment has been shown to correlate with the patient's likelihood of progression to cancer. These findings suggest that patients with "focal" high-grade dysplasia (ie, involving five or fewer crypts) on a single biopsy may be surveyed endoscopically, and more invasive treatment may be optimal only for patients who progress to frank adenocarcinoma.

If a patient is found to have high-grade dysplasia in a nodule or a focal, discrete lesion, endoscopic mucosal resection (EMR) should be considered. This is a method of endoscopically resecting the mucosal layer of the esophagus after separating it from the muscular layer with a submucosal injection of saline (Plates 13 and 14) or band ligation. The main risks of EMR include bleeding and perforation. An endoscopic ultrasound should be performed prior to considering EMR to confirm that the stage of the lesion is superficial and appropriate for endoscopic resection. If the resected specimen is removed en bloc, the completeness of cancer resection may be assessed pathologically. Frequently EMR is combined with an endoscopic ablative technique, such as radiofrequency ablation or photodynamic therapy, to treat high-grade dysplasia and intramucosal carcinoma.

Photodynamic therapy is a mucosal ablation technique whereby a patient is given a photosensitizer intravenously that is preferentially taken up by dysplastic cells. After a time delay, laser light of a certain wavelength is used to illuminate the tissue and activate the photosensitizer, which then interacts with oxygen to mediate cell injury (Plates 15, 16, and 17). The lining of the esophagus is ablated with a transmural burn, which can cause odynophagia and chest pain immediately following illumination. The risks of photodynamic therapy include posttreatment strictures, atrial fibrillation, and pleural effusions. This therapy is typically used alone in patients who are not operative candidates with extensive, diffuse high-grade dysplasia or intramucosal carcinoma. The overall mortality and long-term survival in patients with high-grade dysplasia who are treated with photodynamic therapy appears to be comparable to that of those treated with esophagectomy.

Various other endoscopic ablative techniques have been developed to treat dysplastic Barrett esophagus epithelium, including radiofrequency ablation, focal thermal, and cryoablation methods. Long-term comparative studies are needed to determine which method is the safest and most effective; however, it appears that radiofrequency ablation holds significant promise, with a recent study demonstrating a 90% eradication rate for high-grade dysplasia. This has been corroborated in a randomized, sham-controlled trial of radiofrequency ablation in 127 patients that demonstrated eradication rates of 90% and 81% for low-grade and high-grade dysplasia, respectively.

The treatment of high-grade dysplasia has evolved over time from a standard recommendation of esophagectomy for all patients to a more case-specific, less-invasive approach. Once the diagnosis has been confirmed by two expert GI pathologists, the patient's operative risk, the focality of the dysplasia, and the local surgical and endoscopic expertise should be considered before deciding on intensive surveillance, endoscopic ablation, or a surgical approach.

Buttar NS, Wang KK, Sebo TJ, et al. Extent of high-grade dysplasia in Barrett's esophagus correlated with risk of adenocarcinoma. *Gastroenterology.* 2001;120:1630–1639. [PMID: 11375945]

Ganz RA, Overholt BF, Sharma VK, et al. Circumferential ablation of Barrett's esophagus that contains high-grade dysplasia: a U.S. Multicenter Registry. *Gastrointest Endosc.* 2008;68:35–40. [PMID: 18355819]

Prasad GA, Wang KK, Buttar NS, et al. Long-term survival following endoscopic and surgical treatment of high-grade dysplasia in Barrett's esophagus. *Gastroenterology.* 2007;132:1226–1233. [PMID: 17408660]

Schnell TG, Sontag SJ, Chejfec G, et al. Long-term nonsurgical management of Barrett's esophagus with high-grade dysplasia. *Gastroenterology.* 2001;120:1608–1619. [PMID: 11375943]

Shaheen NJ, Sharma P, Overholt BF, et al. Radiofrequency ablation in Barrett's esophagus with dysplasia. *N Engl J Med.* 2009;360: 2277–2288. [PMID: 19474425]

Spechler SJ, Lee A, Ahnen D, et al. Long-term outcome of medical and surgical therapies for gastroesophageal reflux disease: a follow-up of a randomized controlled trial. *JAMA.* 2001;285: 2331–2338. [PMID: 11343480]

Wang VS, Hornick JL, Sepulveda JA, et al. Low prevalence of submucosal invasive carcinoma at esophagectomy for high-grade dysplasia or intramucosal adenocarcinoma in Barrett's esophagus: a 20-year experience. *Gastrointest Endosc.* 2009;69:777–783. [PMID: 19136106]

Weston AP, Sharma P, Topalovski M, et al. Long-term follow-up of Barrett's high-grade dysplasia. *Am J Gastroenterol.* 2000;95: 1888–1893. [PMID: 10950031]

Course & Prognosis

The vast majority of patients with Barrett esophagus have no long-term sequelae from the presence of metaplastic esophageal epithelium other than the inconvenience of undergoing surveillance endoscopy. Patients should be reassured that despite the increased risk of progression to adenocarcinoma, the number of patients who progress is very small. Surveillance protocols result in detection of earlier stage adenocarcinoma. The goal of treatment of patients with Barrett esophagus is to adequately control their GERD, which empiric evidence suggests may prevent progression to malignancy. If patients require antireflux surgery to control their GERD, the risk of adenocarcinoma is not reduced and continued surveillance is required, even if the patient is asymptomatic.

As mentioned previously, there have been attempts to justify treating nondysplastic Barrett esophagus by endoscopic ablative therapies. Currently there are no long-term studies regarding the cost-effectiveness, safety, and efficacy of this practice. A decrease in the incidence of esophageal cancer in patients who have undergone ablative therapies of nondysplastic Barrett esophagus has not been demonstrated. Despite this, the demonstrated safety of radiofrequency ablation and malignant potential of dysplastic Barrett esophagus has led some investigators to strongly advocate for radio frequency ablation in patients with nondysplastic Barrett esophagus. At present, ablating nondysplastic Barrett esophagus cannot be recommended.

The course and prognosis for the majority of patients with Barrett esophagus are benign, and despite the anxiety that this diagnosis can provoke in patients, the disease can be managed effectively by appropriate surveillance, acid suppression therapy, and patient reassurance.

Corey KE, Schmitz SM, Shaheen NJ. Does a surgical antireflux procedure decrease the incidence of esophageal adenocarcinoma in Barrett's esophagus? A meta-analysis. *Am J Gastroenterol.* 2003;98:2390–2394. [PMID: 14638338]

Fleischer DE, Odze R, Overholt BF, et al. The case for endoscopic treatment of non-dysplastic and low-grade dysplastic Barrett's esophagus. *Dig Dis Sci.* 2010;55:1918–1931. [PMID: 20405211]

This chapter is a revised version of the chapter by Dr. John M. Poneros that was in the previous edition of Current Diagnosis & Treatment: Gastroenterology, Hepatology, & Endoscopy.

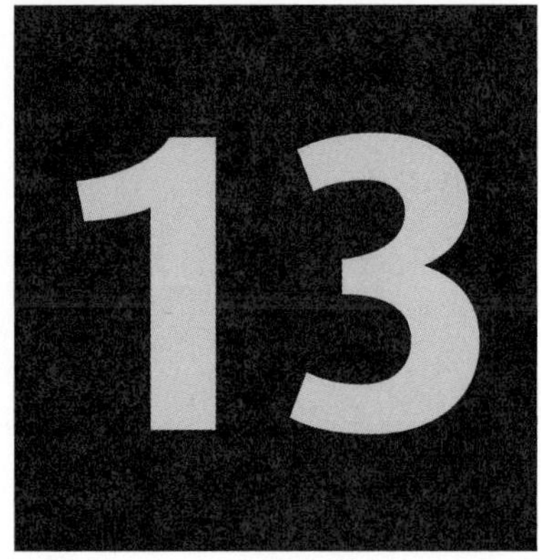

Oropharyngeal & Esophageal Motility Disorders

Arun Chaudhury, MD
Hiroshi Mashimo, MD, PhD

General Considerations

Oropharyngeal and esophageal motility disorders have significant impact on patients' quality of life. Mechanical and functional problems may interact to cause symptoms; thus, diagnosis of these disorders can be challenging.

Dysphagia (difficulty swallowing) must be distinguished from other symptoms such as odynophagia (pain on swallowing, suggestive of a defect in mucosal integrity, eg, from irradiation, inflammation, or infection) and aphagia (inability to swallow, generally suggestive of mechanical obstruction in patients presenting acutely). Symptoms that do not necessarily correlate with the immediate process of swallowing, such as rumination and globus sensation, should also be discerned.

Dysphagia can be differentiated into two categories: (1) oropharyngeal (also called transfer dysphagia), arising from disorders affecting the oropharynx, larynx, and upper esophageal sphincter (UES); and (2) esophageal, arising from the esophagus, lower esophageal sphincter (LES), or gastroesophageal junction. The causes of dysphagia are many, and specific entities are considered here.

Massey BT, Shaker R. Oral pharyngeal and upper esophageal sphincter motility disorders. GI Motility Online. Available at: http://www.nature.com/gimo/index.html; doi: 10.1038/gimo19, 2006.

Paterson WG, Goyal RK, Habib FI. Esophageal motility disorders. GI Motility Online. Available at: http://www.nature.com/gimo/index.html; doi: 10.1038/gimo20, 2006.

Wise JL, Murray IA. Oral, pharyngeal and esophageal motility disorders in systemic diseases. GI Motility Online. Available at: http://www.nature.com/gimo/index.html; doi: 10.1038/gimo40, 2006.

OROPHARYNGEAL MOTILITY DISORDERS

OROPHARYNGEAL DYSPHAGIA

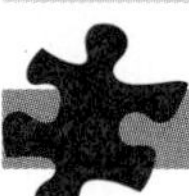

ESSENTIALS OF DIAGNOSIS

- History of poor oral bolus preparation and control, difficulty in initiating a swallow, nasal and oral regurgitation, aspiration and coughing with swallowing, food sticking at the level of the throat.
- Evidence of a generalized neuromuscular disorder.
- Documentation by videofluoroscopic swallowing study (VFSS).

General Considerations

Many neuromuscular disorders can cause dysphagia (Table 13–1). Among these are various disorders causing cortical lesions; supranuclear, nuclear, and cranial nerve lesions; defects of neurotransmission at the motor end plates; and muscular diseases.

Many patients with dysphagia are elderly and hence develop this symptom secondary to other disorders (eg, stroke). History of strokes or other neurologic illnesses, nasal regurgitation and frequent coughing immediately upon swallowing, and poor oral coordination of bolus formation or dysphonia may help suggest the greater likelihood of oropharyngeal dysphagia over esophageal dysmotility, but diagnosis, assessment of severity, and therapeutic intervention are generally guided by VFSS.

Table 13–1. Neuromuscular disorders causing oropharyngeal dysphagia.

1. Diseases of cerebral cortex and brainstem
a. With altered consciousness or dementia
• Dementias, including Alzheimer disease
• Altered consciousness, metabolic encephalopathy, encephalitis, meningitis, cerebrovascular accident, brain injury
b. With normal cognitive functions
• Brain injury
• Cerebral palsy
• Rabies, tetanus, neurosyphilis
• Cerebrovascular disease
• Parkinson disease and other extrapyramidal lesions
• Multiple sclerosis (bulbar and pseudobulbar palsy)
• Amyotrophic lateral sclerosis (motor neuron disease)
• Poliomyelitis and post-poliomyelitis syndrome
2. Diseases of cranial nerves (V, VII, IX, X, XII)
a. Basilar meningitis (chronic inflammatory, neoplastic)
b. Nerve injury
c. Neuropathy (Guillain-Barré syndrome, Bell palsy, afamilial dysautonomia, sarcoid, diabetic, and other causes)
3. Neuromuscular
a. Myasthenia gravis
b. Eaton-Lambert syndrome
c. Botulinum toxin
d. Aminoglycosides and other drugs
4. Muscle disorders
a. Myositis (polymyositis, dermatomyositis, sarcoidosis)
b. Metabolic myopathy (mitochondrial myopathy, thyroid myopathy)
c. Primary myopathies (myotonic dystrophy, oculopharyngeal myopathy)
d. Acute and chronic radiation injury

Adapted, with permission, from Goyal RK. Dysphagia. In: Fauci AS, Braunwald E, Kasper DL, et al (editors). *Harrison's Principles of Internal Medicine*, 17th ed. McGraw-Hill, 2008:237–240.

Clinical Findings

A. Symptoms and Signs

History and physical examination provide the most valuable information in making the diagnosis. Defects in different phases of oropharyngeal swallowing should be identified by careful analysis of symptoms and signs.

Defects in the oral preparatory phase of swallowing manifest as chewing problems, oral stasis of food, inability to form a bolus, and coughing, choking, or aspiration pneumonia from regurgitation and aspiration. These symptoms occur during or immediately after the onset of swallowing. In disorders of neuromuscular dysfunction, liquids are usually more problematic than solids in causing symptoms of misdirection. On the other hand, secondary causes from oral mucosal lesions (eg, aphthous ulcers, herpetic lesions, mucositis), dental problems, or decreased saliva and xerostomia (eg, medications, Sjögren) may lead to poor processing of the bolus and are often less problematic with moistened foods or liquids.

Generally, problems in the pharyngeal phase result in dysphagia, which the patient localizes to the throat. Often the patient makes repeated attempts to clear the throat of food or saliva.

Abnormalities of the UES phase have no distinctive symptoms, but impaired UES opening further impairs pharyngeal transport and may aggravate the symptoms of pharyngeal stasis. On the other hand, a hypotonic UES may lead to esophagopharyngeal reflux and aspiration not related to swallowing.

Because many neuromuscular structures involved in swallowing are also involved in speech, dysarthria and dysphonia are common in these patients. Moreover, patients usually have evidence of neuromuscular defects in other parts of the body. Many patients with oropharyngeal dysphagia have impaired consciousness and cognitive functions that may make evaluation difficult.

B. Videofluoroscopic Swallowing Study (VFSS)

VFSS is the study of choice for the evaluation of oropharyngeal dysphagia (Figure 13–1). VFSS allows slow-motion replay of oropharyngeal swallowing. This aids in identifying defects of the oropharyngeal phase of swallowing, which normally takes less than a second to complete. Different consistencies of food and various swallowing maneuvers can be used during the study to assess for retention or aspiration. Barium swallow or an upper gastrointestinal series is not useful in evaluation of oropharyngeal dysphagia. Plain radiographs and computed tomography (CT) scan of the neck are useful in evaluating structural lesions such as tumors and cysts. Imaging studies should be obtained prior to upper endoscopy, because pharyngeal and upper esophageal abnormalities such as diverticula and malignant strictures can perforate in this poorly visualized region.

Gramigna GD. How to perform videofluoroscopic swallowing studies. GI Motility Online. Available at: http://www.nature.com/gimo/index.html; doi: 10.1038/gimo95, 2006.

C. Manometry

Because of the complex anatomy of the oral and pharyngeal passages and the speed of coordinated contractions, intraluminal manometry is not usually helpful. However, it may be useful in the evaluation of upper esophageal function and resistance to flow across the UES.

D. Videoendoscopy

Regular upper endoscopy is not helpful in the evaluation of oropharyngeal dysphagia; however, videoendoscopy, available at some specialized centers, can provide information about oropharyngeal dysfunction.

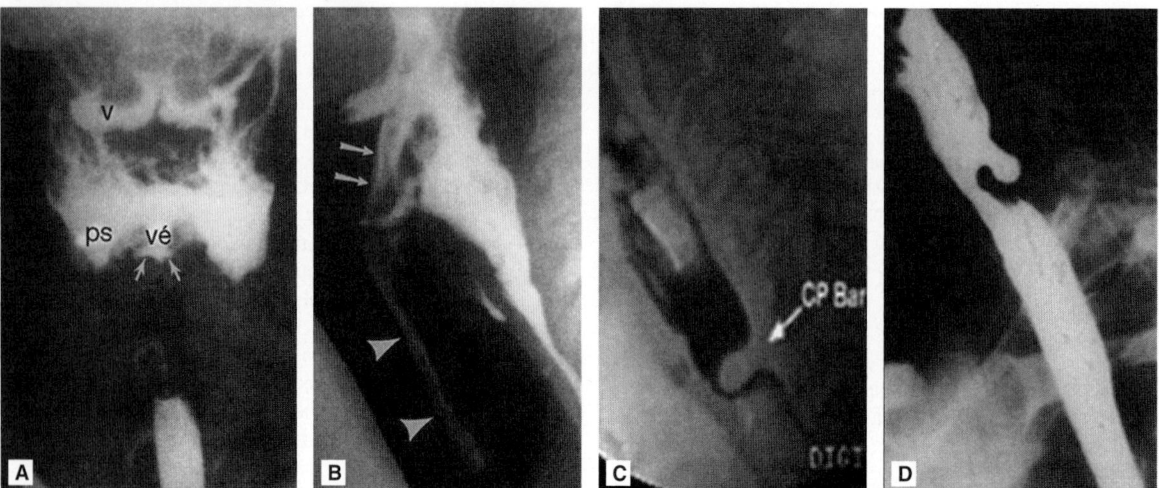

▲ **Figure 13–1.** Radiologic appearance of oropharyngeal motility disorders. **A:** Frontal view of the pharynx demonstrates aspiration of retained bolus. Note that there is retention of contrast in the valleculae (v) and piriform sinuses (ps). No swallow is taking place, yet there is entry of contrast into the laryngeal vestibule (vé) and between the vocal folds and in the ventricle *(arrows)*. **B:** A stop-frame print from a cinepharyngogram in the lateral position shows incomplete laryngeal closure during swallowing with laryngeal penetration *(arrows)* and aspiration *(arrowheads)* down into the trachea. The bolus is passing through the open cricopharyngeus into the cervical esophagus. Degenerative change is noted in the cervical spine. **C:** Cricopharyngeal bar. **D:** Zenker diverticulum. (Reproduced, with permission, from (A) Jones B (editor): *Normal and Abnormal Swallowing: Imaging in Diagnosis and Therapy*, 2nd edition. Springer-Verlag, 2003; (B) Jones B, Donner MW (editors): *Normal and Abnormal Swallowing: Imaging in Diagnosis and Therapy*. Springer-Verlag, 1991.)

Differential Diagnosis

Figure 13–2 is an algorithm outlining an approach to the patient with oropharyngeal dysphagia.

Complications

The major complications of oropharyngeal dysphagia are fatal pulmonary aspiration and pneumonia, malnutrition, and weight loss.

Treatment

Evaluation and management by a deglutition team consisting of a deglutitionist (speech and swallow therapist), radiologist, gastroenterologist, otolaryngologist, and neurologist provide the best outcome in the care of these patients. Deglutitionists assess the risk of aspiration, type of food, and patient posture that is most likely to prevent aspiration and facilitate safe swallowing. Certain rehabilitative exercises to strengthen swallowing muscles may be helpful. Electrical stimulation of muscles is also being explored as a newer avenue of therapy for oropharyngeal dysplasia. Investigations are performed to find the underlying cause of the disorder, and appropriate therapy, if available, is initiated. If safe oral feeding cannot be undertaken, a percutaneous endoscopic gastrostomy (PEG) tube is placed by a gastroenterologist. The overall management of the patient, rather than focused treatment of the swallowing difficulty, is essential for effective management.

Course & Prognosis

Prognosis depends on the underlying cause, compliance with therapy, and prevention of acute pulmonary complications. Patients with recent cerebrovascular accidents may regain their swallowing function after 6–8 weeks. Those with diseases such as myasthenia gravis, metabolic myopathies such as thyroid disorders, polymyositis, and Parkinson disease usually respond to appropriate treatment. Other patients, such as those with muscular dystrophy, amyotrophic lateral sclerosis, and multiple sclerosis, sometimes develop recurrent aspiration pneumonia that may prove fatal.

Achem SR, DeVault KR. Dysphagia in aging. *J Clin Gastroenterol.* 2005;39:357–371. [PMID: 15815202]

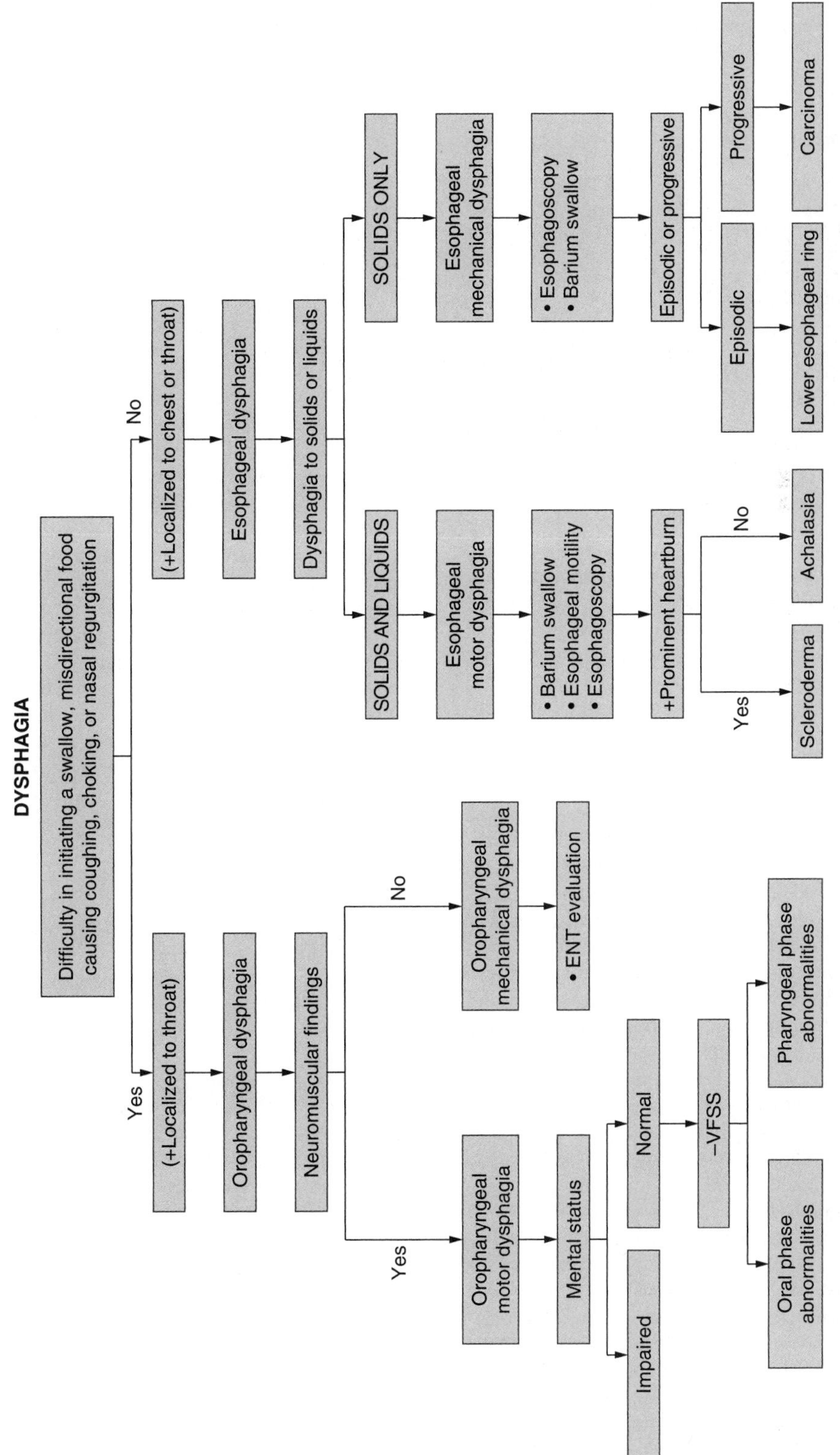

▲ **Figure 13–2.** Algorithm outlining an approach to the patient with dysphagia. ENT, ear, nose, throat; VFSS, videofluoroscopic swallowing study.

Cook IJ. Clinical disorders of the upper esophageal sphincter. GI Motility Online. Available at: http://www.nature.com/gimo/index.html; doi: 10.1038/gimo37, 2006.

Curtis JL. Pulmonary complications of oral-pharyngeal motility disorders. GI Motility Online. Available at: http://www. nature.com/gimo/index.html; doi: 10.1038/gimo33, 2006.

Ford CN. Evaluation and management of laryngopharyngeal reflux. *JAMA*. 2005;28:1534–1540.

Goyal RK. Dysphagia. In: Fauci AS, Braunwald E, Kasper DL, et al (editors). *Harrison's Principles of Internal Medicine*, 17th ed. McGraw-Hill, 2008:237–240.

Logemann JA. Medical and rehabilitative therapy of oral pharyngeal motor disorders. GI Motility Online. Available at: http://www.nature.com/gimo/index.html; doi: 10.1038/gimo50, 2006.

CRICOPHARYNGEAL ACHALASIA & CRICOPHARYNGEAL BAR

UES dysfunction has been variably defined and described. Cricopharyngeal "achalasia" is a confused and often misused term that is best avoided since the diagnosis is rarely made by manometric or electromyographic evidence to demonstrate failure of UES relaxation, but historically used when there is radiographic evidence for failed opening of the UES. UES "achalasia" should be replaced by more specific descriptions such as failed UES relaxation, cricopharyngeal spasms, and cricopharyngeal bar. The clinical presentation of these entities comprising UES dysfunction is variable, but most patients complain of food sticking in the lower third of the neck. Patients may also have heartburn, choking, and odynophagia, and less commonly dysphonia or globus sensation during swallows. These entities are considered primary if the abnormality is confined to the cricopharyngeus muscle without neurologic or systemic cause and secondary if produced by another disease process. Primary UES dysfunction, in turn, is subdivided into idiopathic and intrinsic myopathies (eg, polymyositis, inclusion body myositis, muscular dystrophy, hypothyroidism). Secondary causes include amyotrophic lateral sclerosis, polio, oculopharyngeal dysphagia, stroke, Parkinson disease, fibrosis from prior irradiation, and peripheral nerve disorders such as myasthenia gravis and diabetic neuropathy. Gastroesophageal reflux has also been suggested to cause cricopharyngeal spasm.

The diagnostic criteria for UES dysfunction are subject to much controversy. The plain radiographic appearance is not reliable in making this diagnosis, and some experts advocate highly specialized radiologic (VFSS) and solid-state manometric probe studies. However, lack of data and standardization in measurements (eg, in anteroposterior, lateral, or circumferential pressures) and the possibility of the manometric catheter eliciting cricopharyngeal spasms have thwarted its standard use. Many clinicians base their diagnosis simply on symptoms. Thus, the true incidence of UES dysfunction or UES "achalasia" is unknown but may involve 5–25% of patients being evaluated for dysphagia.

The cricopharyngeal bar is a radiologic abnormality, often equated with UES "achalasia." However, manometric studies in patients with cricopharyngeal bars have demonstrated generally normal UES pressure and relaxation. Thus, they are generally not associated with failed UES relaxation or cricopharyngeal spasm. Barium swallow shows a characteristic prominent projection on the posterior wall of the pharynx at the level of the lower part of the cricoid cartilage (see Figure 13–1C). A transient cricopharyngeal bar is seen in up to 5% of individuals without dysphagia undergoing upper gastrointestinal studies; it can be produced in normal individuals during a Valsalva maneuver. A persistent cricopharyngeal bar may be caused by fibrosis or frank myositis in the cricopharyngeus. Some cases have been reported with dermatomyositis or inclusion body myositis. However, muscle biopsies are not routinely taken.

Failed UES relaxation is poorly responsive to medical therapy including muscle relaxants. Cricopharyngeal myotomy is usually not helpful unless obstruction at the cricopharyngeus is demonstrated by videofluoroscopy in severely symptomatic patients, such as those with significant aspiration or weight loss. Similarly, local injection of botulinum toxin is falling out of favor with recognition that effects are short lived and the injections are rarely well confined to the affected muscles; frequent leakage outside the cricopharyngeus may result in temporary dysphonia or aspiration. However, a trial injection may be considered to aid in making the diagnosis, or for patients who are poor surgical candidates. These procedures are contraindicated in patients with cervical tumors and relatively contraindicated in those who have a fibrotic lesion after neck irradiation or who have a progressive neurologic disorder such as bulbar palsy. One exception appears to be patients with oculopharyngeal dysphagia, who appear to do well with surgical myotomy or with repeated dilations. Myotomy is also contraindicated in the presence of severe gastroesophageal reflux because it may lead to pharyngeal and pulmonary aspiration. In patients with gastroesophageal reflux, aggressive therapy with proton pump inhibitors is warranted in addition to management of the underlying disorder. The classic surgical approach is external cricopharyngeal myotomy.

ZENKER DIVERTICULUM

Zenker diverticulum arises in the posterior wall of the hypopharynx, just above the cricopharyngeus muscle. The pathogenesis of Zenker diverticulum is not fully understood. It may form due to natural weakness of the pharynx (Killian triangle) associated with impaired opening of the cricopharyngeus muscle, which is often fibrotic. Barium swallow or VFSS shows characteristic findings that allow easy diagnosis (see Figure 13–1D). With time, the diverticulum may become very large. Zenker diverticulum may retain food and secretions and classically lead to halitosis, delayed regurgitation, recurrent aspiration, and pneumonia. Dysphagia is usually due to compression of a food-filled diverticulum of the esophagus. Treatment is diverticulectomy with cricopharyngeal myotomy, and transoral approaches have also been introduced as an alternative and minimally invasive treatment.

GLOBUS PHARYNGEUS

Globus pharyngeus is a common functional disorder characterized by the persistent or intermittent nonpainful sensation of a lump or foreign body in the throat, but without any difficulty in swallowing or pain on swallowing. This disorder is more common in women than in men and is often associated with an underlying psychiatric disorder experienced during an emotional event. Some of these patients also have gastroesophageal reflux disease (GERD), and ambulatory pH monitoring or empiric trial of acid suppression is recommended. The latter has been shown to improve symptoms in a third of the patients. Findings on barium swallow are generally normal, but may discern pharyngeal dysfunction or possible cricopharyngeal bar in patients with these symptoms. Esophageal manometry also may reveal achalasia in patients with these symptoms, even when devoid of dysphagia. Results of upper endoscopy, when performed, are generally normal. However, an observational report describes improvement after ablation of cervical inlet patches, and this endoscopically often missed entity located at or just distal to the UES should be sought carefully. In most cases, treatment of globus pharyngeus consists of reassurance. Patients with concurrent psychiatric disorders, such as depression, panic, and somatization disorders, may benefit from tricyclic antidepressant therapy. Relaxation therapy has also been reported as helpful in refractory patients.

ESOPHAGEAL MOTILITY DISORDERS

Three esophageal motility disorders commonly seen in clinical practice are esophageal motor dysphagia, GERD, and esophageal chest pain. In these disorders, symptoms result from dysfunction of one or more of the mechanisms necessary for normal esophageal function.

Esophageal motility disorders are classified, depending on the involvement of one or more of the three components of esophageal peristalsis, as disorders of inhibitory innervation, excitatory innervation, or smooth muscles (Figure 13–3).

The inhibitory innervation to the esophagus consists of vagal preganglionic neurons and the postganglionic neurons in the myenteric plexus, which release vasoactive intestinal peptide (VIP) and nitric oxide. The inhibitory pathway is responsible for relaxation of the LES and the gradient of peristaltic contraction in the esophageal body. Deficiency of inhibitory innervation results in achalasia and diffuse esophageal spasm. In achalasia, both the LES and esophageal body are affected, whereas in diffuse esophageal spasm, the esophageal body is primarily affected. Increased inhibitory nerve activity is responsible for so-called transient LES relaxation (TLESR).

The excitatory innervation consists of vagal preganglionic neurons and postganglionic neurons that release acetylcholine and substance P. The excitatory nerves contribute to basal LES hypertension, hypertensive contraction, and the force of peristaltic contraction. Deficiency of the excitatory nerves causes hypotensive LES and hypotensive peristaltic contractions. The esophageal body and LES consist of phasic and tonic muscles, respectively. Phasic muscles of the esophageal body contract during peristalsis, and tonic muscles of

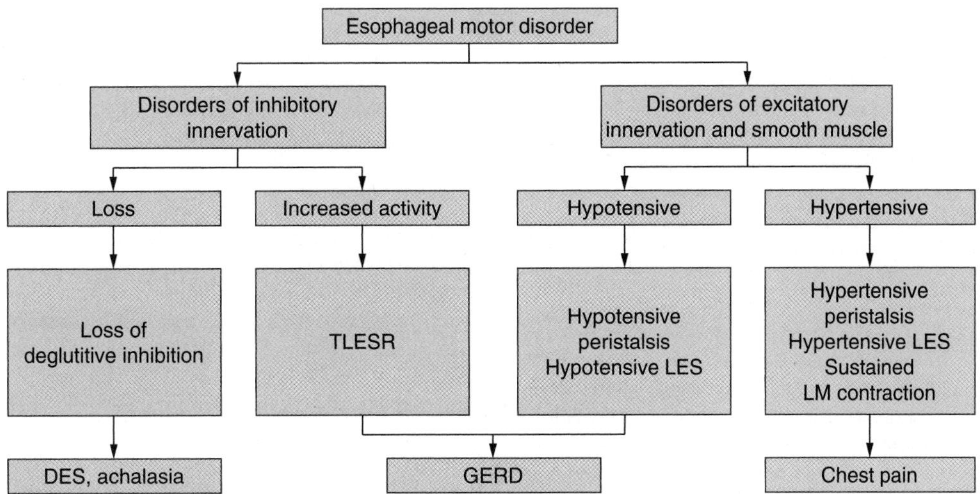

▲ **Figure 13–3.** Pathophysiologic classification of motor disorders of the smooth muscle portion of the esophagus. DES, diffuse esophageal spasm; GERD, gastroesophageal reflux disease; LES, lower esophageal sphincter; LM, longitudinal muscle; TLESR, transient lower esophageal sphincter relaxation.

LES are responsible for tonic contraction. Muscle disorders may lead to hypotensive LES and hypotensive peristalsis.

In most conditions outlined below, a combination of imaging studies and intraluminal pressure measurements helps obtain an accurate clinical diagnosis.

Goyal RK. Diseases of the esophagus. In: Fauci AS, Braunwald E, Kasper DL, et al (editors). *Harrison's Principles of Internal Medicine*, 17th ed. McGraw-Hill, 2008:1847–1855.

Goyal RK, Chaudhury A. Physiology of normal esophageal motility. *J Clin Gastroenterol.* 2008;42:610–619.

Pandolfino JE, Kahrilas PJ. New technologies in the gastrointestinal clinic and research: impedance and high-resolution manometry. *World J Gastroenterol.* 2009;15:131–138.

ESOPHAGEAL MOTOR DYSPHAGIA

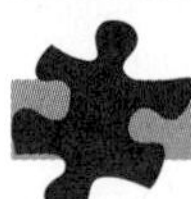

ESSENTIALS OF DIAGNOSIS

- Dysphagia to solids and liquids, localized to the chest or throat.
- Associated symptom of chest pain and regurgitation.
- Coughing and choking spells at night and unrelated to swallowing.
- Symptoms of GERD.
- Confirmation of abnormal motility by barium study and esophageal manometry.

General Considerations

Dysphagia must be distinguished from odynophagia (pain on swallowing); the latter suggests a breach in mucosal integrity by trauma, infection, and inflammation. The role of upper endoscopy is to rule out mucosal abnormalities such as strictures, webs, malignancies, infections, and eosinophilic esophagitis. Full-column barium swallow may reveal muscular rings, which are often missed on endoscopy. Manometric studies differentiate specific motility disorders.

Pathogenesis

Motor dysphagia in the thoracic esophagus occurs when deglutitive inhibition is lacking, due to loss of inhibitory nitrergic nerves, and peristaltic contractions become nonperistaltic; when the LES does not relax properly; or when the peristaltic contractions are weakened due to muscle weakness. Causes of esophageal motor dysphagia are listed in Table 13–2.

Table 13–2. Causes of esophageal motor dysphagia.

1. **Disorders of cervical esophagus**
   (see "Oropharyngeal Motility Disorders" in text)
2. **Disorders of thoracic esophagus**
   a. Disease of smooth muscle or excitatory nerves
      (1) Weak muscle contraction or LES tone
         - Idiopathic
         - Scleroderma and related collagen vascular diseases
         - Hollow visceral myopathy
         - Myotonic dystrophy
         - Metabolic neuromyopathy (amyloid, alcohol, diabetes)
         - Drugs—anticholinergics, smooth muscle relaxants
      (2) Enhanced muscle contraction
         - Hypertensive peristalsis (nutcracker esophagus)
         - Hypertensive LES, hypercontracting LES
   b. Disorders of inhibitory innervation
      (1) Diffuse esophageal spasm
      (2) Achalasia
         - Primary
         - Secondary (Chagas disease, carcinoma, lymphoma, neuropathic intestinal pseudo-obstruction syndrome)
         - Contractile (muscular) lower esophageal ring

LES, lower esophageal sphincter. Adapted, with permission, from Goyal RK. Dysphagia. In: Fauci AS, Braunwald E, Kasper DL, et al (editors). *Harrison's Principles of Internal Medicine*, 17th ed. McGraw-Hill, 2008:237–240.

Clinical Findings

A. Symptoms and Signs

Dysphagia resulting from dysfunction of the esophageal body is described as a feeling that the swallowed bolus becomes "stuck" or "hung up" on the way down. This may be accompanied by pain or discomfort. The patient typically describes difficulty in swallowing both solids and liquids. Although most patients feel as though the bolus stops at the level of the suprasternal notch, the area of obstruction may be well below this. Many patients have associated symptoms of regurgitation and chest pain.

B. Radiography

Chest radiographs may show mediastinal widening and air-fluid level when a food-filled dilated esophagus is present as in long-standing achalasia. Barium swallow may show the characteristic appearance of achalasia or diffuse esophageal spasm (Figure 13–4). Radiographic studies also help in excluding mechanical causes of dysphagia. Videofluoroscopic examination of the esophagus may identify abnormalities in peristaltic sequence and in the force of peristaltic contractions.

C. Manometry and Impedance Manometry

Esophageal manometry can be used to measure the strength (amplitude), duration, and sequential nature of the contractions

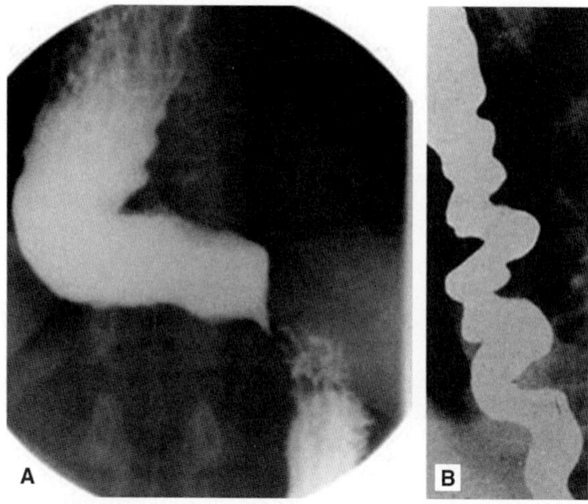

▲ **Figure 13–4.** Radiologic appearance of motor disorders of the smooth muscle portion of the esophagus. **A:** Note the sigmoid-shaped esophagus and "bird-beaking" of the lower end in achalasia. **B:** Corkscrew appearance in diffuse esophageal spasm. (B: Used with permission from Dr. Harvey Goldstein)

of the esophageal body, as well as the resting pressure and relaxation of the LES. This technique involves passage, through the nose and into the esophagus and stomach, of a small, flexible catheter with an array of pressure sensors. Figure 13–5 summarizes patterns of esophageal motility in normal subjects and in a variety of esophageal motility disorders. Newer manometric probes with an array of dozens of sensors (high resolution) have also helped identify some patients with weak or slow contractions near the transition zone (a variable area of interdigitating striated and smooth muscle fibers) that correlate with dysphagia. Impedance sensors in the same catheter assembly have helped correlate functional liquid and viscous bolus clearance in patients with various types of esophageal motility abnormalities, and have allowed new algorithms to analyze pressure waves.

D. Endoscopy

Endoscopy is required in most patients with esophageal motility disorders that cause dysphagia to exclude mechanical causes such as peptic stricture and other complications of an erosive esophagitis, and rule out lesions such as gastroesophageal junction adenocarcinoma that may produce secondary achalasia. Biopsies at multiple levels of the esophageal body are also often obtained to rule out eosinophilic esophagitis.

Differential Diagnosis

Refer to Figure 13–2, which outlines an approach to the patient with dysphagia.

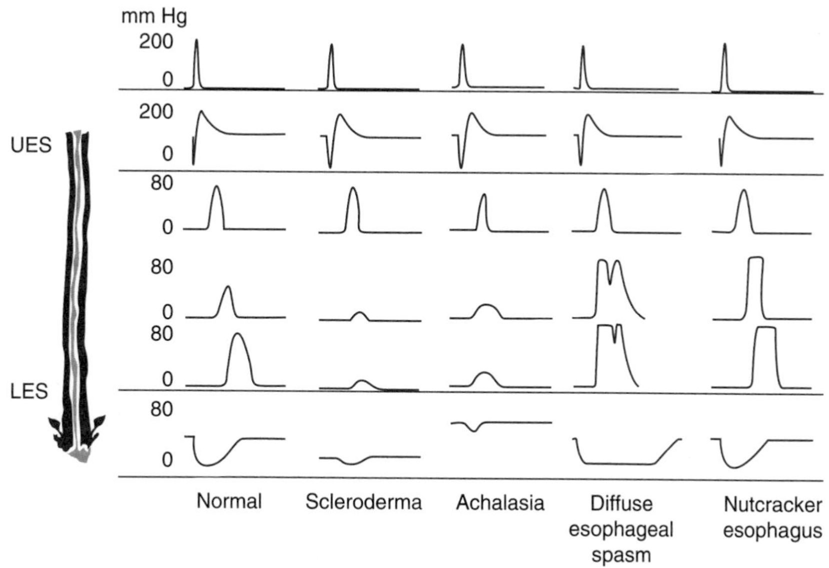

▲ **Figure 13–5.** Motility patterns in esophageal smooth muscle disorders. LES, lower esophageal sphincter; UES, upper esophageal sphincter. (Adapted, with permission, from Goyal RK: Diseases of the Esophagus. In: Fauci AS, Braunwald E, Kasper DL, et al (editors): *Harrison's Principles of Internal Medicine*, 17th ed. McGraw-Hill, 2008.)

Treatment

Management of esophageal motility disorders depends on the type of the disorder and its clinical consequences. (For details, see "Disorders of Inhibitory Innervation" and "Disorders of Excitatory Nerves and Smooth Muscles" later in this chapter.)

Achem SR, DeVault KR. Dysphagia in aging. *J Clin Gastroenterol.* 2005;39:357–371.

Goyal RK. Dysphagia. In: Fauci AS, Braunwald E, Kasper DL, et al (editors). *Harrison's Principles of Internal Medicine,* 17th ed. McGraw-Hill, 2008:237–240.

Hejazi RA, Reddymasu SC, Sostarich S, McCallum RW. Disturbances of esophageal motility in eosinophilic esophagitis: a case series. *Dysphagia.* 2010;25:231–237.

Kahrilas PJ, Ghosh SK, Pandolfino JE. Esophageal motility disorders in terms of pressure topography: the Chicago Classification. *J Clin Gastroenterol.* 2008;42:627–635.

Mulder DJ, Justinich CJ. Understanding eosinophilic esophagitis: the cellular and molecular mechanisms of an emerging disease. *Mucosal Immunol.* 2011;4:139–147.

GASTROESOPHAGEAL REFLUX DISEASE (SEE CHAPTER 11)

GERD is the most common manifestation of impaired esophageal motility and one of the most common disorders seen in clinical practice. The basic cause of GERD is incompetent antireflux barriers at the gastroesophageal junction, which normally prevents backflow of gastric acid into the stomach. Competence of the gastroesophageal barrier is the result of the intra-abdominal location of the LES, mucosal folds at the gastroesophageal junction, LES closure, reflex LES contraction, and the proper position of the diaphragmatic crura, which can be disrupted with the presence of a sliding hiatal hernia. Factors such as increased intra-abdominal pressure (that may arise, for example, from obesity), gastric stasis (that may arise, for example, from chronic diabetes or medications), and inappropriate transient relaxations of the LES can increase the likelihood of developing GERD.

The pathogenesis of gastroesophageal reflux is complicated and multifactorial. Important esophageal motor abnormalities underlying GERD are hypotensive LES, TLESR, or both. Hypotensive esophageal contractions are commonly associated with hypotensive LES and contribute to reflux-associated esophageal mucosal damage.

Although the main clinical manifestations of GERD are heartburn and regurgitation, other manifestations, including development of chronic cough and the premalignant condition of Barrett esophagus, may occur. Moreover, the majority of patients with GERD do not have symptoms. Manifestations and complications of GERD are discussed in detail in Chapter 11.

Diamont NE. Pathophysiology of gastroesophageal reflux disease. GI Motility Online. Available at: http://www.nature.com/gimo/index.html; doi: 10.1038/gimo21, 2006.

Falconer J. Gastro-oesophageal reflux and gastrooesophageal reflux disease in infants and children. J Fam Health Care. 2010;20:175–177.

Harding SM. Gastroesophageal reflux and chronic cough. GI Motility Online. Available at: http://www.nature.com/gimo/index.html; doi: 10.1038/gimo77, 2006.

ESOPHAGEAL CHEST PAIN

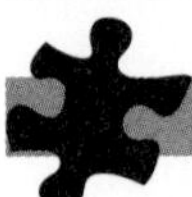

ESSENTIALS OF DIAGNOSIS

- Chronic symptoms.
- Rule out life-threatening conditions (eg, ischemic heart disease).
- Rule out panic disorder, related psychiatric disorders, and musculoskeletal disorders.
- Well-accepted causes are reflux esophagitis, achalasia, and diffuse esophageal spasm.
- Probable causes are hypertensive esophageal motor disorders, cervical inlet patch, sustained longitudinal muscle contraction, and esophageal hypersensitivity.

General Considerations

Heartburn and odynophagia are classical symptoms of esophageal disease. However, some patients with esophageal disorders present with chest pain that is neither typical heartburn nor odynophagia. Esophageal chest pain may resemble cardiac chest pain. This overlap is due to the spinal primary sensory afferent that carries cardiac and esophageal nociceptive information and also innervates common cutaneous segments.

Pathogenesis

For practical purposes, causes of chronic esophageal chest pain can be divided into well-accepted and possible causes.

A. Well-Accepted Causes of Esophageal Chest Pain

Well-established causes of chest pain are reflux esophagitis and motility disorders such as achalasia and diffuse esophageal spasm. Overall, reflux esophagitis is the most common cause of noncardiac chest pain.

B. Probable Causes of Esophageal Chest Pain

Esophageal disorders that have been proposed as causes of chest pain are hypertensive esophageal motility disorders, sustained longitudinal muscle contraction, esophageal hypersensitivity, and esophageal sensory neuropathy.

1. Hypertensive esophageal motility disorders—Some esophageal motility disorders, particularly those associated with hypertensive esophageal peristaltic contractions (so-called nutcracker esophagus), hypertensive LES, and hypercontracting LES, have been identified during manometric evaluation of patients with unexplained chest pain. Therefore, these manometric diagnoses were proposed as causing chest pain. However, a causal relationship has not been established. Moreover, a temporal association between these conditions and chest pain has not been documented, and treatment of the hypercontractile states with smooth muscle relaxants has not proved to be effective in the relief of chest pain.

2. Sustained longitudinal muscle contraction—Dynamic high-resolution endoscopic ultrasound has shown that episodes of chest pain are associated with sustained contraction of the esophageal longitudinal muscle. The longitudinal muscle contraction remains undetected by intraluminal manometry. Therefore, sustained esophageal longitudinal muscle contraction has been proposed as a cause of chest pain in patients with normal esophageal manometry. Further studies are needed to fully establish this sustained contraction as the cause of unexplained chest pain.

3. Defects in sensory nerves and pain perception—Several recent studies have suggested that the esophagus may develop sensory hypersensitivity, in which stimuli that do not normally produce pain are perceived as painful. Esophageal hypersensitivity may be a part of generalized visceral hypersensitivity. The pathophysiology of visceral hypersensitivity is not fully understood but may occur peripherally in the esophageal afferent nerves or centrally in the central nervous system. Esophageal hypersensitivity is demonstrated by showing a reduced threshold to esophageal balloon distention. Esophageal mucosal hypersensitivity can also be tested by the esophageal acid perfusion test (Bernstein test), discussed later.

Lee R, Mittal R. Heartburn and esophageal pain. GI Motility Online. Available at: http://www.nature.com/gimo/index.html; doi: 10.1038/gimo75, 2006.

Miwa H, Kondo T, Oshima T, Fukui H, Tomita T, Watari J. Esophageal sensation and esophageal hypersensitivity: overview from bench to bedside. *J Neurogastroenterol Motil.* 2010;16: 353–362.

Prakash Gyawali C. Esophageal hypersensitivity. *Gastroenterol Hepatol.* 2010;6:497–500.

Remes-Troche JM. The hypersensitive esophagus: pathophysiology, evaluation, and treatment options. *Curr Gastroenterol Rep.* 2010; 12:417–426.

Clinical Findings

Chest pain is a common and alarming symptom. Acute chest pain syndromes are due to life-threatening conditions such as myocardial infarction, aortic dissection, pulmonary embolism, esophageal perforation, acute bolus obstruction, or penetrating esophageal ulcer. Patients with these conditions require emergent care.

Patients presenting with chronic chest pain should undergo careful clinical evaluation to classify them into the following broad groups: cardiac chest pain, musculoskeletal chest pain, psychosomatic chest pain, esophageal chest pain, and miscellaneous causes of chest pain. In the majority of patients, the origin of chest pain is easily identified and treated. However, in some patients, the origin of chest pain remains obscure.

Differential Diagnosis & Treatment

An algorithm outlining an approach to the patient with chest pain of unknown origin (CPUO) is presented in Figure 13–6. A working definition of CPUO has not been developed. However, it is clear that this diagnosis should be used only after careful initial evaluation. For example, cardiac evaluation and treatment should be performed for patients with ischemic heart disease and typical symptoms of cardiac ischemia; a trial of a proton pump inhibitor should be initiated for patients suspected of having heartburn and GERD; a trial of nonsteroidal anti-inflammatory drugs (NSAIDs) and possibly skeletal muscle relaxants should be used for those with musculoskeletal disorders; and a therapeutic trial should be started for those with panic disorder.

A. Chest Pain of Unknown Origin

Patients in whom the initial evaluation does not yield a cause are identified as having CPUO. The first step in the evaluation of a patient with CPUO is to carefully exclude coronary artery disease because of the life-threatening nature of cardiac chest pain. This may require coronary angiography, which remains the gold standard, apart from careful consideration of cardiac causes of chest pain. The speculative cardiac causes of chest pain include microvascular angina or syndrome X. This diagnosis is sometimes considered in patients with atypical anginal symptoms and normal coronary arteries, especially when abnormalities are present on noninvasive tests of cardiac function such as exercise radionuclide angiography or exercise thallium scintigraphy. Similarly, mitral valve prolapse is frequently present in patients with chest pain of undetermined etiology; however, most investigators agree that it does not cause chest pain. CPUO patients in whom cardiac causes of chest pain have been excluded are identified as having noncardiac chest pain. These patients require careful screening for esophageal, musculoskeletal, psychosomatic, and miscellaneous causes of chest pain.

B. Reflux Esophagitis

Reflux esophagitis is one of the most common causes of esophageal chest pain. Among patients with reflux, 10–20% will have chest pain alone, and reflux esophagitis remains the

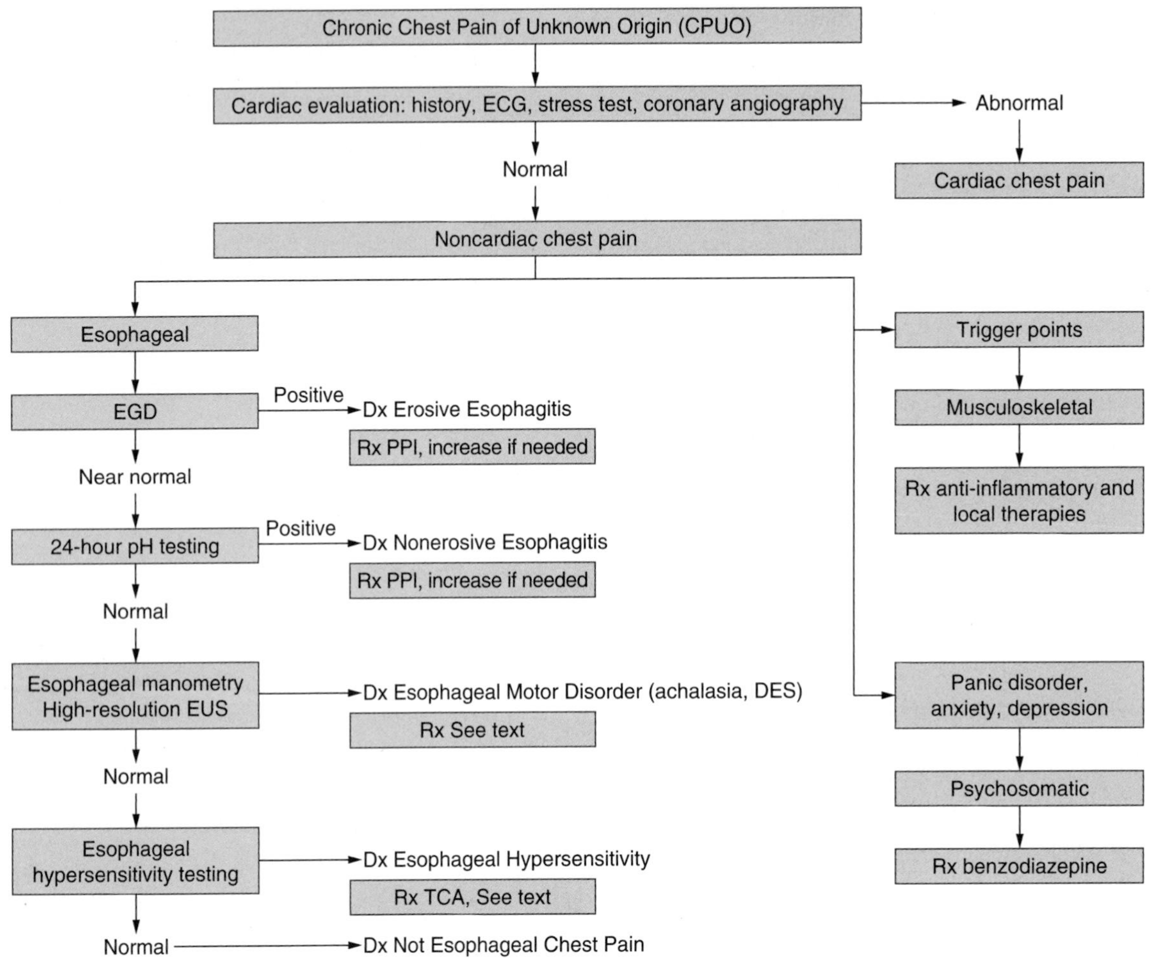

▲ **Figure 13–6.** Algorithm outlining an approach to the patient with unexplained chest pain. CPUO, chest pain of unknown origin; DES, diffuse esophageal spasm; Dx, diagnosis; ECG, electrocardiogram; EGD, esophagogastroduodenoscopy; EUS, esophageal ultrasound; Rx, prescription; PPI, proton pump inhibitor; TCA, tricyclic antidepressant.

most common cause of unexplained chest pain. Therefore, the first step is to prescribe a therapeutic trial of a proton pump inhibitor if this therapy has not already been initiated. If there is no satisfactory response, the patient should undergo endoscopic examination. Esophageal erosions, ulcers, and peptic strictures provide evidence of GERD, which should be treated with a proton pump inhibitor, including high-dose therapy if needed. If no or minimal mucosal abnormalities are found, high-magnification endoscopy or narrow band image endoscopy may be performed to look for microerosions. Mucosal biopsies should be obtained in patients with negative endoscopic results. These patients should undergo pH monitoring by placement of a pH capsule in the distal esophagus. If capsule monitoring is not available, 24-hour ambulatory esophageal pH testing should be performed. Mucosal biopsy specimens may show enlarged intercellular spaces, which are thought to represent very early mucosal damage in reflux esophagitis. Patients having abnormal mucosal biopsy and esophageal pH findings are diagnosed as having nonerosive reflux disease and treated aggressively with proton pump inhibitor therapy. Newer pH catheters with impedance have allowed assessment of volume reflux and distinction of these episodes as acidic or nonacidic.

Cho YK. How to interpret esophageal impedance pH monitoring. *J Neurogastroenterol Motil.* 2010;16:327–330. [PMID: 20680174]

Fass R, Dickman R. Nonerosive reflux disease. GI Motility Online. Available at: http://www.nature.com/gimo/index.html; doi: 10.1038/gimo42, 2006.

C. Esophageal Motility Problems & Esophageal Hypersensitivity

In patients showing no evidence of esophagitis, intraluminal manometry should be performed to evaluate for the presence of motility disorders such as early achalasia, diffuse esophageal spasm, and hypertensive esophageal motility. These disorders comprise only a small number of cases of unexplained chest pain. Patients who have normal esophageal motility should be evaluated for esophageal hypersensitivity by determining the threshold to esophageal distention by intraesophageal balloon inflation. Mucosal sensitivity may be determined by the acid perfusion test (also called the Bernstein test), in which 0.1% hydrochloric acid is perfused by catheter into the distal esophagus.

The antidepressant trazodone (100–150 mg/day), which has no direct effect on esophageal motility, has been effective in decreasing the distress of esophageal symptoms in patients with motility disorders. This suggests that underlying psychiatric problems may play a role in patients with esophageal motility abnormalities. Use of trazodone in men is limited by the side effect of priapism. Surgical myotomy has no role in the management of patients with chest pain and motility disorders other than achalasia.

D. Musculoskeletal Chest Pain

The diagnosis of musculoskeletal chest pain may be overlooked in the initial evaluation of the patient with CPUO. Careful history and physical examination is required. Several musculoskeletal disorders may cause chest pain. Localized myofascial pain, ankylosing spondylitis, fibromyalgia, Tietze syndrome, rheumatoid arthritis, thoracic outlet syndrome, and "slipping rib" syndrome should be considered in the differential diagnosis. The diagnosis of fibromyalgia is based on at least a 3-month history of widespread pain, with more than 10–18 trigger points of tenderness on digital palpation. Patients with musculoskeletal chest pain are treated with reassurance, application of local heat, NSAIDs, and corticosteroid-lidocaine injection when appropriate. Patients with fibromyalgia may benefit from cyclobenzaprine (2.5–10 mg four times daily) or amitriptyline (10–50 mg at bedtime).

E. Psychiatric Disorders

Psychiatric disorders, including depression, anxiety, and panic disorder, may not be recognized initially as a cause of chest pain, in part because these disorders are very common in clinical practice, affecting approximately 5% of the U.S. population. Patients with symptoms of panic and anxiety should be referred to a psychiatric specialist for diagnostic evaluation and treatment. Treatment of these disorders includes antidepressants, anxiolytics, and cognitive-behavioral therapy. Many patients with these disorders require education about their disease, and gentle persuasion and reassurance that effective treatment exists, before they will accept these recommendations.

F. More Than One Cause of Chest Pain

It is important to recognize the various disorders that cause chest pain as they are very common and more than one cause may be present concurrently. For example, the incidence of GERD is markedly increased in patients with ischemic heart disease because of the overlapping risk factors for the two diseases and also because smooth muscle relaxants that are used in the treatment of coronary angina or hypertension may aggravate GERD. Similarly, patients with unexplained chest pain may be diagnosed with esophageal motility disorder, panic disorder, and microvascular angina. Moreover, many of these patients complain of characteristic chest pain during catheterization with right ventricular stimulation, suggesting a heightened visceral nociception.

Course & Prognosis

Patients with CPUO have a normal survival rate. However, their quality of life and functional status are markedly impaired. Most patients continue to experience chest pain and functional impairment even after a diagnosis of CPUO has been made, resulting in high utilization of health care resources and associated medical costs.

Fang J, Bjorkman D. A critical approach to noncardiac chest pain: pathophysiology, diagnosis, and treatment. *Am J Gastroenterol.* 2001;96:958–968.

DISORDERS OF INHIBITORY INNERVATION

1. Achalasia

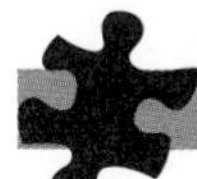

ESSENTIALS OF DIAGNOSIS

- Slowly progressive esophageal dysphagia to both solids and liquids.
- Absence of acid reflux.
- Regurgitation of undigested food without acid or bile; episodes of pneumonia.
- Chest radiograph may show a mediastinal mass with air-fluid levels.
- Barium esophagogram shows a dilated esophagus without peristalsis and a "bird beak" in the distal esophagus.
- Esophageal manometry shows nonperistalsis esophageal contractions and failure of LES relaxation on swallowing.

General Considerations

Achalasia is a disorder of the thoracic esophagus characterized by nonperistaltic esophageal contractions and impaired relaxation of the LES in response to swallowing. It results primarily from degeneration of nitrergic inhibitory neurons in the myenteric plexus. Achalasia is an important but uncommon clinical disorder with an incidence of 1 in 100,000 persons. It most often manifests between the ages of 25 and 50 years but affects patients of all ages and both sexes. Diagnosis is generally established on the basis of radiologic findings and manometric studies, and by ruling out secondary causes such as cancer. Definitive therapy is surgical myotomy, but various medical and endoscopic treatments have been employed for symptomatic relief.

Pathogenesis

Achalasia is associated with degeneration of postganglionic inhibitory neurons, which release nitric oxide and VIP (Figure 13–7). Postganglionic excitatory neurons may also be affected in advanced disease. Preganglionic vagal fibers and vagal nuclei may also be involved.

Most cases in the United States are of no known cause and are classified as idiopathic achalasia. A viral etiology for the inflammation has also been proposed, and elevated antibody titers to measles and varicella zoster have been described in a high proportion of patients with idiopathic achalasia. Autoimmunity has been proposed as contributing to the etiology based on observation of T-lymphocyte infiltration in the myenteric plexus, and there is a higher prevalence of the disorder in patients with certain human leukocyte antigen (HLA) types. Autoantibodies to neurons are also found in many patients with achalasia.

Familial achalasia comprises about 2–5% of all cases and generally involves an autosomal-recessive mode of inheritance, particularly in children younger than 4 years of age. In children, this may be part of the AAA syndrome (achalasia, alacrima, achlorhydria), which may also be associated with adrenocorticotropic hormone insensitivity, microcephaly, and nerve deafness. Additionally, a small percentage of patients have associated neurodegenerative diseases such as Parkinson disease and hereditary cerebellar ataxia.

Secondary achalasia refers to inhibitory neuronal degeneration caused by a known etiologic agent such as *Trypanosoma cruzi* (the causative organism in Chagas disease) and carcinoma.

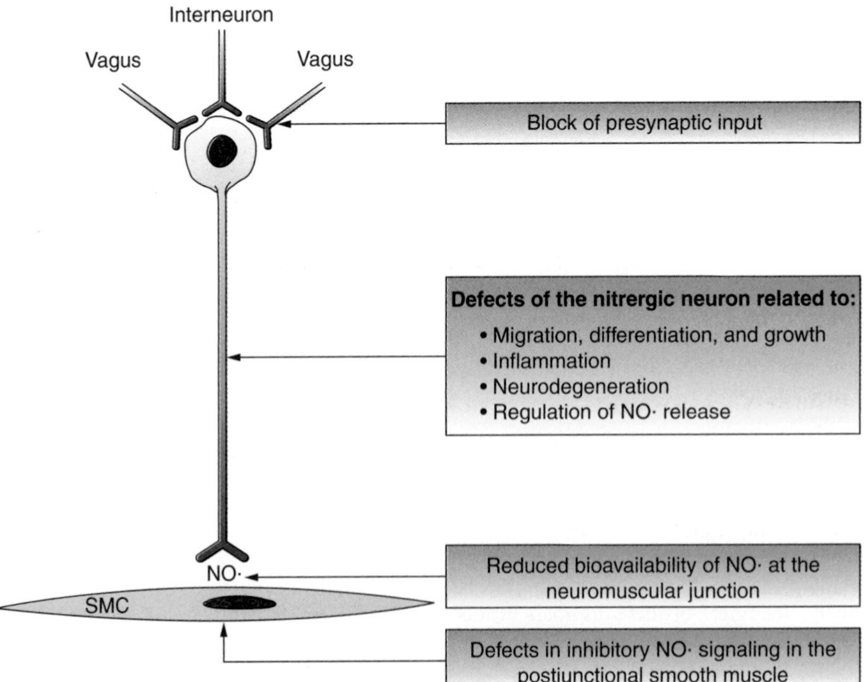

▲ **Figure 13–7.** Schematic diagram of different parts of a nitrergic neuron that may be affected by various kinds of pathology, resulting in esophageal neuromuscular diseases. NO, nitric oxide.

Although the cause of primary achalasia is largely unknown, degenerative changes have been noted in the dorsal motor nucleus (Lewy bodies), along with degeneration of vagal fibers and loss of ganglion cells in the esophageal body and LES. In particular, there may be an inflammatory response, predominantly of T-cell lymphocytes. However, these changes are not consistent and may be secondary to an enteric nervous system disease involving loss of nitrergic and VIP-containing neurons (the main relaxatory mediators of the esophageal smooth muscle) and a decrease in the number of interstitial cells of Cajal. Muscular hypertrophy, possibly secondary to the denervation, and variable extent of muscle degeneration has also been described. However, these muscular and neuronal changes cannot be assessed by evaluation of mucosal biopsies obtained during endoscopy. Newer approaches are being assessed for obtaining full-thickness biopsies to facilitate evaluation of neuromuscular pathology.

Fraser H, Neshev E, Storr M, et al. A novel method of full-thickness gastric biopsy via a percutaneous, endoscopically assisted, transenteric approach. *Gastrointest Endosc.* 2010;71:831–834.

Goyal RK, Chaudhury A. Pathogenesis of achalasia: lessons from mutant mice. *Gastroenterology.* 2010;139:1086–1090.

Hirano I. Pathophysiology of achalasia and diffuse esophageal spasm. GI Motility Online. Available at: http://www.nature.com/gimo/index.html; doi: 10.1038/gimo22, 2006.

Pasricha PJ, Pehlivanov ND, Gomez G, et al. Changes in the gastric enteric nervous system and muscle: a case report on two patients with diabetic gastroparesis. *BMC Gastroenterol.* 2008;8:21.

Clinical Features

A. Symptoms and Signs

Dysphagia is the most common presenting symptom of achalasia and is present in nearly all patients. Dysphagia to both liquids and solids is characteristic of this disease; however, symptoms may initially involve primarily solids, followed by liquids. Dysphagia is mainly localized to the lower chest, although it may be localized to the neck. Generally, it is worsened by emotional stress or hurried eating. Patients often complain of taking longer to eat a meal or of drinking a large amount of liquid to clear the food from the esophagus. They may even describe having to stand up, perform the Valsalva maneuver, or arch their backs to help clear food from the esophagus.

The second most frequent presenting symptom is regurgitation of food, which is generally undigested, nonbilious, and nonacidic. Patients may wake in the middle of the night as a result of coughing or choking after regurgitation, the content of which is often described as white and foamy, arising from an inability to clear saliva from the esophagus. Chest pain and heartburn occur in approximately 40% of patients and can be misdiagnosed as GERD. However, the heartburn is generally not postprandial or responsive to antacids.

Mild weight loss is noted in approximately 85% of patients and may even mimic cancer when profound. However, the interval from the presenting symptom to the point at which the patient seeks medical attention is quite variable, sometimes extending beyond a decade.

B. Laboratory Findings

Some patients with idiopathic achalasia have increased antineuronal antibodies, including anti–Hu-1 antineuronal antibodies. Enzyme-linked immunosorbent assay (ELISA) tests, agglutination tests, and confirmatory assays, including immunofluorescence, immunoblot, Western blot, and radioimmunoprecipitation tests, may aid in identifying *T cruzi* in patients with achalasia caused by Chagas disease.

C. Imaging Studies

Barium esophagogram, the preferred initial method of evaluation in patients with dysphagia, may reveal characteristically smooth, symmetric narrowing or "bird-beaking" of the distal esophagus, and often a dilated esophagus with no peristaltic activity and poor esophageal emptying. In severe achalasia, chest radiographs may reveal a dilated esophagus containing food, possibly air-fluid level within the esophagus in the upright position, absence of gastric air bubble, and sometimes a tubular mediastinal mass beside the aorta. Administration of a smooth muscle relaxant such as sublingual nitroglycerin or inhaled amyl nitrate may cause relaxation of the LES and distinguish achalasia from pseudoachalasia arising from mechanical causes. Severe cases may reveal a markedly dilated and tortuous esophagus, called a sigmoid esophagus (see Figure 13–4).

D. Endoscopy

Esophagogastroduodenoscopy is not sensitive in the diagnosis of esophageal motility disorders. However, it is very useful in excluding mechanical disorders, particularly those that may be the cause of the motility disorder (eg, infiltration by gastroesophageal junction cancer, causing secondary achalasia).

E. Manometry

The diagnosis is confirmed by esophageal manometry, which typically reveals complete absence of peristalsis, incomplete LES relaxation (<50% of baseline pressure), and often but not necessarily increased lower esophageal basal tone (>30 mm Hg). Weak contractions may be noted in the esophageal body, which are simultaneous or appear simultaneous but identical if the esophageal body becomes a single lumen (common cavity effect) (see Figure 13–5). Esophageal pressures may also exceed gastric pressures when the esophagus is filled with food or fluid.

Differential Diagnosis

The differential diagnosis of achalasia begins with the broad differential diagnosis of dysphagia and exclusion of mechanical causes of dysphagia. Strictures, benign neoplasms, vascular rings, webs, foreign bodies, and severe esophagitis (peptic, infectious, chemical, drug induced) are among the frequently encountered entities.

Achalasia must be distinguished from other motility disorders such as diffuse esophageal spasm and scleroderma that has been complicated by a peptic stricture. The next step is to determine whether it is due to an identifiable cause. These cases, termed secondary achalasia, may be due to infection with *T cruzi* (Chagas disease) or neural degeneration as a paraneoplastic syndrome associated with many malignancies. Gastroesophageal junction carcinoma may produce myenteric plexus degeneration by local tumor invasion, resulting in achalasia. The term *pseudoachalasia* is used when there is no functional cause of achalasia but the gastroesophageal junction is narrowed due to outside compression or fibrosis and the esophageal body is dilated due to obstruction. Patients with secondary achalasia due to tumor at the gastroesophageal junction present with more recent and progressive onset of dysphagia or with progressive weight loss. Careful retroflexed inspection of the cardia and gastroesophageal junction by upper endoscopy is necessary.

Treatment

Current options for treatment of achalasia are directed at removing the functional obstruction caused by the nonrelaxing LES. However, these therapeutic modalities do not restore peristalsis. Treatment includes pharmacologic therapy, pneumatic dilation of the LES, surgical myotomy, and botulinum toxin injection therapy.

A. Pharmacologic Therapy

Sublingual nitroglycerin, calcium channel blockers, phosphodiesterase inhibitors, and anticholinergics are used to relieve the symptoms in the subset of patients who have mild symptoms without esophageal dilation, or are unable to undergo dilations or surgery.

B. Pneumatic Dilation

The disruption of muscle requires far larger diameters compared with disruption of mucosal lesions such as strictures. A 3-cm diameter balloon is used initially. Based on patient's response, successive dilations of up to 4 cm can be applied. At each session, a balloon is placed under fluoroscopic guidance to stretch the area of the gastroesophageal junction. In less than 4% of dilations, perforations occur that may require surgical repair. In experienced hands, the efficacy of pneumatic dilation and laparoscopic surgery are nearly equal, and dilation appears to be the more cost-effective initial approach.

C. Surgical Myotomy

A modified Heller cardiomyotomy of the LES and cardia results in good to excellent symptomatic relief in over 85% of patients. GERD is expected to ensue in up to 20% of patients. Myotomy can also be performed using a laparoscopic approach; this is less invasive, reduces postoperative complications, and allows a shorter hospital stay. The success of surgery does not appear to be compromised by prior botulinum or pneumatic dilation treatments.

D. Botulinum Toxin Injection

Botulinum toxin A is injected directly into the LES using an endoscope. Approximately 20–25 units of the toxin are used per injection into four quadrants in the LES. This results in reduction of lower esophageal pressures in 85% of patients. However, approximately 50% of patients relapse with symptoms over the next 6–9 months. Approximately 25% have a sustained response lasting more than 1 year. Approximately 75% of initial responders who relapse have improvement with repeat injection therapy. Because of the lower efficacy and sustained response compared with surgical myotomy, this method is often reserved for elderly patients or those with multiple medical problems.

Course & Prognosis

Untreated, achalasia can lead to severe weight loss mimicking cancer, and respiratory complications such as stridor. Patients may develop distal esophageal diverticulum and bezoars. After surgery, patients may develop GERD, strictures, and Barrett esophagus.

Pehlivanov N, Pasricha PJ. Medical and endoscopic treatment of achalasia. GI Motility Online. Available at: http://www.nature.com/gimo/index.html; doi: 10.1038/gimo52, 2006.

2. Diffuse Esophageal Spasm

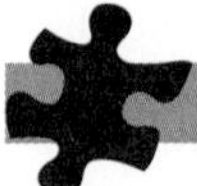

ESSENTIALS OF DIAGNOSIS

- Nonperistaltic simultaneous contractions of the esophagus.
- Dysphagia to solids and liquids and chest pain are common presenting symptoms.
- Some patients may progress to achalasia.

General Considerations

The reported incidence of diffuse esophageal spasm depends on the diagnostic criteria used. When large amplitude of contractions is considered in the diagnosis, only 3–5% of patients undergoing manometry for suspected esophageal motility disorders fit the diagnostic criteria. Diffuse esophageal spasm is a disorder of the thoracic esophagus resulting from impairment of inhibitory innervation. It involves the esophagus but spares the LES, leading to nonperistaltic contractions but normal LES relaxation, as evidenced on manometry. The amplitude of the contractions may be normal, increased, or decreased. Acid suppression and other medical and endoscopic treatments may alleviate symptoms. A subset of patients may progress to achalasia.

Pathogenesis

Nonperistaltic contractions are due to loss of deglutitive inhibition associated with impaired inhibitory nerve function in the esophageal body. The amplitude of contractions involves many components, including the rebound contraction, which is dependent on the inhibitory nerves, cholinergic excitatory nerves, and myogenic factors. Loss of inhibitory nerves alone would be expected to reduce the force of contraction, whereas compensatory cholinergic and myogenic factors may lead to increased force of contraction. However, little is known about the pathology of diffuse esophageal spasm. There appears to be patchy neural degeneration localized to nerve processes rather than degeneration of nerve cell bodies, as evidenced in achalasia. Hypertrophy of the muscularis propria and associated development of distal esophageal diverticula also occur.

Clinical Features

A. Symptoms and Signs

Chest pain, dysphagia, and regurgitation are the main presenting symptoms. Chest pain may be particularly prominent in patients with high-amplitude and protracted contractions and can occur at rest, with swallowing, or with emotional stress. The pain is generally retrosternal but can radiate to the back, sides of the chest, arms, or the jaw. Pain can last from seconds to several minutes and can mimic that of cardiac angina. Dysphagia for solids and liquids can be present. Regurgitation of food that fails to move into the stomach may occur.

B. Imaging Studies

Findings on barium swallow may be normal or show nonpropagated contractions (called tertiary contractions), particularly below the aortic arch, with the appearance of curling or multiple ripples in the wall, sacculations, and pseudodiverticula, leading to the appearance of a "corkscrew" esophagus in severe cases.

C. Manometry

The diagnosis is generally made by esophageal manometry, which reveals more than 20% of wet swallows as simultaneous contractions. However, because the disorder is episodic, manometric findings can be entirely normal at the time of study. Simultaneous contractions must be distinguished from identical contraction patterns suggestive of a common cavity effect from functional or mechanical obstruction in the esophagus during the study. Moreover, occasional nonperistaltic contractions can occur normally. The amplitude of the nonperistaltic contractions can be increased, normal, or even decreased, and sometimes the contractions are multipeaked. However, LES relaxation is normal, and normally conducted peristaltic contraction must be evidenced in at least one swallow.

Methods to provoke esophageal spasm, including cold swallows and edrophonium, can induce chest pain but may not necessarily correlate with motility changes. Thus, provocation tests have limited utility.

Differential Diagnosis

Diffuse esophageal spasm must be distinguished from other causes of chest pain, especially cardiac ischemia. Esophageal motility disorders are an uncommon cause of noncardiac chest pain, which is more commonly caused by reflux esophagitis or visceral hypersensitivity.

Treatment

The mainstay of therapy is reassurance, control of esophageal acidification by proton pump inhibitors or histamine receptor antagonists, and use of smooth muscle relaxants such as nitrates and calcium channel blockers. There are no controlled studies to substantiate any particular treatment modality, although smooth muscle relaxants or anticholinergic agents used for achalasia may be helpful for improving symptoms. Some studies suggest that low-dose tricyclic antidepressant therapy may be a better option for treating chest pain. Empiric bougienage has been advocated, but studies comparing large- versus small-caliber bougies showed no differences in response rate, suggestive of a placebo effect. Similarly, there have been no controlled studies to validate the use of botulinum toxin either into the LES or at intervals along the esophageal body. Long esophageal myotomy is rarely used to treat intractable dysphagia and chest pain, particularly when associated with pulsion diverticula.

Course & Prognosis

Patients may have intermittent dysphagia and chest pain for many years without progression. A small subset of these patients (~5%) develops vigorous or classic achalasia, which should be suspected if patients develop regurgitation with worsening dysphagia.

3. Inappropriate Transient Lower Esophageal Sphincter Relaxation (TLESR)

Transient LES relaxation normally occurs on swallowing, belching, or vomiting reflexes. When it occurs in the absence of such activities, it has been called inappropriate transient LES relaxation or simply transient LES relaxation (TLESR). TLESR is a vagovagal inhibitory reflex that is mediated via the nitrergic inhibitory nerves to the LES. The frequency of TLESR is increased by gastric distention. Increased frequency of TLESR has been shown to be an important cause of GERD. Diagnosis of TLESR can only be made by long-term manometric recordings, which are employed mainly in research but not in common clinical practice.

Basal LES pressure is dependent on the myogenic tone of the sphincter muscle, and superimposed, counterbalancing influence of inhibitory and excitatory nerves. The force of peristaltic contraction is dependent on the contractile ability of the smooth muscle and influence of the excitatory as well as the inhibitory nerves. The inhibitory nerves are responsible not only for inhibition but also for the rebound contraction that follows the inhibition. Therefore, loss of rebound contraction can only occur if the preceding deglutitive inhibition is also lost. Disorders of TLESR that involve normal deglutitive inhibition and peristaltic sequence can be classified into hypotensive and hypertensive esophageal motility disorders and are described in the following sections.

DISORDERS OF EXCITATORY NERVES AND SMOOTH MUSCLES

1. Hypotensive Esophageal Disorders

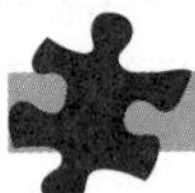

ESSENTIALS OF DIAGNOSIS

- GERD and dysphagia.
- Hypotensive LES (LES pressure <10 mm Hg).
- Hypotensive peristaltic contractions (<30 mm Hg).

General Considerations

Hypotensive esophageal disorders include hypotensive LES, hypotensive peristaltic contraction, or both. Hypotensive LES may lead to GERD, and hypotensive peristaltic contractions may lead to dysphagia, impaired esophageal clearing of refluxed material, and accentuation of GERD.

Pathogenesis

Hypotensive esophageal disorders are due to either impaired excitatory innervation or impaired muscle contractility. Most cases are idiopathic, but a few are secondary to known causes. Secondary causes include anticholinergic agents, smooth muscle relaxants, estrogens, progesterone, and pregnancy. Other important causes are connective tissue disorders, particularly scleroderma and intestinal pseudo-obstruction syndrome. The latter may be caused by muscular atrophy, disease or impairment of the cholinergic neurons, or both. Most cases of hypotensive LES are idiopathic in nature.

Clinical Findings

By esophageal manometry, abnormally hypotensive peristaltic contractions are generally evidenced in the distal esophagus (consisting of smooth muscle). Low-amplitude contractions can be normal in the transition zone between striated and smooth muscle. However, high-resolution manometry and impedance have revealed a small minority of patients with dysphagia (<4% in one series) who have a larger gap of poor contractility (<20 mm Hg) and slower transit (>1 second) over this transition zone that correlated with poor bolus transit and dysphagia.

Refer to GERD and scleroderma esophagus elsewhere in this chapter.

Treatment

Refer to GERD and scleroderma esophagus elsewhere in this chapter.

2. Hypertensive Esophageal Disorders

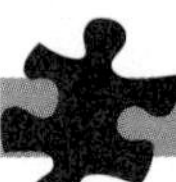

ESSENTIALS OF DIAGNOSIS

- Hypertensive LES, hypercontracting LES, and hypertensive peristalsis identified on intraluminal manometry.
- Sustained longitudinal muscle contraction diagnosed by high-frequency endoscopic ultrasound.
- Usually noted in patients being evaluated for noncardiac chest pain or dysphagia.

General Considerations

Hypercontractile syndromes include entities such as hypertensive LES, hypercontracting LES, hypertensive peristalsis (nutcracker esophagus), and sustained contraction of the esophageal longitudinal muscle.

Pathogenesis

These hypercontractile states may result from overactive excitatory nerves or stress. The cause is unknown, but patients may have esophageal hypersensitivity.

Clinical Findings

A. Symptoms and Signs

When hypertensive peristalsis or nutcracker esophagus was initially described, it was a common manometric abnormality found in patients with noncardiac chest pain. However, it is now appreciated that these episodes of high-amplitude contraction coincide poorly with chest pain and may be an epiphenomenon or perhaps a marker for hypersensitivity or a hyperreactive esophagus. Dysphagia has been reported by some patients with manometric findings of hypercontractile esophagus.

There are no physical findings specific for hypercontractile esophagus.

B. Laboratory, Imaging, and Manometric Studies

Hypertensive peristalsis is the most common manometric finding in patients referred for evaluation of noncardiac angina-like chest pain. Generally, barium studies show normal peristalsis, normal esophageal transit, and no structural esophageal disease. Esophagoscopy is also normal.

Prolonged ambulatory manometric studies reveal that some patients with hypertensive peristalsis have nonperistaltic contractions during mealtime, but not during standard wet swallows of a standard manometric study.

A subset of these patients may have inappropriate contractions of the esophageal longitudinal muscles that are poorly transduced on standard manometric evaluations but may be revealed on esophageal ultrasonography.

Specimens are rarely available for pathologic examination of these hypercontractile states, although a single report has described loss of intramural neurons in the LES of patients with isolated hypertensive LES.

As the names imply, hypertensive peristalsis, hypertensive LES, and hypercontracting LES are diagnosed manometrically. In hypertensive peristalsis, the amplitude of the peristaltic contractions exceeds 180 mm Hg or the duration of contraction exceeds 7.5 seconds. In hypertensive LES, the basal pressure of the LES exceeds 40 mm Hg. Similarly, hypercontracting LES shows prolonged and high-amplitude postrelaxation (rebound) contraction.

Differential Diagnosis

As with achalasia, ischemic heart disease must be excluded in patients presenting with chest pain. GERD is the most common cause of atypical noncardiac chest pain and should be excluded, either with an empiric trial of proton pump inhibitor therapy or through ambulatory pH testing. Other causes of chest pain include chest wall origin, pericarditis, atelectasis, and panic attacks.

Treatment

Anticholinergic drugs and smooth muscle relaxants (nitrates and calcium channel blockers) are often used but have unproven value. Low-dose tricyclic antidepressants may improve chest pain in some patients, perhaps because of their modulation of visceral hypersensitivity. Cognitive-behavioral therapy has also been employed with benefit to some patients.

3. Scleroderma Esophagus

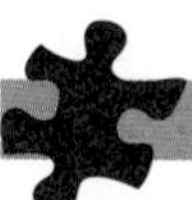

ESSENTIALS OF DIAGNOSIS

- Absent LES tone and esophageal peristalsis.
- Symptoms of GERD or dysphagia, or both.
- Respiratory compromise from aspiration or direct lung involvement.

General Considerations

Esophageal scleroderma occurs as part of a connective tissue disorder and leads to atrophy of esophageal smooth muscle with consequent loss of LES tone and force of esophageal peristalsis. The condition occurs in 75–85% of patients with scleroderma and affects particularly woman in the 30- to 50-year age group. Patients with Raynaud phenomenon frequently have esophageal motor abnormalities.

Pathogenesis

The cause of scleroderma is unknown, but it is thought to involve an autoimmune response. Progressive atrophy and sclerosis of the esophageal smooth muscles lead to poor peristaltic contractions in the distal esophagus and to LES incompetence. Microvessel disease in scleroderma may lead to intramural neuronal dysfunction early in the disease. Subsequently, fibrosis and atrophy of esophageal smooth muscle develop, leading to a markedly hypotensive LES and loss of peristaltic contractions in the smooth muscle segment of the esophagus.

Clinical Findings

Diagnosis is confirmed by the presence of Raynaud phenomenon and cutaneous manifestations of scleroderma along with symptoms of dysphagia and GERD. Physiologic changes in the esophagus contribute to poor esophageal clearance and marked gastroesophageal reflux. This can result in reflux esophagitis and strictures in advanced cases. Pulmonary interstitial fibrosis can result from either direct smooth muscle involvement of the disease or from aspiration of refluxate.

A. Symptoms and Signs

Owing to LES incompetence and lack of esophageal acid clearance from lack of esophageal peristalsis, patients often have severe GERD, leading to heartburn, regurgitation, dysphagia, and chest pain. However, symptoms can be relatively mild despite severe mucosal disease. Dysphagia may occur even in the absence of obvious skin and joint involvement, although Raynaud phenomenon is usually present.

B. Laboratory Findings

Certain autoimmune markers such as the antiendonuclear antigens and anti–ScL-70 and anticentromere antibodies may be present.

C. Imaging Studies

In advanced disease, barium swallow reveals a dilated esophagus with poor esophageal clearance and weak contractions.

D. Manometry

Manometry shows a hypotensive LES and low-amplitude peristaltic contractions in the thoracic esophagus. Sometimes, swallow-induced contractions are nonperistaltic, suggesting additional impairment of the nitrergic inhibitory nerves.

Differential Diagnosis

In the absence of other features of a connective tissue disorder, scleroderma can be confused with primary GERD. Cutaneous manifestations of scleroderma may be absent in up to 5% of patients. History of Raynaud phenomenon may be very useful in the diagnosis. Pulmonary fibrosis may even be attributed to repeated aspiration from GERD. In patients presenting with dysphagia, eosinophilic esophagitis should be excluded by multiple (at least five) mucosal biopsies obtained at different levels of the esophagus. Scleroderma esophagus may sometimes be confused with achalasia, particularly in patients with a dilated esophagus on barium swallow and poor peristaltic contractions in the thoracic esophagus on barium swallow or esophageal manometry. However, patulous and hypotensive LES on endoscopic and manometric findings can distinguish the two. In scleroderma, LES is usually patulous unless complicating peptic stricture is present.

Treatment

There is no specific treatment for esophageal scleroderma. Severe reflux, which is generally the source of the patient's predominant symptoms, is treated with proton pump inhibitors, often requiring double-dose, twice-daily administration. Esophageal bougienage may be required for strictures. Generally, antireflux surgery should be avoided because of the risk of severe postoperative dysphagia. Otherwise, a partial fundoplication, generally with a Collis procedure and esophageal lengthening, is performed.

Eosinophilic Esophagitis

14

Norton J. Greenberger, MD

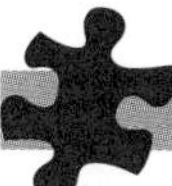

ESSENTIALS OF DIAGNOSIS

- In adults, a major symptom is recurrent dysphagia, often with food impaction; mean duration of symptoms before treatment is 4–6 years.
- Esophageal biopsy shows dense eosinophilic infiltration (≥20 eosinophils per high power field [HPF]).
- Full diagnostic criteria are (1) clinical symptoms of esophageal dysfunction; (2) increased eosinophils in esophageal mucosal biopsies; (3) lack of sustained response to high-dose proton pump inhibition treatment or normal pH monitoring of the distal esophagus.

General Considerations

Eosinophilic esophagitis is a chronic and increasingly recognized inflammatory disorder of the esophagitis characterized by abnormal infiltration of eosinophils of the esophageal mucosa, often resulting in dysphagia and food impaction. The disorder is being diagnosed with much greater frequency, and increased recognition, by virtue of increased endoscopic volume, alone may not be responsible for this trend. Studies have indicated that the incidence has increased more than fourfold in the last 5–10 years. More than 80% of patients diagnosed with eosinophilic esophagitis complain of dysphagia, and between 5% and 16% of patients undergoing endoscopic evaluation for dysphagia are found to have eosinophilic esophagitis. Further, more than 50% of patients presenting with frank food impaction are diagnosed with eosinophilic esophagitis. By contrast, in children and adolescents, gastroesophageal reflux disease (GERD) and esophageal reflux symptoms are as common as food impaction and dysphagia.

Pathogenesis

The pathogenesis of eosinophilic esophagitis is incompletely defined. However, considerable evidence suggests that eosinophilic esophagitis is an allergic disorder induced by antigen sensitization either through foods and/or aeroallergens.

A majority of patients have evidence of food allergies and a concurrent history of respiratory allergies. A seasonal variation has been documented in the diagnosis of eosinophilic esophagitis that correlated with pollen counts. By contrast, food anaphylaxis is uncommon, occurring in less than 15% of pediatric patients with eosinophilic esophagitis.

The recruitment of eosinophils occurs in several inflammatory or infectious conditions and after exposure to inhaled or ingested allergens. Eosinophils also release chemoattractants, such as interleukins, which can perpetuate an inflammatory response. The latter phenomenon has led to trials of leukotriene inhibitors in the treatment of eosinophilic esophagitis.

Rothenberg ME. Biology and treatment of eosinophilic esophagitis. *Gastroenterology.* 2009;137:1238–1249. [PMID: 19596009]

Clinical Findings

A. Symptoms and Signs

The leading symptom in adults is recurrent attacks of dysphagia. Mean duration of symptoms before diagnosis and initiation of treatment in one large series was 4.6 years. Recurrent dysphagia is present in the majority of patients, as is the history of food impaction. A personal history of allergic diseases (ie, airway allergies, food allergies, or skin allergies) is frequently present. Serum immunoglobulin E (IgE) elevations have been documented in one series in two thirds of the patients. However, it should be emphasized that there is no difference in symptoms, endoscopic findings, or histology in patients with increased serum IgE levels versus those with normal IgE levels. Symptoms appear to be more pronounced in patients with peripheral blood eosinophilia. Another clinical feature is the presence of symptoms of GERD, dyspepsia, and xiphisternal and retrosternal discomfort that are seemingly refractory to medical management. In children and adolescents, symptoms include vomiting, regurgitation, GERD symptoms not responding to medical management, upper abdominal pain, and food impaction in the esophagus.

B. Endoscopy

Endoscopic features associated with eosinophilic esophagitis are highly variable. The esophageal mucosa may actually appear to be normal. Other more frequent findings include trachea-like circular rings that can be transient or fixed, white exudates, white nodules with granularity, linear furring, and vertical lines on the esophageal mucosa. In addition, the passage of the endoscope may lead to trauma. Finally, strictures in the proximal, middle, or distal esophagitis are sometimes encountered. Examples of typical endoscopic findings in eosinophilic eosinophils are shown in Plates 18 and 19.

Other disorders also may be associated with increased eosinophilic infiltration of the esophagus (see below). Accordingly, biopsies should be taken in both the distal and mid-esophagus in patients with suspected eosinophilic esophagitis. Characteristic histologic findings in eosinophilic esophagitis are shown in Plate 20.

Dellon ES, Aderju A, Woosley JT, et al. Variability in diagnostic criteria for eosinophilic esophagitis: a systematic review. *Am J Gastroenterol.* 2007;102:2300–2313. [PMID: 17617209]

Furuta GT, Liacouras CA, Collins MH, et al. Eosinophilic esophagitis in children and adults: a systematic review and consensus recommendations for diagnosis and treatment. *Gastroenterology.* 2007;133:1342–1363. [PMID: 17919504]

C. Diagnostic Criteria

The usual criteria for the diagnosis of eosinophilic esophagitis are as follows:

1. Clinical symptoms of esophageal dysfunction, especially dysphagia and a history of food impaction.
2. Biopsies of the esophageal mucosa reveal a dense eosinophilic infiltration (ie, ≥20 eosinophils/HPF).
3. Lack of responsiveness or an incomplete response to treatment of high doses of proton pump inhibitors, or normal pH monitoring of the distal esophagus, or both.

Differential Diagnosis

Data from 151 patients with eosinophilic esophagitis and 126 with GERD were analyzed. Features that independently predicted eosinophilic esophagitis included younger age; symptoms of dysphagia; documented food allergies; observation of esophageal rings, linear furrows, white plaques, or exudates by upper endoscopy; absence of a hiatal hernia; and a higher maximum eosinophil count. Although increased eosinophilic infiltration in the esophagus is characteristic of eosinophilic esophagitis, it is not exclusively found in that disorder. Other disorders that may be associated with increased eosinophilic infiltration of the esophagitis include GERD, Crohn disease, hypereosinophilic syndrome, cardiovascular disease, drug-induced esophagitis, and infectious esophagitis (ie, herpes or *Candida*). Increased eosinophils can be found in the distal esophagus in reflux esophagitis but not in the mid-esophagus.

Dellon ES, Gibbs WB, Fritchie KJ, et al. Clinical, endoscopic, and histologic findings distinguish eosinophilic esophagitis from gastroesophageal reflux disease. *Clin Gastroenterol Hepatol.* 2009;7:1305–1313. [PMID: 19733260]

Rodrigo S, Abboud G, Oh D, et al. High intraepithelial eosinophil counts in esophageal squamous epithelium are not specific for eosinophilic esophagitis in adults. *Am J Gastroenterol.* 2008;103:435–442. [PMID: 18289205]

Treatment

A. Topical Corticosteroids

Several studies that have employed topical fluticasone in doses ranging from 220–440 mcg two to four times daily have demonstrated symptom improvement and complete resolution of symptoms in up to 75% of cases. Patients are generally instructed to swallow rather than inhale the fluticasone and not use a spacer. Twice-daily fluticasone is usually administered for 6–12 weeks, and during this interval, clinical and histologic symptoms are improved in the vast majority of patients. Patients receiving the higher dose of fluticasone are more likely to develop esophageal candidiasis. Furthermore, higher doses of fluticasone (ie, >440 mcg/day) have been associated with systemic side effects, including cataracts and adrenal suppression. Although the use of swallowed corticosteroids is effective in relieving symptoms for a short period of time (4 months or less), long-term efficacy remains controversial. It should be emphasized that symptoms are more likely to recur in a period of 4–18 months after therapy has been discontinued in approximately half the patients.

An alternative to swallowed fluticasone is the use of a suspension of budesonide. Pulmicort Respules are a liquid-based formulation of budesonide containing 0.5 mg of budesonide, and 2 mL of Pulmicort Respules mixed with five packets of sucralose will make a dose of a 10–15 mL slurry that can be taken twice daily. Although data are limited, this preparation may well be a viable alternative to using swallowed fluticasone. This preparation was well tolerated in 20 children and led to histologic improvement in 80% of these patients.

B. Systemic Corticosteroids

Systemic corticosteroids are effective in eosinophilic esophagitis, but side effects limit their use, especially for periods longer than 4 weeks. They may be indicated when urgent symptom relief is required as with patients experiencing severe dysphagia, dehydration, and significant weight loss or esophageal strictures.

C. Esophageal Dilation

Esophageal dilation may be necessary in patients with strictures, but it must be done carefully as it has been associated with deep mucosal tears, esophageal perforation, increased postendoscopic analgesia, and difficulty in inserting the endoscope. Approximately half the patients treated with esophageal dilation will become asymptomatic.

D. Leukotriene Receptor Antagonists

The leukotriene receptor antagonist montelukast has been studied in a small number of patients with eosinophilic esophagitis; eight patients showed a complete resolution of symptoms with a dosage of 20–40 mg/day and maintained this response for a median of 14 months. However, once the medication was discontinued, six of the eight patients had a recurrence of their symptoms. Data are insufficient to recommend leukotriene receptor antagonists for the treatment of eosinophilic esophagitis.

E. Cromolyn Sodium

Cromolyn sodium, a mast cell stabilizer, has not shown any apparent benefit for patients with eosinophilic esophagitis although it has no significant adverse effects.

F. Dietary Therapy

Dietary therapy is an important emerging form of therapy for eosinophilic esophagitis. Three different dietary approaches have been examined.

1. Elemental (amino-based formula)—Although this may be effective in reducing disease manifestations, it is often not well tolerated.

2. Elimination diets—This can be difficult because patients are typically sensitive to multiple food groups that include common and uncommon foods. Efficacy of specific food elimination diets remains controversial. Several studies have demonstrated a poor correlation of diagnostic skin testing, radioallergosorbent testing, and IgE skin prick tests with improvement in either symptoms or tissue inflammation.

3. Empiric elimination diet with removal of common food allergies—One center did report a significant improvement in patients on a specific food elimination diet. Kagalwalla and colleagues demonstrated that eliminating the six most common allergenic foods (dairy, eggs, wheat, soy, peanuts, and fish/shellfish) resulted in significant improvement in 74% of the 35 patients who received the six-food elimination diet.

G. Treatment of Gastroesophageal Reflux Disease

Antireflux therapy with proton pump inhibitors is usually not successful or achieves only a partial response in patients with GERD. However, some patients may have both GERD and eosinophilic esophagitis, and in this setting, treatment with a proton pump inhibitor may be appropriate.

Aceves SS, Bastian JF, Newbury RO, et al. Oral viscous budesonide: a potential new therapy for eosinophilic esophagitis in children. *Am J Gastroenterol.* 2007;102:2271–2275. [PMID: 17581266]

Alexander JA, Katzka DA. Therapeutic options for eosinophilic esophagitis. *Gastroenterol Hepatol.* 2011;7:59–61. [PMID: 21346856]

Bohm M, Richter JE. Treatment of eosinophilic esophagitis: overview, current limitations, and future directions. *Am J Gastroenterol.* 2008;103:2635–2644. [PMID: 18721234]

Furuta GT, Liacouras CA, Collins MH, et al. Eosinophilic esophagitis in children and adults: a systematic review and consensus recommendations for diagnosis and treatment. *Gastroenterology.* 2007;133:1342–1363. [PMID: 17919504]

Kagalwalla AF, Sentongo TA, Ritz S, et al. Effects of six-food elimination diet on clinical and histologic outcomes in eosinophilic esophagitis. *Clin Gastroenterol.* 2006;4:1097–1102. [PMID: 16860614]

Konikoff MR, Noel RJ, Blanchard C, et al. Randomized, double-blind, placebo-controlled trial of fluticasone propionate for pediatric eosinophilic esophagitis. *Gastroenterology.* 2006;131:1381–1391. [PMID: 17101314]

Straumann A, Consus S, Degen L, et al. Budesonide is effective in adolescent and adult patients with active eosinophilic esophagitis. *Gastroenterology.* 2010;139:1526–1537. [PMID: 20682320]

Course & Prognosis

Straumann and coworkers described 30 patients followed for a mean of 7.2 years (range, 1.4–11.5 years); 23% of the patients reported increased dysphagia and 36.7% reported stable symptoms. Mean duration of symptoms before treatment was 4.6 years. Recurrent episodes of dysphagia were documented in 29 of 30 patients, and the symptoms were more pronounced in patients with peripheral eosinophilia. Eosinophilic esophagitis does not seem to be associated with esophageal metaplasia (ie, Barrett esophagus or cardiac metaplasia or esophageal neoplasms).

Straumann A, Spichtin HP, Grize L, et al. Natural history of primary eosinophilic esophagitis: a follow-up of 30 adult patients for 11.5 years. *Gastroenterology.* 2003;125:1660–1669. [PMID: 14724818]

Unresolved Issues

There are several unresolved issues with regard to the natural history and treatment of eosinophilic esophagitis. Treatment end points and maintenance medical management remain incompletely defined. Treatment initiatives are aimed at relieving symptoms, which may or may not be accompanied by histologic response and resolution of eosinophilic esophagitis. In this regard, after treatment, esophageal eosinophilia can persist, and such patients may be asymptomatic or only have minimal symptoms. There is no consensus on how to define histologic remission in response to treatment. It may well be necessary to continue treatment in patients with documented eosinophilic esophagitis and persistent esophageal symptoms in the absence of esophageal abnormalities. The disease almost uniformly recurs when therapy is discontinued (ie, glucocorticosteroids) or dietary modifications are discontinued.

Peptic Ulcer Disease

15

Edward Lew, MD, MPH

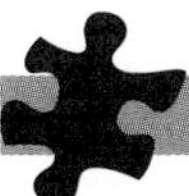

ESSENTIALS OF DIAGNOSIS

- Peptic ulcers are mucosal defects in the stomach or small intestine.
- *Helicobacter pylori* infection, nonsteroidal anti-inflammatory drugs (NSAIDs), and aspirin use are the most common causes.
- Patients may have epigastric pain or complications such as gastrointestinal bleeding, perforation, and obstruction.
- Diagnosis relies on endoscopy or radiologic studies.

General Considerations

Peptic ulcers are defects or breaks in the gastric or small intestinal mucosa that have depth and extend through the muscularis mucosae. In contrast to erosions, which are small and superficial mucosal lesions, peptic ulcers can vary in size from 5 mm to several centimeters and may lead to complications such as gastrointestinal (GI) bleeding, obstruction, penetration, and perforation.

The pathogenesis of ulcers is multifactorial and arises from an imbalance of protective and aggressive factors such as when GI mucosal defense mechanisms are impaired in the presence of gastric acid and pepsin. Peptic ulcer disease was long considered an idiopathic and lifelong disorder. This paradigm changed dramatically in 1984 when Marshall and Warren reported that a curved bacillus, initially named *Campylobacter pyloridis* and subsequently classified as *Helicobacter pylori*, was linked to ulcers. Multiple studies have since shown that eradication of *H pylori* significantly reduces the rate of ulcer recurrence. Another major risk factor for peptic ulcers is the use of nonsteroidal anti-inflammatory drugs (NSAIDs) and aspirin. These medications generally exert their therapeutic and toxic effects by inhibiting the enzymes cyclooxygenase-1 (COX-1) and cyclooxygenase-2 (COX-2), which, in turn, impair mucosal protection and promote ulcers. The treatment of ulcer patients has been revolutionized since the development of the acid-suppressive medications such as the histamine-2 (H_2)-receptor blockers and proton pump inhibitors, the synthetic prostaglandin misoprostol, and the selective COX-2 inhibitors. To date, *H pylori* and the use of NSAIDs and aspirin account for most cases of peptic ulcers. Only a small fraction of ulcers are associated with neoplasia or caused by acid hypersecretory states such as Zollinger-Ellison syndrome and other rare disorders.

The incidence of both gastric and duodenal ulcers in developed countries rapidly increased throughout the 19th century and peaked during the first half of the 20th century. Since the 1950s, however, the incidence and prevalence of both ulcers have steadily declined. There has also been a decrease in the prevalence of *H pylori* over recent decades, attributed to improved hygiene and widespread use of antibiotics in developed countries. Hospital discharge data for the general U.S. population showed that the age-adjusted hospitalization rate for peptic ulcer disease and *H pylori* was highest among adults age 65 years and older and decreased with each subsequent age group. These trends are thought to reflect an underlying birth cohort effect with a decrease in *H pylori* incidence among younger generations.

In the United States, over 4 million individuals are affected by peptic ulcers, and approximately 15,000 die from ulcer complications each year. Over two thirds of ulcer patients develop the disease between the ages of 25 and 64 years. The lifetime prevalence of peptic ulcers is 12% in men and 10% in women. The impact of peptic ulcer disease on U.S. health care costs is substantial, with direct and indirect costs totaling over an estimated $10 billion per year. In addition, peptic ulcer complications adversely affect functional status and quality of life. Over 30% of patients with peptic ulcers have a marked decline in their functional levels or frank disability, whereas 30% also have somatic and psychological symptoms.

Feinstein LB, Holman RC, Yorita Christensen KL, et al. Trends in hospitalizations for peptic ulcer disease, United States, 1998–2005. *Emerg Infect Dis.* 2010;16:1410–1418. [PMID: 20735925]

Sandler RS, Everhart JE, Donowitz M, et al. The burden of selected digestive diseases in the United States. *Gastroenterology.* 2002;122:1500–1511. [PMID: 11984534]

Pathogenesis

A. Causes of Peptic Ulcers

Helicobacter pylori infection and the use of NSAIDs and aspirin have numerous effects on the GI tract and are the most common causes of peptic ulcers (Table 15–1). In general, both factors disrupt normal mucosal defenses and repair, making the mucosa more susceptible to acid. Suppression of gastric acid secretion using pharmacologic agents heals ulcers and reduces future complications. Only a few patients have an underlying acid hypersecretory state causing ulcers. For example, less than 1% of patients with duodenal ulcers have a gastrin-secreting tumor causing profound acid secretion as part of the Zollinger-Ellison syndrome. Approximately 3–5% of gastric ulcers represent malignancy including adenocarcinoma, lymphoma, or metastatic lesions. Other infections and conditions that increase ulcer formation include cytomegalovirus or herpes simplex (especially among immunosuppressed patients), tuberculosis, Crohn disease, the use of other non-NSAID medications, hyperparathyroidism, sarcoidosis, myeloproliferative disorder, and systemic mastocytosis.

Cigarette smoking also promotes the development of ulcers and may interact with *H pylori* and NSAIDs to increase mucosal injury. Smoking also impairs ulcer healing and increases ulcer recurrence. Several studies suggest that alcohol use and diet do not appear to increase ulcer formation, whereas emotional stress may predispose some individuals to ulcers. Critically ill patients with severe burns, physical trauma, or multiple organ failure also have an increased risk of developing gastroduodenal ulcers and associated complications. There is also an association of peptic ulcers with medical conditions such as chronic obstructive lung disease and chronic renal failure, but the mechanisms are unclear. A genetic susceptibility has been reported but now is thought to stem mainly from intra familial infection with *H pylori.* Recent studies also suggest that an increasing proportion of ulcers are idiopathic, as they are not related to *H pylori*, NSAIDs, aspirin, acid hypersecretion, or any other known cause.

Table 15–1. Risk factors for peptic ulcers.

Helicobacter pylori infection
NSAID and aspirin use
Other medications (eg, potassium chloride, concomitant use of steroids with NSAIDs, bisphosphonates, sirolimus, mycophenolate mofetil, fluorouracil)
Neoplasia
Acid hypersecretory disorders (eg, Zollinger-Ellison syndrome)
Hyperparathyroidism
Crohn disease
Sarcoidosis
Myeloproliferative disorder
Systemic mastocytosis
Other rare infections (eg, cytomegalovirus, herpes simplex, tuberculosis)
Critically ill patients with severe burns, head injury, physical trauma, or multiple organ failure

NSAID, nonsteroidal anti-inflammatory drug.

Malfertheiner P, Chan FK, McColl KE. Peptic ulcer disease. *Lancet.* 2009;374:1449–1461. [PMID: 19683340]

B. *Helicobacter pylori* Infection

Helicobacter pylori is a spiral gram-negative urease-producing bacterium that can be found in the mucus coating the gastric mucosa or between the mucus layer and gastric epithelium. Multiple factors enable the bacterium to live in the hostile stomach acid environment, including its ability to produce urease, which helps alkalinize the surrounding pH. *Helicobacter pylori* infection is most commonly acquired in childhood and results in a chronic active gastritis that is usually lifelong without specific treatment. Risk factors for acquiring *H pylori* include low socioeconomic status, household crowding, and country of origin. The prevalence of *H pylori* varies among different countries and is significantly higher in developing than in industrialized countries. The majority of infected persons remain asymptomatic, but approximately 10–15% develop peptic ulcer disease during their lifetime. In addition to causing chronic gastritis and peptic ulcers, *H pylori* has been associated with the development of gastric adenocarcinoma and gastric mucosa-associated lymphoid tissue (MALT) lymphoma. In 1994, the International Agency for Research on Cancer classified *H pylori* as a group 1 carcinogen and a definite cause of gastric cancer in humans.

Infection with *H pylori* increases the risk of peptic ulcers and GI bleeding from threefold to sevenfold. Depending on the population, *H pylori* is present in up to 70–90% of patients with duodenal ulcers and up to 30–60% of gastric ulcers. Multiple clinical studies show that *H pylori* eradication reduces ulcer recurrence to less than 10% as compared with recurrences of 70% with acid suppression alone. *Helicobacter pylori* generally causes mucosal injury and ulcer complications through inflammation and cytokines. Despite a vigorous systemic and mucosal humoral response, antibody production does not lead to eradication of the infection.

Helicobacter pylori is a highly heterogeneous bacterium. A combination of microbial and host factors determines the outcome of *H pylori* infection. The virulence of the organism, host genetics, and environmental factors affect the distribution and severity of gastric inflammation and level of acid secretion. For example, the presence of different *H pylori* virulence factors that affect the induction of proinflammatory cytokine release or adhesion to the epithelial cell partly explain geographic differences in the incidence of gastric cancer. Several of these bacterial virulence factors include the *Cag* pathogenicity island (*cag*PAI), the vacuolating cytotoxin (VacA), and the blood group antigen-binding adhesin (BabA) and are associated with a more severe clinical outcome. Other virulence factors include *H pylori* neutrophil-activating protein and cell-wall polysaccharide. *Helicobacter pylori* that express the cytotoxin-associated gene A (*CagA*-positive strains) reportedly represent virulent strains having greater interactions with humans. Several genes in a genomic fragment that make up a Cag pathogenicity island encode components of a type IV secretion island that translocates CagA in host cells and affects cell growth and cytokine production. CagA is a highly antigenic protein that is associated with a prominent inflammatory response by eliciting interleukin-8 production. *Helicobacter pylori* strains that also express active forms of VacA or the outer membrane proteins BabA and OipA are similarly associated with a higher risk of diseases than are strains that lack these factors.

Blaser MJ, Atherton JC. *Helicobacter pylori* persistence: biology and disease. *J Clin Invest.* 2004;113:321–333. [PMID: 14755326]

Cover TL, Blaser MJ. *Helicobacter pylori* in health and disease. *Gastroenterology.* 2009;136:1863–1873. [PMID: 19457415]

Yamaoka Y. Mechanisms of disease: *Helicobacter pylori* virulence factors. *Nat Rev Gastroenterol Hepatol.* 2010;7:629–641. [PMID: 20938460]

C. Aspirin and NSAIDS

Aspirin and NSAIDs are among the most frequently used drugs worldwide. NSAIDs are used to treat pain and inflammation, whereas aspirin is being increasing used for primary and secondary prevention of cardiovascular events. Unfortunately, these drugs have substantial GI toxicity and are associated with the development of peptic ulcers and life-threatening GI bleeding. Endoscopic studies have shown that up to 15–30% of patients on NSAIDs develop gastric and duodenal ulcers. Epidemiologic studies also suggest that the risks of ulcer complications and death among regular NSAID users are 3–10 times higher as compared with those not taking these drugs. More than 107,000 hospitalizations in the United States are attributed to NSAIDs each year. The elderly are at particularly increased risk, and one study found that the adjusted hospitalization rate for ulcer complications was 16.7 per 1000 person-years among elderly Medicaid patients on NSAIDs, in contrast to a rate of 4.2 among nonusers, with an attributable rate of 12.5 excess hospitalizations for ulcer disease per 1000 person-years among users.

Aspirin and other NSAIDs generally exert their therapeutic and toxic effects by inhibiting COX-1 and COX-2 isoenzymes, which, in turn, decrease prostaglandin synthesis. COX-1 is the rate-limiting enzyme for GI prostaglandins that normally help maintain mucosal blood flow and increase secretion of mucus and bicarbonate. Inhibition of COX-1 impairs mucosal protection and leads to ulcers. The risks of peptic ulcers and GI bleeding are dependent on the dose, duration, and type of NSAID. Several other factors have also been shown to increase the development of peptic ulcers among NSAID users. They include increasing age, a previous history of GI bleeding or ulcers, and concomitant use of steroids. In a meta-analysis, the pooled relative risks for ulcer complications ranged from 1.6–9.2, according to the individual NSAID, with a pooled relative risk of 1.6 for aspirin. Even very low doses of aspirin have been associated with ulcers and GI bleeding, suggesting that there are no true safe doses of aspirin. A case-control study, for example, found that low-dose aspirin and nonaspirin NSAIDs both significantly increased the risk of ulcer bleeding with odds ratios of 2.4 and 7.4, respectively.

Laine L, Curtis SP, Cryer B, et al. Risk factors for NSAID-associated upper GI clinical events in a long-term prospective study of 34 701 arthritis patients. *Aliment Pharmacol Ther.* 2010;32:1240–1248. [PMID: 20955443]

Malfertheiner P, Chan FK, McColl KE. Peptic ulcer disease. *Lancet.* 2009;374:1449–1461. [PMID: 19683340]

Clinical Findings

A. Symptoms and Signs

Epigastric pain is the classic symptom associated with peptic ulcer disease. The pain is often described as a gnawing, dull, aching, "empty," or "hunger-like" sensation. The classic pain associated with duodenal ulcer is sometimes relieved with ingestion of milk, food, or antacids but recurs 2–4 hours after eating and may also awaken the patient at night. In contrast, most patients with gastric ulcers report that eating exacerbates the pain. During fasting, they may have relief of their symptoms, which then recur shortly after eating. As a result, some gastric ulcer patients experience nausea, avoidance of food/anorexia, and even weight loss.

Peptic ulcer symptoms tend to recur at intervals of weeks or months. An acute worsening or change in the pain characteristic such as generalized pain may arise from ulcer penetration or perforation. Alarm symptoms such as melena, hematemesis, guaiac-positive stools, and unexplained anemia suggest possible ulcer bleeding, while persistent vomiting may represent obstruction. Early satiety, anorexia, and unexplained weight loss may arise from a cancer. Patients with upper abdominal pain with radiation to the back may have penetration, while those with severe or worsening abdominal pain may have perforation. However, many ulcer patients present with few or no symptoms until the development of complications such as GI bleeding, perforation, penetration, and obstruction. In one study, abdominal pain was absent in over 30% of older patients with peptic ulcers seen on upper endoscopy. Less common symptoms such as nausea and vomiting may arise from a gastric outlet obstruction with ulcer edema or scarring.

The physical examination is unreliable and often normal, although some ulcer patients have epigastric tenderness to deep palpation. Occult or gross blood may be detected in the setting of bleeding ulcers. Tachycardia and orthostasis may be found in patients with significant bleeding or dehydration, while a rigid abdomen with diffuse rebound tenderness may reflect ulcer perforation with peritonitis. Rarely, a distended abdomen or a succession splash can be noted in patients with an ulcer that is complicated by outlet obstruction.

The majority of duodenal ulcers develop in the bulb or pylori channel. Patients with duodenal ulcers tend to have a younger age of onset, often between 30 and 55 years of age on average. These duodenal ulcer patients also have an increased parietal cell mass and acid secretion (with increased average basal and nocturnal gastric acid secretion). Bicarbonate secretion has been reported to be impaired among patients with active duodenal ulcers. It is thought that the imbalance between duodenal acid load and buffering capacity leads to the development of small islands of gastric metaplasia in the duodenal bulb. Colonization of these islands by *H pylori* subsequently leads to duodenitis and duodenal ulcer.

In the stomach, most benign ulcers are found in the antrum and lesser curvature of the stomach at the junction of the body and antrum. Gastric ulcers often occur later in life, usually among patients between the ages of 55 and 70 years with a peak incidence in the sixth decade. Patients with gastric ulcers often have normal or decreased acid secretion. A few patients present with both gastric and duodenal ulcers are found to have increased acid secretion. The gastric ulcers in these patients tend to be located in the distal antrum or pyloric channel.

B. Endoscopy

Definitive diagnosis of peptic ulcers can be made with upper endoscopy. Endoscopy has a much higher diagnostic yield than barium contrast radiology and enables biopsy specimens to be obtained for evaluation of *H pylori* infection and underlying malignancy. Because up to 5% of gastric ulcers are malignant, it is generally recommended that biopsy samples be taken from the ulcer margin or that a follow-up endoscopy be scheduled 12 weeks after starting acid-suppressive medications to document complete healing. Ulcers greater than 3 cm in size and those that are associated with a mass are more likely to be malignant. In contrast, the incidence of malignant duodenal ulcers is extremely low; thus, they do not routinely require biopsy. Actively bleeding ulcers or ulcers at high risk for rebleeding can also be treated during endoscopy with hemostasis therapy.

Patients suspected of having an ulcer who present with alarm symptoms, such as GI bleeding, early satiety, and unexplained weight loss, and those who are elderly should undergo prompt evaluation with endoscopy. Patients who are found to have multiple ulcers, refractory ulcers, or ulcers in unusual locations, such as postbulbar or jejunum, or who have diarrhea and weight loss should also be considered for evaluation of Zollinger-Ellison syndrome.

In contrast, there is some controversy as to the best approach for initial evaluation and treatment of young patients under the age of 55 years without alarm symptoms who present with ulcer-like symptoms or dyspepsia. Possible options include (1) testing and treating for *H pylori*, (2) treating with acid-suppressive medications and monitoring response, or (3) making a direct referral for evaluation with upper endoscopy. Prompt endoscopy potentially offers a small benefit in terms of finding a specific diagnosis and directing treatment but is not cost effective for the initial management of dyspepsia as compared to the other strategies. Instead, several other studies recommend that young patients with undifferentiated dyspepsia initially undergo noninvasive testing for *H pylori* followed by treatment if this infection is present. Successful cure of *H pylori* potentially reduces the need for endoscopy as well as ulcer recurrence, and clinical studies suggest that this strategy does not adversely affect outcomes. Further evaluation with endoscopy is recommended for patients with persistent symptoms despite therapy. Alternatively, young patients with a presentation suggestive of uncomplicated ulcers may first be given empiric treatment with acid-suppressive medications. Further evaluation is recommended if these patients continue to have persistent or recurrent symptoms 2–4 weeks later. All patients should discontinue aspirin and NSAIDs if possible, as well as stop alcohol, smoking, and use of illicit drugs. In one large clinical trial, patients having dyspepsia without alarm symptoms were randomized to testing and treating for *H pylori* versus empiric proton pump inhibitor therapy. After 1 year of follow-up, patients in the two groups had a similar rate of persistent dyspeptic symptoms, and both strategies were found to be equally cost effective in the initial management of dyspepsia. It is notable that over 80% of these patients continued to experience dyspeptic symptoms despite eradication of *H pylori* (82%) or acid-suppressive therapy (83%).

Delaney BC, Qume M, Moayyedi P, et al. *Helicobacter pylori* test and treat versus proton pump inhibitor in initial management of dyspepsia in primary care: multicentre randomized controlled trial (MRC-CUBE trial). BMJ 2008;336:651–654. [PMID: 18310262]

C. Barium Studies

Barium upper GI studies are widely available and are safer and cheaper than endoscopy, but they have limited accuracy for detecting ulcers and other mucosal lesions. In contrast to endoscopy, barium upper GI studies do not permit biopsy and other specimens to be obtained for histologic evaluation or allow immediate treatment of bleeding ulcers.

Table 15–2. Diagnostic tests for *Helicobacter pylori*.

Test	Sensitivity (%)	Specificity (%)	Comments
Noninvasive			
Serologic ELISA	85	79	Detects exposure to *H pylori* but cannot be used to confirm successful cure after treatment
Urea breath test	95–100	91–98	Recommended for both screening and confirming cure; recent use of antibiotics and PPIs can increase false-negative results
H pylori stool antigen test	91–98	94–99	Can be used for initial diagnosis and to confirm successful cure
Invasive			
Endoscopy with biopsy			
• Histology	>95	95–98	Widely used method of diagnosis during endoscopy; sensitivity is improved by taking at least 2 biopsies from antrum and 1 from body of stomach
• Rapid urease test (CLO test)	93–97	95–100	Reduced accuracy reported among patients with GI bleeding
• Culture	70–80	100	Technically demanding; sensitivity varies among laboratories

CLO, *Campylobacter*-like organism; ELISA, enzyme-linked immunosorbent assay; GI, gastrointestinal; PPI, proton pump inhibitor.

D. Tests to Diagnose *H pylori* Infection

Several methods are available to detect *H pylori* infection (Table 15–2). The noninvasive tests include serologic testing, urea breath test, and stool antigen test. Infection can also be detected during endoscopy in which a biopsy sample is obtained for a rapid urease testing, histologic study, or even culture. Serum immunoassays for immunoglobulin G (IgG) antibodies to *H pylori* are inexpensive but have a reported sensitivity of 85% and specificity of 79%. As a result, the positive predictive value of serologic testing is limited in populations with a low pretest probability of having the infection. Moreover, serologic testing should not be used to determine the success of *H pylori* cure after treatment since antibody titers do not always become negative. The urea breath test or the stool antigen test can be used for both the initial diagnosis and follow-up of eradication therapy because they have sensitivities and specificities of over 90%. Urea breath testing is based on detecting *H pylori*-derived urease activity in the stomach, whereas the stool antigen test uses polyclonal anti-*H pylori* capture antibody adsorbed to microwells. It is generally recommended to wait at least 4 weeks or more after completing eradication therapy to confirm successful cure. To help minimize false-negative results, proton pump inhibitors should be withheld for 1–2 weeks and antibiotics and bismuth compounds for 4 weeks prior to testing.

In patients who undergo endoscopy, an antral biopsy can be obtained for rapid urease testing, which has a sensitivity of 89–100% and specificity of 92–100%. Biopsies can also be performed and specimens sent for histologic examination using routine hematoxylin and eosin staining. The presence of polymorphonuclear leukocytes in inflamed gastric tissue is suggestive of *H pylori* gastritis. In biopsy specimens in which *H pylori* cannot be found, the use of modified Giemsa, Warthin-Starry, Genta, and other stains may be helpful. Culture of *H pylori* from biopsy samples has a specificity of 100% if results are positive, but it is not routinely performed. Because culture is difficult to perform and expensive, it is usually reserved to determine antibiotic susceptibilities for patients who fail to respond to second-line eradication therapy.

Differential Diagnosis

In some studies, only half of patients with peptic ulcer present with classic symptoms. Unfortunately, the history and physical examination are neither sensitive nor specific enough to accurately diagnose peptic ulcers or distinguish between duodenal and gastric ulcers. A diagnosis of a peptic ulcer may be suspected in selected patients presenting with epigastric pain, but the differential is broad and includes gastroesophageal reflux disease, biliary tract disease, hepatitis, pancreatitis, abdominal aortic aneurysm, gastroparesis, functional dyspepsia, neoplasia, mesenteric ischemia, and myocardial ischemic pain, among others.

Although peptic ulcers can be diagnosed during upper endoscopy, laboratory and radiologic tests may help narrow the differential diagnosis. Some ulcer patients are anemic due to acute bleeding or chronic blood loss from benign or malignant ulcers. Liver function tests and levels of amylase and lipase should be checked to help evaluate for hepatitis and pancreatitis. An abdominal ultrasound may show gallstone disease or an abdominal aortic aneurysm. An electrocardiogram and measurement of cardiac enzymes help evaluate myocardial causes of pain. Finally, an acute abdominal series with upright and lateral decubitus views showing free air suggests perforation.

Complications

The most common complication associated with peptic ulcers is the development of GI hemorrhage. Up to 15% of peptic ulcers bleed, and affected patients have an overall mortality rate of 10%. Patients older than 60 years of age have a higher incidence of bleeding ulcers and mortality. Those who also have a large initial bleed, continued or recurrent bleeding, or severe comorbid illnesses have the greatest risk of death. Patients with bleeding ulcers can present with hematemesis or coffee ground emesis, passage of black tarry stool, and rarely, hematochezia.

Up to 7% of ulcer patients have perforation with severe abdominal pain and a rigid abdomen from peritonitis. Owing to the widespread use of NSAIDs among the elderly, they are at increased risk, and many do not present with antecedent ulcer pain or peritoneal findings. Penetration occurs when the ulcer crater erodes into an adjacent organ as, for example, when a duodenal ulcer penetrates into the pancreas leading to pancreatitis or a gastric ulcer penetrates into the left hepatic lobe.

Gastric outlet obstruction occurs in less than 2% of ulcer patients and may arise from ulcer inflammation and edema in the prepyloric area. Chronic ulcer scarring in the prepyloric area can also lead to a fixed mechanical obstruction that may require endoscopic balloon dilation or surgical therapy. This diagnosis should be suspected in patients who complain of nausea, vomiting, early satiety, and weight loss, especially if they also have dehydration and electrolyte imbalances.

Treatment

A. General Principles

Treatment of peptic ulcers consists of healing the ulcer and preventing ulcer recurrences and future complications. All ulcer patients should be tested and treated for *H pylori* even if they have a clear history of NSAID or aspirin use. It is not clinically possible to determine whether ulcers arise directly from *H pylori*, NSAID/aspirin use, or a combination of these factors. Although *H pylori* and NSAID use cause most ulcers, the level of acid secretion still plays a role in pathogenesis and healing. Multiple studies show that the administration of acid-suppressive medications promotes active ulcer healing. Intravenous acid-suppressive therapy should be promptly started in ulcer patients with signs of upper GI bleeding, followed by early endoscopy to improve outcomes. In some studies, the use of an intravenous proton pump inhibitor decreased transfusion requirements, the need for surgery, and even duration of hospitalization. A randomized trial has also showed that administration of an intravenous proton pump inhibitor prior to endoscopy downstages the ulcer lesion and decreases the need for hemostasis therapy as compared to placebo. Use of a promotility agent such as erythromycin or metoclopramide prior to endoscopy is not recommended for routine use but may be considered in patients suspected of having a substantial amount of blood in the upper GI tract. This potentially improves the examination during upper endoscopy.

Endoscopic hemostasis is recommended for high-risk ulcers, based on their endoscopic appearance and likelihood of further bleeding. High-risk ulcers that should be treated include those that are actively spurting or oozing blood, those that have a nonbleeding visible vessel, or those that have an adherent clot. Hemostasis can be performed through a combination of coagulation of bleeding sites (thermocoagulation therapy), placement of hemoclips (mechanical therapy), and injection of epinephrine, alcohol, or a sclerosant (injection therapy). Thermocoagulation or clip placement, either alone or with epinephrine injection, has been shown to be effective, but epinephrine injection alone is not recommended. Intravenous high-dose proton pump inhibitor therapy after successful endoscopic hemostasis therapy has been shown to decrease rebleeding and mortality in patients with high-risk stigmata. Second-look endoscopy may be useful in selected patients but is also not routinely recommended. Nonhealing gastric ulcers should be biopsied or closely followed to exclude underlying neoplasia.

Barkun AN, Bardou M, Kuipers EJ, et al. International consensus recommendations on the management of patients with nonvariceal upper gastrointestinal bleeding. *Ann Intern Med.* 2010;152:101–113. [PMID: 20083829]

Lau JY, Leung WK, Wu JC, et al. Omeprazole before endoscopy in patients with gastrointestinal bleeding. *N Engl J Med.* 2007; 356:1631–1640. [PMID: 17442905]

B. Peptic Ulcers in Patients Requiring Chronic NSAIDs

Patients who develop peptic ulcers while on NSAIDs should be tested and treated for *H pylori* and the NSAID should be discontinued if possible. *Helicobacter pylori* eradication alone is insufficient to completely prevent recurrent GI complications among ulcer patients who continue to take NSAIDs. Acid-suppressive medication, usually with a proton pump inhibitor, should also be administered to help the ulcer. Proton pump inhibitors block acid secretion by irreversibly binding and inhibiting the hydrogen-potassium ATPase that resides on the luminal surface of the parietal cell. The proton pump inhibitors include omeprazole, lansoprazole, pantoprazole, rabeprazole, and esomeprazole.

If patients cannot switch to acetaminophen and require chronic NSAIDs, they should consider taking the lowest effective NSAID dose along with co-therapy with either a proton pump inhibitor or a prostaglandin analog called misoprostol. These drugs have been shown to significantly reduce recurrent ulcer complications among chronic NSAID users. Unfortunately, misoprostol at 200 mcg four times daily is often associated with cramps, diarrhea, and poor patient compliance.

Drugs that selectively inhibit COX-2 were developed to have similar analgesic and anti-inflammatory effects as traditional NSAIDs but with a reduced risk of GI complications. Several studies have suggested that COX-2 inhibitors help treat musculoskeletal as well as arthritic conditions with fewer ulcer complications because they do not inhibit the gastric mucosal prostaglandins. Among healed ulcer patients, the use of a COX-2 inhibitor had a lower rate of adverse upper and lower GI events as compared to the strategy of providing a traditional NSAID with proton pump inhibitor co-therapy. Another trial has also shown that combining a selective COX-2 inhibitor with a proton pump inhibitor was even more effective in preventing recurrent ulcer bleeding than taking a COX-2 inhibitor alone. However, COX-2 inhibitors have been also associated with an increased risk of cardiovascular and thrombotic events. The exact mechanisms for this are not clear but may be related to the fact that thromboxane A2 is a COX-1-mediated product that causes irreversible platelet aggregation, vasoconstriction, and smooth muscle proliferation. In contrast, prostacyclin is synthesized from COX-2 and is an inhibitor of platelet aggregation while causing vasodilation and inhibition of smooth muscle proliferation. Selective inhibition of COX-2 may lead to an imbalance in these products that promotes thrombosis. Thus, clinicians must be judicious when prescribing these drugs. COX-2 inhibitors should be considered for chronic NSAID patients who have a substantial risk of ulcer complications but a low risk of cardiovascular disease. The addition of low-dose aspirin to a COX-2 inhibitor increases the ulcer rate to that seen with nonselective NSAIDs.

Barkun AN, Bardou M, Kuipers EJ, et al. International consensus recommendations on the management of patients with nonvariceal upper gastrointestinal bleeding. *Ann Intern Med.* 2010;152:101–113. [PMID: 20083829]

Chan FK, Lanas A, Scheiman J, et al. Celecoxib versus omeprazole and diclofenac in patients with osteoarthritis and rheumatoid arthritis (CONDOR): a randomized trial. *Lancet.* 2010;376: 173–179. [PMID: 20638563]

Chan FK, Wong VW, Suen BY, et al. Combination of a cyclo-oxygenase-2 inhibitor and a proton-pump inhibitor for prevention of recurrent ulcer bleeding in patients at very high risk: a double-blind, randomized trial. *Lancet.* 2007;369:1621–1626. [PMID: 17499604]

Malfertheiner P, Chan FK, McColl KE. Peptic ulcer disease. *Lancet.* 2009;374:1449–1461. [PMID: 19683340]

C. Peptic Ulcers in Patients Requiring Chronic Antiplatelet Therapy

The use of enteric-coated or buffered aspirin does not substantially reduce the risk of ulcer complications compared to noncoated aspirin due to the systemic effects of these drugs. There are also other widely used antiplatelet drugs such as clopidogrel that selectively and irreversibly block the adenosine diphosphate receptor on platelets. Clopidogrel, with or without aspirin, has been shown to be beneficial in the treatment of acute coronary syndrome and in the prevention of ischemic events among patient with atherosclerotic diseases. As expected, the combined use of clopidogrel with aspirin causes a greater increase in GI bleeding risk compared to aspirin alone.

Patients taking aspirin who present with potential ulcer complications such as GI bleeding should receive intravenous proton pump inhibitor therapy and undergo upper endoscopy. Ulcers that are found to have high-risk bleeding stigmata are then treated with hemostasis therapy. Testing and treating for *H pylori* as well as providing secondary prophylaxis with a proton pump inhibitor have been shown to be effective in reducing recurrent aspirin-induced GI complications. Proton pump inhibitors, for example, are superior to high-dose H_2-receptor antagonists in preventing recurrent aspirin-related ulcers and erosions. Moreover, the coadministration of a proton pump inhibitor with aspirin greatly reduces recurrent ulcer bleeding as compared to switching patients to clopidogrel alone. One study found that up to 13% of patients with a prior history of ulcers who take clopidogrel develop recurrent ulcers during a 6-month follow-up period.

Among patients requiring chronic aspirin therapy who suffer an acute ulcer bleed, it has long been unclear when to safely resume aspirin. Restarting aspirin before the ulcer has adequately healed potentially increases recurrent bleeding, but delayed administration of aspirin may also lead to greater cardiovascular or ischemic events in high-risk patients. This issue has been addressed in a large study of aspirin patients with a bleeding ulcer who underwent endoscopic hemostasis followed by maintenance therapy with a proton pump inhibitor. These patients were then randomized to immediately continuing aspirin versus a delay in resuming aspirin until 8 weeks after endoscopy. Early continuation of aspirin was found to increase recurrent bleeding but significantly reduce the all-cause and specific-cause mortality compared with restarting aspirin 8 weeks later. These data highlight the importance of carefully weighing the short- and long-term risk and benefits of restarting aspirin for prevention of acute coronary syndromes. In this clinical trial, the protective effects of aspirin appear to outweigh its potential for further short-term GI complications that mainly occurred within 5 days after the index bleed. Aspirin should be restarted as soon as the risk for cardiovascular events outweighs the risk for recurrent ulcer complications. The investigators recommended considering holding aspirin for 3–5 days after the index bleed and then resuming after stabilization.

Other studies have also suggested that the use of new drugs such as the nitric oxide-releasing NSAIDs or nitric oxide-releasing aspirin may help reduce ulcer complications, but they are not yet available for clinical use. In small trials, for example, adding a nitric oxide-donating moiety to aspirin was associated with less GI mucosal damage and yet provided similar inhibition of platelet aggregation and thromboxane B2 production as traditional aspirin.

Long-term studies are needed to determine if nitric oxide–releasing aspirin is truly safer and provides the same benefits as traditional aspirin.

Chan FK, Ching JY, Hung LC, et al. Clopidogrel versus aspirin and esomeprazole to prevent recurrent ulcer bleeding. *N Engl J Med.* 2005;352:238–244. [PMID: 15659723]

Sung JJ, Lau JY, Ching JY, et al. Continuation of low-dose aspirin therapy in peptic ulcer bleeding: a randomized trial. *Ann Intern Med.* 2010:152:1–9. [PMID: 19949136]

D. Potential Interaction Between Clopidogrel and Proton Pump Inhibitors

There has been much ongoing controversy about a potential interaction between proton pump inhibitors and clopidogrel. Clopidogrel is a prodrug that requires activation by hepatic metabolism through the cytochrome P450 (CYP) system. The CYP2C19 isoenzyme is an important determinant of the response to clopidogrel. Among patients taking clopidogrel, carriers of a CYP2C19 reduced-function allele were found to have lower levels of active clopidogrel metabolites, diminished platelet inhibition, and a higher rate of major cardiovascular events than noncarriers. Unfortunately, the CYP2C19 isoenzyme is also involved in the metabolism of most proton pump inhibitors. It is thought that proton pump inhibitors potentially decrease conversion of clopidogrel into its active metabolites and diminish the antiplatelet effects because of competitive inhibition of the CYP2C19 isoenzyme. Some studies that test platelet activity support an interaction between clopidogrel and proton pump inhibitors, but the results from clinical studies have been conflicting. A few retrospective observational studies have shown an increased rate of cardiovascular events among patients receiving both clopidogrel and a proton pump inhibitor. However, several other large clinical studies have not confirmed any clinically significant interaction between these drugs. One such report includes a Danish nationwide cohort study of myocardial infarction patients. Another clinical trial randomized patients on aspirin and clopidogrel to receive prophylactic omeprazole or placebo. Concurrent use of omeprazole significantly reduced the rate of upper GI bleeding. Although there was no apparent cardiovascular interaction between clopidogrel and omeprazole, the study was unable to rule out a clinically meaningful difference in cardiovascular events from proton pump inhibitor use. A smaller randomized controlled study similarly found that administration of a proton pump inhibitor to patients on clopidogrel reduced recurrent ulcers. Among a subset of these patients who also underwent platelet aggregation testing, the proton pump inhibitor did not interfere with the effect of clopidogrel on platelet aggregation.

To date, the clinical significance of a clopidogrel and proton pump inhibitor interaction remains unclear. Some have suggested that these drugs be taken during different times of the day to help minimize potential interference. The U.S. Food and Drug Administration and the European Medicines Agency have since posted safety warnings and discouraged the concomitant use of proton pump inhibitor with clopidogrel unless absolutely necessary. Until adequately powered studies are completed, management of these patients should be individualized. The routine use of proton pump inhibitor therapy is not recommended for everyone on chronic antiplatelet therapy. Instead, the risks and benefits must be carefully weighed for each patient to determine the most appropriate treatment. Proton pump inhibitor therapy should be considered for patients on chronic antiplatelet therapy who are at substantial risk for GI complications.

Bhatt DL, Cryer BL, Contant CF, et al. Clopidogrel with or without omeprazole in coronary artery disease. *N Engl J Med.* 2010;363:1909–1917. [PMID: 20925534]

Charlot M, Ahlehoff O, Norgaard ML, et al. Proton-pump inhibitors are associated with increased cardiovascular risk independent of clopidogrel use: a nationwide cohort study. *Ann Intern Med.* 2010;153:378–386. [PMID: 20855802]

Mega JL, Close SL, Wiviott SD, et al. Cytochrome p-450 polymorphisms and response to clopidogrel. *N Engl J Med.* 2009; 360:354–362. [PMID: 19106084]

E. Eradication Therapy for *H pylori* Infection

Patients with active duodenal or gastric ulcers and those with a prior ulcer history should be tested for *H pylori.* Appropriate therapy should be given for eradication. After successful cure, reinfection with *H pylori* is considered rare. In the United States, the estimated incidence is approximately one reinfection per 100 patients per year. Patients with MALT lymphoma should also be tested and treated for *H pylori* since eradication of this infection can induce remission in many patients when the tumor is limited to the stomach. Several consensus conferences, including the Maastricht III Consensus Report, recommend testing and treating several other groups of patients, but there is limited evidence of benefit. This includes patients diagnosed with gastric adenocarcinoma (especially those with early-stage disease who undergo resection), patients found to have atrophic gastritis or intestinal metaplasia, and first-degree relatives of patients with gastric adenocarcinoma since the relatives themselves are at increased risk of gastric cancer partly due to the intra familial transmission of *H pylori.* Although the mechanisms are unknown, a few studies suggest that *H pylori* may play a role in autoimmune disorders such as idiopathic thrombocytopenic purpura. Eradication of *H pylori* has been shown to increase the platelet count in these patients. It is also recommended to consider testing and treating for *H pylori* among patients with unexplained iron deficiency anemia as successful eradication may reverse the anemia in these gastritis patients and improve iron absorption. To date, it remains controversial whether to test and treat all patients with functional dyspepsia, gastroesophageal reflux disease, or other non-GI disorders as well as asymptomatic individuals.

The success of *H pylori* cure depends on the type and duration of therapy, patient compliance, and bacterial factors such as antibiotic resistance. There are multiple treatment regimens for *H pylori* eradication and most include the use of a proton pump inhibitor combined with two antibiotics for 7–14 days (Table 15–3). Some commonly used antibiotics are amoxicillin, clarithromycin, metronidazole, and tetracycline; studies often report cure rates of over 80–90% with these agents. European studies report that 7-day regimens are adequate, but a meta-analysis suggested that a 14-day treatment regimen had a higher eradication rate and was more cost effective compared with 7-day therapy (81% vs 72%). A study conducted in the United States several years ago found that the overall resistance rate to clarithromycin was 10.1%, to metronidazole was 36.9% and to amoxicillin was only 1.4%. It may be possible to predict possible resistance to clarithromycin or to metronidazole by taking a careful history and inquiring about prior use of these drugs. Owing to regional antibiotic resistance differences, a 14-day regimen appears to be more effective in the United States and is recommended by the U.S. Food and Drug Administration. A commonly prescribed regimen, for example, is triple therapy

Table 15–3. Common treatment regimens for *Helicobacter pylori*.

Treatment Regimen	Eradication Rates (%)	Comments
Triple Therapy		
Proton pump inhibitor **Plus** Clarithromycin, 500 mg twice daily, or metronidazole, 500 mg twice daily **Plus** Amoxicillin, 1 g twice daily for 7–14 days	73–86	Often used as first-line therapy; in United States, recommendation is to treat for at least 10 days
Proton pump inhibitor **Plus** Clarithromycin, 500 mg twice daily **Plus** Metronidazole, 500 mg twice daily for 7–14 days	70–85	May be used as first-line therapy in penicillin-allergic patients
Quadruple Therapy		
Bismuth subsalicylate, 525 mg four times daily **Plus** Metronidazole, 250 mg orally four times daily **Plus** Tetracycline, 500 mg orally four times daily **Plus** PPI twice daily (or ranitidine, 150 mg orally twice daily) for 10–14 days	75–90	Usually used as second-line therapy in patients who fail to respond to triple therapy
Levofloxacin-Based Triple Therapy		
PPI twice daily **Plus** Levofloxacin, 250–500 mg twice daily **Plus** Amoxicillin, 1 g twice daily for 10 days	60–80	Often recommended for second-line or rescue therapy
Sequential Therapy		
PPI twice daily **Plus** Amoxicillin, 1 g twice daily for the first 5 days followed by PPI twice daily **Plus** Clarithromycin, 500 mg twice daily, and tinidazole, 500 mg twice daily, for the next 5 days	83–98	Overall eradication rate >90%; recommended for second-line or rescue therapy but may also be considered for initial therapy

PPI, proton pump inhibitor.

using a proton pump inhibitor (given twice daily) along with clarithromycin (500 mg twice daily) and amoxicillin (1 g twice daily) or metronidazole (500 mg twice daily, for penicillin-allergic patients) for 14 days. Ranitidine bismuth citrate (400 mg twice daily) may be substituted for the proton pump inhibitor. A clarithromycin-based regimen should not be used in areas where the resistance rate is known to be greater than 15%. In contrast to metronidazole, *H pylori* resistance to clarithromycin cannot be easily overcome by increasing the dose of the drug. Instead quadruple therapy or another first-line eradication regimen is usually recommended. Quadruple therapy uses a proton pump inhibitor twice daily and four-times-daily dosing of antibiotics with tetracycline (500 mg) and metronidazole (500 mg), along with bismuth subsalicylate or subcitrate (525 mg four times daily).

Patients most often fail to respond to initial *H pylori* eradication therapy because of noncompliance and/or antibiotic resistance. Prior to initiating eradication therapy, patients should be given careful instructions not to arbitrarily miss any doses. They should also be able to contact a clinician if they experience any adverse side effects. After completing therapy, patients should be queried about any side effects, missed doses, and completion of therapy. Since culture with antibiotic sensitivities is not routinely performed when *H pylori* infection is diagnosed, it is generally recommended that different antibiotics be given at higher doses for 14 days. Quadruple therapy has been widely used in the past with cure rates of 70–80%, but more recent studies also suggest the use of either levofloxacin-based triple therapy or sequential therapy (see Table 15–3). These latter two regimens can also be used as primary therapy. Levofloxacin-based triple therapy consists of a proton pump inhibitor twice daily, levofloxacin (250 mg twice daily), and amoxicillin (1 g twice daily) given together for 10 days. Clarithromycin sequential therapy consists of a proton pump inhibitor twice daily throughout the treatment period along with amoxicillin (1 g twice daily) for the first 5 days followed by clarithromycin (500 mg twice daily) and tinidazole (500 mg twice daily) for the next 5 days. Clarithromycin sequential therapy is relatively well tolerated and effective as either first- or second-line therapy even among patients who harbor clarithromycin-resistant strains. Recently, a levofloxacin-based sequential therapy was found to be effective in areas with a greater than 15% prevalence of clarithromycin resistance. This regimen includes use of a proton pump inhibitor twice a day throughout the treatment period along with amoxicillin (1 g twice daily) for the first 5 days followed by levofloxacin (250 or 500 mg twice daily) and tinidazole (500 mg twice daily) for the next 5 days, with an overall reported eradication rate of greater than 95%. However, it is likely that the prevalence of levofloxacin resistance will increase as this antibiotic is being used more often. Patients who fail to respond to second-line eradication may undergo culture for *H pylori* and a determination of antibiotic sensitivities to help direct further therapy.

Malfertheiner P, Megraud F, O'Moran C, et al. Current concepts in the management of *Helicobacter pylori* infection: the Maastricht III Consensus Report. *Gut.* 2007;56:772–781. [PMID: 17170018]

Romano M, Cuomo A, Gravina AG, et al. Empirical levofloxacin-containing versus clarithromycin-containing sequential therapy for *Helicobacter pylori* eradication: a randomized trial. *Gut.* 2010;59:1465–1470. [PMID: 20947881]

Vakil N, Megraud F. Eradication therapy for *Helicobacter pylori*. *Gastroenterology.* 2007;133:985–1001. [PMID: 17854602]

F. *Helicobacter pylori* and Gastric Adenocarcinoma

Up to 5% of gastric ulcers represent underlying neoplasia. Although the incidence of gastric cancer has steadily declined over the past few decades, it still remains a major cause of cancer death worldwide. There is wide regional variation in the incidence of gastric cancer. High incidence rates have been reported in Japan, Eastern Asia, Eastern Europe, and parts of Latin America, while low incidence rates have been reported in the United States and Western Europe. Gastric carcinogenesis is a multistep process, starting from chronic gastritis and progressing over many years to atrophy, intestinal metaplasia, dysplasia, and eventually adenocarcinoma. Three meta-analyses of case-control and cohort studies report summary odds ratios for *H pylori* and gastric adenocarcinoma of 1.92 (95% confidence interval [CI], 1.32–2.78), 2.5 (95% CI, 1.90–3.40), and 2.04 (95% CI, 1.69–2.45). In an animal study, long-term infection with *H pylori* in Mongolian gerbils has been shown to induce gastric adenocarcinoma.

Additional data supporting an association between *H pylori* and gastric cancer in humans comes from a long-term prospective cohort study from Japan by Uemura and colleagues. In this study, 1526 patients with various GI disorders, including duodenal ulcers, gastric ulcers, gastric hyperplasia, and nonulcer dyspepsia, underwent endoscopy with biopsy at enrollment and then 1–3 years after enrollment. There were 1246 *H pylori*-infected and 280 uninfected patients followed for a mean duration of 7.8 years. Among the *H pylori* patients, 253 received eradication therapy at an early stage of follow-up. Gastric cancer developed in approximately 3% of the infected patients but in none of the uninfected patients. In addition, none of the *H pylori* patients who received eradication therapy developed gastric cancer. *Helicobacter pylori* patients with severe gastric atrophy, corpus-predominant gastritis, and intestinal metaplasia were at significantly higher risk for gastric cancer. The risk was also increased in almost all subgroups of *H pylori*-infected patients (those with gastric ulcers, gastric hyperplastic polyps, or nonulcer dyspepsia) but not in those with duodenal ulcers. It is noteworthy that infected patients who received eradication therapy did not develop gastric cancer. These results support the notion that eradication of *H pylori* may potentially prevent or delay the development of cancer.

A meta-analysis of seven randomized studies from areas with a high incidence of gastric cancer showed that *H pylori* eradication treatment reduces gastric cancer risk. Another randomized study has also shown that successful cure of *H pylori* after endoscopic resection of early gastric cancer significantly reduces the development of metachronous gastric carcinoma. It is known that the risk of gastric cancer is greater in patients with low gastric acidity such as those with severe atrophic gastritis with intestinal metaplasia and pernicious anemia. Patients who have had a partial gastrectomy are also at risk for gastric cancer after a long latency period, but their risk appears greater after an additional acid-reducing procedure such as vagotomy. Low acid secretion has been hypothesized to predispose to gastric cancer by affecting vitamin C absorption and overgrowth of salivary and intestinal bacteria in the stomach, which potentially promote the formation of carcinogenic nitrosamines. Chronic inflammation with alterations to DNA or changes in expression of cytokines and chemokines may also affect early progression. Host genetics also play a key role, and studies have shown how human genetic polymorphisms profoundly affect gastric carcinogenesis. For example, interleukin-1β is an important proinflammatory cytokine and a powerful inhibitor of acid secretion. Levels of interleukin-1β within the gastric mucosa are increased by *H pylori* infection. Genetic polymorphisms that promote high expression of interleukin-1β help explain why some *H pylori*–infected patients develop gastric cancer while others do not.

Cover TL, Blaser MJ. *Helicobacter pylori* in health and disease. *Gastroenterology.* 2009;136:1863–1873. [PMID: 19457415]

Fuccio L, Zagari RM, Eusebi LH, et al. Meta-analysis: can *Helicobacter pylori* eradication treatment reduce the risk for gastric cancer? *Ann Intern Med.* 2009;151:121–128. [PMID: 19620164]

Fukase K, Kato M, Kikuchi S, et al. Effect of eradication of *Helicobacter pylori* on incidence of metachronous gastric carcinoma after endoscopic resection of early gastric cancer: an open-label, randomized controlled trial. *Lancet.* 2008;372: 392–397. [PMID: 18675689]

Uemura N, Okamoto S, Yamamoto S, et al. *Helicobacter pylori* infection and the development of gastric cancer. *N Engl J Med.* 2001;345:784–789. [PMID: 11556297]

G. *Helicobacter pylori* and Gastric MALT Lymphoma

There is strong evidence supporting the role of *H pylori* infection in the development of low-grade B-cell MALT lymphoma of the stomach. Epidemiologic studies have shown that patients with gastric MALT lymphomas are significantly more likely than matched control subjects to have had previous *H pylori* infection. There is also direct evidence that MALT lymphomas arise in the presence of *H pylori* gastritis. Some investigators have even been able to detect the lymphoma B-cell clone in the chronic gastritis that preceded the lymphoma. Nevertheless, the strongest evidence of a causal association is that *H pylori* eradication can induce remission in these patients. A pooled data analysis of 34 studies showed that successful cure of *H pylori* infection was associated with remission of gastric MALT lymphoma in 78% of patients. Many of these patients remain in remission for years.

Malfertheiner P, Megraud F, O'Moran C, et al. Current concepts in the management of *Helicobacter pylori* infection: the Maastricht III Consensus Report. *Gut.* 2007;56:772–781. [PMID: 17170018]

Zullo A, Hassan C, Andriani A, et al. Eradication therapy for *Helicobacter pylori* in patients with gastric MALT lymphoma: a pooled data analysis. *Am J Gastroenterol.* 2009;104:1932–1937. [PMID: 19532131]

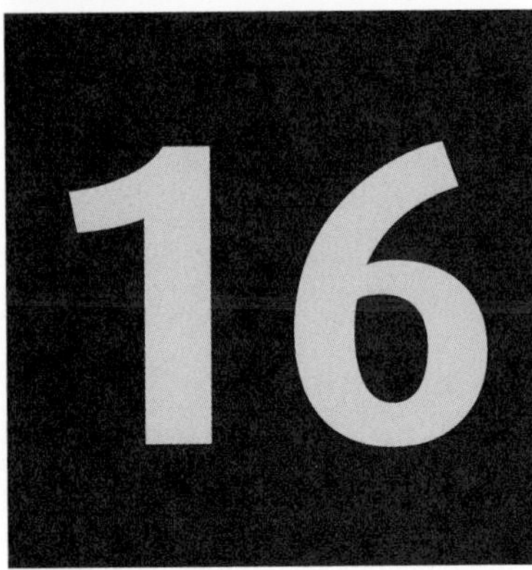

Zollinger-Ellison Syndrome (Gastrinoma)

Edward Lew, MD, MPH

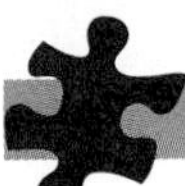

ESSENTIALS OF DIAGNOSIS

- Peptic ulcer disease, abdominal pain, and diarrhea are common presentations.
- Patients have marked gastric acid secretion arising from a gastrin-secreting non-β islet cell tumor.
- Multiple endocrine neoplasia syndrome type 1 (MEN 1) is present in ~20–25% of patients.
- Serum gastrin concentration >1000 pg/mL in combination with acidic stomach pH <2.0 is diagnostic.
- Up to 40% of patients have elevated serum gastrin levels that are <500 pg/mL and warrant a secretin test.
- Significant hypergastrinemia can occur with proton pump inhibitor use, *Helicobacter pylori* infection, or chronic atrophic gastritis and hypochlorhydria.

General Considerations

Zollinger-Ellison syndrome (ZES) is characterized by peptic ulcers, diarrhea, and marked gastric acid hypersecretion in association with a gastrin-secreting non-β islet cell endocrine tumor (gastrinoma). The reported incidence of gastrinomas ranges from 0.5 to 4 cases per million of the population per year. ZES is a rare cause of peptic ulcer disease and accounts for only 0.1–1% of ulcers. The mean age of onset of symptoms is 41 years, and slightly more males than females are affected, with a ratio of 3:2. The diagnosis of ZES is typically delayed by at least 5–7 years. Although the majority of gastrinomas develop as a sporadic tumor, approximately 20–25% of ZES patients have gastrinomas as part of the inherited multiple endocrine neoplasia syndrome type 1 (MEN 1). MEN 1 is an autosomal-dominant inherited syndrome characterized by pancreatic neuroendocrine tumors, pituitary tumors, and hyperparathyroidism, and is caused by mutations of the MEN 1 tumor suppressor gene on chromosome 11q13.

Pathogenesis

Patients with ZES most often present with symptoms arising from excessive gastric acid secretion. The unregulated gastrin production from the gastrinoma binds to CCK-2 receptors located on enterochromaffin-like (ECL) cells causing the release of histamine. Histamine then binds to H_2 receptors on parietal cells to stimulate the release of acid. In addition, gastrin also has trophic effects on gastric epithelial and ECL cells. Chronic hypergastrinemia increases parietal cell mass, which further augments acid hypersecretion. The enteroendocrine cells that make up the gastrinoma are well differentiated and round, with small nuclei and prominent nucleolus. They often contain neuroendocrine tumor markers, including chromogranin A, neurospecific enolase, and synaptophysin.

Clinical Findings

A. Symptoms and Signs

Abdominal pain and diarrhea are the most common symptoms experienced by ZES patients. Gastroesophageal reflux, nausea, weight loss, and bleeding are other typical symptoms. The widespread use of acid-suppressive medications such as proton pump inhibitors (PPIs) may mask symptoms and delay diagnosis. Table 16–1 shows the frequency of these presenting symptoms in ZES patients. Diarrhea arises from the hypersecretion of acid, which inactivates pancreatic enzymes (leading to malabsorption and steatorrhea), damages enterocytes, and causes primary bile acids to become insoluble. Nasogastric suctioning can alleviate the diarrhea. In advanced cases, patients experience symptoms directly from the growth of the gastrinoma. Patients with ZES and MEN 1 syndrome may also present with primary hyperparathyroidism as well as anterior pituitary tumors, and up to 37% develop gastric carcinoids.

Over 70% of ZES patients develop peptic ulcers, which can appear similar to ulcers associated with *H pylori* and

Table 16–1. Clinical symptoms of patients with Zollinger-Ellison syndrome.

Clinical Findings	Percentage Among 261 Patients at NIH	Range of Percentages of Patients in Literature
Abdominal pain	75	26-98
Diarrhea	73	17-73
Gastroesophageal reflux symptoms	44	0-56
Nausea	30	0-37
Vomiting	25	0-51
Bleeding	24	8-75
MEN 1 present	22	10-48
History of peptic ulcer	71	71-93

MEN, multiple endocrine neoplasia; NIH, National Institutes of Health. Data from Roy PK, Venzon DJ, Shojamanesh H, et al. Zollinger-Ellison syndrome. Clinical presentation in 261 patients. *Medicine (Baltimore)*. 2000;79:379; and Jensen RT. Gastrinomas: advances in diagnosis and management. Neuroendocrinology. 2004;80:23.

nonsteroidal anti-inflammatory drug (NSAID) use. ZES patients often also have prominent gastric folds that can be seen on upper endoscopy. Only a small fraction present with a perforated ulcer or esophageal stricture. ZES should be suspected in patients who have had peptic ulcers in unusual locations (eg, second part of the duodenum and jejunum), patients with severe ulcers refractory to acid-suppressive medications, ulcer patients with hypercalcemia, and those with a personal history or family history of MEN 1 syndrome. Clinicians should also consider ZES among patients who present with the triad of abdominal pain, diarrhea, and weight loss as well as patients with prominent gastric rugal folds on endoscopy. ZES may also be considered as a rare cause of ulcers in patients without *H pylori* infection who have not taken any aspirin or NSAIDs.

Morrow EH, Norton JA. Surgical management of Zollinger-Ellison syndrome: state of the art. *Surg Clin North Am.* 2009;89:1091–1103. [PMID: 19836486]

Roy PK, Venzon DJ, Shojamanesh H, et al. Zollinger-Ellison syndrome. Clinical presentation in 261 patients. *Medicine (Baltimore)*. 2000;79:379–411. [PMID: 11144036]

B. Laboratory Findings

The diagnosis of ZES is based on finding an elevated fasting serum gastrin level associated with gastric acid hypersecretion. The upper limit of normal for gastrin is 110 pg/mL. Figure 16–1 is an algorithm outlining an approach to the evaluation of ZES. Patients suspected of having ZES should have a measurement of a fasting serum gastrin level, ideally while they are off all acid-suppressive medications. PPIs should be stopped at least 1 week before testing. Patients who develop significant gastrointestinal symptoms after temporarily stopping their PPIs may require high-dose histamine-2 (H_2)-receptor blockers and frequent antacids. The H_2-receptor blockers should be stopped at least 2 days before testing while the patient continues to frequently take high doses of antacids.

A serum gastrin concentration above 1000 pg/mL in a patient with an acidic stomach pH below 2.0 is considered diagnostic of ZES (in patients who do not have a retained gastric antrum), and no other diagnostic studies are necessary. Unfortunately, this occurs in only 5–9% of ZES patients. Patients with more moderate degrees of hypergastrinemia may require more detailed investigations. Up to 40% of ZES patients actually have elevated serum gastrin levels of less than 500 pg/mL. This range of hypergastrinemia can overlap with non-ZES patients having low acid secretion. Many of these patients without ZES develop a secondary hypergastrinemia in response to high gastric pH and decreased acid feedback inhibition of gastrin release. Patients taking PPIs as well as those with *H pylori* infection or chronic atrophic gastritis/pernicious anemia and hypochlorhydria can develop significant hypergastrinemia. Other causes of hypergastrinemia that are not associated with excessive acid secretion include renal failure or uremia, short gut syndrome, or status post vagotomy. Disorders causing hypergastrinemia with excessive acid secretion include G-cell hyperplasia, retained gastric antrum (eg, intact antrum after Billroth type II partial gastrectomy), and gastric outlet obstruction.

Murugesan SV, Varro A, Pritchard DM. Review article: strategies to determine whether hypergastrinaemia is due to Zollinger-Ellison syndrome rather than a more common benign cause. *Aliment Pharmacol Ther.* 2009;29:1055–1068. [PMID: 19226290]

C. Special Tests

The secretin stimulation test can establish the diagnosis of ZES and is the provocative test of choice because of its high sensitivity, ease of administration, and minimal side effects. Some studies suggest that secretin can stimulate gastrin release by direct interaction with receptors on gastrinoma cells. Intravenous administration of secretin stimulates an exaggerated serum gastrin increase in ZES patients, while the serum gastrin level falls or remains unchanged in other disorders.

During secretin stimulation testing, a baseline serum gastrin is measured and then 2 units/kg of body weight of secretin (Secretin-Kabi) are administered intravenously over 1 minute. Repeated measurements of gastrin are subsequently made 2, 5, 10, 15, and 20 minutes later. A widely used criterion for a positive secretin stimulation test is an absolute increase in serum gastrin by 200 pg/mL or greater after secretin injection. This result has a sensitivity and specificity of over 83%

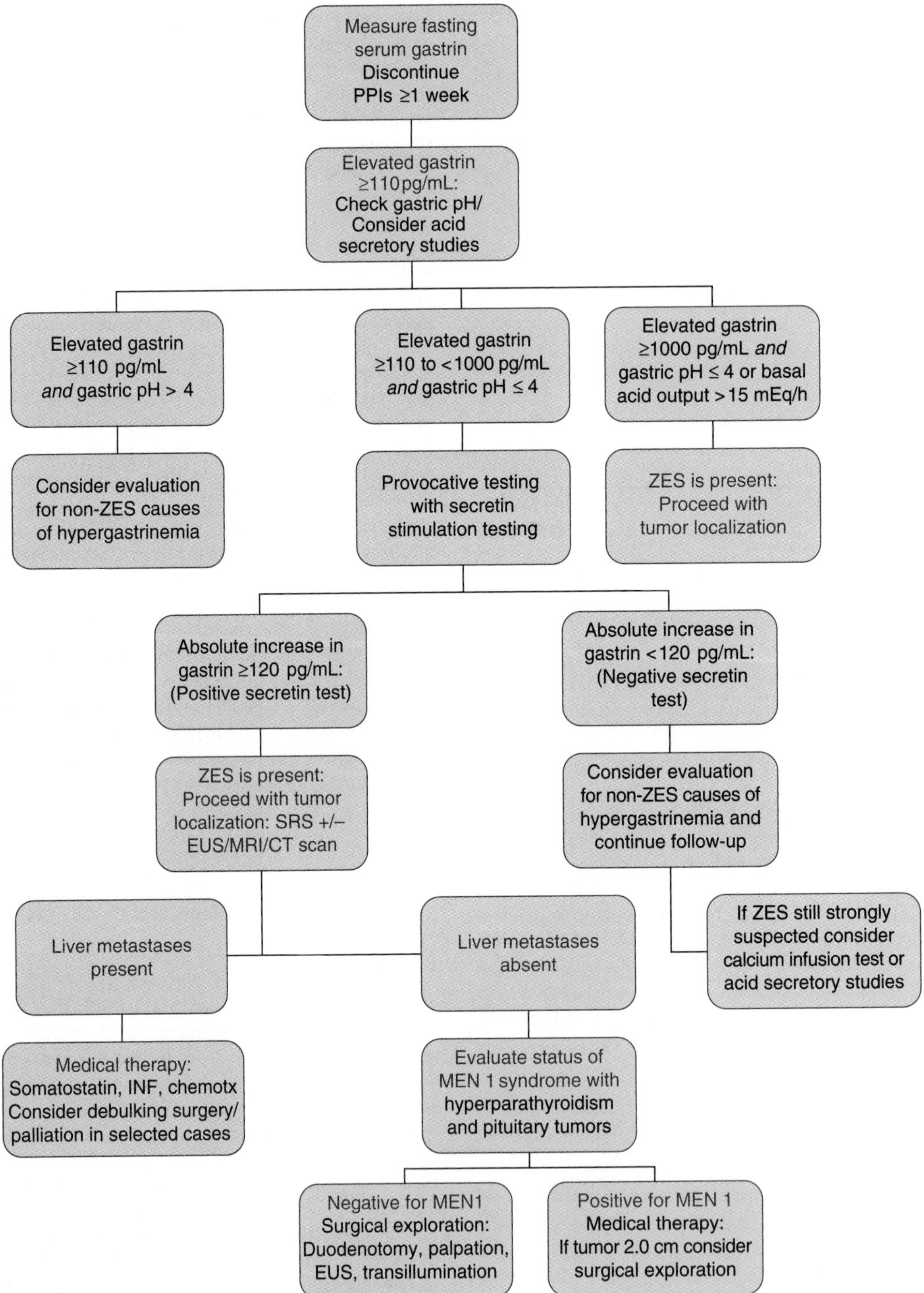

▲ **Figure 16–1.** Algorithm for evaluation of suspected Zollinger-Ellison syndrome (ZES). chemotx, chemotherapy; CT, computed tomography; EUS, endoscopic ultrasound; INF, alfa-interferon; MEN 1, multiple endocrine neoplasia syndrome type 1; PPIs, proton pump inhibitors; MRI, magnetic resonance imaging; somatostatin, somatostatin analog therapy; SRS, somatostatin receptor scintigraphy.

for detecting gastrinomas. However, a new criterion for the diagnosis of ZES has been recommended by Jensen and colleagues as part of a large study involving 293 ZES patients from the National Institutes of Health who were compared with 537 patients in the literature. An absolute increase in gastrin of more than 120 pg/mL was found to have the highest sensitivity (94%) and a specificity of 100%. It is important to note that another preparation of secretin is now also available that is made by the Repligen Corporation (Waltham, MA) and is given at a dose of 0.4 mcg/kg of body weight.

The calcium infusion study has less diagnostic accuracy (with a sensitivity of 62%) and is difficult to perform. It is also associated with adverse side effects but may be positive in the rare gastrinoma patient with a negative or equivocal secretion stimulation result. During meal provocative testing, the gastrin response unfortunately overlaps with those seen in patients with antral syndromes and is thus generally not useful. Gastric acid secretion studies have previously aided in the diagnosis of ZES through a determination of the basal acid output (BAO) and pentagastrin-stimulated acid output (MAO) but are not widely available. Hypergastrinemia with a BAO greater than 15 mEq/h or greater than 5 mEq/h in patients with a prior vagotomy and partial gastrectomy is suggestive of ZES. These acid output studies are mainly reserved to monitor response and determine an adequate dose of acid-suppressive medications. Recent reports suggest that serum levels of chromogranin A may also be helpful, because this value is frequently elevated in patients with neuroendocrine tumors including those with gastrinomas.

Berna MJ, Hoffman KM, Long SH, et al. Serum gastrin in Zollinger-Ellison syndrome: II. Prospective study of gastrin provocative testing in 293 patients from the National Institutes of Health and comparison with 537 cases from the literature. Evaluation of diagnostic criteria, proposal of new criteria, and correlations with clinical and tumoral features. *Medicine (Baltimore).* 2006;85:331–364. [PMID: 17108779]

D. Imaging Studies

More than 80% of gastrinomas are localized in a gastrinoma triangle area that is defined by the convergence of the cystic duct and common bile duct, the junction of the second and third portion of the head and body of the duodenum, and the junction of the head and body of the pancreas. Over 80% of duodenal gastrinomas are located in the first and second portion of the duodenum. Duodenal gastrinomas tend to be small and multiple, whereas pancreatic gastrinomas are often larger than 1 cm. The gastrinomas associated with MEN 1 syndrome are also multiple and localized in the duodenum. Rare extrapancreatic sites include the gastric antrum-pyloric area, ovaries, bones, mesentery, liver, bile duct, heart, and lymph nodes.

Gastrinomas express somatostatin receptors that bind octreotide, and this can be used for tumor imaging. Most gastrinomas can now be localized through the use of somatostatin receptor scintigraphy (SRS) with 111-Indium pentetreotide (OctreoScan) and single photon emission computed tomography. Although computed tomography (CT) scanning and magnetic resonance imaging are widely available and may be helpful, SRS is more sensitive than all conventional imaging studies combined and should be considered as the first imaging method used because of its sensitivity (85%) and cost effectiveness. The sensitivity of CT scans ranges from 54–56%, and sensitivity of magnetic resonance imaging ranges from 25–30%. SRS is extremely useful for diagnosing primary and metastatic liver lesions as well as bone metastasis in affected patients. Endoscopic ultrasound is also useful for preoperative tumor localization (with a sensitivity of 67%) and staging in ZES patients, especially for tumors in the head and body of the pancreas. The combined use of SRS and endoscopic ultrasound has an overall sensitivity of 93% for detecting gastrinomas.

Morrow EH, Norton JA. Surgical management of Zollinger-Ellison syndrome: state of the art. *Surg Clin North Am.* 2009;89: 1091–1103. [PMID: 19836486]

E. Special Examinations

The more invasive localization methods such as portal venous sampling and selective intra-arterial injection of secretin combined with venous sampling have high sensitivity but only provide for a regionalization and not an exact localization of the tumor. During exploratory surgery, duodenotomy is the method of choice to find duodenal gastrinomas. The addition of endoscopic transillumination of the duodenal wall and intraoperative ultrasonography may increase detection of small duodenal tumors not seen on other imaging studies.

Treatment

The principal goals of treating ZES patients are to medically control gastric acid hypersecretion (which reduces symptoms and complications) and attempt surgical cure (ie, removal) in selected patients or control tumor growth. The acid hypersecretion can be effectively treated both acutely and long term through the use of high doses of oral PPIs such as omeprazole, 60–120 mg/day. Since the development of these powerful acid-suppressive medications, the survival of patients with gastrinomas primarily depends on tumor growth and the extent of disease involvement.

Surgical exploration with possible curative resection is recommended for all ZES patients without MEN 1 syndrome who are also free of liver and distant metastases. This includes sporadic ZES patients with localized resectable tumor in addition to those with no tumor found on imaging studies. Unfortunately, preoperative imaging may miss up to 30% of gastrinomas. Intraoperative methods, such as duodenotomy, palpation, transillumination of the duodenal wall, ultrasonography, or a combination of these techniques, greatly help to localize the gastrinoma. The goal of surgery in sporadic ZES is to cure the disease. Experienced surgeons have recommended an exploratory laparotomy with extended Kocher maneuver and careful palpation of the pancreas and duodenum for nodules. Reports suggest that duodenotomy is very effective in identifying duodenal gastrinomas, which account for 60% of gastrinomas. Appropriate patients should also undergo enucleation of pancreatic head tumors, or distal pancreatectomy for tail lesions, and duodenotomy and regional lymphadenopathy. One study reported an immediate postsurgical cure rate of 60% with a subsequent 10-year cure rate of 34%. Another large study of 195 ZES patients followed for 12 years after diagnosis demonstrated that surgical exploration for gastrinoma removal or cure significantly increased patient survival. Patients undergoing surgery had greater disease-related survival than nonsurgery patients, which was attributed to significant reductions in (the remaining) tumor growth and progression as well as liver metastases.

The role of surgery in patients with ZES as part of the MEN 1 syndrome remains controversial because these gastrinomas are multifocal and surgery is rarely curative. As a result, an individualized approach to these patients should be considered. Several studies have shown that MEN 1 patients with small gastrinomas (<2 cm) usually have an indolent clinical course and excellent long-term prognosis. However, because primary tumor size does affect the subsequent development of liver metastases, surgical exploration should be considered for ZES patients with MEN 1 having tumors greater than 2–2.5 cm in an attempt to decrease the risk of malignant spread.

As previously indicated, ZES patients with diffuse liver metastases, especially those that are rapidly increasing in size, have substantially reduced survival. Aggressive surgical resection or cytoreductive surgery in patients with advanced disease may be considered to improve outcomes. Embolization, chemoembolization, and cryoablation of liver lesions are alternative approaches for palliation. Somatostatin analogs are often used alone or with alfa-interferon as the initial antitumor therapy. Somatostatin analogs such as octreotide and lanreotide, as well as the long-acting depot form lanreotide-SR, not only help control acid secretion but may also decrease tumor size or slow its growth. Systemic chemotherapy with streptozotocin, doxorubicin, or 5-fluorouracil potentially decreases the tumor size in a small proportion of patients but does not appear to improve survival. These agents also have substantial toxicity and are reserved for patients with diffuse metastatic disease. Cytotoxic chemotherapy with temozolomide has also been reportedly effective in a small series of patients with malignant neuroendocrine tumors. The role of liver transplant is still under investigation but may be considered for younger patients with metastases limited to the liver.

Somatostatin analogs are often used alone or with alfa-interferon as the initial antitumor therapy. This includes the long-acting somatostatin analogs such as octreotide-LAR or lanreotide-SR or the auto-gel preparations that not only help control acid secretion but may also decrease tumor size or slow its growth. Systemic chemotherapy with streptozotocin, doxorubicin, or 5-fluorouracil potentially decreases the tumor size in a small proportion of patients but does not appear to improve survival. These agents also have substantial toxicity and are reserved for patients with diffuse metastatic disease. The role of liver transplantation is still under investigation but may be considered for younger patients with metastases limited to the liver.

Fendrich V, Langer P, Waldmann J, et al. Management of sporadic and multiple endocrine neoplasia type 1 gastrinomas. *Br J Surg.* 2007;94:1331–1341. [PMID: 17939142]

Morrow EH, Norton JA. Surgical management of Zollinger-Ellison syndrome: state of the art. *Surg Clin North Am.* 2009;89: 1091–1103. [PMID: 19836486]

Mortellaro VE, Hochwald SN, McGuigan JE, et al. Long-term results of a selective surgical approach to management of Zollinger-Ellison syndrome in patients with MEN-1. *Am Surg.* 2009;75:730–733. [PMID: 19725300]

Norton JA, Fraker DL, Alexander HR, et al. Surgery increases survival in patients with gastrinoma. *Ann Surg.* 2006;244:410–419. [PMID: 16926567]

Norton JA, Jensen RT. Role of surgery in Zollinger-Ellison syndrome. *J Am Coll Surg.* 2007;205:S34–37. [PMID: 17916516]

Tomassetti P, Campana D, Piscitelli L, et al. Treatment of Zollinger-Ellison syndrome. *World J Gastroenterol.* 2005;11:5423–5432. [PMID: 16222731]

Prognosis

Several reports suggest that 60–90% of gastrinomas are malignant. Tumor progression and the presence of metastases are the main determinants of survival. Patients with a gastrinoma and diffuse liver metastases have a 10-year survival rate of 15%, whereas gastrinoma patients without liver metastases have a much better prognosis with a 20-year survival of 95%. In part due to a larger tumor size and hence a greater propensity for liver metastases, the survival rate of patients with pancreatic gastrinomas tends to be lower than that of patients with duodenal gastrinomas. The 10-year survival rate was 57% in patients with sporadic pancreatic gastrinomas and 84% in patients with duodenal gastrinomas. An aggressive form of gastrinoma develops more commonly among female ZES patients without the MEN 1 syndrome who have shorter disease duration but large pancreatic tumors with liver metastases.

Fendrich V, Langer P, Waldmann J, et al. Management of sporadic and multiple endocrine neoplasia type 1 gastrinomas. *Br J Surg.* 2007;94:1331–1341. [PMID: 17939142]

Morrow EH, Norton JA. Surgical management of Zollinger-Ellison syndrome: state of the art. *Surg Clin North Am.* 2009;89: 1091–1103. [PMID: 19836486]

Functional (Nonulcer) Dyspepsia

17

Walter W. Chan, MD, MPH
Robert Burakoff, MD, MPH

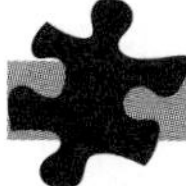

ESSENTIALS OF DIAGNOSIS

- Dyspepsia is a common symptom having either an organic or a functional cause; distinguishing between the two can be a challenge.
- Clinical features of functional dyspepsia, gastroesophageal reflux disease, and gastrointestinal motility disorders overlap, making diagnosis difficult.
- Most patients with functional dyspepsia have normal esophagogastroduodenoscopy (EGD) findings.
- Endoscopy is indicated for patients with new-onset symptoms who are >55 years of age or have alarm features.
- Functional dyspepsia remains a diagnosis of exclusion.

General Considerations

This chapter outlines the evaluation and management of dyspepsia, with a primary focus on functional dyspepsia, also interchangeably called nonulcer dyspepsia. The term *dyspepsia* derives from the Greek "dys," meaning bad, and "pepsis," meaning digestion. Dyspepsia is a symptom, not a diagnosis. The term encompasses a broad spectrum of symptoms that include upper abdominal pain or discomfort, bloating, early satiety, postprandial fullness, nausea with or without vomiting, anorexia, symptoms of gastroesophageal reflux disease (GERD), regurgitation, and belching.

A. Classification

The multiple causes of dyspepsia can be classified as organic or functional. Among the organic causes are esophagitis, gastritis, peptic ulcer disease, benign esophageal strictures, upper gastrointestinal malignancies, chronic intestinal ischemia, and pancreaticobiliary disease. In addition, several medications can cause dyspeptic symptoms (Table 17–1). Most notable are nonsteroidal anti-inflammatory drugs (NSAIDs), which can cause mucosal injury leading to gastritis. Functional dyspepsia excludes all organic causes.

Previously, the Rome II criteria defined functional dyspepsia as pain centered in the upper abdomen in the setting of a normal endoscopy, with three main subtypes: ulcer-like, dysmotility-like, and unspecified (nonspecific). Recognizing that patients with functional dyspepsia may present with epigastric symptoms other than pain, the revised Rome III criteria in 2006 added bothersome postprandial fullness, early satiation, and epigastric burning to the diagnostic criteria (Table 17–2). Therefore, functional dyspepsia is now defined as "the presence of symptoms thought to originate from the gastroduodenal region, in the absence of any organic, systemic, or metabolic disease that is likely to explain the symptoms." In addition, the prior subtypes were revised to improve their clinical utility. Per Rome III criteria, functional dyspepsia symptoms fall into two main, distinctively defined disorders: postprandial distress syndrome and epigastric pain syndrome. Postprandial distress syndrome includes bloating, fullness, or early satiety with meals, while epigastric pain syndrome is defined by focal burning or pain localized to the epigastric region not relating to gallbladder or biliary causes. Postprandial distress syndrome and epigastric pain syndrome may coexist in patients with functional dyspepsia.

Tack J, Talley NJ, Camilleri M, et al. Functional gastroduodenal disorders. *Gastroenterology.* 2006;130:1466–1479. [PMID: 16678560]

B. Epidemiology

Prior studies estimated that 20–30% of community patients report dyspeptic symptoms each year, with the majority believed to be related to functional dyspepsia. In prospective studies, the incidence of patients reporting dyspeptic symptoms for the first time is approximately 1% per year. It is believed that only about half of the patients with dyspeptic

Table 17–1. Medications that can cause dyspepsia.

Acarbose
Aspirin, nonsteroidal anti-inflammatory drugs
Colchicine
Digitalis preparations
Estrogens
Gemfibrozil
Glucocorticoids
Iron
Levodopa
Narcotics
Niacin
Nitrates
Orlistat
Potassium chloride
Quinidine
Sildenafil
Theophylline

symptoms ultimately seek medical care, with severity of pain and anxiety being the significant predictive factors. Of patients who have not been worked up, 40% may have an organic cause for their dyspepsia. The prevalence of functional dyspepsia is about 12–15%.

Table 17–2. Rome III criteria for functional dyspepsia.

Functional Dyspepsia—at least 3 months, with onset at least 6 months previously of 1 or more of the following:
- Bothersome postprandial fullness
- Early satiation
- Epigastric pain
- Epigastric burning

  And
- No evidence of structural disease (including at upper endoscopy) that is likely to explain the symptoms

Subtypes

a. Postprandial Distress Syndrome—at least 3 months, with onset at least 5 months previously of 1 or more of the following:
   - Bothersome postprandial fullness
     1. Occurring after ordinary-sized meals
     2. At least several times a week

     Or
   - Early satiation
     1. That prevents finishing a regular meal
     2. And occurs at least several times a week

b. Epigastric Pain Syndrome—at least 3 months, with onset at least 6 months previously, with all of the following:
   - Pain and burning that is:
     1. Intermittent
     2. Localized to the epigastrium of at least moderate severity, at least once per week
   - And *not*
     1. Generalized or localized to other abdominal or chest regions
     2. Relieved by defecation or flatulence
   - Fulfilling criteria for gallbladder or sphincter of Oddi disorders

Dyspepsia has led to sizeable health care burden, with new cases accounting for 5–7% of primary care office visits. Dyspeptic symptoms can account for up to 40–70% of gastrointestinal complaints in a general gastroenterology practice. The cost of treatment is substantial.

El-Serag HB, Talley NJ. Systematic review: the prevalence and clinical course of functional dyspepsia. *Aliment Pharmacol Ther.* 2004;19:643–654. [PMID: 15023166]

Fraser A, Delaney B, Moayyedi P. Symptom-based outcome measures for dyspepsia GERD trials: a systematic review. *Am J Gastroenterol.* 2005;100:442–452. [PMID: 15667506]

Pathogenesis

Organic dyspepsia can develop as a consequence of the varied disease processes mentioned in this chapter and described elsewhere in this text. The pathogenesis of functional dyspepsia is unclear. Factors that play a role in causation include altered visceral sensitivity, disturbances in motility, alterations in gastric accommodation, dietary factors, and psychosomatic factors. The role of *Helicobacter pylori* in the genesis of symptoms is controversial.

A. Altered Gastrointestinal Motility

Disturbances in gastrointestinal motility may be associated with dyspepsia symptoms and represent the underlying causative factor in functional dyspepsia. Motor disorders such as gastroesophageal reflux, gastroparesis, small bowel dysmotility, and biliary dyskinesia may cause dyspeptic symptoms. Disturbances in gastric emptying and gastrointestinal motor function occur in subgroups of patients with functional dyspepsia, and studies of these patients show female sex predominance. The prevalence of motility disorders has varied markedly between studies, likely due to subject selection criteria and study methodology. A meta-analysis of studies investigating functional dyspepsia and disturbed solid phase gastric emptying found 40% of patients with functional dyspepsia had slower emptying, and the pooled estimate of slowing was 1.5 times that of normal patients. On the other hand, a prospective study using a liquid test meal demonstrated that decreased maximum-tolerated meal volume and increased postprandial symptoms were associated with faster gastric emptying.

As mentioned, symptoms of GERD often overlap with dyspepsia symptoms. Poor visceral localization of symptoms can often cause a reflux event to be confused with other upper gastrointestinal sources of discomfort. A study of patients with diagnosis of functional dyspepsia per Rome III criteria revealed that almost one third had pathologic signs of acid reflux. In addition, both acid and nonacid reflux can cause symptoms. A report noted that patients with functional dyspepsia swallow air more frequently than controls; this finding was associated with an increase in nonacid reflux, which can also cause epigastric symptoms.

Conchillo JM, Selimah M, Bredenoord AJ, et al. Air swallowing, belching, acid and non-acid reflux in patients with functional dyspepsia. *Aliment Pharm Ther.* 2007;25:965–971. [PMID: 17403001]

Talley NJ, Locke GR, Lahr BD, et al. Functional dyspepsia, delayed gastric emptying, and impaired quality of life. *Gut.* 2006;55:933–939. [PMID: 16322108]

XiaoYL, Peng S, Tao J, et al. Prevalence and symptom pattern of pathologic esophageal acid reflux in patients with functional dyspepsia based on the Rome III criteria. *Am J Gastroenterol.* 2010;105:2626–2631. [PMID: 20823838]

B. Altered Gastric Accommodation

Alterations in gastric accommodation or compliance have been hypothesized to be a cause of functional dyspepsia. During normal ingestion of food, the gastric fundus relaxes to "accommodate" the food particles. This accommodation is mediated by serotonin (5-HT_{1p}) and nitric oxide via vagal inhibitory neurons of the enteric nervous system. The accommodation reflex may be impaired in as many as 40% of patients with functional dyspepsia, as demonstrated by gastric scintigraphy and ultrasound. Measurement of gastric pressure by a barostat, or a polyethylene balloon inflated in the stomach, connected to a pressure monitor has shown impaired meal-induced accommodation as well.

Kindt S, Tack J. Impaired gastric accommodation and its role in dyspepsia. *Gut.* 2006;55:1685–1691. [PMID: 16854999]

C. Visceral Hypersensitivity

While poor gastric compliance may result in dyspepsia symptoms, some patients may instead have normal gastric compliance but a lowered pain threshold. With visceral hypersensitivity or hyperalgesia, patients begin to experience pain or discomfort at a level of gastric distention normally not associated with symptoms in healthy individuals., resulting from increased sensory input to and from the stomach. Such enhanced perception is not limited to mechanical distention, but may also occur in response to temperature stress, acid exposure, chemical or nutrient stimuli, or hormones, such as cholecystokinin and glucagons-like peptide 1. In patients with visceral hypersensitivity, there may be altered central nervous system processing of these stimuli. Studies have demonstrated hypersensitivity to balloon distention in the stomach in as many as 50% of patients with functional dyspepsia. Compared with controls, patients with functional dyspepsia had a significantly lower threshold to both initial sensation of balloon distention and to sensation of pain. Some have suggested that such alteration in perception may be the main distinguishing factor between functional and organic dyspepsia. A similar mechanism of pathogenesis has also been proposed for irritable bowel syndrome.

Mertz H, Fullerton S, Naliboff B, et al. Symptoms and visceral perception in severe functional and organic dyspepsia. *Gut.* 1998;42:814–822. [PMID: 9691920]

D. Dietary Factors

Dietary factors may be a potential cause of symptoms in functional dyspepsia. Patients with functional dyspepsia appear to have altered eating patterns as well as food intolerances. They frequently report being able to tolerate only small quantities of food, with a high prevalence of snacking and low prevalence of eating large meals. Food intolerances are also high in prevalence among these patients. Fatty foods, in particular, have been linked to dyspepsia. Other intolerances with a reported prevalence greater than 40% include spices, alcohol, spicy foods, chocolate, peppers, citrus fruits, and fish. However, a recent epidemiologic study found no difference in total caloric, protein, fat, and carbohydrate intake between patients with dyspepsia and healthy controls. In particular, the percentages of protein, fat, and carbohydrate in their diet were also similar. In the same study, alcohol and nicotine use were not found to be risk factors for dyspepsia.

Food allergy has been cited as a possible mechanism for development of dyspeptic symptoms, especially postprandial symptoms. Some common food-specific immunoglobulin G antibody titers have been found to be elevated in functional dyspepsia patients compared to controls.

Feinle-Bisset C, Horowitz M. Review article: dietary factors in functional dyspepsia. *Neurogastroenterol Motil.* 2006;18: 608–618. [PMID: 16918725]

Gathaiya N, Locke GR, Camilleri M, et al. Novel associations with dyspepsia: a community-based study of familial aggregation, sleep dysfunction and somatization. *Neurogastroenterol Motil.* 2009;21:922–e69. [PMID: 19496951]

Zuo XL, Li YQ, Li WJ, et al. Alterations of food antigen-specific serum immunoglobulins G and E antibodies in patients with irritable bowel syndrome and functional dyspepsia. *Clin Exp Allergy.* 2007;37:823–830. [PMID: 17517095]

E. *Helicobacter pylori* Infection

The role of *H pylori* in functional dyspepsia is controversial, and no clear causal relationship has been established. This is true for both the symptom profile and pathophysiology of functional dyspepsia. Although some epidemiologic studies have suggested an association between *H pylori* infection and functional dyspepsia, others have not. The discrepancy may stem in part from differences in methodology and lack of adequate consideration of confounding factors such as past history of peptic ulcer disease and socioeconomic status. Controlled trials disagree about whether or not *H pylori* eradication is beneficial in functional dyspepsia, with roughly half of the trials showing improvement and the other half no improvement. A prior systematic review in the *Annals of Internal Medicine* on the benefit of eradicating *H pylori* in functional dyspepsia suggested no statistically significant effect, with an odds ratio (OR) for treatment success versus control of 1.29 (95% confidence interval [CI], 0.89–1.89; $P = .18$). However, the most recent update of a Cochrane Database review showed a small but statistically significant effect in curing symptoms (*H pylori* cure vs placebo, 36% vs 30%, respectively; relative risk reduction [RRR], 8%; 95% CI, 3–18%; number needed to treat [NNT] = 18). Despite the conflicting results, current guidelines by both major gastroenterological societies in the United States recommend eradication of *H pylori* in patients with functional dyspepsia.

Laine L, Schoenfeld P, Fennerty MB. Therapy for *Helicobacter pylori* in patients with nonulcer dyspepsia. A meta-analysis of randomized, controlled trials. *Ann Intern Med.* 2001;134: 361–369. [PMID: 11242496]

Moayyedi P, Deeks J, Talley NJ, et al. An update of the Cochrane systematic review of *Helicobacter pylori* eradication therapy in nonulcer dyspepsia: resolving the discrepancy between systematic reviews. *Am J Gastroenterol.* 2003;98:2621–2626. [PMID: 14687807]

Talley NJ, Quan C. Review article: *Helicobacter pylori* and nonulcer dyspepsia. *Aliment Pharmacol Ther.* 2002;16(Suppl 1):58–65. [PMID: 11849130]

F. Duodenal Eosinophilia

In recent years, some have hypothesized that duodenal eosinophilia may play a role in a subset of patients with functional dyspepsia. Several recent studies have shown significantly greater eosinophil counts in duodenal biopsies from patients with functional dyspepsia compared to those from healthy controls. These studies suggest that duodenal eosinophils may play a role in functional dyspepsia. However, eosinophilic infiltration has also been described in many different clinical scenarios, including healthy individuals. Therefore, the role of duodenal eosinophils in functional dyspepsia remains to be elucidated.

Talley NJ, Walker MM, Aro P, et al. Non-ulcer dyspepsia and duodenal eosinophilia: an adult endoscopic population-based case-control study. *Clin Gastroenterol Hepatol.* 2007;5:1175–1183. [PMID: 17686660]

G. Psychological Factors

Psychosomatic and cognitive factors are important in the evaluation of patients with chronic dyspepsia. The psychiatric hypothesis holds that the symptoms of dyspepsia maybe due to depression, increased anxiety, or a somatization disorder. Epidemiologic studies suggest there is an association between functional dyspepsia and psychological disorders. Symptoms of neurosis, anxiety, hypochondriasis, and depression are more common in patients being evaluated for unexplained gastrointestinal complaints than in healthy controls. In addition, prior studies have demonstrated significant associations between dyspepsia symptoms and a history of abuse in childhood or adulthood. Comparisons of functional and organic dyspepsia have shown that patients with functional dyspepsia are less likely to have decreased stress or anxiety at 1-year follow-up after being reassured of having no serious disease. This suggests that functional dyspepsia symptoms are long-lasting, compared with those of organic dyspepsia, and that the emotional ties are strong.

Castillo EJ, Camilleri M, Locke GR, et al. A community-based, controlled study of the epidemiology and pathophysiology of dyspepsia. *Clin Gastroenterol Hepatol.* 2004;2:985–996. [PMID: 15551251]

Pajala M, Heikkinen M, Hintikka J. A prospective 1-year follow-up study in patients with functional or organic dyspepsia: changes in gastrointestinal symptoms, mental distress and fear of serious illness. *Aliment Pharmacol Ther.* 2006;24:1241–1246. [PMID: 17014583]

Talley NJ, Fett SL, Zinsmeister R, et al. Gastrointestinal tract symptoms and self-reported abuse: a population-based study. *Gastroenterology.* 1994;107:1040–1049. [PMID: 7926457]

Clinical Findings

A. Symptoms and Signs

The initial clinical evaluation should focus on symptom characteristics, onset, and chronicity. The clinician should try to interpret the symptoms in order to identify possible etiologies such as GERD, gallstones, medications side effects (particularly NSAIDs), chronic pancreatitis, diabetic gastroparesis, or obstruction. The patient should be asked about comorbidities, surgical history, family history of upper gastrointestinal malignancy, alcohol and tobacco use, dietary changes or allergies, stressful life events, and psychological factors.

In most cases, however, the clinical history is of limited use in distinguishing organic causes from functional dyspepsia. A large systematic review of the literature was performed to evaluate the effectiveness of diagnosing organic dyspepsia by clinical opinion versus computer models in patients referred for upper endoscopy. The computer models were based on patient demographics, risk factors, historical items, and symptoms. The study showed that neither clinical impression nor computer models were able to adequately distinguish organic from functional disease.

In a recent study, patients with peptic ulcer disease were compared with patients with functional dyspepsia in an age- and sex-matched study. Although the functional dyspepsia group reported more upper abdominal fullness and nausea and overall greater distress and anxiety, almost all the same symptoms were seen in both groups.

Therefore, it is the clinician's challenging task to separate patients who may have an organic disorder, and thus warrant further diagnostic testing, from patients who have functional dyspepsia, who are given empiric symptomatic treatment. The workup should be targeted to identify or rule out specific causes. Traditionally, high-risk patients have been identified by "alarm" features, which are listed in Table 17–3. However, the utility of these features in identifying

Table 17–3. "Alarm" features suggestive of the presence of upper gastrointestinal malignancy.

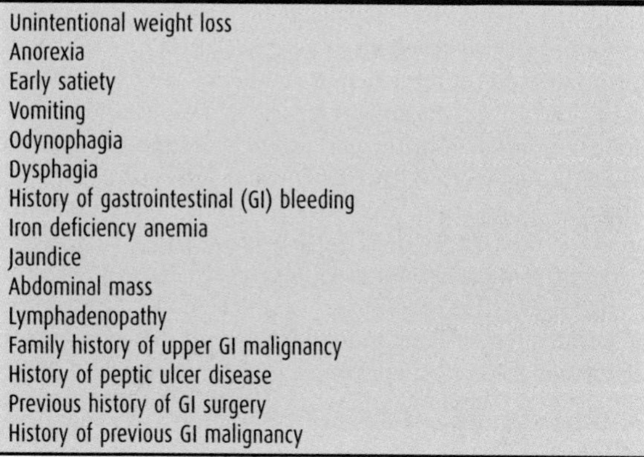

Unintentional weight loss
Anorexia
Early satiety
Vomiting
Odynophagia
Dysphagia
History of gastrointestinal (GI) bleeding
Iron deficiency anemia
Jaundice
Abdominal mass
Lymphadenopathy
Family history of upper GI malignancy
History of peptic ulcer disease
Previous history of GI surgery
History of previous GI malignancy

the presence of upper gastrointestinal malignancy has been debated. A meta-analysis looking at the sensitivity and specificity of alarm features found a range of 0–80% and 40–98%, respectively. However, there was high heterogeneity between studies.

The physical examination may elicit abdominal tenderness. Although this finding is nonspecific, several features may shed lights on possible underlying etiologies. A positive Carnett sign, or focal tenderness that increases with abdominal wall contraction and palpation, suggests an etiology involving the abdominal wall musculature. Cutaneous dermatomal distribution of pain may suggest a thoracic polyradiculopathy. Thump tenderness over the right upper quadrant may suggest chronic cholecystitis. Most commonly, however, the physical examination is normal.

Flier SN, Rose S. Is functional dyspepsia of particular concern in women? A review of gender differences in epidemiology, pathophysiologic mechanism, clinical presentation and management. *Am J Gastroenterol.* 2006;101:S644–S653. [PMID: 17177870]

Moayyedi P, Talley NJ, Fennerty MB, et al. Can the clinical history distinguish between organic and functional dyspepsia? *JAMA.* 2006;295:1566–1576. [PMID: 1659759]

B. Diagnostic Evaluation

If a careful history and physical examination, along with judicious use of screening laboratory tests, does not lead to the diagnosis, then other studies with specific management strategies are recommended. Strategic algorithms have been suggested by the American Gastroenterology Association (Figures 17–1 and 17–2) and the American College of Gastroenterology.

There are several main strategies for new-onset dyspepsia, which include (1) empirical histamine-2 (H_2)-receptor blocker therapy; (2) empirical proton pump inhibitor (PPI)

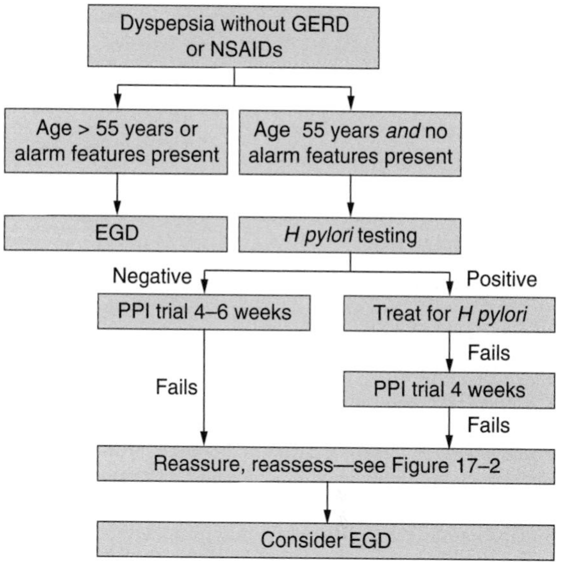

▲ **Figure 17–1.** Management of dyspepsia based on age and alarm features. EGD, esophagogastroduodenoscopy; GERD, gastroesophageal reflux disease; NSAIDs, nonsteroidal anti-inflammatory drugs; PPI, proton pump inhibitor. (Adapted, with permission, from Talley NJ; American Gastroenterological Association. American Gastroenterological Association medical position statement: evaluation of dyspepsia. *Gastroenterology.* 2005;129:1753–1755.)

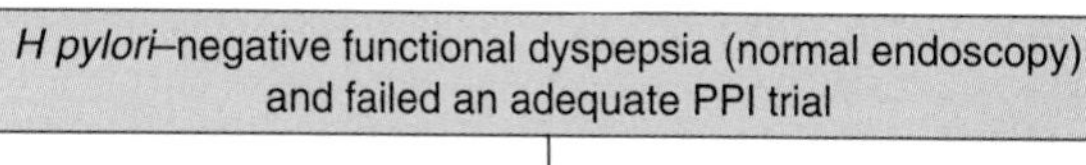

▲ **Figure 17–2.** Management of functional dyspepsia. IBS, irritable bowel syndrome; PPI, proton pump inhibitor. (Adapted, with permission, from Talley NJ; American Gastroenterological Association. American Gastroenterological Association medical position statement: evaluation of dyspepsia. *Gastroenterology.* 2005;129:1753–1755.)

therapy; (3) *H pylori* testing and treatment of positive cases, followed by acid suppression if the patient remains symptomatic; (4) early endoscopy; (5) early endoscopy with biopsy for *H pylori* and treatment, if positive; (6) acid suppression, followed by endoscopy and biopsy if the patient remains symptomatic; or (7) *H pylori* testing and treatment, if positive, followed by endoscopy if the patient remains symptomatic.

Several considerations, outlined below, should guide the selection of a strategy.

1. Esophagogastroduodenoscopy (EGD)—Patients who have not been previously worked up for dyspepsia should be scheduled for EGD if they demonstrate alarm features or are older than 55 years of age. Special consideration also should be given to patients whose country of origin is a region where stomach cancer is more prevalent (eg, Japan, China, and Chile). EGD is the gold standard for evaluating the upper gastrointestinal tract, as it can provide direct visualization and allows the endoscopist to obtain a biopsy specimen of the mucosa if needed. Thus, EGD has essentially replaced the upper gastrointestinal radiologic series as the diagnostic test of choice. Cost effectiveness of early endoscopy in patients older than 50 years of age has been studied in the United Kingdom, with findings of improvement in symptom scores, quality of life, and 48% reduction in use of PPIs. A recent study of 2741 dyspeptic patients without alarm features in the United States found a low prevalence of cancer (0.2%) and an age cut-off of 50 years old for early endoscopy to be adequate for detection of occult malignancy.

Patient's age is an important consideration with regard to endoscopy. The timing of upper endoscopy in younger patients (<55 years) is debatable. Patients who respond to the *H pylori* testing and treatment strategy, outlined below, can be managed without further investigation. In younger patients with continued symptoms despite this strategy, endoscopy usually adds little more to the diagnostic workup. Furthermore, the utility of endoscopy in reassuring patients with functional dyspepsia has been studied and has been deemed questionable as measured by anxiety and depression, which did not change before and after the procedure in these patients.

Vakil N, Talley N, van Zanten SV, et al. Cost of detecting malignant lesions by endoscopy in 2741 primary care dyspeptic patients without alarm symptoms. *Clin Gastroenterol Hepatol.* 2009;7:756–761. [PMID: 19364542]

Van Kerkhoven LA, van Rossum LG, van Oijen MG, et al. Upper gastrointestinal endoscopy does not reassure patients with functional dyspepsia. *Endoscopy.* 2006;38:879–885. [PMID: 16981103]

2. *Helicobacter pylori* testing—For patients younger than 55 years of age and without alarm features, the clinician should first consider testing for *H pylori* and treating, if positive. The optimal test for *H pylori* is a ^{13}C-urea breath test or stool antigen test. *Helicobacter pylori* is the main cause of peptic ulcer disease not associated with NSAID use, and it may be associated with functional dyspepsia in a small fraction of patients. Treatment usually consists of two antibiotics of different classes (eg, amoxicillin and clarithromycin), with a double dose of a PPI (eg, omeprazole, 40 mg twice daily). Many other regimens are available for use if the patient has a history of allergic reactions to a particular class or has previously failed one of the standard regimens (Table 17–4). If the patient is *H pylori*–negative, a trial of acid suppression is suggested; the most optimal approach to acid suppression is use of a PPI. As the prevalence of *H pylori* varies widely among different population, this strategy of *H pylori* test-and-treat followed by PPI trial is particularly recommended for patients from backgrounds with high prevalence of *H pylori* (>10%). On the other hand, empirical PPI therapy for 4–8 weeks before *H pylori* testing has been shown to be cost effective in patients with a low prevalence of *H pylori* (≤10%).

3. Other studies—If a patient's symptoms are suggestive of biliary pain, an ultrasound of the abdomen should be obtained to evaluate the gallbladder for cholelithiasis or cholecystitis. Classic biliary colic is characterized by sudden onset of right upper quadrant pain that is constant, lasting 2–6 hours, associated with nausea, and worsened postprandially. Because of the visceral nature of the pain, it is poorly localizable. Patients with biliary-type pain with findings of gallstones should be considered for cholecystectomy. A quantitative cholescintigraphy scan with cholecystokinin challenge may suggest chronic cholecystitis as the diagnosis if the ejection fraction is less than 50%.

Abdominal computed tomography (CT) can also provide diagnostic clues in patients with chronic unexplained abdominal pain to the presence of chronic pancreatitis, pancreatic cystic lesions, or abdominal tumors such as carcinoid or gastrointestinal stromal tumors (GISTs). CT enterography can visualize the small bowel to aid in looking for undiagnosed Crohn disease or rare small bowel polyps or tumors.

A 24-hour pH test, using a catheter with multichannel intraluminal impedance, can demonstrate acid or nonacid reflux in patients with symptoms likely attributable to GERD. However, in most cases, empiric treatment with PPI therapy is more cost effective and practical. Gastric scintigraphy usually does not add much more information to the diagnostic picture. Although scintigraphy findings may be abnormal in up to 40–50% of cases, they do not help establish the diagnosis or provide therapeutic guidance.

Talley NJ; American Gastroenterological Association. American Gastroenterological Association medical position statement: evaluation of dyspepsia. *Gastroenterology.* 2005;129:1753–1755. [PMID: 16285970]

Talley NJ, Vakil N; Practice Parameter Committee of the American College of Gastroenterology. Guidelines for the management of dyspepsia. *Am J Gastroenterol.* 2005;100:2324–2337. [PMID: 16181387]

Vakil N, Moayyedi P, Fennerty MB, et al. Limited value of alarm features in the diagnosis of upper gastrointestinal malignancy: systematic review and meta-analysis. *Gastroenterology.* 2006;131:390–401. [PMID: 15890692]

Table 17–4. *Helicobacter pylori* eradication regimens.

Description	Regimen	Duration
Traditional first-line therapy	Amoxicillin, 1 g twice daily Clarithromycin, 500 mg twice daily PPI twice daily	7–14 days
First line in penicillin-allergic patients	Metronidazole, 500 mg twice daily Clarithromycin, 500 mg twice daily PPI twice daily	7–14 days
First line in macrolide-allergic patients or those who have failed traditional first-line therapy	Amoxicillin, 1 g twice daily Metronidazole, 500 mg twice daily PPI twice daily	14 days
Rescue therapy for patients failing above therapies	Amoxicillin, 1 g twice daily Levofloxacin, 250–500 mg twice daily PPI twice daily	14 days
Quadruple therapy—used for first-line retreatment	Bismuth, 525 mg 4 times daily Metronidazole, 500 mg 4 times daily Tetracycline, 500 mg 4 times daily PPI twice daily	7–14 days for first-line, 14 days for retreatment
Alternative rescue therapies	Rifabutin, 150 mg twice daily Amoxicillin, 1 g twice daily PPI twice daily *Or* Amoxicillin, 1 g three times daily PPI twice daily	14 days

PPI, proton pump inhibitor.

Differential Diagnosis

The differential diagnosis of dyspepsia is broad. The findings from history and physical examination and judicious use of the diagnostic studies outlined in the preceding section can aid in distinguishing the various organic causes of dyspepsia from functional dyspepsia.

A. GERD and Nonerosive Reflux Disease

GERD and dyspepsia overlap frequently, often coexisting in the same patient. Thus, GERD should always be considered in the dyspeptic patient. If the symptoms are predominantly regurgitation, substernal burning, and acid taste, then GERD is more likely to be the cause than other etiologies. Formal reflux testing with a 24-hour pH study with esophageal impendence off antisecretory medications (eg, PPI) can demonstrate whether reflux, acid or nonacid, is present and identify the association between these reflux events and symptoms.

B. Peptic Ulcer Disease

About 15% of patients with dyspeptic symptoms have gastric or duodenal ulcers. Once diagnosed, the possible underlying causes of the ulcers should be investigated, as many risk factors for peptic ulcers may also lead to dyspepsia symptoms themselves, including the use of NSAIDs and the presence of *H pylori* infection.

C. Upper Gastrointestinal Malignancy

Less than 2% of dyspeptic patients have gastric cancer. Older patients carry a much higher risk, with 98% of cancers occurring in patients older than 50 years of age. Other risks for gastric cancer include *H pylori* infection, country of origin in an area endemic for gastric malignancy (Eastern Asia, the Andean regions of South America, and Eastern Europe), excessive salt and nitrate consumption, tobacco use, and family history of gastric cancer.

D. Chronic Intestinal Ischemia

Chronic intestinal ischemia (so-called intestinal angina) is characterized by chronic postprandial pain with marked weight loss due to mesenteric blood flow that is inadequate to the demands required by digestion. Typically the patient has a history of tobacco use or underlying atherosclerotic disease. A diagnosis may be made by magnetic resonance angiography or CT angiography.

E. Pancreaticobiliary Disease

The pain associated with chronic pancreatitis may be epigastric or localized to the central abdomen, classically with radiation to the mid back. Weight loss may occur. Pancreatic endocrine or exocrine insufficiency (eg, diabetes, steatorrhea) may or may not be present. Cholelithiasis usually is distinguishable from dyspepsia in being more localizable to the right upper quadrant.

F. Motility Disorders

Upper gastrointestinal motility disorders also overlap with dyspepsia. Many patients with functional dyspepsia have gastroparetic-type symptoms, which led to the Rome II classification of "dysmotility-like dyspepsia." This classification was of debatable clinical value, and has now been dropped from the Rome III criteria. Nonetheless, there is a preponderance of symptoms of bloating, early satiety, and nausea with vomiting in patients with functional dyspepsia. Causes of motility disturbance may include diabetic gastroparesis, chronic intestinal pseudo-obstruction, scleroderma, or post-vagotomy syndromes.

G. Systemic Disorders

Dyspepsia may exist in a number of systemic disorders such as diabetes mellitus, coronary artery disease, thyroid disease, hyperparathyroidism, adrenal insufficiency, and collagen vascular diseases.

H. Infections

Gastric infections other than *H pylori* can cause dyspepsia. These include cytomegalovirus, tuberculosis, or fungal infections. Parasites to consider include *Giardia lamblia* and *Strongyloides stercoralis.* Small intestinal bacterial overgrowth is associated with nonspecific symptoms such as bloating, gassiness, and abdominal discomfort that may emulate dyspepsia and is increasingly identified. It is often associated with more lower gastrointestinal symptoms such as diarrhea that may distinguish it from classic dyspepsia. Diagnosis can be established by breath testing or a trial of antibiotics, if suspected.

I. Other Considerations

Other conditions to consider in the differential diagnosis include chronic gastric volvulus, infiltrative diseases (sarcoidosis, amyloidosis, eosinophilic gastroenteritis, Ménétrier disease), undiagnosed inflammatory bowel disease, celiac sprue, and idiopathic cause.

Treatment

The treatment of organic dyspepsia is targeted to the cause. Specific treatment regimens for GERD, peptic ulcer disease, and other disorders that may cause dyspepsia can be found in their respective chapters in this book.

The treatment of functional dyspepsia primarily targets symptom relief. Studies have shown high placebo effect rates, and moderate success in response to PPIs, motility agents, and antidepressants. An effective physician-patient relationship is vital to treatment success.

Longstreth GF. Functional dyspepsia—managing the conundrum. *N Engl J Med.* 2006;354:791–793. [PMID: 16495391]

McNally MA, Talley NJ. Current treatments in functional dyspepsia. *Curr Treat Options Gastroenterol.* 2007;10:157–168. [PMID: 17391631]

Panganamamula KV, Fisher RS, Parkman HP. Functional (nonulcer) dyspepsia. *Curr Treat Options Gastroenterol.* 2002;5:153–160. [PMID: 11879596]

A. General Measures

The physician-patient relationship is crucial to the treatment of functional dyspepsia. Earnest efforts to accurately assess the extent and chronicity of the patient's symptoms will engender trust and reassurance. Fears of having cancer or a life-threatening condition, anxiety levels, and stressful factors in the patient's life should be assessed and addressed early in the evaluation.

Reassuring patients that the cause of their symptoms is non–life threatening and not cancer related is often therapeutic in itself. Nevertheless, reviewing the workup and the differential diagnosis remains important, so that patients have an understanding of where they are in the treatment process. The diagnosis of functional dyspepsia should also be explained as a recognized clinical entity with the emphasis on the understood pathophysiology of the problem and perhaps, more importantly, what is not known about it.

Due to the chronicity of the problem, many patients have already tried different remedies to alleviate their symptoms. Often patients understand what works for them and what does not prior to the office visit, such as meal content and quantity, positional factors, and home remedies. It is important to recognize the variability of symptoms, exacerbators and alleviators, and response to treatment in patients with dyspeptic symptoms.

B. Lifestyle Modifications

No trials have been done to formally evaluate the efficacy of dietary or lifestyle modifications in functional dyspepsia. The current understanding of dietary contributors stems from observation in clinical settings or epidemiologic studies. Foods generally reported to cause symptoms include onions, peppers, citrus fruit, coffee, carbonated beverages, and spices. General dietary recommendations are to avoid fatty or heavily spiced foods and excessively large meals. Smaller, more frequent meals are beneficial in patients with GERD, impaired gastric accommodation, and delayed gastric emptying. Food allergies should be noted and avoided. A food diary can help identify triggers. A trial of dairy product avoidance may be helpful in identifying lactose intolerance, with a hydrogen breath test performed to formally make the diagnosis. Caffeine intake and alcohol should be minimized, although a recent epidemiologic study did not identify a link between alcohol and functional dyspepsia. Regular exercise and adequate restful sleep are also important and can be helpful in alleviating stress.

C. Pharmacotherapy

If reassurance and lifestyle changes do not alleviate symptoms, medications can be tried. However, drug therapy trials in functional dyspepsia have yielded conflicting results and conclusions, possibly owing to several factors. Placebo response rates are known to be high in functional dyspepsia, ranging from 32–85%. Studies are often limited by insufficient sample size, single-center trials, and variability in the definition of functional dyspepsia. Furthermore, enrollment of patients from tertiary referral centers into drug trials may not represent the general population in primary care. Patients with GERD may inadvertently be included in trials, which would bias response rates in antisecretory trials.

In addition to *H pylori* eradication therapy, the pharmacologic therapy for dyspepsia includes antisecretory agents, promotility agents, antidepressants and anxiolytics, and other classes of drugs.

1. Antisecretory agents—PPIs have been extensively studied in several large, carefully designed, randomized controlled trials. A systematic review of eight studies with a total of 3293 patients who received PPI therapy for 2–8 weeks found a significant effect over placebo. PPI therapy relieved or eliminated symptoms in 33% of patients compared with 23% of those receiving placebo. The relative risk (RR) of remaining symptomatic on PPI versus placebo was significantly protective (RR = 0.86; 95% CI, 0.78–0.95; $P = .003$; NNT = 9).

Analysis of the subtypes of functional dyspepsia showed that patients with reflux-like and epigastric pain had a significant favorable response with PPI therapy, but those with dysmotility-type dyspepsia did not. Similarly, another meta-analysis of seven randomized placebo-controlled trials of PPIs with a total of 3725 patients found PPIs to be effective for patients with ulcer-like dyspepsia (RRR = 12.8%; 95% CI, 7.2–18.1%) and reflux-like dyspepsia (RRR = 19.7%; 95% CI, 1.8–34.3%), but not dysmotility-like dyspepsia and unspecified dyspepsia. As for H_2-receptor blockers, the evidence supporting their use is generally modestly beneficial. Systematic reviews on H_2-blockers versus placebo have shown improvement in epigastric pain, but not global symptoms.

Peura DA, Gudmundson J, Siepman N, et al. Proton pump inhibitors: effective first-line treatment for management of dyspepsia. *Dig Dis Sci.* 2007;52:983–987. [PMID: 17342402]

2. Promotility agents—Promotility agents are drugs that accelerate peristalsis by interacting with receptors for serotonin, acetylcholine, dopamine, and motilin (Table 17–5). The focus of drug development is now on serotonergic and dopaminergic drugs. Among the prokinetic agents available in the United States are metoclopramide and macrolide antibiotics, most commonly, erythromycin.

The use of these drugs has shown no clear relationship between pharmacologic enhancement of motility and improvement in symptoms of functional dyspepsia. Therefore, the benefit of prokinetics cannot be attributed solely to accelerated peristalsis. In fact, some drugs may actually worsen symptoms. An example is the negative influence that many drugs (eg, erythromycin and metoclopramide) have on postprandial fundic relaxation, or accommodation.

A systematic review of 14 randomized controlled trials reported prokinetics to be more effective than placebo in functional dyspepsia. However, the majority of the studies looked at cisapride, a serotonin 5-HT_4 agonist and 5-HT_3 antagonist that was taken off the market in the United States due to its association with adverse cardiac arrhythmia events. Another systematic review of 17 studies looked at cisapride and domperidone (also not available in the United States, again due to cardiac arrhythmia risk) and found both agents to be superior to placebo, but only by a global assessment of improvement by the investigator. Both agents are available through compassionate use protocols. A more recent systematic analysis of prokinetics showed that the effect over placebo was lost when only high-quality studies were included in the meta-analysis.

Table 17–5. Mechanism of action of promotility agents.

	Serotonin (5-HT_4) Agonist	5-HT_3 Antagonist	Dopamine (D_2) Antagonist	Motilin Receptor Agonist
Cisapride*	√	√		
Metoclopramide	√	√	√	
Tegaserod*	√			
Domperidone*			√	
Itopride*			√	
Levosulpiride*			√	
Erythromycin				√

*Available only on approval by the U.S. Food and Drug Administration.

Metoclopramide was found to be more effective than placebo in two older studies. However, there are medicolegal concerns about long-term use of metoclopramide due to potential neurologic side effects, particularly movement disorders.

Among the more recently tested agents are tegaserod, a 5-HT_4 agonist, and itopride, a dopaminergic antagonist. Neither drug is currently available in the United States. Tegaserod was previously approved for treatment of women with irritable bowel syndrome–predominant constipation and for men and women younger than 65 years with chronic constipation. It has been shown to increase gastric emptying and mildly improve symptoms in functional dyspepsia in phase III randomized controlled trials. However, in response to adverse events related to cardiac ischemia and stroke, tegaserod was removed from the market in early 2007. Itopride, which is available in Japan, is a dopaminergic antagonist that also acts as a weak muscarinic agonist. A recent phase II randomized controlled study of itopride versus placebo showed a dose-dependent improvement in the global assessment of patients with functional dyspepsia without significant differences in adverse events between treatment and placebo groups. The most frequent adverse events were abdominal pain, diarrhea, nausea, and constipation. A study of itopride in healthy subjects found that it reduces total postprandial volume without significantly accelerating gastric emptying or altering gastric motor or sensory function. This suggests that itopride, if efficacious in functional dyspepsia, is likely therapeutic in ways other than altering gastrointestinal motility. More recently, two phase III multicenter, randomized, double-blind, placebo-controlled studies have shown no benefit over placebo in a global patient assessment. Safety was comparable to placebo in these studies, with the rare occurrence of prolactin elevation in the patients receiving itopride (3.1% vs 0.2%).

Choung RS, Talley NJ, Peterson J, et al. A double-blind, randomized, placebo-controlled trial of itopride (100 and 200 mg three times daily) on gastric motor and sensory function in healthy volunteers. *Neurogastroenterol Motil.* 2007;19:180–187. [PMID: 17300287]

Hiyama T, Yoshihara M, Matsuo K, et al. Meta-analysis of the effects of prokinetic agents in patients with functional dyspepsia. *J Gastroenterol Hepatol.* 2007;22:304–310. [PMID: 17295768]

Holtmann G, Talley NJ, Liebregts T, et al. A placebo-controlled trial of itopride in functional dyspepsia. *N Engl J Med.* 2006;254:832–840. [PMID: 16495395]

Talley NJ, Tack J, Ptak T et al. Itopride in functional dyspepsia: results of two phase III multicenter, randomized, double-blind, placebo-controlled trials. *Gut.* 2007;57:740–746. [PMID: 17965059]

Vakil N, Laine L, Talley NJ, et al. Tegaserod treatment for dysmotility-like functional dyspepsia: results of two randomized, controlled trials. *Am J Gastroenterol.* 2008;103:1906–1919. [PMID: 18616658]

Veldhuyzen van Zanten SJ, Jones MJ, Verlinden M, et al. Efficacy of cisapride and domperidone in functional (nonulcer) dyspepsia: a meta-analysis. *Am J Gastroenterol.* 2001;96:689–696. [PMID: 11280535]

3. Antidepressants and anxiolytic agents—The efficacy of antidepressants and anxiolytics is based largely on clinical observation and anecdotal data. Low-dose tricyclic antidepressants (TCAs), such as amitriptyline or desipramine, have been used in patients with various functional disorders, including functional dyspepsia and irritable bowel syndrome. Typically much lower doses (10–100 mg/day) are given for functional dyspepsia than for depression. As TCAs can slow gastric emptying due to their anticholinergic effect, they should be avoided in patients with gastroparesis–functional dyspepsia overlap syndrome. A high-quality randomized trial investigating the use of TCAs in treating functional gastrointestinal disorders (including irritable bowel syndrome and functional dyspepsia) showed that patients who could tolerate the therapy might show a benefit with desipramine over placebo (73% vs 49%, $P = .0005$, NNT = 4). However, 28% of patients dropped out because of adverse reactions, with the most commonly reported adverse effects being dry mouth, sleep disturbance, constipation, and confusion. The side effects are related to the anticholinergic activity of TCAs, and patients should be warned about the possible occurrence of these effects prior to use.

Use of selective serotonin reuptake inhibitors in functional dyspepsia has not been studied in randomized controlled trials. These drugs may be helpful in patients with concurrent depression.

4. Other drugs—Antacids and bismuth have each been evaluated in a few trials for functional dyspepsia and have been consistently found to be no better than placebo. Sucralfate has been studied in several limited trials and found to be no more effective than placebo. Consequently, all of these agents play no major role in the treatment of functional dyspepsia.

5. Recommendations for pharmacotherapy—To summarize, if, after providing reassurance and basic dietary and lifestyle interventions, symptoms persist, the clinician can consider a trial of pharmacologic agents. If *H pylori* testing yields a positive result, treatment is recommended with the understanding that eradication may or may not improve symptoms. Antisecretory medications can then be added, such as H_2-blockers (ranitidine, 150 mg twice daily; cimetidine, 400 mg twice daily; or famotidine, 20 mg twice daily) or PPIs (omeprazole, 20 mg daily; esomeprazole, 40 mg daily; pantoprazole, 40 mg daily; lansoprazole, 30 mg daily; or rabeprazole, 20 mg daily). Antisecretory medications most likely benefit those with GERD symptoms or ulcer-like dyspepsia. If there is a response, a course of 2–6 weeks can be tried, with assessment of resolution of symptoms. If prokinetics are used, short courses of metoclopramide can be considered (5–10 mg prior to meals). Metoclopramide elixir is preferable to pill form. If symptoms are refractory and persist, low-dose TCAs (amitriptyline, imipramine, nortriptyline, or desipramine at 10–25 mg at bedtime) can be tried even in those without depression.

Van Zanten SV, Armstrong D, Chiba N, et al. Esomeprazole 40 mg once a day in patients with functional dyspepsia: the randomized placebo-controlled "ENTER" trial. *Am J Gastroenterol.* 2006;101:2096–2106. [PMID: 16817845]

D. Psychological Therapy

Psychological therapy addresses the cognitive aspects of the pathophysiology of functional dyspepsia. Several modalities have been used, including cognitive-behavioral therapy, biofeedback, hypnotherapy, relaxation therapy, and insight-oriented psychotherapy. A systematic review of randomized controlled trials of psychological therapies found four eligible trials on applied relaxation therapy, psychodynamic psychotherapy, cognitive therapy, and hypnotherapy that all reported symptomatic improvement at 1 year. However, the studies were of small sample size and had other technical limitations to provide adequate evidence for efficacy.

E. Complementary and Alternative Medical Therapy

Nonprescription therapies have been tried in functional dyspepsia, often being self-prescribed. These therapies are not regulated by the U.S. Food and Drug Administration (FDA); therefore, standardization of purity and potency is not enforced. Safety and efficacy are also not regulated. Nevertheless, studies have been conducted with several of these agents. A systematic review of herbal remedies was published examining 17 studies that evaluated agents such as Angelica, artichoke, boldo, gentian, ginger, lemon balm, milk thistle, peppermint, and turmeric. Although the definitions of functional dyspepsia and study methodologies had significant heterogeneity, the symptom improvement scores ranged from 60% to 90% favoring treatment over placebo. Few adverse reactions were associated with the remedies, but formal safety reporting was not routinely available. Short-term use is likely safe.

Thompson Coon J, Ernst E. Systematic review: herbal medicinal products for non-ulcer dyspepsia. *Aliment Pharmacol Ther.* 2002;16:1689–1699. [PMID: 12269960]

Course & Prognosis

The clinical course of functional dyspepsia has been evaluated in retrospective and prospective studies, with follow-up of 1.5–10 years for prospective studies and 5–27 years for retrospective studies. In general, a significant number of patients with functional dyspepsia became asymptomatic or improved overall after 1 to several years. History of GERD treatment during follow-up, prior history of peptic ulcer disease, use of aspirin, longer clinical history (>2 years), lower education, and psychological vulnerability were found to be associated with poorer prognosis in these studies. One study in Taiwan reported that patients with *H pylori* infection and functional dyspepsia were less likely to be symptom free at 2 years compared to those without *H pylori* (49% vs 58%).

This chapter is a revised version of the chapter by Dr. Victor S. Wang and Dr. Robert Burakoff that was in the previous edition of Current Diagnosis & Treatment: Gastroenterology, Hepatology, & Endoscopy.

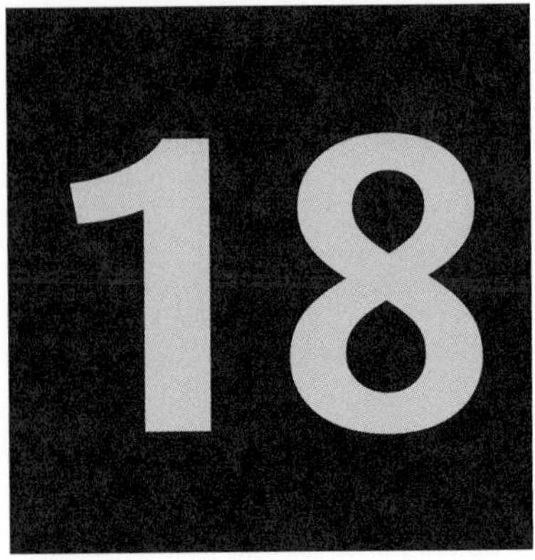

Disorders of Gastric & Small Bowel Motility

Walter W. Chan, MD, MPH
Robert Burakoff, MD, MPH

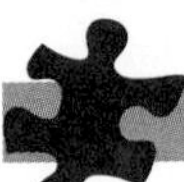

ESSENTIALS OF DIAGNOSIS

- The three most common causes of gastroparesis are idiopathic, diabetic, and postsurgical.
- Chronic intestinal pseudo-obstruction (CIPO) involves intermittent failure of intestinal peristalsis in the small or large intestine, or both.
- Noninvasive imaging or endoscopy, or both, should be used to rule out mechanical obstruction in patients being worked up for gastroparesis or CIPO.
- The 4-hour gastric emptying scintigraphy scan using a low-fat, egg-white meal is the best test for gastroparesis.
- Accelerated gastric emptying and dumping syndrome are often related to postgastric surgery.

General Considerations

Altered gastric and small bowel motility result in either delayed gastric emptying or rapid transit. Among the disorders of gastric and small bowel motility discussed in this chapter are gastroparesis, chronic intestinal pseudo-obstruction (CIPO), dumping syndrome, and rapid transit dysmotility of the small bowel.

Gastroparesis and CIPO are chronic long-term problems that have a variety of causes and can be neuropathic or myopathic. Treatment of these conditions includes dietary, medical, and, rarely, surgical therapies. Research in gastroparesis is ongoing with a focus on improving diagnostics and newer therapeutic agents. Dumping syndrome is a postsurgical iatrogenic problem that is occurring less often in relation to gastric ulcer surgery, but may be increasing among bariatric surgery patients in tandem with the increase in surgical treatment of obesity. Patient education, dietary change, and management of underlying medical problems are important factors in the overall management of these motility disorders.

Pathogenesis

Normal gastric emptying requires coordinated efforts by the muscles that control the four regions of the stomach, nerves that modulate the actions of these muscles, and chemical mediators. Important events that occur during gastric filling and emptying include fundic relaxation (accommodation) in response to food ingestion, antral contractions and churning (trituration) of large food particles, and finally pyloric relaxation.

The neurogenic network of the stomach includes elements of both the central nervous system (CNS) and the enteric nervous system (ENS). The CNS elements involve both sympathetic fibers and parasympathetic fibers. Sympathetic fibers arise from the thoracic spinal nerves, extending to postganglionic nerves that run along the celiac plexus and the vascular supply to the stomach. The sympathetic innervation includes afferent pain fibers that arise from the stomach, as well as motor fibers that innervate the pyloric sphincter. The parasympathetic innervation stems from the right and left vagal trunks, which eventually divide into multiple branches that course throughout the stomach wall and synapse with the ENS.

The ENS is an independent branch of the peripheral nervous system that is divided into two plexuses: the submucosal (Meissner) and the myenteric (Auerbach) plexuses. The submucosal plexus receives only parasympathetic input and innervates the cells of epithelial layer and muscular externa. The myenteric plexus, on the other hand, is situated between the middle circular and the outer longitudinal muscle layers, receiving both sympathetic and parasympathetic input. It mediates the motor function of both muscle layers and the secretory functions of the mucosa.

The interstitial cells of Cajal (ICCs) are the "pacemaker cells" of the stomach. They are located in the myenteric plexus and are responsible for basal slow-wave activity, which occurs at 3 cycles per minute. This slow-wave activity is also called the electronic control activity or the pacesetter potential. The ICCs are also responsible for bridging the myogenic and neurogenic control mechanisms.

The migrating motor complex (MMC) is the pattern of motility activity that occurs in the fasted state. It is a 1–2 hour cycle beginning in the stomach or small intestine and divided into three phases. Phase I (45–60 minutes) is a quiescent period. Phase II (30 minutes) is a period of random intermittent contractions. Lastly, phase III (5–15 minutes), also called the activity front, is a period in which bursts of rapid, even-paced uninterrupted peristaltic contractions occur.

Upon ingesting a meal, the MMC is abolished. Gastric accommodation occurs with distention of the fundus to make room for the incoming ingested contents. This response is mediated by the parasympathetic activity from the vagal nerve through cholinergic neurotransmitters, and inhibitory input by neurotransmitters such as nitric oxide, vasointestinal peptide, and serotonin.

The ingested contents upon entering the stomach are distributed, triturated, and then emptied into the duodenum. Liquids are usually dispersed and emptied immediately. The rate of liquid emptying is slowed by high osmolarity, high nutrient content, and carbonation. Solids, on the other hand, are stored in the fundus, churned in the antrum, and emptied in two phases: a lag period and a linear emptying period. The two periods occur over 3–4 hours, with the lag period lasting 1–3 hours. During the lag period, food particles move proximally to distally and undergo trituration and redistribution. Trituration occurs in the antrum with high-amplitude contraction waves that propagate proximally to distally. The food particles are reduced to a size of approximately 1–2 mm in diameter prior to emptying. The pylorus ultimately regulates how much content is emptied into the duodenal bulb by coordinated contractions and maintenance of the lumen with fixed tone.

Besides mechanical factors, neurohormonal factors also control the rate of emptying. Glucagon and incretins (eg, amylin and glucagon-like peptide 1) slow gastric emptying. The vagus provides both excitatory and inhibitory innervation. The presence of chyme in the duodenum provides negative feedback on the rate of emptying as mediated by duodenal distention, acidification, or perfusion with fats and protein. The regulation of duodenal intake controls the level of postprandial hyperglycemia from nutrient absorption.

Camilleri M. Integrated upper gastrointestinal response to food intake. *Gastroenterology.* 2006;131:640–658. [PMID: 16890616]

Kindt S, Tack J. Impaired gastric accommodation and its role in dyspepsia. *Gut.* 2006;55:1685–1691. [PMID: 16854999]

GASTROPARESIS & CHRONIC INTESTINAL PSEUDO-OBSTRUCTION

General Considerations

Gastroparesis is characterized by delayed gastric emptying that is not associated with the presence of an obstructing structural lesion in the stomach or distally in the gastrointestinal tract.

Table 18–1. Causes of gastroparesis.

Gastroesophageal diseases
Gastroesophageal reflux
Gastritis (chronic or acute)
Acute gastroenteritis (cytomegalovirus)
Atrophic gastritis
Peptic ulcer disease
Neuromuscular disorders
Muscular dystrophy
Parkinson disease
Systemic disorders
Diabetes mellitus
Hypothyroidism
Uremia
Chronic liver disease
Anorexia nervosa
Rheumatologic disorders
Scleroderma
Surgical procedures
Gastrectomy
Roux-en-Y syndrome
Vagotomy
Pyloromyotomy
Pancreatectomy
Antireflux operations
Combined heart-lung transplantation
Trauma
Head injuries
Spinal cord injuries
Other etiologies
Idiopathic
Medications
Idiopathic pseudo-obstruction
Amyloidosis

Many disorders that interfere with the normal neuromuscular coordination of the stomach can lead to gastroparesis (Table 18–1). The three most common causes are idiopathic, diabetic, and postsurgical. A tertiary referral series of 146 patients showed the causes of gastroparesis to be 36% idiopathic, 29% diabetic, 14% postgastric surgery, 7.5% Parkinson disease, 4.8% collagen vascular disorders, 4.1% intestinal pseudo-obstruction, and 6% miscellaneous causes (eg, paraneoplastic syndrome, superior mesenteric artery syndrome, and median arcuate ligament syndrome). The idiopathic causes included acute viral-like gastroenteritis (23%), gastroesophageal reflux disease (GERD) and nonulcer dyspepsia (19%), and cholecystectomy.

CIPO is characterized by obstructive symptoms generated from the small or large bowel occurring in the absence of anatomic obstruction. It is a severe form of dysmotility that is considered a failure or insufficiency of the "intestinal pump." Like gastroparesis, CIPO has a wide variety of causes (Table 18–2). These can generally be separated into congenital versus acquired causes, and myopathic versus neuropathic processes. Because gastroparesis and CIPO have very similar

Table 18–2. Causes of chronic intestinal pseudo-obstruction.

Myopathic processes
Myotonic dystrophy
Duchenne muscular dystrophy
Postoperative states
Ileus
Ogilvie syndrome (colonic pseudo-obstruction)
Autoimmune disorders
Systemic lupus erythematosus
Scleroderma
Dermatomyositis
Polymyositis
Celiac disease
Autoimmune myositis or ganglionitis
Oncologic disorders
Pheochromocytoma
Paraneoplastic syndrome (small cell cancer, ganglioneuroblastoma)
Multiple myeloma
Hematologic disorders
Sickle cell disease
Infectious/postinfectious disorders
Chagas disease
Cytomegalovirus
Varicella-zoster virus
Epstein-Barr virus
Kawasaki disease
Endocrine disorders
Diabetes mellitus
Hypoparathyroidism
Hypothyroidism
Metabolic disorders
Mitochondrial cytopathies
Toxins
Fetal alcohol syndrome
Jellyfish envenomation
Drugs
Chemotherapy
Diltiazem and nifedipine
Developmental disorders
Delayed maturation of interstitial cells of Cajal
Other etiologies
Ehlers-Danlos syndrome
Eosinophilic gastroenteritis
Angioedema
Crohn disease
Radiation enteritis

clinical approaches, this section discusses the assessment and treatment of these conditions together.

The true prevalence of gastroparesis has been difficult to study due to underdiagnosis and the lack of inexpensive diagnostic testing that is also widely available. A large population-based study in Olmsted County, Minnesota, estimated the age-adjusted prevalence of definite gastroparesis, defined as delayed gastric emptying on scintigraphy and typical symptoms for more than 3 months, to be 24.4 per 100,000 persons (95% confidence interval [CI], 15.7–32.6). Other population studies have shown upper gastrointestinal symptoms to be present in 11–18% of diabetic patients, with 50–65% of them having delayed gastric emptying. The mean age of gastroparetic patients in one study was 45 years old, with a mean age of onset of 33.7 years. The prevalence of gastroparesis per 100,000 persons was 9.6 among men versus 37.8 among women. It is unclear whether gender influences the pathophysiology of gastroparesis or if this represents a difference in health care–seeking behavior between men and women. An overlap syndrome of gastroparesis and functional dyspepsia has been noted, and 25–42% of patients with functional dyspepsia have concomitant gastroparesis.

Bytzer P, Talley NJ, Leemon M, et al. Prevalence of gastrointestinal symptoms associated with diabetes mellitus: a population-based survey of 15000 adults. *Arch Intern Med.* 2001;10:1989–1096. [PMID: 11525701]

Jung HK, Choung RS, Locke GR 3rd, et al. The incidence, prevalence, and outcomes of patients with gastroparesis in Olmsted County, Minnesota, from 1996 to 2006. *Gastroenterology.* 2009; 136:1225–1233. [PMID: 19249393]

Maleki D, Locke GR 3rd, Camilleri M, et al. Gastrointestinal tract symptoms among persons with diabetes mellitus in the community. *Arch Intern Med.* 2000;9:2808–2816. [PMID: 11025791]

Clinical Findings

A. Symptoms and Signs

Typical complaints of gastroparesis include postprandial nausea, vomiting, belching, early satiety, bloating, discomfort, or pain. Reflux symptoms are also common. Chronic symptoms include weight loss or electrolyte disturbances, or both. Signs and symptoms of nutritional and vitamin deficiencies that may be noted include temporal wasting and loss of subcutaneous fat (malnutrition), gum bleeding (vitamin C), visual changes with night blindness (vitamin A), neuropathy, or impaired memory and confusion (folate, vitamin B_{12}). Dysphagia or odynophagia may occur as a result of reflux esophagitis. Diarrhea and malabsorption may be a consequence of bacterial overgrowth caused by altered peristalsis. Symptoms to look for include dry mouth, eyes, or vagina; difficulties with visual accommodation in bright light; anhidrosis (absence of sweating); impotence; dizziness on standing; scleroderma symptoms such as Raynaud phenomenon, skin tightening, and peripheral paresthesia; and numbness or focal weaknesses. A medication history can elicit drugs that may contribute to altered gastric motility (Table 18–3).

The examination should include assessment of volume status for dehydration (eg, orthostasis, pallor, and poor skin turgor) and signs of metabolic alkalosis, such as decreased respirations. Abdominal examination may reveal distention or surgical scars. The examiner should auscultate for obstructive high-pitched or absent bowel sounds, and palpate for focal tenderness or mass. A succussion splash may be

Table 18–3. Common medications that may affect gastric emptying.

Delay Gastric Emptying	Accelerate Gastric Emptying
Calcium channel blockers (nifedipine diltiazem, verapamil, others) Potassium Dopamine Sucralfate Aluminum hydroxide Opiates Tricyclic antidepressants (imipramine, amitriptyline, desipramine) L-Dopa	Bulk laxatives Diazepam Macrolide antibiotics (erythromycin, clarithromycin, azithromycin) Antiemetics (metoclopramide)

heard when auscultating over the stomach while shaking the abdomen from side to side 1 hour or more postprandially. The examiner should also test for abdominal wall–related pain by observing for Carnett sign (positive when tenderness is increased upon tensing of the abdominal muscles). Findings suggesting diabetic microvascular complications should be noted (eg, retinopathy and sensory or autonomic neuropathy). Signs of recurrent vomiting may include worn tooth enamel. Nutritional deficiencies may manifest as brittle hair and nails, cheilosis, glossitis, and tetany.

Symptoms can also be assessed by a validated instrument, the Gastroparesis Cardinal Symptom Index (GCSI), which was developed for measurement of three subsets of symptoms, including postprandial fullness/early satiety, nausea/vomiting, and bloating. The GCSI has been validated for measuring symptom severity.

B. Imaging and Endoscopic Studies

Radiologic studies include plain film abdominal radiographs, computed tomography of the abdomen, small bowel follow-through examination, and magnetic resonance imaging (MRI). Oral contrast should be water soluble to prevent formation of barium concretions in the gastrointestinal tract with dysmotility. Gastroparesis may be demonstrated by retained contrast in the stomach or its slow gastric transit into the small bowel. In CIPO, abdominal films may show dilated loops of small bowel and air-fluid levels (Figure 18–1), and small bowel follow-through studies may help rule out obstructive lesions. MRI can measure gastric emptying and may provide additional information including gastroduodenal motility. However, its use in the evaluation for gastroparesis is still limited to the research setting.

Upper endoscopy is useful for ruling out a mechanical obstruction of the upper gastrointestinal tract (eg, masses, peptic ulcer disease [PUD], complications of pyloric stenosis, or acute PUD with antral edema). Retained food despite overnight fast may also be seen in the stomach during upper endoscopy in patients with gastroparesis.

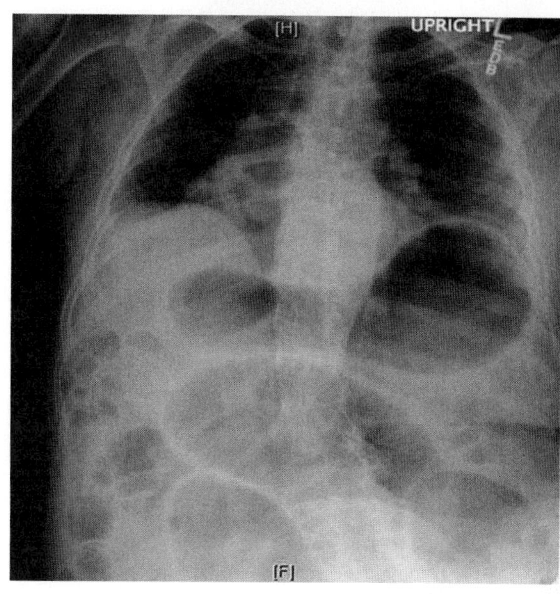

▲ **Figure 18–1.** Chronic intestinal pseudo-obstruction seen on plain upright abdominal film. The stomach and small bowel are distended with intestinal gas.

C. Scintigraphy

The best current clinical test for delayed gastric emptying is gastric emptying scintigraphy using radionuclide technetium 99–labeled food. The test involves ingestion of a radiolabeled meal prepared by cooking radioisotope into the solid portion, which is usually a soft-textured food such as eggs. Scintigraphy is then performed 1–4 hours after ingestion (Figures 18–2A and 18–2B). Retention is abnormal when more than 90% of the tracer remains in the stomach at 1 hour, more than 60% at 2 hours, or more than 10% at 4 hours.

Tests shorter than 4 hours are less accurate for several reasons, including reduced sensitivity. Furthermore, the lag period is variable; some patients with prolonged lag phases have apparently normal 4-hour tests due to a "catch-up" in gastric emptying. Gastric residual measured at 4 hours after ingestion has a 100% sensitivity and 70% specificity for gastroparesis.

There had been some concerns about the lack of standardization of the procedure, and several proposed protocols have been suggested. Most recently, a consensus statement from experts of the American Neurogastroenterology and Motility Society and the Society of Nuclear Medicine recommends a standardized protocol with a 4-hour test using low-fat, egg-white meal. Scintigraphy measurements are then taken at 0, 1, 2, and 4 hours after ingestion.

Another use of scintigraphy is the assessment of gastric accommodation. By dividing the area of interest into a distal and proximal segment and radiographically measuring the

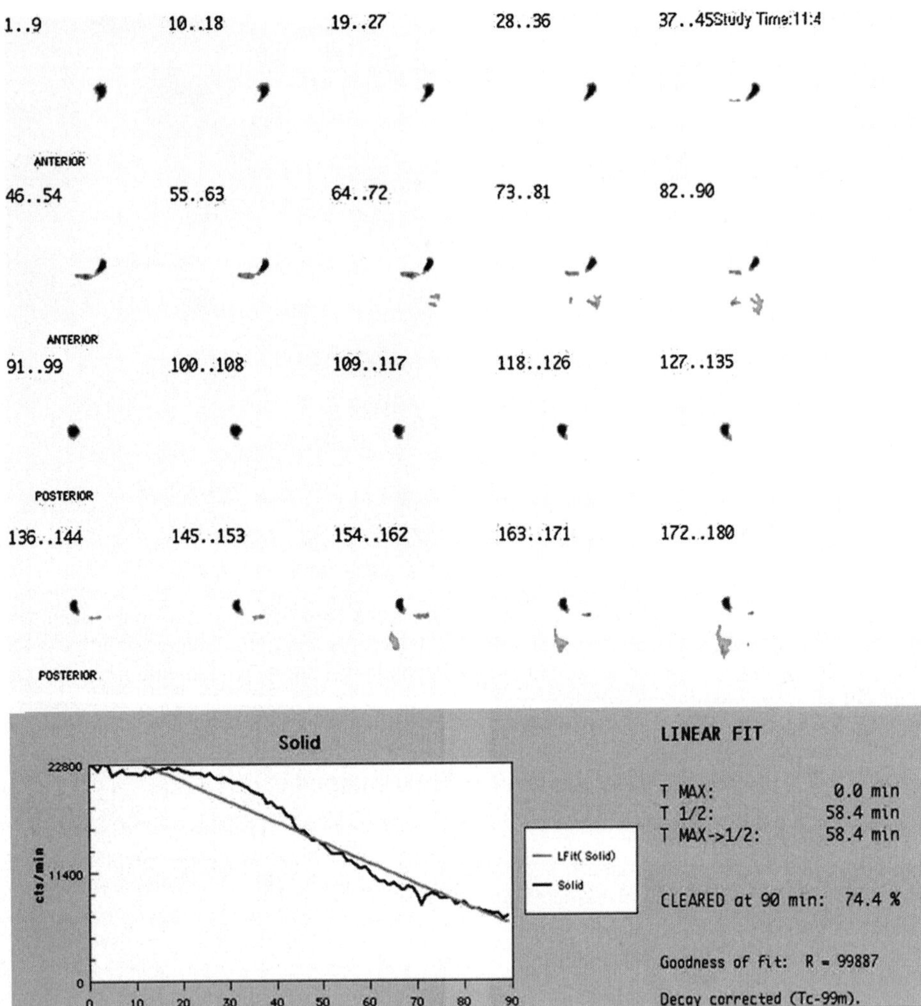

▲ **Figure 18–2A.** A normal ^{99m}Tc-labeled solid-phase gastric emptying scan showing 74.4% clearance at 90 minutes.

gastric volume in each segment, the regional changes over time can be assessed. A normal stomach with appropriate accommodation usually shows redistribution of the meal to the distal segment after accumulation in the proximal segment. Impaired gastric accommodation can be seen in diabetic vagal neuropathy, postvagotomy surgery, post-fundoplication dyspepsia, and functional dyspepsia.

Abell TL, Camilleri M, Donohoe K, et al. Consensus recommendations for gastric emptying scintigraphy: a joint report of the American Neurogastroenterology and Motility Society and the Society of Nuclear Medicine. *Am J Gastroenterol.* 2008;103: 753–763. [PMID: 18028513]

Guo JP, Maurer AH, Fisher RS, et al. Extending gastric emptying scintigraphy from 2 to 4 hours detects more patients with gastroparesis. *Dig Dis Sci.* 2001;46:24–29. [PMID: 11270790]

Tougas G, Eaker EY, Abell TL, et al. Assessment of gastric emptying using a low fat meal: establishment of international control values. *Am J Gastroenterol.* 2000;95:1456–1462. [PMID: 10894578]

Ziessman HA, Bonta DV, Goetze S, et al. Experience with a simplified, standardized 4-hour gastric-emptying protocol. *J Nucl Med.* 2007;48:568–572. [PMID: 17401093]

D. Breath Testing

Another tool to measure gastric emptying is breath testing using a solid meal with nonradioactive isotope ^{13}C-labeled medium-chain triglycerides, octanoate, or spirulina. When ingested, the ^{13}C-labeled octanoate or spirulina is rapidly absorbed in the small intestine and metabolized into $^{13}CO_2$, which can then be measured in breath samples to indirectly estimate the rate of gastric emptying. This test has been

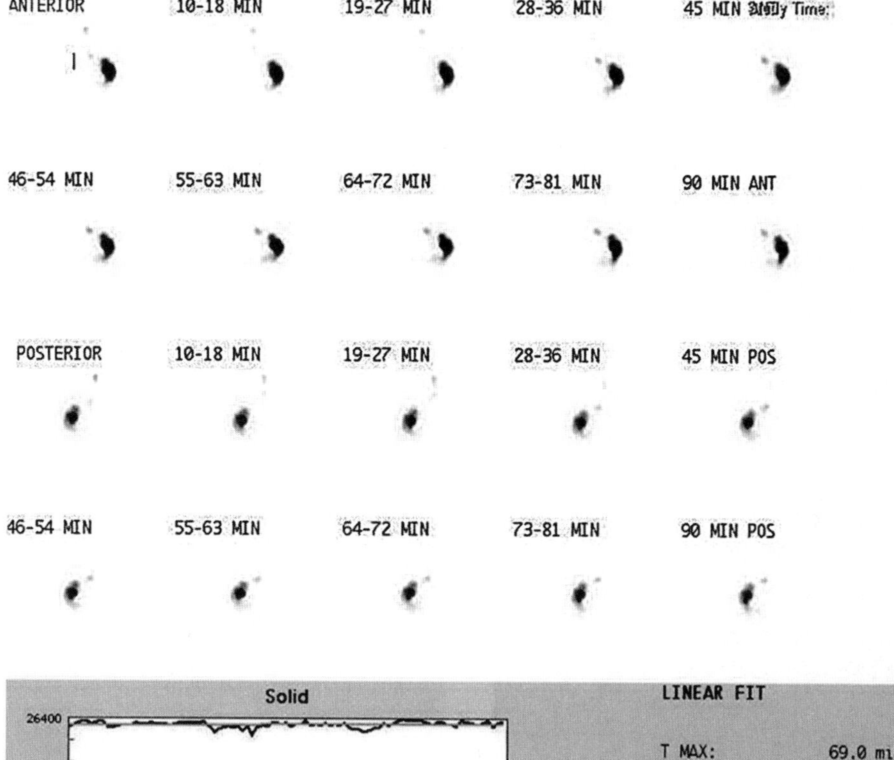

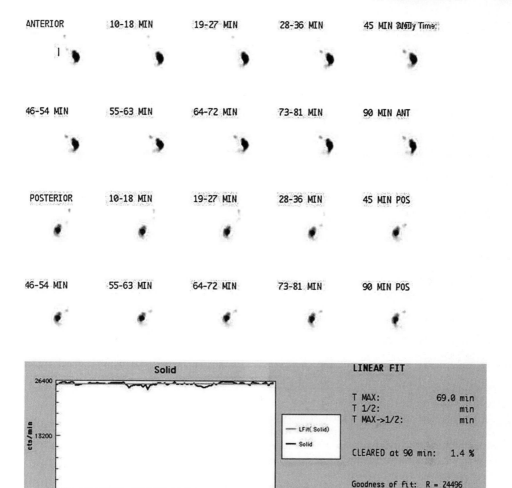

▲ **Figure 18–2B.** An abnormal ^{99m}Tc-labeled solid-phase gastric emptying scan showing 1.4% clearance (or 98.6% retention) at 90 minutes.

shown to correlate strongly with scintigraphy by some clinical studies, and its execution has been simplified with recent development of a standardized test meal for octanoate. Further research in this method of measuring gastric emptying is ongoing with the goal of using breath testing possibly as an office-based test in the future.

E. Special Tests of Motility

Ingestion and counting of radiopaque markers at 6 hours has been used to help identify the location of functional dysmotility. However, the clinical utility of this test is limited due to lack of standardization and possible uncertainty about whether markers are located in the stomach or within a segment of small bowel that overlaps the stomach.

For evaluation of small bowel motility, upper gastrointestinal and small bowel film series provide rough assessments at best. Quantification can be done by scintigraphy.

Antroduodenal manometry, which is not widely available, can provide information about the coordination of gastric and duodenal motility and can help differentiate between a neuropathic and a myopathic motility problem in CIPO. It involves inserting a large catheter with multiple manometric sensors down to the antrum and the proximal small bowel, usually with the aid of fluoroscopy. The test is then performed over several hours in the fasting state, with a test meal, and sometimes with motility agents such as erythromycin. A neuropathic process that is intrinsic or visceral is usually characterized by uncoordinated contractions of normal amplitude, and abnormal or even absent phase III contractions of the MMC. The presence of phase III of the MMC is associated with a favorable prognosis, with better tolerance of enteral feedings and response to prokinetic drugs. In contrast, contraction amplitudes are reduced with myopathic processes, while spatial and temporal organization is preserved. Other antroduodenal manometric findings in CIPO may include simultaneous waveforms, retrograde propagation of phase III of the MMC, high-amplitude and high-frequency bursts during both fasting and fed periods, and sustained high-pressure zones in limited small bowel segments, or inability of a meal to initiate the fed period activity pattern.

F. Electrogastrography

Electrogastrography can record gastric muscular activity waveforms via cutaneously placed pads, similar to an electrocardiogram for the myocardium. Abnormal electrogastrograms are defined as observed dysrhythmia for more than 30% of the recording time or failure of an ingested meal to elicit increased amplitude in gastric signals. However, the electrogastrogram has not been widely used clinically. Furthermore, there has been little evidence that electrogastrography aids in the management of patients with gastroparesis.

G. SmartPill Capsule Monitoring

The SmartPill GI Monitoring System is an ingested capsule that can deliver information on pressure, pH, and temperature wirelessly to a data recorder worn by the patient. The pill is swallowed after ingesting a standard 220-kcal meal. The data permit estimates of gastric emptying time, combined small and large bowel transit time, and total transit time, as well as study of pressure patterns from the gastrointestinal tract in the stomach, small bowel, and colon. The capsule has been approved by the U.S. Food and Drug Administration (FDA) for use in studying gastroparesis. The device has been compared with gastric scintigraphy at a 2-hour emptying time ($r = 0.63$) and at a 4-hour emptying time ($r = 0.73$). The better correlation with 4-hour emptying time is likely due to the capsule, a nondigestible solid, being emptied from the stomach after the emptying of most of the test meal in the subject. The device is a reasonable alternative to conventional scintigraphy for gastroparesis. The utility of SmartPill in the study of small and large intestinal dysmotility in the clinical setting remains unclear, given the current lack of standard parameters.

Differential Diagnosis

Once mechanical obstruction is ruled out, vomiting related to gastroparesis must be distinguished from regurgitation, rumination syndrome, and the eating disorders of anorexia nervosa and bulimia. Rumination syndrome is characterized by daily, early postprandial regurgitation of food that occurs effortlessly without nausea, likely as a learned behavior. Daily vomiting is seen only in severe gastroparesis. In addition, associated symptoms of abdominal pain, discomfort, and bloating are more suggestive of gastroparesis. Other nonobstructive disorders with symptoms that may mimic gastroparesis include functional dyspepsia (postprandial distress syndrome subtype), accelerated gastric emptying, and esophageal dysmotility.

Treatment

Treatment should be tailored for each individual. The general approach to management involves correction of dehydration, malnutrition, and nutritional deficiencies; dietary modifications; use of pharmacologic motility agents, including prokinetics and antiemetics; and normalization of hyperglycemia in diabetic gastroparesis. For patients with refractory gastroparesis, more aggressive therapies include decompression by gastrostomy tubes, consideration of gastric pacing, pyloric injection with botulinum toxin, and surgical treatment.

Camilleri M. Clinical practice. Diabetic gastroparesis. *N Engl J Med.* 2007;356:820–829. [PMID: 17314341]

Camilleri M, Bharucha AE, Farrugia G. Epidemiology, mechanisms, and management of diabetic gastroparesis. *Clin Gastroenterol Hepatol.* 2011;9:5–12. [PMID: 20951838]

Connor FL, Di Lorenzo C. Chronic intestinal pseudo-obstruction: assessment and management. *Gastroenterology.* 2006;130:S29–S36. [PMID: 16473068]

Park MI, Camilleri M. Gastroparesis: clinical update. *Am J Gastroenterol.* 2006;101:1129–1139. [PMID: 16696789]

Parkman HP, Hasler WL, Fisher RS. American Gastroenterological Association. American Gastroenterological Association medical position statement: diagnosis and treatment of gastroparesis. *Gastroenterology.* 2004;127:1589–1591. [PMID: 15521025]

A. Correction of Dehydration and Nutritional Deficiencies

During acute exacerbation of gastroparesis, dehydration and electrolyte imbalances should be corrected promptly. Hypokalemia and metabolic alkalosis are common in patients with persistent vomiting. Repletion can be instituted orally, enterally through feeding tubes, or parenterally. If the gastrointestinal tract is severely impaired, parenteral nutrition should be considered. Prolonged enteral feeding may require a jejunostomy tube to bypass the pylorus.

B. Dietary Modifications

Dietary recommendations include eating frequent, smaller sized meals. Solid foods can also be substituted for those that are pureed or liquid, such as soups. High-fat foods delay gastric emptying, as do high-fiber foods.

C. Pharmacotherapy

1. Prokinetics—Prokinetics available in the United States include metoclopramide and erythromycin, both of which can be administered orally and intravenously. Erythromycin

(40–250 mg three times daily) is a macrolide antibiotic that has activity on motilin receptors on both neurons and smooth muscles. Metoclopramide (starting with 5 mg twice daily to 10–20 mg two to three times daily) is a 5-HT_4 agonist and dopamine antagonist, and, therefore, contains both antiemetic and prokinetic activity. Both of these drugs have been shown in randomized controlled trials to improve symptoms by 25–68% and to increase gastric emptying in objective tests by 25–72%. Elixir forms of both drugs may have better absorption and subsequent bioavailability than pill forms. Intravenous erythromycin at 3 mg/kg (given at 125–250 mg three to four times daily) is more effective than placebo in hospitalized patients with gastroparesis and has been demonstrated to decrease symptoms, with positive objective measures of improved emptying. Unfortunately, the beneficial effect of erythromycin is often short-lived due to tachyphylaxis, or tolerance to the medication. Rapid development of tolerance to the medication may be due to saturation of motilin receptors and their subsequent down regulation. The treatment effect of erythromycin significantly drops after 4 weeks, although some patients may continue to experience benefit. Therefore, erythromycin may be best used during exacerbations of symptoms or on an intermittent basis in those unable to tolerate, those who need a holiday from, or those unresponsive to metoclopramide.

Several other prokinetics have been used clinically for gastroparesis but are not widely available in the United States. Other agents include cisapride, a parasympathomimetic that acts as a serotonin 5-HT_4 agonist, and domperidone, a dopamine (D_2) receptor antagonist. Both drugs are available in Canada, Mexico, and Europe. Domperidone is available in the United States through an FDA investigational new drug (IND) program. Cisapride has been associated with long QT syndrome, which can predispose to torsades de pointes, causing the drug to be taken off the U.S. market in March 2000. Likewise, domperidone has not been approved by the FDA due to risk of cardiac arrhythmia and its bioavailability in breast milk. However, both drugs have been found to be efficacious in treating gastroparesis. Additional concerns with metoclopramide and domperidone relate to CNS side effects, which include somnolence, mental function, anxiety, and depression. There are also medicolegal concerns about the chronic use of metoclopramide owing to adverse reactions (ie, neurologic effects and movement disorders). Early effects include akathisia (a sensation of "inner restlessness") and dystonia, and later effects may include tardive dyskinesia and parkinsonism. Because domperidone does not cross the blood-brain barrier, its CNS effects are notably less compared to metoclopramide. On the other hand, both domperidone and metoclopramide are equally effective in controlling symptoms of diabetic gastroparesis in comparative trials.

2. Antiemetics—Antiemetics such as diphenhydramine, phenothiazine compounds, and even metoclopramide can help control symptoms of nausea. The more commonly used agents include prochlorperazine, trimethobenzamide, and promethazine. Serotonin (5-HT_3) antagonists, such as granisetron and ondansetron, are frequently used in chemotherapy patients but are also useful in gastroparesis. They act on the area postrema and peripheral afferent nerves. Other agents used in clinical practice, albeit without strong supportive data, include benzodiazepines, synthetic cannabinoids, and transdermal scopolamine.

3. Alternative agents—Multiple other agents with different mechanisms have also been tried. Tegaserod (Zelnorm; 2–6 mg twice daily) is a partial 5-HT_4 receptor agonist that enhances gastric emptying, but no clinical trials have been undertaken specifically in patients with gastroparesis. It has been used with anecdotal success, but was removed from the market in early 2007 due to concerns about increased risk of myocardial infarction and stroke. Agents with limited success and also with notable adverse cholinergic side effects include bethanechol (10–20 mg two to three times daily), a muscarinic cholinergic agent, and pyridostigmine (30 mg four times daily), an anticholinesterase.

4. Pain management—The management of pain in gastroparesis has not been specifically addressed in clinical studies. Currently, the most commonly used agents are tricyclic antidepressants (nortriptyline, amitriptyline), which have been shown to be effective in treating functional bowel disorders. Other approaches to pain management in gastroparesis include the use of tramadol, a weak μ-opioid receptor agonist, and gabapentin, a γ-aminobutyric acid analog. Opioids commonly prescribed for chronic pain syndromes should be avoided given their effects on gastrointestinal motility.

5. Other drugs—Pharmacologic treatment for disorders associated with CIPO include antibiotic regimens for bacterial overgrowth, which is usually treated with common antibiotics such as doxycycline, ciprofloxacin, metronidazole, or double-strength trimethoprim–sulfamethoxazole for 7–10 days. More recently, rifaximin (400–1200 mg/day), a nonabsorbable antibiotic approved for use in traveler's diarrhea, has been effective for small bowel bacterial overgrowth and normalizing hydrogen breath tests.

Short-acting subcutaneous octreotide (50 mcg subcutaneously at night) has been tried in patients with CIPO, and studies have shown that it increases MMCs in the small bowel. This therapy should be avoided in patients with concomitant bacterial overgrowth.

6. Investigational drugs—Some of the drugs currently under investigation include other prokinetics such as itopride, a dopamine receptor antagonist, and mosapride, a 5-HT_4 receptor agonist. Ghrelin agonists are also under investigation. Several motilitides, which are motilin receptor agonists without some of the undesirable features of erythromycin, are also being studied. Azithromycin given intravenously has been compared with erythromycin and was found to result in higher antral contraction amplitude and motility index. Further study of its effects on symptom improvement is needed.

D. Normalization of Hyperglycemia

There is little evidence that controlling hyperglycemia has a direct relationship to symptom improvement. However, there is a well-established inverse relationship between blood glucose levels and rate of gastric emptying. Hyperglycemia is associated with delayed gastric emptying, as are euglycemia with normal gastric emptying and hypoglycemia with accelerated gastric emptying. Moreover, acute changes in blood glucose concentration have an effect on both gastric motor function and upper gastrointestinal symptoms. Evidence also suggests that response to prokinetics is partially determined by hyperglycemia. With regard to practical care of diabetic patients with gastroparesis, short-acting insulin should be dosed after, rather than prior, to eating to ensure that the patient tolerates the entire meal and to avoid hypoglycemia.

E. Decompression Gastrostomy Tubes and Jejunal Feeding Tubes

Advanced gastroparesis or CIPO may require decompression. Venting can be accomplished by a nasogastric tube or by a percutaneous endoscopic gastrostomy (PEG) or jejunostomy tube. Several feeding tubes have both a venting port upstream and a feeding port downstream. However, before placing the tube in a patient with severe symptoms, it is prudent to try nasal jejunal tube feeding first to test whether the patient can tolerate enteral feeding. Criteria for tube feeding include severe weight loss, multiple hospitalizations, and malnutrition.

F. Gastric Electrical Stimulation (GES)

Electrical stimulation of the stomach for treatment of gastroparesis is done laparoscopically by implanting a device into the antral muscular wall, with electrodes that connect to a pacemaker pocketed into the abdominal wall. The stimulation is classified based on the frequency of the electrical stimulus (high or low frequency). A high-frequency electrical stimulation device (Enterra, Medtronic) has been approved by the FDA through a humanitarian device exemption. A crossover controlled trial of 33 patients with idiopathic or diabetic gastroparesis showed that the frequency of vomiting was decreased significantly, but overall effect on symptoms was not significant. Open-label long-term studies with follow-up of 3.4–3.7 years have shown relief of symptoms and decreased need for nutritional supplementation. Predictors of treatment success in patients receiving GES include diabetic gastroparesis, symptoms that are predominantly nausea and vomiting, and symptoms that do not require narcotic therapy. Although GES is a promising therapy, further studies are needed in this area.

Abell T, McCallum R, Hocking M, et al. Gastric electrical stimulation for medically refractory gastroparesis. *Gastroenterology.* 2003;125:421–428. [PMID: 12891544]

Abidi N, Starkebaum WL, Abell TL. An energy algorithm improves symptoms in some patients with gastroparesis and treated with gastric electrical stimulation. *Neurogastroenterol Motil.* 2006;18:334–338. [PMID: 16553589]

G. Pyloric Injection with Botulinum Toxin

Gastric emptying may be facilitated by keeping the pylorus relaxed. Injection of botulinum A toxin into the pyloric sphincter has been thought to paralyze the smooth muscle of the pylorus and antrum by inhibiting acetylcholine release. Several uncontrolled open-label trials have previously reported its efficacy in gastroparesis. However, two randomized, controlled trials have shown no treatment benefit in both subjective (symptoms) and objective (gastric emptying) endpoints. These results suggest no role for pyloric sphincter botulinum toxin injection in the treatment of gastroparesis.

Arts J, Holvoet L, Caenepeel P, et al. Clinical trial: a randomized-controlled crossover study of intrapyloric injection of botulinum toxin in gastroparesis. *Aliment Pharmacol Ther.* 2007;26: 1251–1258. [PMID: 17944739]

Friedenberg FK, Palit A, Parkman HP, et al. Botulinum toxin A for the treatment of delayed gastric emptying. *Am J Gastroenterol.* 2008;103:416–423. [PMID: 18070232]

H. Surgical Treatment

Surgical treatment is the last resort for both gastroparesis and CIPO and is rarely indicated. For gastroparesis, surgical placement of gastrostomy and jejunostomy tubes may be done for feeding and decompression. Definitive surgical treatment for gastroparesis includes a subtotal or complete gastrectomy. A systematic review of surgical therapy for gastroparesis found that gastrectomy may help postsurgical gastroparesis, but issued caution on surgical therapy for diabetic or idiopathic gastroparesis.

For CIPO, the surgical therapy aims to bypass areas of localized disease in the small intestine, or resect the colon for severe constipation. Again, caution is warranted when considering surgery in this condition as the original problem may manifest itself in unresected portions of the gut. If the disease is within the upper and lower intestinal tract, colectomy is less likely to be beneficial. Gastrostomy, jejunostomy, or loop enterostomy may be done to shorten the gut, facilitate transit, and vent the bowel. Percutaneous colonoscopy in adult CIPO patients has shown success in reducing distention.

Small bowel transplantation is indicated for patients with end-stage parenteral nutrition–dependant pseudo-obstruction and complications of prolonged parenteral nutrition or line access.

Prognosis

Little is known about either the overall prognosis or the quality of life of patients with gastroparesis and CIPO. The disease can be long-standing and have a substantial impact on well-being. Symptom severity scales have been developed and validated and may be useful in clinical and research settings. The overall long-term prognosis is determined by the underlying disease process, if known.

DUMPING SYNDROME & ACCELERATED GASTRIC EMPTYING

General Considerations

Dumping syndrome and accelerated gastric emptying are diseases that can occur after gastric surgery when a truncal vagotomy or gastrectomy has been performed. With the onset of medical treatment for PUD and *Helicobacter pylori* eradication, gastric ulcer surgery has significantly decreased, and expectedly, these postoperative accelerated gastric states have also decreased. Presently, bariatric surgery with Roux-en-Y gastric bypasses causes dumping syndrome in as many as 50% of patients. Aside from the iatrogenic causes, diabetes with vagal dysfunction and Zollinger-Ellison syndrome can also be associated with rapid gastric emptying. Rapid gastric emptying is caused by high gastric pressures, impaired gastric accommodation, and the lack of a regulating pyloric sphincter.

Clinical Findings

A. Symptoms and Signs

Dumping syndrome can be characterized as early or late, each with different symptoms. Both types of dumping syndrome can occur in the same patient. Early dumping syndrome occurs during or immediately after a meal and is characterized by nausea, vomiting, bloating, cramping, diarrhea, dizziness, and fatigue. These early symptoms are hypothesized to be due to a hyperosmolar load in the small bowel. Some of the postprandial upper abdominal symptoms associated with early dumping syndrome can be indistinguishable from those of delayed gastric emptying. Late dumping happens 1–3 hours after a meal and is characterized by hypoglycemia, weakness, sweating, and dizziness. Hypoglycemia occurs because a high carbohydrate content absorption into the small bowel evokes a strong insulin response with secondary hypoglycemia.

B. Diagnostic Tests

Dual-phase gastric scintigraphy using radiolabeled solids and liquids is the best diagnostic test. Hydrogen breath tests can be diagnostic in the appropriate clinical scenario. If early dumping is suspected, an early peak will be noted, usually within 1 hour of ingestion.

Treatment

The treatment of dumping syndrome involves mainly dietary modifications. These include switching to smaller, more frequent meals; minimizing ingestion of simple carbohydrates; avoiding simultaneous fluid intake with solids; and adding supplemental fiber (pectin, guar gum) to increase the viscosity of the ingested food and delay gastric emptying. Medical therapy includes acarbose (50–100 mg three times daily), an α-glucosidase inhibitor that blunts the rapid absorption of glucose. Short-acting (50 mcg subcutaneously three times daily) or long-acting (10 mg intramuscularly every 4 weeks) octreotide acts by inhibiting effects on insulin and gut hormone release, as well as decreasing intestinal transit time. Short-term use is initially effective, but response is less optimal with longer use.

Didden P, Penning C, Masclee AA. Octreotide therapy in dumping syndrome: analysis of long-term results. *Aliment Pharmacol Ther.* 2006;24:1367–1375. [PMID: 17059518]

Hasler WL. Dumping syndrome. *Curr Treat Options Gastroenterol.* 2002;5:139–145. [PMID: 11879594]

RAPID TRANSIT DYSMOTILITY OF THE SMALL BOWEL

Rapid transit of small bowel contents occurs in postvagotomy diarrhea, short bowel syndrome, irritable bowel, diabetic enteropathy, or carcinoid syndrome. These syndromes, except for irritable bowel syndrome, can cause severe dehydration and electrolyte disturbances.

Scintigraphy or the lactulose hydrogen breath test can be diagnostic. Small bowel manometry is not widely available but may show high-amplitude contractions, rapid peristalsis, and prolonged duration.

Treatment

The initial focus of treatment is on correction of dehydration and electrolyte imbalance. Patients, once stabilized, should avoid hyperosmolar drinks and receive rehydration with isoosmolar fluids. Parenteral support with intravenous fluids or even parenteral nutrition may be necessary for patients with less than 1 meter of small bowel.

Loperamide (4 mg, 30 minutes prior to meals and bedtime) can decrease the gastrocolic reflex and slow motility. Verapamil (40 mg twice daily) or clonidine (0.1 mg twice daily), or both, may be used in conjunction with loperamide. Subcutaneous octreotide (50 mcg twice daily) can be considered if other drugs fail.

This chapter is a revised version of the chapter by Dr. Victor S. Wang and Dr. Robert Burakoff that was in the previous edition of Current Diagnosis & Treatment: Gastroenterology, Hepatology, & Endoscopy.

Treatment of Obesity: The Impact of Bariatric Surgery

Malcolm K. Robinson, MD
Norton J. Greenberger, MD

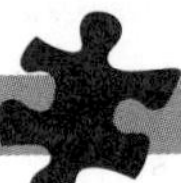

ESSENTIAL CONCEPTS

- Body mass index (BMI) >25 is considered overweight; >30, grade I obesity; >35, grade II obesity; >40, grade III obesity; and >50, "super obesity."
- Using these criteria, two thirds of Americans are overweight or obese.
- Diet, pharmacotherapy, and behavior modification are the available nonsurgical treatment options and are of limited efficacy, with durable weight loss rarely exceeding 10 kg.
- Patients with a BMI >35 can be considered for bariatric surgery if they have severe weight-related comorbid conditions (eg, diabetes, hypertension, disabling arthritis, or sleep apnea).
- Patients with a BMI >40 may be appropriate surgical candidates, with or without weight-related comorbid conditions.
- Two long-term studies of the efficacy of bariatric surgery noted a 29–40% reduction in all causes of death, with decreased mortality from coronary artery disease, stroke, diabetes, and cancer.

General Considerations

Obesity has reached epidemic proportions worldwide and continues to exact a high cost in human and monetary terms within the United States. This disease is second only to cigarette smoking as a preventable cause of death, and deaths attributable to obesity far outnumber colon cancer. Three hundred thousand people die annually from obesity-related disorders in the United States. In addition, health care costs to treat obesity and weight-related conditions exceed $100 billion annually. This problem is of particular concern because upwards of one third of adult Americans are obese, with 5% of the population meeting the criteria for the most severe form of the disease. In short, obesity is a major public health problem that requires aggressive prevention and treatment.

Weight loss surgery has been recognized for decades as an effective treatment of obese individuals. This has resulted in a dramatic increase in such procedures. Over a 5-year period, there was a 113% increase in such procedure in the United States and Canada, and currently over 220,000 bariatric operations are performed each year in this region alone. Surgical treatment of obesity is routinely associated with loss of greater than 100 pounds. Hence, it is not surprising that patients who undergo such operations can have substantial amelioration of comorbid conditions.

Bariatric surgery may not be the ideal obesity treatment. However, surgery is currently the most effective and durable treatment of the obese compared with any other available therapy in terms of weight loss, alleviation of comorbid conditions, reduction in mortality risk, and decreased long-term health care costs.

Buchwald H, Oien DM. Metabolic/bariatric surgery worldwide 2008. *Obes Surg.* 2009;19:1605–1611. [PMID: 19885707]

Hedley AA, Ogden CL, Johnson CL, et al. Prevalence of overweight and obesity among US children, adolescents, and adults, 1999–2002. *JAMA.* 2004;291:2847–2850. [PMID: 15199035]

Maggard MA, Shugarman LR, Suttorp M, et al. Meta-analysis: surgical treatment of obesity. *Ann Intern Med.* 2005;142:547–559. [PMID: 15809466]

Mokdad AH, Marks JS, Stroup DF, et al. Actual causes of death in the United States. *JAMA.* 2000;291:1238–1245. [PMID: 15010446]

TREATMENT OF OVERWEIGHT & OBESE PATIENTS

Treatment of overweight and obese individuals is based on the degree of excess body weight and the presence or absence of weight-related conditions. The degree and categorization of excess body weight is routinely based on body mass index (BMI).

Table 19–1. Classification and health risks of overweight individuals.[a]

Category	Body Mass Index (BMI)	Health Risk	Risk with Comorbidities
Normal	18.5–25	Minimal	Low
Overweight	25–26.9	Low	Moderate
	27–29.9	Moderate	High
Obese			
Class I	30–34.9	High	Very high
Class II	35–39.9	Very high	Extremely high
Class III	>40	Extremely high	Extremely high

[a]Based on NIH recommendations for the treatment of overweight and obesity in adults.

A patient's BMI is calculated by dividing weight in kilograms by the height in meters squared. This index normalizes weight for a given height and is independent of gender. The BMI is generally considered a better classification scheme of excess body weight than the outdated Metropolitan Life tables, which are gender-dependent and require a rough estimate of body frame size.

A BMI of 18.5–25 kg/m^2 is considered "normal." A BMI greater than 25 kg/m^2 is considered "overweight" or "obese" (Table 19–1). Based on these criteria an astounding two thirds of adult Americans are overweight or obese. A person is considered obese when his or her BMI is 30 kg/m^2 or higher, and obesity is divided into at least three categories, classes I, II, and III. Bariatric surgeons have defined an additional "super obese" category, which is a BMI greater than 50 kg/m^2. This extra surgical category has been used in clinical studies when analyzing data and correlating outcomes with preoperative weight class.

Although BMI correlates with excess body fat, it is possible for a highly trained, muscular athlete who in fact is quite lean to have a high BMI. In addition, the association between obesity and mortality appears to be weaker for African Americans as compared with Anglo-Americans. Although the validity of BMI may vary in some patient populations according to their demographic characteristics, including ethnicity, the index has proven to be a clinically relevant measure of obesity that can be linked to disease and mortality risk. For example, the BMI associated with the lowest risk of death is within the normal range for most men and lies within the normal to overweight range for most women (see Table 19–1).

Once BMI is determined, health risk is based on the BMI classification and the presence or absence of weight-related comorbid conditions. The National Institutes of Health (NIH) treatment recommendations start with "healthy eating, exercise, and lifestyle changes" for those with minimal and low health risks and then recommend the addition of diet, pharmacotherapy, or bariatric surgery as health risk increases to the "extremely high health risk" category (Table 19–2). These weight loss treatment recommendations are theoretically based on three parameters: (1) the assessment of the risk of not treating an overweight or obese individual; (2) the risk of a particular weight loss treatment; and (3) the likelihood and degree of benefit from the treatment.

The preceding risk-benefit calculation can be done for those with class III obesity (ie, BMI >40 kg/m^2) to determine the treatment of choice. Untreated obesity of this degree is well known to be associated with several conditions, including diabetes, hypertension, sleep apnea, and cardiovascular disease, that lead to increased mortality and years of life lost. Fontaine and colleagues calculated the years of life lost for obese individuals, and found that 30-year-old white men and women with a BMI of 30 can expect to lose 10 years and 8 years of life expectancy, respectively, if their obesity goes untreated. A 20-year-old black male with a BMI of 45 can expect to lose 20 years of his life expectancy if untreated. Hence, the natural history of class III obesity is clearly associated with both increased morbidity and mortality risk, and thus mandates aggressive intervention.

Diets, pharmacotherapy, and behavior modification with or without exercise are the available nonsurgical treatment options for obesity. Diet therapy is the most common self- and primary care provider–prescribed therapy. There is no doubt that diets are highly effective and generally safe—for

Table 19–2. Risk-based treatment in obese individuals.[a]

Health Risk[b]	Treatment
Minimal or low	Healthy eating, exercise, and lifestyle changes
Moderate	All of the above, plus low-calorie diet
High or very high	All of the above, plus pharmacotherapy or very low-calorie diet
Extremely high	All of the above, plus bariatric surgery

[a]Based on NIH recommendations for the treatment of overweight and obesity in adults.
[b]See Table 19–1.

those who adhere to dietary guidelines. This, unfortunately, is a very small number of individuals. Average weight loss at 12 months is generally quite modest, and the long-term recidivism rate of obesity for those who use diet therapy exceeds 95%. A recent trial compared four popular diets on weight loss and cardiovascular risk reduction. The investigators randomly assigned patients to the Atkins low-carbohydrate, high-protein, high-fat diet; the Zone balanced carbohydrate and protein diet; the Ornish vegetarian, low-fat diet; or the commercially popular Weight Watchers diet. They found that average weight loss at 1 year was 3 kg and BMI was reduced by 1 kg/m^2. There was no difference among the diets. The limited efficacy may be due, in part, to the fact that the patients reported that they adhered to the diets 70% of the time during the first month of intervention but only 30% of the time by the 12th month.

Although the efficacy of pharmacotherapy for weight loss is better than diet alone, it is still considered modest compared with the weight loss efficacy of surgery. Two diet drugs are currently approved by the U.S. Food and Drug Administration (FDA): sibutramine (Meridia) and orlistat (Xenical). At 12 months sibutramine is associated with a mean weight loss of 4 kg for obese individuals while orlistat is associated with a 3-kg placebo-subtracted effect. In addition, FDA approval for drugs is usually limited to 12–24 months, and it is expected that weight gain will occur with drug cessation. This scenario has led several obesity experts to believe that pharmacotherapy has a limited role for those with severe obesity.

Behavior modification appears to have limited efficacy and durability as well. For example, Christiansen and colleagues conducted an intensive lifestyle intervention trial in which 249 subjects underwent a 21-week intensive treatment with exercise, diet, and psychological counseling. Although subjects had lost 22 kg at the end of the treatment phase, the average weight loss was reduced to 7 kg 4 years after treatment. In addition, two thirds of subjects had reduced their weight by less than 5% at the 4-year mark after intensive treatment, with only 28% achieving a weight loss of greater than 10%—the authors' definition of "success"—at 4 years. The XENDOS trial (XENical in the prevention of diabetes in obese subjects) compared orlistat (trade name Xenical) versus placebo plus behavior modification. This 4-year double-blind trial found a 2.7% weight loss in the placebo plus behavior modification group versus 5.4% in the Xenical group.

Overall, the long-term benefit of nonsurgical treatment of those with class III obesity is likely to be quite limited except for a very small percentage of individuals. In contrast, surgical intervention, as detailed below, has an acceptable risk profile and clear, long-term benefits in terms of weight loss, resolution of comorbid conditions, and reduction in mortality risk. As such, bariatric surgery has the best cost-benefit ratio and is therefore considered the weight loss treatment of choice by the NIH for those with severe obesity.

Christiansen T, Bruun JM, Madsen EL, et al. Weight loss maintenance in severely obese adults after an intensive lifestyle intervention: 2- to 4-year follow-up. *Obesity (Silver Spring).* 2007;15:413–420. [PMID: 17299115]

Clinical guidelines on the identification, evaluation, and treatment of overweight and obesity in adults—the evidence report. National Institutes of Health. *Obes Res.* 1998;6(Suppl 2): 51S–209S. [PMID: 9813653]

Dansinger ML, Gleason JA, Griffith JL, et al. Comparison of Atkins, Ornish, Weight Watchers and Zone diets for weight loss and heart disease risk reduction: a randomized trial. *JAMA.* 2005;293:43–53. [PMID: 15632335]

Fontaine KR, Redden DT, Wang C, et al. Years of life lost due to obesity. *JAMA.* 2003;289:187–193. [PMID: 12517229]

McTigue KM, Harris R, Hemphill B, et al. Screening and interventions for obesity in adults: summary of the evidence for the U.S. preventive services task force. *Ann Intern Med.* 2003; 139:933–949. [PMID: 14644897]

Rucker D, Padwal R, Li SK, et al. Long term pharmacotherapy for obesity and overweight: updated meta-analysis. *BMJ.* 2007;335:1194–1203. [PMID: 18006966]

Torgerson JS, Hauptman J, Boldrin MN, et al. XENical in the prevention of diabetes in obese subjects (XENDOS) study: a randomized study of orlistat as an adjunct to lifestyle changes for prevention of type 2 diabetes in obese patients. *Diabetes Care.* 2004;27:155–161. [PMID: 14693982]

INDICATIONS FOR BARIATRIC SURGERY

The indications for surgical treatment of severe obesity are based on the recommendations of the NIH Consensus Development Conference on Gastrointestinal Surgery for Severe Obesity. The first criterion that must be met before considering a patient for bariatric surgery is weight as assessed by BMI. Patients with a BMI of 35–39.9 kg/m^2 (ie, class II obesity) can be considered for surgical intervention if they have severe weight-related conditions such as diabetes, hypertension, debilitating osteoarthritis, or sleep apnea. Those with a BMI of 40 kg/m^2 or greater (ie, class III obesity) may be appropriate candidates for bariatric surgery with or without weight-related comorbid conditions. Approval for surgery based on the preceding BMI criteria assumes there are no contraindications to surgery.

Of note, an FDA advisory panel voted to lower the acceptable weight limits for certain types of weight loss surgery in December of 2010. They recommended that patients with a BMI of 30–35 kg/m^2 with weight-related comorbid conditions and those with a BMI greater than 35 kg/m^2 even without weight related comorbid conditions may be acceptable for adjustable gastric banding. Full approval of the FDA and approval of insurance companies for such surgery may follow in the near future. If approved, this could increase the potential number of people eligible for some type of bariatric surgery by 50–100%.

If a patient satisfies the BMI criteria for bariatric surgery, he or she is more fully evaluated. The patient should have an extensive history of previous weight loss attempts prior to seeking surgery. Most patients in this weight category have undergone a wide variety of nonsurgical interventions over several years. There should be no unstable psychological conditions or substance abuse. Many surgeons operate on patients with depression, but decline to operate on those with unstable conditions. For example, a recent suicide attempt may preclude surgery for at least 1 year or more depending on the ability to demonstrate psychological stability. Patients are routinely screened for such psychiatric issues before proceeding with surgery.

Additional consideration is given to the status of major organs. The bariatric surgical patient should not have severe organ dysfunction, which would make perioperative morbidity and mortality risk unacceptably high. Patients with unstable angina, end-stage pulmonary disease, or cirrhosis may have relative or absolute contraindications to bariatric surgery. However, optimization of treatment of such conditions may improve a patient to the point where he or she may become a bariatric surgical candidate. Generally speaking, there are no guidelines regarding bariatric surgery in those with chronic conditions such as HIV/AIDS or a history of treated cancer. The decision to operate on such individuals must be individualized after careful consultation with the patient, primary care provider, and other specialists who are caring for the individual.

The appropriate age limit for patients considering bariatric surgery is an area of controversy. Adults in the 21–60-year age range are generally deemed appropriate candidates assuming they have no contraindications to surgery. Several articles have explored operative risk in individuals older than 55 years who undergo bariatric surgery. Although it is generally accepted that operative risk is higher in older compared with younger individuals, it does not seem prohibitive. Accordingly, some surgeons believe that operating on severely obese patients up to age 70 to induce weight loss may be appropriate. In general, a firm age cutoff is not necessary if patients are selected carefully and comorbid medical conditions are brought under optimal control before surgical intervention for weight loss. It should be recognized, however, that older patients require a more extensive evaluation looking for silent organ disease, such as asymptomatic atherosclerotic heart disease. Although such a workup may not prevent a bariatric surgical complication, it will theoretically select for those who have the physiologic reserve to better tolerate and survive a complication if one were to occur. In short, the ultimate decision to proceed in older patients should be based on the specific individual's risks relative to the potential benefits, and not just age alone.

Adolescent bariatric surgery is being studied as well, given the rise in type 2 diabetes and other weight-related comorbidities in this age group. Initial studies indicate significant benefits in this age group, which is slowly increasing the medical community's comfort level with having adolescents be considered for bariatric surgery. As with operating in individuals at the other end of the age spectrum, there are special considerations. It is recommended that surgery be reserved for those adolescents with class III obesity (ie, BMI >40 kg/m^2) who have weight-related conditions. This is stricter than the adult criterion of class II obesity with weight-related comorbidities. Adolescents should have documented evidence of failure of at least a 6-month nonsurgical weight loss program. In addition, surgery should not be considered in adolescents until the epiphyseal plates are closed and mature bone length has been achieved. Rapid weight loss may adversely affect bone growth due to restricted caloric intake during this critical time of development. Finally, the family support system takes on an especially important role when operating on younger individuals. It is the extremely rare individual who at so young an age does not absolutely require the full support of family. Thus, patient evaluation in the very young essentially mandates extensive evaluation of the patient's family and support network as well.

One final consideration of bariatric surgery in adolescents is the relative advisability of gastric bypass versus adjustable gastric banding (see the description of these procedures in the next section). The gastric bypass requires cutting and rerouting of the intestines, permanently altering the patient's anatomy with unknown long-term effects in adolescents. The laparoscopic adjustable band does not permanently alter patient anatomy and can be removed, thereby returning the anatomy to normal if necessary. However, the long-term (ie, 50 or more years) effects of a band in young individuals are completely unknown, and this approach may or may not be more appropriate for the very young. Although there is a great deal to learn about adolescent bariatric surgery, some form of such surgery may take on an important role given the rapid rise of obesity and obesity-related conditions in this age group.

In general, the decision to proceed with bariatric surgery requires careful evaluation of the patient and analysis of both physical and psychological well-being of the patient. This usually requires a multidisciplinary team with a comprehensive program to support patients preoperatively, during hospitalization, and for a lifetime postoperatively. Procedures available for the treatment of obesity are outlined next.

Horgan S, Holterman MJ, Jacobsen GR, et al. Laparoscopic adjustable gastric banding for the treatment of adolescent morbid obesity in the United States: a safe alternative to gastric bypass. *J Pediatr Surg.* 2005;40:86–90. [PMID: 15868564]

Inge TH, Krebs NF, Garcia VF, et al. Bariatric surgery for severely overweight adolescents: concerns and recommendations. *Pediatrics.* 2004;217–223. [PMID: 15231931]

O'Brien PE, Sawyer SM, Laurie C, et al. Laparoscopic adjustable gastric banding in severely obese adolescents: a randomized trial. *JAMA.* 2010;303:519–526. [PMID: 20145228]

Papasavas PK, Gagne DJ, Kelly J, et al. Laparoscopic Roux-en-Y gastric bypass is a safe and effective operation for the treatment of morbid obesity in patients older than 55 years. *Obes Surg.* 2004;14:1056–1061. [PMID: 15479593]

Sjöström L, Narbro K, Sjöström CD, et al; Swedish Obese Subjects Study. Effects of bariatric surgery on mortality in Swedish obese subjects. *N Engl J Med.* 2007;357:741–752. [PMID: 17715408]

Sugerman HJ, DeMaria EJ, Kellum JM, et al. Effects of bariatric surgery in older patients. *Ann Surg.* 2004;240:243–247. [PMID: 15273547]

BARIATRIC SURGICAL PROCEDURES

Surgical treatment of obesity began in the early 1950s when several groups proposed shortening the intestinal tract via "bypass" procedures to produce substantial decreases in absorptive area. This proposal was based on the observation that massive small bowel resections for treatment of other pathologic conditions resulted in weight loss followed by weight stabilization. Since that time, more than 30 different surgical techniques have been described for treating obesity. The field underwent a recent revolution with the introduction of minimally invasive laparoscopic techniques to produce surgical weight loss. In general, the surgical approach to obesity treatment is designed to create negative energy balance by (1) reducing caloric absorption by way of a small intestinal bypass; (2) reducing caloric consumption by severely restricting gastric capacity; or (3) producing weight loss through a procedure that combines both malabsorption and restriction of caloric intake. The description of every type of bariatric procedure is beyond the scope of this chapter. However, the commonly used, well-known, and emerging procedures are described.

Kim JJ, Tarnoff ME, Shikora SA. Surgical treatment for extreme obesity: evolution of a rapidly growing field. *Nutr Clin Pract.* 2003;18:109–123. [PMID: 16215028]

1. Roux-en-Y Gastric Bypass

Currently, the most frequently performed operation and the gold standard of bariatric procedures in the United States is the Roux-en-Y gastric bypass (GBP) (Figure 19–1). Approximately two thirds of bariatric procedures worldwide are the GBP. In this procedure, a 30-mL pouch is constructed to which a Roux loop of jejunum is anastomosed. This creates a short biliopancreatic limb through which bile and pancreatic secretions flow; an alimentary limb of 100–200 cm, depending on a patient's preoperative weight, in which food from the gastric pouch travels; and a common limb that consists of the remainder of the small bowel just distal to the anastomosis of the alimentary and biliopancreatic limbs. The majority of the stomach, the duodenum, and several centimeters of proximal jejunum are bypassed in this configuration. Thus, the procedure is traditionally said to combine both restrictive and malabsorptive features. In reality, however, the importance of malabsorption in contributing to the weight loss produced by GBP has been questioned. Most now believe that there is very little, if any, macronutrient malabsorption. Other neuroendocrine alterations, such as the reduction in the orexigenic gastric peptide, ghrelin, may contribute to the weight loss efficacy of this procedure. Clearly, much more study is needed before the physiologic alterations associated with GBP can be definitively attributed to this hormone or any other neuroendocrine change.

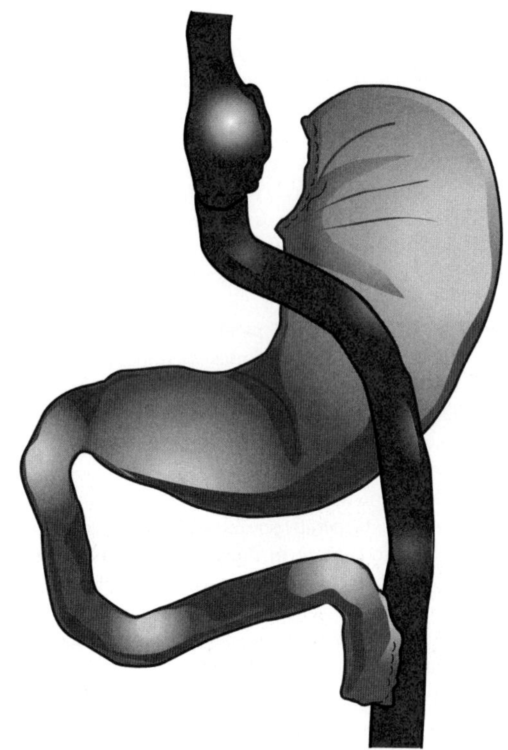

▲ **Figure 19–1.** Roux-en-Y gastric bypass.

The GBP procedure can be performed either laparoscopically or "open," with equivalent weight loss effectiveness. The majority of academic medical centers now perform the GBP laparoscopically, believing that complications and outcome other than weight loss may be superior with this approach versus the open approach. However, a recent publication has challenged this notion and suggests that the open approach is of equivalent, if not superior, benefit compared with the laparoscopic approach. The in-depth analysis of this controversy is beyond the scope of this chapter. Regardless of whether the laparoscopic or open approach is employed, the gastric bypass is the bariatric surgical procedure to which all other bariatric procedures are compared in terms of efficacy, morbidity, and mortality.

Buchwald H, Oien DM. Metabolic/bariatric surgery worldwide 2008. *Obes Surg.* 2009;19:1605–1611. [PMID: 19885707]

Cummings DE, Weigle DS, Frayo RS, et al. Plasma ghrelin levels after diet induced weight loss or gastric bypass surgery. *N Engl J Med.* 2002;346:1623–1630. [PMID: 12023994]

Jones KB Jr, Afram JD, Benotti PN, et al. Open versus laparoscopic Roux-en-Y gastric bypass: a comparative study of over 25,000 open cases and the major laparoscopic bariatric reported series. *Obes Surg.* 2006;16:721–727. [PMID: 16756731]

Nguyen NT, Hinojosa M, Fayad C, et al. Use and outcomes of laparoscopic versus open gastric bypass at academic medical centers. *J Am Coll Surg.* 2007;205:248–255. [PMID: 17660071]

2. Biliopancreatic Diversion

More recently, another type of malabsorptive procedure, originally described by Scopinaro of Genoa, Italy, has been gaining popularity in the United States (Figure 19–2). Known as the biliopancreatic diversion (BPD), the procedure consists of a subtotal gastrectomy leaving a gastric remnant of 200–400 mL. The small bowel is divided 250 cm proximal to the ileocecal valve. The distal small bowel limb is then anastomosed to the gastric remnant. The end of the proximal small bowel limb is anastomosed to the side of the distal small bowel limb 50 cm proximal to the ileocecal valve. This construction results in three small bowel limbs similar to that described with the GBP: a long biliopancreatic limb, a 200-cm alimentary limb, and a 50-cm common limb in which food and biliopancreatic secretions mix and most of the digestion and absorption of consumed food occurs. This operation produces weight loss by inducing malabsorption. The relatively large gastric remnant does little to restrict food intake. Similar to the GBP, the BPD can be done open or laparoscopically. This procedure is popular in certain parts of Europe, although only 5% of bariatric procedures done worldwide are of this type. Some believe that the malabsorption induced by the BPD can be overly harsh and lead to debilitating diarrhea as a result of the typical, high-fat American diet compared with the high-in-complex-carbohydrate diet characteristic of Italy.

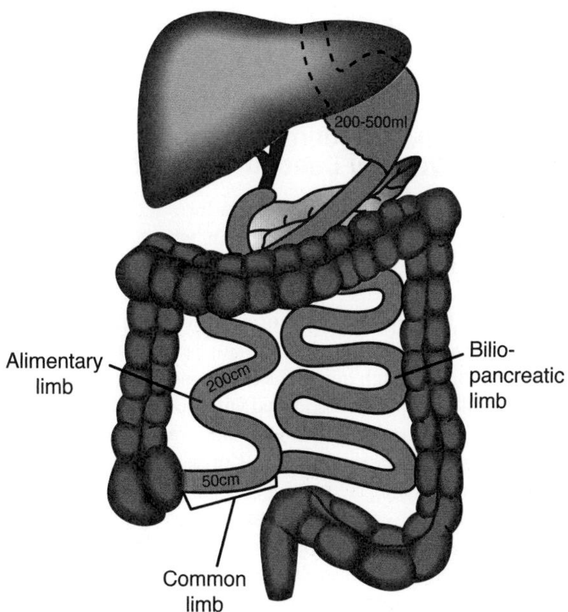

▲ **Figure 19–2.** Biliopancreatic diversion procedure.

Scopinaro N, Gianetta E, Gianetta E, et al. Bilio-pancreatic bypass for obesity: II. Initial experience in man. *Br J Surg.* 1979;66: 618–620. [PMID: 497645]

Weber M, Müller MK, Bucher T, et al. Laparoscopic gastric bypass is superior to laparoscopic gastric banding for treatment of morbid obesity. *Ann Surg.* 2004;240:975–982. [PMID: 15570103]

3. Adjustable Silicone Gastric Banding

Adjustable silicone gastric banding (ASGB) is a relatively new restrictive procedure gaining popularity among patients, surgeons, and primary care physicians alike and approved by the FDA for use in the United States in 2001. Overall about a quarter of bariatric procedures worldwide are of this type and are now almost exclusively placed laparoscopically. In the laparoscopic adjustable silicone gastric banding (LASGB) procedure, a silicone-jacketed, beltlike device (ie, the band) is wrapped around the upper part of the stomach near the angle of His. This results in partitioning of the stomach into a small 30-mL proximal pouch and a larger distal stomach remnant in continuity with the pouch. The inner part of the band has an inflatable fluid-filled sack to which a catheter is attached. The catheter, in turn, is attached to a port, which sits just beneath the skin of the abdominal wall. The port can be accessed through the skin with a syringe and a needle to either add or remove saline from the sack, thereby tightening or loosening the band, respectively. Thus, the band is "adjustable." Patients have their bands adjusted depending on adequacy of weight loss or symptoms suggesting that it is too tight.

The advantage of the LASGB is that it is a fast, relatively safe procedure that requires no cutting or stapling of the stomach. The adjustability of the band is also thought to be an advantage, allowing increased durability of weight loss. The downside of the LASGB is that weight loss is significantly slower than that achieved using other bariatric procedures; with the LASGB, up to 2–3 years may be needed to achieve weight loss equal to that observed at 12–18 months with the GBP and BPD. Some experts feel that those who undergo LASGB will never achieve a maximal weight loss equivalent to GBP or BPD. This, however, is controversial, with some investigators suggesting that although weight loss is slower with LASGB compared with GBP, long-term weight loss is the same.

Buchwald H, Oien DM. Metabolic/bariatric surgery worldwide 2008. *Obes Surg.* 2009;19:1605–1611. [PMID: 19885707]

Jan JC, Hong D, Pereira N, et al. Laparoscopic adjustable gastric banding versus laparoscopic gastric bypass for morbid obesity: a single-institution comparison study of early results. *J Gastrointest Surg.* 2005;9:30–39. [PMID: 15623442]

Mognol P, Chosidow D, Marmuse JP. Laparoscopic gastric bypass versus laparoscopic adjustable banding in the super-obese: a comparative study of 290 patients. *Obes Surg.* 2005;15:76–81. [PMID: 15760503]

Weber M, Müller MK, Bucher T, et al. Laparoscopic gastric bypass is superior to laparoscopic gastric banding for treatment of morbid obesity. *Ann Surg.* 2004;240:975–982. [PMID: 15570103]

4. Sleeve Gastrectomy

Recently a new procedure known as the sleeve gastrectomy has been used in some centers. This was first described by Ren and colleagues and was born out of the notion that the morbidity and mortality risk for a laparoscopically performed BDP would be improved if the procedure was performed in two stages. In the first stage, the sleeve gastrectomy is performed. The majority of the stomach on the greater curve side is removed, leaving a "sleeve" of stomach based on the lesser curve (Figure 19–3). After 6–12 months of weight loss, resolution or improvement of comorbid conditions, and presumably marked decrease in operative risk, the second stage is performed. In this stage, the sleeve procedure is converted to a GBP or a BPD laparoscopically. This is thought to be particularly appropriate for the high-risk, high-BMI patient in whom a one-stage GBP or BPD is considered prohibitively risky.

The two-stage procedure has an obvious drawback in that it requires two separate operations. Hence, such an approach must be balanced against the relative risks of the one-stage, longer operation performed in a poorer surgical candidate. Early experience with the sleeve gastrectomy has suggested that the weight loss induced by this procedure alone (ie, without performing the second stage) is significant enough to be used as a definitive one-stage procedure. This evidence includes a recent prospective, double-blind study in which the sleeve gastrectomy was compared with a GBP. The authors found that weight loss for the sleeve was better than the GBP (69.7% vs 60.5% excess body weight lost at 1 year, $P = .05$ sleeve vs GBP). This result was associated with the finding that the orexigenic gastric peptide, ghrelin, was significantly lower in the sleeve group, as was appetite, compared with that of the GBP group. It is important to note, however, that these data are relatively short term and several experts have expressed concern that the gastric pouch of the sleeve will dilate over time and weight loss efficacy may be lost. However medium- and longer-term results are confirming the initial enthusiasm for this procedure. Further study is needed before determining the appropriate place of the sleeve gastrectomy in the armamentarium of the bariatric surgeon.

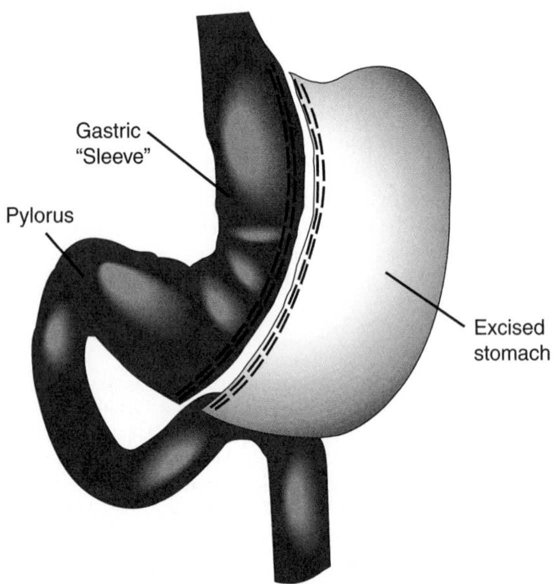

▲ **Figure 19–3.** Sleeve gastrectomy.

Bellanger DE, Greenway FL. Laparoscopic sleeve gastrectomy, 529 cases without a leak: short-term results and technical considerations. *Obes Surg.* 2011;21:146–150. [PMID: 21132397]

Bohdjalian A, Langer FB, Shakeri-Leidenmuler S, et al: Sleeve gastrectomy as sole and definitive bariatric procedure: 5-year results for weight loss and ghrelin. *Obes Surg.* 2010;20:535–540. [PMID: 20094819]

Frezza EE. Laparoscopic vertical sleeve gastrectomy for morbid obesity. The future procedure of choice? *Surg Today.* 2007;37: 275–281. [PMID: 17387557]

Karamanakos SN, Vagenas K, Kalfarentzos F, et al. Weight loss, appetite suppression, and changes in fasting and postprandial ghrelin and peptide-YY levels after Roux-en-Y gastric bypass and sleeve gastrectomy. *Ann Surg.* 2008;247:401–407. [PMID: 18376181]

Ren CJ, Patterson E, Gagner M. Early results of laparoscopic biliopancreatic diversion with duodenal switch: a case series of 40 consecutive patients. *Obes Surg.* 2000;10:514–523. [PMID: 11175958]

5. Outdated Procedures: Jejunoileal Bypass & Vertical Banded Gastroplasty

Two outdated bariatric surgical procedures require mention. The first is the jejunoileal bypass, in which the proximal jejunum is divided 35 cm distal to the ligament of Treitz and anastomosed to the distal ileum, 10 cm proximal to the ileocecal valve. The long bypassed or excluded segment of small intestine is vented to the colon or small intestine to prevent obstruction. Although quite effective in inducing weight loss, the jejunoileal bypass is associated with debilitating diarrhea, electrolyte imbalances, vitamin and mineral deficiencies, and life-threatening liver dysfunction. Consequently, this procedure has been abandoned.

The other well-known but outdated bariatric procedure is the vertical banded gastroplasty (VBG) originally described by the "father" of bariatric surgery, Edward Mason. It is a purely restrictive procedure in which a vertically oriented 15–30 mL gastric pouch is created along the lesser curve of the proximal stomach. The outlet of this pouch, which leads to the remaining stomach, is encircled with a band of Marlex mesh to prevent dilation of the outlet over time. The advantage of this procedure is that it is technically easier and faster to perform than malabsorptive procedures and avoids issues with severe diarrhea, vitamin and mineral deficiencies, and liver dysfunction. However, the long-term weight loss is less effective than that achieved with the GBP and BPD, and the LASGB has supplanted VBG use by bariatric surgeons. This is largely due to the adjustability feature of the LASGB, which is thought to improve weight loss efficacy and durability relative to the VBG.

POSTOPERATIVE CARE & COMPLICATIONS

In high-volume centers, hospital stay for bariatric surgery patients varies from 1 to 3 days depending on the type of procedure performed. LASGB patients are usually discharged within 24 hours of surgery, although some centers are moving to day surgery for LASGB in which patients are sent home on the same day of the procedure. GBP patients who have surgery performed laparoscopically are generally discharged from the hospital in 2–3 days. Patients who have an open GBP are generally discharged from the hospital after 2–3 days as well. Routine care during hospitalization focuses on providing adequate pain control and ensuring adequate oral intake. Once these are achieved, the patient can be safely discharged to home. The diet is advanced through various "stages" over several weeks, and patients receive extensive education about maintaining hydration status and consuming adequate protein.

The most common "complication" in bariatric surgical patients is nausea and vomiting, which may occur in as many as 30–40% of patients. This can lead to rehospitalization to treat dehydration, despite no identifiable anatomic obstruction of the gastrointestinal tract. Patients usually receive intravenous hydration and are discharged to home in 24–48 hours in good condition. Other complications include wound infections, which affect from 1–2% of patients undergoing laparoscopic procedures to as high as 10–15% of those undergoing open procedures. Long-term complications include ventral hernia formation, which is more common in the open approach than the laparoscopic approach. Less common issues include pouch ulcer formation, internal hernia formation, and small bowel obstruction from adhesion formation.

The most common life-threatening complications from bariatric surgery include peritonitis and intra-abdominal abscess associated with an anastomotic leak or iatrogenic, unrecognized perforation of a viscus. Bariatric patients are notorious for having a paucity of classic signs of peritonitis. Instead of abdominal pain and rebound tenderness, these patients may complain of back and left shoulder pain and have a relatively "benign" abdominal examination until impending death. They may also have tachypnea, tachycardia, and hypoxia without clear etiology. The surgeon should have a low threshold for obtaining radiologic evaluation with water-soluble contrast agents if any of these symptoms should occur without clear explanation. However, radiologic studies may be falsely negative given the patient's body habitus and technical difficulties associated with obtaining and interpreting radiographs in the morbidly obese. Thus, a patient requires surgical reexploration even in the face of negative studies if he or she is clinically unstable and without an identifiable source of pathology. The reported incidence of leaks is 1–2% and may be higher in those undergoing laparoscopic procedures, especially in the first 100 cases of a surgeon's experience.

Pulmonary embolism, although feared and often discussed, is relatively uncommon in bariatric surgery patients. It occurs less than 1% of the time in those who receive appropriate prophylaxis against pulmonary embolism, which is generally "double coverage" (eg, low molecular weight heparin and pneumatic compression boots). Pulmonary embolism can be hard to diagnose in the morbidly obese. Persistent tachypnea and hypoxia may be suggestive, but many obese patients have a preoperative history of pulmonary issues with such symptoms, which may lull practitioners into a false sense of security. Hence, there should be a low threshold to work up bariatric patients with ventilation-perfusion scans or spiral chest computed tomography (CT) for even subtle changes in pulmonary status.

High-volume centers report a mortality rate of 1 in 200–500 patients for GBP. Data from the State of Washington suggest that the rate may be higher, at 1–2%, if one collects data from all centers conducting bariatric surgery, which includes those with less experience and higher mortality rates. LASGB has a very low mortality rate of 1 in 2000. Data are limited for emerging procedures such as the sleeve gastrectomy, but it is believed the mortality risk is lower compared with the GBP but higher than the LASGB.

The "perfect" bariatric procedure has yet to be identified. Although, it is generally accepted that the LASGB is the "safest" procedure, it is not clear that it is the most efficacious. Gastric bypass generally is thought to have the best weight loss, but clearly has a higher complication rate. Sleeve gastrectomy is thought to be an intermediate operation in that it has better weight loss than the LASGB and better safety profile than the GBP. However, it is unclear whether the early favorable results of the sleeve procedure will be confirmed in the long run.

Bellanger DE, Greenway FL. Laparoscopic sleeve gastrectomy, 529 cases without a leak: short-term results and technical considerations. *Obes Surg.* 2011;21:146–150. [PMID: 21132397]

Bohdjalian A, Langer FB, Shakeri-Leidenmuler S, et al: Sleeve gastrectomy as sole and definitive bariatric procedure: 5-year results for weight loss and ghrelin. *Obes Surg.* 2010;20:535–540. [PMID: 20094819]

Chapman AE, Kiroff G, Game P, et al. Laparoscopic adjustable gastric banding in the treatment of obesity: a systematic literature review. *Surgery.* 2004;135:326–351. [PMID: 14976485]

Flum DR, Dellinger EP. Impact of gastric bypass operation on survival: a population-based analysis. *J Am Coll Surg.* 2004; 199:543–551. [PMID: 15454136]

Nguyen NT, Paya M, Stevens CM, et al. The relationship between hospital volume and outcome in bariatric surgery at academic medical centers. *Ann Surg.* 2004;240:586–594. [PMID: 15383786]

Nguyen NT, Silver M, Robinson M, et al. Result of a national audit of bariatric surgery performed at academic centers: a 2004 University Health System Consortium Benchmarking Project. *Arch Surg.* 2006;141:445–450. [PMID: 16702515]

Robinson MK. Surgical treatment of obesity–weighing the facts. *N Engl J Med.* 2009;361:520–521. [PMID: 19641209]

Sapala JA, Wood MH, Schuhknecht MP, et al. Fatal pulmonary embolism after bariatric operations for morbid obesity: a 24-year retrospective analysis. *Obes Surg.* 2003;13:819–825. [PMID: 14738663]

Shikora SA, Kim JJ, Tarnoff ME, et al. Laparoscopic Roux-en-Y gastric bypass: results and learning curve of a high-volume academic program. *Arch Surg.* 2005;140:362–367. [PMID: 15837887]

Smith SC, Edwards CB, Goodman GN, et al. Open vs laparoscopic Roux-en-Y gastric bypass: comparison of operative morbidity and mortality. *Obes Surg.* 2004;14:73–76. [PMID: 14980037]

The Longitudinal Assessment of Bariatric Surgery Consortium. Perioperative safety in the longitudinal assessment of bariatric surgery. *N Engl J Med.* 2009;361:445–454. [PMID: 19641201]

GASTROENTEROLOGY EVALUATION & TREATMENT

1. Nausea & Vomiting

Nausea and vomiting with or without abdominal pain is a common complaint after bariatric surgery. Hence, it is not uncommon for gastroenterologists, particularly those based at bariatric surgical centers, to be asked to evaluate patients with these symptoms. The most common cause of nausea and vomiting in the early postoperative period is dehydration and dietary noncompliance, as previously noted. Red meat, bread (particularly doughy breads such as bagels), pasta, and dry chicken are poorly tolerated and can lead to nausea, vomiting, and subsequent dehydration. Patients may also be lactose intolerant, and the consumption of milk-based liquid supplements, which are frequently prescribed in the immediate postoperative period, can precipitate symptoms. Nausea and vomiting purely related to dehydration and dietary indiscretion quickly resolve with rehydration and consultation with a knowledgeable bariatric dietitian. However, one must be on guard when evaluating nausea and vomiting in bariatric surgical patients; the list of differential diagnoses is long and varies from the self-limited to the life threatening.

The first step in evaluating the bariatric surgery patient with nausea and vomiting is determining the type of procedure the patient had. Nomenclature of procedures is variable around the country, and those unfamiliar with bariatric surgical procedures (eg, patients and primary care providers) may use terms incorrectly to convey what procedure was performed. Hence, it is advisable to obtain an operative report if possible and time permits.

The most common patient that the gastroenterologist will be called to evaluate is one who has had a laparoscopic or open GBP, as this is the most commonly performed procedure. Although dehydration and dietary noncompliance may be immediately evident, it is possible that there are other concomitant problems that need to be ruled out. Regurgitation of food and epigastric pain that occur when eating, are absent when not eating, and may be described as the sensation of a "knot" or "ball" in the epigastrium, all suggest a problem with the gastrojejunal anastomosis. Initial evaluation usually includes an upper gastrointestinal (UGI) radiocontrast series to rule out an anastomotic stricture and gastrogastric fistula with or without an anastomotic ulcer. If the UGI series rules in one of these findings, or the patient has persistent epigastric pain without a known etiology, an upper endoscopy (esophagogastroduodenoscopy [EGD]) is indicated.

The EGD will identify a stricture, ulcer, and possible gastrogastric fistula if present virtually 100% of the time. Strictures can successfully be dilated to avoid revisional surgery greater than 95% of the time by an experienced gastroenterologist. Some strictures may require serial dilation at planned intervals to achieve durable results. Narrow strictures (eg, 5 mm or less) should be redilated two times at 2-week intervals for a total of three successive dilations to ensure long-term relief of the stricture. Although dilation may be attempted up to six times, the average number of dilations required for durable success is two to three. Ulcers are treated with standard medical therapy and must be treated aggressively, particularly if associated with a stricture or upper gastrointestinal bleeding. Similarly, gastrogastric fistulae (ie, a channel between the gastric pouch and bypassed stomach) should be treated for symptoms such as ulcer formation and weight regain.

A new subspecialty within gastroenterology is emerging in which the preceding complications and others are being treated endoscopically by gastroenterologists who specialize in the treatment and evaluation of the postoperative bariatric surgical patient. Conditions that formerly were thought to mandate surgical exploration and revision are now being treated successfully with outpatient, low-morbidity—although complex—endoscopic procedures. For example, patients who have weight regain or nonhealing ulcers associated with gastrogastric fistulae have been treated successfully with endoscopic suturing to close the orifice leading to the bypassed stomach pouch. Similarly, patients who have weight gain secondary to a dilated gastrojejunal anastomosis and pouch dilation may benefit from an attempt at endoscopic suturing to reduce anastomotic and pouch size. Preliminary results suggest that this approach can restore weight loss efficacy of the GBP without surgical revision. Finally, a small series of hemodynamically stable patients, *without* diffuse peritonitis and chronic gastrojejunal anastomotic leaks, have been treated successfully by endoscopic techniques. These initial results, while encouraging, must be viewed carefully. First, such procedures should be done only by those with advanced endoscopic therapeutic technical skills and most likely in a specialty center. Second, long-term follow-up studies (currently under way) are necessary to determine if these procedures can be recommended on a regular basis.

Nausea and vomiting may also occur with more distal pathology such as jejunojejunal anastomotic stricture, jejunal intussusception, and an internal hernia. Usually patients present with abdominal pain as well as vomiting with these conditions, and the initial evaluation includes abdominal CT scanning. The CT scan may miss the diagnosis, in which case persistent symptoms may prompt EGD interrogation down to the jejunojejunal anastomosis. Pathology may be identified by endoscopic interrogation and may identify a diagnosis missed on CT scan. Chronic vomiting, particularly with abdominal pain and unknown etiology or in the acutely ill patient, should prompt exploratory laparotomy to rule out internal hernias, intussusception, or jejunojejunal stricture. Such diagnoses can be hard to make short of surgery, and missing an internal hernia, for example, can be fatal in the postoperative bariatric surgical patient.

The causes of nausea and vomiting in the lap band patient include dehydration and dietary indiscretion, similar to that observed in the GBP patient. Band-related causes include overtightening of the band and band slippage. Patients may find they can tolerate liquids but not solids immediately after band tightening. This suggests overtightening of the band and can be relieved by simple withdrawal of saline from the port. In contrast, acute or slowly progressive dysphagia to solid and liquids in a patient in whom band tightening has not recently occurred should prompt a UGI study to rule out band slippage. Band slippage is the anterior or posterior herniation of the stomach through the band ring. Pain and inability to swallow food and liquids should prompt urgent evaluation to rule out band slip. Withdrawal of saline from the port may alleviate the pain associated with this complication and should be done to alleviate any stomach ischemia even before obtaining a UGI to confirm the diagnosis. The acute onset of pain and inability to swallow food and liquids should be evaluated urgently to rule out band slip. An acute slip with pain is indicative of stomach ischemia and can lead to frank stomach necrosis if not treated promptly. Finally, LASGB port site infection, which does not occur in the immediate postoperative period, should prompt local treatment of the port site as well as EGD to rule out band erosion. Band erosion may allow tracking of gastric bacteria along the catheter retrograde to the port.

2. Cholelithiasis & Cholecystitis

It is well known that rapid weight loss is associated with the development of cholelithiasis and cholecystitis. Controversy still exists among bariatric surgeons regarding whether the gallbladder, if present, should be removed in all bariatric surgical patients. It is clear, however, that the gastroenterologist will occasionally be asked to assist with treatment of those patients who have choledocholithiasis. This is generally straightforward in band patients, although one should consider complete deflation of the band to assist with endoscopic retrograde cholangiopancreatography (ERCP) if indicated.

In contrast, ERCP in the GBP patient can be quite challenging, although possible, by performing an EGD down to the jejunojejunal anastomosis and going retrograde up the biliopancreatic limb to access the duodenal ampulla of Vater. ShapeLock technology can assist with negotiating the route to the duodenum. If peroral ERCP is unsuccessful, laparoscopic gastrotomy and transabdominal passage of a sterile endoscope into the stomach and antegrade down the duodenum to the ampulla can be done. This procedure requires general anesthesia but generally causes less morbidity than an open or laparoscopic common bile duct exploration, and the gallbladder can be removed at the same time if appropriate.

3. Constipation

Finally, constipation is common after bariatric surgery, and the gastroenterologist may be asked to evaluate and treat this complex condition. The condition may be due to one or several factors, among them:

- A history of infrequent bowel movements that antedates the surgery. It is not generally appreciated that 2% of U.S. women have two or fewer bowel motions per week.
- Insufficient intake of "laxative"-type foods, which may induce bowel motions. Such foods include peaches, pears, cherries, apples, apple juice, orange juice, milk and milk products, cola beverages, other high-fructose beverages, pastries, candy, chocolate, salads, Brassica vegetables (cabbage, cauliflower, asparagus, broccoli, Brussels sprouts), bran cereal, and muffins. Although such foods can alleviate constipation, they may also produce "dumping" syndrome in GBP patients—a syndrome characterized by crampy abdominal pain, nausea, vomiting, perspiration, and diarrhea—related to rapid transit of a high osmotic load through the small gastric pouch to the jejunum. One must balance the goal of treating constipation with avoiding this syndrome through dietary intervention.
- Insufficient fluid intake. Bariatric patients should ingest at least 1½–2 quarts of fluids a day, which can be challenging given the limited size of their newly created gastric reservoirs. Patients can achieve this goal by drinking small quantities of fluid throughout the day.
- Concurrent use of medications with anticholinergic or antimotility effects such as antihistamines, tricyclic antidepressants, calcium channel blockers, calcium supplements, iron supplements such as ferrous sulfate, and selective serotonin reuptake inhibitors.
- Antecedent hysterectomy. Five percent of patients undergoing a hysterectomy develop refractory constipation.

Accordingly, the approach to patients with constipation is to take a detailed history and determine what the patient actually means by the term "constipation." This may mean infrequent stools (<3 per week) or unusually hard stools difficult to pass. The next step is to assess fluid intake to ensure adequate fluid intake, as discussed previously. The third step is to review the patients' medications and consider discontinuation of those who constipate unless clearly needed. The fourth step is to prescribe a stool softener. The most useful preparations are those that contain both docusate and sorbitol. If patients do not respond to these steps, one can add a medicine such as lubiprostone (Amitiza).

Most bariatric patients respond to the aforementioned treatments. However, for those who do not, a Sitz marker study can be ordered to rule out colonic inertia, or anorectal manometry, or magnetic resonance imaging defecography to rule out pelvic floor muscle dysfunction. Patients may also have a combination of colonic inertia and pelvic floor muscle dysfunction. Treatment can be rendered depending on the severity of constipation and the diagnoses made by these studies.

Go MR, Muscarella P, Needleman BJ, et al. Endoscopic management of stomal stenosis after Roux-en-Y gastric bypass. *Surg Endosc.* 2004;18:56–59. [PMID: 14625732]

Merrifield BF, Lautz D, Thompson CC. Endoscopic repair of gastric leaks after Roux-en-Y gastric bypass: a less invasive approach. *Gastrointest Endosc.* 2006;63:710–714. [PMID: 16564884]

Moore KA, Ouyang DW, Whang EE. Maternal and fetal deaths after gastric bypass surgery for treatment of morbid obesity. *N Engl J Med.* 2004;351:721–722. [PMID: 15306679]

Nguyen NT, Hinojosa MW, Slone J, et al. Laparoscopic transgastric access to the biliary tree after Roux-en-Y gastric bypass. *Obes Surg.* 2007;17:416–419. [PMID: 17546853]

Pai RD, Carr-Locke DL, Thompson CC. Endoscopic evaluation of the defunctionalized stomach by using ShapeLock technology (with video). *Gastrointest Endosc.* 2007;66:578–581. [PMID: 17725949]

Thompson CC, Carr-Locke DL, Saltzman J, et al. Per oral repair of staple-line dehiscence in roux-en-Y gastric bypass: a less invasive approach. Presented at the 45th annual meeting of the Society for Surgery of the Alimentary Tract, 2004.

Thompson C, Robinson MK, Lautz D. FACS. Enteroscopic diagnosis of internal hernia after roux-en gastric bypass, a case study. Presented at the annual meeting of the Society of American Gastrointestinal and Endoscopic Surgeons, 2006.

Thompson CC, Slattery J, Bundga ME, et al. Peroral endoscopic reduction of dilated gastrojejunal anastomosis after Roux-en-Y gastric bypass: a possible new option for patients with weight regain. *Surg Endosc.* 2006;20:1744–1748. [PMID: 17024527]

LONG-TERM OUTCOME OF BARIATRIC SURGERY

Current weight loss surgical procedures are associated with significant weight loss and resolution of weight-related conditions. The Swedish Obese Subjects (SOS) study, which examined weight reduction, reduction in cardiovascular risk factors, and mortality over a 10-year period, is probably the best-known study of bariatric surgery outcome. In this study, 2010 obese subjects who underwent bariatric surgery were contemporaneously matched with 2037 control obese subjects who received nonsurgical treatment. Patients were followed for up to 15 years, and the investigators found that weight loss for all patients undergoing surgery was significantly greater compared with that observed in the control patients (Figure 19–4). GBP patients lost 32% of initial body weight at 1 year, which was maintained at a level of 28% loss of initial body weight at 15 years. Band patients lost less than the GBP patients but still a significant amount: 21% of initial body weight at the 1-year mark and 13% at the 15-year mark after surgical intervention. In contrast, conventionally treated patients essentially had no change in weight over the 15 years of study.

When the surgical patients in the SOS study were compared with the control patients, a marked, statistically significant improvement was seen in lipid profile, diabetes, hypertension, and hyperuricemia, as well as a decrease in the risk of developing these conditions if not present at the time of surgery. The authors concluded that, as compared with conventional, nonsurgical treatment, bariatric surgery results in long-term weight loss, improved lifestyle, and amelioration of a variety of cardiovascular risk factors.

Others have also reported positive findings similar to those of the SOS study. For example, Dixon and colleagues randomized patients to LASGB or nonsurgical treatment and found that not only was weight loss greater in the surgical group, but 76% of the surgical patients also had complete resolution of diabetes compared with 15% for the nonsurgical group. Others have demonstrated that the beneficial effects of weight loss surgery extend to noncardiac risk factors such as pregnancy and neonatal outcomes in obese women who undergo bariatric surgery prior to conceiving. Maggard and colleagues performed a meta-analysis of 147 published studies comparing surgical with nonsurgical treatment. They concluded that "surgery is more effective than nonsurgical treatment for weight loss and control of some comorbid conditions in patients with a BMI of 40 kg/m^2 or greater."

The impact of surgical treatment of the obese is not just limited to alleviation of comorbid conditions. The SOS study found a statistically significant (29%) reduction in death in patients undergoing surgery compared with conventionally treated individuals. In another study, Adams and colleagues assessed mortality risk in 7925 gastric bypass patients compared with 7925 control patients matched for age, gender, and BMI. The adjusted long-term mortality in the surgery group decreased by 40% compared with that in the control group.

A final question regarding use of surgery to treat morbid obesity is the financial cost. Can we as a nation afford to offer such treatment given the high number of patients who potentially qualify for surgery? It is clear that initial health care costs for obese individuals who undergo surgery are higher than the costs for obese individuals who receive

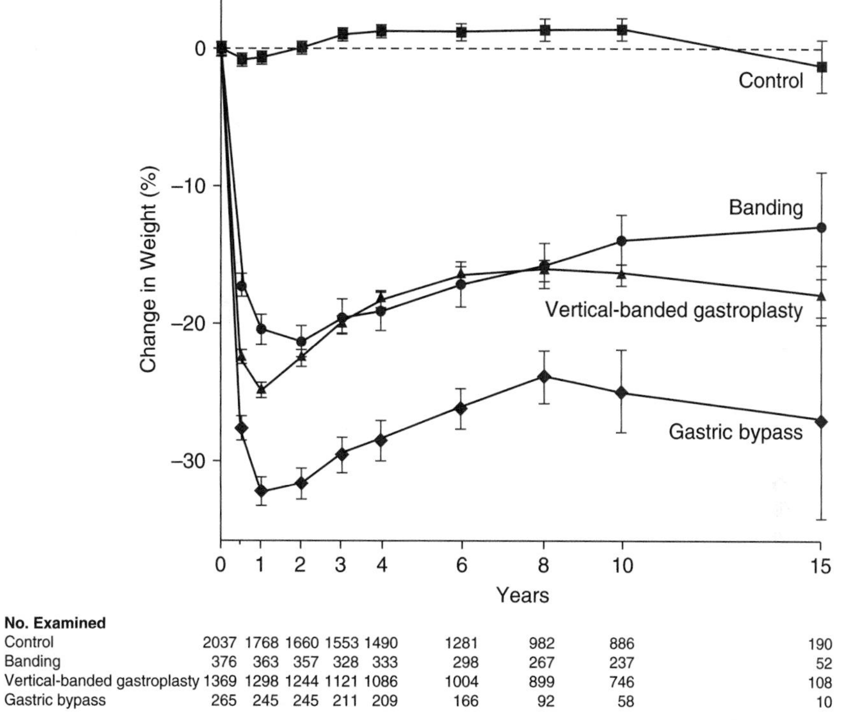

No. Examined	0					6	8	10	15
Control	2037	1768	1660	1553	1490	1281	982	886	190
Banding	376	363	357	328	333	298	267	237	52
Vertical-banded gastroplasty	1369	1298	1244	1121	1086	1004	899	746	108
Gastric bypass	265	245	245	211	209	166	92	58	10

▲ **Figure 19–4.** Mean percentage of weight loss in control subjects versus patients undergoing gastric bypass, vertical banded gastroplasty, and adjustable gastric banding in the Swedish Obese Subjects (SOS) study. (Data from Sjöström L, Narbro K, Sjöström CD, et al; Swedish Obese Subjects Study. Effects of bariatric surgery on mortality in Swedish obese subjects. *N Engl J Med.* 2007;357:741–752.)

nonsurgical treatments or go untreated. However, 3 years after surgery, the health care costs of surgical patients are less than those of patients who do not undergo obesity surgery. Over a 5-year period, the number of hospitalizations, total hospital days, physician visits, and prescription costs are less in surgically treated obese individuals. This is associated with up to a 25% reduction in health care costs in these individuals compared with obese patients who receive nonsurgical or no treatment for their weight condition. Hence, bariatric surgery is also cost-effective compared with nonsurgical treatments.

Although it makes intuitive sense that massive weight loss leads to improved health and decreased mortality, the mechanism through which surgery exerts its salubrious effects has yet to be fully identified. One theory is that surgery has a beneficial effect on the inflammatory mediators associated with obesity. Initial work has suggested that inflammatory mediators such as angiotensinogen, transforming growth factor-β, tumor necrosis factor-α, and interleukin-6 are all elevated in obesity. These mediators may in part lead to the development of several cardiovascular risk factors, such as hypertension, diabetes, dyslipidemia, and thromboembolic phenomena. Weight loss surgery is associated with reduction of these factors, possibly through reduction of adipocyte mass, and therefore may be the mechanism through which weight loss surgery so effectively reduces cardiovascular risk and prolongs life. Clearly, much more study is needed to examine how weight loss in general, and obesity surgery in particular, improves outcome. However, at this time, the evidence is quite strong in favor of surgery for treatment of severely obese individuals compared with prolonged efforts at nonsurgical treatment.

Adams TD, Gress RE, Smith SC, et al. Long-term mortality after gastric bypass surgery. *N Engl J Med.* 2007;357:753–761. [PMID: 17715409]

Cottam DR, Mattar SG, Barinas-Mitchell E, et al. The chronic inflammatory hypothesis for the morbidity associated with morbid obesity: implications and effects of weight loss. *Obes Surg.* 2004;14:589–600. [PMID: 15186624]

Dixon JB, Dixon ME, O'Brien PE. Birth outcomes in obese women after laparoscopic adjustable gastric banding. *Obstet Gynecol.* 2005;106:965–972. [PMID: 1626013]

Dixon JB, O'Brien PE, Playfair J, et al. Adjustable gastric banding and conventional therapy for type 2 diabetes: a randomized controlled trial. *JAMA.* 2008;299:316–323. [PMID: 18212316]

Maggard MA, Shugarman LR, Suttorp M, et al. Meta-analysis: surgical treatment of obesity. *Ann Intern Med.* 2005;142:547–559. [PMID: 15809466]

Patel JA, Colella JJ, Esaka E, et al. Improvement in infertility and pregnancy outcomes after weight loss surgery. *Med Clin North Am.* 2007;91:515–528. [PMID: 17509393]

Ramos EJ, Xu Y, Romanova I, et al. Is obesity an inflammatory disease? *Surgery.* 2003;134:329–335. [PMID: 12947337]

Sampalis JS, Liberman M, Auger S, et al. The impact of weight reduction surgery on health-care costs in morbidly obese patients. *Obes Surg.* 2004;14:939–947. [PMID: 15329183]

Sjöström L, Lindroos AK, Peltonen M, et al. Lifestyle, diabetes, and cardiovascular risk factors 10 years after bariatric surgery. *N Engl J Med.* 2004;351:2683–2693. [PMID: 15616203]

Sjöström L, Narbro K, Sjöström D, et al; Swedish Obese Subjects Study. Effects of bariatric surgery on mortality in Swedish obese subjects. *N Engl J Med.* 2007;357:741–752. [PMID: 17715408]

RECOMMENDATIONS & CAVEATS

Weight loss surgery is the treatment of choice for appropriately selected individuals who have class II obesity with weight-related comorbid conditions and patients with class III obesity with or without comorbid conditions. Several surgical procedures designed to treat obese individuals and current procedures are quite effective in inducing long-term weight loss. However, patients require a careful, comprehensive evaluation before proceeding with such treatment to minimize surgical risks and justify such an invasive treatment. In appropriately selected individuals, bariatric surgery is associated with reduced cardiovascular and other weight-related risks, reduced mortality, and reduced health care costs, making such surgery appropriate in this group of individuals until equally or more effective weight loss treatments are developed.

Intestinal Malabsorption

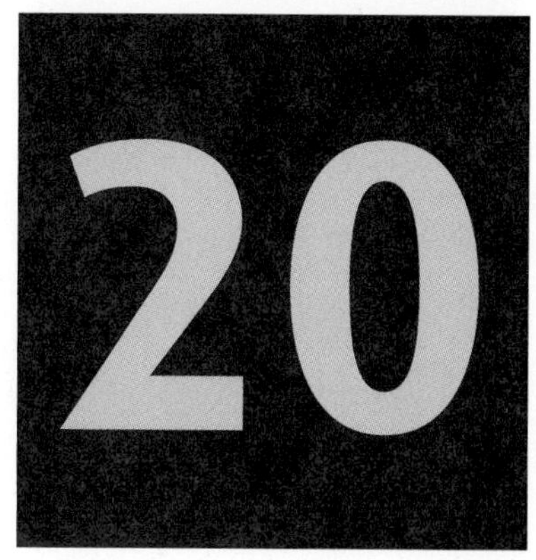

Jerry S. Trier, MD

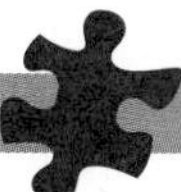

ESSENTIALS OF DIAGNOSIS

- Celiac disease—characteristic though not specific small bowel mucosal lesion, positive anti–tissue transglutaminase test (anti-tTGA) or antiendomysial antibody test (anti-EMA), and clinical response to gluten withdrawal.
- Tropical sprue—appropriate geographic exposure; exclude other mucosal diseases (eg, celiac disease and protozoal infections), exclude small intestinal bacterial overgrowth, and assess response to antibiotics and folate.
- Eosinophilic gastroenteritis—histologic demonstration of increased gastric, intestinal, or colonic mucosal or mural eosinophilic infiltration or eosinophilic ascites.
- Systemic mastocytosis—demonstration of increased mucosal mast cells (>20 per high-power field) in stomach, small bowel, colon; elevated serum tryptase.
- Radiation enteritis—history of radiation with mucosal telangiectasias, obliterative endarteriolitis, fibrosis, and strictures; small intestinal bacterial overgrowth may develop.
- Whipple disease—demonstrate *Tropheryma whipplei* and characteristic periodic acid–Schiff-positive macrophages in intestinal mucosa or other tissue.
- Small intestinal bacterial overgrowth—document evidence of malabsorption, positive breath test (lactulose, glucose), response to antibiotics.
- Short bowel syndrome—history of small bowel resection and confirmation by imaging (barium contrast small bowel series or computed tomographic enterography).
- Intestinal lymphangiectasia—hypoproteinemia, lymphopenia, evidence of protein-losing enteropathy, increased fecal loss of α_1-antitrypsin.

General Considerations

Normally the human gastrointestinal tract digests and absorbs dietary nutrients with remarkable efficiency. A typical Western diet ingested by an adult includes approximately 100 g of fat, 400 g of carbohydrate, 100 g of protein, 2 L of fluid, and the required sodium, potassium, chloride, calcium, vitamins, and other elements. Salivary, gastric, intestinal, hepatic, and pancreatic secretions add an additional 7–8 L of protein-, lipid-, and electrolyte-containing fluid to intestinal contents. This massive load is reduced by the small and large intestines to less than 200 g of stool that contains less than 8 g of fat, 1–2 g of nitrogen, and less than 20 mM each of Na^+, K^+, Cl^-, HCO_3^-, Ca^{2+}, or Mg^{2+}.

If there is impairment of any of the many steps involved in the complex process of nutrient digestion and absorption, intestinal malabsorption may ensue. If the abnormality involves a single step in the absorptive process, as in primary lactase deficiency, or if the disease process is limited to the very proximal small intestine, *selective malabsorption* of only a single nutrient (iron or folate) may occur. However, *generalized malabsorption* of multiple dietary nutrients develops when the disease process is extensive, thus disturbing several digestive and absorptive processes, as occurs in celiac disease with extensive involvement of the small intestine.

Pathogenesis

Many authors classify diseases associated with malabsorption into three major categories: (1) those associated with impaired intraluminal digestion; (2) those associated with impaired mucosal digestion and absorption; and (3) those associated with impaired postmucosal nutrient transport (Table 20–1). Indeed, these are the major mechanisms of intestinal absorption and some disease entities fit neatly into these specific categories. For example, impaired delivery of

Table 20–1. Classification of causes of intestinal malabsorption.

1. **Diseases in which impaired intraluminal digestion is dominant**
   - Pancreatic diseases (see Chapter 26)
   - Hepatobiliary disease
   - Postgastrectomy malabsorption
2. **Diseases in which impaired mucosal digestion, uptake, and transport are dominant**
   - Celiac disease
   - Refractory sprue
   - Immunoproliferative small intestinal disease (IPSID) and lymphoma
   - Tropical sprue
   - Eosinophilic gastroenteritis
   - Systemic mastocytosis
   - Radiation enteritis
   - Amyloidosis
   - Whipple disease
   - Crohn disease (see Chapter 3)
   - Abetalipoproteinemia
   - Parasitic infestations
   - Carbohydrate intolerance
3. **Diseases and syndromes in which both impaired intraluminal digestion and mucosal function are often operative**
   - Intestinal bacterial overgrowth
   - Short bowel syndrome
   - Gastrinoma (Zollinger-Ellison syndrome)
4. **Diseases or syndromes in which impaired postmucosal transport is dominant**
   - Primary intestinal lymphangiectasia
   - Secondary intestinal lymphangiectasia

pancreatic lipase, proteases, and bicarbonate in pancreatic insufficiency and impaired delivery of hepatobiliary secretions, notably bile salts in biliary obstruction, into the intestinal lumen may result in profound intraluminal maldigestion and may induce malabsorption, especially steatorrhea. In diseases such as abetalipoproteinemia or lactase deficiency, in which the evident pathology is confined to the intestinal mucosa, deficient mucosal digestion or absorption, or both, produce nutrient malabsorption. Impaired intestinal lymphatic drainage, whether due to primary or secondary postmucosal obstruction of intestinal lymphatics, results in impaired fat absorption and fecal protein loss.

However, such a classification of malabsorption diseases has its limitations; although one mechanism may dominate in any given disease, in many instances, others contribute. For example, in short bowel syndrome, the marked reduction in mucosal surface and brush border hydrolases results in impaired mucosal absorption and digestion, but if the ileum is absent, bile salt deficiency results in impaired intraluminal digestion; in small intestinal bacterial overgrowth, bacteria impair intraluminal lipid digestion but also damage brush border hydrolases and may induce significant mucosal inflammation impairing mucosal digestion and absorption; in Whipple disease, the mucosal infiltration by macrophages and *T whipplei* impair mucosal absorption, but mesenteric and retroperitoneal lymph node involvement may produce lymphatic obstruction, impairing postmucosal delivery and systemic distribution of absorbed dietary lipids.

Clinical Findings (Table 20–2)

A. Signs and Symptoms

1. Gastrointestinal manifestations—Depending on the nature of the disease process causing malabsorption and its extent, gastrointestinal symptoms may range from severe to subtle or may even be totally absent. Diarrhea, weight loss, flatulence, abdominal bloating, abdominal cramps, and pain may be present. Although diarrhea is a common complaint, the character and frequency of stools may vary considerably, ranging from over 10 watery stools per day to less than one voluminous putty-like stool, the latter causing some patients to complain of constipation. On the other hand, stool mass is invariably increased above the normal of 150–200 g/day in patients with generalized malabsorption and significant steatorrhea. Not only do unabsorbed nutrients contribute to stool mass, but mucosal fluid and electrolyte secretion is also increased in diseases associated with mucosal inflammation such as celiac disease. In addition, unabsorbed fatty acids, converted to hydroxy-fatty acids by colonic flora, as well as unabsorbed bile acids impair absorption and induce secretion of water and electrolytes by the colon adding to stool mass.

Weight loss is common among patients with significant intestinal malabsorption but must be evaluated in the context of caloric intake. Some patients compensate for fecal wastage of unabsorbed nutrients by significantly increasing their oral intake. Eliciting a careful dietary history from patients with suspected malabsorption is therefore crucial.

Excessive flatus and abdominal bloating may reflect excessive gas production due to fermentation of unabsorbed carbohydrate, especially among patients with primary or secondary disaccharidase deficiency. Malabsorption of dietary nutrients and excessive fluid secretion by inflamed small intestine also contribute to abdominal distention and bloating.

Prevalence, severity, and character of abdominal pain vary considerably among the various disease processes associated with intestinal malabsorption. For example, pain is common in patients with chronic pancreatitis or pancreatic cancer and Crohn disease, but it is absent in many patients with celiac disease or postgastrectomy malabsorption.

2. Extraintestinal manifestations—Substantial number of patients with intestinal malabsorption present initially with symptoms or laboratory abnormalities that point to other organ systems in the absence of or overshadowing symptoms referable to the gastrointestinal tract (see Table 20–2). For example, there is increasing epidemiologic evidence that

Table 20–2. Clinical findings in intestinal malabsorption.

Organ System	Clinical Feature	Cause
Gastrointestinal tract	Diarrhea	Nutrient malabsorption; small intestinal secretion of fluid and electrolytes; action of unabsorbed bile acids and hydroxy-fatty acids on colonic mucosa
	Weight loss	Nutrient malabsorption; decreased dietary intake
	Flatus	Bacterial fermentation of unabsorbed dietary carbohydrates
	Abdominal pain	Distention of bowel, muscle spasm, serosal and peritoneal involvement by disease process
	Glossitis, stomatitis, cheilosis	Iron, riboflavin, niacin deficiency
Hematopoietic system	Anemia, microcytic	Iron, pyridoxine deficiency
	Anemia, macrocytic	Folate, vitamin B_{12} deficiency
	Bleeding	Vitamin K deficiency
Musculoskeletal system	Osteopenic bone disease	Calcium, vitamin D malabsorption
	Osteoarthropathy	Not known
	Tetany	Calcium, magnesium, and vitamin D deficiency
Endocrine system	Amenorrhea, impotence, infertility	Generalized malabsorption and malnutrition
	Secondary hyperparathyroidism	Protracted calcium and vitamin D deficiency
Skin	Purpura	Vitamin K deficiency
	Follicular hyperkeratosis and dermatitis	Vitamin A, zinc, essential fatty acids, niacin deficiency
	Edema	Protein-losing enteropathy, malabsorption of dietary protein
	Hyperpigmentation	Secondary hypopituitarism and adrenal insufficiency
	Vesicular eruption	Dermatitis herpetiformis
Nervous system	Xerophthalmia, night blindness	Vitamin A deficiency
	Peripheral neuropathy	Vitamin B_{12}, thiamine deficiency

more patients with celiac disease present with anemia and osteopenic bone disease in the absence of significant gastrointestinal symptoms than present with classic gastrointestinal symptomatology. Microcytic, macrocytic, or dimorphic anemia may reflect impaired iron, folate, or vitamin B_{12} malabsorption. Purpura, subconjunctival hemorrhage, or even frank bleeding may reflect hypoprothrombinemia secondary to vitamin K malabsorption. Osteopenic bone disease is common, especially in the presence of steatorrhea. Impaired calcium and vitamin D absorption and chelation of calcium by unabsorbed fatty acids resulting in fecal loss of calcium may all contribute. If calcium deficiency is prolonged, secondary hyperparathyroidism may develop. Prolonged malnutrition may induce amenorrhea, infertility, and impotence. Edema and even ascites may reflect hypoproteinemia associated with protein-losing enteropathy caused by lymphatic obstruction or extensive mucosal inflammation. Dermatitis and peripheral neuropathy may be caused by malabsorption of specific vitamins or micronutrients and essential fatty acids.

Bernstein CN, Leslie WD, Leboff MS. AGA technical review on osteoporosis in gastrointestinal disease. *Gastroenterology.* 2003;124:795–841. [PMID: 12612917]

Fine KD, Schiller LR. AGA technical review on the evaluation and management of chronic diarrhea. *Gastroenterology.* 1999;116:1464–1486. [PMID: 10348832]

B. Laboratory and Imaging Studies (Table 20–3)

1. Stool studies—Descriptions of bowel movements by patients are subjective and often inaccurate. Therefore, careful inspection of the stool by the physician is an important component of the malabsorption evaluation. Steatorrheic stool may be loose or formed but is usually pale, greasy, often bulky, and has a characteristic rancid odor. Sudan stain of a spot stool sample for fat is a simple and useful screening test for steatorrhea. Although some fat is present in normal stool, the number and size of fat droplets are markedly increased if there is substantial steatorrhea. Quantitative determination of fat in a pooled 48- or 72-hour stool collection, although

Table 20–3. Useful laboratory tests in evaluation of intestinal malabsorption.

Test	Impaired Intraluminal Digestion	Mucosal Disease	Lymphatic Obstruction	Limitations
Stool fat (qualitative, quantitative)	Increased (concentration usually >9.5%)	Increased (concentration usually <9.5%)	Increased	False-negative result if inadequate ingestion of dietary fat or recent barium ingestion; false-positive result with castor oil or mineral oil ingestion
Stool elastase	Low in moderate and severe pancreatic exocrine insufficiency	May be low due to dilution	Usually normal	Low specificity for pancreatic disease if small intestinal disease is present
Stool ova and parasites and specific parasitic antigens	May be positive in parasitic biliary cholangiopathy	May diagnose *Giardia, Isospora*, cryptosporidia, microsporidia, tapeworms.	Negative	False-negative result may occur if recent barium ingestion
Serum carotene	Decreased	Decreased	Decreased	Low values may occur in normal subjects who ingest little dietary carotene
Serum cholesterol	Decreased	Decreased	Decreased	May be normal or increased in patients with untreated lipoprotein abnormality
Serum albumin	Usually normal, except with bacterial overgrowth	Often decreased	Often decreased	Hypoalbuminemia may reflect impaired synthesis in liver disease
Prothrombin activity	Decreased if severe	Decreased if severe	Decreased if severe	May also be decreased in liver disease but parenterally administered vitamin K should induce normalization if caused by malabsorption
Serum calcium	Usually normal if pancreas is the cause	Decreased	Decreased	May reflect hypoalbuminemia
Serum 25-OH vitamin D	Decreased	Decreased	Decreased	
Serum iron	Normal	Often decreased	Normal	
Serum folate	Normal	Often decreased	Normal	
Xylose absorption	Normal, except with bacterial overgrowth	Abnormal, unless disease confined to distal small intestine	Normal	Requires normal gastric emptying and renal function
Lactose absorption (lactose tolerance test or breath hydrogen after lactose load)	Normal, except in some instances of bacterial overgrowth	Increase in plasma glucose <20 mg/dL; increase in breath H_2 >20 ppm above fasting baseline	Normal	May be abnormal in all categories if patient has primary intestinal lactase deficiency; requires normal gastric emptying
Vitamin B_{12} absorption (Schilling test)	Decreased in bacterial overgrowth and exocrine pancreatic insufficiency	Decreased in extensive ileal disease	Normal	Requires good renal function
Lactulose and glucose breath hydrogen test	Early appearance of H_2 in breath in bacterial overgrowth	Normal	Normal	Requires normal gastric emptying; false-positive results may occur in patients with rapid small intestinal transit
Secretin/cholecystokinin stimulation tests	Abnormal in chronic pancreatic exocrine insufficiency	Normal	Normal	Relatively low sensitivity, cumbersome and labor intensive
IgA anti-tissue transglutaminase and IgA antiendomysial antibody	Absent	Present in celiac disease	Absent	Lower sensitivity in infants and all ages in mild disease, false-negative results in IgA deficiency
Endoscopic intestinal biopsy	Normal except in severe bacterial overgrowth	Often abnormal	Often abnormal	May miss patchy mucosal disease
Wireless capsule endoscopy	Usually normal	Often abnormal	Often abnormal	Labor intensive, cannot biopsy lesions, may obstruct strictured intestine

cumbersome, remains the definitive test for steatorrhea. Ideally the patient should be placed on an 80–100-g fat diet for a day or two before the stool collection is begun and maintain that intake throughout the collection period. Unabsorbable fat, such as mineral oil, Olestra, and fat-based suppositories, must be avoided. The collection should be refrigerated until assay to minimize bacterial metabolism of long-chain fatty acids. Excretion of more than 7–8% of fat intake connotes steatorrhea. The collection should be weighed so that stool fat concentration can be calculated; a stool fat concentration over 9.5% suggests intraluminal maldigestion, whereas a stool fat concentration less than 9.5% suggests mucosal disease as intestinal fluid secretion and malabsorptions of other nutrients dilute stool fat in the latter situation.

Measurements of the pancreatic enzyme, elastase, in the stool assayed using a monoclonal or polyclonal enzyme-linked immunosorbent assay (ELISA) is useful for detecting severe pancreatic exocrine deficiency, but its role in detecting milder disease is limited due to its lack of sensitivity. The secretin/cholecystokinin stimulation test, although cumbersome and rarely done nowadays, remains the gold standard for detecting pancreatic insufficiency (see Chapter 26).

Stool samples should be evaluated for ova and parasites and for specific parasitic antigens in patients with suspected malabsorption, especially if diarrhea is present. Several protozoal diseases, including giardiasis, cryptosporidiosis, microsporidiosis, and *Isospora belli* infection, can produce significant malabsorption.

Bo-Linn GW, Fordtran JS. Fecal fat concentration in patients with steatorrhea. *Gastroenterology.* 1984;87:318–322. [PMID: 6735076]

Simko V. Fecal fat microscopy. Acceptable predictive value in screening for steatorrhea. *Am J Gastroenterol.* 1981;75:204–208. [PMID: 7234842]

2. Blood studies—Abnormalities in the formed elements of the peripheral blood are quite common in patients with diseases that produce malabsorption. Anemia is common. Diffuse lesions of the proximal intestine as occurring in celiac disease or Whipple disease interfere with iron absorption and folate absorption resulting in microcytic (iron deficiency or blood loss), macrocytic (folate or B_{12} deficiency), or dimorphic anemia (combined iron and folate deficiency). Ileal resection or severe ileal disease as well as intraluminal bacterial overgrowth and, rarely, severe pancreatic exocrine insufficiency interfere with vitamin B_{12} absorption and may produce macrocytic anemia. Concomitantly, serum iron saturation, serum ferritin, iron, folate, and B_{12} levels are decreased. Normocytic anemia may reflect acute or subacute blood loss as may occur in Crohn disease, intestinal lymphoma, or Whipple disease. Peripheral leukocytosis is unusual, but the differential count may reveal eosinophilia in eosinophilic enteritis or some parasitic diseases or profound lymphopenia in patients with intestinal lymphangiectasia. Thrombocytosis, if present, may reflect hyposplenism, which occurs in some adults with celiac disease.

A number of other blood chemistries and serologies may be abnormal and may provide clues that malabsorption is present and, in some instances, help define a specific diagnosis. Low serum carotene and cholesterol are nonspecific indicators of fat malabsorption, but the serum carotene also largely reflects recent dietary carotene intake. Low serum calcium in patients with malabsorption may reflect poor absorption in mucosal disease, intraluminal formation of insoluble calcium soaps by interaction with unabsorbed fatty acids, as well as coexistent vitamin D deficiency, all resulting in fecal wastage of calcium. Low serum calcium may also accompany hypoalbuminemia, especially in patients with mucosal disease or lymphangiectasia, causing exudative enteric protein loss. The prothrombin time may be prolonged as vitamin K is fat soluble, but in the absence of liver disease, the international normalized ratio (INR) should normalize following intravenous vitamin K replacement. Levels of immunoglobulin A (IgA) anti–tissue transglutaminase or IgA antiendomysial antibody, or both, should be obtained if celiac disease is suspected.

3. Specific oral absorption tests and breath tests—Where available, the D-xylose absorption test may help to differentiate malabsorption caused by small intestinal mucosal disease from malabsorption due to impaired intraluminal digestion or lymphatic obstruction. This pentose sugar requires no intraluminal processing and is absorbed by facilitated diffusion. After administration of a 25-g dose orally to a well-hydrated patient, 5 g or more are normally excreted in the urine over 5 hours, and blood levels should reach 25 mg/dL 2 hours after the test dose. Low urine excretion and blood levels suggest disease of the mucosa of the proximal small intestine such as celiac disease. However, the test has significant limitations. It is dependent on normal gastric emptying and normal renal function; delayed gastric emptying will lower both urine xylose excretion and blood xylose levels giving a potentially false-positive result; impaired renal function will reduce urine xylose excretion but not blood xylose levels in the face of normal gastric emptying. Ascites and edema may result in sequestration of absorbed xylose and produce a false-positive test result. Additionally, in patients with bacterial overgrowth in the proximal small intestine, the xylose absorption test may be positive as some bacterial species metabolize xylose.

To screen for intestinal lactase or, less commonly, sucrase deficiency, either breath hydrogen excretion or blood glucose can be measured following an orally administered test dose of lactose or sucrose. Determination of breath hydrogen excretion has virtually supplanted measurement of blood glucose when testing for lactase deficiency because of its simplicity and because no venipuncture is needed. If lactose is malabsorbed, it travels to the distal small intestine where the bacterial flora metabolize the sugar releasing hydrogen, which is excreted by the lungs and can be readily measured in the breath. After a test dose of 2 g/kg (25 g maximum), a rise of less than 10 parts per million (PPM) is normal, whereas a rise to 20 PPM suggests lactase deficiency. Limitations include impaired gastric emptying, chronic pulmonary disease, recent antibiotic usage, or absence of hydrogen-producing bacteria, all of which reduce breath hydrogen excretion, potentially giving rise to falsely negative results. On the other hand, proximal small bacterial overgrowth may result in a false-positive result, causing hydrogen release before the sugar can be normally absorbed. Disaccharidase enzyme levels can also be directly measured biochemically if fresh mucosal biopsy tissue is available for this purpose; however, this is rarely done in the clinical setting today. It is important to emphasize that neither oral absorption tests nor hydrogen breath tests, nor direct measurements of disaccharidase enzymes in mucosal tissues, distinguish primary enzyme deficiency from secondary enzyme deficiency caused by other disease processes that damage the epithelium mucosa of the small intestine.

Several substrates have been used in breath tests to screen for small intestinal intraluminal bacterial overgrowth. These include ^{14}C-xylose, glucose, and lactulose. In all instances, the presence of bacteria in the proximal small intestine should result in rapid bacterial metabolism of the sugars and hence appearance in the breath of $^{14}CO_2$ after ^{14}C-xylose and of hydrogen after glucose as well as early peak breath hydrogen levels after lactulose administration. Under normal circumstances, lactulose is not metabolized until it reaches the distal ileal and colonic flora, resulting in later peak hydrogen levels, whereas glucose and xylose are fully absorbed in the proximal intestine before there is opportunity for bacterial metabolism. All three tests have significant limitations. Delayed gastric emptying, rapid small intestinal transit, absence of hydrogen-producing colonic flora, and significant pulmonary disease all reduce sensitivity or specificity when compared with the gold standard for diagnosing intraluminal bacterial overgrowth, namely, quantitative culture of an aspirate of proximal jejunal intraluminal contents.

Abdelshaheed NN, Goldberg DM. Biochemical tests in diseases of the intestinal tract: their contribution to diagnosis, management, and understanding the pathophysiology of specific disease states. *Crit Rev Clin Lab Sci.* 1997;34:141–223. [PMID: 9143817]

Craig RM, Ehrenpreis ED. D-xylose testing. *J Clin Gastroenterol.* 1999;29:143–150. [PMID: 10478874]

Thomas PD, Forbes A, Green J, et al. Guidelines for the investigation of chronic diarrhoea, 2nd edition. *Gut.* 2003;52(Suppl 5): 1–15. [PMID: 12801941]

4. Imaging studies—Various imaging studies are available to help clarify the nature of pancreatic and hepatobiliary disease that may cause or contribute to intestinal malabsorption. These include endoscopic retrograde cholangiopancreatography (ERCP), magnetic resonance cholangio pancreatography (MRCP), abdominal computed tomography (CT), abdominal magnetic resonance imaging (MRI), and abdominal and endoscopic ultrasonography. They are discussed in some detail in Chapter 9 of this text.

For many years, conventional barium contrast studies of the small intestine were the standard for evaluating the gross structure of the small intestine in suspected or proven malabsorption. However, both sensitivity and specificity of the conventional small intestinal contrast series are low. Sensitivity, especially for detection of focal lesions, can be improved by utilizing double-contrast enteroclysis performed by instilling both barium and carboxymethyl cellulose into the duodenal lumen and fluoroscopically following the contrast material as it transits the small intestine. However, enteroclysis is labor intensive and results in substantial exposure of the patient to radiation. More recently, computed tomographic enterography (CTE), where available, is very promising for detecting small intestinal abnormalities. CTE is performed with ingestion of a large volume of neutral contrast material after which both sagittal and cross-sectional images are obtained. This technique has been especially useful in the evaluation of patients with Crohn disease and is also useful in assessing the length of remaining small intestine in patients after major intestinal resections and in the detection of focal abnormalities such as intestinal strictures and neoplasms, including lymphoma. MRI enterography, though less available and somewhat more costly, provides similar information as CTE with the benefit of avoidance of exposure to ionizing radiation.

5. Endoscopic and biopsy studies—Visualization of the mucosal surface of the small intestine within the reach of the endoscope allows the detection of abnormal gross mucosal surface features. These include the diminution and scalloping of mucosal folds, absence or apparent blunting of villi (common in celiac disease), and whitish-appearing dilated lymphatic lacteals within villi commonly found in Whipple disease and intestinal lymphangiectasia. However, both the sensitivity and specificity of such endoscopic findings are low. Rather, the greatest contribution of direct endoscopy to the evaluation of patients with malabsorption is its facilitation of mucosal biopsy under direct vision. As indicated in Table 20–4, some diseases, such as Whipple disease, amyloidosis, and giardiasis, are associated with a specific lesion, and biopsy is often diagnostic. Other diseases are characterized by histologic features that, although abnormal, lack specificity and require additional clinical information for a definitive diagnosis. However, even when the biopsy specimen is not in and of itself diagnostic, it is often of great value as it establishes unequivocally the presence of mucosal disease. The definitive diagnosis is then established by additional diagnostic studies or by a response to specific therapy.

Because intestinal malabsorption may occur in a number of diseases in which mucosal involvement may be patchy (see Table 20–4), multiple biopsy specimens should be obtained from several sites in the duodenum or proximal

Table 20–4. Information provided by mucosal biopsy of the small intestine.

1. **Disorders in which biopsy result is diagnostic: diffuse lesions**
   a. Whipple disease
      - Lamina propria infiltrated with periodic acid–Schiff-positive macrophages
      - Characteristic bacilli in mucosa

   b. *Mycobacterium avium–intracellulare* enteritis: similar to Whipple disease but bacilli are acid fast
   c. Severe immunoglobulin deficiency
      - Mucosal architecture from normal to flat
      - Plasma cells absent or markedly diminished in lamina propria
      - *Giardia* trophozoites may be present

   d. Abetalipoproteinemia
      - Mucosal architecture normal
      - Lipid-laden absorptive cells appear vacuolated
2. **Disorders in which biopsy result may be diagnostic: patchy lesions**
   a. Intestinal lymphoma
      - Villi widened, shortened, or absent
      - Malignant lymphoma cells infiltrate epithelium lamina propria and submucosa

   b. Intestinal lymphangiectasia
      - Mucosal architecture normal
      - Dilated lymphatics in lamina propria and submucosa

   c. Eosinophilic enteritis
      - Mucosal architecture from normal to flat
      - Patchy infiltration of lamina propria with aggregates of eosinophils

   d. Mastocytosis
      - Mucosal architecture from normal to flat
      - Patchy infiltration of lamina propria with mast cells, eosinophils, and neutrophils

   e. Amyloidosis
      - Mucosal architecture normal
      - Amyloid in lamina propria and submucosa, often in blood vessel walls, shown with Congo red stain and polarized light

   f. Crohn disease
      - Mucosal architecture variable
      - Noncaseating granulomata and inflammation in lamina propria and submucosa

   g. Giardiasis
      - Mucosal architecture from normal to flat
      - Trophozoites in lumen and on surface of absorptive cells
      - Minimal to severe inflammation in lamina propria

   h. Coccidiosis
      - Villi shortened
      - Crypts hyperplastic
      - Coccidial forms on surface of (cryptosporidiosis) or within (*Isospora*) absorptive cells
      - Inflammation of lamina propria
3. **Disorders in which biopsy result is abnormal but not diagnostic**
   a. Celiac disease
      - Villi shortened or absent
      - Crypts hyperplastic
      - Damaged absorptive cells
      - Increased intraepithelial lymphocytes (IELs)
      - Inflammation of lamina propria

   b. Refractory sprue: histology indistinguishable from celiac sprue; immunocytochemistry may show phenotypically abnormal IELs
   c. Tropical sprue
      - Mucosal architecture from nearly normal to flat mucosa (as in celiac sprue)
      - Absorptive cell damage mild
      - Inflammation of lamina propria

   d. Viral gastroenteritis: indistinguishable from mild to moderate tropical sprue or celiac disease lesion
   e. Intraluminal bacterial overgrowth: may be normal or indistinguishable from mild to moderate tropical sprue or celiac disease lesion.
   f. Folate or vitamin B_{12} deficiency, acute radiation enteritis
      - Shortened villi
      - Hypoplastic crypts
      - Megalocytic epithelium
      - Diminished mitoses
      - Inflammation of lamina propria

jejunum. Samples of luminal fluid can also be obtained at the time of endoscopy, facilitating the diagnosis of parasitic infestation such as giardiasis and coccidioses and, if sophisticated culture facilities are available, intestinal intraluminal bacterial overgrowth.

Wireless capsule endoscopy using a swallowed camera that transmits color images of reasonable quality of the mucosal surface as it tumbles through the gastrointestinal tract is a relatively new modality for imaging of the intestinal mucosa, including that of the mid and distal small intestine (see Chapter 33). It has been particularly useful in detecting focal lesions beyond the reach of the endoscope, especially among patients with gastrointestinal bleeding of previously unknown cause. Like direct endoscopy, it also provides useful views of the gross structure of the mucosa and detects the fold scalloping, flat mucosa, and distended lymphatic lacteals when these lesions are well developed. A limitation of capsule endoscopy is that it provides no tissue for pathologic evaluation. Hence, its role in the diagnosis of intestinal malabsorption is complementary to endoscopy and biopsy. The capsule camera may cause intestinal obstruction if tight strictures are present; hence, it must be used with caution in patients with suspected malignancy or Crohn disease unless the absence of strictures has previously been documented by other imaging techniques.

Babbin BA, Crawford K, Sitaraman SV. Malabsorption work-up: utility of small bowel biopsy. *Clin Gastroenterol Hepatol.* 2006; 4:1193–1198. [PMID: 16979950]

Siddika HA, Fidler JL, Fletcher JG, et al. Prospective comparison of state-of the-art MR enterography and CT enterography in small-bowel Crohn's disease. *Am J Roentgenol.* 2009;193:113–121. [PMID: 19542402]

SPECIFIC CONDITIONS RESULTING IN INTESTINAL MALABSORPTION

DISEASES ASSOCIATED WITH INTRALUMINAL MALDIGESTION

1. Pancreatic & Hepatobiliary Diseases

Delivery of adequate amounts of pancreatic lipase, colipase, proteases, and amylases as well as bicarbonate into the proximal intestine is essential for normal intraluminal digestion of dietary lipids, proteins, and complex carbohydrates. Pancreatic reserve is substantial, and significant malabsorption generally does not occur unless there is 85–90% reduction in pancreatic enzyme secretion. The diagnostic and clinical ramifications of chronic pancreatic insufficiency are discussed in detail in the chapters that deal with pancreatitis (see Chapter 25) and pancreatic neoplasms (see Chapter 28). As described earlier, determination of stool fat concentration (see Table 20–3) is useful in distinguishing malabsorption caused by pancreatic insufficiency resulting in impaired intraluminal digestion from malabsorption caused by mucosal disease. In malabsorption caused by pancreatic disease, tests of mucosal absorption, such as oral tolerance tests and intestinal mucosal structure as assessed by biopsy and imaging studies, are usually normal unless there is coexisting mucosal disease.

Delivery of bile salts into the proximal intestinal lumen is essential for normal dispersion and intraluminal digestion of dietary lipids prior to their absorption by the intestinal mucosa. Hence, hepatobiliary disease that reduces significantly bile salt synthesis and delivery of bile salts into the proximal intestinal lumen causes significant malabsorption as does fecal bile salt loss caused by ileal disease or resection sufficient to deplete the circulating bile salt pool. (See the discussion of "short bowel syndrome," later.)

2. Postgastrectomy Malabsorption

With the recognition of gastric *Helicobacter pylori* colonization as a cause of peptic ulcer disease, the development of histamine-2 (H_2) blockers and proton pump inhibitors for therapy of peptic ulcer disease, and endoscopic interventional techniques to control ulcer bleeding, the need for surgical intervention to treat peptic ulcer disease has diminished strikingly in recent decades. However, occasionally patients still require surgery to control ulcer bleeding and others require partial or total gastric resection for malignancy, vascular compromise, or gastric infections. Hence, a pool of individuals at risk for malabsorption after gastric surgery persists. The risk of significant malabsorption correlates with the extent of alteration of normal anatomy. Thus, the risk is greatest after total gastrectomy and progressively decreases after partial gastrectomy and gastrojejunal anastomoses (Billroth II), antrectomy and gastric duodenal anastomoses (Billroth I), and vagotomy and pyloroplasty and is virtually nonexistent after selective proximal vagotomy.

Several mechanisms may cause malabsorption after gastric surgery, and treatment varies depending on the causes (Table 20–5). The most common has been termed "poor mixing and poor timing." Rapid gastric emptying coupled with decreased release of secretin and cholecystokinin results in suboptimal exposure of the nutrient bolus to both bile salts and pancreatic enzyme as it traverses the small intestine. This diagnosis is made after excluding more treatable causes of postgastrectomy malabsorption.

Intraluminal bacterial overgrowth should be excluded as a cause of postgastrectomy malabsorption. Reduced acid secretion and intraluminal stasis, especially in patients with an afferent loop following total gastrectomy or a Billroth II operation, are predisposing causes.

Patients with silent or latent celiac disease may develop symptomatic celiac disease after gastrectomy most likely caused by the rapid delivery of gluten to the small intestine and its impaired digestion in the remaining gastric remnant and proximal intestine.

Recurrent ulcer disease, especially in patients who have undergone a gastrojejunostomy, may cause a gastrocolic

Table 20–5. Malabsorption associated with gastric surgery.

Cause	Onset	Diagnosis	Treatment
"Poor mixing, poor timing"	Immediate	Exclusion of other causes	Antimotility agents, supplemental pancreatic enzymes
Intraluminal bacterial overgrowth	Delayed	Vitamin B_{12} absorption tests, breath tests, cultures of luminal contents	Antibiotics, surgical revision if refractory to antibiotics
Unmasked latent celiac disease	Immediate	Anti-tissue transglutaminase or antiendomysial antibodies, intestinal mucosal biopsy	Dietary gluten withdrawal
Gastrocolic or jejunocolic fistula	Delayed	Barium enema	Antibiotics and surgery
Inadvertent gastroileostomy	Immediate	Upper gastrointestinal series	Surgery

or jejunocolic fistula. Reflux of colonic contents into the gastric remnant and proximal intestine through the fistula results in massive bacterial overgrowth. As intracolonic pressure exceeds intrajejunal pressure, a barium enema is the diagnostic procedure of choice as infused barium will flow through the fistula into the stomach or proximal bowel, bypassing the distal small intestine. Control with antibiotics is usually unsuccessful, and further surgery is indicated to correct the cause of the recurrent ulcer and to remove or repair the fistula.

Severe malabsorption immediately after surgery has been reported if a surgeon inadvertently creates a gastroileostomy rather than a gastrojejunostomy. Fortunately, such surgical misadventure is very rare, and treatment is surgical revision of the anastomoses.

Malabsorption of specific vitamins and minerals may occur. For example, calcium and vitamin D malabsorption may result in osteopenia and iron malabsorption may result in anemia, especially among those in whom the duodenum and proximal jejunum have been bypassed. Vitamin B_{12} malabsorption may result from major gastric resections or atrophy of the remaining gastric mucosa. Specific therapy for these deficiencies should be provided as indicated.

Lactose intolerance may be aggravated or first become evident after gastric surgery due to rapid delivery of lactase-containing nutrients into the small intestine. Treatment with supplemental lactase or low-lactose dairy products is usually effective.

DISEASES ASSOCIATED WITH IMPAIRED MUCOSAL DIGESTION & ABSORPTION

1. Celiac Disease (Celiac Sprue)

Celiac disease is a T-cell–mediated gluten intolerance in genetically predisposed individuals in whom exposure to wheat, barley, or rye induces a characteristic mucosal lesion that responds to dietary gluten withdrawal. With the increase in availability during the past 20 years of reliable serologic screening tests, it has become evident that the disease is far more common than was previously appreciated. Whereas the disease is rare among those of Chinese, Japanese, Korean, and African heritage, it occurs in 0.3–1.0% of Caucasians of European extraction. Symptoms may initially present at virtually any age, ranging from infancy (upon addition of gluten-containing cereal to feedings) to late adulthood.

Pathogenesis

Genetic factors and altered immune function both play a major role in the pathogenesis of celiac disease. The disease has a prevalence of 8–12% in first-order relatives (parents, children, and siblings) of affected individuals. Concordance is approximately 70–85% among identical twins, and approximately 30% among HLA-identical siblings. Ninety to 95% of affected individuals carry the HLA-DQ2 heterodimer; over 90% of the remaining 5–10% carry the HLA-DQ8 heterodimer.

Because of their high proline content, the gluten proteins in wheat, barley, and rye resist intraluminal proteolytic digestive processes. This results in the accumulation of large peptide fragments, some of which have been shown to damage the mucosa of individuals with celiac disease both in vivo and in vitro. Mucosal tissue transglutaminase diamidates glutamine residues on the immunogenic peptide fragments. These fragments bind to the antigen-binding grooves of intestinal antigen-presenting cells from individuals with celiac disease which, in turn, present these dietary gluten peptides to and thus activate DQ2-restricted or DQ8-restricted gluten peptide–specific mucosal T lymphocytes. Once activated, the T lymphocytes release cytokines that likely contribute to the development of mucosal damage.

More recently evidence has been obtained that activation of the innate immune system may participate in the pathogenesis of celiac disease in concert with the acquired immune system. Upregulation of mucosal interleukin-15 expression during gluten exposure ultimately imparts natural killer cell–like properties to the lymphocytes residing among the mucosal epithelial cells (intraepithelial lymphocytes [IELs]), resulting in epithelial cell damage and increased mucosal permeability. This, in turn, likely facilitates the exposure of mucosal antigen-presenting cells to toxic gluten peptides and the resulting T-cell activation of the adaptive immune response.

Jabri B, Sollid LV. Tissue-mediated control of immunopathology in celiac disease. *Nat Rev Immunol.* 2009;9:858–871. [PMID: 19935805]

Clinical Findings

A. Symptoms and Signs

The clinical spectrum of celiac disease is very broad. In those with a mild lesion involving only the proximal small intestine, the disease may be completely silent with no evident clinical manifestations. In others with a lesion limited to the proximal intestine, selected nutrient deficiencies, which may include iron, folate, or calcium, may be present with resultant anemia or osteopenia but with no significant gastrointestinal symptoms. On the other hand, if a more severe lesion extends to the more distal intestine, panmalabsorption with gastrointestinal symptoms, including weight loss, diarrhea, excess flatus, and abdominal discomfort, may all be present in concert with evidence of involvement of other systems (see Table 20–2). The severity of the mucosal lesion and the extent of the intestinal involvement by the lesion are likely important factors in the clinical presentation of any given patient.

B. Laboratory Findings

Laboratory findings, like the clinical manifestations, may vary enormously depending on extent of disease, ranging from no abnormalities or only isolated iron or folate deficiency to multiple abnormalities including steatorrhea, hypoalbuminemia, hypoprothrombinemia, hypocalcemia, and so on (see Table 20–3). Elevated serum transaminase levels may be the presenting finding in some patients with celiac disease.

To correctly diagnose celiac disease, the clinician obviously must suspect that the disease may be present. This is simple enough in those in whom gastrointestinal symptoms and malabsorption are obvious. It is more of a challenge if only subtle symptoms or a nonspecific laboratory abnormality is present. Such patients are often diagnosed as having irritable bowel syndrome, unexplained osteopenia, or unexplained iron deficiency or folate deficiency anemia. A high index of suspicion is essential for the correct diagnosis of the many patients who present with subtle findings.

Serologic tests are useful screening tests for celiac disease. Both the IgA anti–tissue transglutaminase test (anti-tTGA) and the IgA antiendomysial antibody test (anti-EMA) are useful and have reported sensitivities of 80–95% and specificities of 95–99%, although recent reports suggest somewhat lower sensitivities and specificities in nonresearch settings, especially among infants, toddlers, and patients with mild or silent disease. Both tests measure the autoantibody directed against the enzyme, tissue transglutaminase. Tissue transglutaminase is found in many body tissues including the intestinal mucosa. Whereas the role of the autoantibody in the pathogenesis of celiac sprue is unknown, tissue transglutaminase itself deamidates and cross-links immunogenic gluten peptides facilitating their presentation to T lymphocytes by mucosal antigen-presenting cells.

Both conventional anti-tTGA and anti-EMA measure IgA class antibodies; therefore, some false-negative tests are inevitable as the prevalence of selective IgA deficiency among celiac sprue patients is 2–4%. Thus, if an anticipated positive test is reported as negative, the serum IgA level should be quantitated. IgG anti-tTGA and IgG anti-EMA can be determined, but in limited studies, the sensitivity of these tests appears substantially lower than that of their IgA counterparts. Recently, both IgA and IgG anti–deamidated gliadin peptide (DGP) antibody tests have become available. However, it has not been demonstrated that IgA anti-DGP provides a significant advantage over IgA anti-tTGA. On the other hand, IgG anti-DGP has higher sensitivity and specificity than IgG anti-TGA and may become the test of choice in IgA deficient individuals.

Mucosal intestinal biopsy of the bulb, the distal duodenum or proximal jejunum, coupled with a clinical response to the dietary withdrawal of gluten, remains the gold standard for the diagnosis of celiac disease. Because dietary gluten withdrawal is a lifetime commitment with substantial cost and social liability, a diagnostic trial of a gluten-free diet should not be undertaken without first obtaining biopsy evidence consistent with celiac sprue. Villi may be blunted or the mucosal surface may appear to be flat with complete absence of villi (Plate 21). Crypts are hyperplastic, with increased numbers of mitotic figures. Surface absorptive cells are damaged and infiltrated by increased numbers of IELs (Plate 22). There is also extensive infiltration of the lamina propria by a lymphoplasmacytic infiltrate. The mucosal lesion, although characteristic, is not specific. Other diseases that may have similar clinical manifestations and may have similar mucosal histology include refractory sprue, tropical sprue, viral gastroenteritis (especially when caused by rotavirus in children), intraluminal bacterial overgrowth, and eosinophilic gastroenteritis. Hence, a clinical response to gluten withdrawal is a crucial step in establishing the diagnosis.

HLA testing is of value in patients with atypical features or incongruent serologic and biopsy results for excluding celiac disease. The absence of both HLA-DQ2 and HLA-DQ8 makes the likelihood of the diagnosis extremely low (<1%). On the other hand, the test is expensive, and detection of either of these haplotypes is of no direct diagnostic value in establishing the diagnosis of celiac disease as they are present in approximately 25–35% of Caucasians of European heritage.

Table 20–6. Initial treatment of celiac disease.

• Avoid all wheat, barley, rye, and oat gluten
• Rice, corn, millet, potato, buckwheat, and soybeans are safe
• Read all labels of processed foods; be suspicious of all additives such as hydrolyzed vegetable protein
• Limit intake of dairy products until diarrhea disappears
• Replace all deficient micronutrients with specific supplements as needed (calcium, iron, folate, vitamins)
• Join a local celiac disease lay support group

Leffler DA, Schuppan D. Update on Serological Testing in Celiac Disease. *Am J Gastroenterol.* 2010;105:2520-2524. [PMID: 21131921]

Treatment

The cornerstone of treatment of celiac disease is the elimination of products containing wheat, barley, and rye from the diet (Table 20–6). There is convincing evidence that at least moderate quantities of oats (50 g/day) are well tolerated by celiac patients, but some brands of commercially available oats may be contaminated with wheat and other cereal grains during processing and shipping. Hence, it is wise, at least initially, to avoid oats unless obtained from a reliable source that is known to supply oats free of other contaminating cereal grains. Many other dietary carbohydrate staples including rice, corn, potatoes, and soybeans are well tolerated by celiac patients. Micronutrient deficiencies including iron and folate deficiencies should be treated. If osteopenia is present (bone density should be determined), calcium and vitamin D should be prescribed. Pneumococcal vaccine should be administered to those with evidence of hyposplenism.

Although implementation of a gluten-free diet sounds simple, it is not. Wheat is ubiquitous in the Western diet and is particularly hard to spot in processed foods such as ice cream, sauces, and candies. For example, an additive as benign sounding as "hydrolyzed vegetable protein" is often derived from wheat and therefore may be rich in gluten. Hence, counseling by a knowledgeable dietician and physician as well as participation in local celiac disease lay support groups are important facets in the education of celiac patients and facilitation of long-term dietary compliance.

If diarrhea and steatorrhea are present, lactose restriction may be needed initially as clinically significant secondary lactase deficiency is often present. However, dairy products are a good source of many nutrients, including calcium and protein, and should be encouraged as symptoms disappear unless primary lactase deficiency is also present. Pure oats from a reliable source can be added if desired by the patients once symptoms have cleared with gluten withdrawal. Dietary compliance should be monitored on follow-up visits every 6–12 months. A repeat serologic test (IgA anti-tTGA or IgA anti-EMA) is helpful 12 or so months after initiation of gluten withdrawal as the antibodies disappear in fully compliant celiac patients. With those exceptions and perhaps an annual hemoglobin or hematocrit, stool for occult blood, and monitoring of bone density, no other specific follow-up beyond routine medical care is needed in the absence of symptoms and signs.

Course & Prognosis

By and large, the prognosis of patients with celiac disease is excellent. There is a higher incidence of lymphoma, especially of the T-cell type derived from IELs (see next section), among celiac patients (see Figure 9–14). But the risk is greatest among symptomatic patients who have had many years of gluten exposure. In contrast, the risk is very low among those with latent or silent disease. Most of the celiac disease–associated lymphomas that do develop occur in the intestine, but lymphoma at distant sites may also develop, including B-cell lymphomas. There is increasing evidence that strict adherence to a gluten-free diet substantially reduces the risk of subsequent lymphoma development. Screening for lymphoma is not recommended unless suggestive symptoms develop. The incidence of small intestinal, esophageal, and pharyngeal carcinomas may also be increased in celiac disease, but available evidence is less convincing than for lymphomas.

Rarely, celiac patients develop recurrent symptoms while adhering strictly to a gluten-free diet. Then, thorough evaluation is needed to exclude other gastrointestinal diseases such as lymphoma, refractory sprue (see next section), microscopic colitis, and irritable bowel syndrome (Table 20–7).

Given the known high prevalence of celiac disease in first-order relatives or patients with the disease, all immediate family members should be screened for celiac disease. The prevalence of celiac disease also is high in several other diseases, many of which are associated with autoimmunity (Table 20–8). Although studies of the cost-effectiveness of screening for celiac disease in these conditions are limited, evidence that persistent gluten ingestion increases the risk of malignancy and that clinical manifestations of celiac disease are often subtle yet damaging (eg, osteopenia) provides a strong argument for increased serologic screening.

Table 20–7. Considerations in patients unresponsive to a gluten-free diet.

Poor dietary compliance
Coexistent irritable bowel syndrome
Microscopic colitis
Primary lactase deficiency
Small intestinal bacterial overgrowth (SIBO)
Lymphoma
Refractory sprue

Table 20–8. Prevalence of celiac sprue in selected diseases.

Disease or Finding	Prevalence of Celiac Sprue
Dermatitis herpetiformis	>90%
Diabetes mellitus type 1	2–8%
Autoimmune thyroid disease	~3%
Down syndrome	3–12%
Turner syndrome	2–10%
Unexplained infertility	2–4%
Unexplained osteopenia	2–3%
Unexplained anemia	2–8%
Irritable bowel syndrome	Up to 10%
↑ Liver function tests	1.5–9.0%
Selective IgA deficiency	Up to 8%

Green PHR, Cellier C. Celiac disease. *N Engl J Med.* 2007;357: 1731–1743. [PMID: 17960014]

Rostom A, Murray JA, Kagnoff MF. American Gastroenterological Association (AGA) Institute technical review on the diagnosis and management of celiac disease. *Gastroenterology.* 2006;131: 1981–2002. [PMID: 17087937]

Tack GJ, Verbeek WHM, Schruers MWJ, et al. The spectrum of celiac disease: epidemiology, clinical aspects and treatment. *Nat Rev Gastroenterol Hepatol.* 2010;7:204–213. [PMID: 20212505]

2. Refractory Sprue

The clinical picture and small intestinal mucosal histology of refractory sprue mimic those of severe untreated celiac disease. Generalized malabsorption and its complications and a severe mucosal lesion of the intestine with blunted villi or absent villi, crypt hyperplasia, mucosal inflammation, and increased IELs are all present. However, unlike celiac disease, there is no or, at best, an incomplete response to dietary gluten withdrawal. Some patients initially respond like classical celiac disease patients to gluten withdrawal and have serologic tests that are consistent with celiac disease and then, after months or years, become refractory to gluten withdrawal. Others are refractory to gluten elimination at presentation and may lack the serologic celiac markers even before a trial of gluten withdrawal. In all, other potential causes for the symptoms, including poor dietary compliance or other diseases such as lymphoma, lymphocytic colitis, tropical sprue, intraluminal bacterial overgrowth, and eosinophilic enteritis, must be excluded as refractory sprue is a diagnosis of exclusion.

There are two major categories of refractory sprue. In the first (type 1), the expanded population of IELs consists of phenotypically normal polyclonal T cells. Many patients in this category improve with corticosteroids or other immunosuppressive treatments. Gluten withdrawal should also be maintained. Oral budesonide should be tried first, and systemic corticosteroids or other immunosuppressant agents such as azathioprine should be reserved for those who fail budesonide, given the need for long-term treatment and potential side effects. In the second category (type 2), epithelial cell interleukin-15 overexpression promotes the emergence of clonal populations of phenotypically aberrant IELs, which may represent prelymphoma. These abnormal T cells express CD3 in their cytoplasm but fail to express surface CD3, CD8, or the T-cell receptor for β-chain. Patients with type 1 refractory sprue may, with time, progress to type 2.

The prognosis is guarded for patients with refractory sprue, especially those with type 2 disease. Many develop intractable nutritional deficiencies requiring long-term parenteral alimentation that may lead to complicating infections. Some ultimately progress to T-cell lymphoma. Attempts at treatment when conventional immunosuppression fails have included infliximab, cladribine, and autologous stem cell transplantation resulting in anecdotal reports of responses in some but not all patients, but there is concern that these treatments may hasten progression to lymphoma.

Lui H, Brais R, Lavergne-Slove A, et al. Continual monitoring of intraepithelial lymphocyte immunophenotype and clonality is more important than snapshot analysis in the surveillance of refractory celiac disease. *Gut.* 2010;59:452–460. [PMID: 19996326]

Malamut G, Afchain P, Verkarre V, et al. Presentation and long-term follow-up of refractory celiac disease: comparison of type I with type II. *Gastroenterology.* 2009;136:81–90. [PMID: 19014942]

3. Immunoproliferative Small Intestinal Disease (IPSID) & Intestinal Lymphoma

Primary small intestinal lymphoma is uncommon in developed countries, occurring most often in middle-aged men with focal involvement and with a predilection for the ileum. As primary focal intestinal lymphomas are not usually associated with diarrhea and malabsorption but usually present as bleeding or mass-related abdominal pain and obstruction, they will not be considered further in this chapter. In contrast, two variants of small intestinal lymphoma regularly cause malabsorption, IPSID-associated lymphoma and enteropathy-associated T-cell lymphoma (EATL).

IPSID occurs primarily in young adults among native Middle-Eastern populations as well as in South Africa and Pakistan. It is exceedingly rare in more industrialized nations. Its cause is unknown, but because IPSID occurs where hygiene is poor, it has been suggested that bacteria or other antigens cause excessive proliferation of lamina propria immunocompetent cells and that poor nutrition in the at-risk population plays a permissive role. However no specific causative pathogen has been identified, although an association of IPSID with *Campylobacter jejuni* has been suggested.

In the early stages of the disease, there is diffuse infiltration of the mucosa and submucosa with B lymphocytes and plasma cells. As the disease progresses, the infiltrating cells develop histologically malignant characteristics, and mesenteric nodes become involved. Clinical features include anorexia, weight loss, diarrhea, steatorrhea, and abdominal pain. As the disease progresses, edema, ascites, and hepatic splenomegaly and palpable abdominal masses may become evident.

A distinctive laboratory feature found in the majority of patients with IPSID and IPSID-associated lymphoma is the presence of a paraprotein consisting of the Fc portion of IgA, devoid of light chains, that migrates as a broad band on protein electrophoresis in the $\alpha2$ and β regions.

Early in the disease before frankly malignant cells are observed, prolonged treatment (6 months or more) with antibiotics such as tetracycline, ampicillin, and metronidazole has induced prolonged remission and even cures. Hence, this stage of the disease has been likened to *H pylori*–associated gastric early mucosa-associated lymphoid tissue (MALT) lymphomas. If the process fails to respond to antibiotics, or once frank lymphoma has been established, either by endoscopic biopsy or staging laparotomy, combination chemotherapy with or without radiotherapy and nutritional support are the only therapeutic options as the extent of intestinal involvement usually precludes surgical resection.

EATL is a complication of celiac disease, as mentioned earlier in the chapter. It occurs primarily in patients over the age of 50 years who have had prolonged gluten exposure and symptomatic celiac disease, although occasionally celiac disease may be undiagnosed until the initial presentation of EATL. Clinical deterioration in a patient with established celiac disease despite strict compliance with a gluten-free diet or failure of a patient recently diagnosed with celiac disease to respond to a strict gluten-free diet should raise suspicion and trigger further diagnostic evaluation (see Table 20–7). Symptoms and signs are similar to those seen in IPSID and include anorexia, weight loss, diarrhea, steatorrhea, and abdominal pain. Rarely, perforation with resultant peritonitis may occur. Useful studies include push enteroscopy with mucosal biopsies from multiple levels of the small intestine, capsule endoscopy, conventional abdominal CT, and CTE or MRI enterography. If suspicious lesions are detected or if results of studies are negative but the suspicion of EATL is high, laparoscopy or laparotomy with full-thickness small intestine biopsies and mesenteric lymph node biopsies must be considered.

The prognosis is dismal. With few exceptions, responses to intensive chemotherapy have been transient. Recently, autologous stem cell transplantation following intensive chemotherapy has shown some promise, but further studies are needed.

Catassi C, Bearzi I, Holmes GK. Association of celiac disease and intestinal lymphomas and other cancers. *Gastroenterology.* 2005;128:S79–S86. [PMID: 15825131]

Salem PA, Estephan FF. Immunoproliferative small intestinal disease: current concepts. *Cancer J.* 2005;11:374–382. [PMID: 16259867]

4. Tropical Sprue

Tropical sprue occurs among natives of, visitors to, and expatriates from selected countries located, by and large, between the Tropic of Cancer and the Tropic of Capricorn. Major epidemics have been described in south Indian villages. Sporadic cases seen in the United States are largely among immigrants and visitors from the Caribbean or tropical Asia as well as returning tourists who have spent at least several weeks in endemic areas. The cause of tropical sprue remains obscure, but its epidemiology and its response to antibiotic therapy strongly suggest that colonization of the intestine by an infectious agent or alteration in the intestinal bacterial flora induced by the exposure to another environmental agent is important. It must be stressed that no single causative infectious agent has been identified.

Clinical symptoms and signs are nonspecific and include diarrhea, steatorrhea, weight loss, nausea, and anorexia. Anemia is common and most often megaloblastic, reflecting vitamin B_{12} or folate deficiency, or both, although coexistent iron deficiency may result in a dimorphic anemia. Mucosal biopsy of the small intestine reveals a nonspecific lesion of variable severity, which may involve the length of the small intestine in patchy fashion. Architectural changes range from minimal villous blunting to complete absence of villi. Lamina propria mononuclear cells are increased, as are IELs. Thus, the histologic lesion cannot be distinguished with certainty from that observed in celiac sprue, viral gastroenteritis, or intraluminal bacterial overgrowth. As there is no specific diagnostic test for tropical sprue, the diagnosis relies on excluding celiac disease (Table 20–9) and other diseases such as protozoal infections, which can cause similar symptoms and are also endemic to the tropics where sanitation may be suboptimal.

Recommended treatment is based on observational studies and includes an antibiotic such as tetracycline and high-dose folic acid. The optimal duration of treatment is unclear, although treatment for 1 to 3 months appears to be sufficient for most travelers and expatriates. Treatment lasting 6 months to 1 year is recommended for chronically ill residents

Table 20–9. Features that distinguish tropical sprue from celiac disease.

History of exposure to an endemic region
Anti-tissue transglutaminase and antiendomysial antibodies are absent
Vitamin B_{12} deficiency more common
No response to gluten-free diet
Response to treatment with folic acid and antibiotics in most cases
Biopsy histology does not distinguish between tropical sprue and celiac disease

in the tropics. Specific nutritional deficiencies such as vitamin B_{12}, vitamin D, and calcium deficiencies should also be corrected. The response to treatment is usually prompt; hence, the prognosis with proper treatment is excellent, although relapses occurring months to years after treatment have been noted. It has been suggested that overall the response among those with tropical sprue acquired in the Caribbean is more predictable than that observed among those with tropical sprue acquired in Asia, but rigorous comparative studies are not available, and this perception may be confounded by the presence of other causes of gastrointestinal symptoms among Asian populations.

Nath SK. Tropical sprue. *Curr Gastroenterol Rep.* 2005;7:343–349. [PMID: 16168231]

5. Eosinophilic Gastroenteritis

Eosinophilic gastroenteritis is an uncommon, poorly understood disease characterized by infiltration of the stomach, small intestine, or colon with mature eosinophils and, in about 80% of those affected, pronounced peripheral eosinophilia. More than 50% of patients have a history of significant atopy or specific food intolerances. The pathogenesis is poorly understood. Presumably, chemokines such as eotaxin-1 and eotaxin-2 recruit eosinophils to the gut where they are activated to release proinflammatory mediators, including major basic protein, eosinophilic peroxidase, eosinophilic cationic protein, and leukotrienes, but the initiating trigger is not known. Deposits of eosinophilic major basic protein have been noted in the intestinal mucosa.

Clinical Findings

Three major patterns of eosinophilic infiltration can generally induce distinctive clinical features, although the features are not necessarily syndromic and there may be substantial overlap. The most common is associated with mucosal and submucosal eosinophilic infiltration most pronounced in the small intestine. Characteristic clinical features of this subset include diarrhea, steatorrhea (usually mild), abdominal pain, nausea, and, in some cases, vomiting. Iron deficiency and hypoalbuminemia associated with protein-losing enteropathy may be present. Imaging of the small intestine may reveal small bowel wall thickening and mucosal nodularity.

The second pattern is associated primarily with submucosal and visceral muscle wall eosinophil infiltration sometimes sufficient to produce mass lesions evident on imaging studies of the stomach, small intestine, and, rarely, colon. Obstructive symptoms including nausea and vomiting are often accompanied by abdominal pain. These findings may mimic those of malignancy. Weight loss is common, and diarrhea may be present.

The third and least common pattern, in which there is primarily serosal and subserosal eosinophilic infiltration, is associated with ascites containing large numbers of eosinophils as well as with abdominal discomfort, nausea, and diarrhea.

The diagnosis rests on the presence of gastrointestinal symptoms, the histologic demonstration of visceral eosinophil infiltration or eosinophilic ascites, and the exclusion of other entities that produce eosinophilia and gastrointestinal symptoms. These include parasitic disease, food or drug hypersensitivities, mastocytosis, polyarteritis nodosa, Churg-Strauss syndrome, lymphoma, inflammatory bowel disease, and the hypereosinophilic syndrome. In patients with mucosal involvement of the small intestine, eosinophilic infiltration is often patchy, and the mucosa from adjacent areas can be normal or have the features of a nonspecific enteritis. Hence, multiple biopsies should be obtained at endoscopy from several intestinal levels. Even then, while the observation of extensive eosinophilic infiltration helps to establish the diagnosis, its absence does not exclude it given the patchy nature of mucosal involvement. Correct diagnosis is especially important in patients with muscle wall eosinophilic infiltration mimicking malignancy and may require full-thickness biopsy at laparoscopy or laparotomy to avoid unnecessary radical resective surgery.

Treatment

Although controlled therapeutic studies are lacking, treatment with corticosteroids is remarkably effective in the majority of patients regardless of the pattern of clinical presentation. Hence, the overall prognosis in this disease is very good. In most patients, sustained symptomatic remission is induced with a 2–4 week course at moderate corticosteroid dosages (prednisone, 20–40 mg/day) followed by a gradual taper. Recently, non–enteric-coated budesonide has been used successfully. A minority of patients may relapse and require repeated courses of corticosteroids. A few unfortunate patients require continuous steroid maintenance or fail to respond to corticosteroids. Whereas dietary avoidance of poorly tolerated foods is obviously desired, elimination diets based on skin sensitivity and radioallergosorbent testing have been disappointing in that sustained responses are uncommon. There are anecdotal reports of responses to oral cromolyn, ketotifen, and montelukast in some but not all refractory patients.

Chang JY, Choung RJ, Lee RM, et al. A shift in the clinical spectrum of eosinophilic gastroenteritis toward the mucosal disease type. *Clin Gastroenterol Hepatol.* 2010;8:669–675. [PMID: 20451664]

Rothenberg ME. Eosinophilic gastrointestinal disorders (EGID). *J Allergy Clin Immunol.* 2004;113:11–28. [PMID: 14713902]

6. Systemic Mastocytosis

Given the multiple forms of systemic mastocytosis and its diverse clinical features, comprehensive discussion of the disease is beyond the scope of this chapter and the focus will be on the small intestinal involvement, which may produce malabsorption.

Although many patients with systemic mastocytosis have gastrointestinal symptoms, in selected patients with systemic mastocytosis, there is extensive infiltration of the intestinal mucosa and submucosa with mast cells, occasionally in the absence of the obvious skin lesions usually associated with this disease. The mast cell infiltration can be focal or quite diffuse. In and of itself, it may produce malabsorption and can contribute to the gastrointestinal symptoms, which may include weight loss, diarrhea, steatorrhea, nausea, vomiting, and abdominal pain. In addition, excessive gastric acid secretion related to mast cell histamine release may inactivate pancreatic lipase and cause intestinal mucosal damage, predisposing to malabsorption. Release of mediators such as prostaglandin D_2 from local or distant mast cells may increase motility, contributing to diarrhea, malabsorption, and abdominal discomfort.

The presence of classic skin manifestations of mastocytosis, including dermatographia and urticaria pigmentosa, coexistent splenomegaly, or peptic ulcer disease, the latter caused by mast cell histamine release, should arouse suspicion and facilitate the diagnosis of symptomatic intestinal mast cell disease. Serum tryptase concentration and serum and urinary histamine levels are elevated. Small bowel imaging studies reveal an infiltrative pattern with thickened or nodular folds. Increased mast cells and eosinophil infiltration of the mucosa and submucosa in biopsy specimens are diagnostic if present in the appropriate clinical setting.

Sodium cromoglycate, ketotifen, antileukotrienes, oral prednisone, H_2-blockers, proton pump inhibitors, and low-dose aspirin have been reported as being beneficial in relieving diarrhea, abdominal pain, and other symptoms, but treatment is empiric as suitable controlled trials are lacking. Direct treatment of the mast cell proliferation with tyrosine kinase inhibitors such as imatinib mesylate has been disappointing as resistance is conferred by the D816V mutation in the tyrosine kinase domain of c-kit. This mutation is present in 90% or more of systemic mastocytosis patients.

Sokol H, Georgin-Lavialle S, Grandpeix-Guyodo C, et al. Gastrointestinal involvement and manifestations in systemic mastocytosis. *Inflamm Bowel Dis.* 2010;16:1247–1253. [PMID: 20162539]

7. Radiation Enteritis & Colitis

The small intestine and colon are especially susceptible to the acute effects of radiation, given the rapid renewal rate of their epithelia. Radiation inhibits epithelial cell renewal in the exposed intestine. In the small intestine and colon, this results in true mucosal atrophy with decreased villus and crypt height in the small intestine and decreased crypt height in the colon and the rectum. In addition, substantial mucosal inflammation occurs in the mucosa of both organs that lie within the field of radiation. Although the damaged segment of the small intestine is functionally impaired, clinically evident malabsorption is unusual as there is sufficient unexposed small intestine to compensate and the mucosal lesion heals rapidly once radiation exposure ceases. On the other hand, diarrhea and hematochezia are common features of the colitis and proctitis that accompanies radiation therapy. These symptoms also remit promptly, in most instances, after radiation therapy has been completed.

In contrast, the delayed effect of radiation therapy to the intestine can cause serious debilitating disease and may manifest months to many years after radiation exposure. The threshold dose is in the range of 4000–5000 cGy and is influenced by associated risk factors, including concomitant chemotherapy and prior surgery causing fixation of the intestine in the radiation field through adhesions, and by radiation technique. An obliterative endarteriolitis of submucosal arterioles develops producing fibrosis, strictures, fistula formation, and telangiectasias and ulceration of the overlying mucosa largely on an ischemic basis. Malabsorption develops in some patients due to (1) bacterial overgrowth caused by stricture-induced stasis and impaired motility if there is neuromuscular involvement, (2) bile salt deficiency if ileal involvement is severe, (3) lymphatic obstruction, or (4) enterocolic fistula formation.

Symptoms include diarrhea, abdominal pain, melena, and hematochezia. Strictures may produce partial or even complete intestinal obstruction with nausea, vomiting, and painful abdominal distention. Imaging studies such as CT or MRI enterography, barium enema, and small intestinal series help to characterize the extent of disease and localize the site of stricture, but the images may resemble closely the features of other ischemic or inflammatory lesions. If the involved intestine is within the reach of an endoscope, biopsy is usually diagnostic with demonstration of the endarteriolaritis, fibrosis, and the presence of bizarre-appearing submucosal fibroblasts.

Overall, treatment is disappointing. If there is associated bacterial overgrowth caused by stasis and strictures, treatment with antibiotics as detailed in the later section dealing with that entity is often beneficial. If ileal disease is present, bile salt–binding resins may reduce the bile salt–induced diarrhea but may also aggravate steatorrhea by further reducing the bile salt pool. Supportive measures such as polymeric dietary supplements containing medium-chain triglycerides or even parenteral nutrition may be needed. Dilation of strictures within endoscopic reach may be helpful.

Surgery should be reserved for severe intestinal or colonic strictures and enterocolic, enterovesical, or rectovesical fistulas. Surgery is associated with substantial morbidity because the compromised circulation of the affected bowel interferes with normal healing. For bleeding rectal and colonic telangiectatic lesions, laser or argon plasma coagulation is often helpful, but treatments used for idiopathic inflammatory bowel disease including local or oral corticosteroids or 5-aminosalicylate have not shown consistent benefit. Radiation enteritis and colitis are often progressive; hence, the prognosis is guarded.

Theis VS, Sripadam R, Ramani V, et al. Chronic radiation enteritis. *Clin Oncol.* 2010;22:70–83. [PMID: 19897345]

8. Intestinal Amyloidosis

Intestinal amyloid deposits are most often seen among patients with secondary amyloidosis (acute phase serum amyloid A [AA type]) but have also been noted among patients with primary amyloidosis (monoclonal immunoglobulin light chains [AL type]) and dialysis-associated amyloidosis (β_2-microglobulin retention). Several mechanisms may contribute to the malabsorption that may accompany intestinal amyloid deposition. Neuromuscular infiltration results in impaired motility predisposing to stasis, resulting in intestinal pseudo-obstruction often with associated intraluminal bacterial overgrowth. Vascular infiltration may induce small vessel ischemia. In advanced disease, mucosal amyloid deposits may impair enterocyte function and diffusion of absorbed nutrients from the lumen to the mucosal vasculature and lymphatics.

Symptoms and signs vary from patient to patient. In some, a pseudo-obstruction-like picture may predominate with abdominal distension, nausea, anorexia, constipation, or diarrhea. Weight loss may be severe, resulting from impaired oral intake and malabsorption. Orthostasis may be prominent. In other patients, gastrointestinal bleeding from ulcerated mucosa usually related to vascular amyloid deposition may be the presenting feature. Protein-losing enteropathy may produce edema and ascites. The diagnosis should be suggested by the presence of conditions known to be associated with secondary amyloidosis. Examples include rheumatoid or psoriatic arthritis, tuberculosis or other chronic infections, amyloid deposition in other organs such as the kidney or liver, or a history of chronic dialysis. Imaging studies suggesting intestinal stasis and pseudo-obstruction or mucosal infiltrative disease are helpful but not specific. Demonstration of amyloid deposition by biopsy of the rectum or small intestine is definitive. Congo red stains should be obtained and examined with polarized light as the vascular amyloid infiltration can be subtle.

Treatment of secondary amyloidosis should be directed at the underlying cause to minimize progression or even induce improvement. Bacterial overgrowth, if present, should be treated with antibiotics. Prokinetic agents may be useful. Other treatment of malabsorption is generally supportive, with dietary and, if needed, parenteral nutrition.

Petre S, Shah IA, Gilani N. Review article: gastrointestinal amyloidosis-clinical features, diagnosis and therapy. *Aliment Pharmacol Ther.* 2008;27:1006–1016. [PMID: 18363891]

9. Whipple Disease

Whipple disease is an unusual and uncommon systemic infectious disease with protean clinical manifestations. The small intestine is almost always involved, producing malabsorption in the majority of patients. Although the disease was described in 1907, the role of bacterial infection in its pathogenesis was not recognized until more than 50 years later. Identification, culture, and molecular characterization of the organism, the actinobacteria *Tropheryma whipplei,* was finally achieved two decades ago.

Despite characterization of *T whipplei,* many aspects of the pathogenesis of Whipple disease remain enigmatic. There is evidence that *T whipplei* is widely present in the environment. *T whipplei* DNA has been found in the saliva and feces of up to 30% of healthy individuals, and up to 70% have IgG serum antibodies directed against *T whipplei.* Yet the scarcity of the disease and the lack of documented person-to-person transmission are most unusual for a disease that is caused by an infectious agent. Host factors no doubt play an important pathogenic role as suggested by a two- to threefold increase in the frequency of HLA-B27 antigen among affected individuals. There is some evidence of altered macrophage function and activation and an impaired type 1 T-cell response but, interestingly, little to suggest increased susceptibility to other infections among successfully treated Whipple disease patients.

Clinical Findings

As suggested above, the clinical features may include virtually any of the body's organ systems. In the classic presentation, gastrointestinal symptoms are usually striking and resemble those seen in other diseases with generalized malabsorption. Weight loss, diarrhea, steatorrhea, and abdominal distention are present in 80–90% of patients, and both peripheral edema reflecting hypoproteinemia from protein-losing enteropathy and poor nutrition are common. Fever is present in 30–50% of patients and occasionally is the sole presenting symptom. Arthralgia and arthritis occur in 60–75%, often involving multiple joints and often preceding the onset of gastrointestinal symptoms by months to even years. Patients with Whipple disease may present with extraintestinal symptoms in the absence of or overshadowing gastrointestinal manifestations. In addition to the joint symptoms mentioned earlier, central nervous system (CNS) symptoms such as cognitive deterioration, ophthalmoplegia, hypothalamic dysfunction, oculomasticatory or oculofacial myorhythmia, or ataxia may be the presenting complaints. In other patients, cardiac manifestations, including pericarditis and culture-negative endocarditis, or pleuropulmonary involvement, including pleural effusions, cough, and sarcoid-like pulmonary infiltrates, may be the initial manifestations. Occasional patients have presented with fever of unknown origin.

In addition to the physical findings characteristic of malabsorption, skin hyperpigmentation, peripheral lymphadenopathy, cardiac murmurs, signs of arthritis, and neurologic abnormalities may be present. Anemia with or without occult gastrointestinal bleeding, hypoalbuminemia, and hypocalcemia are relatively common.

The diagnosis is established by demonstration of *T whipplei* in involved tissues by microscopy together with the characteristic infiltration of periodic acid–Schiff (PAS)-positive macrophages (Plate 23). In the small intestine, mucosal architecture is distorted by the macrophage infiltrate, and mucosal and submucosal lymphatics are dilated. Electron microscopy reveals the characteristic bacteria in the mucosa. Biopsy of the mucosa of the proximal intestine is the diagnostic procedure of choice because the small intestinal mucosa is involved in the vast majority of patients. Care must be taken to exclude *Mycobacterium avium* infection in immunocompromised patients, which mimics the intestinal histologic features of Whipple disease but can easily be distinguished with Ziehl-Nielson staining, as *M avium* is acid fast whereas *T whipplei* is not. Alternatively, polymerase chain reaction (PCR) amplification of involved tissues can be used for diagnosis, although its availability is limited. In suspected CNS involvement, PCR and cytology of cerebral spinal fluid sediment are of major diagnostic value.

Treatment

Empiric treatment with antibiotics results in prompt improvement in most patients and in permanent cure in many. Because of the danger of CNS involvement even in the absence of symptoms, use of antibiotics that penetrate the blood-brain barrier is desirable. One recommended regimen is ceftriaxone, 2 g/day for 2 weeks followed by twice daily trimethoprim, 160 mg, and sulfamethoxazole, 800 mg, for 1–3 years, but trimethoprim–sulfamethoxazole alone has been successful in most patients. There are no evidence-based studies that establish the optimal duration of antibiotic treatment to prevent relapses. Replacement therapy to correct specific nutritional deficiencies is also indicated.

The overall prognosis in the absence of CNS involvement is excellent, although patients should be carefully monitored indefinitely for signs of relapse that may occur even years after apparently successful treatment. CNS symptoms may be the first sign of relapse.

Fenollar F, Puéchal X, Raoult D. Whipple's disease. *N Engl J Med.* 2007;356:55–66. [PMID: 17202456]

Fuerle GE, Junga NS, Marth T. Efficacy of ceftriaxone or meropenem as initial therapies in Whipple's disease. *Gastroenterology* 2010;138:478–486. [PMID: 19879276]

10. Crohn Disease

Crohn disease patients with extensive ileal involvement, extensive intestinal resections, enterocolic fistulas, and strictures leading to small intestinal bacterial overgrowth may develop significant and occasionally devastating malabsorption (see Chapter 3).

11. Abetalipoproteinemia

In this rare autosomal-recessive disease, mutations in the gene encoding microsomal triglyceride transfer protein interfere with posttranslational processing of apoprotein B, resulting ultimately in the absence of apoprotein B–containing lipoproteins in the circulating blood. Absorptive cells of the small intestine are packed with huge lipid droplets reflecting the impaired export of lipid from the epithelium following its uptake from the gut lumen.

The disease is usually evident in infancy or childhood when diarrhea and steatorrhea are noted. Acanthocytic red blood cells, reflecting their altered membrane lipid content, appear early, whereas the onset of retinitis pigmentosa and neurologic manifestations, including ataxia, tremors, peripheral neuropathy, and nystagmus, appear later in childhood or adolescence in untreated patients. Hepatic steatosis and, in a few cases, cirrhosis have been described. Laboratory features in addition to acanthocytosis and steatorrhea include absent serum β-lipoproteins and very low serum cholesterol and triglycerides, abnormal liver chemistries, and, in untreated patients, low levels of vitamin E and other fat-soluble vitamins.

Although specific treatment of the genetic defect is not available, prompt institution of high-dose oral vitamin E and A replacement at an early age markedly attenuates and sometimes prevents the development of the retinal lesions and the neurologic complications. Other fat-soluble vitamins should also be replaced. Cautious substitution of long-chain dietary fats with medium-chain triglycerides can be tried to improve nutrition, but in a few individuals, cirrhosis has been attributed to medium-chain triglyceride use.

Gregg RE, Wetterau JR. The molecular basis of abetalipoproteinemia. *Curr Opin Lipidol.* 1994;5:81–86. [PMID: 8044420]

Zamel R, Khan R, Pollex, RL, et al. Abetalipoproteinemia: two case reports and literature review. *Orphanet J Rare Dis.* 2008;3:19. [PMID: 18611256]

12. Parasitic Infestations

Whereas mild infestation of the intestine with *Strongyloides stercoralis* usually causes no symptoms, heavy infestation may induce fever, nausea, vomiting, weight loss, abdominal pain, and steatorrhea. The clinical picture may resemble tropical sprue, but eosinophilia is usually evident in severe infestations. If stool studies are negative, duodenal aspiration is indicated. A highly specific ELISA serology is available but may remain positive for years after parasitic eradication and may be negative in immunocompromised hosts. Ivermectin is the most effective therapy; in severe infestations, it can be combined with albendazole for greatest efficacy.

Giardia and coccidial infestations produce malabsorption. These protozoal infestations are discussed in Chapter 5.

13. Carbohydrate Intolerance

The terminal phase of digestion of ingested complex carbohydrates such as starch as well as disaccharides, including lactose, sucrose, maltose, and trehalose, occurs at the brush border membrane of intestinal absorptive cells where glycoprotein enzymes including lactase, sucrase-isomaltase, maltase-glucoamylase, and trehalase are located. Deficiency of any of these enzymes or defects in the monosaccharide transport process produces retention of unabsorbed sugars in the gut lumen. These, if present in sufficient quantity, produce osmotic diarrhea and flatulence, the latter caused by intraluminal bacterial fermentation of the unabsorbed sugars. In addition, approximately 50% of healthy individuals are unable to absorb completely 25 g of free fructose. Ingestion of nonabsorbable sugars such as sorbitol, used to sweeten dietary foods, or of excessive amounts of fruit juices or of high-fructose corn syrup–containing carbonated beverages may cause gastrointestinal symptoms in some individuals.

Congenital disaccharidase deficiencies and monosaccharide transport defects are uncommon and produce symptoms in infancy upon introduction of the offending carbohydrate into the diet. Isolated lactase deficiency is the most common cause of carbohydrate intolerance and may become symptomatic after the age of 5 years. Low mucosal lactase levels are observed in 5–20% of adult North American and Western European Caucasians, 50–95% of African Americans and Africans, 50% of Hispanics, and over 90% of Asians. The diagnosis is suggested by a history of the induction of diarrhea, abdominal discomfort, bloating, and flatulence following the ingestion of dairy products or other foods rich in lactose. However, as these symptoms lack specificity, it is not uncommon to ascribe the symptoms of another clinical entity, such as irritable bowel syndrome, to lactase deficiency. The diagnosis is confirmed by the lactose breath hydrogen test. An alternative is the oral lactose tolerance test.

Diseases that are associated with substantial mucosal damage such as celiac disease may produce clinically significant carbohydrate intolerance caused by impaired mucosal digestion and absorption of carbohydrates. Unless the individual also has isolated lactase deficiency, carbohydrate digestion and absorption should normalize as the mucosa heals with effective therapy of the underlying disorder.

Treatment of carbohydrate intolerance consists of decreasing or removing the offending carbohydrate from the diet. For lactase deficiency, reduction of dietary lactose by limiting dairy products and lactose-rich baked or processed foods is usually sufficient. A completely lactose-free diet is rarely necessary. Indeed, elegant studies have demonstrated unequivocally that most individuals with isolated acquired lactase deficiency can tolerate moderate amounts of lactose (the equivalent of 8 oz of milk twice daily) in their diet. Alternatively, commercially available lactase preparations can be ingested in concert with lactose-containing foods or foods pretreated with lactase can be utilized. Supplemental calcium and vitamin D should be recommended if there is significant dietary restriction of dairy products.

Gibson PR, Newnham E, Barrett JS, et al. Fructose malabsorption and the bigger picture. *Aliment Pharmacol Ther.* 2007;25:349–363 [PMID: 17217453]

Suchy FJ, Brannon PM, Carpenter TO, et al. National Institutes of Health Consensus Development Conference: lactose intolerance and health. *Ann Intern Med.* 2010;152:792–796. [PMID: 20404261]

DISEASES CAUSED BY IMPAIRMENT OF BOTH INTRALUMINAL DIGESTION & MUCOSAL DIGESTION/ABSORPTION

1. Small Intestinal Bacterial Overgrowth (SIBO)

Under normal circumstances, the proximal small intestinal lumen harbors less than 10^5 bacteria per milliliter of intestinal contents, most of which are derived from the oropharyngeal flora. The major mechanisms limiting excessive bacterial growth in the proximal intestine are normal intestinal motor function and normal gastric acid secretion. Secretion of immunoglobulins into the gut lumen also inhibits proximal bacterial proliferation. The presence of any condition that interferes with these protective mechanisms, notably impaired intestinal motility, structural lesions predisposing to intestinal stasis, profound reduction or absence of gastric acid secretion, and immunodeficiency syndromes, may precipitate SIBO (Table 20–10).

Table 20–10. Causes of bacterial overgrowth in the proximal intestine.

1. **Motility disorders**
    a. Scleroderma
    b. Amyloidosis
    c. Pseudo-obstruction
    d. Vagotomy
    e. Diabetes with visceral neuropathy
    f. Irritable bowel syndrome
2. **Structural abnormalities**
    a. Diverticula
    b. Strictures
        - Crohn disease
        - Vascular disease
        - Radiation enteritis
    c. Adhesions causing partial obstruction
    d. Afferent loop stasis after Billroth II gastrectomy
    e. Fistulas
        - Gastrocolic
        - Jejunocolic
        - Jejunoileal
3. **Hypochlorhydria or achlorhydria**
    a. Gastric atrophy with or without pernicious anemia
    b. Vagotomy or gastric resection
    c. Prolonged use of high-dose proton pump inhibitors
4. **Hypogammaglobulinemia or agammaglobulinemia**

Pathogenesis

Several mechanisms contribute to the malabsorption that develops in SIBO. Normally, bile salts secreted by the liver are conjugated to glycine or taurine and are absorbed by a specific active transport process in the distal ileum. In SIBO, the bacteria produce enzymes that deconjugate the bile salts. The more lipid-soluble deconjugated bile salts are absorbed prematurely in the proximal gut by passive nonionic diffusion resulting in their decreased availability intraluminally. Moreover, the deconjugated bile salts are poorly soluble at the normal intraluminal pH and are less effective detergents, resulting in less effective intraluminal dispersion of dietary lipids for absorption. Additionally, the bacteria produce proteases and glycosidases and, in some instances, toxins that damage the epithelium, especially brush border hydrolases, interfering with the terminal phase of carbohydrate and protein digestion. The interaction of the bacteria with the mucosa may also produce an inflammatory mucosal lesion further contributing to impaired absorption. Finally, within the gut lumen, the bacteria bind and metabolize vitamin B_{12}, preventing its absorption in the distal ileum.

Clinical Findings

The clinical features of SIBO that are caused by bacterial overgrowth are typical of those seen in other malabsorptive states, with weight loss, diarrhea, steatorrhea, flatulence, and abdominal distention being common. Extraintestinal manifestations may be prominent. In the elderly, SIBO is probably an under recognized cause of poor nutrition; weight loss and mild diarrhea may be the major features. If the condition has persisted long enough to deplete vitamin B_{12} stores, megaloblastic anemia and neurologic manifestations identical to those observed in pernicious anemia may develop. In addition, a spectrum of additional symptoms, such as abdominal pain, nausea, and vomiting, may reflect the primary disease process predisposing to SIBO.

Quantitative culture of the duodenal fluid is the diagnostic gold standard for documenting SIBO but is not generally available, as it is invasive and costly, and the fastidious growth requirements of the gut flora require the use of multiple media and growth conditions not available in most clinical microbiology laboratories. Breath tests utilizing lactulose, xylose, and glucose are reasonable surrogates but are subject to major limitations described earlier in this chapter. If there is no ileal disease, the two-stage radiolabeled vitamin B_{12} absorption test (Schilling test) is helpful if available; the bacteria impair absorption both of free vitamin B_{12} and intrinsic factor-bound vitamin B_{12}; hence urinary excretion is low. Tissue retrieved by small intestinal mucosal biopsy may range from normal histology to a severe but nonspecific lesion with villus blunting, crypt hyperplasia, damaged absorptive cells, and substantial mucosal inflammation. Often a clinical response to antibiotic treatment is used diagnostically.

Treatment

If a correctable lesion such as a gastrocolic fistula or a discrete intestinal stricture is the cause of SIBO, surgical repair is the treatment of choice. If SIBO is associated with chronic motor abnormalities, achlorhydria, or noncorrectable anatomic abnormalities such as multiple jejunal diverticula, antibiotics are the treatments of choice. Some patients respond to amoxicillin–clavulanate alone; others require broader coverage with the addition of metronidazole. Promising responses have been obtained with rifaximin, a poorly absorbed although costly antibiotic. A single 2-week course of therapy may effect a prolonged remission in some patients; others require frequent intermittent courses of antibiotics when symptomatic or even continuous treatment for maximum benefit. Use of prokinetic agents has shown little or no benefit. As with all diseases associated with malabsorption, nutritional deficiencies, including vitamin B_{12} deficiency, should be corrected.

Recently, SIBO has been incriminated in some patients with irritable bowel syndrome, especially in the subset with diarrhea. In this group of patients, clinical improvement with antibiotic treatment has been reported, although considerable controversy remains.

Ford AC, Speigel BM, Talley NJ, et al. Small intestinal bacterial overgrowth in irritable bowel syndrome: systematic review and meta-analysis. *Clin Gastroenterol Hepatol.* 2009;7:1279–1286. [PMID: 19602448]

Quigley EM, Quera R. Small intestinal bacterial overgrowth: roles of antibiotics, prebiotics, and probiotics. *Gastroenterology.* 2006;130:S78–S90. [PMID: 16473077]

Rana SV, Bhardwaj SB. Small intestinal bacterial overgrowth. *Scand J Gastroenterol.* 2008;43:1030–1037. [PMID: 186091656]

2. Short Bowel Syndrome

The small intestine has sufficient reserve so that resection of 50% is well-tolerated provided that the duodenum and proximal jejunum and the distal 100 cm of the ileum are not removed and are free of disease. Resection of smaller lengths that include the proximal or distal segments often produce symptoms and signs related to their selective absorptive functions (iron, folate, and calcium malabsorption for the proximal intestine and bile salt and vitamin B_{12} malabsorption for the distal ileum). On the other hand, resection of 70–80% of the small intestine often produces catastrophic malabsorption with massive diarrhea with severe electrolyte imbalances and steatorrhea, especially if the distal ileum, ileocecal valve, and colon have been lost. Factors contributing to the malabsorption include the reduction of the available absorptive surface, acid hypersecretion that can induce intestinal mucosal damage and that can inactive pancreatic lipase, depletion of the bile salt pool, and SIBO. Conditions that may require small bowel resection of significant magnitude to result in short bowel syndrome include vascular catastrophes involving the mesenteric circulation, refractory long-standing Crohn disease, radiation enterocolitis, severe trauma, and malignant disease. In the past, bariatric jejunoileal bypass and inadvertent gastroileal anastomosis at the time of partial gastrectomy were uncommon causes.

Prompt and vigorous fluid and electrolyte replacement based on careful monitoring of losses is essential, as is early implementation of parenteral alimentation with meticulous vitamin and mineral supplementation. Early initiation of continuous enteral feedings is desirable to minimize intestinal mucosal atrophy and maximize adaptive mucosal hyperplasia. Protein hydrolysate–based polymeric supplements, which contain more fat and less carbohydrates and less of an osmotic load, are usually better tolerated than elemental supplements after the first few weeks. Acid hypersecretion during the early period following massive resection should be controlled with liberal proton pump inhibitor administration. Although growth hormone and glutamine have been advocated to facilitate adaptive changes in the residual small intestine, their use is controversial due to conflicting evidence as to their efficacy. Liberal use of agents to increase intestinal transit time, including loperamide or codeine, and hence contact of nutrients with the intestinal mucosa is desirable. Octreotide has been beneficial, although tachyphylaxis develops and high doses reduce secretion of pancreatic enzymes and may predispose to gallstones. SIBO, if suspected, should be treated with antibiotics (see above). Transition to oral feedings, starting with multiple small meals while tapering parenteral nutrition, is a major goal and is often feasible as intestinal adaptation progresses over time. Bowel lengthening procedures such as serial transverse enteroplasty may be beneficial in selected patients, especially young children. In patients in whom adaptation is not adequate and long-term parenteral nutrition is not feasible due to loss of venous access, recurrent line sepsis, or progressive liver disease, small intestinal transplantation is an alternative. Two-year survival is now in excess of 50% in expert hands, but the shortage of organ donors and the relatively few centers with the requisite surgical skills and experience limit this option to a selected few.

There are a number of complications that may develop with time in patients with short bowel syndrome. Cholelithiasis may form, especially if long-term parenteral alimentation is required and the enterohepatic bile salt circulation is interrupted. Prophylactic ursodeoxycholate may be useful. If feasible, some surgeons perform prophylactic cholecystectomy at the time of bowel resection. Renal calculi, often composed of calcium oxalate, may develop if colon is retained. Unabsorbed fatty acids bind calcium, reducing its availability to form calcium oxalate in the gut lumen. Free oxalate is then absorbed in the colon, especially if bile acids also spill, increasing colonic permeability to oxalate. Supplemental calcium, low-oxalate diet, and high fluid intake are therapeutic approaches. Steatotic and cholestatic liver disease may develop and progress to cirrhosis and its complications, especially if long-term parenteral nutrition is required and the distal ileum is absent. D-Lactic acidosis, likely reflecting bacterial metabolism of unabsorbed carbohydrates to D-lactic acid, may develop, especially in children.

Buchman AL. Etiology and initial management of short bowel syndrome. *Gastroenterology.* 2006;130:S5–S15. [PMID: 16473072]

DiBaise JK, Young RJ, Vanderhoof JA. Enteric microbial flora, bacterial overgrowth, and short-bowel syndrome. *Clin Gastroenterol Hepatol.* 2006;4:11–20. [PMID: 16431299]

Fishbein TM. Intestinal transplantation. *N Engl J Med.* 2009;361: 998–1008. [PMID: 19726774]

3. Gastrinoma & Zollinger-Ellison Syndrome (See also Chapter 16)

Patients with Zollinger-Ellison syndrome frequently present with symptoms and signs of malabsorption, including weight loss, diarrhea, and steatorrhea in the absence of or overshadowing acid peptic symptoms. The massive gastric acid secretion inactivates pancreatic lipase and impairs lipid emulsification by bile salts resulting in impairment of intraluminal lipid dispersion, which is required for efficient absorption. Moreover, the persistent and intense exposure to acid damages the mucosa of the proximal small intestine, impairing absorptive function. Biopsy specimens can demonstrate a striking architectural lesion with blunting or absence of villi and profound inflammation of the lamina propria. Diagnosis requires a high index of suspicion and is established by the demonstration of an elevated serum gastrin, a positive secretin stimulation test, and the presence of a gastrinoma by imaging studies. Treatment includes inhibition of gastric secretion with proton pump inhibitors and surgical resection of the gastrinoma, if feasible (see Chapter 16).

Roy PK, Venzon DJ, Shojamanesh H, et al. Zollinger-Ellison syndrome. Clinical presentation in 261 patients. *Medicine* (Baltimore). 2000;79:379–411. [PMID: 11144036]

DISEASES CAUSED BY IMPAIRED POSTMUCOSAL TRANSPORT

Intestinal Lymphangiectasia

Intestinal lymphangiectasia may be primary or secondary. The primary form usually presents in infancy or childhood and is associated with focal or diffuse ectasia of the mucosal intestinal lymphatics, most likely reflecting impaired lymphatic formation during development. Concomitant defects in lymphatics at other body sites such as the extremities support this concept. Familial clustering of cases suggests a genetic basis in some. Secondary intestinal lymphangiectasia results from acquired obstruction of mesenteric or more proximal lymphatics. Disruption of intestinal lymphatic drainage may reflect trauma, retroperitoneal fibrosis, neoplasms, infections such as tuberculosis, congestive heart failure, or severe portal hypertension. Rupture of the lymphatics results in leakage of protein and lymphocyte-rich lymph into the gut lumen as well as impaired transport of dietary lipids to the systemic circulation by the damaged lymphatics.

Clinical features in both primary and secondary types include weight loss, growth failure in children, steatorrhea, and diarrhea if disease is extensive. Edema, chylous ascites, and chylous pleural effusions reflect associated protein-losing enteropathy and impaired transport and leakage of dietary lipids. Helpful laboratory findings include lymphopenia, which may be striking, and low serum albumin, immunoglobulins, transferrin, and ceruloplasmin. Increased clearance of α_1-antitrypsin pinpoints the intestinal tract as the source of protein loss, but the evaluation of the test requires adjustment in patients with diarrhea; clearance greater than 24 mL/day in the absence of diarrhea or greater than 56 mL/day in the presence of diarrhea indicates increased enteric protein loss. Imaging studies such as CT scan of the abdomen can help to localize anatomic abnormalities such as fibrosis and adenopathy and often reveal thickening and edema of the abdominal wall. Contrast or magnetic resonance lymphangiography, if available, may localize the site of lymphatic obstruction or leakage. Endoscopy may reveal whitish villi due to distended ectatic mucosal lymphatics. Mucosal biopsy characteristically shows tall villi, dilated lymphatics, and mucosal edema, but involvement may be patchy; hence, absence of lymphatic dilation in available biopsy specimens does not exclude the diagnosis.

Treatment includes reduction of dietary long-chain triglycerides that stimulate lymph formation, increasing intralymphatic pressure and predisposing to lymphatic rupture and lymph leakage. Addition of medium-chain triglyceride–containing supplements and use of medium-chain triglyceride oil benefit nutrition as they are transported in the portal blood, not the lymphatics. A high-protein diet utilizing supplements as needed helps counter enteric protein loss. If the responsible disease process involves a limited segment of the intestine, resection can be beneficial. Likewise, if a surgically correctable focal obstruction of a major lymphatic is found, surgery should be considered. Obviously, treatment of underlying specific diseases such as retroperineal neoplasm or infection is indicated.

Diverticular Disease of the Colon

21

Anne C. Travis, MD, MSc, FACG
Richard S. Blumberg, MD

DIVERTICULOSIS

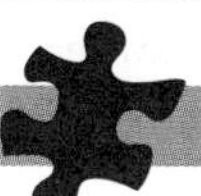

ESSENTIALS OF DIAGNOSIS

- Radiographic or endoscopic demonstration of diverticula.
- Normal vital signs and laboratory evaluation.
- Absence of complications (diverticulitis, diverticular hemorrhage).

General Considerations

Diverticula are acquired herniations of the colonic mucosa and submucosa through the muscularis propria. They occur most commonly in the sigmoid colon and can vary in size and number, although typically they are between 5 and 10 mm in diameter. Diverticulosis refers to the presence of diverticula in an individual who is asymptomatic, whereas diverticular disease refers to the presence of diverticula associated with symptoms, which occurs in 20% of individuals with diverticula.

Diverticular disease is the most common structural abnormality of the colon and, in terms of health care expenditures (both direct and indirect costs), it is the fifth most important gastrointestinal disease in Western countries, representing total annual expenditures of over $2.6 billion. It accounts for almost 2.2 million office visits and for more than 230,000 hospital admissions annually in the United States, with a mortality rate of 2.5 per 100,000 per year.

Although diverticula were described as early as 1700, diverticulosis was uncommon until the 20th century. Currently, it is estimated that diverticulosis affects less than 5% of people at age 40, 30% of people by age 60, and 50–65% of people by age 80. An exception to this is in vegetarians, in whom the prevalence of diverticula is much lower, presumably due to diets that are higher in fiber. Men and women are affected equally. The prevalence and distribution of diverticula vary throughout the world. Whereas diverticula are common and predominantly left-sided in Western countries (95% involve the sigmoid colon), in urbanized areas of Asia, such as Japan, Hong Kong, and Singapore, the prevalence is only 20% and the diverticula are predominantly right-sided, even among those who have adopted a Western-style, low-fiber diet.

Pathogenesis

A. Colonic Motility

Segmentation within the colon is thought to play an important role in the development of diverticula. Segmentation refers to the process by which a short segment of the circular muscle of the colon contracts in a nonpropulsive manner. This produces a closed segment of colon with increased intraluminal pressure, and likely serves to increase water and electrolyte absorption from the colon. These elevated intraluminal pressures may ultimately result in herniation of the mucosa and submucosa at sites of weakness (namely, where the vasa recta penetrates the muscularis propria between the taeniae coli), resulting in the formation of diverticula. Diverticula are not seen in the rectum because the taeniae coalesce at the rectum to form the circumferential longitudinal muscle layer.

The *law of Laplace* (transmural pressure gradient equals the wall tension divided by the radius, $\Delta P = T/r$) may help to explain why diverticula are so common in the sigmoid colon. Compared with the remainder of the colon, the sigmoid has a smaller radius. Because the transmural pressure gradient is inversely proportional to the bowel radius, it will be highest at the level of the sigmoid, potentially favoring the formation of diverticula in this region. Additionally, myochosis (thickening of the circular muscle layer, shortening of the taeniae coli, and narrowing of the lumen, Figure 21–1) is seen in most patients with sigmoid diverticula. These changes result from increased deposition of collagen and elastin within

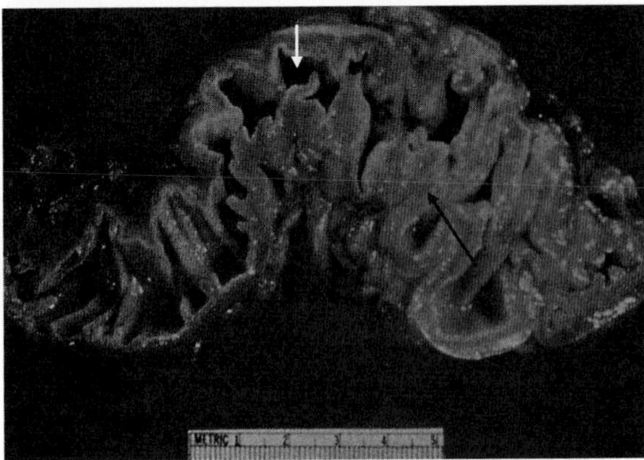

▲ **Figure 21–1.** Myochosis. Note marked thickening of muscle layer (*lower arrow*) and resultant lumina narrowing (*top arrow*) in a patient with myochosis and left lower quadrant abdominal pain.

the taeniae, and not from hypertrophy or hyperplasia of the bowel wall. In addition to increasing intraluminal pressure by narrowing the lumen, these changes may also decrease the resistance of the colon wall (see below).

Alterations in myoelectrical activity may also contribute to the development of diverticulosis. The interstitial cells of Cajal are thought to be responsible for the generation of slow waves. Extracellular electrodes show that these slow waves correspond to muscle contractions within the colon. Some studies have shown increased slow-wave activity in patients with diverticulosis, which could result in increased segmental contractions. However, one study found that there were significantly reduced numbers of interstitial cells of Cajal in patients with diverticulosis, possibly leading to delayed transit.

B. Colonic Wall Changes

As individuals age, the tensile strength of the collagen and muscle fibers of the colonic wall decreases due to increased cross-linking of abnormal collagen fibers and deposition of elastin in all layers of the colonic wall. The colonic wall may be weakened by the breakdown and damage of mature collagen, as well as by the synthesis of immature collagen. This may also contribute to the creation of more distensible muscle fibers. The importance of structural changes in the colonic wall is suggested by the early formation of diverticula in patients with connective tissue disorders, such as Marfan syndrome, Ehlers-Danlos syndrome, and polycystic kidney disease.

Collagen fibers vary in conformation throughout the colon. With increasing age, the collagen fibrils in the left colon become smaller and more tightly packed compared with those in the right, changes that are accentuated in diverticular disease. This may explain why colonic compliance is lower in the sigmoid colon and descending colon compared with the transverse and ascending colon, and may also explain why diverticular disease is more common in the left colon.

Extracellular matrix degradation and remodeling is mediated in part by matrix metalloproteinases. Activation of matrix metalloproteinases results in the degradation of the extracellular matrix, including collagens, noncollagenous glycoproteins, and proteoglycans. Tissue inhibitors of metalloproteinases serve as local regulators by blocking the effects of matrix metalloproteinases. Patients with diverticular disease have been shown to have an increase in collagen synthesis, an increase in tissue inhibitors of metalloproteinases, and a decrease in the expression of a matrix metalloproteinase subtype that is responsible for the degradation of collagen. These changes may contribute to the changes in the structure of the colonic wall seen in patients with diverticulosis.

C. Visceral Hypersensitivity

Patients who have symptoms from uncomplicated diverticular disease resemble patients with irritable bowel syndrome. In both groups, visceral hypersensitivity has been demonstrated in response to rectosigmoid distention. Patients with asymptomatic diverticulosis, however, do not demonstrate increased pain perception with rectal distention. The visceral hypersensitivity seen in patients with symptomatic diverticular disease is not limited to areas of the sigmoid with diverticula and is not associated with altered colonic wall compliance. This suggests that there is a generalized state of visceral hypersensitivity in symptomatic diverticular disease that is similar to that seen in irritable bowel syndrome.

D. Inflammation

Patients with diverticulosis may exhibit low-grade colonic inflammation that may resemble inflammatory bowel disease histologically, a condition known as *segmental colitis*. Segmental colitis is characterized by a chronic inflammatory process that is localized to the portion of the colon with diverticula, sparing the rectum and right colon.

While the exact prevalence is not known, retrospective studies have found segmental colitis in 0.25–1.48% of patients undergoing colonoscopy. In patients with diverticular disease, the prevalence is 1.15–11.4%.

The pathophysiology of segmental colitis is unknown. Multiple theories have been put forth, including that it is an atypical form of inflammatory bowel disease, that it is the result of mucosal redundancy and prolapsed mucosa, and that it results from changes in bacterial floral and bacterial enzyme activity due to fecal stasis within diverticula. There is evidence to support the theory that segmental colitis is a form of inflammatory bowel disease. Patients with segmental colitis have higher levels of tumor necrosis factor-α than controls with irritable bowel syndrome, segmental colitis often behaves similarly to ulcerative colitis or Crohn disease, it often has an endoscopic and histologic appearance that is similar to inflammatory bowel disease, and in one case report, it responded to treatment with infliximab.

E. Fiber

The role of fiber in the development of diverticulosis was first suggested by epidemiologic evidence. Diverticula rarely develop in rural Asia or Africa (prevalence of <0.2%), where diets are high in fiber. However, in areas that have developed economically and have adopted Western dietary habits, diverticula become more prevalent. In addition, populations that have moved from rural to urban environments show an increased prevalence of diverticulosis.

Higher fiber in the diet leads to increased stool bulk and decreased colonic transit times. Individuals from countries with high-fiber diets tend to have larger diameter colons, compared with those from countries with low fiber intake. Having a larger colonic diameter may impair the segmental contractions of the colon that lead to higher intraluminal pressures.

Clinical Findings

A. Symptoms and Signs

The majority of patients with diverticulosis are asymptomatic, with only 20% developing symptoms over their life span. Abdominal pain is the most common symptom, and is usually localized in the left lower quadrant. It is important to emphasize that left lower quadrant pain may be the result of myochosis (thickening of the circular muscle layer, shortening of the taeniae coli, and narrowing of the lumen often seen in patients with diverticular disease). In patients with right-sided diverticula, the pain can be felt in the right lower quadrant. The pain may worsen after eating and in some is relieved with the passage of stool or flatus. Patients may also complain of nausea, cramping, irregular bowel movements (intermittent diarrhea or constipation), bloating, and flatulence. Patients with segmental colitis may present with chronic diarrhea, abdominal pain, or rectal bleeding.

Patients do not demonstrate abnormal vital signs, such as tachycardia or fever, in uncomplicated diverticulosis. With palpation of the left lower quadrant, mild tenderness and voluntary guarding may be present.

B. Laboratory Findings

In uncomplicated diverticulosis, laboratory values, including the hematocrit, hemoglobin, and white blood cell count, are normal, and Hemoccult testing of the stool is negative.

C. Imaging Studies

A double-contrast barium enema will demonstrate the presence, localization, and number of diverticula (Figure 21–2). If segmental spasm is present, a transient saw-tooth pattern

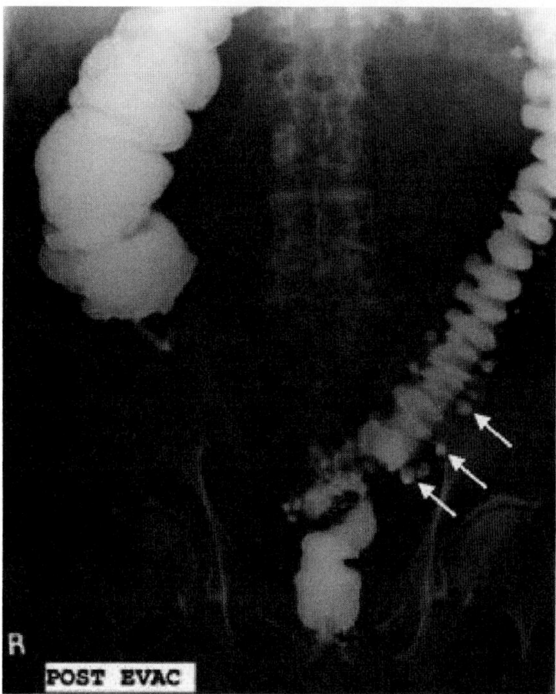

▲ **Figure 21–2.** Barium enema showing the presence of diverticula (*arrows*).

may be seen. In uncomplicated diverticulosis, there should be no extravasation of contrast, nor should there be evidence of fistulae, strictures, or persistent spasm, all of which suggest diverticulitis. Diverticulosis can also be seen on abdominal computed tomography (CT) with oral or rectal contrast.

In patients with myochosis, a plain abdominal x-ray may show scalloping in the left colon due to muscle hypertrophy (Figures 21–1 and 21–3).

D. Endoscopy

Diverticulosis is frequently discovered during colonoscopy as an incidental finding (Plate 24). Additionally, because disorders such as colorectal cancer, inflammatory bowel disease, and ischemic colitis are included in the differential diagnosis for patients with abdominal pain related to diverticulosis, colonoscopy is the preferred diagnostic study. Colonoscopy, however, can be difficult to perform in patients with diverticulosis due to narrowing of the colonic lumen and possible colonic fixation from prior episodes of diverticulitis resulting in inflammation and pericolic fibrosis. Colonoscopy is relatively contraindicated in patients in whom acute diverticulitis is suspected, due to an increased risk of colonic perforation.

In patients with segmental colitis, endoscopy reveals inflammation of the interdiverticular mucosa, characterized by erythema, granularity, and friability. The involvement may be diffuse or patchy. The inflammation is only seen in areas

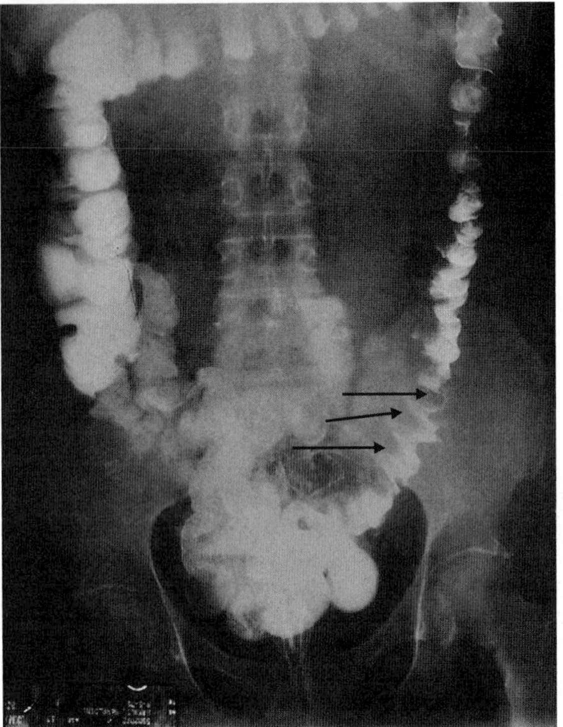

▲ **Figure 21–3.** Scalloping and luminal narrowing due to muscle enlargement (myochosis) and luminal narrowing.

with diverticula and spares the rectum. The rectal sparing is particularly important when attempting to differentiate segmental colitis from ulcerative colitis, since the two entities can appear very similar both endoscopically and histologically. Histologic findings include nonspecific mucosal inflammation, crypt abscesses, a mononuclear cell infiltrate in the lamina propria, and occasional submucosal inflammation.

Differential Diagnosis

The nonspecific symptoms of uncomplicated diverticulosis can mimic many other conditions, and differentiation can be difficult. Many of the signs and symptoms of symptomatic diverticulosis are also seen in irritable bowel syndrome. The fact that both disorders are common, and can coexist, makes differentiation even more difficult. Irritable bowel syndrome frequently causes diffuse abdominal pain; thus, pain localized to the left lower quadrant in the setting of demonstrated diverticula supports a diagnosis of uncomplicated diverticulosis.

Mild diverticulitis can manifest similarly and is not ruled out by the absence of a fever, elevated white blood cell count, or other signs of infection. Other pelvic infections, such as appendicitis and pelvic inflammatory disease, can also mimic diverticulosis. Other causes of lower abdominal pain that need to be considered are infectious colitis, inflammatory bowel disease, ischemic colitis, colorectal cancer, and endometriosis.

Complications

Diverticulosis can be complicated by acute diverticulitis, which results from the perforation of a diverticulum, as well as by hemorrhage, which occurs when the arteriole associated with the diverticulum erodes.

Treatment

Most patients with diverticulosis do not require any specific treatment, and there are no medical treatments that will lead to the regression of diverticula, once present. The treatment of patients with recurrent uncomplicated diverticular disease focuses on relieving symptoms. Therapies used to treat uncomplicated diverticular disease include fiber-rich diets, nonabsorbable antibiotics, mesalazine, probiotics, and prebiotics. Contrary to popular teaching, there is no strong evidence that seeds, nuts, or popcorn lead to an increase in the frequency of complications from diverticulosis. Patients with myochosis may get symptom relief with the addition of a fiber supplement.

Treatment approaches for segmental colitis have only been studied in small groups of patients or presented as case reports. Treatments include oral and topical mesalazine, topical steroids, high-fiber diets, antibiotics, oral steroids, probiotics, and infliximab. Patients with severe disease may require segmental or total colectomy. Patients with mild to moderate disease often respond well to medical therapy (most often with a 5-aminosalicylate), while patients with more severe disease may require topical and/or oral steroids.

A. Fiber

Fiber is slowly or completely fermented by gut microflora, resulting in the production of short-chain fatty acids and gas. This in turn results in shortened gut transit time, which reduces intracolonic pressure and helps with constipation. The recommended daily fiber intake for adults is 20–35 g/day, and fiber supplements are available to help meet this requirement. Supplements contain either soluble fiber (psyllium, ispaghula, calcium polycarbophil) or insoluble fiber (corn fiber, wheat bran). Soluble fiber is more readily fermented by gut microflora, whereas insoluble fiber undergoes minimal fermentation, and likely exerts its effects by increasing stool mass and thus increasing the luminal diameter, which in turn decreases the transmural pressure gradient. (Recall that, according to the law of Laplace, $\Delta P = T/r$.) Studies looking at the effect of high-fiber diets on symptoms from uncomplicated diverticular disease, however, have not been conclusive, with some studies showing a benefit, while others do not. Despite this, increasing dietary fiber, often with fiber supplements, is currently the mainstay of treating uncomplicated diverticular disease.

B. Nonabsorbable Antibiotics

Rifaximin is a broad-spectrum antibiotic that acts by binding to the β-subunit of bacterial DNA-dependent RNA polymerase. Eighty to 90% of rifaximin remains within the gut. Although the exact mechanism is unknown, rifaximin has been shown in a few studies to improve the symptoms of uncomplicated diverticular disease. Symptom improvement may be due to the ability of rifaximin to influence the metabolic activity of gut flora that degrade dietary fiber and produce gas. The drug may also influence the gut flora responsible for chronic, low-grade mucosal inflammation. Two studies in which patients were randomized either to rifaximin plus a fiber supplement or to placebo plus a fiber supplement for 1 year demonstrated symptom improvement in those who received rifaximin. In one study, the number of patients reporting no or only mild symptoms at the end of the study was 69% in the group that received rifaximin and 39% in the group that received placebo. Another study showed that in patients treated over the course of 10 years with rifaximin, 5% had a relapse of symptoms, with 1% developing complications.

C. Mesalazine

Mesalazine is an anti-inflammatory drug that acts topically on the gut mucosa and is typically used in the treatment of inflammatory bowel disease. Because some of the symptoms of diverticular disease may be related to chronic mucosal inflammation, mesalazine may have a role in the treatment of patients with symptoms related to diverticular disease. In a 2004 study, 90 patients were treated with rifaximin plus mesalazine (800 mg three times daily) for 10 days and then received mesalazine alone (800 mg twice daily) for another 8 weeks. At the end of the study, 81% of patients reported being asymptomatic. From this, the investigators concluded that mesalazine may help to maintain clinical remission.

D. Probiotics and Prebiotics

Probiotics contain microorganisms with beneficial properties, and the goal in using them is to alter the gut's microflora to reestablish the normal bacterial flora. *Bifidobacteria* and *Lactobacilli* are used most frequently. Some preparations also contain other bacteria and nonbacterial organisms, such as *Escherichia coli* and *Saccharomyces boulardii*. In diverticular disease, the normal bacterial flora may be altered by slowed colonic transit and stool stasis, so it is theorized that reestablishing normal gut flora may lead to symptomatic improvement. In a study of patients with colonic stenosis following an episode of diverticulitis, the combination of rifaximin and lactobacilli for 12 months was effective in preventing symptom recurrence and complications. In a second study, a small group of patients with uncomplicated diverticular disease were given an intestinal antimicrobial agent and an absorbent. That was followed by administration of a nonpathogenic *E coli* strain for a mean period of 5 weeks. These patients showed improvement in all abdominal symptoms.

Prebiotics are substances that promote the growth and metabolic activity of beneficial bacteria, especially *Bifidobacteria* and *Lactobacilli*. Prebiotics are frequently indigestible complex carbohydrates. Bacteria ferment these substances, leading to a more acidic luminal environment, which suppresses the growth of harmful bacteria. Substances that have been shown to promote the growth of *Bifidobacteria* and *Lactobacilli* include psyllium fiber, lactulose, fructose, oligosaccharides, germinated barley extracts, and inulin.

Prognosis

Twenty percent of patients with diverticula will develop symptoms of uncomplicated diverticular disease, while 10–25% of patients with diverticulosis will go on to develop a complication (75% of whom will have had no preceding symptoms). Fortunately, most episodes of diverticulitis and diverticular hemorrhage are self-limited and can be managed medically. An additional small subset of patients will develop severe pain and colonic dysmotility. Although not life-threatening, the symptoms can be debilitating.

Di Mario F, Comparato G, Fanigliulo L, et al. Use of mesalazine in diverticular disease. *J Clin Gastroenterol.* 2006;40:S155–S159. [PMID: 16885700]

Petruzziello L, Iacopini F, Bulajic M, et al. Review article: uncomplicated diverticular disease of the colon. *Aliment Pharmacol Ther.* 2006;23:1379–1391. [PMID: 16669953]

Sandler RS, Everhart JE, Donowitz M, et al. The burden of selected digestive diseases in the United States. *Gastroenterology.* 2002;122:1500–1511. [PMID: 11984534]

Sands BE. From symptom to diagnosis: clinical distinctions among various forms of inflammation. *Gastroenterology.* 2004;126:1518–1532. [PMID: 15168364]

Shaheen NJ, Hansen RA, Morgan DR, et al. The burden of gastrointestinal and liver diseases, 2006. *Am J Gastroenterol.* 2006;101:2128–2138. [PMID: 16848807]

Simpson J, Scholefield JH, Spiller RC. Origin of symptoms in diverticular disease. *Br J Surg.* 2003;90:899–908. [PMID: 12905541]

Tursi A. Segmental colitis associated with diverticulosis: complication of diverticular disease or autonomous entity? *Dig Dis Sci.* 2011;56:27–34. [PMID: 20411418]

ACUTE DIVERTICULITIS

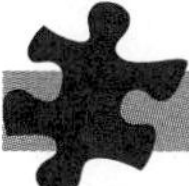

ESSENTIALS OF DIAGNOSIS

- Abdominal pain and tenderness (typically left lower quadrant).
- Fever or leukocytosis, or both.
- Characteristic radiographic findings.

General Considerations

First described in 1849, diverticulitis results from the micro- or macroperforation of a diverticulum, resulting in anything from subclinical inflammation to feculent peritonitis. It affects 10–25% of patients with diverticulosis and can be associated with significant complications (abscess, fistula, obstruction, phlegmon, bleeding, or macroperforation). There is a male predominance in patients younger than 50 years of age, with equal gender distribution after age 60 years. Hospital admissions for diverticulitis have been increasing. In a study from Scotland, the rate of hospitalization from diverticulitis increased from 12.8 per 100,000 for 1958–1961, to 23.5 per 100,000 for 1968–1971. A study from England demonstrated a 16% increase in hospital admissions for diverticulitis among males, and a 12% increase among females between 1990 and 2000.

Acute diverticulitis can be either complicated or uncomplicated. The severity of diverticulitis is often described using the Hinchey classification, which categorizes diverticulitis into four stages based on clinical and operative findings. Modifications of the classification have also been developed that take into account CT findings (Table 21–1).

Pathogenesis

A. Elevated Colonic Pressure

Previously it was thought that diverticulitis was the result of obstruction of a diverticulum by a fecalith leading to increased pressure within the diverticulum, with subsequent perforation. Currently, it is thought that diverticular obstruction is a rare event and that most cases of diverticulitis are the result of erosion of the diverticular wall due to increased intraluminal pressure or inspissated food particles. This then leads to inflammation and focal necrosis, with resultant perforation of the thin-walled diverticulum. The role of increased pressure is supported by the observation that most perforations occur in the sigmoid colon, where pressures are the highest. Factors that favor increased colonic pressures are altered autonomic activity (seen with decreased exercise and neostigmine), activation of opioid receptors, and decreased mechanical stretching of the colon due to a low-fiber diet. Recall that the transmural pressure gradient decreases with an increase in luminal diameter, which explains why a decrease in stool bulk is associated with an increased transmural pressure gradient. (Refer to the law of Laplace, $\Delta P = T/r$, discussed earlier.)

B. Changes in Bacterial Flora

Altered microbial composition within the gut, possibly due to effects on the innate immune system that allow normal commensal flora to act pathologically, may impair the mucosal barrier, resulting in chronic low-grade inflammation. Secretion of mucus and bacterial overgrowth can occur when food particles become inspissated within a diverticulum. It has also been demonstrated that the composition of gut flora differs between rural and urban populations. One study comparing a rural African population with a low prevalence of diverticulitis to an English population found that there were lower levels of *Bifidobacteria* and higher levels of *Bacteroides* in the English population. The growth of *Bifidobacteria* is promoted by soluble fiber, the fermentation of which leads to the generation of short-chain fatty acids, the preferred energy source for colonocytes. The increased production of short-chain fatty acids may aid in maintaining the colonic barrier.

C. Nonsteroidal Anti-Inflammatory Drugs

Nonsteroidal anti-inflammatory drugs (NSAIDs) have been associated with diverticulitis and perforation. In one study, patients with complicated diverticular disease (defined as bleeding or perforation) were more likely to have used

Table 21–1. Hinchey classification and modified Hinchey classification of acute diverticulitis.

Stage	Hinchey Classification	Stage	Modified Hinchey Classification
		0	Mild clinical diverticulitis
I	Pericolic abscess or phlegmon	Ia	Confined pericolic inflammation or phlegmon
		Ib	Confined pericolic abscess
II	Pelvic, intra-abdominal, or retroperitoneal abscess	II	Pelvic, distant intra-abdominal, or retroperitoneal abscess
III	Generalized purulent peritonitis	III	Generalized purulent peritonitis
IV	Generalized feculent peritonitis	IV	Fecal peritonitis
		Fistula	Colovesical, vaginal, enteric, cutaneous
		Obstruction	Large or small bowel obstruction, or both

Adapted, with permission, from Kaiser AM, Jiang JK, Lake JP, et al. The management of complicated diverticulitis and the role of computed tomography. *Am J Gastroenterol*. 2005;100:910–917.

NSAIDs than a matched control group from the community (34% vs 4%). In a second study, 48% of patients with complicated diverticular disease (fistula, extracolonic abscess, purulent peritonitis, feculent peritonitis, septicemia, portal pyemia) had used NSAIDs, compared with 20% of patients with uncomplicated diverticular disease. A third study compared 115 patients with complicated diverticulitis (fistula, abscess, peritonitis) to 77 with uncomplicated diverticulitis (peridiverticulitis or an inflammatory mass) and found that NSAIDs were associated with the severe complications of peritonitis and abscess formation. The association of NSAIDs with diverticulitis is postulated to be related to decreased prostaglandin synthesis and direct topical mucosal damage. By stimulating mucin and bicarbonate secretion and increasing mucosal blood flow, prostaglandins aid in maintaining the colonic mucosal barrier. In addition, NSAIDs are weak acids that may denude epithelial cells, resulting in increased mucosal permeability, ulceration, and the translocation of bacteria and toxins.

D. Diet

As previously mentioned, a diet low in fiber may not only predispose to the formation of diverticula, but may also predispose to the development of diverticulitis. By increasing stool weight and water content, fiber helps reduce colonic segmentation pressures, which may protect against perforation.

Red meat intake has also been associated with diverticulitis. Heterocyclic amines are products of cooking meat and have been associated with apoptosis of colonic epithelial cells. Heme has also been shown to produce a cytotoxic factor in rat colons. These effects on the colonic epithelial cells may predispose to perforation.

E. Smoking, Alcohol, Coffee, and Caffeine

The data supporting smoking as a risk factor for diverticulitis are contradictory. In one study, smoking increased the odds for diverticular complications threefold. A large cohort study, however, found no association between complicated diverticular disease and smoking. Alcohol, coffee, and caffeine have not been shown to increase the risk for diverticulitis.

Clinical Findings

A. Symptoms and Signs

Diverticulitis should be suspected in a patient presenting with lower abdominal pain, fever, and leukocytosis. In the West, left lower quadrant pain is the most common complaint (70%). The onset is usually gradual, and the pain may be present for several days prior to the patient's seeking medical attention. The pain is constant, with intermittent exacerbations that are associated with colonic spasms and are followed by loose bowel movements. Patients may also complain of nausea and vomiting (20–62%), constipation (50%), diarrhea (25–35%), and urinary symptoms (10–15%).

The patient's presentation is associated with the stage of disease. The pain is typically localized in patients with Hinchey stage I and II disease, as the inflammation is confined to the pericolic tissue. Although typically in the left lower quadrant, in patients with a large sigmoid loop or with right-sided diverticulitis, it may extend to the mid or right abdomen. In stage II disease, patients have developed pelvic, intra-abdominal, or retroperitoneal abscesses. These patients often complain of anorexia, nausea, and vomiting. This is especially common if the abscess is large. Urinary symptoms (urgency, frequency) can result if the abscess is near the bladder. An area of localized tenderness with swelling and erythema of the abdominal wall suggests an underlying abscess progressing to form a colocutaneous fistula. Patients with stage III and IV disease have symptoms of generalized peritonitis, including severe, diffuse abdominal pain. Patients may be reluctant to move. It is common for an ileus to develop, resulting in bloating, nausea, and vomiting. In stage IV disease, because free perforation has occurred, the onset of the pain is often acute and severe.

It is important to remember that patients who are immunosuppressed (eg, the elderly, those with cancer, HIV infection, or who have received an organ transplant) are much more likely to have an atypical presentation.

On examination, tenderness is usually present in the left lower quadrant, with a tender mass being present in 20%. Tenderness in the right lower quadrant can result from either a large sigmoid loop or from right-sided diverticulitis. A low-grade or high-grade fever is common. Diffuse tenderness suggests free perforation and peritonitis. Abdominal distention and hypoactive bowel sounds may be present if an ileus has developed. In cases of free perforation, hemodynamic instability may develop, along with a rigid abdomen.

B. Laboratory Findings

The most common finding is a leukocytosis, but it is not required to make the diagnosis. In one series, a normal white blood cell count was noted in 45% of patients. Marked leukocytosis is suggestive of peritonitis or abscess formation. Liver function tests are usually normal. The serum amylase is either normal or mildly elevated. If the amylase is elevated, it is suggestive of possible peritonitis or a perforation. Severe episodes may also be associated with hyponatremia, impaired renal function, and acidosis as a result of sepsis. If the urinary bladder is involved, pyuria or hematuria may result, and polymicrobial urinary tract infections can be seen with a colovesical fistula.

C. Imaging Studies

Plain abdominal radiographs are typically normal in patients with mild diverticulitis, but in the setting of severe disease, there may be an ileus pattern or, if obstruction is present, proximal bowel dilation. A large abscess may be associated with an air-fluid level on upright films. If there is perforation into the retroperitoneal space, the psoas shadow may be obliterated due to air diffusing along the psoas muscle. Free air under the diaphragm may be seen on upright films in the setting of intraperitoneal perforation, especially if there is feculent peritonitis.

Ultrasound is a noninvasive method with limited utility. It is highly operator dependent, and in the setting of an ileus may be limited due to distention of the bowel by gas. It may identify a phlegmon, abscess, or bowel wall thickening. It can be helpful in guiding the drainage of intra-abdominal abscesses.

Barium enema, although used in the past to diagnose acute diverticulitis, has largely been replaced by CT scanning. Findings on barium enema in the setting of acute diverticulitis include persistent spasm, saw-tooth pattern of the involved segment, deformed diverticulum, sinus tract or fistula, extravasation of contrast, abscess, stricture, obstruction, mass effect from extraluminal compression, and pneumoperitoneum.

CT scanning is currently the radiographic test of choice for diagnosing diverticulitis. Its sensitivity is as high as 97%, and specificity is reported to be as high as 100%. The following findings are seen with diverticulitis: soft tissue density of the pericolic fat (98%), diverticula (84%), bowel wall thickening of more than 4 mm (70%), and phlegmon or pericolic fluid (35%). CT scanning is also helpful in classifying patients as having mild, moderate, or severe disease; in guiding therapeutic decisions; and in diagnosing the complications of diverticulitis, such as abscess formation, fistula formation, peritonitis, or obstruction. Because CT scans cannot reliably exclude cancer, patients who have not previously had a colonoscopy should have one 6–8 weeks after their diverticulitis has resolved.

D. Endoscopy

During an acute episode of suspected diverticulitis, rigid proctoscopy, flexible sigmoidoscopy, and colonoscopy are relatively contraindicated. This is due to the fact that the required air insufflation can unseal or worsen a perforation. However, as mentioned above, patients who have not previously had a colonoscopy should have one to exclude an underlying malignancy or other disorder, with a waiting period of 6–8 weeks following resolution of the episode of diverticulitis. If an endoscopy is to be performed in order to differentiate between acute diverticulitis and cancer or colitis prior to surgery, it should only be attempted by an experienced endoscopist, with minimal insufflation. Findings of diverticulitis on endoscopy include edema, erythema, strictures, and (rarely) purulent drainage from a diverticulum. Following resolution of an episode of diverticulitis, endoscopic findings are often minimal.

Differential Diagnosis

Because of the proximity of the colon to other intra-abdominal organs, and because of the varied presentations of diverticulitis, many other diagnoses need to be considered. The differential diagnosis includes inflammatory bowel disease, ischemic colitis, infectious colitis, appendicitis, cancer, complicated peptic ulcer disease, pyelonephritis, pelvic inflammatory disease, ovarian cyst or torsion, and ectopic pregnancy. In patients with AIDS and colonic perforation, cytomegalovirus infection and Kaposi sarcoma should also be considered.

Complications

Complications of acute diverticulitis are seen in 15–20% of patients and include pericolic or pelvic abscess formation, perforation with purulent or feculent peritonitis, fistula formation to adjacent organs, colon obstruction, and sepsis. Fistulas most frequently arise from the sigmoid colon and involve adjacent organs. The common fistulas are colovesical fistulas (65%) and colovaginal fistulas (25%). Peritonitis is associated with a significant mortality rate. Mortality is approximately 6% if there is purulent peritonitis and 35% if there is feculent peritonitis.

Treatment

A. Medical Therapy

For patients with uncomplicated diverticulitis, medical therapy is successful in 70–100%. Patients who are candidates for outpatient therapy have pain that is mild, minimal evidence of systemic infection, no signs of paralytic ileus, and good functional status. Inpatient treatment should be considered for patients with more severe presentations, inability to tolerate oral intake, or comorbid illnesses. Additional considerations include the lack of available support, poor patient reliability, and poor patient comprehension of the indications for seeking medical attention (fever, worsening pain, inability to take in adequate fluids). Hospitalization and intravenous administration of antibiotics is usually recommended for the elderly, immunosuppressed, those with significant comorbid illnesses, and those with a high fever or significant leukocytosis.

Therapy consists of bowel rest and antibiotics. Antibiotic choice is dictated by the typical bacteria associated with diverticulitis, namely gram-negative rods and anaerobes. Single antibiotic coverage using an antibiotic with activity against colonic flora is as effective as combination therapy. Examples of treatment regimens are shown in Table 21–2. The choice of antibiotics should take into account medication allergies and prior antibiotic use. Antibiotics are typically given for 7–10 days.

Table 21–2. Common antibiotic regimens for acute diverticulitis.

Antibiotic(s)	Dose	Route of Administration
Outpatient Regimens (choose one regimen from the two listed)		
Metronidazole plus	500 mg three times daily	Oral
ciprofloxacin	500 mg twice daily	Oral
Amoxicillin-clavulanate	875/125 mg twice daily	Oral
Inpatient Regimens (choose one regimen from the six listed)		
Metronidazole plus	500 mg every 8 hours	IV
ciprofloxacin or	400 mg every 12 hours	IV
levofloxacin or	500 mg daily	IV
ceftriaxone or	1–2 g daily	IV
cefotaxime	1–2 g every 6 hours	IV
Ampicillin-sulbactam	3 g every 6 hours	IV
Piperacillin-tazobactam	3.75 or 4.5 g every 6 hours	IV
Ticarcillin-clavulanate	3.1 g every 8 hours	IV
Imipenem	500 mg every 6 hours	IV
Meropenem	1 g every 8 hours	IV

IV, intravenous.

Outpatients should be put on a clear liquid diet, with slow advancement of the diet once clinical improvement is seen. Patients who fail to show signs of improvement in 2–3 days, develop increasing pain or fever, or are no longer able to tolerate fluids should be hospitalized and investigated for possible complications.

B. Radiologically Guided Therapy

Abscesses traditionally were treated with surgery, but with advances in CT-guided drainage, some patients can be managed with percutaneously placed catheters. Drains are usually placed through the anterior abdominal wall, although transgluteal, transrectal, or transvaginal approaches are also used for abscesses deep within the pelvis. Catheters are left in place until the daily output drops to less than 10 mL, which may take up to 30 days. Patients who fail to improve with catheter drainage require surgery. CT-guided drainage has also been used to bridge patients from emergent to elective surgery.

C. Surgical Therapy

Fifteen to 30% of patients will require surgery for their first episode of diverticulitis. Indications for surgery during an episode of diverticulitis include diffuse peritonitis, obstruction, and failure of medical therapy. Elective surgery is also recommended for patients with fistulas, which result from the spontaneous drainage of an abscess. When this occurs, the inflammation usually resolves. Fistulas, therefore, are rarely an indication for emergency surgery.

Whether to perform elective surgery for the 20–30% of patients with recurrent episodes of diverticulitis is controversial. Based on data from 1969, it was previously recommended that patients undergo elective surgery after two episodes of uncomplicated diverticulitis. In the 1969 study, it was noted that 7–45% of patients will have recurrent symptoms following the first attack of diverticulitis, and that the response rate to therapy drops with each subsequent attack, from 70% for the first episode, to 6% for the third episode. Other more recent studies, however, have failed to show an increased risk of complications with subsequent attacks. In a 2005 study of 25,058 patients hospitalized for an initial episode of diverticulitis, 80% were managed without surgery, 19% had recurrent diverticulitis, and 5.5% underwent emergent colectomy. The study noted that patients younger than age 50 were more likely to have a recurrence (27% vs 17%) and were more likely to require an emergent colectomy (7.5% vs 5%). It may therefore be more appropriate to individualize recommendations about elective colectomy, instead of recommending surgery for all patients after two episodes of diverticulitis. For example, patients who live or work in remote locations or travel to areas where there is decreased access to health care may be appropriate candidates for elective surgery.

Prior to surgery, all patients should receive antibiotics. If possible, bowel preparation is carried out, although in emergent situations, it often is not feasible. For sigmoid diverticulitis, the proximal resection margin should be in an area of healthy (soft, nonedematous) colon. The distal resection margin is in the upper third of rectum, where the taeniae coli coalesce. If part of the distal sigmoid colon is retained, the recurrence rate of diverticulitis doubles. It is not necessary to remove all of the diverticula, because recurrence proximal to the anastomosis is unlikely.

When time allows for a bowel preparation, a one-stage procedure can be performed. Most patients with Hinchey stage I and II disease are able to undergo a bowel preparation prior to surgery. Placement of an endoluminal stent may allow for bowel preparation in a patient with an obstruction. In a one-stage procedure, the diseased colon is resected and a primary anastomosis is created. In order to create a primary anastomosis, the bowel being joined must be well vascularized, without edema or tension, and well prepared. Fecal peritonitis and purulent peritonitis are contraindications to a one-stage procedure, as are poor nutrition, immunosuppression, and other associated medical comorbidities.

Patients requiring emergency surgery usually undergo a two-stage procedure. In the case of sigmoid diverticulitis, in the first stage, the diseased sigmoid is removed and an end colostomy and a rectal stump (Hartmann pouch) are created. An alternative approach is to resect the diseased colon, perform a primary anastomosis, and create a diverting colostomy or ileostomy proximal to the anastomosis. If the diverticulitis is right-sided, the first stage is a right hemicolectomy with formation of an ileostomy and a mucous fistula (a mucous fistula is formed by bringing the distal resection margin through the abdominal wall). The second stage for all of these surgical approaches occurs 3 months later, when the colostomy or ileostomy is taken down and an anastomosis (if not already created) is formed.

An alternative to a two-stage procedure is an on-table lavage, in which the colon is lavaged with 3–6 L of warm saline, with povidone–iodine being added to the last liter of saline. This allows for resection of the diseased colon with a primary anastomosis (a one-stage procedure). The infection rate associated with a one-stage procedure following an on-table lavage is less than 20%, with an anastomotic leakage rate of less than 6%.

A three-stage procedure is the classic approach but is rarely used because of its higher mortality rate (26% vs 7% for other procedures). In the first stage, the diseased segment is drained and a proximal diverting stoma is created, but no resection is carried out. During the second stage, the diseased colon is resected and a primary anastomosis is created. Finally, in the third stage, the stoma is closed. The first stage of the procedure can be carried out to stabilize a patient who is unstable prior to transfer to a larger medical center, or when inflammation prevents safe dissection of the ureters or iliac vessels.

Many surgeons are now employing laparoscopic techniques to carry out the resections. Laparoscopic techniques have been associated with decreased rates of postoperative ileus, shorter hospital stays, and decreased postoperative pain.

Prognosis

Patients requiring surgery for free perforation have a mortality rate of 30% compared with 1% for those undergoing elective surgery. Following resolution of an initial episode of diverticulitis, up to 30% of patients will go on to develop recurrent diverticulitis. Four to 30% of patients will have episodic cramps, without clinical signs of diverticulitis, and 30–40% will be asymptomatic. Patients who have recovered after having peritonitis may develop small bowel obstructions due to adhesions. Patients with colovesical fistulas may develop urosepsis, and those with coloenteric fistulas may develop malabsorption due to bacterial overgrowth or due to short gut syndrome (as a result of the bypassing of segments of small bowel). Local irritation of the perineum or abdominal wall skin can be seen with colovaginal and colocutaneous fistulas, respectively. These fistulas can also be associated with fluid losses.

For patients who have undergone a surgical resection, 1.0–10.4% will develop recurrent diverticulitis, with 0–3.1% requiring an additional resection. Twenty-seven to 33% will complain of persisting symptoms.

Frattini J, Longo WE. Diagnosis and treatment of chronic and recurrent diverticulitis. *J Clin Gastroenterol.* 2006;40:S145–S149. [PMID: 16885698]

Gervaz P, Ianan I, Perneger T, et al. A prospective, randomized, single-blind comparison of laparoscopic versus open sigmoid colectomy for diverticulitis. *Ann Surg.* 2010;252:3–8. [PMID: 20505508]

Janes S, Meagher A, Frizelle FA. Elective surgery after acute diverticulitis. *Br J Surg.* 2005;92:133–142. [PMID: 15685694]

Kaiser AM, Jiang JK, Lake JP, et al. The management of complicated diverticulitis and the role of computed tomography. *Am J Gastroenterol.* 2005;100:910–917. [PMID: 15784040]

Korzenik JR. Case closed? Diverticulitis: epidemiology and fiber. *J Clin Gastroenterol.* 2006;40:S112–S116. [PMID: 16885692]

Morris CR, Harvey IM, Stebbings WS, et al. Epidemiology of perforated colonic diverticular disease. *Postgrad Med J.* 2002;78: 654–659. [PMID: 12496319]

Touzios JG, Dozois EJ. Diverticulosis and diverticulitis. *Gastroenterol Clin N Am.* 2009;38:513–525. [PMID: 19699411]

DIVERTICULAR HEMORRHAGE

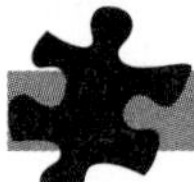

ESSENTIALS OF DIAGNOSIS

- Hematochezia, maroon stool, or melena.
- Nasogastric lavage that is negative for blood.
- Endoscopic or radiographic demonstration of diverticula.
- Exclusion of other bleeding sources.

General Considerations

Up to 15% of patients with diverticulosis will develop diverticular bleeding, bleeding that will be massive in approximately one third of the patients. Mortality rates for massive hemorrhage are significant, at 10–20%, in large part because many patients with diverticular hemorrhage are elderly with comorbid illnesses.

Pathogenesis

Diverticula form at the site of penetration of the vasa recta through the muscularis propria. Thus, each diverticulum has an associated arteriole, and mucosa is all that separates the vessel from the bowel lumen. Over time, due to recurrent exposure to injury, eccentric intimal thickening and thinning of the media may develop, leading to segmental weakness, predisposing the artery to rupture along its luminal aspect. In 50–90% of patients, the source of bleeding is right-sided diverticula (despite the fact that 75% of diverticula are located on the left). This markedly increased propensity for right-sided diverticula to bleed may occur because right-sided diverticula have wider necks and domes, so a longer portion of the vasa recta is exposed to injury. In addition, the wall of the right colon is thinner, which may also contribute.

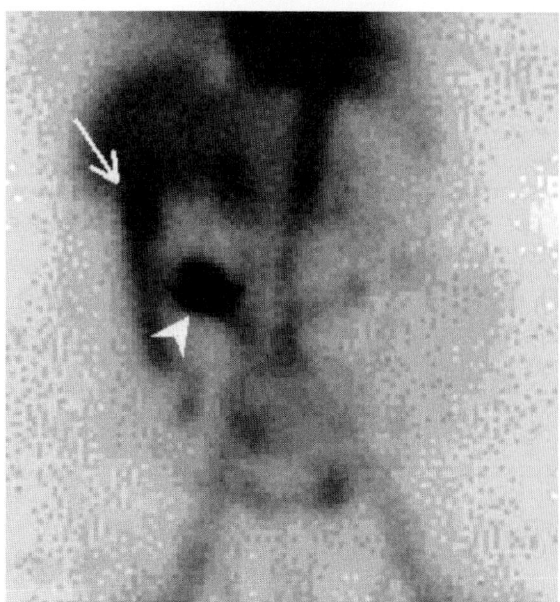

▲ **Figure 21–4.** Tagged red blood cell scan demonstrating bleeding originating in the right upper quadrant (*arrow*) along with pooling of the tagged red blood cells (*arrowhead*).

Clinical Findings

A. Symptoms and Signs

Patients typically present with moderate to large amounts of maroon stool or hematochezia. Clots are more commonly seen with a distal source, as is bright red blood. Melena may occasionally be seen in cases of right-sided bleeding. The bleeding is typically painless, although patients may report cramping due to the cathartic effects of blood within the bowel.

On examination, pallor, tachycardia, orthostatic hypotension, or shock may be noted with massive hemorrhage. However, in one study of patients with bleeding demonstrated on arteriogram, only 30% were tachycardic. The abdomen may be mildly distended with active bowel sounds. Rectal examination shows gross blood, which can range from bright red to melenic. Nasogastric lavage should be considered to evaluate for a possible upper gastrointestinal source of bleeding.

B. Laboratory Findings

Upon initial presentation, a normal hemoglobin is not uncommon because sufficient time may not have elapsed for hemodilution and equilibration to have occurred. Low hemoglobin at presentation is suggestive of either anemia that predated the bleed or bleeding that has been present for hours to days. Once equilibration has occurred, red cell indices should indicate a normochromic, normocytic anemia. The presence of a hypochromic, microcytic anemia suggests chronic blood loss from another source. Associated medical conditions or drug therapy may lead to an altered platelet count, coagulation parameters, or liver function tests. These conditions, while not responsible for diverticular bleeding, may contribute to its severity.

C. Imaging Studies

Radionuclide scanning using technetium sulfur colloid or ^{99m}Tc pertechnetate–labeled red blood cells can be used to identify acute bleeding and to localize the site of bleeding (Figure 21–4). These techniques can detect bleeding at a rate of 0.1 mL/min. Technetium sulfur colloid has a short half-life and thus can only detect bleeding that occurs within a few minutes of injection. ^{99m}Tc pertechnetate–labeled red blood cells, which have a longer half-life and can be used to detect bleeding up to 24 hours after injection, are now being used instead of technetium sulfur colloid. This allows for repeated scanning of patients with intermittent bleeding over 24 hours. In one series, ^{99m}Tc pertechnetate–labeled red blood cell scanning demonstrated a sensitivity of 97% and a specificity of 83% for active bleeding. The major limitation of radionuclide scanning is that localization is imprecise and can only identify an area of the abdomen where the bleeding is occurring and not an exact site. The accuracy of localization ranges from 24% to 91%. Blood can move from the site of extravasation due to peristaltic or antiperistaltic motion, which can lead to inaccurate localization. In addition, because localization is to an area of the abdomen, and not an area of colon, incorrect assumptions can be made about localization. For example, bleeding from a redundant sigmoid colon may incorrectly be attributed to the right colon. Although radionuclide scanning does not allow for therapeutic maneuvers, it can aid in directing subsequent angiography.

An alternative to nuclear imaging is dynamic enhanced helical CT scan. In a study of five patients, intravenous contrast was given, followed by scans at 30 seconds and 5 minutes.

In four of the patients, contrast pooling was detected, and all studies were completed within 15 minutes.

Angiography has the advantage of being both diagnostic and therapeutic. It requires a brisker rate of bleeding than radionuclide scans of 0.5 mL/min. If a prior study has suggested a possible location for the bleed, angiography starts with the injection of the appropriate feeding vessels. However, if prior localization is not available, sequential injection of the mesenteric arteries is performed, starting with the superior mesenteric artery, because the majority of bleeds arise from the right colon. If results are negative, the inferior mesenteric artery and, finally, the celiac artery are studied. Angiography is successful in identifying a source of bleeding in 14–85% of cases. The success rate is influenced by both the timing of the study relative to an episode of active bleeding and by the expertise of the radiologist performing the study. Angiography is 100% specific, but only 47% sensitive for an acute bleed (30% for a recurrent bleed). Performing a radionuclide scan prior to angiography may decrease the rate of negative examinations, but this may be counterbalanced by an increased rate of negative tests because of the delay introduced by performing the radionuclide scan prior to the angiography. If the initial study result is negative, the angiography catheter can be left in place for a short period to allow for rapid imaging if rebleeding occurs. Complications of angiography, which occur in 9% of patients, include arterial thrombosis, embolization, and renal failure.

Plain abdominal films are not helpful in identifying a source of lower gastrointestinal hemorrhage, and barium enemas are contraindicated because the presence of barium interferes with the performance of angiography and colonoscopy.

D. Endoscopy

Colonoscopy is the initial examination of choice in the evaluation of lower gastrointestinal bleeding. Like angiography, it allows for both diagnosis and treatment. Colonoscopy can be limited, however, by poor visualization due to retained blood and by the risks of sedation in an actively bleeding patient. Although some physicians will perform a colonoscopy in an unprepared bowel, relying on the cathartic properties of blood to empty the colon, many attempt to cleanse the colon either with enemas or with polyethylene glycol. A common regimen is to rapidly administer 4–8 L of polyethylene glycol, often via a nasogastric tube. A median dose of 5.5 L over 3–4 hours is needed to cleanse the colon. Metoclopramide (10 mg intravenously) may help to control nausea and to increase gastric emptying. Urgent colonoscopy will lead to a definite or presumptive diagnosis in 74–90% of patients (50% of these will be diverticular). Although visualizing active bleeding is uncommon, a presumptive source can be identified through the visualization of an adherent clot or a mucosal lesion. Forty percent of patients with presumed diverticular bleeds demonstrate stigmata of recent hemorrhage, including a bleeding diverticulum, accumulation of fresh blood after clearing the colon, a nonbleeding visible vessel at the mouth of a diverticulum, or an adherent clot that cannot be dislodged with vigorous irrigation.

Differential Diagnosis

The differential diagnosis for massive lower gastrointestinal bleeding is broad. Diverticular bleeding is the most common cause of maroon stool or hematochezia, and accounts for 42–56% of acute lower gastrointestinal bleeding. Angiodysplasias are responsible for 20–30% of cases of hematochezia. Colon cancer is the most common cause of lower gastrointestinal blood loss, but accounts for less than 10% of lower gastrointestinal hemorrhage. Although most hematochezia results from lower gastrointestinal bleeding, massive upper gastrointestinal hemorrhage or small bowel hemorrhage can also manifest with hematochezia (11% and 9%, respectively, in one study). Rectal causes of lower gastrointestinal hemorrhage include ulcers, radiation proctopathy, varices, and Dieulafoy lesions. Massive hemorrhoidal bleeding is rare. Rarely, inflammatory bowel disease can result in massive lower gastrointestinal hemorrhage. Although rectal bleeding is more common with ulcerative colitis, massive lower gastrointestinal hemorrhage is more common with Crohn disease. This observation may stem from the fact that Crohn disease is a transmural process and thus may involve larger submucosal vessels. Unlike patients with other causes of lower gastrointestinal hemorrhage, patients with inflammatory bowel disease usually have severe abdominal pain and tenderness.

Complications

Complications of diverticular hemorrhage are the result of massive blood loss, including death from exsanguination. Ischemic injuries to the heart, brain, or kidneys are the most common manifestations, especially in the elderly.

Treatment

A. Medical Therapy

A general treatment algorithm is shown in Figure 21–5. In 75–90% of patients, bleeding stops spontaneously; in those with a transfusion requirement of less than 4 units/day, the rate of spontaneous resolution increases to 99%. Initial therapy focuses on resuscitation. Patients should have large-bore intravenous access, such as a central venous catheter, or two 18-gauge peripheral intravenous lines. Patients should initially receive saline solutions while blood is cross-matched. Antiplatelet and anticoagulant agents should be discontinued, if possible. Any coagulopathies should be reversed. Patients with hemodynamic instability or with underlying cardiopulmonary disease should receive care in an intensive care unit.

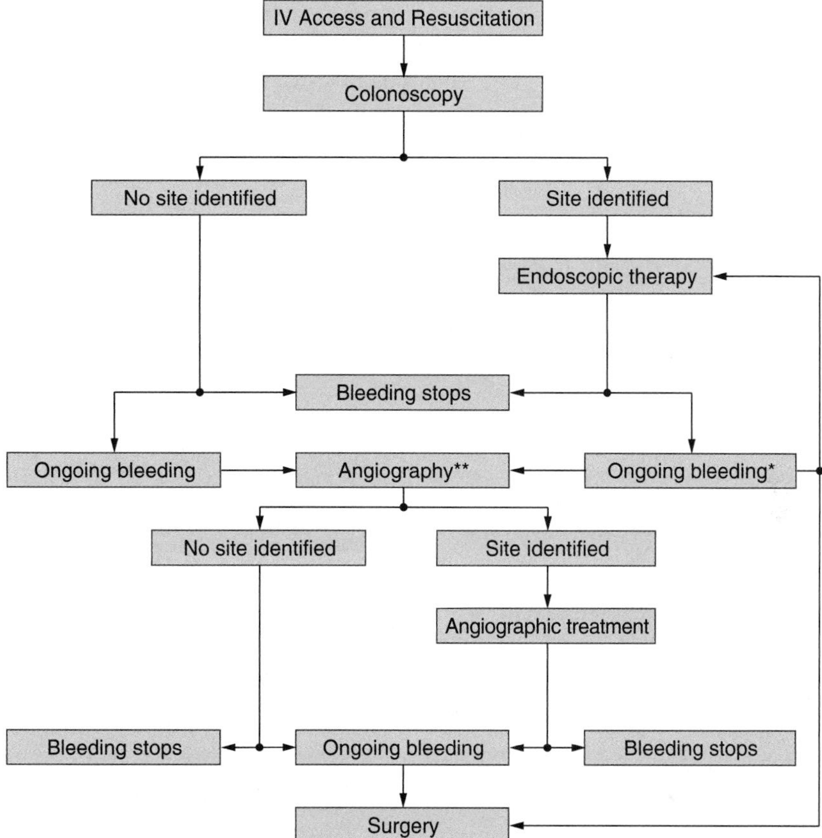

▲ **Figure 21–5.** Management algorithm for diverticular hemorrhage. IV, intravenous.

Endoscopic or angiographic interventions are then employed in an attempt to provide definitive therapy. If a bleeding source is identified endoscopically, therapy with injection of epinephrine (1:10,000 to 1:20,000) followed by thermal coagulation is recommended; if a nonbleeding visible vessel is seen, electrocautery alone can be applied. It is recommended that the multipolar electrocautery probe be applied to the vessel with mild to moderate pressure. It should be set at 10–15 watts, and the pulses should last 1–2 seconds. An alternative to electrocautery is the placement of hemoclips. If an adherent clot is noted, it is recommended that it be removed after the base is injected with epinephrine. The clot is then shaved down using a cold guillotine technique.

The pedicle of the clot, once visualized, should be treated with electrocautery if active bleeding or a visible vessel is seen. If the bleeding vessel within a diverticulum cannot be identified, blind injection therapy with epinephrine can be carried out, or the mouth of the diverticulum can be closed with hemostatic clips. It is recommended that a tattoo or a hemoclip be placed at the site of the bleed in case there is recurrent hemorrhage requiring either repeat endoscopy or surgery. Patients treated with electrocautery should be monitored for signs of perforation.

If a bleeding source is identified with angiography, therapy can be carried out. Vasopressin infusion will stop bleeding in 90% of patients, but 50% will rebleed when the vasopressin is stopped. Despite the significant rate of rebleeding, the use of vasopressin may allow for resuscitation and preparation for semi elective surgery. Vasopressin is started at a rate of 0.2 units/min. Angiography is then repeated after 20 minutes, and the rate is increased to 0.4–0.6 units/min if bleeding persists. Once bleeding ceases, the infusion is continued for 12–36 hours and subsequently tapered over 24 hours. Patients receiving vasopressin should be monitored in an intensive care setting. Complications of vasopressin include cardiac ischemia and fluid and electrolyte abnormalities. Transcatheter embolization using polyvinyl alcohol particles or microcoils is a potentially more definitive method for controlling hemorrhage; however, it is complicated by intestinal infarction in up to 20% of patients.

B. Surgical Therapy

Surgery is required for patients in whom bleeding persists and cannot be controlled through medical means and in those with recurrent bleeding. Persistent hemodynamic instability will necessitate surgery in 18–25% of patients who have required blood transfusions. Operative morbidity ranges from 37% for emergent colectomy to 8.6% for semi elective surgery. Operative mortality, which is often related to comorbid conditions, is approximately 10%. For patients who lack preoperative localization, exploratory laparotomy will be successful in identifying a source in 78% of patients. During exploratory laparotomy, the small bowel should be examined, and if a significant portion of the small bowel contains blood, intraoperative enteroscopy should be performed to evaluate for a possible small bowel source. Once the source of bleeding has been localized (either preoperatively or intraoperatively), segmental colectomy is performed. A primary anastomosis is possible in most cases due to the cathartic effects of blood. It is not necessary to remove all diverticula in patients with extensive diverticular disease.

Blind segmental resection is contraindicated due to its high rebleeding rate (30–42%), morbidity (83%), and mortality (57%). Thus, if a bleeding source cannot be identified, a subtotal colectomy should be performed. Although the rebleeding rate following a subtotal colectomy is less than 10%, the morbidity and mortality rates for the procedure are high (37% and 11–33%, respectively).

Prognosis

Seventy-five to 92% of patients will stop bleeding spontaneously. However, following an initial episode of diverticular hemorrhage, the risk of recurrent bleeding is 10–40% (often within 48 hours of the initial bleed). NSAIDs may increase the risk of early rebleeding. After a second episode, the risk of recurrent hemorrhage increases to 21–50%. Mortality is low in patients whose bleeding stops spontaneously (2% in one study). However, the overall mortality rate for those with massive hemorrhage is 10–20% and is related to comorbid illnesses. In those requiring surgery, the overall operative mortality rate is approximately 10% and is often related to comorbid illnesses.

Buttenschoen K, Buttenschoen DC, Odermath R, et al. Diverticular disease-associated hemorrhage in the elderly. *Langenbecks Arch Surg.* 2001;386:1:8–16. [PMID: 11405093]

DeBarros J, Rosas L, Cohen J, et al. The changing paradigm for the treatment of colonic hemorrhage: superselective angiographic embolization. *Dis Colon Rectum.* 2002;45:802-808. [PMID: 12072634]

Elta GH. Urgent colonoscopy for acute lower-GI bleeding. *Gastrointest Endosc.* 2004;59:402–408. [PMID: 14997144]

Jensen DM, Machicado GA, Jutabha R, et al. Urgent colonoscopy for the diagnosis and treatment of severe diverticular hemorrhage. *N Engl J Med.* 2000;342:78–82. [PMID: 10631275]

Yamaguchi T, Yoshikawa K. Enhanced CT for initial localization of active lower gastrointestinal bleeding. *Abdom Imaging.* 2003;28:634–636. [PMID: 14628865]

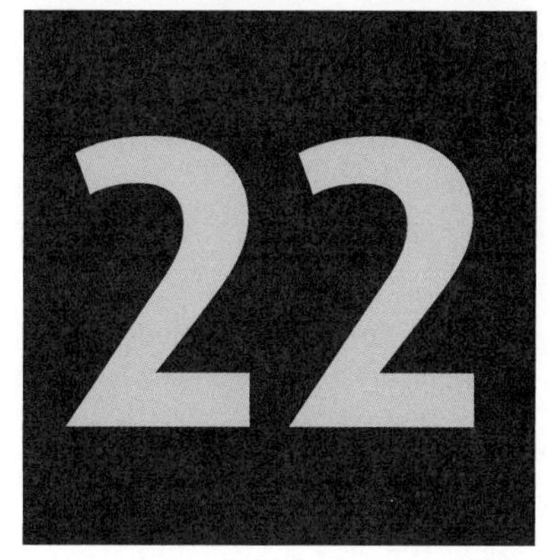

Colorectal Cancer Screening

Sapna Syngal, MD, MPH
Fay Kastrinos, MD, MPH

Screening for colorectal cancer (CRC) can reduce disease-related morbidity and mortality. The existing evidence has led to the recommendation of CRC screening as a standard component of preventive health care.

General Considerations

CRC is the second leading cause of cancer death in the United States and Western Europe. The lifetime risk of CRC in the United States is approximately 6%. In 2010, it was estimated that 72,090 men and 70,480 women would be diagnosed and 51,370 individuals would die of CRC. However, overall disease survival has improved from 51.4% in the 1970s to 64.9% in early 2000. Increased knowledge about the pathogenesis, advances in medical and surgical care, and the increasing emphasis on CRC screening programs have contributed to these substantial gains.

CRC can be prevented through readily available screening. Prevention efforts rely on the long time interval required for a benign adenomatous polyp to progress into an invasive cancer. It is estimated that the adenoma to carcinoma sequence unfolds over a 7- to 10-year period. In addition, CRC-related deaths are preventable if the disease is detected early. When diagnosed early, the 5-year survival rate for CRC that is still confined to the primary site (localized stage) is approximately 90%. Conversely, the corresponding 5-year survival for patients with known distant metastases is only 10%. Unfortunately, only 39% of cancers are diagnosed at an early stage and up to 19% of patients have distant metastases.

Nevertheless, CRC screening is presently underutilized in the United States. Approximately half of the population is currently compliant with standard screening recommendations, despite the array of available choices. CRC screening lags far behind screening for other common malignancies, such as breast, cervical, and prostate cancer. According to recent results by the National Center for Health Statistics, only 54% of Americans aged 50 years or older had undergone any type of CRC screening and only 42% had undergone screening within the recommended time interval. At present, issues of sensitivity, specificity, and patient acceptance limit existing CRC screening methods. Several factors contribute to the lack of compliance with CRC screening, including inappropriate perception of risk (particularly if patients are asymptomatic and without a family history of CRC), dietary restrictions or burdensome cathartic preparations, the invasiveness of procedures, and perceived discomfort, pain, and embarrassment related to certain screening techniques.

American Cancer Society. Cancer Statistics 2006 Presentation. Available at: http://www.cancer.org/downloads/STT/Cancer_Statistics_2006_Presentation.ppt#257,2, US Mortality, 2003. Accessed June 28, 2007.

Centers for Disease Control and Prevention. Colorectal cancer screening rates. Available at: http://www.cdc.gov/cancer/colorectal/statistics/screening_rates.html. Accessed July 3, 2007.

Edwards BK, Ward E, Kohler BA, et al. Annual report to the nation on the status of cancer, 1975–2006, featuring colorectal cancer trends and impact of interventions (risk factors, screening, and treatment) to reduce future rates. *Cancer.* 2010;116:544–573. [PMID: 19998273]

Jemal A, Siegel R, Xu J, et al. Cancer statistics, 2010. *CA Cancer J Clin.* 2010;60:277–300. [PMID: 20610543]

Ries LA, Melbert D, Krapcho M, et al. Surveillance Epidemiology and End Results (SEER) Cancer Statistics Review, 1975–2005, National Cancer Institute. Available at: http://seer.cancer.gov/csr/1975_2005/results_single/sect_01_table.01.pdf. Accessed September 8, 2008.

Seeff LC, Nadel MR, Klabunde CN, et al. Patterns and predictors of colorectal cancer test use in the adult U.S. population. *Cancer.* 2004;100:2093–2103. [PMID: 15139050]

Pathogenesis

In 1990, a stepwise, chronologic model for colorectal tumorigenesis was proposed. It outlined sequential alterations in key growth regulatory genes, such as *APC, K-ras,* and *tp53,* culminating in the development of a malignant neoplasm.

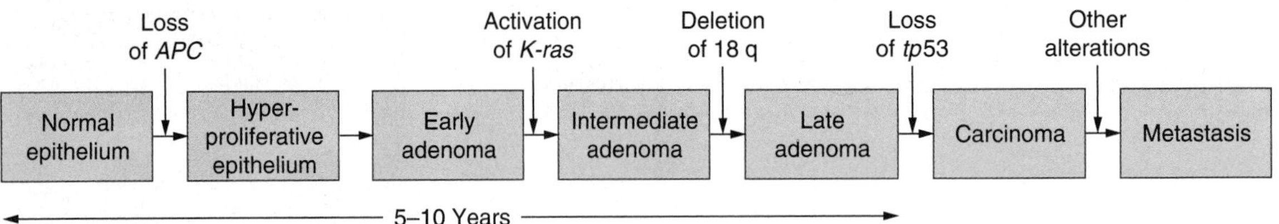

▲ **Figure 22–1.** Genetic model for colorectal tumorigenesis. (Adapted, with permission, from Fearon ER, Volgelstein B. A genetic model for colorectal tumorigenesis. *Cell.* 1990;61:759.)

This pathway contributes to the development of 85% of colorectal tumors that arise from preexisting adenomatous polyps. When adenomas accumulate the necessary combination of genetic mutations in the suggested stepwise manner, the end result is cancer (Figure 22–1).

The genes implicated in CRC can be divided into three categories: (1) tumor-suppressor genes, (2) proto-oncogenes, and (3) DNA repair genes.

The function of tumor-suppressor genes is to down-regulate normal growth stimulatory pathways. In CRC, the genes most frequently inactivated are *APC, tp53,* and *p16.* Consistent with the Knudson "two-hit hypothesis," acquired (or somatic) mutations in both alleles of the tumor-suppressor gene are required to fully inactivate gene function and cause cancer. In autosomal-dominant CRC syndromes, a preexisting germline mutation in one allele ("first hit") is inherited and a "second hit" occurs when an acquired mutation inactivates the other allele.

Proto-oncogenes, such as *K-ras,* are components of signaling pathways that promote normal cellular growth and proliferation. A mutation in a proto-oncogene leads to an active gene product with a resulting tumorigenic effect.

DNA repair genes function to maintain the integrity of the genome. Individual nucleotides can be modified by biochemical reactions such as oxidation, alkylation, spontaneous deamination, and ultraviolet cross-linking. When errors occur, they are corrected through a sophisticated process known as "base excision repair." Another manner in which errors are introduced into the genome is through mispairing of nucleotides, which can occur during normal DNA replication. These errors are corrected by a DNA "mismatch repair" system. When either of these DNA repair processes is dysfunctional, deleterious mutations can accumulate in genes that directly control cellular growth and proliferation.

Fearon ER, Vogelstein B. A genetic model for colorectal tumorigenesis. *Cell.* 1990;61:759–767. [PMID: 2188735]

RISK STRATIFICATION

The approach to CRC screening in asymptomatic individuals depends on risk stratification and the likelihood of developing the disease. Screening for CRC takes place in persons who have no personal or family history of adenomatous polyps or cancer. Surveillance takes place in persons with a personal history of either adenomatous polyps or CRC, or one of the genetic syndromes that requires more intensive monitoring. Individuals who have signs or symptoms suggestive of CRC fall outside the domain of screening and should be offered appropriate diagnostic evaluation.

CRC screening programs begin by classifying an individual's level of risk based on age, as well as personal and family medical history (Figure 22–2). This vital information helps determine when screening should be initiated, with what appropriate tests, and the frequency of subsequent examinations. CRC risk is commonly stratified into three broad categories: average risk, moderate risk, and high risk.

SCREENING & SURVEILLANCE RECOMMENDATIONS

1. Average Risk

An average-risk individual is defined as an asymptomatic person without a personal or family history of colonic polyps or cancer. The majority of the general population is considered to be at average risk for CRC. Given that age is the strongest risk factor for the development of CRC and adenomatous polyps, men and women at average risk should be offered screening beginning at age 50 years.

Available screening options for average-risk individuals fall into two broad categories: (1) tests that primarily detect CRC, and (2) those that detect precancerous adenomatous polyps and CRC (Table 22–1). Tests that primarily detect cancer are fecal tests, including guaiac-based and immunochemical occult blood tests, and fecal DNA tests. These modalities provide limited opportunity for prevention because detection of premalignant adenomatous polyps is most often incidental. Tests that detect both adenomatous polyps and cancer include flexible sigmoidoscopy (FS), colonoscopy, double-contrast barium enema (DCBE), and computed tomography colonography (CTC). Because prevention is the primary goal of CRC screening, recent guidelines from the American Cancer Society, the U.S. Multisociety Task Force on Colorectal Cancer, and the American College of Radiology strongly encourage clinicians to offer those tests

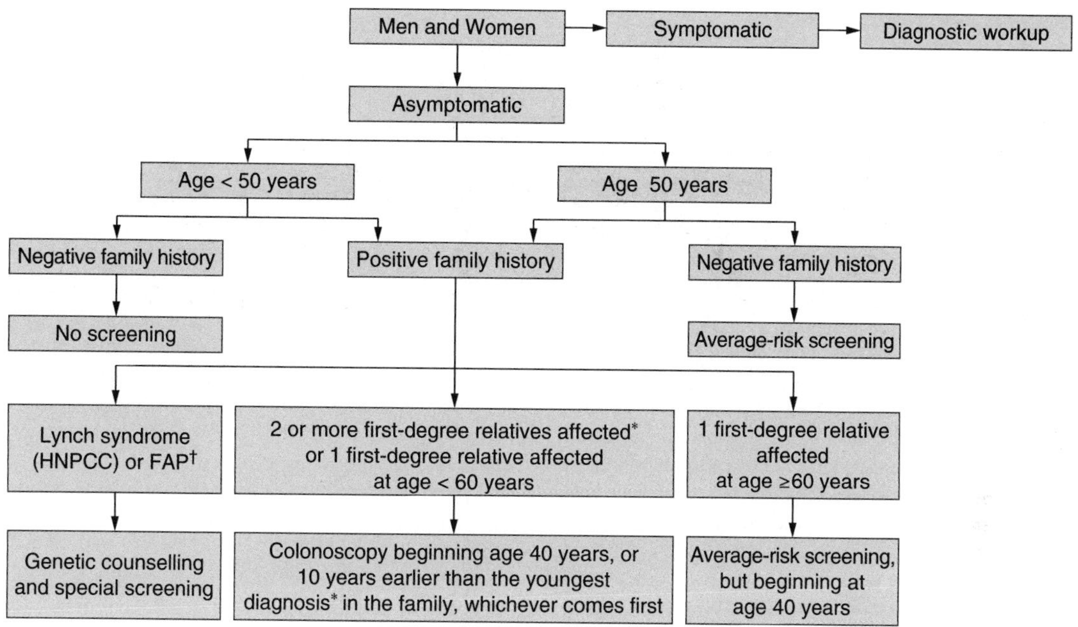

▲ **Figure 22–2.** Algorithm for colorectal cancer screening. FAP, familial adenomatous polyposis; HNPCC, hereditary non-polyposis colorectal cancer; *, either colorectal cancer or adenomatous polyps; †, see text. (Adapted, with permission, from Winawer SJ, Fletcher R, Rex D, et al. Gastrointestinal Consortium Panel. Colorectal cancer screening and surveillance: clinical guidelines and rational–update based on new evidence. *Gastroenterology.* 2003;124:546.)

that are designed to detect both early cancer and adenomatous polyps if resources are available and if patients are willing to undergo an invasive examination. Noninvasive tests must be repeated at regular intervals to be effective, are less likely to prevent CRC than invasive examinations, and, if abnormal, require colonoscopy.

Table 22–1. Testing options for asymptomatic adults aged 50 years and older.

Tests that detect adenomatous polyps and CRC
Flexible sigmoidoscopy
Colonoscopy
Double-contrast barium enema
Computed tomography colonography
Tests that primarily detect CRC
Guaiac-based fecal occult blood testing
Fecal immunochemical tests
Stool DNA

CRC, colorectal cancer.
Adapted, with permission, from Levin B, Lieberman DA, McFarland B, et al. Screening and surveillance for the early detection of colorectal cancer and adenomatous polyps, 2008: a joint guideline from the American Cancer Society, the US Multisociety Task Force on Colorectal Cancer, and the American College of Radiology. *Gastroenterology.* 2008;134:1570–1595.

Nevertheless, health care providers are encouraged to focus on increasing screening rates through periodic use of any of the recommended modalities. Providers should present their patients with information about the advantages and disadvantages associated with the multiple available screening tests. In turn, patients have the opportunity to select how they wish to be screened based on their own preferences. The rationale for such an approach is that it may increase the likelihood that screening will occur. Even though the currently available screening techniques are not equal in effectiveness, cost, or associated risks, they all have been demonstrated to be cost-effective compared with no screening at all.

Levin B, Lieberman DA, McFarland B, et al. Screening and surveillance for the early detection of colorectal cancer and adenomatous polyps, 2008: a joint guideline from the American Cancer Society, the US Multisociety Task Force on Colorectal Cancer, and the American College of Radiology. *Gastroenterology.* 2008;134:1570–1595. [PMID: 18384785]

Smith RA, Mettlin CJ, Davis KJ, et al. American Cancer Society guidelines for the early detection of cancer. *CA Cancer J Clin.* 2000;50:34–49. [PMID: 10735014]

Winawer S, Fletcher R, Rex D, et al. Gastrointestinal Consortium Panel. Colorectal cancer screening and surveillance: clinical guidelines and rationale–update based on new evidence. *Gastroenterology.* 2003;124:544–560. [PMID: 12557258]

2. Moderate Risk

Individuals with a personal or family history of adenomatous polyps or CRC are considered to be at intermediate risk for the development of CRC. For these patients, colonoscopy is the recommended screening method. Other conventional screening modalities are not typically recommended in this setting.

A. Personal History of Adenomatous Polyps

Certain characteristics of colorectal adenomas at baseline colonoscopy are the basis for decisions about surveillance intervals. Existing data from the National Polyp Study (NPS), a pooled analysis of chemoprevention studies, as well as observational cohort studies support the presence of the following predictors for the development of future advanced adenomas or cancers: (1) three or more adenomas, (2) adenoma size greater than 1 cm, and (3) adenoma with villous features or high-grade dysplasia. A proximal location of adenomas (ascending colon or cecum) may also predict metachronous advanced adenomas, but this has not been well studied to date. In addition, there is a general consensus among many of the studies that individuals with adenomas with lesser findings (eg, one or two subcentimeter adenomas without high-grade dysplasia or villous features) are at lower risk for subsequent advanced adenomas.

By stratifying patients into "lower risk" and "higher risk" groups for future advanced adenoma development based on findings from initial colonoscopy, the NPS has provided evidence-based guidelines for surveillance of postpolypectomy patients. In a randomized comparison of surveillance intervals after colonoscopic removal of newly diagnosed adenomatous polyps, there was no better detection of advanced lesions with surveillance examination 1 year after the initial colonoscopy than with follow-up examination in 3 years. The inference made is that the rate of developing metachronous adenomas with advanced pathology is slow; therefore, the current recommendation for patients with a personal history of three or more adenomas, adenomas of 1 cm or larger, or adenomas with villous or high-grade dysplasia, or any combination of these findings, is surveillance colonoscopy in 3 years. In addition, patients who have more than 10 adenomas removed during one endoscopic examination should be examined in a shorter time interval (<3 years) based on clinical judgment and should be considered for the possibility of an underlying familial syndrome. The standard of care for a sessile, malignant polyp removed by piecemeal fashion is 3–6 months after the initial endoscopic resection.

However, it is important to acknowledge that the timing of surveillance colonoscopy in patients with a history of adenomatous polyps is still evolving. The existing studies assessing subsequent risk for neoplasia after colonoscopic polypectomy have only followed patients for 5–6 years. This is a significant limitation and has led to the current projection that patients without advanced adenomas can wait at least 5 years (and perhaps up to 10 years) for repeat colonoscopy. As a result, further studies are needed to evaluate this "low risk" group in order to confirm the strategy of these intervals.

Winawer SJ, Zauber AG, Ho MN, et al. Prevention of colorectal cancer by colonoscopic polypectomy. The National Polyp Study Workgroup. *N Engl J Med.* 1993;329:1977–1981. [PMID: 8247072]

B. Personal History of CRC

Individuals with a history of CRC are at risk for recurrent cancer and metachronous neoplasms and require endoscopic surveillance after surgical resection. Anywhere from 2% to 7% of patients with CRC have one or more synchronous cancers in the colon or rectum at the time of initial diagnosis; it is therefore important to perform a complete colonoscopy in the preoperative period. In cases where an obstructing colonic or rectal lesion is detected, CTC or DBCE should be considered perioperatively, and a complete colonoscopy should be performed 3–6 months after surgery. Once the colon is cleared of any synchronous lesions, a postoperative surveillance colonoscopy is recommended at 1 year to evaluate for any metachronous lesions. If the examination at 1 year is normal, the subsequent examination should be at 3 years. If this examination is also found to be normal, surveillance colonoscopy can thereafter be extended to every 5 years. Neither individual randomized controlled clinical trials of intense surveillance with annual colonoscopy nor a meta-analysis of these trials for the purpose of detecting recurrent disease have shown a survival benefit for patients with CRC.

Colonoscopy at 1 year after surgical resection is recommended based on reports of a high incidence of metachronous second cancers noted within the first 2 years after resection. Among an aggregate of studies reporting results from post-cancer surveillance colonoscopy, there was an incidence rate of 0.7% metachronous cancers in the first 2 years after resection of the initial primary cancer. This estimate is consistent with data from a tumor registry review in Nebraska, which calculated an annual incidence of 0.35% per year for metachronous cancers. This is considered sufficient information to warrant a colonoscopy at 1 year following surgical resection. However, this should not diminish the importance of a high-quality colonoscopic examination in the perioperative period to exclude synchronous neoplasms.

In addition, it is important to distinguish between rectal and colon cancer because of the differing rates of local recurrence. The recurrence of colon cancer at the anastomotic site occurs in only 2–4% of patients. In contrast, local recurrence rates of rectal cancer when patients have undergone a low anterior resection can be 10 or more times higher. High recurrence rates of rectal cancer are partly a function of surgical technique. Local recurrence rates of cancer can be reduced by using a surgical technique called mesorectal excision, as well as administering radiation and chemotherapy in the neoadjuvant, preoperative setting to patients with locally advanced disease. However, because reported local recurrence rates for rectal cancer across the United States are generally higher than those achieved in case series using total mesorectal excision, there is a rationale for performing periodic examinations of the rectum. Although effectiveness has not been proven, performing proctoscopy at 6-month intervals for the first 2 years after surgical resection can be considered for the detection of a surgically curable recurrence of the original rectal cancer.

When colon or rectal cancer is endoscopically resected and surgery is not needed, follow-up endoscopic examination to inspect the biopsy site within 1 year is a reasonable strategy. As previously noted, colonoscopy is considered the test of choice for the detection of metachronous neoplasms in patients with a history of CRC. CTC has not been evaluated adequately in this setting, and guaiac-based fecal occult blood testing (FOBT) has been considered to have a very low positive predictive value after colonoscopic evaluation.

Rex D, Kahi CJ, Levin B, et al. Guidelines for colonoscopy surveillance after cancer resection: a consensus update by the American Cancer Society and the US Multisociety Task Force on Colorectal Cancer. *Gastroenterology.* 2006;130:1865–1871. [PMID: 16737948]

Winawer SJ, Zauber AG, Fletcher RH, et al. Guidelines for colonoscopy surveillance after polypectomy: a consensus update by the US Multisociety Task Force on Colorectal Cancer and the American Cancer Society. *Gastroenterology.* 2006;130: 1872–1885. [PMID: 16697750]

C. Family History of CRC or Adenomatous Polyps

An individual's risk of CRC is increased if there is a family history of adenomatous polyps or CRC. The screening recommendations based on familial risk are derived largely from the observed colon cancer risk in relatives of patients with CRC and adenomas diagnosed before age 60 years (Table 22–2).

Table 22–2. Relative risk of colorectal cancer (CRC) based on family history.[a]

	Relative Risk
One FDR with CRC	2–3
One FDR with CRC diagnosed at ≤50 years	3–4
Two FDR with CRC	3–4
Two SDR with CRC	2–3
One FDR with an adenomatous polyp	2

FDR, first-degree relative; SDR, second-degree relative.
[a]Compares individuals at moderate risk with individuals at average risk based on family history.

Data from a meta-analysis of 27 studies assessing familial risk of CRC and adenomatous polyps report a relative risk of CRC when a first-degree relative was affected with CRC to be 2.4. The relative risk for CRC if the first-degree relative had an adenomatous polyp was 1.9, with age effects similar to those observed for cancer. In addition, if more than one relative was affected and CRC was diagnosed before age 45 years, the relative risk increased to 4.2 and diminished to 2.2 and 1.8 for ages 45–59 years and older than 59 years, respectively. Therefore, familial risk needs to be readily identified and should prompt the early initiation of screening with colonoscopy.

At present, the U.S. Multisociety Task Force on Colorectal Cancer recommends that for patients who report one first-degree relative under 60 years or two first-degree relatives of any age with adenomatous polyps or CRC, screening colonoscopy should start at age 40 years or 10 years younger than the earliest diagnosis of an affected relative (whichever one comes first) and continue every 5 years (Figure 22–2, Table 22–3). Screening should start at the same time for those patients with a single first-degree relative with CRC or adenomas diagnosed after age 60 years, but surveillance should be performed as for average-risk individuals. The rationale for starting screening at age 40 years is that the incidence of CRC in these patients resembles the risk in persons with no family history but precedes it by approximately 10 years. In addition, a patient reporting a second- or third-degree relative with adenomatous polyps or CRC does not confer additional risk, and therefore, average-risk screening recommendations are sufficient.

However, it is important to note that no studies to date have reported a reduction in mortality in persons with a family history of CRC or adenomatous polyps who undergo screening. Therefore, the present screening recommendations are considered provisional, and further evidence is needed to better delineate the CRC risk in relatives with adenomatous polyps or CRC as this information continues to evolve.

Johns LE, Houlston, RS. A systematic review and meta-analysis of familial colorectal cancer risk. *Am J Gastroenterol.* 2001;96:2992–3003. [PMID: 11693338]

3. High Risk

For individuals with a hereditary CRC syndrome, such as familial adenomatous polyposis (FAP) or Lynch syndrome (also known as hereditary nonpolyposis colorectal cancer, or HNPCC), genetic counseling and special screening protocols are recommended (Table 22–4). Readily identifying these individuals is of great importance given the known benefit of intensive endoscopic surveillance and prophylactic surgery on morbidity and mortality. Recognizing these syndromes also has an impact on referral for predictive genetic testing, wherein identifying gene carriers improves the efficiency of cancer surveillance and helps identify family members who

Table 22–3. Colorectal cancer screening recommendations.

Assessed Risk	Age to Initiate	Test	Interval
Average	50 y	Colonoscopy FOBT sDNA FS FOBT + FS DCBE[a]	10 y or Annually or Uncertain[b] 5 y or Annual FOBT + FS every 5 y or 5 y
		CTC	5 y[c]
Moderate			
Personal history of:			
CRC		Colonoscopy	3 y; if normal, every 5 y
1-2 adenomas <1 cm		Colonoscopy	5 y
≥3 adenomas <1 cm[d]		Colonoscopy	3 y
Adenoma ≥1 cm		Colonoscopy	3 y
Adenoma with villous features		Colonoscopy	3 y
Adenomas with HGD complete resection		Colonoscopy	3 y
Piecemeal resection		Colonoscopy	3-6 mo[e]; 3 y
Normal exam with prior adenoma resected		Colonoscopy	5 y
Family history:			
FDR with CRC/adenoma <60 y	40 y	Colonoscopy	5 y
FDR with CRC/adenoma >60 y	40 y	Colonoscopy	10 y
≥2 FDR with CRC/adenoma[f]	40 y	Colonoscopy	5 y
High			
FAP[g]			
Classic	10-12 y	Flexible Sigmoidoscopy	Annually[h]
Attenuated	10 y earlier than first polyps/CRC diagnosed in family	Colonoscopy	1-2 y
Lynch syndrome[g]	20-25 years	Colonoscopy	1-2 y
Crohn or ulcerative colitis			
Pancolitis	8 y after diagnosis	Colonoscopy	1-2 y
Left-sided colitis	15 y after diagnosis	Colonoscopy	1-2 y

CRC, colorectal cancer; CTC, computed tomography colonography; DCBE, double-contrast barium enema; FAP, familial adenomatous polyposis; FDR, first-degree relative; FOBT, fecal occult blood test; FS, flexible sigmoidoscopy; HGD, high-grade dysplasia; sDNA, stool DNA.
[a]DCBE not endorsed by all professional gastroenterologic societies.
[b]Interval for sDNA testing to be determined.
[c]Interval for CTC testing to be determined.
[d]If ≥10 adenomatous polyps consider attenuated FAP diagnosis.
[e]Short interval of 3–6 months to ensure complete resection.
[f]Consider clinical diagnosis of Lynch syndrome.
[g]Consider germline genetic testing.
[h]If polyposis has not formed by age 35 y, extend colonoscopy to every 3 y.
Reproduced, with permission, from Levin B, Lieberman DA, McFarland B, et al. Screening and surveillance for the early detection of colorectal cancer and adenomatous polyps, 2008. *Gastroenterology*. 2008;134(5):26.

require intense management versus those who can receive the standard of care. Additionally, for patients with long-standing inflammatory bowel disease such as Crohn disease or ulcerative colitis, surveillance colonoscopy with systematic biopsies should be performed because the risk of CRC is increased in both conditions.

Engelsgjerd M, Farraye FA, Odze RD. Polypectomy may be adequate treatment for adenoma-like dysplastic lesions in chronic ulcerative colitis. *Gastroenterology*. 1999;117:1288–1294. [PMID: 10579969]

Jo WS, Chung DC. Genetics of hereditary colorectal cancer. *Semin Oncol*. 2005;32:11–23. [PMID: 15726502]

Table 22–4. Colon cancer screening recommendations for people with familial or inherited risk.

Familial Risk Category	Screening Recommendation
First-degree relative affected with colorectal cancer or an adenomatous polyp at age ≥60 y, or 2 second-degree relatives affected with colorectal cancer	Same as average risk but starting at age 40 y
Two or more first-degree relatives[a] with colon cancer, or a single first-degree relative with colon cancer or adenomatous polyps diagnosed at an age <60 y	Colonoscopy every 5 y, beginning at age 40 y or 10 y younger than the earliest diagnosis in the family, whichever comes first
One second-degree or any third-degree relative[b,c] with colorectal cancer	Same as average risk

[a]First-degree relatives include patients, siblings, and children.
[b]Second-degree relatives include grandparents, aunts, and uncles.
[c]Third-degree relatives include great-grandparents and cousins.
Adapted, with permission, from Winawer SJ, Fletcher R, Rex D, et al. Gastrointestinal Consortium Panel. Colorectal cancer screening and surveillance: clinical guidelines and rational-update based on new evidence. *Gastroenterology.* 2003;124:544–560.

Ullman T, Croog V, Harpaz N, et al. Progression of flat low-grade dysplasia to advanced neoplasia in patients with ulcerative colitis. *Gastroenterology.* 2003;125:1311–1319. [PMID: 14598247]

A. Familial Adenomatous Polyposis

FAP is an autosomal-dominant syndrome that is associated with mutations in the *adenomatous polyposis coli* (*APC*) gene. Affected individuals classically develop hundreds to thousands of colorectal adenomas at a young age and have a risk of CRC approaching 100% in the absence of prophylactic colectomy. Annual sigmoidoscopy beginning at age 10–12 years is recommended for persons who have a genetic diagnosis or are at risk of having FAP in order to determine if they are expressing the genetic abnormality. Germline genetic testing should be recommended in persons with an FAP phenotype and should be performed after patients (or parents of children) undergo genetic counseling. If a mutation is identified, other family members can be tested to discern the presence or absence of the same mutation with nearly 100% accuracy. Sigmoidoscopy is performed until affected individuals develop polyps, at which point total colectomy is recommended. Family members who test negative for the gene mutation are considered to be at average risk for CRC.

Although classic FAP can be readily identified, a subset of patients has a less obvious phenotype. Patients with 10 or more cumulative colorectal adenomas but less than 100, are at risk for a variant of FAP called attenuated FAP (AFAP). In these patients, the age of onset of adenomas is approximately 10 years later than with classic FAP. AFAP also has an autosomal-dominant mode of inheritance and, as with classic FAP, is due to mutations in the *APC* gene. The true incidence and frequency of AFAP is unknown; however, it may account for up to 10% of adenomatous polyposis families and should be considered in individuals with multiple adenomas. Colonoscopy should be used as the initial screening modality in patients suspected of having AFAP, and the age to initiate screening is based on the age of polyp expression or CRC diagnosis in the family. It is reasonable to start colonoscopic screening 10 years earlier than the earliest age of known polyp or CRC diagnosis in the family. As with FAP, germline genetic testing should be considered in persons presenting with the AFAP phenotype.

B. Lynch Syndrome

Lynch syndrome exhibits an autosomal-dominant pattern of inheritance, and affected individuals have a near 80% lifetime risk of developing CRC without intervention. It is predominantly caused by a mutation in one of four of the DNA mismatch repair genes, *MSH2, MLH1, MSH6,* and *PMS2.* There are several classification systems for the clinical diagnosis of Lynch syndrome, ranging from the most exclusive Amsterdam Classification to the most inclusive revised Bethesda Guidelines, all relying on personal or family medical histories, or both. Commercial genetic testing is currently available for individuals suspected of having Lynch syndrome, as well as for family members who are at risk for the condition.

Once Lynch syndrome has been diagnosed based on clinical criteria or through genetic testing, an intensive screening program should be instituted. Screening colonoscopy should be recommended every 1–2 years beginning at age 20 and 25 years, or 10 years prior to the youngest CRC case diagnosed within the family (whichever occurs earlier). Annual colonoscopy is recommended after the age of 40 years.

C. Inflammatory Bowel Disease

The CRC risk is similar in both Crohn colitis and ulcerative colitis, with an estimated lifetime risk of 15–40%. Although direct supporting evidence is lacking, an expert consensus panel has recommended colonoscopic surveillance every 1–2 years for patients after 8 years of pancolitis or after 15 years in those with limited left-sided colitis. If the extent of disease cannot be accurately assessed, patients should undergo surveillance colonoscopy beginning within 8–10 years of disease.

To consider surveillance effective, an extensive biopsy protocol during colonoscopy should be followed. Experts have recommended that biopsy specimens should be taken every 10 cm in all four quadrants and that additional biopsy specimens should be obtained from anastomotic sites (in cases of previous colonic resections), strictures, and mass lesions (other than pseudopolyps). Polyps should be removed by polypectomy, with biopsies of the adjacent flat mucosa to discern if dysplasia is present. In cases where high-grade dysplasia or multifocal dysplasia is found in flat mucosa, patients should be advised to undergo colectomy. However, it is imperative that pathologic confirmation be made by an experienced pathologist in the field of dysplasia in inflammatory bowel disease prior to colectomy. Controversy exists in cases of low-grade dysplasia in flat mucosa and the need for colectomy. If low-grade dysplasia is unifocal or found in areas of inflammation, attempts should first be made to treat the active colitis.

In cases where a mass lesion is detected, it is important to differentiate whether it is a dysplasia-associated lesion or mass (DALM) or if it has arisen from a sporadic adenoma. A DALM is a dysplastic lesion believed to have arisen because of the cancer potential of the colitis and is an indication for colectomy. In contrast, a lesion arising from a sporadic adenoma should be removed in its entirety during colonoscopy and does not require colectomy unless the lesion is not amenable to complete endoscopic resection. Differentiating between DALMs and adenoma-related masses can be difficult and requires extensive review of the endoscopic appearance, histologic findings, presence of dysplasia in the surrounding flat mucosa, patient's age, and duration of disease.

The decision for colectomy should be individualized in cases of long-standing disease based on a number of concomitant factors known to increase CRC risk. These factors include extensive active colitis or ongoing colitis-related symptoms, personal history of primary sclerosing cholangitis, a family history of CRC, age, and life expectancy.

4. Special Considerations: Hyperplastic & Serrated Polyps

At this time, there is no evidence to suggest that patients with a few small, distally located hyperplastic polyps are at increased risk for CRC. Therefore, such patients should undergo surveillance for CRC similar to that of average-risk individuals.

However, there has been recent literature to suggest that all hyperplastic polyps are not histologically similar and that some variants of hyperplastic polyps may evolve into a unique type of adenoma, called a serrated adenoma. Serrated adenomas resemble hyperplastic polyps with dysplasia and have been linked to the development of sporadic adenocarcinoma with microsatellite instability. Polyps of this type are often large, sessile, and located in the proximal colon. It is important for these neoplastic lesions to be completely removed, and surveillance should follow those recommendations as for typical adenomas.

In addition, there is a recently described syndrome of "hyperplastic polyposis." The following features have been used to define this entity: (1) at least five histologically diagnosed hyperplastic polyps proximal to the sigmoid colon, of which two are greater than 1 cm in diameter, or (2) any number of hyperplastic polyps occurring proximal to the sigmoid colon in an individual who has a first-degree relative with hyperplastic polyposis, or (3) more than 30 hyperplastic polyps of any size distributed throughout the colon. A limited number of studies have suggested an increased risk of CRC in such individuals, although the magnitude of risk has not been determined. A case series of 15 patients fulfilling the preceding criteria did not find any CRC cases within 3 years of follow-up colonoscopic evaluation. Presently, the optimal management for these patients is unclear and requires further study.

Fernández A, Samowitz W, DiSario JA, et al. Phenotypic characteristics and risk of cancer development in hyperplastic polyposis: case series and literature review. *Am J Gastroenterol.* 2004;99:2012–2018. [PMID: 15447765]

Leggett BA, Devereaux B, Biden K, et al. Hyperplastic polyposis: association with colorectal cancer. *Am J Surg Pathol.* 2001;25: 177–184. [PMID: 11176066]

Terdiman JP, McQuaid KR. Surveillance guidelines should be updated to recognize the importance of serrated polyps. *Gastroenterology.* 2010;139:1444–1447. [PMID: 20875785]

SCREENING MODALITIES

1. Fecal Occult Blood Testing

Fecal occult blood testing (FOBT) is the most widely available screening modality for CRC. It is a noninvasive and inexpensive test used to detect the presence of occult blood in the stool of asymptomatic persons. FOBT is recommended as an annual examination and is the only screening test for which randomized controlled trials have shown a reduction in CRC-related incidence by 33%, and mortality benefits ranging from 15% to 20%. This is due primarily to the detection of CRC at an earlier stage or the detection of adenomatous polyps with the ability to remove these lesions during colonoscopy. It is important to emphasize that positive FOBT results need to be appropriately followed by complete visualization of the colon through colonoscopy.

Two types of FOBT exist: the standard guaiac test and the newer immunochemical tests (see following section). Guaiac-based FOBT is widely used for CRC screening worldwide. It is performed by the patient at home and requires the collection of six stool samples from three consecutive stools. The guaiac test detects blood by reacting with peroxidase activity of the heme portion of hemoglobin. As a result, false-positive tests may result from the ingestion of red meat or peroxidase-containing foods, and patients must be made aware of the necessary dietary restrictions. In addition, rehydration results in an increase in the false-positive rate, and should not be performed.

When FOBT is used alone as a screening strategy, it is only 33–50% sensitive in one-time testing, with some improvement if testing is repeated every 1–2 years. The specificity of FOBT as a screening modality is high (estimated to be >95%). False-positive results can stem from other causes of gastrointestinal blood loss or other substances in the stool that might cause a positive guaiac reaction. Patients are instructed to avoid ingestion of vitamin C, iron, aspirin, and nonsteroidal anti-inflammatory medications for 3 days prior to performing FOBT as these substances may interfere with the accuracy of the test. False-negative results can also occur because colorectal lesions can bleed intermittently and blood may not always be present throughout the entire stool. Therefore, a single test of a stool sample during digital rectal examination is not an adequate substitute for FOBT. There is an estimated fivefold decrease in sensitivity with a single test performed during digital rectal examination, and a higher yield has been noted when sampling three consecutive stools for occult blood.

The disadvantages related to FOBT are that current tests fail to detect many polyps and some cancers. Also, individuals who have a false-positive result will subsequently need to undergo the discomfort, cost, and risk of colonoscopy without benefit. In addition, there is reported evidence of low referral rates for colonoscopy following an abnormal FOBT. In the United States, one survey found that up to 30% of patients with positive FOBT did not receive a recommendation for colonoscopy.

In evaluating an FOBT screening program, it is also important to measure programmatic adherence and performance over time. FOBT is ineffective if patients have one test but do not return for repeat testing or do not have colonoscopy for positive tests. When FOBT is recommended, patients must be informed that the test needs to be repeated every 1–2 years if negative and that colonoscopy should be performed if the test is positive.

Collins JF, Lieberman DA, Durbin TE, et al. Accuracy of screening for fecal occult blood on a single stool sample obtained by digital rectal exam: a comparison with recommended sampling practice. *Ann Intern Med.* 2005;142:81–85. [PMID: 15657155]

Leiberman DA, Weiss DG. Veteran's Affairs Cooperative Study Group 380. One-time screening for colorectal cancer with combined fecal occult blood testing and examination of the distal colon. *N Engl J Med.* 2001;345:555–560. [PMID: 11529208]

Mandel JS, Bond JH, Church TR, et al. Reducing mortality from colorectal cancer by screening for fecal occult blood. Minnesota Colon Cancer Control Study. *N Engl J Med.* 1993;328:1365–1371. [PMID: 8474513]

Mandel JS, Church TR, Bond JH, et al. The effect of fecal occult blood screening on the incidence of colorectal cancer. *N Engl J Med.* 2000;343:1603–1607. [PMID: 11096167]

2. Fecal Immunochemical Testing

Newer fecal immunochemical testing (FIT) reacts with antibodies that are specific for the globin portion of the human hemoglobin molecule, and therefore, special dietary restrictions to avoid false-positive tests are not needed. Multiple studies have reported that FIT has a better sensitivity and specificity than guaiac-based FOBT for the detection of CRC, in which the sensitivity ranged from 47.1% to 69% and the specificity ranged from 88.2% to 97.1%; in contrast, the sensitivity of the guaiac test for detecting CRC has been reported to be as low as 37.1%, with a specificity of 86.7%. In addition, the effectiveness of FIT for CRC screening has been shown using "gold standard" endoscopy results for FIT-negative patients. However, given the wide variability in detecting advanced adenomas, which ranges from 25% to 72% based on the type of immunochemical test used, FIT should be best regarded as an early cancer detection test.

There are a number of unresolved issues regarding FIT that require further study, including the number of samples needed for optimal sensitivity and specificity, the cutoff point for hemoglobin detection that provides the best sensitivity and specificity, how to ensure hemoglobin stability in collected samples, and whether there is an advantage of a quantitative FIT over a qualitative test.

Allison JE, Sakoda LC, Levine TR, et al. Screening for colorectal neoplasms with new fecal occult blood tests: update on performance characteristics. *J Natl Cancer Inst.* 2007;99:1462–1490. [PMID: 17895475]

Hundt S, Haug U, Brenner H, et al. Comparative evaluation of immunochemical fecal occult blood tests for colorectal adenoma detection. *Ann Intern Med.* 2009;150:162–169. [PMID: 19189905]

Morikawa T, Kato J, Yamaji Y, et al. A comparison of the immunochemical fecal occult blood test and total colonoscopy in the asymptomatic population. *Gastroenterology.* 2005;129:422–428. [PMID: 16083699]

Park D, Ryu S, Kim Y, et al. Comparison of guaiac-based and quantitative immunochemical fecal occult blood testing in a population at average-risk undergoing colorectal cancer screening. *Am J Gastroenterol.* 2010;105:2017–2025. [PMID: 20502450]

Van Rossum LG, Van Rijn AF, Laheij RJ, et al. Random comparison of guaiac and fecal immunochemical blood tests for colorectal cancer in a screening population. *Gastroenterology.* 2008;135:82–90. [PMID: 18482589]

3. Flexible Sigmoidoscopy

FS allows for direct visualization of the distal third of the colon, ideally from the rectum to the splenic flexure. Several retrospective, case-controlled studies have suggested that FS is associated with a near 70% reduction in cancer mortality resulting from tumors found within reach of the endoscope. A recent multicenter, randomized controlled trial conducted in the United Kingdom found that in an 11-year follow-up of individuals undergoing a single FS for screening initiated between the ages of 55 and 64 years, FS substantially reduced colorectal cancer incidence and mortality by 33% and 43%, respectively. The reduction noted in this study was less compared to results from prior case-control studies and is attributed to the dominance of screen-detected prevalent cancers within the first 4 years of follow-up. The magnitude of reduction in cumulative incidence will likely increase as this cohort is followed in order to examine the important issue of the long-term effects of one screening examination using FS.

FS is recommended every 5 years for average-risk individuals. A 5-year interval is supported by a number of case-controlled trials and cohort studies reporting a mortality benefit from the use of FS up to 10 years from the last screening examination. In a recent study comparing the appropriateness of a 5-year interval with a 3-year interval, there was no difference in the detection of advanced neoplasia (0.9% vs 1.1% at 3- and 5-year intervals, respectively). In addition, multiple studies have reported a low frequency of low-risk and advanced lesions, and there is some speculation that an even longer interval than 5 years between sigmoidoscopic examinations may be reasonable.

To improve the use of FS as a screening modality, certain clinical factors as well as endoscopic findings noted on FS have been considered important predictors of proximal colonic disease. These predictors include the presence of multiple adenomas, any adenoma with villous histology or dysplasia, age older than 65 years, male gender, and a family history of CRC. Hyperplastic polyps detected on FS are not associated with increased adenoma detection elsewhere in the colon.

The advantages cited for FS are that it is inexpensive, requires no sedation, involves a simple bowel preparation, and can be performed by primary care physicians and non-physicians, including physician assistants and nurse practitioners. In addition, the risk of perforation is lower than that associated with colonoscopy. However, the interval for surveillance is shorter with FS than with colonoscopy because FS is a less sensitive examination. This reduced sensitivity is partly due to variable operator experience as a wider variation in adenoma detection rates among different providers has been reported. In addition, the preparation used for colon cleansing prior to FS may be less than optimal, and discomfort in a nonsedated patient may interfere with the completeness of the examination.

Currently, any adenomatous polyp found on FS warrants complete colonic visualization by colonoscopy to exclude the presence of proximal lesions. Such a strategy has been associated with an increase in the adenoma detection rate to approximately 70%. However, these findings highlight a major drawback of FS in that it can miss anywhere from 30% to 65% of advanced neoplasia located proximally. This may be a particular concern for the use of FS in older patients and women, in whom higher rates of proximal neoplasia have been reported. Recent data comparing the performance of FS to colonoscopy in the detection of advanced neoplasia reported that in subjects between 55 and 59 years of age, the incremental benefit of colonoscopy over FS was very small and statistically insignificant. In contrast, for patients 60 years of age or older, the detection rate for colonoscopy was significantly higher than for FS (odds ratio [OR], 2.00; 95% confidence interval, 1.30–3.09). When considered with prior studies, these results suggest that FS could achieve high detection of advanced neoplasia in patients younger than 60 years and is less effective with those older than 60 years. Future studies to determine a combined approach for CRC screening using FS for persons in the sixth decade followed by colonoscopy once subjects are older than 60 years may provide valuable information that may, in turn, conserve colonoscopy resources.

A second shortcoming of FS is that patient compliance with this screening modality is poor. Only 15–30% of eligible persons regularly undergo FS, and this invariably limits its utility in CRC prevention. Lastly, low rates of referral for colonoscopy and colonoscopy completion have been reported, and better measures to assure appropriate follow-up are warranted.

Atkins WS, Edwards R, Kralj-Hans I, et al. Once-only flexible sigmoidoscopy screening in prevention of colorectal cancer: a multicentre randomised controlled trial. *Lancet.* 2010;375: 1624–1633. [PMID: 20430429]

Burke CA, Elder K, Lopez R. Screening for colorectal cancer with flexible sigmoidoscopy: Is a 5-yr interval appropriate? A comparison of the detection of neoplasia 3 yr versus 5 yr after a normal examination. *Am J Gastroenterol.* 2006;101:1329–1332. [PMID: 16771957]

Newcomb PA, Norfleet RG, Storer BE, et al. Screening sigmoidoscopy and colorectal cancer mortality. *J Natl Cancer Inst.* 1992;84:1572–1575. [PMID: 1404450]

Selby JV, Friedman GD, Quesenberry CP, et al. A case-control study of screening sigmoidoscopy and mortality from colorectal cancer. *N Engl J Med.* 1992;326:653–657. [PMID: 1736103]

4. Combined Fecal Occult Blood Test & Flexible Sigmoidoscopy

This combined approach couples annual FOBT with sigmoidoscopy every 5 years. The occult blood test is performed prior to sigmoidoscopy given that a positive result would warrant colonoscopy. A single nonrandomized study reported a 43% reduction in CRC-related deaths by this combination approach compared with sigmoidoscopy alone. In addition, this approach can increase the yield of adenoma detection fourfold compared with FOBT alone. However, more recent studies have not shown such promising results. The addition of FOBT to FS was estimated to increase the adenoma detection rate only from 70% to 75%. Additionally, undergoing a single FS and FOBT was not as effective as biennial FOBT in detecting CRC over a 16-year period. The lack of improvement in detection noted in this long-term case-control study may have been due to lack of compliance associated with undergoing FS.

Rasmussen M, Fenger C, Kronborg O. Diagnostic yield in biennial Hemoccult-II screening program compared to a once-only screening with flexible sigmoidoscopy and Hemoccult-II. *Scand J Gastroenterol.* 2003;38:114–118. [PMID: 12608473]

Segnan N, Senore NC, Andreoni B, et al. Comparing attendance and detection rate of colonoscopy to sigmoidoscopy and FIT for colorectal cancer screening. *Gastroenterology.* 2007;132: 2304–2312. [PMID: 17570205]

5. Double-Contrast Barium Enema

DCBE has not been studied as a screening test for CRC in prospective randomized trials, and several recent studies have highlighted some major limitations associated with the examination. In a number of comparative studies of colonoscopy and DCBE in screening and surveillance populations, DCBE detected only 45–48% of polyps greater than 1 cm. In a large prospective study, the sensitivity for detecting CRC was 83% for DCBE versus 95% for colonoscopy. Overall, DCBE is less sensitive than colonoscopy for the detection of large lesions, and this examination has fallen out of favor among certain endorsing societies as a primary screening strategy in average-risk persons.

However, given the number of deterrents to the widespread use of colonoscopy, DBCE is considered an alternative CRC screening modality to be performed every 5 years. It is a radiologic examination of the colon that requires a cathartic preparation similar to that given prior to colonoscopy and requires the instillation of barium and air to define the contour of the colon. It is included as a screening option because it can evaluate the entire colon, is generally widely available, and has a low risk of serious adverse events. However, this procedure does not allow for polyp removal or biopsy of cancer if detected. Artifact, such as stool appearing as polyps, is common and causes many false-positive tests. All patients with an abnormal barium examination need to undergo colonoscopy.

Although DCBE is an acceptable option for CRC screening in average-risk adults, its utilization has declined over the past few years. This has had an impact on radiology training programs as fewer trainees are able to acquire the necessary skills needed to perform the labor-intensive procedure properly due to the low volume of DBCE studies being requested. This trend is expected to continue as increased efforts are being made to provide training related to computed tomography colonography (CTC) among radiologists.

Winawer SJ, Stewart ET, Zauber AG, et al. A comparison of colonoscopy and double-contrast barium enema for surveillance after polypectomy. National Polyp Study Work Group. *N Engl J Med.* 2000;342:1766–1772. [PMID: 10852998]

6. Colonoscopy

Colonoscopy is considered by many to be the gold standard for CRC screening. Despite the lack of evidence from large-scale randomized trials of screening colonoscopy, the procedure has been shown in cohort studies to decrease the expected incidence of CRC through the removal of adenomatous polyps. The NPS demonstrated that the removal of adenomas led to the decreased incidence of CRC and that colonoscopy was the only single test that could provide screening, diagnosis, and treatment. In the NPS, a group of patients who underwent colonoscopy with clearing of colonic adenomas yielded a 76–90% reduction in CRC compared with reference populations. Given the potential benefits of colonoscopy, multiple gastroenterologic professional societies have recommended colonoscopy as the preferred modality among the menu of screening options.

However, several published studies have addressed the shortcomings of colonoscopy as currently practiced. Indirect evidence from several studies has questioned the accuracy of colonoscopy. In one study, an audit of CRC cases revealed that 5% of subjects with CRC had undergone screening colonoscopy within 3 years of diagnosis. Chemoprevention studies that included follow-up colonoscopy as a means of measuring the efficacy of chemoprevention on polyp recurrence have also demonstrated a higher rate of developing interval cancers (1.7–2.2 cases per 1000 person-years) when compared with NPS results (0.6 cases per 1000 person-years). Recent studies have also questioned the effectiveness of colonoscopy in detecting proximal colonic neoplasia. A large population-based, case-control study using administrative claims data from Ontario, Canada, evaluated the association between colonoscopy and CRC deaths and found that colonoscopy was associated with lower CRC mortality rates. However, the association was primarily limited to deaths from cancer developing in the left side of the colon. The question arises whether CRCs in the proximal colon are more frequently missed due to the variability in endoscopists' performance of colonoscopy or because these lesions have different biologic features compared to distal CRCs, including higher rates of microsatellite instability and the CpG island methylator phenotype (CIMP), and perhaps these biologic features are overrepresented in interval CRCs. The performance of colonoscopy has been shown to vary by endoscopist, and the individual endoscopist may be a powerful predictor of adenomatous polyps detected during colonoscopy. To improve the accuracy (sensitivity) of colonoscopy for adenoma and CRC detection and standardize its performance among endoscopists, the U.S. Multisociety Task Force on Colorectal Cancer and the American Society for Gastrointestinal Endoscopy/American College of Gastroenterology Taskforce on Quality in Endoscopy have proposed several measurable factors of routine colonoscopy to serve as quality indicators. They include appropriate cecal intubation rates, adequate colonic cleansing with minimal fecal residue, a minimum withdrawal time from the cecum of 6 minutes, and goal adenoma detection rates for men and women undergoing screening colonoscopy. It is anticipated that the accuracy of colonoscopy can be increased through quality improvement initiatives for enhanced performance of colonoscopy.

Additionally, characteristics of the baseline colonoscopy are an important predictor for subsequent neoplasia. A population-based, case-control study using administrative claims data reports that the risk of developing CRC in patients following a negative result from a colonoscopy performed in the usual clinical practice is at most 60–70% of the risk of developing CRC in the general population and the duration of decreased CRC risk persists for more than

10 years. A recent prospective study examining the incidence of advanced neoplasia within 5.5 years of screening colonoscopy revealed a strong association between baseline colonoscopy results and the rate of serious incident lesions detected during the surveillance period. It has been shown that the baseline colonoscopy is the most beneficial in that it is responsible for the major benefit of polypectomy and that subsequent examinations may not add significant benefit except in people at high risk for future advanced adenomas. This supports the need to ensure that the baseline colonoscopy is of the highest quality in order to best detect adenomas.

Even though colonoscopy can fail to detect lesions, it is still considered the most sensitive of the screening methods. The advantages of this approach, in addition to the diagnosis and treatment of a lesion in a single session, include a long interval of "protection" in the setting of polypectomy and improved patient satisfaction due to the use of intravenous conscious sedation. However, colonoscopy involves greater cost and risk than other screening modalities. Serious complications associated with colonoscopy include bleeding and perforation and, while extremely rare, these occur at higher rates than with other screening options.

Colonoscopy may be the "preferred" screening modality for some, but it is important to emphasize that the evidence for its efficacy is indirect and that there are no randomized controlled trials demonstrating the superiority of colonoscopy to other screening modalities. In addition, no direct information indicates that a program of periodic colonoscopic surveillance leads to a reduction in CRC incidence or mortality in average-risk individuals. Large-scale, comparative effectiveness studies are needed to determine the impact of colonoscopy and other screening modalities on CRC incidence and mortality and whether the burden of right-sided neoplasia can be affected by colonoscopy to justify the associated extra cost and morbidity.

Barclay RL, Vicari JJ, Doughty AS, et al. Colonoscopic withdrawal times and adenoma detection during screening colonoscopy. *N Engl J Med.* 2006;355:2533–2541. [PMID: 17167136]

Baxter NN, Goldwassser MA, Paszat LF, et al. Association of colonoscopy and death from colorectal cancer. *Ann Intern Med.* 2009;150:1–8. [PMID: 19075198]

Chen SC, Rex DK. Endoscopist can be more powerful than age and male gender in predicting adenoma detection at colonoscopy. *Am J Gastroenterol.* 2007;102:856–861. [PMID: 17222317]

Imperiale TF, Wagner DR, Lin CY, et al. Risk of advanced proximal neoplasms in asymptomatic adults according to the distal colorectal findings. *N Engl J Med.* 2000;343:169–174. [PMID: 10900275]

Lieberman DA, Weiss DG, Bond JH, et al. Use of colonoscopy to screen asymptomatic adults for colorectal cancer. Veterans Affairs Cooperative Study Group 380. *New Engl J Med.* 2000;343:162–168. [PMID: 10900274]

Lieberman DA, Weiss DG, Harford WV, et al. Five-year colon surveillance after screening colonoscopy. *Gastroenterology.* 2007; 133:1077–1085. [PMID: 17698067]

Rex D. Maximizing detection of adenomas and cancers during colonoscopy. *Am J Gastroenterol.* 2006;101:2866–2877. [PMID: 17227527]

Rex DK, Cutler CS, Lemmel GT, et al. Colonoscopy miss rates of adenomas determined by back-to-back colonoscopies. *Gastroenterology.* 1997;112:24–28. [PMID: 8978338]

Robertson DJ, Greenberg ER, Beach M, et al. Colorectal cancer in patients under close colonoscopic surveillance. *Gastroenterology.* 2005;129:34–41. [PMID: 16012932]

Singh H, Turner D, Xue L, et al. Risk of developing colorectal cancer following a negative colonoscopy examination. *JAMA.* 2006;295:2366–2373. [PMID: 16720822]

NOVEL SCREENING MODALITIES

Noninvasive procedures to screen for CRC have been promoted as possible ways to increase compliance with CRC screening strategies. The 2008 consensus guidelines from the American Cancer Society, the U.S. Multisociety Task Force on Colorectal Cancer, and the American College of Radiology include CTC and fecal DNA in the testing options for CRC screening in asymptomatic, average-risk adults aged 50 years and older.

Bromer MQ, Weinberg DS. Screening for colorectal cancer–now and the near future. *Semin Oncol.* 2005;32:3–10. [PMID: 15726501]

Levin B, Lieberman DA, McFarland B, et al. Screening and surveillance for the early detection of colorectal cancer and adenomatous polyps, 2008: a joint guideline from the American Cancer Society, the US Multi Society Task Force on Colorectal Cancer, and the American College of Radiology. *Gastroenterology.* 2008;134:1570–1595. [PMID: 18384785]

1. Computed Tomographic Colonography

Over the last decade, CTC (or virtual colonoscopy) was introduced as a possible alternative noninvasive test for the examination of the colon. It provides a two- and three-dimensional image of the colon using computer programming to combine data from multiple helical CT scans. CTC requires a colon preparation similar to that used for conventional colonoscopy and involves air insufflation through a rectal tube to distend the colon to enhance imaging. After the examination, a radiologist examines the scans; if an abnormality is noted, patients should undergo colonoscopy.

Results from early studies assessing the accuracy of CTC have found it to be comparable to that of conventional colonoscopy for the detection of polyps greater than 1 cm, with a high sensitivity and specificity of 94% and 96%, respectively. Similar results have not been reproduced in other studies, and subsequent sensitivities of approximately 50% have been reported. The inconsistency in the examination's efficacy is likely related to the selection bias of the population studied, because most studies on CTC have been performed in patient populations at increased risk for colorectal neoplasia and more likely to have occult disease.

In addition, only highly trained radiologists were involved in interpreting the results of CTC in the majority of these studies. Therefore, the generalizability of the results of these studies remains unclear.

The technology related to CTC has improved over the past few years, and several screening trials using advanced CTC techniques have demonstrated its favorable performance. In a meta-analysis reviewing the cumulative published CTC performance data (including high-risk and screening cohorts), the pooled sensitivity and specificity for large (>1 cm) polyps were 85–93% and 97%, respectively, and for small polyps (6–9 mm) were 70–86% and 86–93%, respectively. The overall sensitivity for invasive CRC was comparable to that of conventional colonoscopy (96%).

There are a number of limitations and unresolved issues related to CTC. The examination is not widely available and most often is performed at large, academic centers, usually in the setting of research studies. In addition, the false-positive rate is estimated to be about 15% and is related to retained stool mistaken for polyps, diverticular disease that limits colon distensibility, and thickened colonic folds mistaken for lesions. CTC is also not therapeutic, as polyps cannot be removed and masses cannot be sampled for tissue diagnosis during the procedure. Lastly, it is estimated that 27% of patients undergoing CTC will have an incidental finding warranting further diagnostic evaluation. This may increase patient anxiety and lead to an increase in medical costs, because most incidental findings are expected to be benign. It is estimated that there is only a 2% potential clinical benefit to an extensive evaluation for incidental findings noted on CTC.

Although there is variability regarding the optimal manner in which to perform the examination, as well as inconsistent radiology training and competency, the available data supporting its efficacy have rendered CTC an acceptable option for CRC screening in average-risk adults age 50 years and older. However, the interval for repeat examinations is uncertain, and future studies are warranted to determine the appropriate surveillance interval following an initial negative CTC. Presently, there is consensus that all patients with one or more polyps greater than 1 cm or three or more polyps greater than 6 mm should be referred for conventional colonoscopy. The management of patients with fewer than three polyps or polyps of 6–9 mm remains controversial. Research studies using CTC surveillance to evaluate the natural history of polyps in this size range are ongoing. At this time, a reasonable approach for patients with 6–9 mm polyps identified by CTC is to offer therapeutic colonoscopy. There is also a need for multidisciplinary consensus regarding the management of polyps smaller than 6 mm.

For effective implementation of CRC screening, the evolving technology needs to be standardized along with the reporting of findings. Additional information is also needed regarding the safety profile of CTC, including the radiation dose effects for computed tomography examinations for average-risk CRC screening. At present, experts have differing opinions about when and how CTC should be used. The U.S. Preventive Services Task Force decided that there was not enough evidence to recommend it as an option for CRC screening, and the federal Medicare program does not currently provide reimbursement for the use of CTC for routine screening. In a recent cost-effectiveness analysis of CRC screening tests that have been recommended by the U.S. Preventive Services Task Force, American Cancer Society, U.S. Multisociety Task Force on Colorectal Cancer, American College of Radiology, and American College of Gastroenterology, CTC was not deemed a cost-effective strategy for average-risk CRC screening.

Chin M, Mendelson R, Edwards J, et al. Computed tomographic colonography: prevalence, nature, and clinical significance of extracolonic findings in a community screening program. *Am J Gastroenterol.* 2005;100:2271–2276. [PMID: 16393234]

Cotton PB, Durkalski VL, Pineau BC, et al. Computed tomographic colonography (virtual colonoscopy): a multicenter comparison with standard colonoscopy for detection of colorectal neoplasia. *JAMA.* 2004;291:1713–1719. [PMID: 15082698]

Halligan S, Altman DG, Taylor SA, et al. CTC in the detection of colorectal polyps and cancer: systematic review, meta-analysis, and proposed minimum data set for study level reporting. *Radiology.* 2005;237:893–904. [PMID: 16304111]

Johnson CD, Harmsen WS, Wilson LA, et al. Comparison of the relative sensitivity of CT colonography and double-contrast barium enema for screen detection of colorectal polyps. *Clin Gastroenterol Hepatol.* 2004;2:314–321. [PMID: 15067626]

Johnson CD, Harmsen WS, Wilson LA, et al. Prospective blinded evaluation of computed tomographic colonography for screen detection of colorectal polyps. *Gastroenterology.* 2003;125: 311–319. [PMID: 12891530]

Mulhall BP, Veerappan GR, Jackson JL. Metaanalysis: computed tomographic colonography. *Ann Intern Med* 2005;142:635–650. [PMID: 15838071]

Pickhardt PJ, Choi JR, Hwand I, et al. Computed tomographic virtual colonoscopy to screen for colorectal neoplasia in asymptomatic adults. *N Eng J Med.* 2003;349:2191–2200. [PMID: 1465426]

Rockey DC, Paulson E, Niedzwiecki D, et al. Analysis of air contrast barium enema, computed tomographic colonography, and colonoscopy: prospective comparison. *Lancet.* 2005;354:305–311. [PMID: 15664225]

Zauber AG. Cost-effectiveness of colonoscopy. *Gastrointest Endosc Clin N Am.* 2010;20:751–770.

2. Fecal DNA Testing

Testing to detect genetic abnormalities (somatic mutations) in fecal samples has been proposed as a potential screening test for CRC screening. Colorectal epithelial cells are shed in stool, and stable DNA can be extracted from stool and amplified using polymerase chain reaction (PCR). This process allows for the detection of mutations in several genes, including *K-ras*, *APC*, *BAT-26*, and *tp53*.

Early data from a small cohort revealed a sensitivity of 91% for cancer, sensitivity of 82% for adenomatous polyps greater than 1 cm, and specificity of over 90% for either, whereas other studies have reported sensitivities between 52% and 91% for cancer and 27% and 82% for adenomatous polyps. Variable results assessing the sensitivity of fecal DNA testing have been related in large part to the test's evolving technology. In a recent study using a newer fecal DNA test aimed at detecting methylated genes in CRC (Cologuard), 1187 specimens from patients with and without colorectal neoplasia were blindly evaluated, and the accuracy of the fecal DNA test was 85.3% for CRC and 63.8% for adenomas greater than 1 cm, with a specificity of 88% for either. CRCs and adenomas were detected equally well in the proximal and distal colon with higher accuracy for early-stage CRCs and adenomas of increasing size. In addition, the sensitivity of the test was unaffected by patient gender, age, or race.

As fecal DNA testing is able to identify the majority of CRC cases and large adenomas, there has been an expert consensus to include this modality as an acceptable option for CRC screening in average-risk adults. However, newer fecal DNA tests (whether they involve technologic advances made on existing tests or are new variants) warrant careful evaluation in future studies evaluating screening cohorts. At this time, the interval for routine screening between normal examinations is unclear, and there is no societal recommendations given the insufficient data. Nevertheless, the effectiveness of any screening program utilizing fecal DNA will depend on quality, adherence, and cost, as well as the sensitivity and specificity of the test.

Ahlquist DA, Skoletsky JE, Boynton KA, et al. Colorectal cancer screening by detection of altered human DNA in stool: feasibility of a multitarget assay panel. *Gastroenterology.* 2000;119: 1219–1227. [PMID: 11054379]

Alquist DA. American Association for Cancer Research Colorectal Cancer Conference: Biology to Therapy. Philadelphia, PA, October 27–30, 2010.

Imperiale TF, Ransohoff DF, Itzkowitz SH, et al. Fecal DNA versus fecal occult blood for colorectal cancer screening in an average risk population. *N Engl J Med.* 2004;351:2704–2714. [PMID: 15616205]

Itzkowitz SH, Jandorf L, Brand R, et al. Improved fecal DNA test for colorectal cancer screening. *Clin Gastroenterol Hepatol.* 2007;5:111–117. [PMID: 17161655]

Osborn NK, Ahlquist DA. Stool screening for colorectal cancer: molecular approaches. *Gastroenterology.* 2005;128:192–206. [PMID: 15633136]

SUMMARY OF RECOMMENDATIONS

CRC is a preventable cancer. The appropriate identification of individuals at risk dictates the necessary screening and surveillance approach and plays an important role in decreasing CRC mortality. There are several acceptable options presently available for CRC screening, and they provide the means to improving screening compliance. Although a number of randomized trials provide evidence to support the use of FOBT and FS for CRC screening, high-quality colonoscopy is considered the current gold standard given its ability to detect and remove adenomatous polyps, which in turn decreases CRC incidence and related mortality.

Hereditary Gastrointestinal Cancer Syndromes

23

Elena M. Stoffel, MD, MPH
Sapna Syngal, MD, MPH

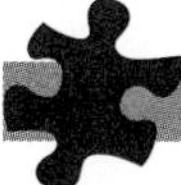

ESSENTIALS OF DIAGNOSIS

- ▶ Approximately 3–5% of colorectal cancers are caused by inherited gene mutations associated with hereditary nonpolyposis colorectal cancer (Lynch syndrome) or familial adenomatous polyposis.
- ▶ Genetic testing is clinically available for several hereditary gastrointestinal cancer syndromes and can be used to guide cancer screening recommendations.

General Considerations

The majority of cases of gastrointestinal cancer are believed to be sporadic events; however, inherited factors play a role in development of some tumors, with an estimated 5% being attributable to a single gene mutation. Hereditary gastrointestinal cancer syndromes convey a markedly increased risk for developing cancer and require specific strategies for diagnosis and management.

Identification of hereditary gastrointestinal cancer syndromes requires a thorough evaluation of patients' personal and family history of cancer. Clinical genetic testing can be useful in confirming the diagnosis of certain hereditary cancer syndromes and guiding cancer screening for family members. Tables 23–1 and 23–2 summarize clinical characteristics and cancer screening recommendations for the hereditary gastrointestinal cancer syndromes discussed in detail in this chapter.

American Society of Clinical Oncology. American Society of Clinical Oncology policy statement update: genetic testing for cancer susceptibility. *J Clin Oncol.* 2003;21:2397–2406. [PMID: 12692171]

Giardiello FM, Brensinger JD, Petersen GM. AGA technical review on hereditary colorectal cancer and genetic testing. *Gastroenterology.* 2001;121:198–213. [PMID: 11438509]

HEREDITARY COLORECTAL CANCER SYNDROMES

Colorectal cancer (CRC) is the most common gastrointestinal malignancy, with more than 150,000 cases diagnosed each year in the United States. Although most CRC patients do not have a striking family history of CRC, approximately 30% report having one or more family members with a diagnosis of CRC. The lifetime risk of developing CRC is approximately 5% for the average American; however, individuals who have a first-degree relative with CRC have a twofold higher risk for developing colorectal neoplasia compared with individuals who have no family history of CRC. For individuals with numerous relatives with CRC, the cancer risk may be markedly higher; those who have inherited mutations in genes involved in mismatch repair or tumor suppression have a lifetime risk of CRC of 70–100% in the absence of medical intervention.

Identification of patients at risk for hereditary CRC syndromes relies on careful family history evaluation, because many individuals may not demonstrate a characteristic phenotype. Cancer risk stratification for every patient should involve eliciting a family history of cancers, including type of cancer and age of onset as well as family history of colorectal adenomas. Individuals whose family history includes multiple individuals with cancer, individuals diagnosed with two or more primary cancers, or with tumors diagnosed at young ages, should undergo more extensive family history evaluation of first-, second-, and third-degree relatives to determine whether there is evidence of an autosomal-dominant or autosomal-recessive pattern of inheritance.

1. Lynch Syndrome (Hereditary Nonpolyposis Colorectal Cancer)

Lynch syndrome, also known as hereditary nonpolyposis colorectal cancer (HNPCC), is the most common hereditary CRC syndrome and is estimated to account for 3–5% of CRC cases. This syndrome was first described by Dr Henry Lynch in families in which multiple cases of CRC were diagnosed

Table 23–1. Clinical characteristics of hereditary gastrointestinal cancer syndromes.

Syndrome	Clinical Features	Gene(s)	Genetic Testing Available
Lynch syndrome (HNPCC)	High risk for colorectal and extracolonic cancers (endometrial, ovarian, urinary tract, sebaceous skin tumors) Young ages at cancer diagnosis Accelerated adenoma–carcinoma sequence CRC tumors demonstrate microsatellite instability	DNA mismatch repair (MMR) genes (*MLH1, MSH2, MSH6, PMS2, TACSTD1/EPCAM*)	Yes
Familial adenomatous polyposis (FAP)	100s–1000s colorectal adenomas appearing in second or third decade CRC risk 100% if colon is not removed Increased risk for duodenal and ampullary adenocarcinoma Risk of desmoid tumors	Tumor-suppressor gene *APC* or base excision repair gene *MYH* biallelic mutations (autosomal recessive)	Yes
Attenuated adenomatous polyposis/multiple adenomas	10–100 colorectal adenomas High risk for CRC ± Upper gastrointestinal adenomas	Tumor-suppressor gene *APC* Base excision repair gene *MYH* (autosomal recessive)	Yes[a]
Peutz-Jeghers syndrome (PJS)	Hamartomatous polyps in GI tract (symptoms of bleeding, intussusception) Pigmented lesions on lips Increased risk for breast cancer, pancreatic cancer, sex cord tumors	Tumor-suppressor gene *STK-11*	Yes[a]
Juvenile polyposis	5+ juvenile polyps in GI tract Family history of GI cancers Increased risk for CRC and other GI cancers Associated with congenital cardiac abnormalities	Tumor-suppressor genes *SMAD-4, BMPR1A*	Yes[a]
Cowden syndrome	Hamartomatous polyps Increased risk for breast and thyroid cancers Macrocephaly	*PTEN*	Yes[a]
Hereditary diffuse gastric cancer	Diffuse infiltrative adenocarcinoma of the stomach (linitis plastica) Increased risk for breast cancer	Tumor suppressor gene *e-cadherin/CDH1*	Yes[a]
Familial pancreatic cancer	3 or more family members with pancreatic cancer May be present as part of other hereditary cancer syndromes, eg, breast/ovarian cancer (HBOC), melanoma (FAMMM), or colorectal/gynecologic cancers (Lynch syndrome)	*BRCA1/2* (HBOC) *P16* (FAMMM) MMR genes (Lynch syndrome) *PRSS1, SPINK1* (hereditary pancreatitis)	Yes[a]

CRC, colorectal cancer; FAMMM, familiar atypical multiple mole melanoma; GI, gastrointestinal; HBOC, hereditary breast/ovarian cancer; HNPCC, hereditary nonpolyposis colorectal cancer.
[a]Genetic testing has limited sensitivity, with mutations detected in 50–70% of affected individuals.

at young ages. The original Lynch syndrome families were identified as having three or more cases of CRC with at least one diagnosed before age 50 years, as described by the Amsterdam criteria; however, additional studies have demonstrated that the cancer spectrum in these families includes other cancers, such as gastrointestinal, gynecologic, urinary tract, and sebaceous neoplasms of the skin. Because as many as 50% of families with Lynch syndrome do not meet the classic Amsterdam criteria, clinical diagnostic criteria have been expanded and modified to improve diagnostic sensitivity. As outlined by the Revised Bethesda guidelines (Table 23–3), Lynch syndrome should be suspected in families that have multiple relatives affected with CRC or related extracolonic tumors, or both, and in individuals who are diagnosed with CRC at a young age, have synchronous or metachronous colorectal cancers, or develop multiple Lynch-associated tumors. Figure 23–1 shows a pedigree of a family fulfilling criteria for Lynch syndrome.

Table 23–2. Cancer screening recommendations for hereditary gastrointestinal cancer syndromes.

Syndrome	Screening Test	Frequency
Lynch syndrome/HNPCC	1. Colonoscopy	1. Every 1–2 y beginning at age 20–25 y
	2. Urine cytology	2. Annually
	3. Transvaginal ultrasound ± endometrial biopsy (women)	3. Annually, beginning between ages 30 and 35 y
Familial adenomatous polyposis (FAP)	1. Sigmoidoscopy or colonoscopy until polyps are too numerous to remove, then surgical colectomy	1. Annually, beginning at age 10–12 y
	2. Upper endoscopy	2. Every 1–3 y, depending on polyp burden, beginning when colonic polyps develop
	3. Thyroid ultrasound	3. Every 1–3 y
Attenuated adenomatous polyposis/multiple adenomas	1. Colonoscopy	1. Frequency varies, depending on number of polyps
	2. Upper endoscopy	2. At diagnosis of colonic polyps
Peutz-Jeghers syndrome (PJS)	1. Upper endoscopy	1. Every 2–3 y, beginning at age 8 y
	2. Small bowel imaging (capsule endoscopy, CT or MRI enterography, or barium study)	2. Every 2–3 y, beginning at age 8 y
	3. Colonoscopy	3. Every 2–3 y, beginning at age 18 y
	4. Imaging of pancreas (endoscopic ultrasound vs secretin-enhanced MRI/MRCP)	4. Every 1–2 y, beginning at age 30–35 y
	5. Mammogram or MRI of breasts	5. Annually, starting at age 25 y (women)
	6. Transvaginal ultrasound and CA-125	6. Annually, starting at age 25 y (women)
	7. Testicular ultrasound	7. Every 2 y until age 12 y (males)
Juvenile polyposis	1. Colonoscopy	1. Every 3 y beginning at puberty, then annually after polyps develop
	2. Upper endoscopy	2. Every 1–3 y after polyps develop
Cowden syndrome	1. Colonoscopy	1. Consider baseline exam between age 35 and 50 y, with intervals depending on polyp burden
	2. Thyroid ultrasound	2. Annually beginning at age 18 y
	3. Mammogram ± breast MRI	3. Annually for women beginning at age 30–35 y
	4. Transvaginal ultrasound	4. Annually for postmenopausal women
	5. Urinalysis	5. Consider annually
Hereditary diffuse gastric cancer	1. Upper endoscopy starting in teens, until prophylactic gastrectomy	1. Evidence suggests endoscopy has poor sensitivity, gastrectomy favored after age 30 y
	2. Mammogram ± breast MRI	2. Annually beginning at age 25 y
Familial pancreatic cancer	1. Various: endoscopic ultrasound, CT, or MRI may be considered	1. To be determined

CT, computed tomography; HNPCC, hereditary nonpolyposis colorectal cancer; MRCP, magnetic resonance cholangiopancreatography; MRI, magnetic resonance imaging.

Clinical Findings

A. Physical Features

CRC is usually the predominant cancer in most families with Lynch syndrome. Initial studies suggested that the mean age of onset of CRC is 44 years; however, there is wide variation in ages of diagnosis among families. Although colonic tumors in Lynch syndrome are often right-sided, many patients develop tumors in the left colon and rectum. Synchronous or metachronous tumors are common, and any individual diagnosed with two primary colon cancers warrants evaluation for Lynch syndrome. Although Lynch

Table 23–3. Revised Bethesda guidelines for Lynch syndrome (HNPCC).[a]

1. Colorectal cancer diagnosed at age <50 y
2. Synchronous or metachronous colorectal or other HNPCC-associated tumors[b] regardless of age
3. Colorectal cancer diagnosed at age <60 y with histologic findings of infiltrating lymphocytes, Crohn-like lymphocytic reaction, mucinous/signet ring differentiation, or medullary growth pattern
4. Colorectal cancer in >1 first-degree relative(s) with an HNPCC-related tumor[b], with one of the cancers being diagnosed at age <50 y
5. Colorectal cancer diagnosed in >2 first- or second- degree relatives with HNPCC-related tumors[b], regardless of age

HNPCC, hereditary nonpolyposis colorectal cancer.
[a]Any one criterion met.
[b]HNPCC-related tumors include the following cancers: colorectal, endometrial/uterine, ovarian, urinary tract, gastric, and sebaceous skin neoplasms.
Data from Umar A, Boland CR, Terdiman JP, et al. Revised Bethesda Guidelines for hereditary nonpolyposis colorectal cancer (Lynch syndrome) and microsatellite instability. *J Natl Cancer Inst.* 2004; 96:261–268.

syndrome is also referred to as hereditary nonpolyposis colorectal cancer (HNPCC), most of the colorectal cancers do appear to arise from adenomatous polyps, although these polyps may be few in number and are often small and flat. The colorectal adenoma–carcinoma sequence appears to be accelerated in Lynch syndrome, and there are many reports of tumors arising within 3 years of a normal colonoscopy.

Endometrial (uterine) cancer is the second most common cancer described in Lynch syndrome families; however in some families, cases of endometrial cancers may outnumber CRC. Women with Lynch syndrome have a 40–60% lifetime risk for developing this malignancy, which is an unusual cancer in the general population. The lifetime risks for developing other Lynch-associated cancers, such as urinary tract cancers, ovarian cancer, and other gastrointestinal cancers (stomach, pancreas, small intestine), are also increased for individuals with Lynch syndrome and are estimated to be between 10% and 20%. Brain tumors (eg, glioblastomas and astrocytomas) have been described in the Turcot syndrome variant of Lynch syndrome. Cutaneous sebaceous adenomas and sebaceous carcinomas are rare skin tumors seen in the Muir-Torre variant, and it is currently recommended that any individual affected with sebaceous neoplasms of the skin undergo evaluation for Lynch syndrome regardless of his or her family history.

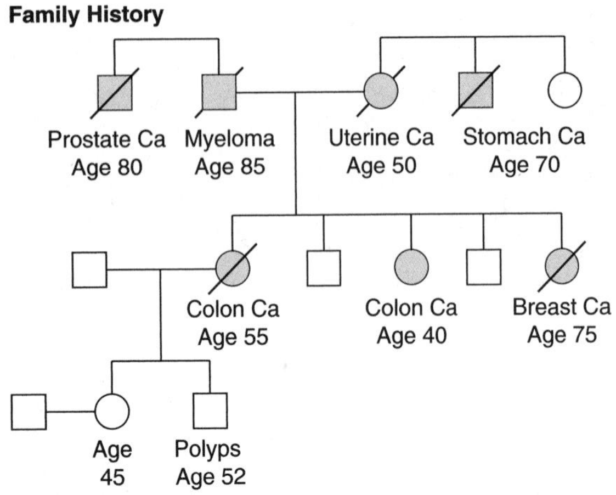

▲ **Figure 23–1.** Pedigree of a family fulfilling modified Amsterdam criteria for hereditary nonpolyposis colorectal cancer (HNPCC)/Lynch syndrome. Ca, cancer.

B. Genetic Features

The increased predisposition to developing cancer in Lynch syndrome is the result of autosomal dominantly inherited mutations in genes involved in DNA mismatch repair (MMR). Mutations in the genes *hMLH1* and *hMSH2* account for more than 80% of the identified MMR alterations in Lynch syndrome families. Mutations in the MMR gene *hMSH6* have been identified in approximately 10% of Lynch syndrome families, and in *hPMS2* in rare families. Recently, mutations in the gene *TACSTD1/EPCAM*, which regulates expression of *MSH2*, were also found in families with a clinical diagnosis of Lynch syndrome.

The protein products of MMR genes are involved in identifying and repairing errors that arise during DNA replication. In the setting of defective MMR gene function, these errors accumulate in segments of DNA containing repeated sequences known as microsatellites. DNA errors that disrupt the function of genes involved in growth regulation can lead to the development of tumors. Approximately 85% of the colorectal tumors in Lynch syndrome patients demonstrate high levels of microsatellite instability (MSI), a characteristic of defective MMR gene function. Immunohistochemical (IHC) analysis of colorectal tumors for expression of MMR proteins MLH1, MSH2, MSH6, and PMS2 frequently reveals loss of staining of the protein corresponding to the gene with the mutation. Since only 15% of sporadic CRC tumors demonstrate high levels of MSI, testing CRC tumors for MSI and loss of expression of MMR proteins has been proposed as a strategy to identify which patients with CRC may be at risk for Lynch syndrome and require additional genetic evaluation.

Approximately 60% of families that meet classic Amsterdam criteria are found to have germline mutations in one of the DNA MMR genes. However, recent studies suggest that classic Amsterdam families with multiple CRC diagnoses may include not only Lynch syndrome families, but also families with familial colorectal cancer syndrome X, which may or may not have a genetic basis. Like Lynch syndrome, familial colorectal cancer syndrome X families have multiple cases of CRC with apparent autosomal-dominant pattern of inheritance; however, the colorectal tumors in patients with familial colorectal cancer syndrome X do not have features of microsatellite instability and affected individuals do not appear to be at increased risk for extracolonic cancers.

Management

The high lifetime risk of colorectal and other extracolonic cancers, the accelerated progression of adenomas to adenocarcinomas, and the young age of onset of colorectal neoplasia require specialized strategies for cancer prevention.

A. Colorectal Cancer Screening

Individuals who are at risk for Lynch syndrome should begin having colonoscopies at age 20–25 years, with repeat examinations every 1–2 years. The need for a shorter interval between examinations became evident from European studies that demonstrated a reduction in CRC mortality for individuals who had colonoscopies every 3 years; however, cancers were still detected during that screening interval. The endoscopist should be vigilant for small or flat lesions, which may be associated with higher malignant potential in Lynch syndrome patients than in the general population.

B. Endometrial Cancer Screening

Expert panels recommend that women at risk for Lynch syndrome undergo endometrial cancer screening with annual transvaginal ultrasound and endometrial biopsy beginning at ages 30–35 years. At present, there are no data to support the efficacy of this endometrial cancer screening regimen, and women who have completed childbearing should be counseled to consider prophylactic hysterectomy as a more definitive measure to reduce their cancer risk.

C. Screening for Other Cancers

Although the risk for other extracolonic cancers is increased in Lynch syndrome, there is insufficient evidence to definitively recommend screening for many of these other cancers. For urinary tract cancer screening, annual urine cytology has been suggested, although its efficacy remains unproven. Screening for ovarian cancer includes transvaginal ultrasound and checking serum CA-125 levels once yearly. Screening for gastric cancer and small intestinal cancer using upper endoscopy has been proposed by some experts, but this has not been recommended by most guidelines. Individuals with Lynch syndrome from families with Muir-Torre should have annual dermatologic examinations to screen for cutaneous sebaceous neoplasms. At present, there are no recommendations for screening for pancreatic or central nervous system tumors because of lack of evidence to support effectiveness.

D. Prophylactic Surgery

Prophylactic surgery may be considered as an alternative to annual screening. For the majority of Lynch syndrome patients who are compliant with surveillance colonoscopies, prophylactic surgery is unlikely to be necessary. For some who develop early or multiple adenomas or for whom colonoscopy is painful, prophylactic colectomy may be a good option. Individuals who develop colorectal neoplasms requiring surgical resection should be offered extended resections with a subtotal colectomy, because the risk for metachronous lesions is high. Individuals who have had subtotal colectomies can then have screening of their residual colonic mucosa via flexible sigmoidoscopy.

Women should be counseled that there is limited evidence regarding the impact of endometrial screening on morbidity and mortality from endometrial cancer and that prophylactic hysterectomy and oophorectomy may be the most effective way to reduce risks of gynecologic cancer.

E. Clinical Genetic Testing

Genetic testing for MMR gene mutations associated with Lynch syndrome is increasingly available in clinical settings and provides the opportunity to confirm the diagnosis of Lynch syndrome in a family and to test other individuals in order to stratify their cancer risk. Cost-effectiveness models support the use of genetic testing for cancer risk stratification in Lynch syndrome families, and evidence suggests knowledge of a gene mutation makes individuals more likely to comply with the intense cancer screening required for cancer prevention.

The most efficient strategy for genetic testing is to begin the genetic evaluation with an individual who has a cancer diagnosis. For individuals who meet the Bethesda guidelines, the American Gastroenterological Association recommends starting with evaluation of a CRC tumor specimen to test for features of MSI and loss of staining for MLH1, MSH2, MSH6, and PMS2 proteins by IHC. As 85% of the CRC tumors in MMR gene mutation carriers demonstrate high levels of MSI or abnormal staining for MMR proteins, this pathologic testing can serve as a prescreening method to select individuals who should undergo germline testing for MMR mutations. Many clinical centers are implementing routine MSI and IHC testing for CRC tumors diagnosed in individuals age 50 and under, and some are advocating for universal tumor testing, as many cases of Lynch-associated CRC are diagnosed at age greater than 50 years.

For individuals who do not have a cancer diagnosis or tumor specimens available for MSI or IHC testing, there are risk assessment models that can be used to estimate the likelihood of Lynch syndrome. The PREMM(1,2,6) model is a Web-based clinical prediction rule that uses data from patients' personal and family history to estimate the probability that an individual carries a mutation in the *MLH1*, *MSH2*, or *MSH6* genes (available from the Dana-Farber

Cancer Institute, at http://www.dfci.org/premm). Individuals whose personal and family history produces a PREMM(1,2,6) model score of more than 5% should undergo additional evaluation for Lynch syndrome. MMRpro is another Web-based model that can be used for similar risk stratification to identify individuals who would benefit from genetic testing.

Clinical genetic testing for germline mutations in the *MLH1, MSH2, MSH6, PMS2,* and *TACSTD1/EPCAM* genes can be performed on DNA extracted from a peripheral blood sample. Clinical laboratories specializing in genetic testing perform full gene sequencing and southern blot analysis for large genomic deletions in these MMR genes. If testing reveals a pathogenic mutation in any of these genes, then testing is considered informative, and mutation-specific testing can be offered (at greatly reduced cost) to other family members to determine who has and has not inherited the genetic predisposition to cancer. If testing in a cancer-affected individual fails to reveal a mutation, then genetic testing is considered uninformative, and a clinical determination must be made about whether the suspicion for Lynch syndrome is sufficiently high to recommend Lynch syndrome cancer surveillance to all members of the family.

The high cost of commercial genetic testing for germline MMR mutations (at present, approximately U.S. $2000–$3000), the difficulties in interpreting and explaining uninformative genetic testing results, and the complexities of family dynamics are challenges in clinical genetic testing. The American Society for Clinical Oncology recommends that genetic testing be performed in conjunction with genetic counseling, which is available through most major cancer centers.

Aarnio M, Mecklin JP, Aaltonen LA, et al. Life-time risk of different cancers in hereditary non-polyposis colorectal cancer (HNPCC) syndrome. *Int J Cancer.* 1995;64:430–433. [PMID: 8550246]

Chen S, Wang W, Lee S, et al. Prediction of germline mutations and cancer risk in the Lynch syndrome. *JAMA.* 2006;296:1479–1487. [PMID: 17003396]

Dinh TA, Rosner BI, Atwood JC, et al. Health benefits and cost-effectiveness of primary genetic screening for Lynch syndrome in the general population. *Cancer Prev Res.* 2011;4:9–22. [PMID: 21088223]

Kastrinos F, Steyerberg E, Mercado R, et al. The PREMM(1,2,6) model predicts risk of germline MLH1, MSH2, and MSH6 germline mutations based on cancer history. *Gastroenterology.* 2011;140:73–81. [PMID: 20727894]

Lindor NM, Petersen GM, Hadley DW, et al. Recommendations for the care of individuals with an inherited predisposition to Lynch syndrome: a systematic review. *JAMA.* 2006;296: 1507–1517. [PMID: 17003399]

Lindor NM, Rabe K, Petersen GM, et al. Lower cancer incidence in Amsterdam-I criteria families without mismatch repair deficiency: familial colorectal cancer type X. *JAMA.* 2005;293: 1979–1985. [PMID: 15855431]

Stoffel EM, Mercado RC, Kohlmann W, et al. Prevalence and predictors of appropriate colorectal cancer surveillance in Lynch syndrome. *Am J Gastroenterol.* 2010;105:1851–1860. [PMID: 20354509]

Umar A, Boland CR, Terdiman JP, et al. Revised Bethesda Guidelines for hereditary nonpolyposis colorectal cancer (Lynch syndrome) and microsatellite instability. *J Natl Cancer Inst.* 2004;96:261–268. [PMID: 14970275]

2. Familial Adenomatous Polyposis

Familial adenomatous polyposis (FAP) is the second most common inherited CRC syndrome. The classic FAP phenotype is one of hundreds to thousands of adenomatous polyps in the colon, with a nearly 100% risk of developing CRC by middle age if the affected individual's colon is not surgically removed. FAP accounts for approximately 1% of CRC cases. The incidence of FAP is approximately 1 in 10,000 persons. Although most cases arise in families with a known history through autosomal-dominant inheritance, approximately 30% of cases emerge as de novo gene mutations in the *APC* gene, and biallelic mutations in the base excision repair gene *MYH* can produce an autosomal-recessive inheritance pattern. Consequently, absence of a family history of polyposis does not exclude FAP.

Clinical Finding

A. Physical Features

Most individuals with classic familial polyposis develop numerous (hundreds to thousands) colorectal adenomas by the second or third decade of life. These adenomas are usually discovered during endoscopic evaluation for symptoms such as bleeding or diarrhea, or during routine screening in individuals with a known family history of FAP. Unfortunately, affected individuals who do not undergo early endoscopic evaluation and prophylactic colectomy often present with CRC by the fifth decade of life.

More than half of individuals affected with colonic polyposis develop adenomatous polyps in the upper gastrointestinal tract. After adenocarcinoma of the colorectum, duodenal and ampullary adenocarcinoma is the second leading cause of cancer death for FAP patients. Fundic gland polyps are common in the stomach; however, these are not known to have significant potential for malignant transformation.

Extracolonic malignancies associated with FAP include papillary thyroid cancer, adrenal carcinomas, and central nervous system tumors (Turcot syndrome). Children have an increased risk of developing hepatoblastomas and require screening with liver ultrasound scans and serum α-fetoprotein during the first 7 years of life. Intra-abdominal desmoid tumors can appear in some individuals with FAP, often arising after abdominal surgery. Although not considered malignancies, desmoid tumors can result in significant morbidity when they involve the mesentery and vasculature. Desmoid tumors define the Gardner syndrome variant of FAP and may be associated with mutations in a certain region of the *APC* gene.

Other physical findings associated with FAP include the presence of extra teeth, osteomas of the jaw and skull, and epidermoid cysts. Congenital hypertrophy of the retinal pigment epithelium (CHRPE) is an ophthalmologic finding that should prompt evaluation for FAP.

B. Genetic Features

Most cases of FAP are caused by germline mutations in the *adenomatous polyposis coli* (*APC*) gene. Although most individuals with *APC* gene mutations inherited them from an affected parent, approximately one third of patients with FAP have new mutations in the *APC* gene and consequently do not have a family history of the disease.

The *APC* gene functions as a tumor suppressor. Loss of *APC* function in colonic epithelial cells is the first step toward neoplastic transformation, and somatic mutations in *APC* can be found in 80% of sporadic colon cancer tumors. Germline mutations in *APC* are believed to be highly penetrant, and most mutation carriers develop hundreds to thousands of colorectal adenomas.

Mutations in the *APC* gene are detected in more than 80% of patients with the classic FAP phenotype of hundreds to thousands of adenomas. Recent reports indicate that up to 30% of individuals with classic polyposis phenotypes without detectable *APC* mutations may have biallelic mutations in *MYH*, a base excision repair gene. Patients with *MYH*-associated polyposis can present with a similar phenotype to classic *APC*-associated FAP, but with an autosomal-recessive pattern of inheritance.

Management

A. Screening

Patients at risk of developing FAP should begin annual colorectal screening for polyps with flexible sigmoidoscopy or colonoscopy by age 11. Most affected individuals will develop colorectal adenomas during their teenage years or early twenties. Once colorectal adenomas are too numerous to be removed endoscopically, surgical removal of the colon is required. Total proctocolectomy with ileoanal anastomosis is the preferred operation. Other less-extensive surgeries, such as total colectomy with ileorectal anastomosis, leave some colonic mucosa behind that is at risk for neoplastic transformation and requires frequent endoscopies or use of chemo-preventive agents (eg, cyclooxygenase-2 [COX-2] inhibitors or sulindac) to control the growth of polyps.

Once patients are found to have colorectal adenomas, upper endoscopy is recommended to assess for adenomas in the duodenum and ampulla. A side-viewing upper endoscope should be used to examine the ampulla and perform biopsies. Duodenal or ampullary adenomas can be managed through endoscopic resection or medications (COX-2 inhibitors, sulindac) to reduce polyp burden. In rare cases, extensive adenomatous involvement, severe dysplasia, or adenocarcinoma is present, which requires surgical resection of the duodenum.

Patients with FAP are at increased risk for papillary thyroid cancer, and some guidelines recommend screening with annual thyroid examinations or thyroid ultrasound scans, or both.

Family members of individuals with FAP should be offered genetic testing for the gene mutation identified in the family in order to stratify their risk. In cases in which an individual does not undergo genetic testing or a genetic mutation cannot be identified in the family, at-risk family members should undergo colorectal screening with flexible sigmoidoscopy or colonoscopy every 1–2 years starting at age 10–12.

National Comprehensive Cancer Network. Clinical Practice Guidelines in Oncology: colorectal cancer screening. Available at: http://www.nccn.org/professionals/physician_gls/f_guidelines.asp. Accessed May 16, 2011.

B. Clinical Genetic Testing

Genetic testing is now part of standard of care for risk stratification of family members of patients with a clinical diagnosis of FAP. Genetic evaluation should start with the proband with the polyposis phenotype, and should begin with testing for mutations in the *APC* gene. Full gene sequencing tests identify *APC* gene mutations in more than 80% of patients with classic polyposis phenotypes. If an *APC* mutation is not identified, then testing for biallelic mutations in the *MYH* gene may be considered. Y165C and G382D are the two most common mutations in the *MYH* gene found in individuals of western European ancestry. Full gene sequencing of *MYH* is performed for individuals who are found to have one of these two mutations or whose racial/ethnic ancestry is not western European. When genetic testing for *APC* and *MYH* in patients with classic polyposis fails to identify a genetic mutation, all family members must be considered at risk for developing FAP and should undergo colorectal screening as previously described.

Sieber OM, Lipton L, Crabtree M, et al. Multiple colorectal adenomas, classic adenomatous polyposis, and germ-line mutations in MYH. *N Engl J Med.* 2003;348:791–799. [PMID: 12606733]

3. Multiple Adenomas or Attenuated Adenomatous Polyposis

Individuals with 10–100 colorectal adenomas are considered to have a phenotype of multiple or attenuated polyposis. There is marked phenotypic and genotypic heterogeneity among patients with attenuated polyposis, and estimates of the risk of CRC vary widely, ranging from two times above population risk to as high as 80% for some patients. Some individuals with *APC* gene mutations in the 3′ or 5′ ends of the gene or with biallelic *MYH* mutations present with an attenuated polyposis phenotype, rather than with classic FAP. Current practice guidelines recommend genetic evaluation for patients with more than 20 colorectal adenomas; however, genetic testing for *APC* and *MYH* mutations is uninformative for many individuals with fewer than 100 adenomas, suggesting that other genetic or environmental factors may be involved in the pathogenesis.

Cancer prevention in patients with attenuated polyposis focuses on frequent endoscopic surveillance with polypectomies to clear the colonic mucosa of adenomas; if adenomas are too numerous or recur too quickly to be managed endoscopically, then surgical colectomy may be indicated. Individuals with attenuated polyposis may require colonoscopies every 1–2 years, with the option to increase or shorten the surveillance interval based on the rate of polyp growth. In cases of attenuated polyposis associated with an *APC* mutation, it is recommended that at-risk individuals follow FAP screening guidelines (see earlier discussion) as phenotypes may change over time and severity of polyposis can vary among family members. For individuals with biallelic *MYH* gene mutations, it is reasonable to begin colonoscopies and upper endoscopies early and repeat exams every 1–2 years, depending on the polyp burden. In cases in which genetic testing is uninformative, family members of affected individuals should begin colonoscopic screening 5–10 years younger than the age at which polyps appeared in the proband (or by age 40, whichever is earlier).

HAMARTOMATOUS POLYPOSIS SYNDROMES

1. Peutz-Jeghers Syndrome

Peutz-Jeghers syndrome (PJS) is characterized by multiple intestinal hamartomatous polyps; mucocutaneous pigmentation, which characteristically involves the lips; and a high lifetime risk of gastrointestinal, pancreatic, and breast cancers.

Clinical Findings

A. Physical Features

Individuals with PJS develop hamartomatous polyps throughout their gastrointestinal tract and can typically present with abdominal pain, stool that is positive for occult blood, obstruction, or intussusception. The clinical diagnosis of PJS can be made in individuals who have hamartomatous polyps and two of the following features: (1) labial melanin deposits, (2) small bowel polyps, or (3) family history of PJS.

PJS is also associated with increased risk for gastrointestinal cancers (colon, small intestine, stomach, pancreas), breast cancer, and sex cord tumors. Recent reports suggest patients with PJS have greater than 85% risk of developing cancer by age 70. Lifetime risks for colon, pancreatic, and breast cancers are estimated at 39%, 36%, and 54%, respectively.

B. Genetic Features

PJS demonstrates an autosomal-dominant pattern of inheritance. Mutations in *STK-11*, a serene/threonine kinase gene with tumor-suppressor function, have been found in approximately 70% of PJS patients. Research is ongoing to identify other genes that may be implicated in PJS patients.

Management

Patients with PJS require careful endoscopic surveillance for removal of polyps and screening for extraintestinal cancers. Recommendations include upper endoscopy, colonoscopy, and small bowel imaging (with small bowel series or capsule endoscopy) every 2–3 years, with removal of all polyps greater than 1–1.5 cm, which may require double-balloon enteroscopy or intraoperative enteroscopy. Women should have annual transvaginal ultrasound scans and serum CA-125 to screen for sex cord tumors and mammograms annually starting at age 25. Boys may be offered annual testicular ultrasound scans from ages 2–12 years. Recent studies have suggested that patients with PJS may benefit from pancreatic cancer screening with endoscopic ultrasound every 1–2 years.

Giardiello FM, Trimbath JD. Peutz-Jeghers syndrome and management recommendations. *Clin Gastroenterol Hepatol.* 2006;4:408–415. [PMID: 16616343]

Van Lier MGF, Wagner A, Mathus-Vliegen MD, et al. High cancer risk in Peutz-Jeghers syndrome: a systematic review and surveillance recommendations. *Am J Gastroenterol.* 2010;105:158–164. [PMID: 20051941]

Wirtzfeld DA, Petrelli NJ, Rodriguez-Bigas MA. Hamartomatous polyposis syndromes: molecular genetics, neoplastic risk, and surveillance recommendations. *Ann Surg Oncol.* 2001;8: 319–327. [PMID: 11352305]

2. Juvenile Polyposis

Juvenile polyposis is characterized by the appearance of multiple juvenile polyps and increased risk for gastrointestinal cancers.

Clinical Findings

A. Physical Features

Patients with juvenile polyposis typically have multiple (more than five) juvenile polyps and a family history of gastrointestinal cancer. Many affected individuals present with symptoms such as anemia, bleeding, or abdominal pain during childhood. There is also an association with cardiac abnormalities and other congenital anomalies. Patients are at increased risk for colorectal, gastric, duodenal, and pancreatic cancers, many of which appear at young ages.

B. Genetic Features

Juvenile polyposis has an autosomal-dominant pattern of inheritance. Mutations in the *SMAD4* and *BMPR1a* genes, as well as in the *PTEN* gene, have been identified in some patients. Clinical genetic testing is available, but is often uninformative, because many affected individuals do not have detectable mutations.

Management

Patients with a family history of juvenile polyposis should undergo colorectal screening every 1–3 years starting at puberty. Affected individuals should have frequent upper endoscopy and colonoscopy for removal of polyps; in some cases, colectomy is required for management of polyp burden.

3. Cowden Syndrome

This hereditary syndrome is characterized by skin lesions (trichilemmomas), macrocephaly, and increased risk for breast, thyroid, and endometrial cancers. Cowden syndrome is associated with mutations in the *PTEN* gene. Although hamartomas of the gastrointestinal tract are described, the risk for gastrointestinal cancers does not appear to be as high for patients with Cowden syndrome as compared with other polyposis syndromes. However, recent data suggest there is some increase in risk for early-onset CRC, and early colonoscopic screening should be considered.

Heald B, Mester J. Rybicki L, et al. Frequent gastrointestinal polyps and colorectal adenocarcinomas in a prospective series of PTEN mutation carriers. *Gastroenterology.* 2010;139:1927–1933. [PMID: 20600018]

OTHER GASTROINTESTINAL CANCER SYNDROMES

1. Hereditary Diffuse Gastric Cancer

Hereditary diffuse gastric cancer (HDGC) manifests as diffuse infiltrative adenocarcinoma of the stomach occurring in families in a pattern of autosomal-dominant inheritance, often affecting young individuals.

Clinical Findings

A. Physical Features

In contrast to most gastric cancers, which appear as ulcers or masses, diffuse gastric cancer usually presents as diffuse thickening of the stomach wall or linitis plastica, without an obvious endoscopic lesion. The International Gastric Cancer Linkage Consortium has defined HDGC as (1) two or more relatives with diffuse gastric cancer diagnosed before age 50 or (2) three or more relatives with diffuse gastric cancer diagnosed at any age. The lifetime risk of gastric cancer for individuals in these families has been estimated to be as high as 70%, and there are numerous reports of cancer diagnoses in individuals younger than 18 years of age. Studies have suggested there is also an increased risk of breast cancer in affected families.

B. Genetic Features

One third of families who meet criteria for HDGC have germline mutations in the *E-cadherin/CDH1* tumor-suppressor gene. *E-cadherin/CDH1* gene mutations were first identified in Maori families with gastric cancer in New Zealand. Genetic testing for HDGC is clinically available; however, it is informative in fewer than 50% of cases. If a pathogenic mutation is identified in a proband, testing can be offered to other family members.

Management

Prevention of gastric cancer among individuals at increased risk is challenging because endoscopic screening has been shown to have poor sensitivity for detecting diffuse gastric cancer. Consequently, prophylactic gastrectomy is recommended for mutation carriers and other patients at highest risk. Prophylactic gastrectomy carries with it considerable morbidity; however, expert panels have concluded that the 70% risk of developing gastric cancer among *CDH1* mutation carriers justifies prophylactic gastrectomy. Given the increased risk of breast cancer among *CDH1* mutation carriers, early screening with mammography or breast magnetic resonance imaging scan, or both, is recommended.

Blair V, Martin I, Shaw D, et al. Hereditary diffuse gastric cancer: diagnosis and management. *Clin Gastroenterol Hepatol.* 2006; 4:262–275. [PMID: 11561603]

2. Familial Pancreatic Cancer

Although the vast majority of cases of pancreatic adenocarcinoma are sporadic, 3–10% seem to have a hereditary component. Risk varies from twofold to as high as 18–57-fold for families with two or three affected relatives. FPC is most often defined as families in which there are two or more first-degree relatives or three or more relatives with pancreatic adenocarcinoma.

Studies of FPC kindreds have identified pathogenic genetic mutations in approximately 20% of cases; thus, for the majority of families, a genetic cause of the pancreatic cancer cannot be found. FPC families may benefit from genetic evaluation for the following hereditary cancer syndromes:

1. Hereditary breast/ovarian cancer (HBOC; *BRCA1/BRCA2*)—Mutations in the *BRCA1* and *BRCA2* genes account for the great majority of genetic mutations identified among pancreatic cancer families. Several studies have reported that prevalence of pancreatic cancer among families with HBOC is increased. The relative risk of developing pancreatic cancer for mutation carriers has been estimated as 2.26 for *BRCA1* and 3.5–8 for *BRCA2*. In some HBOC families, the pancreatic cancer history overshadows the breast cancers. Consequently, it is recommended that evaluations for FPC begin with testing for mutations in *BRCA1* and *BRCA2*.

2. Familial atypical multiple mole melanoma (FAMMM; *P16/CDKN2A*)—FAMMM is defined as more than 50 atypical nevi and malignant melanoma in two or more first- or second-degree relatives. Pancreatic cancer has been reported in nearly one fourth of FAMMM families. Many of these FAMMM families with pancreatic cancer appear to have germline mutations in the gene *P16/CDKN2A* (*cyclin dependent kinase 2A*). Carriers of a specific type of *CDKN2A* mutation appear to have a cumulative risk of pancreatic cancer of approximately 17% by age 75.

3. Peutz-Jeghers syndrome—Individuals with PJS are most commonly characterized by their hamartomatous gastrointestinal polyps and mucocutaneous pigmentation, and approximately half are found to have germline mutations in the *STK11* gene. In addition to conferring increased risk for breast cancer, PJS also confers an increased predisposition to pancreatic adenocarcinoma, with a lifetime risk of 36%.

4. Lynch syndrome (HNPCC)—Pancreatic cancer is one of the gastrointestinal cancers that has been reported in HNPCC, and lifetime risk appears to be approximately 4% for MMR gene mutation carriers.

5. Hereditary pancreatitis—Hereditary pancreatitis often presents as repeated episodes of pancreatic inflammation, ultimately resulting in chronic pancreatitis. In familial cases, there is evidence of autosomal-dominant inheritance, and mutations of the cationic trypsinogen gene (*PRSS1*) are found in 70% of kindreds. Mutations in the *serene protease inhibitor Kazal 1* (*SPINK1*) gene have also been identified in some families. These mutations cause failure to inactivate trypsin, resulting in chronic pancreatitis, and confer a lifetime risk of pancreatic cancer of 40% by age 70.

6. *PALB2*—Mutations in the *PALB2* gene have recently been identified in a small number of familial pancreatic cancer families. The PALB2 protein product binds to *BRCA2*, and *PALB2* mutations have been described in association with inherited predisposition to breast cancer.

Management

Genetic counseling in patients with a genetic predisposition for pancreatic cancer should emphasize that in the majority of cases genetic testing does not reveal mutations in any of the genes known to be associated with pancreatic cancer. Advantages of pursuing genetic testing include the potential for identifying a mutation so that at-risk family members can undergo predisposition genetic testing and risk stratification. Also, identifying a mutation may affect cancer screening recommendations for the affected proband, as well as for the at-risk family members. Disadvantages include the fact that genetic testing may need to be repeated for many different genes, may be costly, and may not identify a genetic cause.

Patients with a family history of pancreatic cancer should be advised to stop cigarette smoking, as this has been found consistently to be an important risk factor for pancreatic cancer. At present, there is limited evidence that pancreatic cancer screening is effective in reducing morbidity and mortality from pancreatic cancer. Studies are ongoing to assess the utility of specialized pancreatic cancer screening for early detection and prevention of pancreatic cancer in individuals at increased risk; however, there are few data regarding which cystic lesions might have higher risk for neoplastic progression. However, experts have suggested considering pancreatic screening for patients in certain high-risk groups (such as those with PJS, those with two or more close relatives with pancreatic cancer, and *BRCA2* mutation carriers with a family history of pancreatic cancer). Endoscopic ultrasound, helical computed tomography scanning, secretin-enhanced magnetic resonance cholangiopancreatography, and endoscopic retrograde cholangiopancreatography have been used alone and in combination to try to detect abnormalities that may be precursors to pancreatic cancer, with the goal of timely pancreatic resection for high-risk lesions.

Canto M, Goggins M, Hruban RH, et al. Screening for early pancreatic neoplasia in high-risk individuals: a prospective controlled study. *Clin Gastroenterol Hepatol.* 2006;4:766–781. [PMID: 16682259]

Jones S, Hruban RH, Kamiyama M, et al. Exomic sequencing identifies PALB2 as a pancreatic cancer susceptibility gene. *Science.* 2009;324:217. [PMID: 19264984]

Kastrinos F, Mukherjee B, Tayob N, et al. Risk of pancreatic cancer in families with Lynch syndrome. *JAMA.* 2009;302:1790–1795. [PMID: 19861671]

Klein AP, Hruban RH, Brune KA, et al. Familial pancreatic cancer. *Cancer J.* 2001;7:266–273. [PMID: 11561603]

Irritable Bowel Syndrome

24

Sonia Friedman, MD

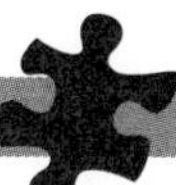

ESSENTIALS OF DIAGNOSIS

- In the United States, irritable bowel syndrome (IBS) is most common in young women.
- Rome III criteria include recurrent abdominal pain or discomfort at least 3 days per month in the last 3 months associated with two or more of the following:
- Improvement with defecation.
- Onset associated with a change in frequency of stool.
- Onset associated with a change in form (appearance) of stool.
- Criteria fulfilled for the past 3 months, with symptom onset at least 6 months prior to diagnosis.
- Rule out "red flag" symptoms before making a diagnosis of IBS.
- IBS can be mild, moderate, or severe; four different subtypes are constipation predominant, diarrhea predominant, mixed, and unsubtyped.
- The Bristol Stool Form Scale is helpful clinically in defining the spectrum of diarrhea to constipation.

General Considerations

IBS affects 10–20% of the adult U.S. population, is the most common diagnosis made by gastroenterologists, and is one of the top 10 reasons for visits to primary care physicians. IBS is the most common functional bowel disorder and affects predominantly women (70% of patients). This may be due to the fact that women more easily report their symptoms of abdominal pain, gas, bloating, and altered bowel movements. It may also be due to hormonal differences between men and women that may affect gut function and alter perception of pain related to abdominal distention. IBS can cause great discomfort, sometimes intermittent or continuous, for many decades in a patient's life and can have a significantly negative impact on quality of life.

The prevalence of IBS in a typical primary care practice is 12% and in a typical gastroenterology practice, 28%. The estimated total yearly cost of IBS in the United States is $21 billion. One billion dollars is spent in direct costs such as diagnostic tests, physician and emergency department visits, hospitalizations, surgeries, and medications; $20 billion is spent on intangible costs such as reduced work productivity, absenteeism, and travel to consultations. The intangible costs of IBS are human suffering and impaired quality of life. IBS sufferers incur 74% more health care costs than non-IBS sufferers.

IBS primarily affects people in the prime of their lives, mostly between the ages of 20 and 40 years. Patient surveys from both the United States and the United Kingdom report an average disease duration of 11 years, with one third of patients having symptoms for much longer. For many patients, symptoms occur frequently and significantly impair emotional, physical, and social well-being. Almost three fourths of patients report symptoms more than once a week and about half report daily symptoms. In a telephone survey of female IBS sufferers in the United States, almost 40% reported pain and discomfort as intolerable without relief. Women with IBS reported 71% more abdominal surgeries than women without IBS (58% vs 34%). The rates of gallbladder operations, hysterectomies, and appendectomies were twice as high or higher among women with IBS. Twenty-five percent had been hospitalized overnight due to symptoms. Seventy-eight percent of women had limits on what they ate, 43% had limits on sports and recreational activity, 43% on social activity, 40% on vacation or travel, and 28% on sexual activity. Two thirds of women were concerned about restroom availability wherever they went, one third avoided group meetings, and 25% got up earlier for work. Even more frustrating was that only 39% of women were diagnosed with IBS by the first physician they saw; 3% saw eight or more physicians before receiving a diagnosis. Time from onset to diagnosis took an average of 3 years, and patients saw an average of three physicians before getting a diagnosis.

Patients with IBS were absent from work or school an average of 13 days per year compared with 5 days per year ($P < .001$) in patients without IBS. In another study, the quality of life of patients with IBS was significantly worse than that of patients with migraines, asthma, or gastroesophageal reflux disease. For this study, quality of life was measured in multiple domains, including physical functioning, pain, general health, vitality, social functioning, emotional functioning, and mental health.

Only about 25% of IBS patients actually consult a physician for their symptoms. Of these, only a small percentage visit a gastroenterologist. Patients who consult a primary care physician for their symptoms usually have mild symptoms and effective coping skills and social support. Of IBS patients who consult subspecialists, 60% or more may have psychological disturbances, including anxiety, somatoform or personality disorders, or chronic pain syndromes. Up to 35% of women who consult subspecialists for IBS have a history of sexual abuse.

Creed F, Ratcliffe J, Fernandez L, et al. Health-related quality of life and health care costs in severe, refractory irritable bowel syndrome. *Ann Intern Med.* 2001;134:860–868. [PMID: 11346322]

Drossman DA. The functional gastrointestinal disorders and the Rome III process. *Gastroenterology.* 2006;130:1377–1390. [PMID: 16678553]

Drossman DA, Morris CB, Hu Y, et al. A prospective assessment of bowel habit in irritable bowel syndrome in women: defining an alternator. *Gastroenterology.* 2005;128:580–589. [PMID: 15765393]

Faresjö A, Grodzinsky E, Johansson S, et al. A population-based case-control study of work and psychological problems in patients with irritable bowel syndrome–women are more seriously affected than men. *Am J Gastroenterol.* 2007;102:371–379. [PMID: 17156145]

Houghton LA, Lea R, Agrawal A, et al. Relationship of abdominal bloating to distention in irritable bowel syndrome and effect of bowel habit. *Gastroenterology.* 2006;131:1003–1010. [PMID: 17030170]

Locke GR III, Zinsmeister AR, Fett SL, et al. Overlap of gastrointestinal symptom complexes in a US community. *Neurogastroenterol Motil.* 2005;17:29–34. [PMID: 15670261]

Longstreth GF, Thompson WG, Chey WD, et al. Functional bowel disorders. *Gastroenterology.* 2006;130:1480–1491. [PMID: 16678561]

Pathogenesis

A. Motility

Although disturbances in small bowel motility have been reported in IBS, none appear specific for the condition. Small bowel motility shows marked diurnal variability, and hence, consistent results can only be obtained with prolonged (at least 24 hour) recordings and large numbers of subjects. Small bowel motor disturbances reported include increased frequency and duration of discrete cluster contractions (DCC), increased frequency of the migrating motor complex (MMC), more retrograde duodenal and jejunal contractions, and an exaggerated motor response to meal ingestion, ileal distention, and cholecystokinin (CCK). Corticotrophin-releasing hormone (CRH) has been reported to increase the number of DCCs. Small bowel transit is faster in IBS patients with diarrhea (IBS-D) compared with constipation (IBS-C), and unlike in healthy controls, colonic distention does not appear to reduce duodenal motility in IBS patients, suggesting an impaired intestine-intestinal inhibitory reflex. The most consistent abnormality in the colon is an exaggerated motility response to meal ingestion. Rectal compliance or increased tension, or both, has also been reported in some studies in patients with IBS. This has been proposed as a possible mechanism for enhanced visceral sensation to balloon distention in IBS.

B. Visceral Hypersensitivity

Abdominal pain and discomfort cause considerable morbidity in IBS patients and are essential components of the Rome III criteria for diagnosis of IBS. Approximately two thirds of IBS patients demonstrate heightened pain sensitivity to experimental gut stimulation, a phenomenon known as visceral hypersensitivity. Visceral hypersensitivity is thought to play an important role in the development of chronic pain and discomfort in IBS patients. It results from a combination of factors that involve both the peripheral and central nervous systems. During tissue injury, peripheral nociceptor terminals are exposed to a mixture of immune and inflammatory mediators, such as prostaglandins, leukotrienes, serotonin, histamine, cytokines, neurotrophic factors, and reactive metabolites. These inflammatory mediators act on nociceptor terminals, leading to the activation of intracellular signaling pathways, which in turn upregulate their sensitivity and excitability. This phenomenon has been termed peripheral sensitization. Peripheral sensitization is believed to cause pain hypersensitivity at the site of injury or inflammation, also known as primary hyperalgesia (increased sensitivity to painful stimuli) and allodynia (nonpainful stimuli are perceived as painful).

A secondary consequence of peripheral sensitization is the development of an area of hypersensitivity in the surrounding uninjured tissue (secondary hyperalgesia or allodynia). This phenomenon occurs due to an increase in the excitability and receptive fields of spinal neurons and results in recruitment and amplification of both non-nociceptive and nociceptive inputs from the adjacent healthy tissue.

Depending on the setting, about 6–17% of patients with IBS report their symptoms began with an episode of gut inflammation due to gastroenteritis. In addition, an increase in mucosal T lymphocytes has been reported in patients with IBS. Therefore, the environment of nociceptor terminals in the gut of IBS patients is likely to be altered, suggesting a role for peripheral sensitization. Evidence for central sensitization as an important mechanism for the development of visceral hypersensitivity in IBS patients comes from three main observations. First, in response to colon stimulation, patients with IBS have greater radiation of pain to somatic structures in comparison with healthy subjects. Second, a proportion of IBS patients also suffer from fibromyalgia, a condition characterized by somatic hyperalgesia. Finally, patients with IBS also often demonstrate hypersensitivity of proximal areas of the gut. The innervation of the different gut organs overlaps and converges with that of the somatic structures at the level of the spinal cord, and these phenomena can be explained by central sensitization of the spinal segments that demonstrate viscerovisceral and viscerosomatic convergence.

Alterations in brain processing in IBS patients can also contribute to visceral hypersensitivity. Brain imaging studies have begun to address the possible neural mechanisms of hypersensitivity in IBS patients, and a common finding has been compared with healthy controls; patients with IBS exhibit altered or enhanced activation of regions involved in pain processing, such as the anterior cingulated cortex, thalamus, insula, and prefrontal cortices, in response to experimental rectal pain.

C. Postinfective IBS

The prevalence of postinfective IBS varies from 17% in primary care in the United Kingdom to as little as 6% in tertiary care in the United States. Population surveys indicate a relative risk of 11.1–11.9% of developing IBS in the year following a bout of gastroenteritis. Known risk factors include the severity of the initial illness; bacterial toxigenicity; female sex; a range of adverse psychological factors, including neuroticism, hypochondriasis, anxiety, and depression; and adverse life events. Postinfective IBS has been reported after *Shigella*, *Salmonella*, and *Campylobacter* infections and does not appear specific to any organism.

The Walkerton Health Study followed the long-term effects of a large outbreak of acute gastroenteritis related to municipal water contamination involving a population of 5000 people in May 2000. In the initial study, all participants were divided into three strata: (1) those who reported no illness during the outbreak (controls); (2) those who reported an acute illness not substantiated by health records; and (3) those with an acute illness documented by health records (gastrointestinal symptoms, diarrhea lasting ≥3 days, or positive stool culture). Of 4561 participants who enrolled in the study in 2002–2003, 3200 returned in 2004, 2572 returned in 2006, and 2451 returned for their 8-year assessment. At years 2–3, the prevalence of diarrhea-predominant IBS was 28.3%, at year 4, 21.4%, at year 6, 14.3%, and at year 8, 15.4%. The risk factors for developing IBS were female sex, younger age, and fever or weight loss during the acute illness. This remarkable study shows that a substantial number of people will develop IBS, with symptoms that can persist for as long as 8 years, after an acute episode of gastroenteritis. Specific host characteristics and the acute enteritis illness can predict the long-term risk of postinfective IBS.

Histologic studies indicate that postinfective IBS is characterized by increased lymphocyte numbers in mucosal biopsies, an effect that is seen throughout the colon. Where the terminal ileum has been biopsied, increased mast cells have also been noted. Another change following inflammation is enterochromaffin cell hyperplasia. Whereas in most subjects, these changes resolve within 3 months, in IBS patients, the levels of both lymphocytes and enteroendocrine cells remain elevated. Increased enterochromaffin cell numbers are associated with an increase in postprandial 5-HT release, an abnormality shown in both postinfective IBS and in diarrhea-predominant IBS without an obvious postinfective origin. Immediately after gastroenteritis affecting the small bowel, there may be transient lactose intolerance, which is particularly obvious in young children. However, in adults with postinfective IBS, who by definition have had symptoms for over 6 months, the incidence of lactose malabsorption is no different from uninfected controls.

D. Stress Response

The response of an organism to external stressors is mediated through the integration of the hypothalamic-pituitary-adrenal axis (HPA) and the sympathetic branch of the autonomic nervous system with the host immune system. A recent model for the pathogenesis of IBS proposes altered stress circuits in predisposed individuals, which are triggered by external stressors resulting in the development of gut symptoms. In postinfective IBS, the persistence of chronic inflammatory mucosal changes and enterochromaffin cell hyperplasia that persists after eradication of the infectious organism are consistent with an inadequate physiologic response to gut inflammation, in particular, an inadequate cortisol or altered sympathetic response. The key interplay between the autonomic nervous system and the HPA axis in regulating gut mucosal immunology has been explored through research looking at how the stress response, which activates both of these systems, may be important in IBS. Environmental stressors are important in predisposing toward IBS and in perpetuating the symptoms of IBS. Prior life stressors and a history of childhood abuse predispose toward developing IBS in later life. Psychiatric illness episodes or anxiety-provoking situations preceded the onset of bowel symptoms in two thirds of IBS patients being treated in tertiary care centers; in addition, IBS patients report significantly more negative life events than matched peptic ulcer patients. In addition, psychological traits such as hypochondriasis, anxiety, and depression predispose previously healthy individuals who develop gastroenteritis to go on to develop symptoms of IBS. In fact, a subgroup of IBS patients have an exaggerated endocrine stress response, as shown by a heightened release of adrenocorticotropic hormone and cortisol in response to exogenous corticotropin-releasing factor administration. This exaggerated stress response seems to be associated with mucosal immune activation.

Arroll B, Goodyear-Smith F, Kerse N, et al. Effect of the addition of a "help" question to two screening questions on specificity for diagnosis of depression in general practice: diagnostic validity study. *BMJ.* 2005;331:884. [PMID: 16166106]

Bengtson MB, Rønning T, Vatn MH, et al. Irritable bowel syndrome in twins: genes and environment. *Gut.* 2006;55:1754–1759. [PMID: 17008364]

Braun T, Voland P, Kunz L, et al. Enterochromaffin cells of the human gut: sensors for spices and odorants. *Gastroenterology.* 2007;132:1890–1901. [PMID: 17484882]

Creed F, Ratcliffe J, Fernandez L, et al. Outcome in severe irritable bowel syndrome with and without accompanying depressive, panic, and neurasthenic disorders. *Br J Psychiatry.* 2005;186:507–515. [PMID: 11346322]

Dickhaus B, Mayer EA, Firooz N, et al. Irritable bowel syndrome patients show enhanced modulation of visceral perception by auditory stress. *Am J Gastroenterol.* 2003;98:135–143. [PMID: 12526949]

Dinan TG, Quigley EM, Ahmed SM, et al. Hypothalamic-pituitary-gut axis dysregulation in irritable bowel syndrome: plasma cytokines as a potential marker? *Gastroenterology.* 2006;130:304–311. [PMID: 16472586]

Guilarte M, Santos J, de Torres I, et al. Diarrhoea-predominant IBS patients show mast cell activation and hyperplasia in the jejunum. *Gut.* 2007;56:203–209. [PMID: 17005763]

Liegregts T, Adam B, Bredack C, et al. Immune activation in patients with irritable bowel syndrome. *Gastroenterology.* 2007;132:913–920. [PMID: 17383420]

Marshall JK, Thabane M, Borgaonkar MR, et al. Postinfectious irritable bowel syndrome after a food-borne outbreak of acute gastroenteritis attributed to a viral pathogen. *Clin Gastroenterol Hepatol.* 2007;5:457–460. [PMID: 17289440]

Marshall JK, Thabane M, Garg AX, et al. Eight year prognosis of postinfectious irritable bowel syndrome following waterborne bacterial dysentery. *Gut.* 2010;59:605–611. [PMID: 20427395]

Naliboff BD, Berman S, Suyenobu B, et al. Longitudinal change in perceptual and brain activation response to visceral stimuli in irritable bowel syndrome patients. *Gastroenterology.* 2006;131:352–365. [PMID: 16890589]

Clinical Findings

IBS is a disease that can be caused by many factors. Disturbed bowel motility, visceral hypersensitivity, bacterial overgrowth, and psychological problems can all contribute to causing or exacerbating IBS. There are several important, take-home points in treating IBS. First, clinicians must take a good history and rule out "red flags." Celiac sprue, bacterial overgrowth, and microscopic colitis, among many other conditions, can masquerade as IBS. Second, clinicians should provide reassurance and close follow-up at first to make sure the diagnosis is correct. Recall that the Rome III criteria have high specificity in making the diagnosis of IBS. Third, despite the lack of evidence-based studies, diet plays a role in exacerbating gastrointestinal symptoms, and a good dietary history should be taken. Fourth, clinicians should not forget the psychological component of IBS. Many patients with IBS have coexisting depression and anxiety, and patients with severe IBS often have a history of physical and sexual abuse.

Table 24–1. Rome III diagnostic criteria[a] for irritable bowel syndrome.

Recurrent abdominal pain or discomfort[b] at least 3 days per month in the last 3 months associated with 2 or more of the following:
• Improvement with defecation • Onset associated with a change in frequency of stool • Onset associated with a change in form (appearance) of stool

[a]Criteria fulfilled for the last 3 months with symptoms onset at least 6 months prior to diagnosis.
[b]Discomfort means an uncomfortable sensation not described as pain. In pathophysiology research and clinical trials, pain or discomfort frequency of at least 2 days a week during screening evaluation was required for subject eligibility.

Lastly, there are only a few newer medications with good data from randomized controlled trials. Given the paucity of specific medicines with positive results in the evidence-based medical literature, treatment is often a trial and error process. However, a combination of dietary and lifestyle changes, relaxation training or psychotherapy, and individualized IBS medicines tailored to each patient's symptoms usually improves quality of life.

A. Symptoms and Signs

As the Rome III criteria indicate (Table 24–1), the key features are abdominal pain or discomfort that is clearly linked to bowel function, either being relieved by defecation or associated with a change in stool form or consistency. These symptoms are not explained by biochemical or structural abnormalities. Symptoms should be present for at least 6 months to clearly distinguish those from other conditions such as infections, which often pass quickly, or progressive diseases such as bowel cancer that are usually diagnosed within 6 months of symptom onset. Symptoms that are common in IBS but are not part of the Rome III criteria include bloating, abnormal stool form (hard, loose, or both), abnormal stool frequency (<3 times/week or >3 times/week), straining at defecation, urgency, feeling of incomplete evacuation, and the passage of mucus per rectum. Most patients experience flares intermittently, with symptoms lasting 2–4 days followed by periods of remission. In women, symptoms can be worse at the time of menstruation and can cycle with the menstrual cycle. One common symptom of IBS not part of the Rome III criteria is repeated defecation in the morning (morning rush) when stool consistency changes from solid to liquid as the colon contents are evacuated.

One important exception to the Rome III criteria is patients who feel abdominal pain continuously. The diagnosis in this case is likely functional abdominal pain, an unusual, particularly severe condition in which patients respond poorly to treatment and often have severe underlying psychological disturbances.

IBS is considered a painful condition, and those with painless bowel dysfunction are labeled as having "functional

Table 24–2. Comparison of irritable bowel syndrome with constipation (IBS-C) with functional constipation.

Symptom	IBS-C	Functional Constipation
Abdominal pain or discomfort	+++	±
Bloating or abdominal distention	+++	+
Sense of anorectal obstruction	+	+++
Manual maneuvers	+	+++
<3 bowel movements/week	+++	+++
Hard, lumpy stools	+++	+++
Straining	+++	+++
Feeling of incomplete evacuation	+++	+++

constipation" or "functional diarrhea." Some of the distinguishing characteristics of IBS-C and functional constipation are detailed in Table 24–2.

1. IBS subtype classification—The Rome III subclassification is based solely on stool consistency and not frequency, urgency, and straining and is thus easy to use (Table 24–3). To better differentiate the different IBS subtypes, the Bristol Stool Form Scale is very helpful clinically in defining the spectrum of diarrhea to constipation (Table 24–4). Patients with hard stools more than 25% of the time and loose stools less than 25% of the time are classified as IBS-C, whereas patients classified as having IBS with diarrhea (IBS-D) have loose stools more than 25% of the time and hard stools less than 25% of the time. About one third to one half of patients are termed IBS-mixed (IBS-M) and have hard stools more than 25% of the time and loose stools more than 25% of the time. A small (4%) group of patients has unclassified IBS (IBS-U), with neither loose nor hard stools more than 25% of the time. Patients whose bowel habits change from one subtype to another over months or years are known as "alternators."

Table 24–3. Subtyping of irritable bowel syndrome by predominant stool pattern.

Subtype	Description
IBS with constipation (IBS-C)	Hard or lumpy stools >25% and loose (mushy) or watery stools <25% of bowel movements
IBS with diarrhea (IBS-D)	Loose (mushy) or watery stools >25% of the time and hard or lumpy stool <25% of bowel movements
Mixed IBS (IBS-M)	Hard or lumpy stools >25% and loose (mushy) or watery stools >25% of bowel movements
Unsubtyped IBS	Insufficient abnormality of stool consistency to meet criteria for IBS-C, D, or M

Table 24–4. Bristol Stool Form Scale.

Type	Description
1	Separate hard lumps like nuts (difficult to pass)
2	Sausage shaped but lumpy
3	Like a sausage but with cracks in its surface
4	Like a sausage or snake, smooth and soft
5	Soft blobs with clear-cut edges (passed easily)
6	Fluffy pieces with ragged edges, a mushy stool
7	Watery, no solid pieces, entirely liquid

2. IBS-associated nongastrointestinal symptoms and comorbidity with other diseases—Nongastrointestinal symptoms associated with IBS include backache; headache; urinary symptoms such as nocturia, frequency, and urgency of micturition; incomplete bladder emptying; and, in women, dyspareunia. Helpful diagnostic behavioral features of IBS in general practice include symptoms present for more than 6 months, frequent consultations for nongastrointestinal symptoms, previous medically unexplained symptoms, and patient reports that stress aggravates symptoms.

Between 20% and 50% of IBS patients also have fibromyalgia. IBS is common in several other chronic pain disorders, being found in 51% of patients with chronic fatigue syndrome, 64% of those with temporomandibular joint disorder, and 50% of those with chronic pelvic pain. The lifetime rates of IBS in patients with these syndromes are even higher: 77% in fibromyalgia, 92% in chronic fatigue syndrome, and 64% in temporomandibular joint disorder. In addition, those with overlap syndromes tend to have more severe IBS. IBS patients in primary care with numerous other somatic complaints report high levels of mood disorder, health anxiety, neuroticism, adverse life events, and reduced quality of life and increased health care seeking.

3. Psychological features—At least half of IBS patients can be described as depressed, anxious, or hypochondriacal. Studies from tertiary care centers suggest that up to two thirds have a psychiatric disorder—most commonly depressive or anxiety disorder. The clinician should always ask the patients about any psychological problems, as well as take a history of physical and sexual abuse. Suggested questions to help assess mood include the following:

- "During the past month, have you often been bothered by feeling down, depressed, or hopeless?"
- "During the past month, have you been bothered by little interest or pleasure in doing things?"
- "Is this something with which you would like help?"

Table 24–5. "Alarm" features in a patient with possible IBS.

Age >50 years
Short history of symptoms
Documented weight loss
Nocturnal symptoms
Male sex
Family history of colon cancer
Anemia
Rectal bleeding
Recent antibiotic usage
New-onset symptoms after age 45

4. "Alarm" features—Certain "alarm" features indicate that the diagnosis might not be IBS. It is very important to take a careful history and perform a thorough physical examination to rule out any such red flag symptoms, which are detailed in Table 24–5. A follow-up observational study lasting 24 months found that, in the absence of alarm features, after full history, examination, and investigation, no IBS patients meeting Rome II criteria (the prior Rome criteria) had another diagnosis. By contrast, a substantial number of those not meeting the Rome II criteria were left with a final diagnosis of IBS, suggesting that the Rome criteria in the absence of alarm symptoms were highly specific but not highly sensitive. A more recent study, which looked at a range of alarm features, found that age greater than 50 years at onset of symptoms, male sex, blood mixed in the stool, and blood on the toilet paper were all predictors for an organic diagnosis. Characteristic features of IBS in this study were pain more than six times in the last year, pain that radiated outside the abdomen, and pain that was associated with looser bowel movements, all of which were much more common in IBS than in organic disease. Other features more common in IBS included a childhood history of abdominal pain, which was found in a quarter of subjects.

5. Physical findings—Physical examination of the patient with IBS usually reveals no relevant abnormality. Important red flags to look for are thyroid abnormalities, lymphadenopathy, abdominal masses, and perianal disease such as anal fistulas, fissures, or skin tags. Abdominal wall pain originating from a hernia, local muscle injury, or a trapped nerve can be elucidated by the Carnett test. This involves asking patients to fold their arms across their chest and raise their head off the pillow against gentle resistance from the physician's hand. Exacerbation of pain indicates a positive Carnett test. Painful rib syndrome is characterized by point tenderness and pain upon springing the rib cage and has a benign cause. Checking for both of these common musculoskeletal problems can save a lot of time and money on diagnostic testing.

B. Laboratory Findings

Basic laboratory screening should include compete blood count, thyroid-stimulating hormone, and serologies for celiac disease. All patients should have stool tested by fecal occult blood testing (FOBT).

C. Colonoscopy

The basic indications for colonoscopy in this setting are age 50 or greater, positive FOBT or frank rectal bleeding, and a family history of colon cancer.

Differential Diagnosis

A. Lactose Intolerance

Lactose intolerance is very common and has similar symptoms to IBS. It is seen in 7–20% of Caucasians, as high as 80–95% of Native Americans, 65–75% of Africans and African Americans, and 50% of Hispanics. The prevalence is greater than 90% in some populations in East Asia. The preferred method of testing is a hydrogen breath test. For patients who are lactose intolerant, lactase preparations such as Lactaid, Lactase, and Dairy Ease may help, but many patients still have symptoms and will have to avoid all lactose-containing food products.

B. Fructose Intolerance

Fructose is another carbohydrate that is poorly absorbed in a number of individuals. The consumption of fructose in the United States has greatly increased over the past two decades and is due in large part to the increase of over 1000% in the consumption of high-fructose corn syrup. A retrospective study of 80 IBS patients found that 38% were fructose intolerant. This same study reported that a fructose-restricted diet results in a significant improvement ($P < .02$) in symptoms including pain, belching, bloating, fullness, indigestion, and diarrhea. In a double-blind, randomized, placebo-controlled trial, 25 IBS patients who had responded to a change in diet (consisting of food low in free fructose and fructans) were rechallenged by graded-dose introduction of fructose or fructans (alone or in combination) or glucose. Patients who were rechallenged with fructose, fructans, or the combination had worse control over their IBS symptoms (70%, 77%, and 79%, respectively) than those rechallenged only with glucose (14%; $P \leq .02$). Because fructose intolerance or malabsorption can occur simultaneously with IBS, fructose should be restricted over a trial period to see if IBS patients respond.

C. Carbohydrates

Because of the evidence of carbohydrate intolerance in patients with IBS-D, a trial of a very low carbohydrate diet (VLCD) in 17 IBS patients was initiated. All patients had moderate to severe IBS-D and were provided a 2-week standard diet and then 4 weeks of a VLCD (20 g of carbohydrate). Thirteen of 17 patients completed the study, with 10 patients (77%) reporting adequate relief for all 4 VLCD weeks. Stool frequency decreased (2.6 ± 0.8 to 1.4 ± 1.2 stools per day; $P < .001$), stool consistency improved from diarrheal to normal form (Bristol Stool Scale score: 5.3 ± 0.7 to 3.8 ± 1.2; $P < .001$), and pain scores and quality of life measures significantly improved. Outcomes were independent of weight loss.

D. Bile Acid Malabsorption

Idiopathic adult-onset bile acid malabsorption is not rare and could contribute to the watery diarrhea of patients with IBS-D. In a pooled analysis of 18 relevant studies in IBS patients, bile acid malabsorption was determined by excessive secretion of an artificial bile salt, selenium homocholic acid taurine (SeHCAT), at 7 days. Five studies (429 patients) indicated that 10% of patients (95% confidence interval [CI], 7–13%) had severe bile acid malabsorption (SeHCAT <5%). Seventeen studies (1073 patients) indicated that 32% of patients (95% CI, 29–35%) had moderate bile acid malabsorption (SeHCAT <10%), and seven studies (618 patients) indicated that 26% of patients (95% CI, 23–30%) had mild bile acid malabsorption (SeHCAT <15%). Pooled data from 15 studies showed a dose-response relationship according to severity of malabsorption to treatment with a bile acid binder. A response to cholestyramine occurred in 96% of severe patients, 80% of moderate patients, and 70% of mild patients. One of the mechanisms for bile acid diarrhea may be defective feedback inhibition of bile acid biosynthesis via fibroblast growth factor-19.

E. Food Intolerances

Although there have been no controlled trials on diet and IBS, certain foods can cause or exacerbate IBS symptoms, and a physicians should not forget to take a dietary history. Once lactose intolerance is excluded, the biggest offenders are sugar-free and carbohydrate-free or low-carbohydrate foods. These foods contain sugar alcohols such as sorbitol, maltitol, and xylitol. They are meant to be indigestible and as such can cause cramping, flatulence, and diarrhea. Sorbitol is even commercially available as a laxative. Diet soft drinks, flavored water, chewing gum, and candies often contain these sugar alcohols. Monosodium glutamate (MSG) can cause symptoms in sensitive individuals and is used as a flavoring in Chinese food and other preparations commonly purchased at the supermarket. Carbonated beverages contribute to gas and bloating, and alcohol can cause gastritis and diarrhea. Caffeine found in coffee, tea, soft drinks, or chocolate can exacerbate abdominal cramps and diarrhea. Other specific diets should be individualized, keeping in mind that there is no evidence-based literature. A suggested diet plan created by Christine Frissora, MD, and successful with her IBS patients at Columbia University is detailed in Table 24–6. Foods likely to cause loose bowel movements and excessive gas and foods likely to cause constipation are detailed in Tables 24–7 and 24–8, respectively. True food allergies are rare in adults, and particular patients in whom there is a high suspicion should be referred to an allergist.

F. Infections

Most bowel infections should be transient, and symptoms will not be present for 6 months in order to meet the Rome III criteria. Broad-spectrum antibiotics lead to transient diarrhea in 10% of cases which, if severe and persistent, should lead to consideration of testing for *Clostridium difficile* toxin or sigmoidoscopy to exclude pseudomembranous colitis. Chronic giardiasis can last for months and manifest with bloating, abdominal pain, and diarrhea. Stool enzyme-linked immunosorbent assay testing for *Giardia* antigen is the most sensitive (90–100%) and specific (95–100%) method to test for *Giardia* and should be considered in patients who have histories of exposure to poor sanitary conditions.

G. Celiac Disease

Celiac disease occurs in about 1 in 250 people in the United States. It can be identified through blood analysis of immunoglobulin A (IgA) level, anti-endomysial antibody, and anti-transglutaminase antibody. IgA level should be checked, because IgA deficiency is more common in patients with celiac disease. Patients who are antibody positive or in whom there is a high suspicion should undergo upper endoscopy and biopsy. Genetic testing is helpful in certain cases. More than 99% of patients with celiac disease have HLA DQ2, DQ8, or both, compared with about 40% of the general population. Thus, celiac disease is highly unlikely in patients without these haplotypes. The treatment of celiac disease is a strict gluten-free diet.

Celiac disease may present with symptoms of IBS. In a study by Sanders et al, 66 of 300 IBS patients has anti-gliadin (IgA) or IgG antibodies and/or anti-endomysial antibodies and 14 (4.7%) had celiac disease confirmed by duodenal biopsy. Three of these 14 patients were anti-endomysial antibody negative (21.4%). In another study with 105 IBS patients and 105 controls, celiac disease was diagnosed in 12 IBS patients and no controls. All 12 had positive tests for anti-endomysial antibody, and all had compatible histologic findings. Of the 12 patients, 3 presented with diarrhea, 4 with constipation, and 5 with alternating diarrhea and constipation. The current serologic test most commonly used in the diagnosis of celiac disease is the tissue transglutaminase antibody, which has a sensitivity of greater than 90% and specificity of greater than 95%.

H. Tropical Sprue

The key diagnostic test in tropical sprue is small intestinal mucosal biopsy, which is usually obtained at esophagogastroduodenoscopy. Gross findings at endoscopy include flattening of duodenal folds and so-called scalloping. The latter finding was originally thought to be pathognomonic of celiac disease but also occurs in tropical sprue and other small bowel diseases. The major histologic findings are shortened, blunted villi and elongated crypts with increased inflammatory cells in the lamina propria. These histologic

Table 24–6. Dr Frissora's diet for the sensitive stomach.

Foods Usually Tolerated	Foods to Use with Caution	Foods to Avoid
Soluble fiber in moderation (oatmeal, berries, beets, cooked lentils, legumes, split pea soup, chick peas, peas, carrots, yams, peaches, blueberries, strawberries, grits, Cream of Wheat, papaya, mango, kiwi)	Citrus and tomatoes (acid)	Crude fiber (residue)—eggplant skin, bell peppers, cucumber skin
Corn Flakes, Rice Krispies, and Special K	Diet sugar-free and carbohydrate-free products	MSG (pain and diarrhea)
Waffles, pancakes	Alcohol	Large seeds
Crackers (graham crackers, low-salt Wheat Thins, rice crackers, unsalted saltines)	Grapes	Nuts
Organic yogurt (Greek: Total, Stonyfield Farm)	Chocolate	Potato skins
Fish and shrimp	Raw broccoli and cauliflower	Fats
Egg whites	Cabbage	Fried foods
Stewed, tender meat, beef Bourguignon	Coleslaw	Carbonated beverages
Lentil soup, homemade chicken and vegetable soups	Cold cuts	High-fructose corn syrup
Rice, pasta, couscous, noodles	Iceberg lettuce	Snapple, Gatorade
Pastina	Popcorn	Garlic, onions
Mashed potatoes	Dairy (lactose)	All artificial sweeteners (Splenda, Equal, Sweet 'N Low)
Cooked, tender baby spinach and turnips	Caffeine	Diet Snapple, diet soda
Banana, plantain, polenta		Sugar-free gum and candy
Nectarines, apricots		
Watermelon, honeydew, and cantaloupe		
Avocado, olive oil		
Chamomile and herbal teas		

Tips and advice

- Chew food well, eat slowly, eat small meals (6 per day), and take in liquids between meals, don't use a straw
- Use chewable vitamins
- Broccoli and cauliflower are best tolerated in a puree soup
- Eat baby leaf/red leaf lettuce in small amounts
- Eat small pieces of cooked carrots, celery, or zucchini with rice, pasta, or couscous

Recommended daily calcium intake

In women:

- Premenopausal women: 1200 mg
- Postmenopausal women (no estrogen): 1500 mg
- Postmenopausal women on hormone replacement: 1000 mg
- Also recommended: Vitamin D, 400 IU daily

Normal healthy men: 1000–1200 mg

Reproduced, with permission, from Frissora CL. Nuances in treating irritable bowel syndrome. *Rev Gastroenterol Disord.* 2007;7:89–96.

Table 24–7. Foods likely to cause loose bowel movements and excessive gas.

All caffeine-containing beverages especially coffee with chicory
Peaches, pears, cherries, apples
Fruit juices, orange, cranberry, apple
Cola beverages that are not caffeine-free, sugar-free
Brassica vegetables such as broccoli, asparagus, cauliflower, cabbage, Brussels sprouts
Bran cereal, whole-wheat bread, high-fiber foods
Pastries, candy, chocolate
Waffle syrup, donuts
Wine (>3 glasses in susceptible individuals)
Milk and milk products if one is sensitive to lactose

changes are similar but not identical to those occurring in patients with untreated celiac disease. Most authorities recommend tetracycline (250 mg orally, four times daily) plus folic acid (5 mg/day) for 3–6 months for the treatment of

Table 24–8. Foods likely to cause constipation or at least help control bowel movements.

Rice, bread
Potatoes, pasta
Meat, veal, poultry, fish
Cooked vegetables
Bananas

tropical sprue. Even on this regimen, relapses or reinfection occur in up to 20% of patients living in the tropics.

I. Small Bowel Bacterial Overgrowth

Small bowel bacterial overgrowth is characterized by nutrient malabsorption associated with an increased number or type of bacteria in the upper gastrointestinal tract. Affected patients can have abdominal pain, watery diarrhea, dyspepsia, and weight loss. The most frequent presenting symptoms in one series of 100 adult patients were diarrhea, weight loss, bloating, and excess flatulence. A [^{14}C]-D-xylose breath test is helpful in making the diagnosis. Xylose is a pentose sugar that is catabolized by gram-negative aerobes, which are invariably part of the microflora implicated in bacterial overgrowth. Bacterial action on the sugar releases the radioactive isotope $^{14}CO_2$, which, after absorption, is detectable in breath samples. Breath hydrogen testing is performed by administering a test dose of carbohydrate (usually lactose or glucose), which, in patients with bacterial overgrowth, is associated with a rise in breath hydrogen levels. It is possible to have no rise in hydrogen production during a lactulose breath hydrogen test if hydrogen is converted to methane or hydrogen sulfide by hydrogen consumptive microbes. Concurrent testing with methane may enhance sensitivity.

Most patients with bacterial overgrowth require treatment with antibiotics. Effective antibiotic treatment should cover both aerobic and anaerobic enteric bacteria, and adequate antimicrobial coverage can be achieved with the following combinations: amoxicillin–clavulanate plus metronidazole or a combination of a cephalosporin with metronidazole, norfloxacin, or rifaximin. A single course of therapy for 7–10 days may improve symptoms and have an effect lasting for months. However, some patients require prolonged therapy (eg, 1–2 months) before a response is seen. It is usually unnecessary to repeat diagnostic testing if symptoms or objective measures of malabsorption respond to treatment. In one paper, rifaximin has been shown to help symptoms of bloating and flatulence. One hundred and twenty-four patients received rifaximin (400 mg twice daily) versus placebo for 10 days. Patients reported decreased bloating and flatulence after 10 days ($P = .03$) and 20 days ($P = .02$). There was decreased hydrogen breath excretion among responders ($P = .01$). The differential diagnosis of IBS-D is detailed in Table 24–9.

Table 24–9. Differential diagnosis of irritable bowel syndrome with diarrhea (IBS-D).

Microscopic colitis
Celiac disease
Giardiasis
Lactose malabsorption
Tropical sprue
Small bowel bacterial overgrowth
Bile salt malabsorption
Colon cancer

J. Inflammatory Bowel Disease

Crohn disease and ulcerative colitis are fairly easy to distinguish from IBS with modern diagnostic testing. Most patients with inflammatory bowel disease present with weight loss, bleeding, and abdominal pain. Laboratory studies often reveal anemia, increased sedimentation rate, and sometimes leukocytosis. Colonoscopy in patients with colitis reveals inflammation, erythema, exudates, and sometimes ulcerations. Pathologic examination shows chronic changes in the mucosa. Subtle Crohn disease of the small bowel is almost always found by computed tomographic enterography or capsule endoscopy in cases that are difficult to diagnose.

K. Microscopic Colitis

Collagenous and lymphocytic colitis are more difficult to distinguish from IBS because patients present with chronic watery diarrhea and often no weight loss. In addition, these forms of colitis have completely normal endoscopic appearances. Collagenous colitis has two main histologic components: increased subepithelial collagen deposition and colitis with increased intraepithelial lymphocytes. The female-to-male ratio is 9:1, and most patients present in the sixth or seventh decades of life. Treatments range from sulfasalazine or mesalamine and diphenoxylate hydrochloride–atropine sulfate (Lomotil) to bismuth, budesonide, and prednisone for refractory disease.

Lymphocytic colitis has features similar to collagenous colitis, including age at onset and clinical presentation, but it has almost equal incidence in men and women and no subepithelial collagen deposition on pathologic section. However, intraepithelial lymphocytes are increased. The frequency of celiac disease is increased in lymphocytic colitis and ranges from 9% to 27%. Celiac disease should be excluded in all patients with lymphocytic colitis, particularly if diarrhea does not respond to conventional therapy. Treatment is similar to that of collagenous colitis with the exception of a gluten-free diet for those who have celiac disease.

L. Fecal Incontinence

Fecal incontinence may masquerade as diarrhea and is a symptom patients are reluctant to report because it is embarrassing. In a study of symptomatic pelvic floor disorders in U.S. women, 9.0% reported fecal incontinence. The prevalence of fecal incontinence increased with age. Obesity and poverty increased the likelihood of symptoms. Other causes of fecal incontinence are a history of a forceps delivery, a total abdominal hysterectomy, diabetes, pelvic radiation, an errant episiotomy, and a perianal fistula repair.

Austin GL, Dalton CB, Hu Y, et al. A very low carbohydrate diet improves symptoms and quality of life in diarrhea predominant irritable bowel syndrome. *Clin Gastroenterol Hepatol.* 2009;7:706–708. [PMID: 19281859]

Frissora CL. Nuances in treating irritable bowel syndrome. *Rev Gastroenterol Disord.* 2007;7:89–96. [PMID: 17597676]

Hammer J, Eslick GD, Howell SC, et al. Diagnostic yield of alarm features in irritable bowel syndrome and functional dyspepsia. *Gut.* 2004;53:666–672. [PMID: 15082584]

Nygaard I, Barber MD, Burgio KL, et al. Prevalence of symptomatic pelvic floor disorders in US women. *JAMA.* 2008;300:1311–1316. [PMID: 18799443]

Pimentel M, Park S, Mirocha J, et al. The effect of a nonabsorbed oral antibiotic (rifaximin) on the symptoms of the irritable bowel syndrome. *Ann Intern Med.* 2006;145:557–563. [PMID: 17043337]

Posserud I, Stotzer PO, Björnsson ES, et al. Small intestinal bacterial overgrowth in patients with irritable bowel syndrome. *Gut.* 2007;56:802–808. [PMID: 17148502]

Sanders DS, Carter MJ, Hurlstone DP, et al. Association of adult coeliac disease with irritable bowel syndrome: a case-control study in patients fulfilling ROME II criteria referred to secondary care. *Lancet.* 2001;358:1504–1508. [PMID: 11705563]

Scarpellini E, Gabrielli M, Lauritano CE, et al. High dosage rifaximin for the treatment of small intestinal bacterial over-growth. *Aliment Pharmacol Ther.* 2007;25:781–786. [PMID: 17373916]

Shahbazkhani B, Forootan M, Merat S, et al. Coeliac disease presenting with symptoms of irritable bowel syndrome. *Aliment Pharmacol Ther.* 2003;18:231–235. [PMID: 12869084]

Sharara AI, Aoun E, Adbul-Baki H, et al. A randomized double-blind placebo-controlled trial of rifaximin in patients with abdominal bloating and flatulence. *Am J Gastroenterol.* 2006;101:326–333. [PMID: 16454838]

Shepherd SJ, Parker FC, Muir JG, et al. Dietary triggers of abdominal symptoms in patients with irritable bowel syndrome; randomized placebo-controlled evidence. *Clin Gastroenterol Hepatol.* 2008; 6:765–771. [PMID: 18456565]

Walters JR, Tasleem AM, Omer OS, et al. A new mechanism for bile acid diarrhea: defective feedback inhibition of bile acid biosynthesis. *Clin Gastroenterol Hepatol.* 2009;7:1189–1194. [PMID: 19426836]

Wedlake L, A'Hern R, Russell D, et al. Systematic review: the prevalence of idiopathic bile acid malabsorption as diagnosed by SeHCAT scanning in patients with diarrhea-predominant irritable bowel syndrome. *Aliment Pharmacol Ther.* 2009;30: 707–717. [PMID: 19570102]

Complications

The complications of IBS are decreased quality of life, time off from work and school, personal expenses of medications and physician visits, and psychological problems such as depression and anxiety. It is commonplace for IBS patients to undergo unnecessary procedures and surgeries, and it is the role of the treating physician to avoid these complications. Comprehensive patient appointments, close follow-up, and much reassurance by the physician are recommended. When asked what they want from their health care professional, IBS patients in England offered their 10 top requests, which are listed in Table 24–10.

Treatment

Current treatment options for IBS are limited and include dietary modification, fiber supplements, pharmacologic agents (Table 24–11), and psychotherapy.

Table 24–10. Top 10 patient requests compiled by the IBS Network in the United Kingdom.

"When I visit my health professional about my IBS I would like them to give me ..."

1. A clear knowledgeable explanation of what IBS is
2. A statement there is no miracle cure
3. A clear indication that it is my body, my illness and that it is up to me to take control
4. A clear explanation that there will be good days and bad days but there will be light at the end of the tunnel
5. An explanation of the different treatment options
6. Recognition that IBS is an illness
7. Consider and discuss complementary/alternative therapies
8. Offer at least one complementary/alternative therapy
9. Offer support and understanding
10. Be aware of conflicting emotion in someone who is newly diagnosed

A. Fiber

Fiber found in whole grains, fruits, nuts, seeds, and vegetables and also in the form of fiber supplements containing psyllium (Metamucil), guar gum (Benefiber), calcium polycarbophil (FiberCon), and methylcellulose (Citrucel) helps to regulate bowel movements and improve stool consistency. Although it may help individual patients and is used commonly for patients with IBS-M disease or alternators, there is no high-quality evidence-based literature supporting the benefits of fiber in treating IBS.

B. Antidiarrheal Agents

Loperamide (Imodium) and diphenoxylate hydrochloride–atropine sulfate (Lomotil) decrease diarrhea but they have no effect on bloating or abdominal pain. Cholestyramine resin binds bile salts and slows down diarrhea but similarly has no effect on abdominal pain or bloating. These agents can be helpful for IBS in combination with other antispasmodics or can be used to provide as-needed therapy for diarrhea.

C. Enemas and Suppositories

Among patients who need these agents for intractable constipation, the majority will use them only occasionally. The safest suppository to use is a glycerin suppository because it is not a stimulant laxative and has no lasting ill effects on the gut. Fleets, tap water, or mineral oil enemas can be used occasionally for refractory constipation but insertion of air that comes with the enema fluid will only exacerbate bloating and abdominal pain.

D. Laxatives

Various laxatives are available for the constipation component of IBS. They include the stimulant laxatives (senna, bisacodyl, cascara) and the osmotic laxatives (polyethylene glycol, lactulose, sorbitol). The stimulant laxatives may cause

Table 24–11. Possible drugs for dominant symptoms in irritable bowel syndrome.

Symptom	Drug	Dose
Diarrhea	Loperamide	2–4 mg as needed, maximum 12 mg/day
	Cholestyramine resin	4 g with meals
	Alosetron	0.5–1 mg twice daily (for severe IBS in women)
Constipation	Psyllium husk	3.4 g twice daily with meals, then adjust
	Methylcellulose	2 g twice daily with meals, then adjust
	Calcium polycarbophil	1 g daily to 4 times daily
	Lactulose syrup	10–20 g twice daily
	70% Sorbitol	15 mL twice daily
	Polyethylene glycol	17 g in 8 oz water daily
	Tegaserod	2–6 mg twice daily for women but now off the market
	Lubiprostone	24 mcg twice daily (for chronic constipation), 8 mcg twice daily (for IBS-C)
	Magnesium hydroxide	2–4 tbsp daily
Abdominal pain	Smooth muscle relaxant	Daily to 4 times daily before meals
	Tricyclic antidepressant	Start 25–50 mg at bedtime, then adjust
	Selective serotonin reuptake inhibitors	Begin small dose, increase as needed

permanent damage to the myenteric plexus but studies are conflicting. In any case, they do exacerbate abdominal cramps and bloating when used chronically. Abdominal cramps and excess gas and bloating are seen with the osmotic laxative, but MiraLax was deemed effective for chronic constipation in one long-term study.

E. Antispasmodics

There is only minimal evidence-based literature that antispasmodics are effective in treating the pain component of IBS. Antispasmodics relax the smooth muscle of the gut and include dicyclomine hydrochloride (Bentyl), hyoscyamine sulfate (Levsin), scopolamine and phenobarbital (Donnatal), and clidinium bromide with chlordiazepoxide (Librax). These medicines are usually given before meals to inhibit abdominal pain and immediate, uncontrolled bowel movements.

F. Tricyclic Antidepressants

Tricyclic antidepressants, such as amitriptyline hydrochloride (Elavil) and nortriptyline hydrochloride (Pamelor), prescribed at low doses, are beneficial in patients with and without diagnosed depression and anxiety because their benefit derives more from pain reduction than depression. There is some evidence-based literature favoring amitriptyline in treating visceral hypersensitivity. Side effects of both antispasmodics and tricyclics include dry mouth, dry eyes, and fatigue. Weight gain is a side effect particular to tricyclics.

G. Selective Serotonin Reuptake Inhibitors (SSRIs)

More recently, citalopram hydrobromide (Celexa) has been tested in patients with IBS. One study found that this SSRI, which is commonly used for depression, was effective in patients with IBS. Citalopram significantly improved symptoms of abdominal pain and bloating and improved quality of life and overall well-being. Fluoxetine hydrochloride (Prozac), an SSRI commonly used in the treatment of depression, is also effective in treating IBS. In a recent study in patients with IBS-C, fluoxetine decreased abdominal discomfort and bloating and increased bowel movements.

H. Newer Medical Therapies for IBS

Two newer medical therapies for inflammatory bowel disease focus on the serotonin receptor in the gut. Alosetron (Lotronex) is a 5-HT_3 antagonist approved for use in women with severe IBS-D who have failed conventional therapy. Alosetron slows colonic transit, decreases rectal urgency, and decreases abdominal pain. The drug was launched in February of 2000 and temporarily withdrawn from the market in November of that year due to isolated reports of constipation and ischemic colitis. There were 3 deaths and 77 hospitalizations. Public outcry resulted in approval by the U.S. Food and Drug Administration (FDA) to allow the reintroduction of alosetron on a limited basis, and the drug was reintroduced in November 2002 under a new risk-management program. Restrictions on the use of alosetron include updated warnings in the complete Prescribing Information; including a Medication Guide for patients that explains what to do if they become constipated or have signs of ischemic colitis; a lower starting dose than previously approved; and a prescribing program for physicians to be enrolled in, based on self-attestation of qualifications and acceptance of certain responsibilities in prescribing alosetron. There is significant evidence-based literature to recommend use of alosetron in women with severe IBS-D, and it is an important drug in the IBS armamentarium. Studies show a statistically significant increase in global improvement in IBS symptoms, adequate relief of IBS pain and discomfort, and improvement in bowel symptoms.

I. Tegaserod

Tegaserod maleate (Zelnorm) is a partial 5-HT_4 receptor agonist. It stimulates the peristaltic reflex, increases velocity of propulsion through the colon, reduces the firing rate of rectal afferent nerves, alters chloride secretion in the intestine, and reduces visceral sensitivity. Tegaserod normalizes bowel function and relieves abdominal pain and discomfort in IBS patients. It is indicated for IBS-C in women and chronic constipation in men and women.

On March 30, 2007, Novartis announced it was complying with a request from the FDA to suspend U.S. marketing and sales of tegaserod due to an analysis of clinical trial data identifying a small but statistically significant imbalance in the number of cardiovascular ischemic events in patients taking tegaserod. The data showed that events occurred in 13 out of 11,614 patients treated with tegaserod (0.11%), compared with one case in 7031 placebo-treated patients (0.01%). These events included heart attack, stroke, and unstable angina. The cardiovascular ischemic events occurred in patients who had preexisting cardiovascular disease or cardiovascular risk factors, or both. No causal relationship has been demonstrated between tegaserod and these events, and on July 27, 2007, tegaserod again become available through a special FDA Investigational New Drug program restricted to gastroenterologists prescribing this medication for female patients younger than 55 years with IBS-C or chronic constipation.

High-quality, evidence-based literature supports the efficacy of tegaserod in IBS. In several randomized-controlled trials, tegaserod was superior to placebo for relief of abdominal discomfort or pain, bloating, and constipation. Patients taking tegaserod had a statistically significant increase in stool frequency and consistency. In one study, a response to tegaserod was observed within the first treatment week. In addition, tegaserod produced greater satisfaction, work productivity, and improved quality of life than placebo ($P < .05$).

J. Lubiprostone

Lubiprostone (Amitiza) is specific chloride channel-2 activator that enhances intestinal fluid secretion to facilitate increased motility. It is currently indicated for the treatment of chronic constipation and has recently been approved for IBS-C. Lubiprostone increases weekly spontaneous bowel movements, and a significant number of patients respond within 24 hours. It is the only medicine for constipation with an indication for patients 65 years of age and older. There is one high-quality study published on lubiprostone in chronic constipation, and the rest of the data are in abstract form only. The main side effect is nausea, which can be alleviated by taking the medicine with food.

K. Rifaximin

Rifaximin (Xifaxan) is a nonsystemic (<0.4%) semisynthetic antibiotic whose spectrum includes most gram-positive and gram-negative bacteria, both aerobes and anaerobes. In one questionnaire study in patients with IBS, there was a statistically significant improvement in overall symptoms and less bloating ($P = .020$) over placebo. There was no difference in pain, diarrhea, or constipation. The dosage of rifaximin used in this study (400 mg orally, three times daily for 10 days) is higher than that approved by the FDA for traveler's diarrhea.

L. Probiotics

In a recent study, *Bifidobacterium infantis* 35624 was shown to alleviate abdominal pain and bloating and bowel movement difficulty. Another probiotic, which contains eight different strains of bacteria including lactobacillus and bifidobacteria, alleviated flatulence and slowed down stools in IBS patients.

Chey WD, Chey WY, Heath AT, et al. Long-term safety and efficacy of alosetron in women with severe diarrhea-predominant irritable bowel syndrome. *Am J Gastroenterol.* 2004;99:2195–2203. [PMID: 15555002]

DiPalma JA, Cleveland MB, McGowan J, et al. A randomized, multicenter, placebo-controlled trial of polyethylene glycol laxative for chronic treatment of chronic constipation. *Am J Gastroenterol.* 2007;102:1436–1441. [PMID: 17984738]

Johanson JF, Ueno R. Lubiprostone, a locally acting chloride channel activator, in adult patients with chronic constipation: a double-blind, placebo-controlled, dose-ranging study to evaluate efficacy and safety. *Aliment Pharmacol Ther.* 2007;25: 1351–1361. [PMID: 17509103]

Johanson JF, Wald A, Tougas G, et al. Effect of tegaserod in chronic constipation: a randomized double-blind, controlled trial. *Clin Gastroenterol Hepatol.* 2004;2:796–805. [PMID: 15354280]

Krause R, Ameen V, Gordon SH, et al. A randomized, double-blind, placebo-controlled study to assess efficacy and safety of 0.5 mg and 1 mg alosetron in women with severe diarrhea-predominant IBS. *Am J Gastroenterol.* 2007;102:1709–1719. [PMID: 17509028]

Morgan V, Pickens D, Gautam S, et al. Amitriptyline reduces rectal pain related activation of the anterior cingulate cortex in patients with irritable bowel syndrome. *Gut.* 2005;54:601–607. [PMID: 15831901]

Müller-Lissner S, Holtmann G, Rueegg P, et al. Tegaserod is effective in the initial and retreatment of irritable bowel syndrome with constipation. *Aliment Pharmacol Ther.* 2005;21:11–20. [PMID: 15644040]

Müller-Lissner S, Kamm MA, Musoglu A, et al. Safety, tolerability, and efficacy of tegaserod over 13 months in patients with chronic constipation. *Am J Gastroenterol.* 2006;101:2558–2569. [PMID: 17090282]

Novick J, Miner P, Krause R, et al. A randomized double-blind, placebo-controlled trial of tegaserod in female patients suffering from irritable bowel syndrome with constipation. *Aliment Pharmacol Ther.* 2002;16:1877–1888. [PMID: 12390096]

O'Mahoney L, McCarthy J, Kelly P, et al. Lactobacillus and Bifidobacterium in irritable bowel syndrome: symptom responses and relationship to cytokine profiles. *Gastroenterology.* 2005;128:541–551. [PMID: 15765388]

Tack J, Broekaert D, Fischler B, et al. A controlled crossover study of the selective serotonin reuptake inhibitor citalopram in irritable bowel syndrome. *Gut.* 2006;55:1096–1103. [PMID: 16401691]

Tougas G, Snape WJ Jr, Otten MH, et al. Long-term safety of tegaserod in patients with constipation-predominant irritable bowel syndrome. *Aliment Pharmacol Ther.* 2002;16:1701–1708. [PMID: 12269961]

Vahedi H, Merat S, Rashidioon A, et al. The effect of fluoxetine in patients with pain and constipation-predominant irritable bowel syndrome: a double-blind randomized-controlled study. *Aliment Pharmacol Ther.* 2005;22:381–385. [PMID: 16128675]

Acute Pancreatitis

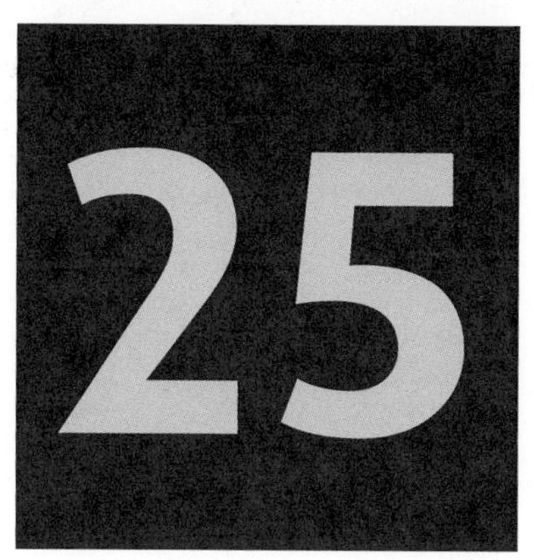

Bechien U Wu, MD, MPH
Darwin L. Conwell, MD, MS
Peter A. Banks, MD

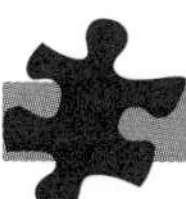

ESSENTIALS OF DIAGNOSIS

- Gallstone disease and alcohol are the most common causes of acute pancreatitis; other causes include hypertriglyceridemia, drugs, and specific disorders of the biliary tree and pancreas.
- Diagnosis is usually made based on a history of acute abdominal pain; a threefold elevation in serum amylase or lipase, or both; or an abnormal abdominal computed tomography (CT) scan showing changes of acute pancreatitis.
- Severe acute pancreatitis is characterized by persistent (>48 hours) organ failure (systemic blood pressure <90 mm Hg, PaO_2 <60 mm Hg, creatinine >2.0 mg/dL) or pancreatic necrosis.
- Diagnosis of necrotizing pancreatitis is confirmed by contrast-enhanced abdominal CT scan.

General Considerations

Acute pancreatitis is an acute inflammatory disorder of the pancreas that involves the pancreas and peri-pancreatic tissues but can sometimes affect other organ systems. The initial evaluation of patients with acute pancreatitis involves determining the cause and assessing the severity of disease since this guides subsequent management.

A. Incidence

Acute pancreatitis is the third most common inpatient gastrointestinal diagnosis in the United States. There were 243,332 hospitalizations in 2002 for acute pancreatitis with a median length of stay of 4 days and median charges amounting to $11,402. The incidence rate of acute pancreatitis appears to be increasing without any changes in the short-term or long-term case fatality rates.

B. Causes and Risk Factors

The most common causes of acute pancreatitis in the United States are gallstones and alcohol abuse, accounting for 70–80% of cases. Table 25–1 lists other causes, including hypertriglyceridemia, drug reactions, iatrogenic causes (eg, postsurgical or endoscopic retrograde cholangiopancreatography [ERCP]), hereditary factors, and idiopathic causes.

The first attack of alcohol-induced acute pancreatitis typically occurs after many (eg, 8–10) years of heavy alcohol consumption, and recurrent episodes can be anticipated if alcohol abuse continues. Gallstone-induced pancreatitis occurs in the setting of choledocholithiasis and is believed to be related to transient or complete obstruction of pancreatic ductal flow or reflux of bile into the pancreatic duct. Hypertriglyceridemia associated acute pancreatitis does not typically occur unless the triglyceride level exceeds 1000 mg/dL and is often seen in patients with type I and V hyperlipidemia as well as in alcoholics. Because triglyceride levels fall by one half in patients who have been fasting for 24 hours, levels are best assessed after an episode of acute pancreatitis with a fasting lipid profile in patients who are consuming a normal diet.

Although many drugs have been associated with acute pancreatitis, the strength of association between the use of a particular drug and the development of acute pancreatitis warrants careful scrutiny. Table 25–2 lists drugs that have a strong association with acute pancreatitis based on a recent review.

ERCP-induced acute pancreatitis is another cause of pancreatic injury. Acute pancreatitis is seen in 5–7% of ERCP cases and, despite extensive research into the medical and endoscopic prevention of post-ERCP pancreatitis, there has been little decline in the rates of occurrence. Recently, use of a prophylactic pancreatic duct stent placed after retrograde pancreatography has shown promise but requires further prospective evaluation. Risk factors for post-ERCP pancreatitis based on a recent prospective study, include minor papilla sphincterotomy, sphincter of Oddi dysfunction, prior history of post-ERCP pancreatitis, age younger than 60 years,

Table 25–1. Causes of acute pancreatitis.

Alcohol
Autoimmune
Biliary (eg, gallstones, gallbladder microlithiasis/sludge)
Drug-induced (see Table 25–2)
Iatrogenic
Surgery (eg, common bile duct exploration, sphincterotomy, splenectomy, distal gastrectomy)
ERCP
Idiopathic
Infectious (eg, ascariasis, clonorchiasis, mumps, toxoplasmosis, coxsackievirus, cytomegalovirus, tuberculosis, *Mycobacterium avium* complex)
Inherited
PRSS1 (cationic trypsinogen) mutations: hereditary pancreatitis)
CFTR (cystic fibrosis transmembrane conductance regulator) mutations
SPINK1 (serine protease inhibitor Kazal type 1) mutations
Metabolic (eg, hypercalcemia, hypertriglyceridemia)
Neoplastic (eg, pancreatic or ampullary tumors)
Structural (eg, pancreatic divisum, annular pancreas, sphincter of Oddi dysfunction, periampullary diverticula, duodenal duplication cysts, choledochocele, anomalous pancreaticobiliary junction, regional enteritis
Toxic (eg, organophosphates, scorpion venom)
Traumatic (especially motor vehicle accidents)
Vascular

more than two contrast injections into the pancreatic duct, and involvement of endoscopic trainees in the procedure.

In recent years, molecular genetic techniques have increased our understanding of acute pancreatitis. Hereditary pancreatitis is an autosomal-dominant disease most commonly associated with mutations in the cationic trypsinogen PRSS1 gene that leads to the inability to deactivate intracellular trypsin resulting in acinar cell auto-digestion. Hereditary pancreatitis should be suspected in patients with early-onset (before 20 years of age) acute pancreatitis or those with a strong family history of idiopathic acute pancreatitis in first- or second-degree relatives. Mutations in the cystic fibrosis transmembrane conductance regulator (*CFTR*) gene are increasingly being recognized as a cause of both acute and chronic pancreatitis. The mechanism of injury is not completely known but is most likely related to decreased pancreatic juice flow due to duct cell secretory dysfunction. Patients with a family history of cystic fibrosis or a history of recurrent pulmonary symptoms (eg, bronchitis, asthma) nasal polyps, or sterility among males should be considered for genetic testing.

Badalov N, Baradarian R, Iswara K, et al. Drug-induced acute pancreatitis: an evidence-based review. *Clin Gastroenterol Hepatol.* 2007;5:648–661. [PMID: 17395548]

Cheng CL, Sherman S, Watkins JL, et al. Risk factors for post-ERCP pancreatitis: a prospective multicenter study. *Am J Gastroenterol.* 2006;101:139–147. [PMID: 16405547]

Fagenholz PJ, Castillo CF, Harris NS, Pelletier AJ, Carmago CA JR. Increasing United States hospital admissions for acute pancreatitis. 1998–2003. *Ann Epidemiol.* 2007;17:491–497 [PMID: 17448682]

Frank CD, Adler DG. Post-ERCP pancreatitis and its prevention. *Nat Clin Pract Gastroenterol Hepatol.* 2006;3:680–688. [PMID: 17130878]

Keiles S, Kammesheidt A. Identification of CFTR, PRSS1, and SPINK1 mutations in 381 patients with pancreatitis. *Pancreas.* 2006;33:221–227. [PMID 17003641]

Shaheen NJ, Hansen RA, Morgan DR, et al. The burden of gastrointestinal and liver diseases, 2006. *Am J Gastroenterol.* 2006; 101:2128–2138. [PMID: 16848807]

Pathogenesis

Acute pancreatitis develops in response to premature activation of intracellular trypsinogen (which causes acinar cell injury) and the release of chemokines and cytokines (which results in the recruitment of neutrophils and macrophages). Recent advances in our understanding of hereditary pancreatitis include the discovery of trypsinogen gene mutations, *PRSS1* and *SPINK1*. Mutations in these genes lead to an imbalance of proteases and their inhibitors within the pancreatic parenchyma, resulting in inappropriate activation of pancreatic zymogens with subsequent autodigestion and inflammation. This, in turn, produces further injury to the acinar cells and elevation of proinflammatory mediators.

The exact mechanisms leading to alcoholic and biliary acute pancreatitis remain to be defined. Gallstone pancreatitis, however, is now the most common etiology. Only a small proportion of patients who abuse alcohol develop pancreatitis. Alcohol metabolism is governed by both oxidative and nonoxidative processes. The oxidative pathway lies primarily within the liver while the nonoxidative pathway lies primarily in the pancreas. The nonoxidative pathway leads to the formation of fatty acid ethanol esters (FAEEs). It is postulated that accumulation of FAEEs may result in alcoholic acute pancreatitis. Biliary pancreatitis is most commonly caused by the passage of a stone from the gallbladder through the cystic duct into the common bile duct; impaction at the ampulla of Vater causes either reflux of bile into the pancreatic duct (Opie 1) or outflow obstruction of the pancreatic duct (Opie 2).

Clinical Findings

A. Symptoms and Signs

Abdominal pain is the most common symptom in patients presenting with acute pancreatitis. The pain is typically epigastric and radiates to the back. Patients also often present with nausea and vomiting. In patients with severe acute pancreatitis, signs and symptoms parallel the presence of a systemic inflammatory response and organ dysfunction. Patients with SIRS (temperature >30°C, respiratory rate of >24 per minute, heart rate >90 per minute, white blood count >12,000, or >10% bands), which arises in response to

Table 25–2. Drugs implicated in acute pancreatitis based on class.

Class IA[a]	Class IB[b]	Class II[c]
α-Methyldopa	All-transretinoic acid	Acetaminophen
Arabinoside	Amiodarone	Chlorothiazide
Azodisalicylate	Azathioprine	Clozapine
Bezafibrate	Clomiphene	Dideoxyinosine (DDI)
Cannabis	Dexamethasone	Erythromycin
Carbimazole	Ifosfamide	Estrogen
Codeine	Lamivudine	L-Asparaginase
Cytosine	Losartan	Pegasparaginase
Dapsone	Lynestrenol/methoxyethinylestradiol	Propofol
Enalapril	6-mercaptopurine	Tamoxifen
Furosemide	Meglumine	
Isoniazid	Methimazole	
Mesalamine	Nelfinavir	
Metronidazole	Norethindronate/mestranol	
Pentamidine	Omeprazole	
Pravastatin	Premarin	
Procainamide	Sulfamethoxazole	
Pyritinol	Trimethoprim–sulfamethoxazole	
Simvastatin		
Stibogluconate		
Sulfamethoxazole		
Sulindac		
Tetracycline		
Valproic acid		

[a]Class IA: at least one case report with positive rechallenge, excluding all other causes of acute pancreatitis.
[b]Class IB: at least one case report with positive rechallenge; however, other causes of acute pancreatitis not ruled out.
[c]Class II: at least four cases in the literature, consistent latency in ≥75% of cases (period between initiation of drug and development of acute pancreatitis).
Adapted, with permission, from Badalov N, Baradarian R, Iswara K, et al. Drug-induced acute pancreatitis: an evidence-based review. *Clin Gastroenterol Hepatol.* 2007;5:648–661.

proinflammatory mediators, can present with fever, tachycardia, tachypnea, or a combination of these findings. Other examination findings include respiratory distress, crackles or absent breathe sounds on lung auscultation, cool extremities, impaired mental status, decreased bowel sounds, abdominal distention, oliguria, and anuria. Cullen sign (periumbilical ecchymoses) and Grey Turner sign (flank ecchymoses) are rare but can be seen in cases of acute pancreatitis with hemorrhage and are associated with increased mortality.

B. Laboratory Findings

Serum amylase and lipase are the principle laboratory tests that aid in the diagnosis of acute pancreatitis. Elevations greater than three times the upper limit of normal are typically used to diagnose acute pancreatitis. However, both enzymes can be elevated in other disease states. For example, amylase is also produced by non-pancreatic organs such as salivary glands, ovaries, and fallopian tubes; thus, diseases of these organs can increase the serum amylase level. Pancreatic amylase and lipase can be elevated in other intra-abdominal disease states such as a perforated ulcer, intestinal obstruction, and mesenteric infarction. Both amylase and lipase are elevated in patients with renal insufficiency or critical illness in the absence of acute pancreatitis.

Serum amylase has rapid clearance and a short half-life and therefore is best measured when there is a brief interval between symptom onset and diagnosis. Serum lipase begins to rise later after symptom onset, but its longer half-life makes it useful to measure when there has been a delay in seeking care. Serum lipase is a more sensitive and specific indicator of acute pancreatitis than serum amylase. The combination of both serum amylase and lipase does not appear to increase the accuracy of diagnosis. The degree of elevation of both serum amylase and lipase does not correlate with severity of acute pancreatitis, nor does the daily assessment of serum pancreatic enzymes help to determine clinical deterioration or resolution.

Elevated findings on liver biochemical tests in a patient with suspected acute pancreatitis usually signify a biliary cause. A threefold elevation in alanine aminotransferase in the setting of acute pancreatitis has been shown to have a 95% positive predictive value for gallstone pancreatitis.

C. Imaging Studies

In the early stages of illness, transabdominal ultrasound is the most widely recommended diagnostic imaging test for patients with acute pancreatitis, primarily in order to evaluate for a potential biliary etiology. Contrast-enhanced abdominal-computed tomography (CT) is not recommended for the initial evaluation of acute pancreatitis unless the diagnosis is uncertain. By contrast, in the setting of persistent abdominal pain or clinical deterioration after 48–72 hours, a contrast-enhanced CT can be useful to evaluate for local complications such as necrosis or development of an acute fluid collection. Findings of interstitial acute pancreatitis that are typically seen on CT scan include enlargement of the pancreas with edema, heterogeneous pancreatic parenchyma, peripancreatic fat stranding, and peripancreatic fluid collections (Figure 25–1). Acute pancreatic necrosis typically appears as focal or diffuse areas of non enhanced pancreatic parenchyma (Figure 25–2).

Timing of CT imaging is important. If an admission diagnosis of acute pancreatitis can be made on the basis of history, physical examination, and elevated pancreatic enzymes, a CT scan should generally be deferred. Given that some patients will present with or develop renal failure, aggressive fluid resuscitation with correction of renal function and intravascular volume resuscitation should take place prior to a contrast-enhanced CT due to the risk of inducing renal insufficiency. Alternatively, a non–contrast-enhanced study can be performed.

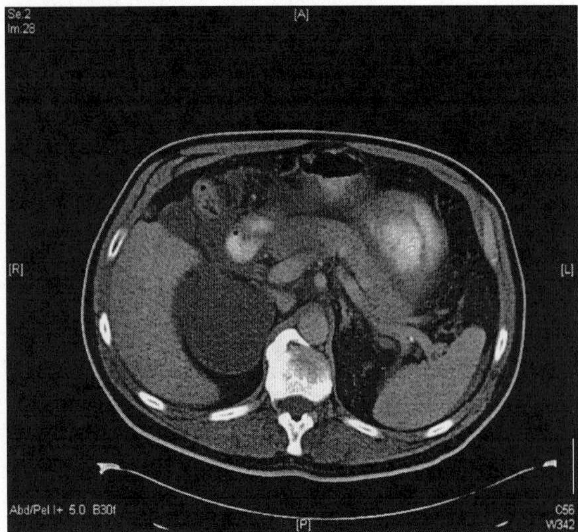

▲ **Figure 25–1.** CT scan showing interstitial acute pancreatitis. There is uniform enhancement of the pancreatic parenchyma, indicating that pancreatic perfusion is preserved. (Benign right renal cyst.)

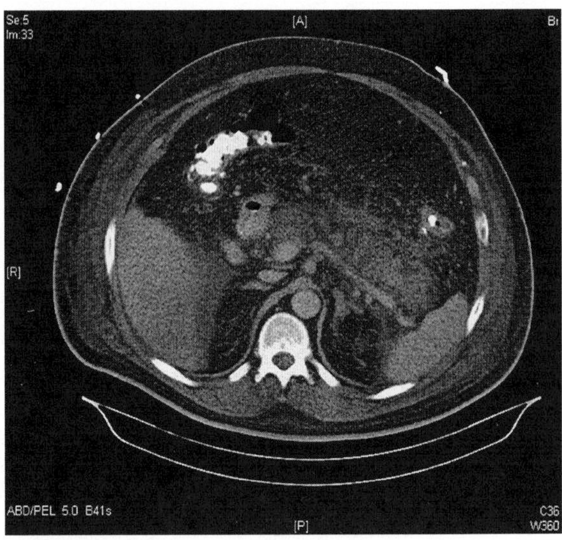

▲ **Figure 25–2.** CT scan showing necrotizing acute pancreatitis. Pancreatic perfusion is diminished on contrast enhancement.

Magnetic resonance cholangiopancreatography (MRCP) can be a helpful modality for further evaluation of a biliary etiology or detection of a retained choledocholith. Gadolinium should not be used in patients with renal impairment.

D. Diagnostic Approach

1. Confirmation of the diagnosis—The diagnosis of acute pancreatitis is usually made when there is a history of acute abdominal pain and a threefold elevation in serum amylase or lipase, or both, or an abnormal abdominal CT scan demonstrating changes consistent with acute pancreatitis.

2. Indications for more extensive evaluation—Even after a careful history and physical examination, laboratory evaluation, abdominal ultrasonography, and CT scan, the cause of 20–30% of cases of acute pancreatitis cannot be elucidated. These cases are termed idiopathic or unexplained. Recent reports suggest that nearly 70% of patient with a single or recurrent episode of idiopathic acute pancreatitis have biliary microlithiasis or sludge from cholesterol monohydrate crystals or calcium bilirubinate granules.

There is considerable debate regarding which subgroup of patients requires more extensive evaluation after being diagnosed with idiopathic acute pancreatitis. It has been suggested that patients younger than age 40, who have had only a single episode of acute pancreatitis, need no further evaluation as the recurrence rate is low. However, patients older than 40 years who have had a single episode and patients who have had two or more episodes of idiopathic pancreatitis require more extensive evaluation. Patients older than 40 years are thought to have an increased risk of pancreatic malignancy. Therefore, a contrast-enhanced CT scan should be part of the evaluation. If the CT scan is negative, then attention is directed at the pancreaticobiliary anatomy. Guidelines from several societies recommend a repeat abdominal ultrasound to evaluate for evidence of biliary sludge that can be missed in the acute setting. In patients with recurrent episodes of idiopathic acute pancreatitis, evaluation by a combination of MRCP and endoscopic ultrasound has been shown to detect additional causes of pancreatitis. Abnormalities noted on either endoscopic ultrasound evaluation or magnetic resonance imaging should prompt consideration of endoscopic or surgical therapy (Figure 25–3). Causes of idiopathic or unexplained acute pancreatitis commonly found during endoscopic evaluation are listed in Table 25–3.

Table 25–3. Causes of idiopathic or unexplained acute pancreatitis diagnosed by endoscopic evaluation.[a]

Ampullary lesions
Choledocholithiasis
Chronic pancreatitis
Gallbladder microlithiasis or sludge
Pancreas divisum
Pancreatic cancer
Sphincter of Oddi dysfunction

[a]Exclusion of hyperlipidemia and medications.

Wilcox CM, Varadarajulu S, Eloubeidi M. Role of endoscopic evaluation in idiopathic pancreatitis: a systematic review. *Gastrointest Endosc.* 2006;63:1037–1045. [PMID: 16733122]

3. Criteria for assessing severity in acute pancreatitis—Assessment of severity in patients with acute pancreatitis is essential for appropriate triage and management. The basis

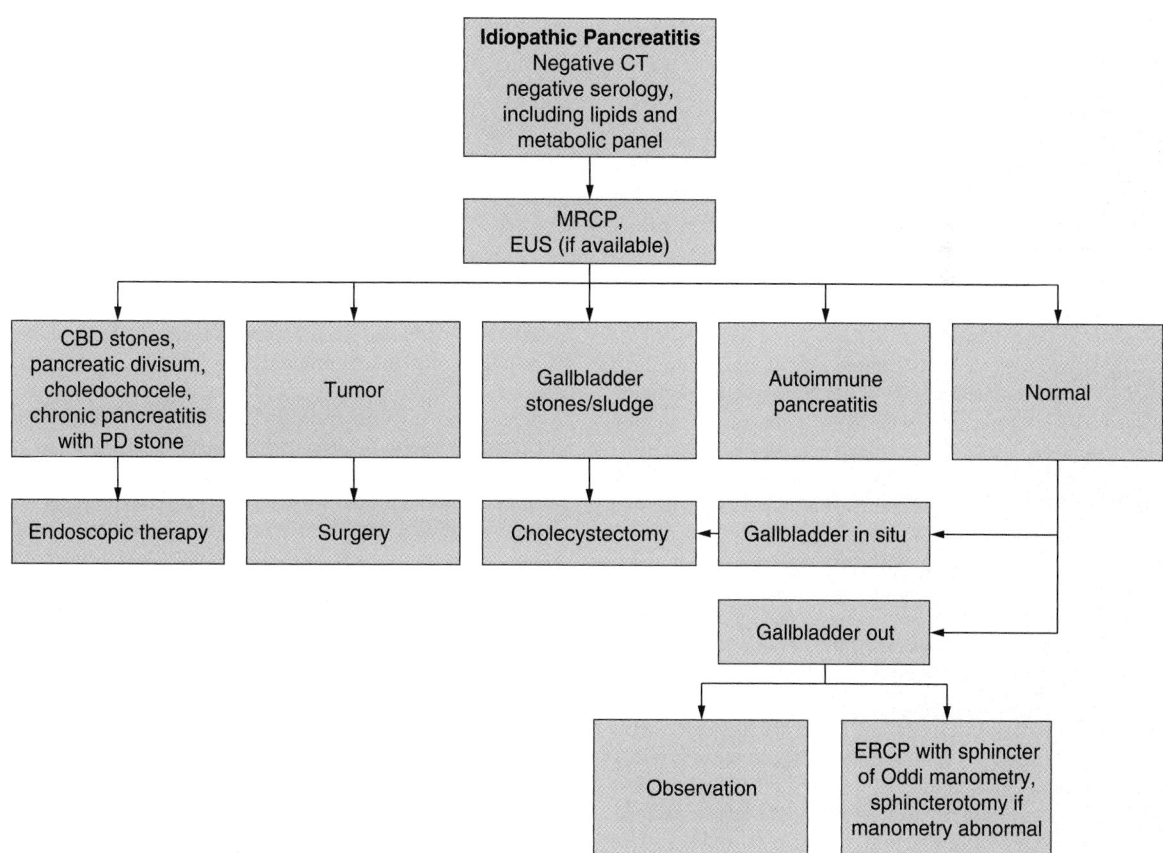

▲ **Figure 25–3.** Algorithm for the evaluation and management of idiopathic pancreatitis. CBD, common bile duct; CT, computed tomography; ERCP, endoscopic retrograde cholangiopancreatography; EUS, endoscopic ultrasound; MRCP, magnetic resonance cholangiopancreatography; PD, pancreatic duct.

for the classification, severity, and complications of acute pancreatitis was established at the International Symposium held in Atlanta in 1992 that is currently undergoing revision. Although the definitions have come under greater scrutiny in recent years, they still serve as the common language for clinical care and research in acute pancreatitis. The criteria for severe acute pancreatitis were defined as organ failure of at least one organ system (systolic blood pressure <90 mm Hg, PaO_2 <60 mm Hg, creatinine >2.0 mg/dL after rehydration, and gastrointestinal bleeding >500 mL/24 h) and the presence of local complications such as necrosis, pseudocyst, and abscess.

Early predictors of severity at 48 hours included 3 or more Ranson signs and an APACHE II score of 8 or higher. However, as illustrated in recent data from a large multicenter study of intensive care units, the vast majority of patients with acute pancreatitis that require admission to an intensive care unit experience clinical deterioration within the first 24 hours of hospitalization. Traditional severity indices such as APACHE II and Ranson criteria have not been as useful clinically because they are cumbersome, require collection of a large number of clinical and laboratory variables over 48 hours, and do not have acceptable positive and negative predictive value for severe acute pancreatitis. A more recently developed and widely validated clinical scoring system for use during the initial 24 hours of hospitalization for acute pancreatitis is the Bedside Index of Severity in Acute Pancreatitis (BISAP). This five-factor scoring system assigns one point for the presence of each of the following, either at admission or during the initial 24 hours of hospitalization: **B**UN >25 mg/dL, **I**mpaired mental status, **S**IRS, **A**ge >60 and a **P**leural effusion. A score of ≥3 points has been associated with increased risk of mortality and complications such as necrosis as well as organ dysfunction.

Apart from the severity indices, additional factors can be used to assess severity in acute pancreatitis. Patient-related risk factors for severe acute pancreatitis include older age (>60 years), obesity (basal metabolic index ≥30), and comorbid disease. In terms of prognostic indices, the persistence of SIRS for >48 hours or any rise in blood urea nitrogen (BUN) during the initial period of resuscitation indicate a poor prognosis marked by increased risk of in-hospital mortality.

The importance of differentiating interstitial from necrotizing acute pancreatitis has led to the development of a CT severity index as another measure of severity. It is best evaluated 2–3 days into hospitalization because it may not be possible to distinguish interstitial from necrotizing pancreatitis on contrast-enhanced CT scan early in the disease course. CT identification of local complications, particularly necrosis, is essential because patients with infected and sterile necrosis are at greatest risk of death, with a median mortality rate of 30% and 12%, respectively. The median prevalence of organ failure is 54% in necrotizing pancreatitis. The prevalence of organ failure is about the same in infected versus sterile necrosis. A recent meta-analysis found that both infected necrosis and organ dysfunction were independent predictors of mortality in severe acute pancreatitis, such that infected necrosis was associated with pooled risk of mortality of 32%, organ failure alone 30% whereas presence of both infected necrosis and organ failure was associated with mortality >40%. Thus, patients with infected necrosis and multisystem organ failure are the most likely to die.

Table 25–4. Differential diagnosis of acute pancreatitis.

Perforated viscus
Cholecystitis
Bowel obstruction
Vascular occlusion (especially mesentery venous disease)
Renal colic
Inferior myocardial infarction
Pneumonia
Diabetic ketoacidosis
Duodenal ulcer

Differential Diagnosis

It is important to exclude other potential intra-abdominal diseases in patients for whom the diagnosis of acute pancreatitis is not certain, especially when management calls for potential surgical intervention. Table 25–4 lists conditions of which the clinician should be particularly aware.

Complications

The complications observed in acute pancreatitis can be related either to local tissue injury or systemically mediated effects. Potential local complications include development of an acute fluid collection, and pancreatic ascites from a pancreas duct disruption. Interventions on pancreatic fluid collections should be considered only in the context of secondary infection or persistence of subsequent symptoms such as abdominal pain or gastric obstruction. Recent literature suggests a benefit of a more conservative approach to even infected necrosis with delayed surgical intervention, temporizing measures such as percutaneous drainage, and in some cases, antibiotic treatment alone. If drainage is considered, this can now be achieved safely by both an endoscopic or surgical approach. Pancreatic ascites or pleural effusion can be managed with endoscopic therapy if the disruption can be "bridged" with a pancreatic stent. Otherwise, surgical therapy may be necessary. Bleeding complications from esophagogastric varices can rarely occur from splenic vein obstruction. In addition, bleeding from a pseudoaneurysm can represent a life-threatening emergency in which angiography is the preferred initial intervention.

Less commonly seen complications include pancreatic encephalopathy, subcutaneous fat necrosis, or splenic complications such as a subcapsular hematoma.

Treatment

A. Mild Acute Pancreatitis

The majority of patients with mild acute pancreatitis respond to supportive care measures that include bowel rest, intravenous hydration with crystalloid, and analgesia. Oral intake can be resumed once the patient is pain free in the absence of parenteral analgesia, has no nausea or vomiting, has normal bowel sounds, and is hungry. Typically, a clear or full liquid diet has been recommended for the initial meal, but a low-fat solid diet is a reasonable choice following recovery from mild acute pancreatitis. Patients discharged with continued pain or tolerating less than a solid diet are at increased risk for early readmission for pancreatitis.

Patients with gallstone pancreatitis are also at increased risk of recurrence. Therefore, following recovery from mild pancreatitis, a laparoscopic cholecystectomy during the same admission is recommended as secondary prevention. An alternative for patients who are not surgical candidates based on comorbid disease or local complications (Figure 25–4) would be to perform an endoscopic biliary sphincterotomy.

B. Severe Acute Pancreatitis

In addition to the aforementioned supportive measures, patients at increased risk of severe acute pancreatitis at admission based on obesity, hemoconcentration, or azotemia should receive vigorous fluid resuscitation. A decrease in hematocrit and/or fall in the BUN by at least 5 mg/dL during the initial 12–24 hours suggests a favorable response to fluid resuscitation. If the hematocrit remains elevated or the BUN rises during resuscitation, the patient may require further hemodynamic monitoring to facilitate adequate resuscitation.

Patients with sustained organ failure that does not respond to increased fluids (to counteract hypotension and increased serum creatinine) or nasal oxygen (to overcome hypoxemia), as well as patients with labored respirations that may herald respiratory failure, should be transferred to an intensive care unit for close monitoring as these patients may require intubation with mechanical ventilation, hemodialysis, and support of blood pressure.

Once it is clear that a patient will not be able to tolerate oral feeding (a determination that can usually be made within 48–72 hours), enteral nutrition (rather than total parenteral nutrition) should be considered. Enteral nutrition maintains gut barrier integrity, thereby preventing bacterial translocation, is less expensive, and is associated with fewer complications than parenteral nutrition. Recent data from a large multicenter randomized-controlled trial has refuted earlier suggestions that probiotics may be helpful in the management of severe acute pancreatitis. Specifically, treatment with probiotics was associated with increased mortality compared to placebo. The best route for administration of enteral nutrition remains controversial. The nasogastric route is easier to establish and may be as safe as the nasojejunal route; however, enteral nutrition that bypasses the stomach and duodenum is believed to produce less pancreatic secretions. Neither route has been shown to alter morbidity and mortality. When patients with necrotizing pancreatitis begin oral intake of food, consideration should also be given to the addition of pancreatic enzyme supplementation to assist with fat digestion, and proton pump inhibitor therapy to reduce gastric acid because of reduced pancreatic bicarbonate secretion.

There is currently no role for prophylactic antibiotics in either interstitial or necrotizing pancreatitis. Although

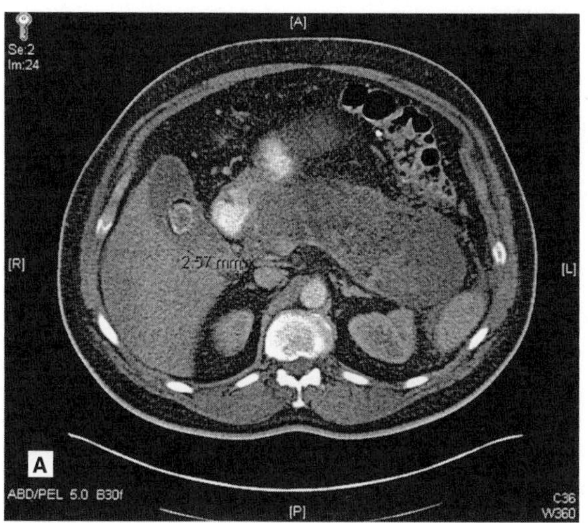

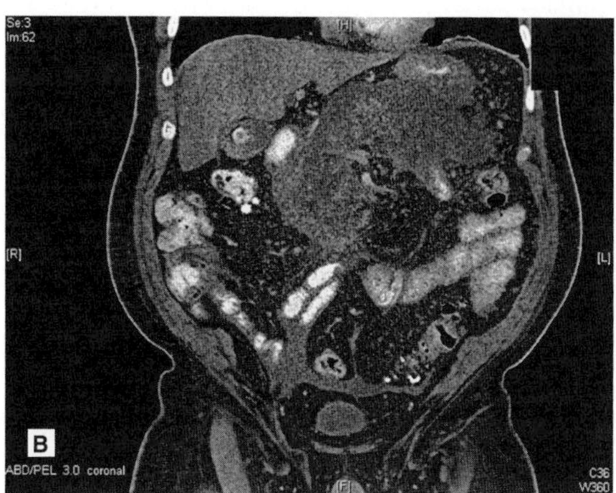

▲ **Figure 25–4.** CT scan in a patient with gallstone pancreatitis. **A:** Axial image with walled-off necrosis and gallbladder stone. **B:** Coronal image showing extent of necrosis and presence of a calcified gallstone.

previous small trials and meta-analyses had suggested benefit, the two most recent adequately powered double-blind randomized controlled trials were unable to demonstrate any impact on the rate of infected necrosis with use of prophylactic carbapenems or fluoroquinolone antibiotics. It is reasonable to start antibiotics in a patient who is clinically unstable while awaiting the results of cultures. If culture results are negative, then antibiotics should be discontinued to minimize the risk of developing fungal superinfection or *Clostridium difficile.*

Percutaneous aspiration of necrosis with Gram stain and culture should generally not be performed until at least 7–10 days after establishing a diagnosis of necrotizing pancreatitis, and then only if there are ongoing signs of possible pancreatic infection such as sustained leukocytosis, fever, or organ failure. Once the diagnosis of infected necrosis is established, appropriate antibiotics should be initiated and surgical debridement should be considered. There exist minimally invasive alternative therapies such as endoscopic, percutaneous catheter, and retroperitoneal techniques for necrosectomy. The optimal approach to management of infected necrosis continues to evolve. There are currently no large randomized studies supporting the use of one modality over another. However, there has been an increasing trend in favor of more conservative, less invasive approaches to management. Temporizing measures such as percutaneous catheter drainage have gained increasing acceptance for management of critically ill patients. For patients with sterile necrosis, medical management is preferred to surgical management unless patients continue to exhibit abdominal pain and are unable to resume oral intake. Surgical debridement should be delayed whenever possible to allow for resolution of inflammation and the development of walled-off necrosis.

There are several clearly defined roles for ERCP in acute pancreatitis. Urgent ERCP (within 24 hours) is indicated in patients who have severe acute biliary pancreatitis with organ failure or cholangitis, or both. Elective ERCP with sphincterotomy can be considered in patients with persistent or incipient biliary obstruction, those deemed to be poor candidates for cholecystectomy, and those in whom there is strong suspicion of bile duct stones after cholecystectomy. ERCP also is indicated for pancreatic ductal disruptions that occur as part of the inflammatory process and result in persistent peripancreatic fluid collections.

Banks PA, Freeman ML. Practice Parameters Committee of the American College of Gastroenterology. Practice guidelines in acute pancreatitis. *Am J Gastroenterol.* 2006;101:2379–2400. [PMID: 17032204]

McClave S. Nutrition support in acute pancreatitis. *Gastroenterol Clin North Am.* 2007;36:65–74. [PMID: 17472875]

Pandol SJ, Saluja AK, Imrie CW, et al. Acute pancreatitis: bench to the bedside. *Gastroenterology.* 2007;132:1127–1151. [PMID: 17854616]

Whitcomb DC. Clinical practice. Acute pancreatitis. *N Engl J Med.* 2006;354:2142–2150. [PMID: 16707751]

Wu BU, Johannes RS, Sun X, Conwell DL, Banks PA. Early changes in blood urea nitrogen predict mortality in acute pancreatitis. *Gastroenterology* 2009; 137:129–135. [PMID: 19344722]

Wu BU, Johannes RS, Sun X, Tabak Y, Conwell DL, Banks PA. The early prediction of mortality in acute pancreatitis: a large population-based study. *Gut* 2008; 57:1698–1703. [PMID: 18519429]

This chapter is a revised version of the chapter by Dr. Vikesh Singh, Dr. Darwin Conwell, and Dr. Peter Banks that was in the previous edition of Current Diagnosis & Treatment: Gastroenterology, Hepatology, & Endoscopy.

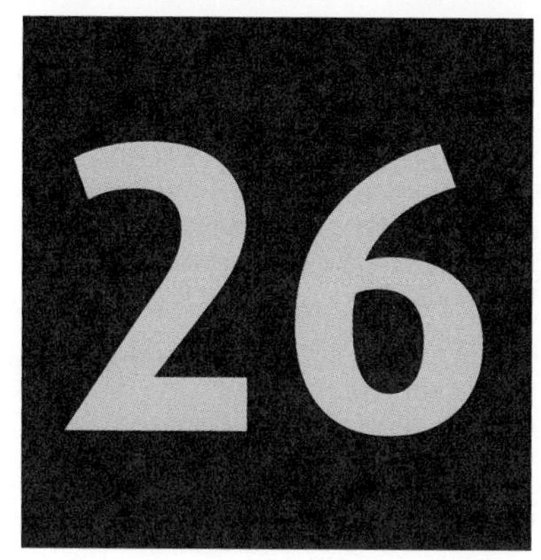

Chronic Pancreatitis

Darwin L. Conwell, MD, MS
Bechien Wu, MD, MPH
Peter A. Banks, MD

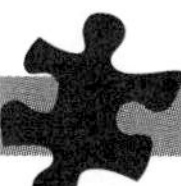

ESSENTIALS OF DIAGNOSIS

- Diagnosis relies on a combination of clinical findings, imaging tests, and pancreatic function testing.
- Pancreatic calcifications, dilated pancreatic ducts, diabetes mellitus, and maldigestion characterize advanced disease.
- Early-stage diagnosis remains a clinical challenge, especially in patients with chronic or episodic abdominal pain and no imaging abnormalities.

General Considerations

Although several risk factors for the development of chronic pancreatitis have been identified, the cause of pancreatitis in some instances remains uncertain. Among established risk factors, alcohol ingestion is associated with up to 60–70% of cases of chronic pancreatitis. In addition, ductal obstruction, autoimmune disease, tropical disease, and an association with further systemic illnesses such as scleroderma and hypertriglyceridemia have been described. Recently new insights have been gained into the genetic and molecular basis associated with hereditary forms of chronic pancreatitis. Recent epidemiologic studies clearly demonstrate that smoking is emerging as an independent risk factor for chronic pancreatitis development. The most widely accepted system of etiologic classification for chronic pancreatitis is the TIGAR-O system, which categorizes risk factors according to mechanism and prevalence (Table 26–1). A more recent M-ANNHEIM multiple risk factor classification system incorporates etiology, different stages of the disease, and various degrees of clinical severity. This system will be helpful for research studies investigating the impact and interaction of various risk factors on the course of the disease and will facilitate the comparison and combination of interinstitutional data.

Cote GA, Yadav D, Slivka A, et al. *Clin Gastroenterol Hepatol.* 2010; [Epub ahead of print].

Etemad B, Whitcomb DC. Chronic pancreatitis: diagnosis, classification, and new genetic developments. *Gastroenterology.* 2001;120: 682–707. [PMID: 11179244]

Schneider A, Lohr JM, Singer MV. The M-ANNHEIM classification of chronic pancreatitis: introduction of a unifying classification system based on a review of previous classifications of the disease. *J Gastroenterol.* 2007;42:101–119. [PMID: 17351799]

Yadav D, Hawes RH, Brand RE, et al. Alcohol consumption, cigarette smoking, and the risk of recurrent acute and chronic pancreatitis. *Arch Intern Med.* 2009;169:1035–1045. [PMID: 19506173]

Yadav D, Whitcomb DC. The role of alcohol and smoking in pancreatitis. *Nat Rev Gastroenterol Hepatol.* 2010;7:131–145. [PMID: 20125091]

Pathogenesis

Morphologic changes associated with chronic pancreatitis include ductal, parenchymal, and nerve changes. Pancreatic ducts may become dilated, irregular, or strictured. Meanwhile, the glandular tissue itself is often characterized by irregular and patchy replacement of normal acinar cell architecture with fibrosis. Morphologic features of neuritis, and hypertrophy may account for part of the pain syndrome.

Several hypotheses have been proposed to explain the mechanisms underlying the pathogenesis of chronic pancreatitis. These focus on (1) the role of oxidative stress, (2) toxic-metabolic causes, (3) obstructive causes, and (4) necrosis-fibrosis (also referred to as the *S*entinel *A*cute *P*ancreatitis *E*vent [SAPE] hypothesis). (Table 26–2). The oxidative-stress hypothesis attributes pancreatic damage to reflux of bile rich in reactive oxidation byproducts. The toxic-metabolic theory involves direct damage to pancreatic acinar cells from noxious stimuli such as alcohol. The obstructive theory attributes the majority of injury to pancreatic ductal injury resulting from obstruction related to increased lithogenicity, the latter, in turn, caused by either genetic or environmental exposures (eg, alcohol). Finally,

Table 26–1. TIGAR-O classification of chronic pancreatitis.

Toxic-Metabolic
Alcoholic
Tobacco smoking
Hypercalcemia (hyperparathyroidism)
Hyperlipidemia (rare and controversial)
Chronic renal failure
Idiopathic
Cause unknown, likely genetic origin
Tropical
Genetic
Autosomal dominant
Cationic trypsinogen
Autosomal recessive/modifier genes
CFTR mutations
SPINK1 mutations
α_1-Antitrypsin deficiency (possible)
Autoimmune
Isolated autoimmune chronic pancreatitis
Associated with:
• Primary sclerosing cholangitis
• Sjögren syndrome
• Primary biliary cirrhosis
• Type 1 diabetes mellitus
Recurrent and Severe Acute Pancreatitis
Postnecrotic (severe acute pancreatitis)
Vascular diseases/ischemia
Postradiation exposure
Obstructive
Pancreas divisum (controversial)
Sphincter of Oddi dysfunction (controversial)
Duct obstruction (tumors, post-traumatic)

the necrosis-fibrosis hypothesis describes chronic pancreatitis as a continuum that is initiated early by an attack of acute pancreatitis; the subsequent recurrent injury and remodeling lead to pancreatic fibrosis. This hypothesis has gained further support with the observation of progression to chronic pancreatitis from childhood through adulthood

Table 26–2. Sentinel Acute Pancreatitis Event (SAPE) hypothesis.

Step 1: Acinar cell stimulation
—Alcohol, gallstone, elevated triglyceride, oxidative stress, smoking, genetic mutations
Step 2: Sentinel event
—Early: pro-inflammatory response
—Late: stellate cells, pro-fibrotic response
Step 3: Removal of stimulus
—Abstinence from alcohol
—Cholecystectomy
—Lipid lowering agents
Step 4: Recurrent stimulation
—Stellate cell mediated periacinar fibrosis
• TGF beta, PDGF, procollagen, matrix proteins

Used with permission from Stevens T, Conwell DL. *Am J Gastroenterol.* 2004;99:2256.

of patients with a rare disorder known as hereditary pancreatitis. This disorder, which is caused by a gain of function mutation in cationic trypsinogen, leads to recurrent bouts of acute pancreatitis with later onset of chronic pancreatitis. These explanations are not necessarily mutually exclusive, and a unifying model explaining the precise mechanisms leading to impaired ductal bicarbonate secretion and the patchy inflammatory changes seen on histopathologic examination remains to be further elucidated.

Recent characterization of pancreatic stellate cells (PSC) has added insight to the underlying cellular responses behind development of chronic pancreatitis. Specifically, PSCs are believed to play a role in maintaining normal pancreatic architecture, which can shift toward fibrogenesis in the case of chronic pancreatitis. It is believed that alcohol or additional stimuli lead to matrix metalloproteinase–mediated destruction of normal collagen in pancreatic parenchyma that later allows for pancreatic remodeling. Proinflammatory cytokines tumor necrosis factor-α (TNFα), interleukin (IL)-1, and IL-6, as well as oxidant complexes, are able to induce PSC activity with subsequent new collagen synthesis. In addition to being stimulated by cytokines, oxidants, or growth factors, PSCs also possess transforming growth factor-β (TGFβ)–mediated self-activating autocrine pathways, which may explain disease progression in chronic pancreatitis even after removal of noxious stimuli.

Ceyhan GC, Bergmann F, Kadihasanoglu M, et al. Pancreatic neuropathy and neuropathic pain: a comprehensive pathomorphological study of 546 cases. *Gastronterology.* 2009;136:177–186. [PMID: 18992743]

Di Sebastiano P, di Mola FF, Di Febbo C, et al. Expression of interleukin 8 (IL-8) and substance P in human chronic pancreatitis. *Gut.* 2000;47:423–428. [PMID: 10940282]

Hoogerwerf WA, Gondesen K, Xiao SY, et al. The role of mast cells in the pathogenesis of pain in chronic pancreatitis. *BMC Gastroenterology.* 2005;5:8. [PMID: 15745445]

Mews P, Phillips P, Fahmy R, et al. Pancreatic stellate cells respond to inflammatory cytokines: potential role in chronic pancreatitis. *Gut.* 2002;50:535–541. [PMID: 11889076]

Omary MB, Lugea A, Lowe AW, Pandol SJ. The pancreatic stellate cell: a star on the rise in pancreatic diseases. *J Clin Invest.* 2007;117: 50–59. [PMID: 17200706]

Schneider A, Whitcomb DC. Hereditary pancreatitis: a model for inflammatory diseases of the pancreas. *Best Pract Res Clin Gastroenterol.* 2002;16:347–363. [PMID: 12079262]

Stevens T, Conwell DL, Zuccaro G. Pathogenesis of chronic pancreatitis: an evidence-based review of past theories and recent developments. *Am J Gastroenterol.* 2004;99:2256–2270. [PMID: 15555009]

Witt H, Apte MV, Keim V, et al. Chronic pancreatitis: challenges and advances in pathogenesis, genetics, diagnosis, and therapy. *Gastroenterology.* 2007;132:1557–1573. [PMID: 17466744]

Clinical Findings

A. Symptoms and Signs

The hallmark features of chronic pancreatitis are abdominal pain and pancreatic insufficiency. Advanced disease can also be associated with weight loss and diabetes. The possibility of chronic pancreatitis should be entertained in any patient with symptoms of chronic abdominal pain. Further supporting features on history include postprandial pain triggered by high-fat or protein-rich meals. In addition, predisposing etiologic factors according to the TIGAR-O classification should be actively sought with attention paid to indicators of possible inherited pancreatic disease such as family history of pancreatitis, pancreatic cancer, or cystic fibrosis.

1. Abdominal pain—The pain associated with chronic pancreatitis is classically described as epigastric, often with radiation to the back. Pain is often unrelenting and difficult to treat. Pain may be postprandial, associated with nausea and vomiting. Early in the disease course, pain is described as occurring in discrete episodes (type A pain). However, as the disease progresses pain may become continuous (type B pain). Ultimately, the pattern and course of pain symptoms is highly variable among patients with chronic pancreatitis. Up to 20–45% of patients having objective evidence of pancreatic endocrine or exocrine dysfunction may not have pain. Thus, pain is not a prerequisite for the diagnosis of chronic pancreatitis.

2. Pancreatic insufficiency—The second cardinal feature of chronic pancreatitis is the development of pancreatic exocrine and endocrine dysfunction with advanced disease. By comparison to the pain of chronic pancreatitis, the symptoms of pancreatic insufficiency are relatively easily managed. Clinically significant protein malabsorption and fat deficiency does not occur until over 90% of pancreatic function is lost. Typically steatorrhea precedes the onset of protein malabsorption. Fat malabsorption can manifest clinically as poorly formed greasy, malodorous stools. Although absorption of fat-soluble vitamins may be reduced, clinically significant vitamin deficiency is rarely reported. There have been numerous small reports of metabolic bone disease in patients with pancreas insufficiency. A recent epidemiologic study reported a high prevalence of low trauma fracture in chronic pancreatitis when compared to age- and gender-matched controls. In fact, the odds of fracture in chronic pancreatitis approached that of other high-risk gastrointestinal illnesses such as inflammatory bowel disease for which osteoporosis screening guidelines exist. Further studies are needed to explore the strength of this association.

Pancreatic endocrine insufficiency presenting as diabetes is a distinctly late occurrence. Patients with chronic calcific pancreatitis or with a family history of diabetes have been observed to be at increased risk of developing this complication. Although diabetes associated with chronic pancreatitis is insulin-requiring, these patients are also at increased risk of hypoglycemia due to impaired glucagon synthesis resulting from pancreatic α cell destruction.

Tignor AS, Wu BU, Whitlock TL, et al. High prevalence of low-trauma fracture in chronic pancreatitis. *Am J Gastroenterol.* 2010;105:2680–2686. [PMID: 20736937]

B. Laboratory Findings

Initial evaluation of chronic pancreatitis should begin with relatively simple and inexpensive testing. Amylase and lipase are often elevated during acute pain episodes early in the natural history of the disease. By contrast, normal or even low levels of amylase or lipase can be found in patients with moderate to advanced chronic pancreatitis. Fecal pancreatic elastase-1 (FPE-1) is a marker of exocrine pancreatic function. FPE-1 is assessed by an enzyme-linked immunosorbent assay (ELISA) performed on stool specimens. A level greater than 200 mcg/g of stool is considered normal, and FPE-1 levels less than 100 mcg/g of stool correlate with severe exocrine pancreatic insufficiency. Of note, pancreatic enzyme supplementation does not interfere with interpretation of test results. The widespread availability of FPE-1 testing has reduced the need for 24-hour fecal fat quantitation as a means of evaluating steatorrhea. A subset of patients with diarrhea predominant irritable bowel syndrome (D-IBS) have abnormal fecal elastase levels suggesting the presence of pancreas exocrine insufficiency. Pancreatic exocrine insufficiency was detected in 6.1% of patients who fulfilled the Rome II criteria for D-IBS in one study. In these patients, pancreatic enzyme therapy might reduce diarrhea and abdominal pain. The authors conclude that pancreatic exocrine insufficiency should be considered in patients with D-IBS. However, diarrhea can cause a falsely low (abnormal) fecal elastase and caution must be taken when interpreting results in this setting.

Additional tests that may be useful in evaluating chronic pancreatitis include hemoglobin A_{1c} (to investigate glucose intolerance) and markers of autoimmune chronic pancreatitis, including immunoglobulin G_4, rheumatoid factor, and antinuclear antibody. Elevation of liver function tests may signal compression of the pancreatic portion of the bile duct from fibrosis, edema, or tumor development.

Leeds JS, Hopper AD, Sidhu R, et al. Some patients with irritable bowel syndrome may have exocrine pancreatic insufficiency. *Clin Gastroenterol Hepatol.* 2010;8:433–438. [PMID: 19835990]

C. Imaging Studies

Plain abdominal radiographs may reveal calcifications within the pancreas (common in alcoholic and tropical pancreatitis). In general, transabdominal ultrasound has been associated with low sensitivity in diagnosing chronic pancreatitis except in patients with severe disease. Contrast-enhanced computed tomography (CT) and magnetic resonance imaging (MRI) offer enhanced visualization of the pancreas and adjoining structures. These latter two imaging modalities have increasingly become the mainstay of noninvasive imaging techniques for the diagnosis of chronic pancreatitis.

In addition to visualizing calcifications, contrast-enhanced CT allows evaluation of the parenchymal architecture (Figure 26–1). Complications such as pseudocysts (Figure 26–2),

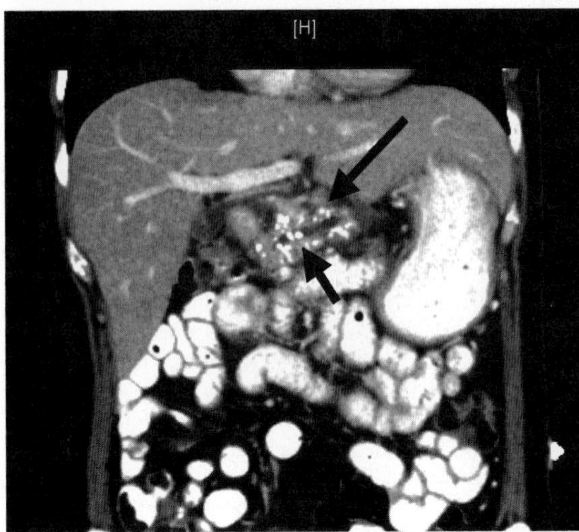

▲ **Figure 26–1.** CT Scan: Chronic calcific p. Coronal view of CT scan with visible calcifications throughout pancreas in a dilated main duct filled with stones.

pseudoaneurysms, and venous thromboses are well characterized by CT.

MRI technology, specifically magnetic resonance cholangiopancreatography (MRCP), has the ability to visualize fluid-filled structures allowing characterization of the pancreatic duct. When compared with endoscopic retrograde cholangiopancreatography (ERCP), MRI demonstrates similar ability to detect main duct abnormalities but is not as accurate in evaluating side branch disease. Although definitive studies have not been published, the administration of secretin has been demonstrated to enhance visualization of both the main pancreatic duct and side branches, which may be particularly useful in patients with early disease prior to the onset of clear ductal dilation (Figure 26–3). Standardization of reports and prospective studies are warranted to determine the diagnostic accuracy of MRI in the assessment of early chronic pancreatitis.

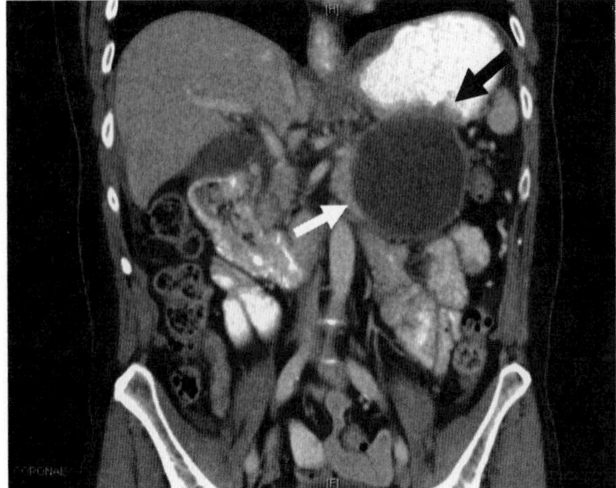

▲ **Figure 26–2.** CT Scan: Chronic symptomatic pseudocyst. Coronal CT scan with large pancreatic pseudocyst with visible compression of stomach (*black arrow*) and distal pancreas parenchyma (*white arrow*).

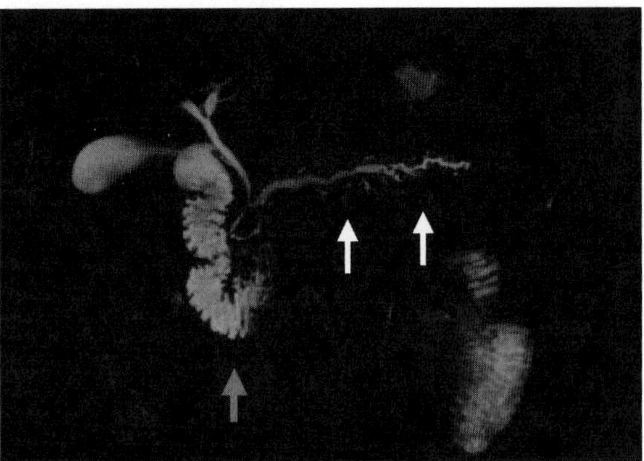

▲ **Figure 26–3.** Secretin enhanced MRCP (sMRCP): Chronic pancreatitis. MRCP/sMRCP with abnormal pancreatic duct with visible side branches (*white arrows*) and fluid-filled duodenum (*gray arrow*) after secretin stimulation.

Czakó L. Diagnosis of early-stage chronic pancreatitis by secretin-enhanced magnetic resonance cholangiopancreatography. *J Gastroenterol.* 2007;42 Suppl 17:113–117. [PMID: 17238039]

Sainani NI, Conwell DL. Secretin-enhanced MRCP: proceed with cautious optimism. *Am J Gastroenterol.* 2009;104:1787–1789. [PMID: 19455128]

Zuccaro P, Stevens T, Repas K, et al. Magnetic resonance cholangiopancreatography reports in the evaluation of chronic pancreatitis: a need for quality improvement. *Pancreatology.* 2009;9:764–769. [PMID: 20110743]

1. Endoscopic ultrasound (EUS)—One of the challenges for noninvasive testing remains the diagnosis of early–mild chronic pancreatitis. Increasingly EUS has played a role in this disease group. Previously established endosonographic criteria for the diagnosis of chronic pancreatitis include parenchymal features (atrophy, hyperechoic foci, stranding, cysts, and lobularity) and ductal features (narrowing, dilation, irregularity, calculi, side branch dilation, and hyperechoic walls) (Figure 26–4). The diagnosis usually requires identification of 5 (or more) of 9–11 criteria. The diagnostic significance of some features may be more important (major criteria) than other (minor) criteria but is an area of active research investigation. EUS also appears to be particularly beneficial when evaluating cystic lesions or neoplasms

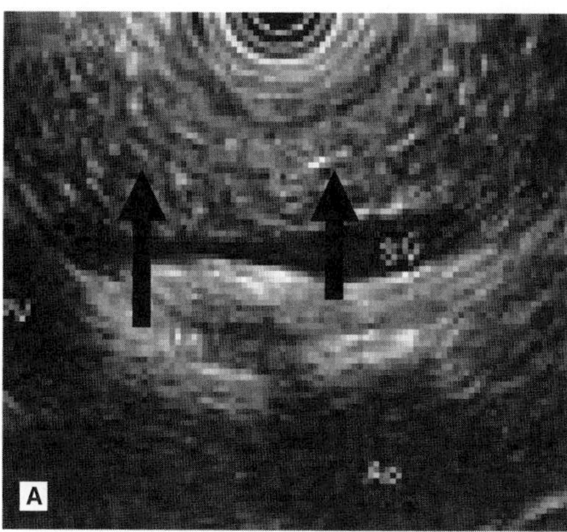

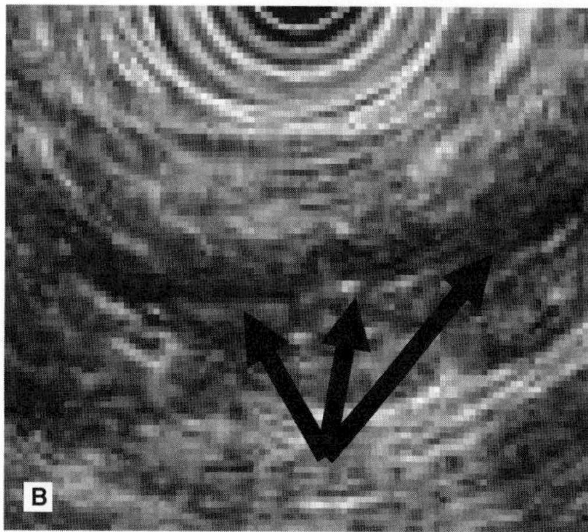

▲ **Figure 26–4.** Endoscopic ultrasound: chronic pancreatitis features. **A.** Parenchymal changes, hyperechoic foci and strands. **B.** Ductal changes, dilated and irregular duct with hyperchoic margins. (Used with permission from Linda S. Lee, MD.)

believed to be arising in the background of chronic pancreatitis as well as examining parenchyma when presence of disease is equivocal. New variations of EUS imaging including elastography and digital imaging enhancement may decrease the subjectivity of image interpretation for early diagnosis.

Albashir S, Bronner MP, Parsi MA, Walsh RM, Stevens T. Endoscopic ultrasound, secretin endoscopic pancreatic function test, and histology: correlation in chronic pancreatitis. *Am J Gastroenterol.* 2010;105:2498–2503. [PMID: 20606675]

Gardner TB, Levy MJ. EUS diagnosis of chronic pancreatitis [review]. *Gastrointest Endosc.* 2010;71:1280–1289. [PMID: 20598255]

Seicean A. Endoscopic ultrasound in chronic pancreatitis: where are we now? *World J Gastroenterol.* 2010;16:4253–4263. [PMID: 20818808]

Stevens T. Update on the role of endoscopic ultrasound in chronic pancreatitis. *Curr Gastroenterol Rep.* 2011;13:117–122. [PMID: 21170612]

Stevens T, Lopez R, Adler DG, et al. Multicenter comparison of the interobserver agreement of standard EUS scoring and Rosemont classification scoring for diagnosis of chronic pancreatitis. *Gastrointest Endosc.* 2010;71:519–526. [PMID: 20189510]

2. Endoscopic retrograde cholangiopancreatography (ERCP)—While providing excellent views of the pancreatic main duct and side branches, ERCP also offers the possibility of therapeutic intervention such as removal of pancreatic duct stones with extracorporeal shock wave lithotripsy (ESWL) assistance (Figure 26–5). However, given the associated risks of inducing acute pancreatitis, ERCP is generally reserved for situations in which therapeutic intervention is likely. Combining EUS with MRI/MRCP is a practical, less invasive, and safe alternative to evaluating the pancreaticobiliary anatomy before attempting ERCP in chronic pancreatitis.

D. Special Tests

1. Gene testing—The role of genetic testing for patients with suspected hereditary forms of chronic pancreatitis continues to evolve. Hereditary and idiopathic forms of chronic pancreatitis account for up to 20–30% of cases. Genetic alterations associated with chronic pancreatitis include mutations in the cationic trypsinogen gene *PRSS1* (carriers bear a markedly increased lifetime risk of pancreatic cancer),

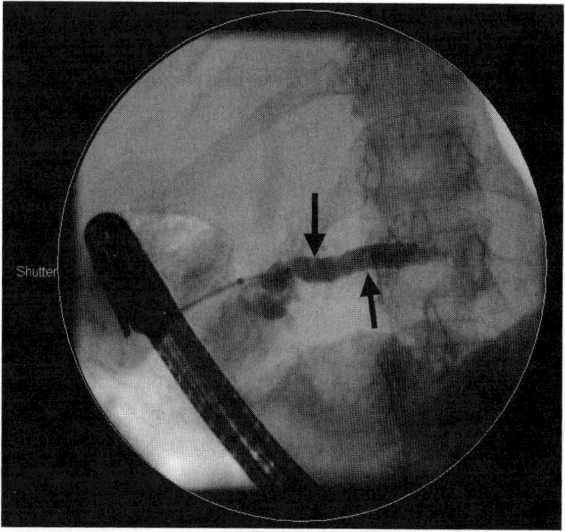

▲ **Figure 26–5.** ERCP: Dilated pancreatic duct with stones. Arrows point to filling defects.

the cystic fibrosis transmembrane conductance regulator (*CFTR*, an apical membrane chloride channel), and the serine protease inhibitor, Kazal type 1 (*SPINK1*). Although widespread screening has yet to come into routine practice, it is indicated in patients with otherwise unexplained onset of chronic pancreatitis or suggestive family history.

Cohn JA. Motion—genetic testing is useful in the diagnosis of nonhereditary pancreatic conditions: arguments against the motion. *Can J Gastroenterol.* 2003;17:53–55. [PMID: 12560856]

Rolston RK, Kant JA. Genetic testing in acute and chronic pancreatitis. *Curr Gastroenterol Rep.* 2001;3:115–120. [PMID: 11276378]

Treiber M, Schlag C, Schmid RM. Genetics of pancreatitis: a guide for clinicians. [Review.] *Curr Gastroenterol Rep.* 2008;10: 122–127. [PMID: 18462597]

Witt H, Luck W, Becker M, et al. Mutation in the SPINK1 trypsin inhibitor gene, alcohol use, and chronic pancreatitis. *JAMA.* 2001;285:2716–2717. [PMID: 11386926]

2. Pancreatic function testing—Sampling of secretin-stimulated pancreatic fluid from duodenal aspirates theoretically allows detection of impaired pancreatic function prior to the onset of structural abnormalities. The most widespread technique consists of aspiration of duodenal juice through a dual lumen (Dreiling tube) every 15 minutes for a total of 60 minutes following administration of secretin. A peak bicarbonate concentration less than 80 mEq/L is consistent with the diagnosis of chronic pancreatitis. More recently endoscopic pancreatic function testing has emerged at specialized centers as an alternative modality for direct sampling of duodenal aspirates. Endoscopic pancreas function testing is very helpful in evaluating patients with chronic pain syndromes and equivocal imaging for early chronic pancreatitis. It can also be combined with EUS to simultaneously assess both structure and secretory physiology (Figure 26–6). Furthermore, breath testing has recently been shown to be equivalent to fecal fat measurements and may allow a noninvasive means of monitoring therapy.

Conwell DL, Zuccaro G Jr, Vargo JJ, et al. An endoscopic pancreatic function test with cholecystokinin-octapeptide for the diagnosis of chronic pancreatitis. *Clin Gastroenterol Hepatol.* 2003;1: 189–194. [PMID: 15017490]

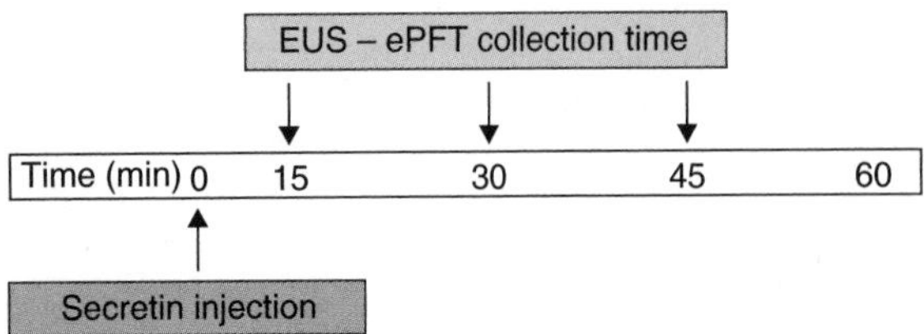

▲ **Figure 26–6.** Combined EUS-ePFT procedure. Timeline of secretin administration and pancreatic fluid collection with endoscopic view of duodenum at selected time points.

Conwell DL, Zuccaro G Jr, Vargo JJ, et al. An endoscopic pancreatic function test with synthetic porcine secretin for the evaluation of chronic abdominal pain and suspected chronic pancreatitis. *Gastrointest Endosc.* 2003;57:37–40. [PMID: 12518128]

Domínguez Muñoz JE. Diagnosis of chronic pancreatitis: functional testing [review]. *Best Pract Res Clin Gastroenterol.* 2010;24:233–241. [PMID: 20510825]

Wu B, Conwell DL. The endoscopic pancreatic function test. *Am J Gastroenterol.* 2009;104:2381–2383. [PMID: 19806083]

3. Mixed triglyceride breath test—The 13C-mixed triglyceride breath test (MTG) has been evaluated as a potential tool for evaluating the effect of enzyme therapy on fat digestion in chronic pancreatitis. The MTG is equivalent to coefficient of fat absorption (CFA) at detecting steatorrhea and can be used to target enzyme therapy to improve nutritional parameters and fat maldigestion. One-year follow-up of patients with chronic pancreatitis using MTG to adjust pancreatic enzyme supplementation showed improvement in body mass index, retinal binding protein, and serum albumin. Of note, MTG-targeted therapy revealed dosages of enzyme requirements were as high as 60,000 units of lipase per meal and in some cases required a proton pump inhibitor.

Domínguez-Muñoz JE, Iglesias-García J, Vilariño-Insua M, et al. 13C-mixed triglyceride breath test to assess oral enzyme substitution therapy in patients with chronic pancreatitis. *Clin Gastroenterol Hepatol.* 2007;5:484–488. [PMID: 17445754]

E. Diagnostic Challenges

The diagnosis of early chronic pancreatitis can be challenging due to overlap with several other chronic pain syndromes and in many cases the late occurrence of objective laboratory or radiographic abnormalities. Moreover, repeated instrumentation (pancreas duct stenting) of the pancreas itself can often lead to significant pathologic changes in the pancreatic parenchyma and duct architecture. Ultimately, a rational approach to diagnosing chronic pancreatitis requires the appropriate use of clinical history, laboratory testing, and radiographic and endoscopic investigation. The role of genetic testing continues to be defined. Molecular biology techniques, such as proteomics analysis, and cytokine or miRNA profiling of biofluids, may provide insight into the pathogenesis of chronic pancreatitis and identify molecular targets for drug therapy.

Paulo JA, Lee LS, Wu B, et al. Optimized sample preparation of endoscopic collected pancreatic fluid for SDS-PAGE analysis. *Electrophoresis.* 2010;31:2377–2387. [PMID: 20589857]

Paulo JA, Lee LS, Wu B, et al. Identification of pancreas-specific proteins in endoscopically (endoscopic pancreatic function test) collected pancreatic fluid with liquid chromatography–tandem mass spectrometry. *Pancreas.* 2010;39:889–896. [PMID: 20182389]

Pungpapong S, Noh KW, Woodward TA, Wallace MB, Al-Haddad M, Raimondo M. Endoscopic ultrasound and IL-8 in pancreatic juice to diagnose chronic pancreatitis. *Pancreatology.* 2007;7:491–496. [PMID: 17912013]

Differential Diagnosis

The differential diagnosis of patients presenting with pain from chronic pancreatitis often includes peptic ulcer disease, inflammatory bowel disease, gastric dysmotility, and irritable bowel syndrome in addition to psychogenic or factitious/drug-seeking disorders. These must be further discriminated through careful clinical evaluation. The maldigestion associated with chronic pancreatitis must be distinguished from other malabsorptive disorders such as carbohydrate malabsorption and celiac disease. It may help to ask about a history of "sticky" or greasy stools as well as the presence of oil drops separating from the main stool. These are features often associated with significant steatorrhea and strongly suggest the diagnosis of pancreatic insufficiency.

Complications

Complications associated with chronic pancreatitis include pseudocyst, biliary ductal or duodenal obstruction, pancreatic ascites or pleural effusion, splenic vein thrombosis, pancreatic fistulae, pseudoaneurysms, and an increased risk of pancreatic cancer.

Treatment

Treatment for chronic pancreatitis begins with lifestyle modifications, including cessation of alcohol, consumption of smaller low-fat meals, and quitting smoking. Further therapy should be directed toward treatment of symptoms and guided by the underlying suspected cause.

A. Pain

By far the most difficult aspect of treatment of chronic pancreatitis relates to management of chronic pain. Treatment should be aimed at analgesia, reducing inflammation, and overcoming intrapancreatic pressure. In addition, investigations are currently under way to evaluate means of altering neural transmission in order to improve analgesia. Increasingly, it has become recognized that many patients labeled with the diagnosis of chronic pancreatitis may not actually have visceral pain. These patients are much less likely to respond to therapy. Another common cause of pain that can be seen in chronic pancreatitis is narcotic bowel syndrome. This is an under recognized source of abdominal discomfort seen in patients on high dosages of narcotics in whom the character or activity of the disease process is not sufficient to fully explain the pain syndrome.

The mechanisms causing pain in pancreatitis have been the focus of intense study due to their enigmatic nature. Likely multifactorial, previously reported factors contributing to pain in chronic pancreatitis have included recurrent tissue inflammation, necrosis, pancreatic ductal hypertension, increased interstitial fluid pressure, pancreatic ischemia, and fibrotic encasement of sensory nerves (Figure 26–7). More recently, attention has focused on pain in chronic

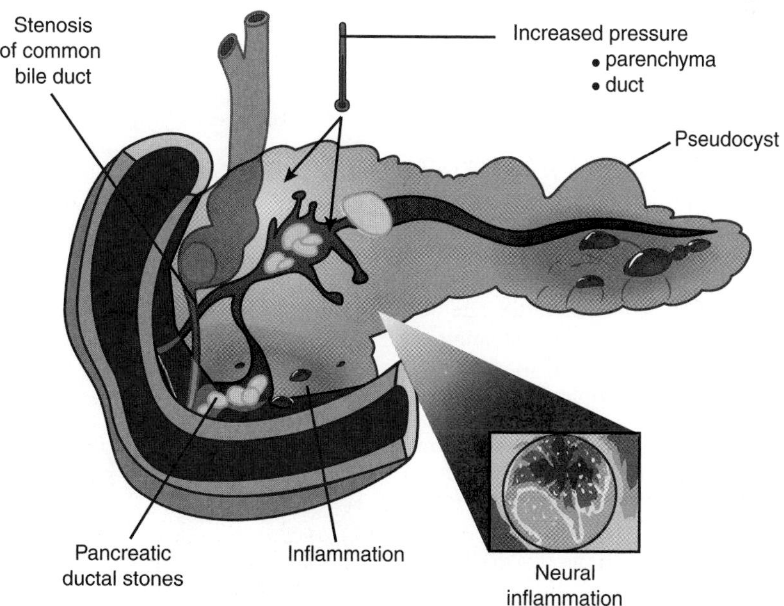

▲ **Figure 26–7.** Sources of pain in chronic pancreatitis. (Reproduced, with permission, from the American Gastroenterological Association Gastroenterology Teaching Project.)

pancreatitis as a neurobiologic phenomenon. Researchers have reported increased changes in the brain cortex of patients with chronic pancreatitis when compared with controls. Recent studies have also demonstrated up-regulation of the pain mediators substance P and calcitonin gene–related peptide in tissue samples from patients with chronic pancreatitis, as well as nerve growth factor–dependent nociceptors. TrkA, a high-affinity receptor for a nerve growth receptor, has been found to be overexpressed in acinar cells in chronic pancreatitis and may serve as a link between inflammation and hyperalgesia. Additional nociceptive pathways implicated in chronic pancreatitis include brain-derived neurotrophic factor as well as proteinase-activated receptor-2 (PAR-2)–mediated stimulation of nociceptive neurons by trypsin activation. Two emerging concepts with respect to pain mediation in chronic pancreatitis include "mechanical allodynia," whereby pain is sensed even in the absence of noxious stimuli given prior sensitization of the nociceptive system, and "inflammatory hyperalgesia," in which relatively minor episodes of inflammation may trigger increased pain response due to already "primed" pancreatic nociceptors.

Analgesics should be administered in conjunction with pain a management center with emphasis on alternative non-narcotic management of the abdominal pain syndrome. The WHO has a suggested stepwise approach to chronic pain management.

Grunkemeier DM, Cassara JE, Dalton CB, Drossman DA. Narcotic bowel syndrome: clinical features, pathophysiology and management. *Clin Gastroenterol and Hepatol.* 2007;5:1120–1139. [PMID: 17916540]

Vargas-Schaffer G. Is the WHO analgesic ladder still valid? Twenty-four years of experience. *Can Fam Physician.* 2010;56:514–517. [PMID: 20547511]

1. Inflammation and pancreatic pressure—Attempts to reduce pancreatic inflammation should include smoking cessation, trial of total parenteral nutrition or enteral feeding, surgery for obstructive pancreatitis, and corticosteroids for autoimmune chronic pancreatitis (Table 26–3). Methods of reducing pancreatic pressure include suppression of secretion via administration of a proton pump inhibitor, pancreatic enzymes, and potentially octreotide. In the rare but now increasingly recognized instance where autoimmune pancreatitis is suspected, therapy with corticosteroids has also been found to be beneficial (see Chapter 27).

Table 26–3. Treatment options for chronic pancreatitis pain.

Proven Benefit	Uncertain Benefit
Smoking cessation Alcohol cessation Corticosteroids for autoimmune pancreatitis (Chapter 27) Analgesics	Pancreatic enzyme supplementation Transcranial magnetic brain stimulation Octreotide Nerve growth factor antibody

2. Obstruction—If ductal obstruction is present due to stricture, stone, or pseudocyst with mass effect, invasive therapy may be necessary. In the case of ductal stones, endoscopic clearance (Plate 25), surgical therapy, or extracorporeal shock wave lithotripsy may be attempted although evidence for individual treatment modalities is limited. Symptomatic pseudocysts may be drained percutaneously, endoscopically (Plates 26 and 27), or surgically. Recent data from randomized head-to-head trials indicate somewhat improved outcomes with surgical drainage over endoscopic therapy. Surgical options for chronic pancreatitis include lateral pancreaticojejunostomy for decompression of a dilated main duct, removal of localized disease by either a Whipple procedure or tail resection, and, finally, total pancreatectomy.

3. Modification of neural transmission—Chronic pain in chronic pancreatitis is complex and may have several origins. Methods of modifying the nociceptive process involved in chronic pancreatitis include EUS-guided celiac plexus block, bilateral thorascopic splanchnicectomy, transcranial magnetic stimulation, as well as additional investigational techniques including medications. One study examining celiac plexus block via EUS found that 55% of subjects had decreased pain after 8 weeks (Figure 26–8), with only 10% experiencing decreased pain after 24 weeks. For the most part, all of these modalities have achieved success only in producing moderate short-term pain relief, with high rates of relapse after long-term follow-up.

Cahen DL, Gouma DJ, Nio Y, et al. Endoscopic versus surgical drainage of the pancreatic duct in chronic pancreatitis. *N Engl J Med.* 2007;356:676–684. [PMID: 17301298]

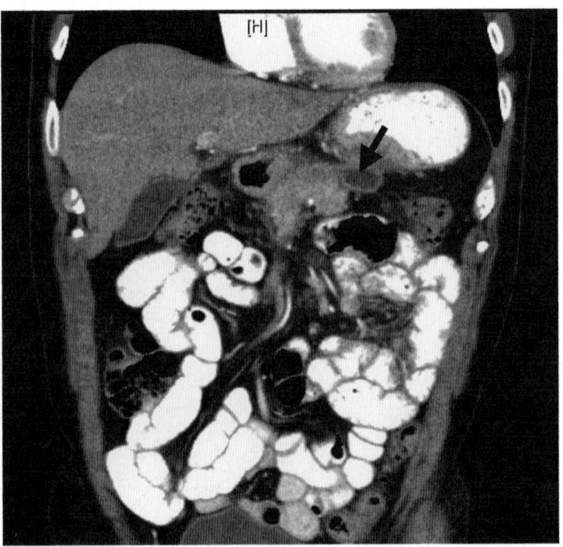

▲ **Figure 26–8.** CT Scan: Residual asymptomatic pseudocyst 6–8 weeks after endoscopic drainage (*arrow*).

Conwell DL, Vargo JJ, Zuccaro G, et al. Role of differential neuroaxial blockade in the evaluation and management of pain in chronic pancreatitis. *Am J Gastroenterol.* 2001;96:431–436. [PMID: 11232686]

Dite P, Ruzicka M, Zboril V, et al. A prospective, randomized trial comparing endoscopic and surgical therapy for chronic pancreatitis. *Endoscopy.* 2003;35:553–558. [PMID: 12822088]

Kaufman M, Singh G, Das S, et al. Efficacy of endoscopic ultrasound-guided celiac plexus block and celiac plexus neurolysis for managing abdominal pain associated with chronic pancreatitis and pancreatic cancer [review]. *J Clin Gastroenterol.* 2010;44:127–134. [PMID: 19826273]

Talamini G, Bassi C. The "natural" history of pain in chronic pancreatitis. *Gastroenterology.* 2000;118:235–237. [PMID: 10644178]

B. Exocrine Insufficiency

Pancreatic enzyme supplementation can aid in addressing the difficulty in digesting protein and lipid products in patients with severe chronic pancreatitis. In addition, it appears that patients with small duct disease may receive an added benefit from high-dose non–enteric-coated pancreatic enzyme supplementation in terms of pain relief, believed to be mediated through reduced duodenal cholecystokinin release. Typically, these enzymes should be given with each meal. Recent evidence suggests that 13C-MTG breath testing may help target appropriate enzyme therapy dosages in chronic pancreatitis.

Whitcomb DC, Lehman GA, Vasileva G, et al. Pancrelipase delayed-release capsules (CREON) for exocrine pancreatic insufficiency due to chronic pancreatitis or pancreatic surgery: a double-blind randomized trial. *Am J Gastroenterol.* 2010;105:2276–2286 [PMID: 20502447]

Course & Prognosis

The natural history of chronic pancreatitis remains poorly defined in part because of its highly variable nature. The relationship between etiologic factors, genetic predisposition, and the pace of disease progression requires further clarification. Modifiable risk factors need to be identified and treated. It appears that discontinuance of alcohol, cessation of smoking, and early administration of corticosteroids in autoimmune disease may affect the natural history and prognosis of the disease. A recent French report on the natural history of hereditary pancreatitis has provided insight that can be extrapolated to chronic pancreatitis of other etiologies. This study documents the time line of initial episodes of abdominal pain and recurrent pancreatitis in childhood that later develop into pancreas insufficiency, diabetes, and, in some, pancreas cancer later as an adult.

Rebours V, Boutron-Ruault MC, Schnee M, et al. The natural history of hereditary pancreatitis: a national series. *Gut.* 2009; 58:97–103. [PMID: 18755888]

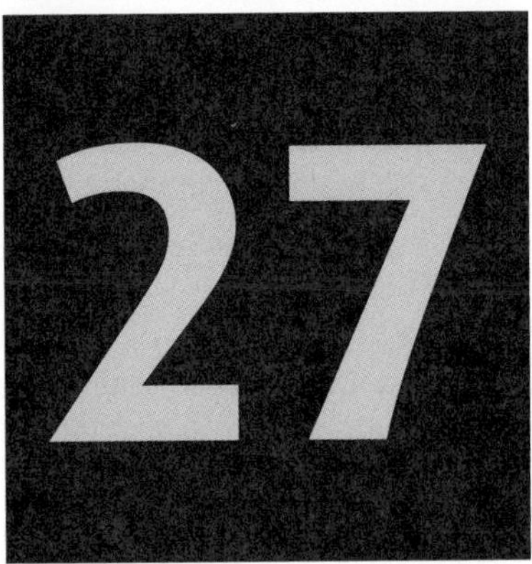

Autoimmune Pancreatitis

Norton J. Greenberger, MD

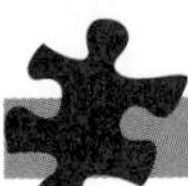

ESSENTIALS OF DIAGNOSIS

- Presentation with obstructive jaundice.
- Diffuse swelling and enlargement of the pancreas, especially the head, the latter mimicking carcinoma of the pancreas.
- Diffuse irregular narrowing of the pancreatic duct on ERCP or MRCP.
- Elevated serum IgG_4 level.
- Extrapancreatic and intrahepatic bile duct strictures.
- Resolution or marked improvement in pancreatic and extrapancreatic manifestations after corticosteroid treatment.
- Pancreatic biopsies reveal extensive fibrosis and lymphoplasmacytic infiltration.
- HISORT criteria used to establish the diagnosis.

General Considerations

Autoimmune pancreatitis is a rare disorder of presumed autoimmune causation with characteristic chemical, histologic, and morphologic findings. It is referred to by various names, including nonalcoholic destructive pancreatitis, tumefactive pancreatitis, and sclerosing pancreatitis, depending in part on specific pathologic findings and on the presence of extrapancreatic manifestations. However, it is believed that the pathologic heterogeneity may reflect different stages or manifestations of the same disease.

Autoimmune pancreatitis has been described as a primary pancreatic disorder and is also associated with other disorders of presumed autoimmune etiology, including primary sclerosing cholangitis, primary biliary sclerosis, retroperitoneal fibrosis, rheumatoid arthritis, and Sjögren syndrome. As a result, it has been proposed that autoimmune pancreatitis represents a systemic autoimmune disease.

Finkelberg DL, Sahani D, Deshpande V, et al. Autoimmune pancreatitis. *N Engl J Med.* 2006;355:2670–2676. [PMID: 17182992]

Clinical Findings

A. Symptoms and Signs

Mild symptoms, usually abdominal pain, are present but attacks of acute pancreatitis are unusual. Furthermore, autoimmune pancreatitis is not a common cause of idiopathic recurrent pancreatitis. In the United States, 50–65% of patients with autoimmune pancreatitis present with obstructive jaundice. Weight loss and new onset of diabetes may also occur. Patients who have associated autoimmune conditions have corresponding clinical features. In this regard, Sjögren syndrome, rheumatoid arthritis, retroperitoneal fibrosis, ulcerative colitis, autoimmune thyroiditis, tubulointerstitial nephritis, and mediastinal adenopathy have all been reported in patients with autoimmune pancreatitis (Tables 27–1 and 27–2).

B. Laboratory Findings

An obstructive pattern on liver tests is common (ie, disproportionately elevated serum alkaline phosphatase and minimally elevated serum aminotransferases). Elevated serum levels of immunoglobulin G_4 (IgG_4) provide a marker for the disease, particularly in Western populations. Serum IgG_4 normally accounts for only 5–6% of the total IgG_4 in healthy patients but is elevated in those with autoimmune pancreatitis.

A large study compared serum IgG_4 levels in 20 patients diagnosed with autoimmune pancreatitis based on clinical features and response to corticosteroids with 20 age- and sex-matched controls and 104 patients with pancreatic cancer, chronic pancreatitis, primary biliary sclerosis, primary cholangitis, and Sjögren syndrome. The median serum IgG_4 concentration in the patients with autoimmune pancreatitis was 663 mg/dL compared with 51 mg/dL in healthy controls

Table 27–1. Clinical features of autoimmune pancreatitis.

- Mild symptoms usually abdominal pain, but without frequent attacks of pancreatitis, are unusual
- Presentation with obstructive jaundice
- Diffuse swelling and enlargement of the pancreas, especially the head, the latter mimicking carcinoma of the pancreas
- Diffuse irregular narrowing of the pancreatic duct in ERCP
- Increased levels of serum gamma globulins especially IgG_4
- Presence of other auto-antibodies, rheumatoid factor
- Can occur with other autoimmune diseases Sjögrens syndrome, primary sclerosing cholangitis, ulcerative colitis, rheumatoid arthritis, autoimmune thyroiditis, tubulointerstitial nephritis
- Extra pancreatic bile duct changes such as stricture of the common bile duct and intrahepatic ducts
- Absence of pancreatic calcifications or cysts
- Pancreatic biopsies reveal extensive fibrosis and lymphoplasmacytic infiltration
- Corticosteroids are effective in alleviating symptoms, decreasing size of the pancreas, and reversing histopathological changes

(in whom normal values ranged from 8–140 mg/dL). Using a cutoff of 280 mg/dL, the sensitivity and specificity of the serum IgG_4 value for distinguishing autoimmune pancreatitis from pancreatic cancer was 95–97%.

It has also been demonstrated that IgG_4 levels may decline during treatment with corticosteroids, and this can be used as a parameter to follow the response of patients to such therapy. These and other observations suggest that serum levels of IgG_4 may be useful to distinguish autoimmune pancreatitis from pancreatic cancer. Additionally, other antibodies such as antinuclear antibodies and rheumatoid factor may be present.

A serologic marker has been identified that is present in most patients with autoimmune pancreatitis. Antibodies against the plasminogen binding protein (PBP) peptide were detected in 19 of 20 patients with autoimmune pancreatitis (95%) but also in 4 of 40 patients with pancreatic cancer (10%). Reactivity was not detected in patients with alcohol-induced chronic pancreatitis or intraductal papillary mucinous neoplasms. While the antibody was detected in most patients with autoimmune pancreatitis, it was also found in 10% of patients with pancreatic cancer making it an imperfect test to distinguish between these two conditions.

Frulloni L, Lunardi C, Simone R, et al. Identification of a novel antibody associated with autoimmune pancreatitis. *N Engl J Med.* 2009;361:2135–2142. [PMID: 19940298]

C. Imaging Studies

Table 27–3 summarizes the imaging findings observed in two large series, one from Massachusetts General Hospital (MGH) and the other from the Mayo Clinic. Pancreatic abnormalities were present in the majority of the patients and included diffuse enlargement, focal enlargement, and a distinct enlargement at the head of the pancreas. Noteworthy was the lack of vascular encasement calcification or pancreatic fluid; however, enlarged pancreatic lymph nodes were noted (Figures 27–1 and 27–2).

Endoscopic retrograde cholangiopancreatography (ERCP) or magnetic resonance pancreatography (MRCP) reveals strictures in the bile duct in over one third of patients with autoimmune pancreatitis; these may be common bile duct strictures, intrahepatic bile duct strictures, or proximal bile duct strictures, with accompanying narrowing of the pancreatic bile duct (Figure 27–3). Rim like enhancement of the pancreatic head can be found on magnetic resonance imaging (MRI) examination. Endoscopic ultrasound is increasingly being used to support a diagnosis of autoimmune pancreatitis, and characteristic findings appear to be diffuse pancreatic enlargement and focal irregular hypoechoic masses.

Chari ST, Smyrk TC, Levy MJ, et al. Diagnosis of autoimmune pancreatitis: the Mayo Clinic experience. *Clin Gastroenterol Hepatol.* 2006;4:1010–1016. [PMID: 16843735]

Hamano H, Kawa S, Horiuchi A, et al. High serum IgG_4 concentrations in patients with sclerosing pancreatitis. *N Engl J Med.* 2001;344:732–738. [PMID: 11236777]

Sahani DV, Kalva SP, Farrell J, et al. Autoimmune pancreatitis: imaging features in 29 patients. *Radiology.* 2004;233:345–352. [PMID: 15459324]

Table 27–2. Characteristic extrapancreatic and histopathologic features in autoimmune pancreatitis.

Extrapancreatic Findings	Histopathologic Findings
Inflammatory bowel disease, primarily ulcerative colitis	Extensive lymphoplasmacytic infiltrate with dense fibrosis
Bile duct strictures, especially long strictures without beading	Inflammatory cells clustered in walls of small veins and nerves
Lung nodules, adenopathy, and infiltrates	PMN infiltrate extending transmurally → obliterative phlebitis
Sjögren syndrome (salivary gland involvement)	Varying degrees of pancreatic parenchymal atrophy
Retroperitoneal fibrosis	Islet cell encasement with intralobular fibrosis
Interstitial nephritis	Pancreatic ducts that are slit-like or star-shaped, but without calcification or plugging
Autoimmune thyroiditis	

PMN, polymorphonuclear neutrophil.

Table 27–3. Imaging features observed in patients with autoimmune pancreatitis.

Computed Tomography	Mayo Clinic (n = 22)[a]	Massachusetts General Hospital (n = 29)[b]
Findings		
Diffuse enlargement	6	14
Focal enlargement	10	7
Distinct mass	3	
Normal	1	
Pancreatic stranding		7
Lack of vascular encasement	22	29
Calcification, peripancreatic fluid		
Enlarged peripancreatic lymph nodes		9
ERCP/MRCP		
Strictures of bile ducts		
• Common bile ducts		12
• Intrahepatic ducts	11	6
• Proximal bile duct		6
Narrowing of pancreatic duct		9
Pancreatic duct stricture		8
Sclerosing cholangitis		1
Magnetic Resonance Imaging		
Rim like enhancement of pancreatic head		2
Endoscopic Ultrasound (n = 14)		
Diffuse hypoechoic pancreatic enlargement		8
Focal irregular hypoechoic mass		6

ERCP, endoscopic retrograde cholangiopancreatography; MRCP, magnetic resonance cholangiopancreatography.

[a]Data from Chari ST, Smyrk TC, Levy MJ, et al. Diagnosis of autoimmune pancreatitis: the Mayo Clinic experience. *Clin Gastroenterol Hepatol*. 2006;4:1010–1016.

[b]Data from Sahani DV, Kalva SP, Farrell J, et al. Autoimmune pancreatitis: imaging features in 29 patients. *Radiology*. 2004;233:345–352.

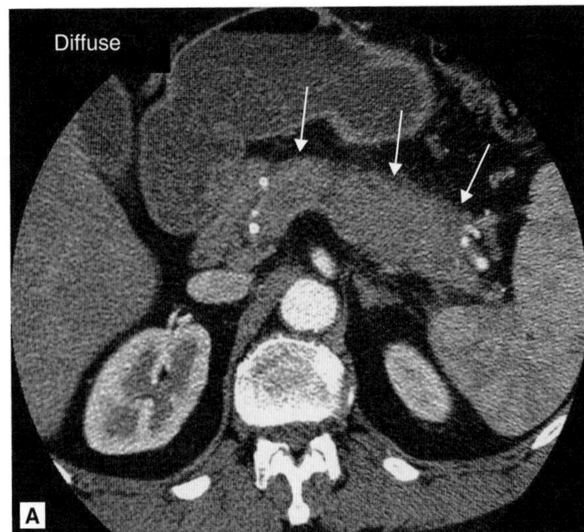

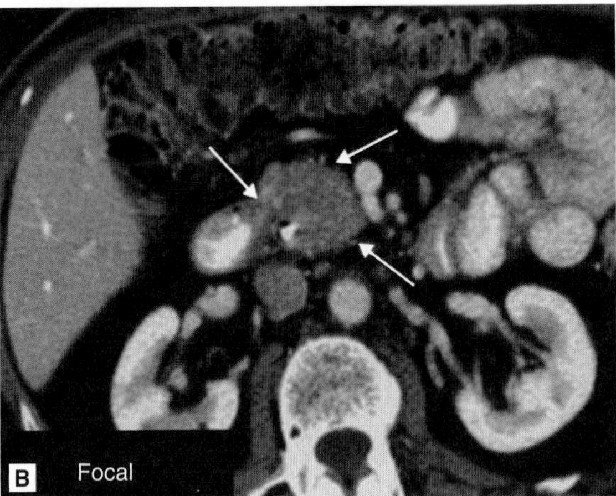

▲ **Figure 27–1.** CT findings in autoimmune pancreatitis. **A:** Diffuse homogenous appearance. **B:** "Halo" around the pancreas (*arrows*), focal enlargement of the head and uncinate, and lack of vascular invasion and peripancreatic changes in all segments. (Used with permission from Dr Dushyant V. Sahani, Massachusetts General Hospital.)

D. Histopathologic Findings

Characteristic findings include extensive lymphoplasmacytic infiltrates with dense fibrosis, and infiltration of polymorphic leukocytes extending transmurally, ultimately resulting in an obliterative phlebitis (see Table 27–1). Inflammatory cells cluster in the walls of the small veins and nerves. Varying degrees of pancreatic parenchymal atrophy may be present, and islets may be encased with intralobular fibrosis. Importantly, pancreatic ducts exhibit no calcification or plugging but are slit like or star shaped.

To date, there have been few published reports describing cytologic diagnosis of autoimmune pancreatitis. It has been suggested that smears rich in inflammatory cells (lymphocytes, plasma cells, and polymorphonuclear leukocytes with sparse epithelial cells lacking atypia) may be useful in

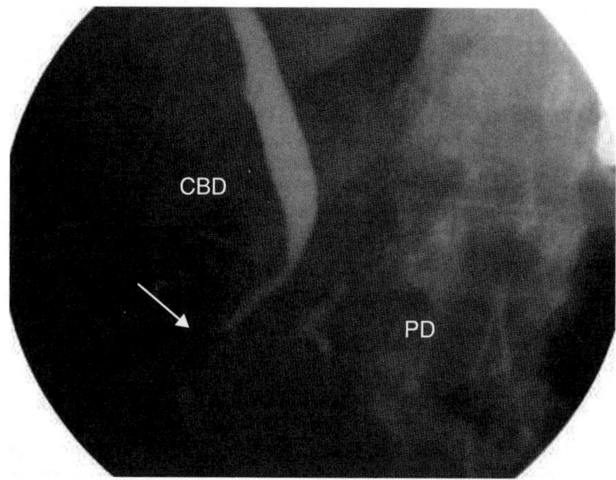

▲ **Figure 27–2.** ERCP findings in autoimmune pancreatitis. Common bile duct stricture, stricture of intrahepatic radicals, diffuse pancreatic duct (PD) narrowing, and PD stenosis.

supporting the diagnosis. It is important to emphasize that the diagnosis of autoimmune pancreatitis can be missed in core biopsies because of the sampling area or patchy involvement of the parenchyma.

Distinct Clinical and Histologic Profile

Autoimmune pancreatitis can be classified as type 1 and type 2 based on histologic patterns and clinical profiles. Type 1 autoimmune pancreatitis is characterized by greater than 10 IgG_4 plasma cells and a lymphoplasmacytic sclerosing pancreatitis with periductal lymphoplasmacytic infiltrate, obliterative phlebitis, and dense fibrosis. Type 2 autoimmune pancreatitis or idiopathic duct centric pancreatitis is characterized by a granulocytic epithelial lesion with minimal IgG_4 plasma cells in the pancreatic parenchyma. In a study of 97 patients with autoimmune pancreatitis, patients with type 1 were found to have a high relapse rate (47%) compared to patients with type 2 (0%) and was more frequently associated with inflammatory bowel disease.

Deheragoda MG, Church NI, Rodriguez-Justo M, et al. The use of immunoglobulin G_4 immunostaining in diagnosis pancreatic and extrapancreatic involvement in autoimmune pancreatitis. *Clin Gastroenterol Hepatol.* 2007;5:1229–1234. [PMID: 17702660]

Sah RP, Chari ST, Pannala R, et al. Differences in clinical and relapse rate of type 1 versus type 2 autoimmune pancreatitis. *Gastroenterology.* 2010;139:140–148. [PMID: 20353791]

Diagnosis and Differential Diagnosis

Autoimmune pancreatitis should be considered in the differential diagnosis of patients presenting with the varied symptoms described earlier that are referable to the pancreas and

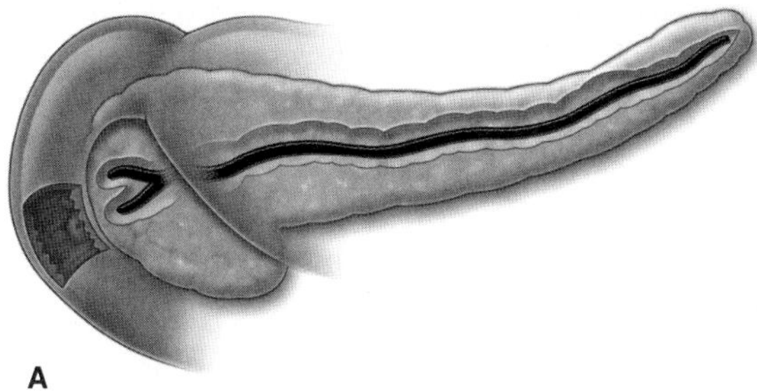

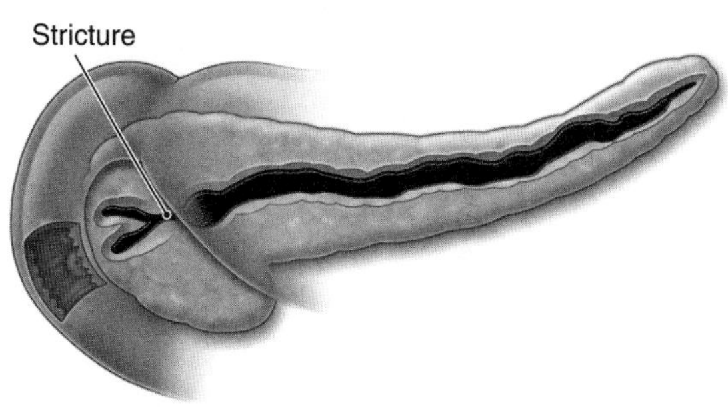

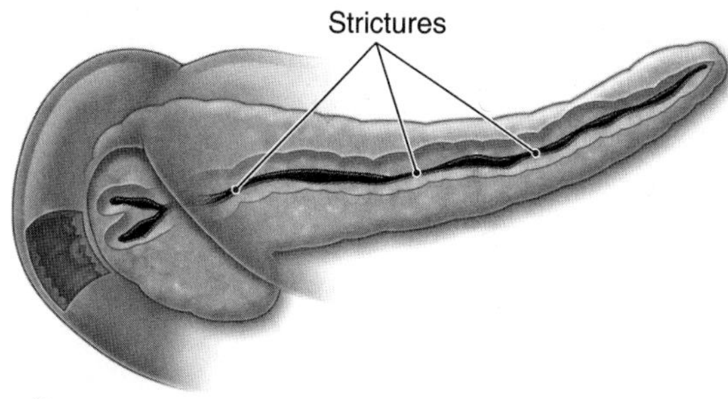

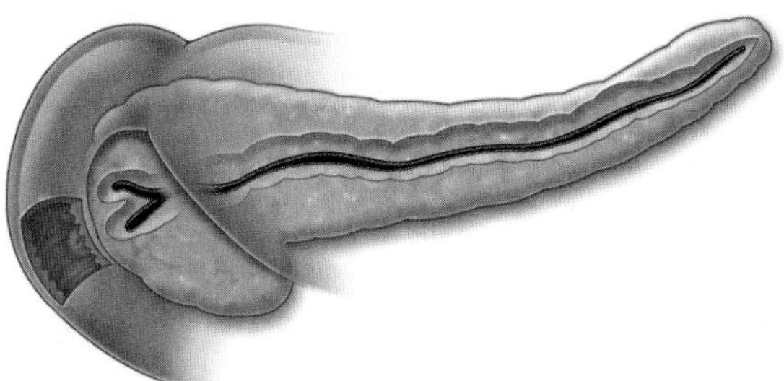

▲ **Figure 27–3.** Pancreatic ductal change in autoimmune pancreatitis. **A:** Normal pancreatic duct. **B:** Focal pancreatic duct stricture. **C:** Segmental pancreatic duct strictures. **D:** Diffuse pancreatic duct narrowing.

biliary tract, particularly in conjunction with other autoimmune conditions. It was formerly believed that the sine qua non for establishing a diagnosis of autoimmune pancreatitis was pancreatic histopathologic abnormalities, including extensive lymphoplasmacytic infiltrates with dense fibrosis. It is now recognized that in addition to histologic findings (H), a diagnosis of autoimmune pancreatitis can be made based on pancreatic imaging (I) and serology (S) (IgG_4 level), other organ involvement (O) and response to corticosteroid treatment (R) have been determined; these have been termed the HISORT criteria. Utilizing this concept, the proposed Mayo Clinic criteria suggest that autoimmune pancreatitis can be diagnosed with at least one of three abnormalities: (1) diagnostic histology, (2) characteristic findings on computed tomography (CT) and pancreatography, with elevated IgG_4 levels; and (3) response to corticosteroid therapy, with improvement in pancreatic and extrapancreatic manifestations (Table 27–4).

Patients with autoimmune pancreatitis sometimes present with features that mimic pancreatic cancer, including a mass on the head of the pancreas. Although autoimmune pancreatitis is diagnosed much less frequently than pancreatic cancer, making the correct diagnosis is necessary to avert the consequences of unnecessary surgery. As detailed in the treatment section, response to corticosteroids within a 2–4 week period is an important parameter by which the diagnosis of autoimmune pancreatitis can be supported. Autoimmune pancreatitis is usually first suggested by imaging procedures such as contrast-enhanced CT or MRI. Of note, characteristic features more suggestive of pancreatic carcinoma (eg, vascular encasement, peripancreatic changes, etc) are usually lacking. Imaging differences between autoimmune pancreatitis and pancreatic cancer are detailed in Table 27–5. A characteristic feature of autoimmune pancreatitis is rim like enhancement of the pancreatic head on MRI. Endoscopic ultrasound is also being used to diagnose autoimmune pancreatitis, and some of the findings that have been noted are listed in Table 27–3.

IgG_4 can also be useful in diagnosing pancreatic and extrapancreatic involvement in autoimmune pancreatitis. In one study that examined both pancreatic and extrapancreatic tissues (gallbladder, stomach, duodenum, colon, salivary glands, and kidney), high levels of IgG_4-immunostaining plasma cells (>10 IgG_4 plasma cells per high-power field [HPF]) were found in 17 of 20 (85%) specimens from patients with autoimmune pancreatitis compared with 1 of 175 (0.6%) specimens from controls. Immunostaining of involved tissue for IgG_4 may be particularly useful when autoimmune pancreatitis is suspected clinically but the serum IgG_4 level is normal.

Table 27–4. Diagnosis of autoimmune pancreatitis based on revised HISORT criteria

Autoimmune pancreatitis can be diagnosed by one of the following:

A. Diagnostic histology: (H)
  - On resection specimen or
  - On pancreatic core biopsy (indicated in a patient with pancreatic mass and/or obstructive jaundice due to distal bile duct obstruction with a negative work-up for cancer
B. Typical imaging (I) + any one of the following:
  - Elevated IgG_4 (S)
  - Other organ involvement (O)
  - Compatible histology
C. Response to steroids (Rt): Resolution/marked improvement in pancreatic/extrapancreatic manifestations in patients meeting criteria for steroid use:
  - Patients in groups A and B
  - Patients without typical imaging findings with negative work-up for cancer and suggestive feature of autoimmune pancreatitis or definitive other organ involvement
  - A steroid trial in the absence of adequate or no collateral evidence of autoimmune pancreatitis must be used with caution

Adapted with permission from Chari ST, Takahashi N, Levy MJ, et al. A diagnostic strategy to distinguish autoimmune pancreatitis from pancreatic cancer. *Clin Gastroenterol Hepatol.* 2009;7:1097–1103. [PMID: 19410017]

Table 27–5. Differences between autoimmune pancreatitis and pancreatic cancer on computed tomography scan.

Structure	Autoimmune Pancreatitis	Pancreatic Cancer
Pancreas	Diffuse enlargement	Focal mass lesion
Ducts	Narrow	Dilated
Pancreatic rim halo	Yes	No
Vessel encasement	No	May be present
Lymphadenopathy	May be present	May be present

Differences between autoimmune pancreatitis and pancreatic cancer on computed tomography scan.

Treatment

A. Caveats

At the outset, several issues should be raised regarding treatment. First, there have been no controlled trials of treatment approaches in autoimmune pancreatitis. Second, patients groups described in existing reports have been heterogeneous, with over 50% of the patients having undergone a Whipple procedure. Third, until recently, uniform diagnostic criteria were lacking, with the exception of typical pathologic changes in resected pancreatic specimens. Fourth, criteria for initiating treatment and assessing response often have not been uniformly delineated. Nonetheless, after a diagnosis of autoimmune pancreatitis has been made based on the previously outlined criteria, treatment with corticosteroids usually is initiated.

B. Corticosteroid Therapy

Corticosteroids have shown efficacy in alleviating symptoms, decreasing the size of the pancreas, and reversing histopathologic features in patients with autoimmune pancreatitis. Patients may respond dramatically to corticosteroid therapy within a 2- to 4-week period. Prednisone is usually administered at an initial dose of 40 mg/day for 4 weeks followed by a taper of the daily dosage by 5 mg/week based on monitoring of clinical parameters. Relief of symptoms, serial changes in abdominal imaging of the pancreas and bile ducts, decreased serum γ-globulin and IgG_4 levels, and improvements in liver tests are suggested parameters to follow.

Improvement in histologic findings after steroid therapy has also been reported. In the Mayo Clinic series mentioned earlier, the median duration of treatment was 12 weeks. A poor response to corticosteroids over a 2- to 4-week period should raise suspicion of pancreatic cancer or other forms of chronic pancreatitis.

In this regard, Moon et al evaluated the utility of a 2-week trial of glucocorticoids in 22 patients who had atypical imaging findings for autoimmune pancreatitis and did not meet characteristic imaging criteria for pancreatic cancer. All patients received prednisolone (0.5 mg/kg per day). At two weeks, steroid responsiveness was defined as a reduction in the pancreatic mass and marked improvement in pancreatic duct narrowing. All 15 patients who responded were confirmed as having autoimmune pancreatitis while the presence of pancreatic cancer was confirmed at operation in 6 of 7 patients who did not respond.

In most reports, 50–70% of patients responded to corticosteroids, but about 25% required a second course of treatment while a smaller number required maintenance treatment with prednisone at a dosage of 5–10 mg/day. In the Mayo Clinic series, 15 of 29 patients had resolution of biliary strictures or pancreatic masses, or both, with steroid treatment.

Kamisawa T, Yoshiike M, Egawa N, et al. Treating patients with autoimmune pancreatitis: results from a long-term follow-up study. *Pancreatology*. 2005;5:234–238. [PMID: 1585582]

Moon SH, Kim MH, Park DH, et al. Is a 2-week steroid trial after initial negative investigation for malignancy useful in differentiating autoimmune pancreatitis from pancreatic cancer? A prospective outcome study. *Gut*. 2008;57:1704–1712. [PMID: 18583399]

Saito T, Tanaka S, Yoshida H, et al. A case of autoimmune pancreatitis responding to steroid therapy. Evidence of histologic recovery. *Pancreatology*. 2002;2:550–556. [PMID: 12435868]

C. Immunomodulatory Drugs

Several recent studies have reported on the use of immunomodulatory drugs (azathioprine, mycophenolate, mofetil, cyclophosphamide) in autoimmune pancreatitis patients who either flared or relapsed while on or after withdrawal of corticosteroid therapy. Raina et al found that 9 of 15 patients who responded initially to corticosteroids relapsed after steroid withdrawal but all 9 responded and are being maintained on azathioprine. In another report by Sandanayake et al, in 10 of 13 patients treated with azathioprine, remission was achieved and maintained by 7 patients with azathioprine monotherapy at a median follow-up of 14 months. Successful treatment with rituximab, a monoclonal antibody, was reported in two patients with autoimmune pancreatitis, one of whom was refractory to glucocorticoid and 6-mercaptopurine. For additional information on immunomodulatory treatment autoimmune pancreatitis see section D below.

Raina A, Yadav D, Krasinskas AM, et al. Evaluation and management of autoimmune pancreatitis: experience at a large US center. *Am J Gastroenterol*. 2009;104:2295–2306. [PMID: 19532132]

Sandanayake NS, Church NI, Chapman MH, et al. Presentation and management of post-treatment relapse in autoimmune pancreatitis/immunoglobulin G_4-associated cholangitis. *Clin Gastroenterol Hepatol*. 2009;7:1089–1096. [PMID: 19345283]

D. Immunoglobulin G_4-Associated Cholangitis

IgG_4-associated cholangitis (IAC), which can mimic primary sclerosing cholangitis, is the biliary manifestation of a steroid-responsive multisystem fibroinflammatory disorder (ie, autoimmune pancreatitis). The affected organs have a lymphoplasmacytic infiltrate rich in IgG_4-positive cells. A recent study described clinical, serologic, and imaging characteristics and treatment response in 53 IAC patients. Among the study participants, 85% were male, 77% presented with obstructive jaundice, 92% had associated autoimmune pancreatitis, 74% showed increased serum IgG_4 levels, and 88% had IgG_4-positive cells in bile duct biopsy specimens (>10/HPF). Bile duct strictures were common, with isolated intrapancreatic bile duct strictures in 51% of patients, proximal extrahepatic or intrahepatic bile duct strictures in 49%, and multifocal structures in 32%.

Thirty patients received prednisone at a dose of 40 mg/day for 4 weeks, which was then tapered to 5 mg/week for a total of 11 weeks; 18 patients underwent surgical resection; and 5 patients were treated conservatively and had spontaneous resolution of their disease. The following treatment responses were observed. Of the 30 patients treated with prednisone, 29 (97%) had an initial response, and 18 (60% of patients) had resolution of strictures and normalization of liver enzymes. Twelve of 17 patients (71%) with proximal bile duct strictures relapsed less than 6 months after prednisone was discontinued; in these patients, the presence of proximal extrahepatic or intrahepatic stricture was predictive of relapse. Fifteen patients were retreated with steroids for relapse, and 7 patients required additional immunomodulating drugs (azathioprine, cyclophosphamide, or mycophenolate mofetil) to remain in steroid-free remission during more than 6 months of follow-up. Eight of the 15 patients retreated with steroids (44%) relapsed.

The authors of the study drew the following conclusions from these findings: first, IAC should be suspected in patients with unexplained biliary strictures associated with increased IgG_4 and unexplained pancreatic disease; second, relapses are common after steroid withdrawal, especially in patients with proximal strictures; and third, the role of immunomodulating drugs for relapses needs to be explored through further study.

Ghazale A, Chari ST, Zhang L, et al. Immunoglobulin G_4-associated cholangitis: clinical profile and response to therapy. *Gastroenterology*. 2008;134:706–715. [PMID: 18222442]

Course & Prognosis

Hirano and colleagues reported outcomes and clinical features in 42 patients with autoimmune pancreatitis. Nineteen patients were treated with corticosteroids (prednisolone) and 23 without. The average observation period was 25 months but ranged up to 7 years. Unfavorable events (sclerosing cholangitis, distal bile duct stenosis, and retroperitoneal fibrosis) developed in 16 of the 23 patients (70%) not treated with corticosteroids but in only 3 of 19 patients (32%) treated with prednisolone. These data support the recommendation that patients with autoimmune pancreatitis, especially those with obstructive jaundice and bile duct strictures, should be treated and maintained on corticosteroids.

Hirano K, Tada M, Isayama H, et al. Long-term prognosis of autoimmune pancreatitis with and without corticosteroid treatment. *Gut.* 2007;56:1719–1724. [PMID: 17525092]

Tumors of the Pancreas

28

Ashish Sharma, MD

PANCREATIC CANCER

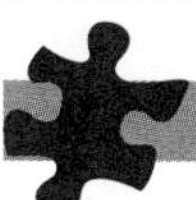

ESSENTIALS OF DIAGNOSIS

- Elevated CA 19-9 in ~80% of patients.
- Helical pancreatic protocol computed tomography (PPCT) is generally the best initial modality for diagnosis and staging.
- Endoscopic ultrasound (EUS) is superior to CT in diagnosing small tumors, and portal and splenic vein invasion.
- Less than 15% of tumors are resectable at the time of diagnosis.

General Considerations

Pancreatic cancer is the second-most-common gastrointestinal malignancy, and the fourth leading cause of cancer-related deaths in the United States. Less than 4% of patients are alive 5 years after diagnosis. Approximately 34,000 new cases were diagnosed in 2006, and 37,000 new cases were expected to be diagnosed in 2008.

The disease is more common in men than in women (1.3:1) and in certain ethnic and racial groups (eg, Blacks, Polynesians, and native New Zealanders). It is rare before the age of 45 years, but the incidence increases sharply after the seventh decade.

Jemal A, Siegel R, Ward E, et al. Cancer statistics, 2008. *CA Cancer J Clin.* 2008;58:71–96. [PMID: 18287387]

Shaib YH, Davila JA, El-Serag HB. The epidemiology of pancreatic cancer in the United States: changes below the surface. *Aliment Pharmacol Ther.* 2006;24:87–94. [PMID: 16803606]

Pathogenesis & Risk Factors

Most pancreatic neoplasms arise from the three different types of the epithelial cells found in the pancreas. Acinar cells account for 80% of the volume of the gland but constitute 1% of exocrine tumors. Ductal cells constitute 10–15% of the volume but give rise to 90% of all tumors. Endocrine cells are 1–2% of volume and account for 1–2% of the tumors. Nonepithelial tumors are very rare.

Approximately 70% of ductal tumors are localized to the head of the pancreas, 5–10% to the body, and 10–15% to the tail. These tumors are hard in consistency due to the strong desmoplastic response they elicit.

Acinar tumors present as large pancreatic masses in the elderly, and distant metastasis is usually present at the time of diagnosis.

A. Molecular Pathogenesis

It has been proposed that pancreatic cancer develops from small intraductal precursor lesions (pancreatic intraepithelial neoplasia), following an evolution similar to the adenoma–carcinoma sequence seen in colorectal tumors. Although the precise mechanism and sequence of genetic mutations responsible for the development of pancreatic cancer remains unclear, genetic alterations found in these tumors can be classified into three categories: (1) activation of oncogenes; (2) inactivation of tumor suppressor genes; and (3) defect in DNA mismatch repair genes. The sonic hedgehog signaling pathway also appears to play a role. The sonic hedgehog gene, which is involved with embryonic development, appears to be unregulated in early and late stages of pancreatic carcinogenesis.

1. Activation of oncogenes—Mutations of the *K-ras* oncogene are seen in 90% of tumors and are the hallmark of pancreatic adenocarcinoma. Although this mutation may be seen in nonmalignant conditions such as chronic pancreatitis, it appears to be an early genetic alteration in pancreatic carcinogenesis.

2. Inactivation of tumor suppressor genes—Inactivation and loss of function of tumor suppressor genes results in critical disruption of the cell cycle involving cellular differentiation, growth inhibition, regulation of transcription, DNA repair, and apoptosis. The genes most frequently involved are *CDKN2A* (95%), *P53* (60%), *DPC4* (50%), *BRCA2,* and *STK11.* About 10% of patients with hereditary pancreatic cancer harbor germline mutations of the *BRCA2* gene.

3. Defect of DNA mismatch repair gene—Mutations of mismatch repair genes, such as *MLH1* and *MSH2,* have been found in 4% of pancreatic tumors.

B. Hereditary Risk Factors

1. Family history of pancreatic cancer—Genetic predisposition is the greatest risk factor for the development of pancreatic cancer. About 8–10% of patients with pancreatic cancer have a first-degree relative with the disease. These patients present at an earlier age, and smoking appears to contribute to the development of the cancer.

2. Hereditary chronic pancreatitis—This autosomal-dominant condition is strongly associated with pancreatic cancer although it accounts for only a small fraction of the total number of cases. It presents as recurrent attacks of acute pancreatitis early in life that may progress to chronic pancreatitis. The risk of an affected family member developing cancer is as high as 40% by age 70 and is highest among those who smoke.

3. Other conditions—The risk of pancreatic cancer is also increased in patients with certain familial cancer syndromes such as Peutz-Jeghers syndrome, ataxia–telangiectasia, familial adenomatous polyposis, and Lynch syndrome II.

Diabetes mellitus is associated with pancreatic cancer, and in most cases there is no family history. In most patients the diagnosis of pancreatic cancer is made within 2 years of the onset of diabetes mellitus. Although some studies have shown that high prediagnosis serum concentrations of glucose and insulin, along with insulin resistance, correlate with an increased risk of pancreatic cancer, other studies suggest that the tumor may be responsible for the diabetogenic state.

C. Environmental Risk Factors

The best-established environmental risk factor associated with pancreatic cancer is cigarette smoking. The relative risk of pancreatic cancer among current smokers is 2.5. The risk increases with the number of cigarettes consumed and returns to baseline 15 years after the patient stops smoking.

Diet appears to be another important environmental factor. Diets high in fat and meat appear to be linked to the development of pancreatic cancer, while consumption of fruits and vegetables seem to have a protective effect. Low levels of selenium and lycopene have been associated with the development of pancreatic cancer.

Data on coffee and alcohol consumption, use of aspirin and other nonsteroidal anti-inflammatory drugs, and the development of pancreatic cancer have been conflicting, and recent studies show no definite relationship. In a recent study, obesity significantly increased the risk of pancreatic cancer. Some studies have shown an association between *Helicobacter pylori* infection, particularly the Cag A strain, and pancreatic cancer.

D. Nonhereditary Risk Factors

The risk of pancreatic adenocarcinoma is about 4% in patients with nonhereditary chronic pancreatitis 20 years after disease onset.

Clinical Findings

A. Symptoms and Signs

Owing to the lack of characteristic signs and symptoms, most patients with pancreatic tumors present late in the course of the disease. As a result, less than 15% of tumors are resectable at the time of diagnosis. Even after surgical resection with negative margins, the 5-year survival rate is between 10% and 25%, with a median survival between 10 and 20 months. Patients may present with vague, low-intensity, dull abdominal discomfort or pain that radiates to the back and may be associated with weight loss, anorexia, weakness, diarrhea, and vomiting (Table 28–1). The pain is primarily due to the invasion of the celiac and superior mesenteric plexus.

Location of the tumor also defines the symptoms and the prognosis. Tumors of the head of the pancreas produce symptoms early, and painless jaundice is seen in more than 50% of cases due to obstruction of the extrahepatic bile duct. In less than one third of patients, obstruction of the bile duct by pancreatic neoplasm is accompanied by a palpable, nontender gallbladder referred to as Courvoisier sign. This finding also may be seen in bile duct obstruction by cholangiocarcinoma, duodenal carcinoma, and carcinoma of the ampulla of Vater.

Table 28–1. Clinical manifestations that may be associated with pancreatic cancer.

Symptoms and Signs	Laboratory Findings
Abdominal pain or discomfort	↑ Serum alkaline phosphatase
Weight loss	↑ Bilirubin
Anorexia	↑ Transaminases
Weakness	↑ Erythrocyte sedimentation rate
Jaundice	↑ Serum CA 19-9
Irritable bowel syndrome (diarrhea)	
New-onset diabetes after age 50 y	
New onset mood changes	

Tumors of the body and tail are either "asymptomatic" or manifest with nonspecific symptoms, such as abdominal discomfort, and the diagnosis is mostly made after metastatic disease has developed.

Obstruction of the pancreatic duct may lead to pancreatic exocrine insufficiency in the form of steatorrhea and malabsorption. New-onset diabetes mellitus after the age of 50 years has been associated with the development of pancreatic cancer, especially in the absence of a family history of diabetes. Other uncommon manifestations of pancreatic neoplasm include acute pancreatitis in the elderly without any obvious cause, thrombophlebitis, psychiatric disturbances, pruritus due to cholestasis, signs and symptoms of gastrointestinal bleeding, and obstruction due to erosion and growth of the pancreatic neoplasm into the duodenal lumen. In patients older than age 50, pancreatic cancer can present with features of irritable bowel syndrome or early-onset diabetes.

B. Laboratory Findings (see Table 28–1)

Malignant obstruction of the distal bile duct by a neoplasm of the pancreatic head characteristically produces an alkaline phosphatase level that is four to five times the upper limits of normal, and the increase is disproportionate to the bilirubin level until late in the course of the disease. The rise in transaminases is usually mild. Despite biliary stasis, cholangitis is uncommon. Lipase and amylase are elevated in tumors that cause pancreatic duct obstruction and present as acute pancreatitis.

1. Tumor markers—CA 19-9 is a sialylated Lewis antigen that has been found to be clinically useful in both diagnosis and monitoring of the treatment response. The sensitivity and specificity, using a cutoff level of 37 units/mL, is 86% and 87%, respectively. Biliary tract obstruction with cholangitis due to a nonmalignant cause can result in high levels of CA 19-9. In one study, levels as high as 32,000 were reported.

C. Imaging and Other Diagnostic Studies (see Chapter 9)

Pancreatic adenocarcinoma is staged using a TNM classification (Table 28–2). It consists of evaluating the characteristics of the primary tumor, namely tumor size and infiltration into major vessels (T stage), regional lymph node involvement (N stage), and the presence and absence of distant metastasis (M stage). Various modalities are available for the diagnosis and staging of pancreatic tumors, including those described below.

1. Computed tomography (CT) scan—Transabdominal ultrasound and the CT scan remain the most common imaging modalities used in patients with suspected pancreatic cancer. A pancreatic protocol helical CT scan is probably the best initial modality for diagnosis and staging of pancreatic adenocarcinoma. Based on the imaging features, a correct diagnosis of pancreatic cancer is made in more than 90% of cases. In addition to detecting metastasis, based on the involvement of adjacent organs, and vascular invasion, the helical CT scan can predict unresectability with more than 90% accuracy. The major drawback is that a significant proportion of patients found to have resectable disease on CT scan have unresectable disease at laparotomy due to small tumor implants in the liver and peritoneum.

Table 28–2. Staging of pancreatic exocrine cancer.

Definition of TNM	
Primary Tumor (T)	
TX	Primary tumor cannot be assessed
T0	No evidence of primary tumor
Tis	In situ carcinoma
T1	Tumor limited to the pancreas, ≤2 cm in greatest dimension
T2	Tumor limited to the pancreas, >2 cm in greatest dimension
T3	Tumor extends beyond pancreas but without involvement of celiac axis or superior mesenteric artery
T4	Tumor involves celiac axis or superior mesenteric artery (unresectable primary tumor)
Regional Lymph Nodes (N)	
NX	Regional lymph nodes cannot be assessed
N0	No regional lymph node metastasis
N1	Regional lymph node metastasis
Distant Metastasis (M)	
MX	Distant metastasis cannot be assessed
M0	No distant metastasis
M1	Distant metastasis
Stage Grouping	
Stage 0	Tis, N0, M0
Stage IA	T1, N0, M0
Stage IB	T2, N0, M0
Stage IIA	T3, N0, M0
Stage IIB	T1-3, N1, M0
Stage III	T4, any N, M0
Stage IV	Any T, any N, M1

Reproduced with permission from the American Joint Committee on Cancer (AJCC), Chicago, Illinois, *AJCC Cancer Screening Manual*, 7th edition, Springer-Verlag, New York, www.springer.com.

2. Endoscopic ultrasound (EUS)—EUS has a diagnostic sensitivity similar to helical CT scan but may be superior in diagnosing small pancreatic tumors, and portal and splenic vein invasion. EUS-guided fine needle aspiration (EUS–FNA) has a diagnostic sensitivity of about 85–90% with a false-negative rate of 10–15%. It is safe procedure with minimal risk of tumor seeding. EUS is less accurate in predicting superior mesenteric vein and superior mesenteric artery involvement by the tumor.

3. Endoscopic retrograde cholangiopancreatography (ERCP)—Pancreatic tumors appear as strictures of the pancreatic duct or the bile duct on ERCP. This stricturing of both the bile duct and the pancreatic duct is referred to as the "double duct sign." Advances in pancreatic imaging such as helical CT have made ERCP unnecessary as an initial test. Major limitations of ERCP are the limited ability to obtain a tissue diagnosis in malignant bile duct obstruction (positive in <50% of cases); limited utility for pancreatic tumor staging, as it provides no information about tumor extent, vascular invasion, or involvement of the lymph nodes; and risk of complications such as pancreatitis, perforation, and rarely, death.

4. Magnetic resonance imaging (MRI)—Accuracy of MRI to determine resectability appears comparable to the dual-phase helical CT scan. Magnetic resonance cholangiopancreatography (MRCP) is as sensitive as ERCP in the diagnosis of pancreatic tumors.

5. Positron emission tomography (PET)—PET scanning is not routinely used in diagnosis of pancreatic cancers. It can be useful in diagnosing tumor reoccurrence after pancreatic resection.

6. Laparoscopy—Studies have shown that standard preoperative imaging modalities, including CT scan in 15–40% cases, are unable to detect small peritoneal and liver metastasis. In select patients, staging laparoscopy along with peritoneal cytologic examination can detect unsuspected metastasis and prevent unwarranted surgery.

D. Diagnostic Approach

Figure 28–1 presents an algorithm for the diagnosis and treatment of suspected pancreatic cancer. The need for tissue to establish a diagnosis in a suspected pancreatic cancer remains controversial. Although consensus on an optimal approach is lacking, any diagnostic strategy should aim to reliably and safely establish a diagnosis, if necessary; determine resectability to avoid costs; and avoid morbidity and mortality associated with unnecessary surgical intervention.

Comparing imaging modalities such as (EUS, MRI, and CT) has methodological limitations, such as patient selection, study design, and quality. EUS has been generally found to be superior to CT and MRI in detection and characterization of smaller lesions. It has been found to be superior to helical CT scan and MRI for tumor and nodal staging, with a sensitivity of greater than 90%. EUS does not offer any advantage over helical CT in determining resectability of preoperatively suspected pancreatic adenocarcinoma, and the two modalities are considered complementary.

Helical pancreatic protocol CT (PPCT) scan is usually the preferred initial test for loco-regional staging and detection of distant metastasis. Based on the CT scan findings, pancreatic masses fall into one of the following four broad categories: (1) no mass, (2) unresectable mass, (3) resectable mass, and (4) equivocal findings.

Based on clinical suspicion and pretest probability, further imaging by MRCP, EUS, ERCP, or a combination of these methods may be necessary, even if the initial CT findings are negative for any mass lesion. EUS can identify lesions not seen on CT or MRI.

If a clearly unresectable mass is identified on CT scan, a tissue diagnosis is usually indicated prior to starting any palliative chemotherapy or radiotherapy. EUS–FNA, or a percutaneous approach using a CT or transabdominal ultrasound, can be used. In patients with pancreatic cancer who experience pain, EUS can be used to perform celiac plexus neurolysis during the initial diagnostic and staging examination.

Patients identified as having a resectable mass on CT scan should be considered for EUS as a complementary test because it is more accurate for local tumor staging and predicting vascular invasion. The need to obtain a tissue diagnosis in this group is controversial. Beyond the patient's desire for a tissue diagnosis, pretest probability of a tumor, and available local expertise, the major consideration determining whether to obtain a tissue diagnosis should be its impact on clinical decision-making and management.

The major drawback of pursuing a tissue diagnosis is that the sensitivity of EUS–FNA is 85–90%, giving it an unacceptably high false-negative rate of 10–15%. If the pretest probability based on the clinical presentation laboratory data and radiological findings for cancer is high, then a negative tissue diagnosis does not influence the decision to proceed with surgery. Although minimal, the potential for complications such as bleeding, pancreatitis, and tumor seeding during fine needle aspiration should also be considered.

Besides confirming the diagnosis of pancreatic cancer in the majority of patients, the advantages of obtaining tissue are that it helps identify other malignancies, such as neuroendocrine tumors, lymphoma, and small-cell carcinoma, as well as nonmalignant conditions such as autoimmune pancreatitis and chronic pancreatitis, resulting in changes in treatment and prognosis.

Complications from surgery are another major concern. Pancreatoduodenectomy is associated with significant morbidity, and the mortality rate can range from less than 1% in a large-volume center to about 15% in centers performing few such surgeries per year. This must be taken into account by the physicians and the patient prior to surgical resection of the pancreas.

Patients with tumors localized to the body and tail of the pancreas and resectable by helical CT criteria should be considered for laparoscopy prior to surgery as these tumors are usually advanced at presentation and frequency of unsuspected spread to the peritoneum can be as high as 50%.

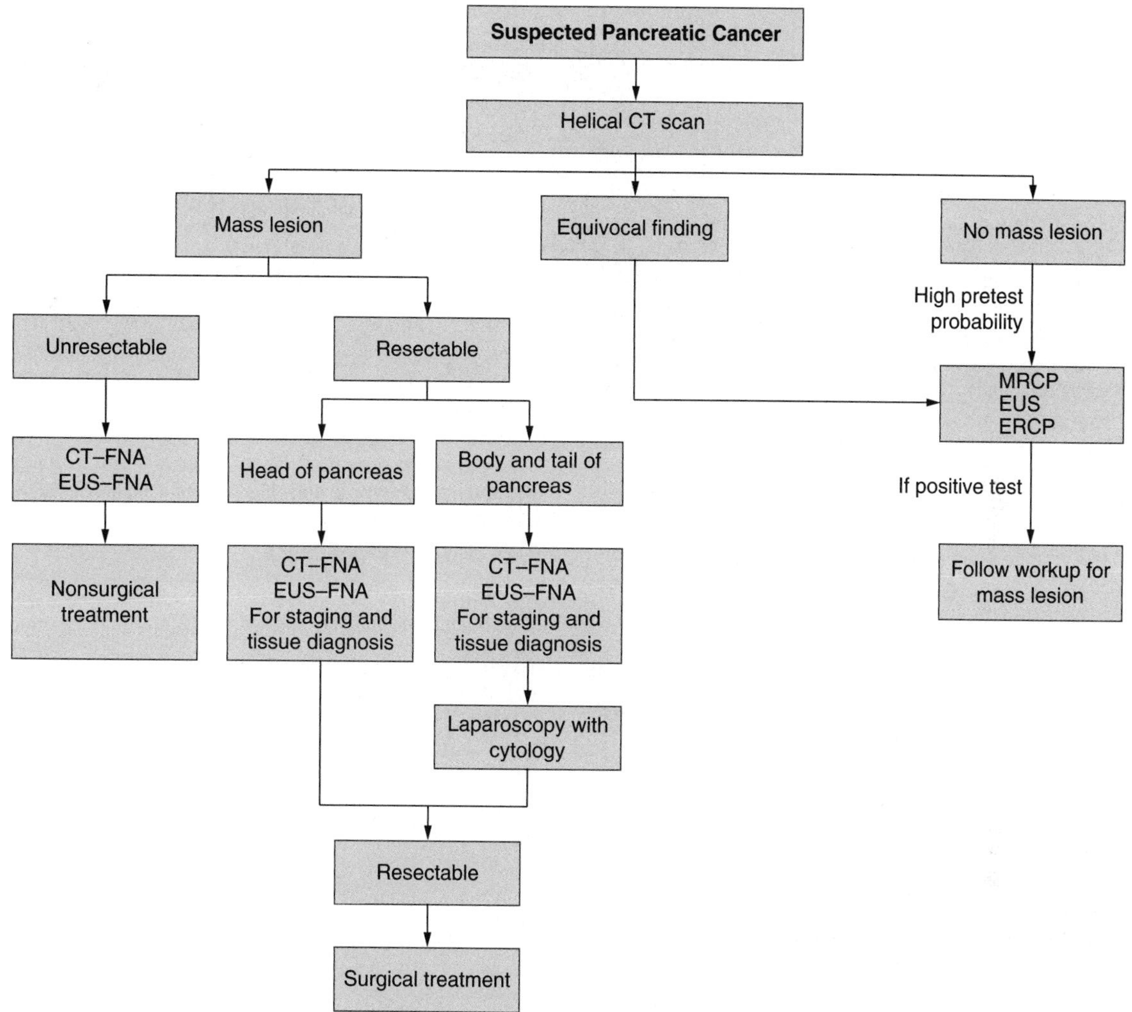

▲ **Figure 28–1.** Algorithm for the diagnosis and treatment of suspected pancreatic carcinoma. CT, computed tomography; ERCP, endoscopic retrograde cholangiopancreatography; EUS, endoscopic ultrasound; FNA, fine needle aspiration; MRCP, magnetic resonance cholangiopancreatography.

In patients whose CT findings are equivocal regarding the presence of a mass or potential for resectability, EUS is indicated, as it is the most sensitive method to detect small tumors of the pancreas and evaluate for vascular invasion.

Adamek HE, Albert J, Breer H, et al. Pancreatic cancer detection with magnetic resonance cholangiopancreatography and endoscopic retrograde cholangiopancreatography: a prospective controlled study. *Lancet.* 2000;356:190–193. [PMID: 10963196]

ASGE Standards of Practice Committee, Gan SI, Rajan E, et al. Role of EUS: communication from the ASGE standards of practice committee. *Gastrointest Endosc.* 2007;66:425–434. [PMID: 17643438]

Dewitt J, Devereaux BM, Lehman GA, et al. Comparison of endoscopic ultrasound and computed tomography for the preoperative evaluation of pancreatic cancer: a systemic review. *Clin Gastroenterol Hepatol.* 2006;4:717–725. [PMID: 16675307]

Mertz HR, Sechopoulos P, Delbeke D, et al. EUS, PET, and CT scanning for evaluation of pancreatic adenocarcinoma. *Gastrointest Endosc.* 2000;52:367–371. [PMID: 10968852]

Soriano A, Castells A, Ayuso C, et al. Preoperative staging and tumor resectability assessment of pancreatic cancer: prospective study comparing endoscopic ultrasonography, helical computed tomography, magnetic resonance imaging, and angiography. *Am J Gastroenterol.* 2004;99:492–501. [PMID: 15056091]

Wiersema MJ, Norton ID, Clain JE. Role of EUS in the evaluation of pancreatic adenocarcinoma. *Gastrointest Endosc.* 2000;52: 578–582. [PMID: 11023593]

Differential Diagnosis

Pancreatic adenocarcinoma must be differentiated from the following conditions of the pancreas that can mimic its symptoms: autoimmune pancreatitis, chronic pancreatitis, pancreatic lymphoma, neuroendocrine tumors of the pancreas, and cystic lesions of the pancreas.

A. Autoimmune Pancreatitis

Autoimmune pancreatitis is a rare disorder of presumed autoimmune etiology that can manifest with obstructive jaundice, weight loss, abdominal pain, and new-onset diabetes. Imaging studies show diffuse enlargement of the pancreas, irregular narrowing of the pancreatic duct, strictures of the common bile duct, and stricture of the intrahepatic radicals similar to that seen in primary sclerosing cholangitis (refer to Table 27–3 in the preceding chapter). Increased levels of serum γ-globulins, especially immunoglobulin G_4, are present. Lymphoplasmacytic infiltration with fibrosis and obliterative phlebitis is seen on histologic examination. Corticosteroids are effective in alleviating symptoms and reversing histopathologic changes (see Chapter 27).

B. Chronic Pancreatitis

The incidence of pancreatic adenocarcinoma in patients with chronic pancreatitis increases about 2% per decade after onset of the disease. Abdominal pain, weight loss, and jaundice may occur in patients with chronic pancreatitis, making it difficult to differentiate chronic pancreatitis complicated by adenocarcinoma.

Imaging studies are not always useful as patients with chronic pancreatitis can present with strictures of the pancreatic and bile duct on ERCP, a mass lesion on CT (variant of AIP), or with changes in the echo texture of pancreatic tissue, making EUS images difficult to interpret. EUS appears to be superior to CT scan for detection of coexistent malignancy.

Although CA 19-9 is elevated in about 80% of patients with adenocarcinoma, it can also be elevated in patients with chronic pancreatitis, and very high values may occur in patients with obstructive jaundice and cholangitis.

K-ras mutations do not seem to be clinically useful in differentiating chronic pancreatitis and pancreatic cancer.

Treatment

Patients with pancreatic cancer can be subdivided into three categories based on the extent of tumor spread: (1) tumor confined to the pancreas (resectable disease at diagnosis), representing approximately 15–20% of patients; (2) locally advanced disease (unresectable), 40%; and (3) metastatic disease, 40%.

A. Resectable Disease

Surgical resection is the only curative treatment for pancreatic cancer. Owing to the characteristically late presentation, only 15% of patients are candidates for pancreatectomy. The most common surgery is the Whipple pancreaticoduodenectomy, used in patients with cancers located in the head of the pancreas. The procedure involves en bloc removal of the gastric antrum, pancreas, and duodenum. Removal of regional lymph nodes has not been shown to be associated with improved survival. Mortality rates for this procedure are about 1–3% at centers that perform a large number of these procedures.

As noted earlier, even after surgical resection with negative margins, patients have a 5-year survival rate of only 10–25%, with median survival of 10–20 months. Involvement of the lymph nodes in resected patients is the most important prognostic factor; 5-year survival after the Whipple procedure is 10% for patients with node-positive disease and 25–30% for those with node-negative disease. Tumor size less than 3 cm, well-differentiated tumors, negative surgical margins, and absence of lymph node metastasis are associated with improved survival.

Surgical resection of tumors located on the body and the tail consists of distal subtotal pancreatectomy along with splenectomy.

Endoscopic stent placement in patients with resectable tumors to relieve jaundice prior to surgery does not alter postoperative morbidity and mortality and is not recommended. If the surgery is scheduled for several weeks later, a plastic stent can be placed to relieve jaundice and reduce the risk of cholangitis.

Birkmeyer JD, Stukel TA, Siewers AE, et al. Surgeon volume and operative mortality in the United States. *N Engl J Med.* 2003; 349:2117–2127. [PMID: 14645640]

Blackstock AW, Mornex F, Partensky C, et al. Adjuvant gemcitabine and concurrent radiation for patients with resected pancreatic cancer: a phase II study. *Br J Cancer.* 2006;95:260–265. [PMID: 16868545]

Neoptolemos JP, Stocken DD, Friess H, et al. A randomized trial of chemoradiotherapy and chemotherapy after resection of pancreatic cancer. *N Engl J Med.* 2004;350:1200–1210. [PMID: 15028824]

Stojadinovic A, Brooks A, Hoos A, et al. An evidence-based approach to the surgical management of resectable pancreatic approach to the surgical management of resectable pancreatic adenocarcinoma. *J Am Coll Surg.* 2003;196:954–964. [PMID: 12788434]

B. Locally Advanced Disease

Optimal treatment in these patients remains controversial. The combination of chemotherapy and radiation is associated with modest improvements in median survival but may produce significant side effects. 5-Fluorouracil, gemcitabine, and paclitaxel are some of the common chemotherapeutic agents used with radiotherapy.

Symptom palliation is an essential component of care for patients with locally advanced disease. Patients with tumors localized to the pancreatic head can develop obstructive jaundice and gastric outlet obstruction; severe abdominal pain is more common with tumors involving the body and tail of the pancreas.

Sohn TA, Yeo CJ, Cameron JL, et al. Do preoperative biliary stents increase post pancreaticoduodenectomy complications? *J Gastrointest Surg.* 2000;4:258–267. [PMID: 10769088]

1. Obstructive jaundice—Compression of the bile duct by the tumor can cause obstructive jaundice. Endoscopic stent placement is the most effective approach to relieve malignant bile duct obstruction. Metal stents are preferred over plastic ones for palliation once the patient is no longer considered a surgical candidate. Unlike plastic stents, which require frequent periodic changes due to occlusion, metal stents have a significantly higher patency rate; however, once placed they cannot be removed endoscopically. The stents may be placed percutaneously if an endoscopic approach is not possible as a result of tumor in-growth or previous surgery. Rarely, a surgical biliary enteric bypass is required to relieve the obstruction.

2. Gastric outlet obstruction—Obstruction of the gastric outlet is caused by extension of the pancreatic cancer and can be treated by gastrojejunostomy or by endoscopically placed expanding metal stents.

3. Pain—Narcotic medications are usually required to control pain associated with pancreatic cancers. Celiac plexus block (chemical neurolysis) can be achieved though a percutaneous approach, or the block can be performed using EUS. Radiation can be used to control intractable pain.

C. Metastatic Disease

Chemotherapy is used for palliation and results in slight survival benefits. Gemcitabine-based combination therapy is the treatment of choice and associated with better pain control, decreased weight loss, and improvement in performance status.

CYSTIC NEOPLASMS OF THE PANCREAS

These lesions represent a spectrum of benign and malignant tumors and account for 1% of pancreatic neoplasms. The most common—mucinous cystic neoplasms, serous cyst adenomas, intraductal papillary mucinous neoplasms (IPMNs), and solid cystic papillary neoplasms (rare)—are described in detail later in this section. Table 28–3 contrasts epidemiologic and biologic characteristics of these and other pancreatic cystic neoplasms.

Clinical Findings

A. Symptoms and Signs

Characteristic manifestations for each lesion are described in detail later in this section.

B. Imaging Studies

CT and MRI are excellent tests for initial detection and characterization of cystic lesions of the pancreas, but differentiation of benign and malignant disease on the basis

Table 28–3. Epidemiologic and biologic characteristics of pancreatic cystic neoplasms.

Type	Sex Predilection	Peak Decade of Life	% of Cystic Neoplasms	Malignant Potential and Natural History
Mucinous cystic neoplasm	Female	5th	10-45	Resection curative, regardless of degree of epithelial dysplasia; poor prognosis when invasive adenocarcinoma present
Serous cyst adenoma (Figure 9–46)	Female	7th	32-39	Resection curative; serous cystadenocarcinoma extremely rare
Intraductal papillary mucinous neoplasm (Figure 9–47, Figure 9–48)	Equal distribution	6th-7th	21-33	Excellent prognosis for lesions showing only adenomatous and borderline cytologic atypia; poor prognosis when invasive carcinoma present
Solid pseudopapillary neoplasm	Female	4th	<10	Indolent neoplasm with rare nodal and extranodal metastases; excellent prognosis when completely resected
Cystic endocrine neoplasm	Equal distribution	5th-6th	<10	Similar to solid neuroendocrine neoplasm
Ductal adenocarcinoma with cystic degeneration	Slight male predominance	6th-7th	<1	Dismal prognosis, similar to solid adenocarcinoma
Acinar-cell cyst-adenocarcinoma	Male	6th-7th	<1	Similar to solid type; aggressive neoplasm with slightly better prognosis than ductal adenocarcinoma

of imaging alone is difficult (see Figures 9–46, 9–47, and 9–48). Besides providing better characterization of the cystic lesion, MRI may also be able to show the communication between the cyst and the pancreatic duct. EUS findings alone are not accurate to determine the type of cystic lesion or its malignant potential. EUS–FNA has emerged as the technique of choice for obtaining cyst fluid for evaluation of tumor makers and cells. It also assists in detecting malignant transformation by providing cells from the cyst walls. EUS–FNA carries a 2–3% risk of pancreatitis. ERCP is useful in detecting intraductal neoplasms, especially IPMN, but its role has become limited by advances in pancreatic imaging.

C. Cytology and Tumor Markers

Cytologic analysis of the cyst fluid has high specificity for mucinous lesions as well as presence of malignancy, but its sensitivity is low (Table 28–4). The yield of cells obtained from EUS–FNA can be insufficient to make a definitive diagnosis or confirm malignant transformation as the lining of the cystic lesions is often denuded. Tumor markers have been shown to improve diagnostic accuracy and differentiation of cystic lesions. Levels of carcinoembryonic antigen (CEA) and CA 72-4 are usually high in mucinous lesions. A CEA cutoff level of 192 ng/mL was found to be most accurate for differentiating between mucinous and nonmucinous cystic lesions with a sensitivity of 73% and specificity of 84%.

Serous cyst adenomas can contain high numbers of glycogen cells whereas mucinous lesions can have fluid high in mucin. The presence of mucin-like antigen as a marker for mucinous tumors has also been used.

Amylase levels are high in both pseudocysts and IPMN, and low in serous cyst adenomas and most mucinous cyst adenomas. CA 19-9 is not elevated in cystic lesions of the pancreas.

Brandwein SL, Farrell JJ, Centeno BA, et al. Detection and tumor staging of malignancy in cystic, intraductal, and solid tumors of the pancreas by EUS. *Gastrointest Endosc.* 2001;53:722–727. [PMID: 11375578]

Brugge WR, Lewandrowski K, Lee-Lewandrowski E, et al. Diagnosis of pancreatic cystic neoplasms: a report of the cooperative pancreatic cyst study. *Gastroenterology.* 2004;126:1330–1336. [PMID: 15131794]

Jacobson BC, Baron TH, Adler DG, et al. ASGE guideline: the role of endoscopy in the diagnosis and the management of cystic lesions and inflammatory fluid collections of the pancreas. *Gastrointest Endosc.* 2005;61:363–370. [PMID: 15758904]

Khalid A, McGrath KM, Zahid M, et al. The role of pancreatic cyst fluid molecular analysis in predicting cyst pathology. *Clin Gastroenterol Hepatol.* 2005;3:967–973. [PMID: 16234041]

Differential Diagnosis

True cystic neoplasms of the pancreas must be differentiated from inflammatory pseudocysts, which are the most common cystic lesions of the pancreas. Pseudocysts are collections of pancreatic secretions without an epithelial lining that occur as a result of inflammation of the pancreas, or obstruction or disruption of the pancreatic duct. Clinical history and associated radiologic findings of acute or chronic pancreatitis, gland atrophy, ductal dilation, and calcification help differentiate pseudocysts from cystic neoplasms. High levels of amylase and low CEA are usually noted in the pseudocyst fluid.

1. Mucinous Cystic Neoplasms

Mucinous cystic neoplasms are the most common cystic tumors of the pancreas, comprising 40–50% of these neoplasms. They occur predominantly in middle-aged women (>80%) and are mostly localized to the body or tail of the pancreas.

Pathogenesis

These tumors are premalignant lesions and are classified as benign (adenomatous), low-grade malignant (borderline), or malignant (carcinoma in situ and invasive cancer) based on the degree of tissue dysplasia. The presence of malignancy in these tumors as estimated in published reports is estimated to be between 10% and 50%.

Table 28–4. Fluid analysis in cystic lesions of the pancreas.

	Mucinous Cystic Neoplasm	Serous Cyst Adenoma	IPMN	Pseudocyst
Viscosity	High	Low	High	Low
CEA	High (>200 ng/mL)	Low (5-20 ng/mL)	High (>250 ng/mL)	Low
Lipase/Amylase	Low	Low	High	High
Cytology	Mucinous epithelial cells ± Malignant cells if adenocarcinoma	Cuboidal cells ± High glycogen content	Mucinous epithelial cells ± Malignant cells if adenocarcinoma	Histiocytes or acellular
DNA analysis	*K-ras* mutations High DNA amount or high amplitude allelic loss in malignancy	Rare abnormalities	*K-ras* mutations High DNA amount or high amplitude allelic loss in malignancy	No abnormalities

CEA: carcinoembryonic antigen. IPMN: intraductal papillary mucinous neoplasm.

These tumors are filled with mesenchymal-like stroma with high viscosity and generally elevated CEA levels. Unlike IPMNs, these tumors do not communicate with the pancreatic ductal system. Larger size, presence of peripheral eggshell calcification on imaging, and association of a solid component with the cystic lesion are features suggestive of malignant progression.

Clinical Findings

A. Symptoms and Signs

Mucinous cystic tumors can be incidental findings on abdominal imaging or can manifest with abdominal pain, palpable mass, recurrent pancreatitis, and vomiting due to gastric outlet obstruction. Jaundice and weight loss are more common with malignant transformation.

B. Imaging Studies

These tumors appear unilocular or multilocular on CT and MRI, with few discrete compartments. EUS can be helpful to further characterize the lesion and obtain cells for evaluation of malignant transformation.

Treatment

Surgical resection is recommended, because of the significant potential for malignant transformation. Resection is associated with an excellent 5-year survival rate (>95% for benign and borderline tumors and 50–75% for malignant tumors with negative margins). As most of these lesions are localized to the tail of the pancreas, distal pancreatectomy is the most common surgery performed.

2. Serous Cyst Adenomas

These tumors, seen mostly in women, are the second most common cystic tumors of the pancreas. About 70% of serous cyst adenomas occur in the body or tail of the pancreas and have a very low potential for malignant transformation.

Clinical Findings

A. Symptoms and Signs

Serous cyst adenomas are usually asymptomatic, but patients can present with abdominal discomfort, a palpable mass, and, if the tumor is large, with bile duct and gastric outlet obstruction.

B. Imaging Studies

On CT scan the tumor consists of multiple tiny cysts separated by delicate fibrous septa arranged around a central stellate scar that may be calcified, giving them a honeycomb appearance. The pathognomonic CT finding of a "sunburst" due to the central scar is seen in 20% of patients.

The cyst fluid has low viscosity (clear and watery), and is high in glycogen, with low CEA levels.

Treatment

Surgery is indicated in symptomatic patients and in those with rapidly enlarging serous cystadenomas. In asymptomatic patients, observation with serial imaging is a valid strategy because of the low risk of malignant transformation.

3. Intraductal Papillary Mucinous Neoplasms

IPMNs are papillary tumors that arise from the pancreatic duct and are associated with mucin hypersecretion. The incidence of IPMN is increasing and they account for 5% of pancreatic neoplasms resected at referral centers. They occur equally in men and women, and the median age at presentation is 65 years. These tumors occur predominantly in the head of the pancreas. IPMNs may involve the main pancreatic duct, a side branch, or both.

Pathogenesis

The role of smoking, alcohol, and genetic predisposition in the development of IPMN remains unclear. Although genetic alterations such as *P53* overexpression, *K-ras* mutations, and *DPC4* overexpression have been identified, their role in the development of IPMN is not understood. Unlike pancreatic cancers, where *DPC4* inactivation is seen in most tumors, *DPC4* is expressed in almost all IPMNs. In 30% of cases IPMN are associated with extra pancreatic tumors. Adenocarcinoma of the colon and stomach being the most common.

Baumagaertner I, Corcos O, Couvelard A, et al. Prevalence of extra pancreatic cancers in patients with histological proven intraductal papillary mucinous neoplasms on the pancreas-A case control study. *Am J Gastroenterol.* 2008,103:2878–2882. [PMID: 18853975]

A. Classification

IPMNs are classified into three types, based on the involvement of the main pancreatic duct (Main duct IPMN) or the side branches (Side Branch IPMN) or both (Mixed IPMN). Side branch IMPN are multifocal in 40% of cases. The main duct type IPMN is more aggressive and has a higher incidence of malignancy.

The WHO (World Health Organization) has histologically classified IPMN into three categories:

- IPMN Adenoma: The cystic lesion is lined by mucin containing columnar cells with no dysplasia.
- IPMN borderline: Lining cells show moderate dysplasia.
- Intraductal Papillary Mucinous Carcinoma: Presence of severe Dysplasia.

The malignant tumors are further classified as noninvasive (carcinoma in situ) or invasive, based on the absence or presence of extension beyond the basement membrane. The location of the IPMN predicts its malignant potential. The risk of malignancy was found to be 57–92% in main duct IPMN, 6–46% in a side branch IPMN and 35–40% in a mixed IPMN in surgically resected specimen. While the prognosis for a benign, borderline, and carcinoma in situ is good, the 5 year survival rate for a invasive malignant lesion is between 30% and 75%.

Brugge WR, Lewandrowski K, Lee-Lewandrowski E, et al. Diagnosis of pancreatic cystic neoplasms: a report of the cooperative pancreatic cyst study. *Gastroenterology.* 2004;126: 1330–1336. [PMID: 15131794]

Maire F, Hammel P, Terris B, et al. Prognosis of malignant intraductal papillary mucinous tumours of the pancreas after surgical resection. Comparison with pancreatic ductal adenocarcinoma. *Gut.* 2002;51:717–722. [PMID: 12377813]

Clinical Findings

A. Symptoms and Signs

About 30% of IPMN are diagnosed on routine imaging studies and are asymptomatic. In symptomatic patients abdominal pain is the most common presenting complaint and is seen in 50–70% patients. About 25% of patients present with acute pancreatitis. Many patients have a history of recurrent bouts of acute pancreatitis, or features of chronic pancreatitis such as diarrhea, new onset diabetes, weight loss/as a result of obstruction of the pancreatic duct by mucus plugs. Weight loss, jaundice, and shorter duration of symptoms are associated with malignant IPMN, though about 40% of malignant IPMN are asymptomatic at presentation.

B. Imaging Studies

Cystic lesions in the pancreas in communication with a dilated pancreatic duct can be seen on CT scan, EUS, and MRI. The sensitivity and specificity of MRCP in diagnosing malignancy in IPMN has been reported to be 70% and 92 % respectively. The presence of mural nodules, segmental or diffuse dilation of the main pancreatic duct greater than 15 mm in diameter, presence of solid component in the cyst is associated with malignant disease. EUS–FNA is also useful in detecting the presence of mucin and provide cells to evaluate for malignant transformation. The cyst fluid aspirate can be useful in distinguishing mucinous lesions from non-mucinous cystic lesions of the pancreas. A CEA (carcinoembryonic antigen) level of 192 g/mL was 79% sensitive in differentiating mucinous tumors from nonmucinous tumors. ERCP is rarely used in the diagnosis of IPMN. The pathognomonic sign on ERCP is a patulous ampulla of Vater with extruding mucus. Pancreatography may also show filling defects due to mucus and communication between the pancreatic duct and cystic areas.

While both IPMN and MCN (mucinous cystic neoplasm) contain mucin and have high CEA levels, MCN do not communicate with the pancreatic duct, and seen mostly in females in the 4–5th decade of life. Unlike IMPN which predominantly occurs in the head of the pancreas, the MCN are seen mostly in the body and tail of the pancreas.

Treatment

Main duct IPMN and mixed IPMN have a significant risk for malignant transformation. About 30–40% of malignant IMPN can be asymptomatic and have a negative cytology on FNA. Surgical resection is recommended in these patients while the prognosis for non malignant IPMN is good, reoccurrence of 50–60% is noted in patients with invasive IPMN with a 5-year survival of 35–75%.

During surgery the resected margins must be examined by frozen section to confirm clearance of the tumor as IPMNs tend to grow longitudinally along the pancreatic ducts rather than radially into the parenchyma.

The risk of malignancy in the side branch IPMN is about 15–25%. In asymptomatic patients with side branch IPMN of size less than 3 cm and no radiological features worrisome for malignancy surveillance is recommended.

Surveillance with periodic imaging is recommended in patients with invasive IPMN, as reoccurrence (most often within the first 3 years) occurs in 50–65% of cases. Patients with carcinoma in situ have a low but significant reoccurrence rate of about 8% and should be followed by yearly CT scan or MRI.

Jang JY, Kim SW, Lee SE, et al. Treatment guidelines for branch duct type intraductal papillary mucinous neoplasms of the pancreas: when can we operate or observe? *Ann Surg Oncol.* 2008;15:199–205. [PMID: 17909912]

Mee J, Jin YJ, Soo JK, et al. Cyst growth rate predicts malignancy in patients with branch duct intraductal papillary mucinous neoplasms. *Clin Gastroenterol Hepatol.* 2011;9:87–93. [PMID: 20851216]

Ohno E, Hirooka Y, Itoh A, et al. Intraductal papillary mucinous neoplasms of the pancreas: differentiation of malignant and benign tumors by endoscopic ultrasound findings of mural nodules. *Ann Surg.* 2009;249:628–634. [PMID: 19300203]

Salvia R, Crippa S, Falconi M, et al. Branch-duct intraductal papillary mucinous neoplasms of the pancreas: to operate or not to operate? *Gut.* 2007;56:1086–1090. [PMID: 17127707]

4. Solid Cystic Papillary Neoplasms

These rare neoplasms with low malignant potential are seen in young women, and are characterized by necrotic and hemorrhagic areas.

PANCREATIC LYMPHOMA

Pancreatic lymphoma represents 1–2% of all pancreatic tumors. It presents as large mass, usually without bile duct obstruction, pain, or weight loss. Treatment consists of combination of chemotherapy and radiation, and is associated with good 5-year survival rates.

29 Polypectomy

Kunal Jajoo, MD

General Considerations

Many epithelial tumors of the gastrointestinal tract develop as benign polyps before becoming malignant, as discussed in detail in earlier sections of this book. These may be symptomatic or asymptomatic, pedunculated or sessile, and range in size from millimeters to many centimeters in diameter. If confined to the mucosa or superficial submucosa, they are nearly all amenable to endoscopic removal by one of a variety of polypectomy techniques, endoscopic mucosal resection (EMR), or endoscopic submucosal dissection (ESD).

The principles of endoscopic polypectomy have evolved to a standardized set of techniques since their introduction almost 40 years ago. EMR and ESD techniques continue to be developed as more recent innovations. Endoscopic resection aims to remove a tumor in its entirety for cure, for complete pathologic assessment, and to reduce or eradicate the risk of recurrence while maintaining the integrity of the wall of the gastrointestinal tract and avoiding procedure-related morbidity. Bleeding is the most common complication of polypectomy, occurring in 0.3– 6.0% of cases. Post-polypectomy hemorrhage can occur immediately (within 12 hours) or can be delayed (up to 30 days) and is more likely to occur with larger polyps, sessile polyps, and polyps with thick stalks. Perforation, the most feared complication of polypectomy, remains rare but relatively unchanged in incidence since the introduction of these techniques. Perforation occurs in 1–2 per 1000 cases and is more likely to occur with piecemeal polypectomy of sessile polyps, cecal polyps and with ESD.

Polypectomy, EMR, and ESD can all be accomplished in the sedated patient as there are no pain receptors in the mucosa and submucosa. The muscularis propria and serosa together with the mesentery are capable of generating pain sensation caused by mechanical forces (eg, stretching) and the thermal effects of electrosurgery. A wide range of accessories is now available for endoscopic polypectomy and the last decade has also seen improvements in electrosurgical generators with respect to ease of use, safety, and efficacy. All endoscopists should be equipped to remove small- to medium-sized sessile polyps and nearly all pedunculated polyps in the colon. Larger sessile polyps (>2 cm in diameter), very large pedunculated polyps in the colon, and polyps of all types in the esophagus, stomach, duodenum, and small bowel require additional expertise and technology and are usually referred to centers with experience in these areas. Such tertiary referral has been demonstrated to be safe and effective and to avoid the risk of unnecessary surgery. It is also cost effective.

EQUIPMENT

Removal of polyps throughout the gastrointestinal tract requires appropriate access with an endoscope bearing an instrumentation channel diameter adequate to take standard accessories. Most of these will pass through a 2.8-mm channel but some may require 3.2 mm or greater. Accessories include biopsy forceps, snares, injection needles, combination devices marrying more than one function in a single instrument, hemostatic clips and loops, bipolar and multipolar probes, and EMR sets providing a spray catheter, injector needle, special snare, and transparent cap, which comes in many shapes and diameters. Accessories for ESD are not yet generally available in the United States. Most accessories designed for colonoscopy will also be long enough for some enteroscopes when therapy in the small bowel is being planned.

Special stains for surface chromoendoscopy (eg, indigo carmine, Lugol iodine, methylene blue, and cresyl violet) may be needed prior to resection in order to optimize visualization of a polyp and its margins. Normal saline is the most common fluid used for submucosal injection during EMR or ESD. Epinephrine can be added to augment immediate hemostasis and methylene blue can be added to enhance visualization. Some experts prefer to inject a fluid of higher viscosity (eg, hyaluronic acid or glycerol), which dissipates less rapidly during resection allowing for a more sustained submucosal cushion during difficult polypectomy. Many endoscopes are capable of imaging with restricted wavelengths of light (eg, narrow band imaging or multiband imaging), which allows visualization of morphology and vasculature in the submucosa, enhancing the endoscopist's ability to recognize the edges of polyps and any malignant features. Marking agents, which are pre-filled vials of a sterile suspension of very fine carbon particles (Spot; GI Supply, Camp Hill, PA); can be used for permanent documentation of a tumor resection site for future endoscopic or surgical reference. With the increasing use of laparoscopic colorectal surgery and the fact that up to 14% of endoscopically identified tumors can be incorrectly localized, endoscopic tattoo marking is essential for subsequent identification.

Many electrosurgical generators are manufactured specifically for endoscopic applications. Most now incorporate computer-controlled outputs modified by feedback through the accessory to achieve the desired tissue effect with the least power necessary. They also incorporate menus for specific endoscopic procedures with defaults set by the manufacturer. All endoscopists and assistants performing electrosurgery must have a thorough knowledge of monopolar high-frequency circuits and their properties in order to understand the safe principles of cutting and coagulation, and to troubleshoot any problems that occur during polypectomy. The concept of current density (power per unit area) is essential to comprehend because this is how snare polypectomy cuts and coagulates tissue as it is being mechanically cut by the closing snare. It is our practice to retain a module for argon plasma coagulation whenever large polyps are being removed as an adjunct for tissue ablation and superficial coagulation. Bowel preparation must be good to excellent both for visibility and to reduce the risk of ignition of bowel gases such as hydrogen and methane. All fluid must be removed from around the polyp to be resected in order to maximize the current density where it is desired at the point of resection.

POLYPECTOMY FOR SESSILE POLYPS

Small polyps less than 5 mm in diameter are often referred to as "diminutive." Irrespective of their site in the gastrointestinal tract, they can usually be removed by any of a number of simple methods that include "cold" biopsy forceps with standard or so-called jumbo forceps, "hot" (ie, combined with electrocautery) biopsy forceps, "cold" snare, and "hot" (ie, combined with electrocautery) snare. A common practice is to place a small diameter snare (eg, 1 cm oval) over the polyp, including a small cuff of normal surrounding mucosa, and then close the snare handle and mechanically cut through the trapped tissue, which will excise the polyp. Because the bleeding risk of simple mechanical cutting and avulsion with cold techniques is minimal, these are favored for such small lesions, which can usually be removed by one pass of the forceps or snare. Such methods are quick and effective and provide the necessary specimen for histopathologic evaluation (Plates 28 and 29) with almost no risk. Resected tissue can be aspirated into the endoscope suction system, to which a specimen trap can be added.

Sessile polyps larger than 5 mm and up to a diameter of 2 cm can usually be removed using electrocautery without additional measures (Plates 30, 31, and 32). Snares are available in many sizes and shapes, with choice being determined by personal or endoscopy unit preference. The principle is to place the snare over the entire polyp and either (1) close it as a cutting or combined cutting and coagulation current is applied until the polyp is detached from the submucosa, or, more commonly, (2) close it as far as possible before applying a pure coagulating current, and then continue closing until the polyp is removed. In both sequences it is important to lift the entrapped tissue away from the wall of the gastrointestinal tract to minimize any deep injury to the gastrointestinal wall. Specimen retrieval is accomplished by suction through the endoscope into a specimen trap. Multiple polyps or those too large for aspiration-retrieval can be collected by a retrieval net.

Several safe methods are available to achieve hemostasis when excessive bleeding occurs immediately after cold or hot snare polypectomy or, very rarely, after forceps removal. Placement of one or more hemostatic clips, injection of diluted epinephrine 1:10,000, application of monopolar coagulation with the snare tip or by argon plasma coagulation, bipolar or multipolar coagulation with a dedicated probe, and band ligation are all used. Endoscopic clips are now readily utilized for immediate hemostasis and for prophylaxis of delayed hemorrhage, likely due to their ease of use. However, there are no studies directly comparing the efficacy of hemoclips and thermal techniques.

Suspected perforation or inadvertent deep submucosal injury can be promptly closed by placing clips to appose the mucosa on either side of the defect.

POLYPECTOMY FOR PEDUNCULATED POLYPS

Pedunculated polyps are so-called because the tumor is situated at the end of a stalk or pedicle and protrudes into the gastrointestinal tract lumen. The principle of polypectomy with these lesions is to resect through the stalk at a sufficient distance from the tumor to ensure its complete removal but not so close to the gut wall as to risk deep thermal injury. A point approximately one-third to one-half way along the stalk from the polyp head is usually chosen for placement of the snare loop (Plate 33); electrocautery is then applied while the snare loop is closed, until the stalk is completely severed. The polyp is then retrieved using either the aspiration method, if small enough, or by snare or net capture.

In contrast to sessile polyps, pedunculated polyps may be so large that the proximal side of the lesion may not be visible endoscopically during snare placement and polypectomy (Plate 34). The endoscopist must then take special precautions (1) to avoid inadvertently trapping normal mucosa in the snare and (2) to avoid injury to the opposite bowel wall if the polyp is touching it. Safe snare position can be confirmed by securing the snare tip on the proximal (further) side first by pulling it toward the endoscope and confirming that the polyp stalk, only, is ensnared before closing it prior to applying cautery. The large polyp extending across the bowel lumen can be removed safely by moving the snare back and forth to prevent any stray current from passing through an undesired site with enough current density to cause injury. This also reduces the power required to achieve the polypectomy. For very large stalks with vessels presumed to be larger than usual, some experts pretreat the stalk with an injection of diluted epinephrine or place an additional mechanical device such as a clip or endoloop before proceeding with polypectomy.

Bleeding from the cut polyp stalk is most readily controlled by resnaring it immediately for tamponade, without applying further cautery, and waiting for natural hemostasis to occur. If this fails, or if the snare has already been removed, any of the methods mentioned earlier can be used. Clips have become popular because of their ease of use and mechanical mechanism of action, which does not risk deep injury to the bowel wall after polypectomy (Plate 35).

Suspected perforation or inadvertent deep submucosal injury can be promptly closed by placing clips to appose the mucosa on either side of the defect.

ENDOSCOPIC MUCOSAL RESECTION

For sessile polyps larger than 2 cm in the colon or duodenum and almost any sized sessile polyp or early cancer in certain anatomic locations, such as the esophagus or stomach, a different set of techniques has been developed, collectively known as EMR. Although there are many technical variations and accessories, the principle of EMR is the same for all. The lesion is lifted or separated from the underlying submucosa before resection is performed either by physical traction or by injecting fluid. One technique employs a two-channel endoscope to lift the lesion first with a grasping device, such as a biopsy forceps passed through one channel of the endoscope, over which is placed a snare, passed through the second channel, to complete the removal. This method, however, has never gained popularity in the United States. A second technique, originally developed in Japan, employs a transparent cap fitted to the tip of an endoscope into which, after submucosal injection of fluid, the lesion is aspirated, and a specially designed ultra-flexible snare placed around the "pseudopolyp" so created. Suction is then released and the polyp resected using the same electrocautery settings as for standard polypectomy (Plates 36 and 37). This method is particularly applicable in the esophagus, stomach, and rectum but is rarely used elsewhere in the gastrointestinal tract.

A third technique employs a band ligation system to raise the lesion into a pseudopolyp before snare resection; this has become popular for small sessile lesions in the upper gastrointestinal tract (Plates 38 and 39). A fourth method, which has become the dominant technique for EMR, is the use of an injection needle to instill fluid around and deep to the polyp to lift it away from the submucosa (Plate 40). Alternative needleless methods for elevation with fluid are also becoming available. This not only ensures that the lesion is safe to resect, as it is not invading deep to the mucosa, but also provides a cushion of safety, protecting the bowel wall from thermal injury. The nonlifting sign after such an attempted injection is an accurate indication of submucosal invasion of carcinoma. After injection, the polyp is snared piecemeal (Plate 41) until the entire area of mucosa has been removed (Plate 42). Any bleeding can be controlled using the methods already outlined. The specimens are retrieved by aspiration, if they are small enough or by a net (Plate 43). The site may be left to heal, or this can be accelerated and possible complications reduced by closing the defect with clips (Plate 44). Although the scar may be visible for follow-up examinations (Plate 45), the site may also be marked with an injection of a permanent ink for future endoscopic surveillance or surgical resection (Plate 46).

ENDOSCOPIC SUBMUCOSAL DISSECTION

A recent extension of EMR developed in Japan is ESD. This collection of techniques aims to remove the sessile lesion as one piece by injecting fluid deep to the lesion, as with EMR, then incising the perimeter of the polyp with a small margin of normal mucosa, followed by careful dissection in the superficial submucosal plane until the resection is complete (Plates 47, 48, and 49). Several accessories are available but none has yet been approved by the U.S. Food and Drug Administration. Although originally intended for removing early gastric cancers, ESD has now been successfully applied to the colon.

This chapter is a revised version of the chapter by Dr. David Carr-Locke that was in the previous edition of Current Diagnosis & Treatment: Gastroenterology, Hepatology, & Endoscopy.

Carpenter S, Petersen BT, Chuttani R, et al. Polypectomy devices. *Gastrointest Endosc.* 2007;65:741–749. [PMID: 17397841]

Fatima H, Rex DK. Minimizing endoscopic complications: colonoscopic polypectomy. *Gastrointest Endosc Clin N Am.* 2007;17: 145–156. [PMID: 17397781]

Fyock CJ, Draganov PV. Colonoscopic polypectomy and associated techniques. *World J Gastroenterol.* 2010;16:3630–3637. [PMID: 20677334]

Kantsevoy SV, Adler DG, Conway JD, et al. ASGE Technology Committee. Endoscopic mucosal resection and endoscopic submucosal dissection. *Gastrointest Endosc.* 2008;68:11–18. [PMID: 18577472]

Kethu SR, Banerjee S, Desilets D, et al; ASGE Technology Committee. Endoscopic tattooing. *Gastrointest Endosc.* 2010;72:681–685. [PMID: 20883844]

Larghi A, Waxman I. State of the art on endoscopic mucosal resection and endoscopic submucosal dissection. *Gastrointest Endosc Clin N Am.* 2007;17:441–469. [PMID: 17640576]

Saito Y, Uraoka T, Matsuda T, et al. Endoscopic treatment of large superficial colorectal tumors: a case series of 200 endoscopic submucosal dissections (with video). *Gastrointest Endosc.* 2007;66: 966–973. [PMID: 17524403]

Swan MP, Bourke MJ, Alexander S, et al. Large refractory colonic polyps: is it time to change our practice? A prospective study of the clinical and economic impact of a tertiary referral colonic mucosal resection and polypectomy service. *Gastrointest Endosc.* 2009;70:1128–1136. [PMID: 19748615]

Tolliver KA, Rex DK. Colonoscopic polypectomy. *Gastroenterol Clin North Am.* 2008;37:229–251. [PMID: 18313548]

Acute Upper Gastrointestinal Bleeding

John R. Saltzman, MD

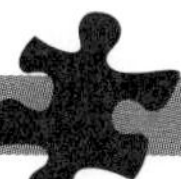

ESSENTIALS OF DIAGNOSIS

- Patients with acute upper GI bleeding can present with hematemesis, melena, or hematochezia
- Clinical guidelines are recommended to predict outcomes, including rebleeding, and mortality
- Stigmata of recent hemorrhage are endoscopic findings that predict outcome
- Endoscopy can provide the diagnosis, prognosis, and the potential for therapy

General Considerations

Nonvariceal upper gastrointestinal (GI) bleeding is a common reason for emergency department visits and admissions to the hospital. It has been estimated that upper GI bleeding is responsible for over 300,000 hospitalizations per year in the United States. An additional 100,000–150,000 patients per year develop upper GI bleeding during hospitalizations for other reasons.

The source of upper GI bleeding is by definition proximal to the ligament of Treitz. The natural history of nonvariceal upper GI bleeding is that approximately 80% of patients will stop bleeding spontaneously and in this group, no further urgent intervention will be needed. However, if a patient rebleeds, there is a tenfold increased mortality rate.

The overall mortality rate is 3–14% for patients with nonvariceal upper GI bleeding. Mortality is typically due to factors other than GI bleeding and occurs primarily in patients who are older and use medications such as nonsteroidal anti-inflammatory drugs (and, more recently, antiplatelet agents such as clopidogrel).

Among patients on long-term, low-dose aspirin, the risk of overt GI bleeding is increased twofold compared to placebo with an annual incidence of major GI bleeding of 0.13%. Compared with aspirin alone, the combination of aspirin and clopidogrel causes a two- to threefold increase in the number of patients with major GI bleeding. Definite risk factors for bleeding in patients taking aspirin and clopidogrel are a history of peptic ulcers and prior GI bleeding, and likely risk factors are male gender, age more than 70 years, and *Helicobacter pylori* infection. Mortality among patients with upper GI bleeding is often due to cardiovascular complications and comorbidities, and not due to uncontrollable GI hemorrhage. In most patients who develop GI bleeding while on aspirin, the aspirin therapy should be restarted once the risk for cardiovascular complications outweighs the risk for bleeding.

Chan FK, Ching JY, Hung LC, et al. Clopidogrel versus aspirin and esomeprazole to prevent recurrent ulcer bleeding. *N Engl J Med.* 2005;352:238–244. [PMID: 15659723]

McQuaid KR, Laine L. Systematic review and meta-analysis of adverse events of low-dose aspirin and clopidogrel in randomized controlled trials. *Am J Med.* 2006;119:624–638. [PMID: 16887404]

Clinical Findings

A. Symptoms and Signs

The clinical presentation of bleeding should be characterized. Hematemesis is overt bleeding with vomiting of fresh blood or clots. Melena refers to dark black and tarry-appearing stool, with a distinctive smell. The term “coffee grounds” describes gastric aspirates or vomitus that contains dark specks of old blood. Hematochezia is the passage of fresh blood or clots per rectum. Although bright red blood per rectum is usually indicative of a lower GI source, it may be seen in patients with brisk upper GI bleeding.

Concurrent with the initial evaluation of patients with suspected upper GI bleeding attention needs to be paid to resuscitation, with the goal of achieving hemodynamic stability. The evaluation must assess vital signs, the presence or absence of shock and hypovolemia, and medical comorbidities (malignancy, chronic obstructive pulmonary disease, coronary

Table 30–1. Risk factors for poor outcome in upper gastrointestinal bleeding.

Age >60 y
Shock (systolic blood pressure <100 mm Hg); pulse >100 beats/min
Malignancy or varices as bleeding source
Onset in hospital
Comorbid illness
Active bleeding (hematemesis, bright red blood in nasogastric tube, or hematochezia)
Recurrent bleeding
Severe coagulopathy

artery disease, etc). Patients with postural hypotension have a significant blood volume loss of at least 10% and those with shock have a blood volume loss of at least 20%, a predictor of poor outcome. Medications used by the patient need to be reviewed with special attention given to anticoagulants (heparin and warfarin), antiplatelet agents (clopidogrel), aspirin, and nonsteroidal anti-inflammatory drugs (NSAIDs).

B. Risk Assessment

1. Clinical predictors—Factors that predict a good or a poor prognosis in patients with nonvariceal upper GI bleeding can be used to appropriately triage and manage patients. The role of nasogastric tube aspiration is controversial. The nasogastric tube aspirate can provide useful information depending on its contents. Nasogastric tube aspirates, however, can be falsely negative; false negatives may occur in patients with bleeding from duodenal ulcers due to spasm of the pylorus and can occur in other conditions, including gastric ulcers and, rarely, esophageal varices (if the tube is positioned in a nondependent area of the stomach).

In patients presenting with upper GI bleeding, several clinical prognostic factors have been shown to be helpful in predicting a poor outcome (Table 30–1). Patients who experience onset of GI bleeding as outpatients have a lower rate of mortality compared with those who are inpatients hospitalized for other reasons. Age of greater than 60 is associated with an increased mortality. The mortality rate increases along with the number of patient comorbidities.

Das A, Wong RC. Prediction of outcome of acute GI hemorrhage: a review of risk scores and predictive models. *Gastrointest Endosc.* 2004;60:85–93. [PMID: 15229431]

Gralnick IM, Dulai GS. Incremental value of upper endoscopy for triage of patients with acute non-variceal upper-GI hemorrhage. *Gastrointest Endosc.* 2004;60:9–14. [PMID: 15229418]

2. Guidelines—Clinical guidelines have been developed to help optimize the management of patients with nonvariceal upper GI bleeding. The aims of these guidelines are to identify low-risk patients who can be discharged either directly from the emergency department or at an early stage of hospitalization, and to identify high-risk patients who will need the most resources. Many clinical guidelines include both clinical data and information obtained at the time of endoscopy. These guidelines can be incorporated as part of routine clinical care to help direct triage decisions. Recent international consensus recommendations on the management of patients with nonvariceal upper GI bleeding recommend the use of prognostic scales for the early risk stratification of patients into low- and high-risk categories of rebleeding and mortality.

The Rockall score is a scoring system used to predict rebleeding and mortality in patients with nonvariceal upper GI bleeding. The Rockall scoring system assigns scores of zero to three to the factors of age, the presence of shock, comorbidity, diagnosis, and endoscopic stigmata (Table 30–2). A low-risk

Table 30–2. Rockall risk assessment score.

Score/Variable	0	1	2	3
Age (y)	<60	70-79	≥80	–
Shock	None	Tachycardia (P >100 beats/min; SBP >100 mm Hg)	Hypotension (P >100 beats/min; SBP >100 mm Hg)	–
Comorbidity	No major comorbidity	–	Congestive heart failure, coronary artery disease, any major comorbidity	Renal or liver failure, metastatic cancer
Diagnosis	Mallory-Weiss tears, no stigmata of recent hemorrhage	All other diagnoses	Upper GI cancer	–
Major stigmata of recent hemorrhage	None or spot	–	Clot, vessel, or spurting	–

GI, gastrointestinal; P, pulse; SBP, systolic blood pressure.
Data from Rockall TA, Logan RFA, Devlin HB, et al. Risk assessment after acute upper gastrointestinal hemorrhage. *Gut.* 1996;38:316–321; and Rockall TA, Logan RF, Devlin HB, et al. Selection of patients for early discharge or outpatient care after acute upper gastrointestinal hemorrhage. National Audit of Acute Upper Gastrointestinal Haemorrhage. *Lancet.* 1996;347:1138–1140.

patient has a score of two or less, which accounted for 29.4% of patients. In this low-risk group, there was a 4.3% risk of rebleeding and 0.1% mortality. Patients with Rockall scores of three to five have intermediate rates of rebleeding and mortality (2.0–7.9%), whereas patients with a score of six or greater have a high rebleeding and mortality rate (15.1–39.1%).

A scoring system that only uses clinical information obtained at the time of presentation, and does not include endoscopic data, has been developed by Blatchford and colleagues. The clinical information incorporated in this scoring system includes hemoglobin, blood urea nitrogen, pulse, systolic blood pressure, presence of syncope, melena, liver disease, and heart failure. This scoring system for upper GI bleeding is valuable because all the information is available at initial presentation, and it does not require endoscopic performance to calculate.

A recently developed risk stratification score for upper GI bleeding also only uses information at the time of the initial presentation and is called the AIMS65 score. This score, which is highly predictive of mortality, uses an equal weighting of its five components: albumin <3.0 g/dL, INR >1.5, mental status changes, systolic blood pressure less than 90 mmHg, and age greater than 65 years. Patients at high risk have two or more of these risk factors present.

The value of clinical guidelines is dependent on treating physicians adhering to the recommendations of the guidelines. Bjorkman and colleagues randomized 93 patients to an urgent endoscopy performed less than 3 hours after presentation with upper GI bleeding or elective endoscopy performed up to 48 hours after presentation. They found the timing of the upper endoscopy did not influence resource utilization or patient outcomes such as overall length of stay or time in the intensive care unit. After urgent upper endoscopy, outpatient care was recommended in 40% of the patients in the study, although actually done in only 9% of the patients, as patients were admitted to the hospital by other treating physicians (not the endoscopists). This finding emphasizes the importance of adherence to guidelines by treating physicians, if there is to be a meaningful impact (Figure 30–1).

Barkun A, Bardou M, Kuipers EJ, et al, for the International Consensus Upper Gastrointestinal Bleeding Conference Group. International consensus recommendations on the management of patients with nonvariceal upper gastrointestinal bleeding. *Ann Intern Med* 2010;152:101–113. [PMID: 20083829]

Bjorkman DJ, Zaman A, Fennerty MB, et al. Urgent vs. elective endoscopy for acute non-variceal upper-GI bleeding: an effectiveness study. *Gastrointest Endosc.* 2004;60:1–8. [PMID: 15229417]

Blatchford O, Murray WR, Blatchford M. A risk score to predict need for treatment for upper-gastrointestinal hemorrhage. *Lancet.* 2000;356:1318–1321. [PMID: 11073021]

Gralnek AM, Barkun AN, Bardou M. Management of acute bleeding from a peptic ulcer. *N Engl J Med.* 2008;359:928–937.

Pang SH, Ching JY, Lau JY, Sung JJ, Graham DY, Chan FK. Comparing the Blatchford and pre-endoscopic Rockall score in predicting the need for endoscopic therapy in patients with upper GI hemorrhage. *Gastrointest Endosc.* 2010;71:1134–1140.

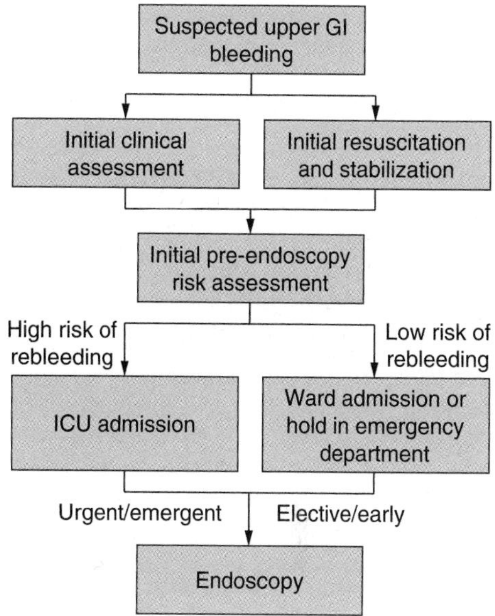

▲ **Figure 30–1.** Algorithm for the management of acute upper gastrointestinal bleeding. ER, emergency room; ICU, intensive care unit. (Adapted, with permission, from Eisen GM, Dominitz JA, Faigel DO, et al. American Society for Gastroenterology. Standards of Practice Committee. An annotated algorithmic approach to upper gastrointestinal bleeding. *Gastrointest Endosc.* 2001;53:853–858.)

Rockall TA, Logan RF, Devlin HB, et al. Risk assessment after acute upper gastrointestinal hemorrhage. *Gut.* 1996;38:316–321. [PMID: 8675081]

Rockall TA, Logan RF, Devlin HB, et al. Selection of patients for early discharge or outpatient care after acute upper gastrointestinal hemorrhage. National Audit of Acute Upper Gastrointestinal Haemorrhage. *Lancet.* 1996;347:1138–1140. [PMID: 8609747]

Treatment of Upper Gastrointestinal Bleeding

A. Medical Therapy

1. Initial therapy—Patients need to have at minimum two large-bore peripheral intravenous access catheters (at least 18 gauge) or central venous access. Crystalloid fluids (normal saline or lactated Ringer) should be initially administered to maintain an adequate blood pressure. Supplemental oxygen should be administered routinely. Patients who are not able to adequately protect their airways or patients with ongoing severe hematemesis and at increased risk for aspiration should be considered for elective endotracheal intubation.

Patients who are at high risk, such as the elderly or those with coronary artery disease, should be transfused to maintain a hematocrit above 30%. Young and healthy patients should be transfused to maintain a hematocrit above 20%.

In patients with a coagulopathy, the coagulopathy should be corrected if possible with transfusion of fresh frozen plasma or administration of vitamin K. In patients with a low platelet count (<50,000), platelet transfusion should be considered.

2. Medications—Various medications have been used to treat patients with nonvariceal upper GI bleeding, including antacids, histamine-2 (H_2)-receptor antagonists, proton pump inhibitors (PPIs), and octreotide. The use of antacids and H_2-receptor antagonists has not been shown to alter the natural history of patients with acute upper GI bleeding.

A. Proton Pump Inhibitors—In studies of PPIs in selected patients with nonvariceal upper GI bleeding, a benefit of medical treatment has been demonstrated. PPIs are the only drugs that can maintain a gastric pH of greater than 6.0 and can thus prevent fibrinolysis of an ulcer clot. The use of PPIs in the treatment of patients with upper GI bleeding has been widely adopted.

An improvement in outcomes with the use of PPIs in nonvariceal upper GI bleeding was first demonstrated by Khuroo and colleagues in a double-blind, placebo-controlled trial of oral omeprazole (40 mg twice daily) versus placebo. Patients enrolled were a select group of 220 patients with peptic ulcers at endoscopy shown to have active bleeding, nonbleeding visible vessels, or adherent clots. Unlike the standard of care in most parts of the world, endoscopic therapy was not performed in this study. Outcomes were further bleeding, surgery, and death. There was a significant advantage to oral omeprazole use in patients who had findings of a visible vessel or an adherent clot. However, there was no advantage to prevent further bleeding in patients who had spurting or oozing lesions. This study, however, did not address whether patients who underwent therapy with endoscopic treatment at the time of endoscopy would attain additional benefit with the use of PPIs.

There have now been several studies showing the benefits of the use of PPIs in patients who have undergone endoscopic therapy with successful hemostasis. Lau and colleagues studied patients who had successful hemostasis using combination therapy of epinephrine injection and application of a bipolar cautery probe. Patients were then randomized to a bolus infusion of omeprazole, 80 mg, followed by a continuous infusion of 8 mg/h, versus a placebo infusion. In these patients, who had all undergone successful endoscopic therapy, the use of omeprazole reduced the rebleeding rates overall and the rebleeding rate within 3 days. There also was a trend toward reduction in surgery and death rates. Thus, with omeprazole use, bleeding is reduced in patients who have undergone endoscopic therapy and receive high-dose PPIs relative to those who undergo endoscopic therapy alone.

Additional studies have been performed that support combined endoscopic and medical management in select patients with upper GI bleeding. Sung and colleagues studied 158 patients with nonvisible vessels or adherent clots receiving omeprazole infusions, randomized to endoscopic therapy or sham therapy. Patients who received both omeprazole infusions and endoscopic therapy had a lower median transfusion rate, less recurrent bleeding, and a trend toward decreased mortality.

In patients initially treated in the emergency department with a bolus infusion of omeprazole followed by a continuous infusion, the need for endoscopic therapy has been shown to be reduced. With the use of initial high-dose PPIs, the number of patients with actively bleeding lesions found at endoscopy is reduced and the number of patients with clean-based ulcers at the time of endoscopy is increased. Thus the early use of PPIs may result in a shift of lesions from high to low risk for further bleeding. However, the natural history of peptic ulcers treated with endoscopic therapies shows that it typically takes 72 hours for most high-risk lesions to become low-risk lesions.

At the present time, there are no studies that compare PPIs to one another in the management of acute upper GI bleeding. The available data suggest that the benefit is a class effect and that dosing should be similar, using the available intravenous PPIs. The current recommendation is for an 80-mg bolus followed by an 8 mg/h infusion for 72 hours in patients who have received successful endoscopic therapy. Patients who remain stable may then be switched to a once-daily standard dose of oral PPIs (unless bleeding was due to severe esophagitis or complicated ulcer disease).

B. Octreotide—Octreotide can be used to treat patients with nonvariceal upper GI bleeding. Although this medication is widely used in patients with variceal bleeding, there is evidence that it may also be helpful in patients with nonvariceal bleeding. In a meta-analysis by Imperiale and Birgisson, 1829 patients from 14 trials using octreotide or somatostatin in nonvariceal upper GI bleeding had a relative risk for further bleeding of 0.53 (0.43–0.63), suggesting that octreotide reduces the risk for continued bleeding from nonvariceal upper GI bleeding. Although a useful adjunctive treatment, octreotide should not, in general, be given as the primary treatment to patients with nonvariceal upper GI bleeding. The use of octreotide should be considered in patients who have persistent bleeding on optimal medical management, including PPIs, and are poor surgical risks (eg, those with multiple comorbidities already in the hospital).

Bianco MA, Rotondano G, Marmo R, et al. Combined epinephrine and bipolar coagulation vs. bipolar probe coagulation alone for bleeding peptic ulcer: a randomized, controlled trial. *Gastrointest Endosc.* 2004;60:910–915. [PMID: 15605005]

Bleau BL, Gostout CJ, Sherman KE, et al. Recurrent bleeding from peptic ulcer associated with adherent clot: a randomized study Comparing endoscopic treatment with medical therapy. *Gastrointest Endosc.* 2002;56:1–6. [PMID: 12085028]

Imperiale TF, Birgisson S. Somatostatin or octreotide compared with H antagonist and placebo in the management of acute nonvariceal upper gastrointestinal hemorrhage: a meta-analysis. *Ann Intern Med.* 1997;127:1062–1071. [PMID: 9412308]

Jensen DM, Kovacs TO, Jutabha R, et al. Randomized trial of medical or endoscopic therapy to prevent recurrent ulcer hemorrhage in patients with adherent clots. *Gastroenterology*. 2002;123: 407–413. [PMID: 12145792]

Khuroo MS, Yatoo GN, Javid G, et al. A comparison of omeprazole and placebo for bleeding peptic ulcer. *N Engl J Med*. 1997;336: 1054–1058. [PMID: 9091801]

Lau JY, Leung WK, Wu JC, et al. Omeprazole before endoscopy in patients with gastrointestinal bleeding. *N Engl J Med*. 2007; 356:1631–1640. [PMID: 17442905]

Lau JY, Sung JJ, Lee KK, et al. Effect of intravenous omeprazole on recurrent bleeding after endoscopic treatment of bleeding peptic ulcers. *N Engl J Med*. 2000;343:310–316. [PMID: 10922420]

Leontiadis GI, Howden CW. The role of proton pump inhibitors in the management of upper gastrointestinal bleeding. *Gastroenterol Clin North Am*. 2009;38:199–213. Review. [PMID: 19446254]

Park CH, Lee SJ, Park JH, et al. Optimal injection volume of epinephrine for endoscopic prevention of recurrent peptic ulcer bleeding. *Gastrointest Endosc*. 2004;60:875–80. [PMID: 15605000]

Sreedharan A, Martin J, Leontiadis GI, et al. Proton pump inhibitor treatment initiated prior to endoscopic diagnosis in upper gastrointestinal bleeding. *Cochrane Database Syst Rev*. 2010;CD005415. [PMID: 20614440]

Sung JJ, Chan FK, Lau JY, et al. The effect of endoscopic therapy in patients receiving omeprazole for bleeding ulcers with nonbleeding visible vessels or adherent clots: a randomized comparison. *Ann Intern Med*. 2003;139:237–243. [PMID: 12965978]

B. Endoscopic Therapy

The goal of endoscopic therapy is to eliminate persistent bleeding and prevent rebleeding. Rebleeding is the greatest contributor to both morbidity and mortality. The ability to achieve sustained hemostasis is dependent on controlled access to the bleeding vessel, a relatively small vessel size, and the absence of significant coagulation defects.

Upper endoscopy provides diagnosis, prognosis, and therapy in patients with acute upper GI bleeding and is reasonably safe to perform in patients with upper GI bleeding (50% of complications are cardiopulmonary). Upper endoscopy is 90–95% sensitive at locating the bleeding site. Sensitivity increases when the procedure is done closer to the onset of the bleeding and decreases with increasing duration from time of onset. Most patients with upper GI bleeding should undergo an upper endoscopy within 24 hours of presentation. Studies have not found an overall advantage of early endoscopy (within 12 hours) in terms of rebleeding rate, need for surgery, or mortality, however patients with active upper GI bleeding may benefit from an early intervention. Endoscopy can offer therapeutic options including injection, cautery, placement of endoclips, or a combination of therapies. Endoscopy can also predict the likelihood of persistent or recurrent bleeding based on recognition of the endoscopic stigmata of recent hemorrhage.

1. Stigmata of recent hemorrhage—It is important to recognize the stigmata of recent hemorrhage, which are endoscopic findings in patients with bleeding peptic ulcers (Table 30–3). Patients with active bleeding seen at the time of upper endoscopy have a very high rate of ongoing bleeding, with rates as high as 90% if no intervention is performed (Plate 50). Patients who have nonbleeding visible vessels are also at high risk of further bleeding, as despite not having active bleeding at the time of endoscopy, rebleeding occurs in approximately 45% (Plates 51 and 52). Patients who have adherent clots that do not easily wash off have an intermediate probability of further bleeding (Plate 53). Approximately 25% of patients with adherent clots will have further bleeding, depending on what is underneath the clot; if there is an underlying non-bleeding visible vessel the rate is much higher, and if the clot base is clean the rate is much lower. Patients who are considered to be at low risk based on endoscopic stigmata of recent hemorrhage include those with flat spots, which have a 10% risk of further bleeding (Plate 54). Patients who have clean ulcer bases (Plate 55) or Mallory-Weiss tears, who do not have concomitant coagulopathies or use of medications that alter clotting, have a very low rate of further bleeding (<5%).

The endoscopic stigmata of hemorrhage can be difficult to interpret. Nonbleeding visible vessels cause the most

Table 30–3. Stigmata of recent hemorrhage: risk of rebleeding, mortality, and prevalence.

Stigmata	Risk of Rebleeding[a] (%)	Mortality (%)	Prevalence (%)
Active arterial bleeding	55-90	11	10
Nonbleeding visible vessel	40-50	11	25
Adherent clot	20-35	7	10
Oozing (without visible vessel)	10-25	NA	10
Flat spot	<10	3	10
Clean ulcer base	<5	2	35

[a]With medical management alone.
NA, not applicable.

difficulty. Nonbleeding visible vessels are raised protuberances from an ulcer bed that can be of any color, but they can be confused with flat spots. These may represent vessels, pseudoaneurysms, or clots and have a variable appearance.

2. Utility of endoscopic therapy—The utility of endoscopic therapy for patients with bleeding peptic ulcers was first shown in 1987 in a sham-controlled trial of multipolar electrocoagulation versus sham endoscopic therapy. Endoscopic therapy resulted in a significant improvement in hemostasis, number of units of blood transfused, number of emergency interventions, hospital stay (in days), and hospital costs. The mortality rate showed a trend toward being lower in the group treated with endoscopic therapy. Since this report, endoscopic therapy has been the standard of care for patients with high-risk stigmata of recent hemorrhage. Patients who have active bleeding or are found to have nonbleeding visible vessels should undergo endoscopic hemostasis to improve outcomes.

Adherent clots are found in about 10% of ulcers and are associated with a rebleeding rate of 20–35%. The optimal management of adherent clots has been controversial. National Institutes of Health consensus guidelines for management of GI bleeding from 1989 recommended against endoscopic treatment of adherent clots. However, this assertion has been challenged by several studies showing the efficacy of endoscopic treatment of adherent clots. The technique to treat an adherent clot starts with the use of epinephrine injection in four quadrants at the pedicle of the clot. A snare is used to cold guillotine the clot 3–4 mm above its base. Care is taken not to shear off the clot, further irritate the area, or provoke bleeding. The base of the ulcer is then vigorously irrigated with fluid to expose any underlying stigmata. This technique appears safe and facilitates endoscopic therapy. Any visible vessel or active bleeding is treated with cautery therapy. The available studies to date show improvement with endoscopic therapy compared to medical therapy using H_2-blockers; however, this technique has not been directly compared to medical therapy with PPIs which has also shown benefit in treatment of patients with adherent clots.

3. Optimizing endoscopic visualization—One of the challenges of managing patients with GI bleeding is visualization due to blood within the GI tract. This problem can be overcome by the use of a variety of techniques, individually or in combination. It is helpful to use double-channel or large channel endoscopes, which allow for vigorous aspiration (Figure 30–2). It is also useful to use a water pump or water jet, which allows for vigorous irrigation. There are several reports of the use of 3% hydrogen peroxide to dissolve clots within the GI tract, although this must be done carefully not to cause excessive bubbles or patient discomfort. It is not necessary to routinely lavage patients with large volumes prior to upper endoscopy, even in those with large upper GI bleeds. However, large tubes placed into the stomach to lavage clots and blood before the endoscopy can improve gastric visualization. Additional suction devices can be placed on the endoscope to facilitate removal of blood and clots directly during endoscopy.

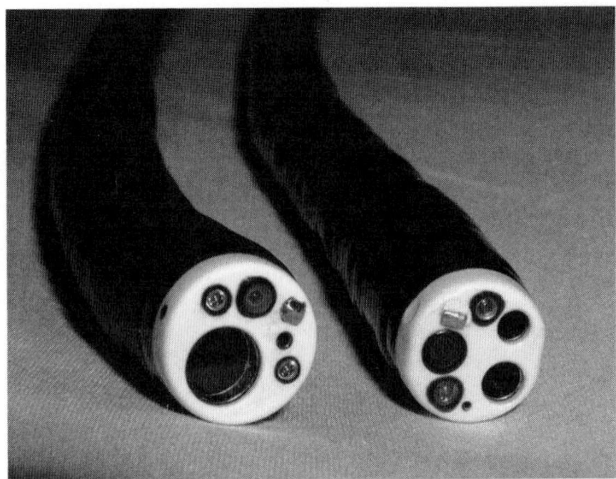

▲ **Figure 30–2.** Large channel therapeutic endoscope (*left*) and double-channel therapeutic endoscope (*right*).

Intravenous erythromycin (250 mg bolus or 3 mg/kg over 30 minutes) can be used as a prokinetic drug to increase gastric emptying and clear the stomach of blood. Erythromycin is given intravenously 30–120 minutes prior to endoscopy. The use of erythromycin significantly improves the quality of the gastric examination. This is a useful adjunctive treatment in patients with large GI bleeds with retained blood in the stomach. It can be used either initially or after an endoscopy shows large amounts of blood remaining in the stomach with withdrawal of the endoscope and the use of erythromycin before proceeding again with endoscopy. There are reports that metoclopramide given before endoscopy can also improve the quality of the gastric exam. In general, promotility agents should not be used routinely before endoscopy to increase the diagnostic yield but should be considered in patients suspected or found to have large amounts of blood or clot in their stomachs.

Coffin B, Pocard M, Panis Y, et al. Erythromycin improves the quality of EGD in patients with upper gastrointestinal bleeding: a randomized controlled study. *Gastrointest Endosc.* 2002; 56:174–179. [PMID: 12145593]

Lee SD, Kearney DJ. A randomized controlled trial of gastric lavage prior to endoscopy for acute upper gastrointestinal bleeding. *J Clin Gastroenterol.* 2004;38:861–865. [PMID: 15492601]

Sridhar S, Chamberlain S, Thiruvaiyaru D, et al. Hydrogen peroxide improves the visibility of ulcer bases in acute non-variceal upper gastrointestinal bleeding: a single-center prospective study. *Dig Dis Sci.* 2009;54:2427–2433. [PMID: 19757051]

4. Methods to control bleeding—The current endoscopic modalities to treat nonvariceal GI bleeding include the use of injection therapies (primarily with dilute epinephrine), contact thermal therapies including heater and bipolar probes, the use of noncontact thermal methods (argon plasma coagulation), mechanical treatments including a variety of endoclips and band ligation techniques, and a combination of the preceding treatment modalities (typically injection therapies combined with one of the other modalities).

Injection therapies reduce blood flow primarily by local tamponade. However, the use of vasoconstricting agents, such as epinephrine (diluted 1:10,000 to 1:100,000), can further reduce blood flow. Several other agents also can be used, including sclerosants such as ethanolamine, and thrombogenic agents, although these are less effective. These therapies may not be beneficial in the setting of active bleeding of fibrotic or penetrating ulcers. Injection therapy as monotherapy is not felt to be as efficacious as other monotherapies and should not be used as the only modality of treatment. A high dose of injection therapy (eg, the use of 20–30 mL of total injectate) may be more beneficial and more efficacious than the lower volumes (<10 mL) traditionally used; however, high doses of injected epinephrine are more likely to cause cardiovascular side effects (especially when injected in the region of the esophagus).

Use of thermal methods to control nonvariceal upper GI bleeding is quite widespread. At the current time, bipolar cautery is the thermal modality used most extensively, as it has the advantage over heater probes of being able to be used perpendicularly or tangentially. The bleeding vessel is compressed and then coagulated to provide "coaptive coagulation." The larger 10 French probes need to be placed via a therapeutic instrument and are generally more effective than the smaller 7 French probes. A relatively low wattage (10–15 watts in the duodenum; 15–20 watts in the stomach) is used for a prolonged time (8- to 12-second pulses) for each treatment pulse. Four to six pulses are typically used to provide effective treatment. The end point of treatment is reached when the involved vessel completely flattens out and there is no further bleeding. Recently, a monopolar probe has become available for treatment of GI bleeding, however its role in the management of patients with acute upper GI bleeding has to be further evaluated before its use can be advocated.

Combination therapies are commonly used and typically involve injection therapies with a dilute 1:10,000 epinephrine, combined with a thermocoagulation technique. Combination therapy is a safe and effective method. Only limited data are available comparing endoscopic therapies directly. Lin and colleagues compared epinephrine injection alone versus bipolar cautery alone versus combination therapy in 96 patients with active bleeding or a nonbleeding visible vessel. Although the rates of initial hemostasis were similar in all three groups, there was a significant reduction in the rebleeding rate in the combination therapy group. Thus combination therapy appears to provide a more durable control of bleeding than monotherapies.

Endoscopic hemoclips (endoclips) are an alternative method of hemostatic control that is widely used and has the theoretical advantage over cautery therapies of not causing further tissue damage or injury (Plates 56 and 57). Comparative studies of endoclip use show a similar primary efficacy at providing initial hemostasis compared with other endoscopic hemostatic modalities; however, the rebleeding rate may be reduced with the use of endoclips. In a study that compared use of combination therapy (dilute epinephrine injection and bipolar cautery) with use of endoclips in the United States, no significant differences were noted in the efficacy of these two therapies. Recent experience using the combination of dilute epinephrine injection with endoclips shows this combination to be an effective endoscopic treatment option. This combination treatment that includes hemoclips may be appropriate in patients with major upper GI bleeding or evidence of persistent bleeding or oozing after the application of endoclips.

At the current time, patients requiring endoscopic control of nonvariceal bleeding should be treated with either combination therapy using an injection of dilute epinephrine combined with a thermocoagulation method or with endoclip use (with or without injection therapy). Because some lesions or locations are better suited to one type of therapy, ideally an endoscopist should be familiar with both treatment options.

Lin HJ, Lo WC, Lee FY, et al. A prospective randomized comparative trial showing that omeprazole prevents rebleeding in patients with bleeding peptic ulcer after successful endoscopic therapy. *Arch Intern Med.* 1998;158:54–58. [PMID: 9437379]

Lin HJ, Tseng GY, Perng CL, et al. Comparison of adrenaline injection and bipolar electrocoagulation for the arrest of peptic ulcer bleeding. *Gut.* 1999;44:715–719. [PMID: 10205211]

Paspatis GA, Charoniti I, Papanikolaou N, et al. A prospective, randomized comparison of 10-Fr versus 7-Fr bipolar electrocoagulation catheter in combination with adrenaline injection in the endoscopic treatment of bleeding peptic ulcers. *Am J Gastroenterol.* 2003;98:2192–2197. [PMID: 14572567]

Saltzman J, Strate L, Di Sena V, et al. Prospective trial of endoscopic clips versus combination therapy in upper GI bleeding (PROTECCT—UGI Bleeding). *Am J Gastroenterol.* 2005;100:1503–1508. [PMID: 15984972]

Yuan Y, Wang C, Hunt RH. Endoscopic clipping for acute nonvariceal upper-GI bleeding: a meta-analysis and critical appraisal of randomized controlled trials. *Gastrointest Endosc.* 2008;68:339–351. [PMID: 18656600]

5. Second-look endoscopy—Second-look endoscopy is the performance of endoscopy at a regularly scheduled interval after a first therapeutic endoscopy. Typically, this is done about 24 hours after the initial endoscopy. During the second endoscopy, any persistent stigmata of hemorrhage are treated, such as the continued presence of a visible vessel. This endoscopic practice is common in many parts of the world, although it has not been widely used in the United States.

There is evidence that second-look endoscopy is beneficial in certain circumstances, especially after injection monotherapy. There has been a randomized trial of second-look endoscopy with a therapeutic procedure performed, if needed, in patients who underwent combination therapy with epinephrine injection followed by heater probe treatment. Chiu and colleagues studied 100 patients who had a second-look endoscopy within 24 hours, and 94 patients who were closely observed. Rebleeding was noted in 5 of the patients randomized to the second-look endoscopy group versus 13 of the control patients ($P = .03$). Only one second-look endoscopy patient needed surgery, compared with six patients randomized to the control group ($P = .05$). Although the group of patients who benefit from a second-look endoscopy and treatment has not been adequately defined in studies in Western populations, a second-look endoscopy may be prudent in select high-risk patients such as those with a suboptimal index endoscopy, due to technical difficulties or poor endoscopic visualization.

Chiu PW, Lam CY, Lee SW, et al. Effect of scheduled second therapeutic endoscopy on peptic ulcer rebleeding: a prospective randomized trial. *Gut.* 2003;52:1403–1407. [PMID: 12970130]

Tsoi KK, Chiu PW, Sung JJ. Endoscopy for upper gastrointestinal bleeding: is routine second-look necessary? *Nat Rev Gastroenterol Hepatol.* 2009;6:717–722. [PMID: 19946305]

C. Treatment of Patients with Recurrent Gastrointestinal Bleeding

The natural history of patients who are treated with endoscopic therapy is that 80–90% of patients will have permanent control of their bleeding (Figure 30–3). However, 10–20% of patients will have recurrent bleeding despite initially successful endoscopic therapy. In these patients, further attempts at endoscopic therapy are less effective at achieving permanent control, as only approximately 50% of those patients will ultimately be controlled by a second endoscopic therapy. In patients who fail a second therapeutic endoscopy, other modalities or treatments should be offered, including angiography and surgery.

In patients with rebleeding after an initially successful therapeutic endoscopy, an important question has been whether a second therapeutic endoscopy should be performed (given the reduced success rates), or whether patients should directly undergo definitive treatment such as surgery. This question was evaluated by Lau and colleagues in a study of 48 patients with rebleeding after endoscopic treatment who were randomized to either endoscopy or surgery. Ultimately, half the patients who were randomized to endoscopic treatment underwent salvage surgery as would be expected.

Patients who were initially randomized to a second endoscopic therapy or surgery showed similar outcomes in terms of mortality, length of hospital stay, and number of blood transfusions. However, there was a higher complication rate in patients who were initially randomized to surgery (16 vs 7 complications, $P = .03$). Predictors of failure of a second endoscopic therapy were an ulcer greater than 2 cm in diameter and the presence of hypotension. Overall, endoscopic treatment for rebleeding reduces the need for surgery without increasing the complication rate. In most patients (with possible exceptions in the situations previously described), a second attempt at endoscopic therapy should be offered before other modalities, such as surgery, are utilized.

It is important to identify patients who will ultimately need angiography or surgery and to proceed to further therapeutic interventions as appropriate. Involve invasive radiologists and surgeons early in the care of patients who may need surgery, such as those who are determined to be at high risk. There is a need for further research in this area to determine which patients would benefit from angiography or surgery at an early stage (who ultimately fail endoscopic treatment).

Lau JY, Sung JJ, Lam YH, et al. Endoscopic retreatment compared with surgery in patients with recurrent bleeding after initial endoscopic control of bleeding ulcers. *N Engl J Med.* 1999;340: 751–756. [PMID: 10072409]

van Vugt R, Bosscha K, van Munster IP, de Jager CP, Rutten MJ. Embolization as treatment of choice for bleeding peptic ulcers in high-risk patients. *Dig Surg.* 2009;26:37–42. [PMID: 19155626]

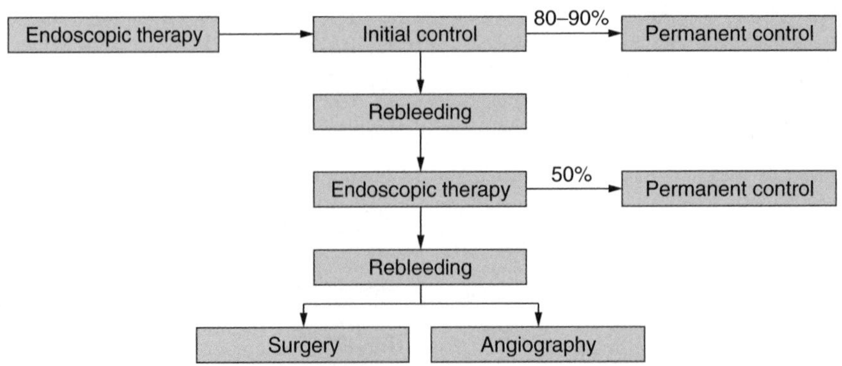

▲ **Figure 30–3.** Natural history of patients undergoing endoscopic therapy.

D. Impact of Anticoagulation on Rebleeding

One factor that has made the management of patients with GI bleeding more difficult in recent years is the increased use of medications that alter coagulation. These include older anticoagulant medications, such as warfarin and heparin, as well as the newer antiplatelet agents, which are widely used in patients with cardiovascular diseases, especially after coronary stent placement. Unfortunately, few data are available to guide management of these patients. In general, anticoagulation is held if possible and the international normalized ratio (INR) is reduced or normalized in these patients.

In a retrospective study of 233 patients with nonvariceal upper GI bleeding receiving endoscopic therapy, the presence of mild to moderate anticoagulation (INR 1.3 to 2.7) did not appear to alter the outcomes of endoscopic therapy. This suggests that upper endoscopy with endoscopic therapy is effective in patients who are mildly to moderately anticoagulated. However, more studies are needed in patients who are on antiplatelet agents. Current recommendations state that endoscopy for non-variceal bleeding should not be delayed in patients receiving anticoagulants unless the INR is supratherapeutic.

Barkun A, Sabbah S, Enns R, et al; RUGBE Investigators. The Canadian Registry on Nonvariceal Upper Gastrointestinal Bleeding and Endoscopy (RUGBE): Endoscopic hemostasis and proton pump inhibition are associated with improved outcomes in a real-life setting. *Am J Gastroenterol.* 2004;99:1238–1246. [PMID: 15233660]

Wolf AT, Wasan SK, Saltzman JR. Impact of anticoagulation on rebleeding following endoscopic therapy for non-variceal upper gastrointestinal hemorrhage. *Am J Gastroenterol.* 2007;102: 290–296. [PMID: 17100959]

E. *Helicobacter pylori* Infection

Patients with acute non-variceal upper GI bleeding should be tested for the presence of *H pylori* infection. Diagnostic tests for *H pylori* include biopsy for histology or rapid urease testing, serology, stool antigen, and urea breath testing, In the setting of acute upper GI bleeding, these tests have a high positive predictive value but a low negative predictive value. Thus initially negative results may need to be repeated at follow-up. Patients who have a positive *H pylori* test should be treated with antibiotics.

Calvet X, Barkun A, Kuipers E, Lanas A, Bardou M, Sung J. Is *H pylori* testing clinically useful in the acute setting of upper gastrointestinal bleeding? A systematic review [Abstract]. *Gastroenterology.* 2009;134.

SPECIFIC CAUSES OF ACUTE UPPER GI BLEEDING

This section discusses the diagnosis and treatment of common (Table 30–4) and uncommon (Table 30–5) sources of upper GI bleeding, including several specific causes of upper GI bleeding, both nonvariceal and variceal in origin.

Table 30–4. Common sources and prevalence of upper gastrointestinal bleeding.[a]

Source	Prevalence (%)
Duodenal ulcer	24.3
Gastric erosions	23.4
Gastric ulcer	21.3
Esophagogastric varices	10.3
Mallory-Weiss tear	7.2
Esophagitis	6.3
Erosive duodenitis	5.8

[a]Frequency >5% in American Society for Gastrointestinal Endoscopy bleeding survey of 2225 patients.

NONVARICEAL BLEEDING

1. Peptic Ulcer Disease

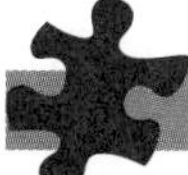

ESSENTIALS OF DIAGNOSIS

- Peptic ulcers are the most common cause of upper GI bleeding
- Most ulcers are caused by *H pylori* infection or NSAID use
- Upper endoscopy is the best test for diagnosis
- Peptic ulcer may not cause symptoms before bleeding

Table 30–5. Uncommon causes of upper gastrointestinal bleeding.[a]

Gastroesophageal reflux disease
Trauma from foreign bodies
Esophageal ulcer
Cameron lesion
Dieulafoy syndrome
Stress ulcer
Drug-induced erosions
Angioma
Watermelon stomach
Portal hypertensive gastropathy
Aortoenteric fistula
Radiation-induced telangiectasia
Benign tumors
Malignant tumors
Blue rubber bleb nevus syndrome
Osler-Weber-Rendu syndrome (hereditary hemorrhagic telangiectasias)
Hemobilia
Hemosuccus pancreatitis
Infections (cytomegalovirus, herpes simplex virus)
Stomal ulcer
Zollinger-Ellison syndrome

[a]Frequency <5%.

General Considerations

The most common cause of acute upper GI bleeding is peptic ulcer disease, which accounts for up to 50% of cases and over 100,000 hospital admissions per year in the United States. The annual incidence of peptic ulcer disease in patients infected with *H pylori* is about 1% per year, which is six to ten times higher than in patients who are uninfected.

Pathogenesis

A variety of conditions can lead to development of erosive or ulcerative diseases of the upper GI tract. In addition to peptic ulcer disease, which develops from an imbalance of protective and disruptive factors of the GI mucosa, medications such as NSAIDs and aspirin, Zollinger-Ellison syndrome, esophagitis, stress-induced gastric injury, and infections can cause erosions or ulcers. Disruptive factors that can damage the mucosa of the GI tract include acid, pepsin, bile salts, ischemia, and *H pylori*. Exogenous causes are predominately medications (NSAIDs and aspirin). Stress-induced ulcers are a common cause of bleeding in patients hospitalized for other severe illnesses. Risk factors for stress-induced ulcers include respiratory failure and coagulopathy. The defensive forces of the upper GI tract include esophageal motility with clearance of refluxed materials, the lower esophageal sphincter to prevent reflux, and salivary secretions that contain bicarbonate. The gastric protective factors include the mucous layer as well as tissue mediators.

Clinical Findings

A. Symptoms and Signs

Clinical manifestations of peptic ulcer disease range from silent, asymptomatic disease to severe abdominal pain with bleeding. Peptic ulcers classically cause dyspepsia with epigastric burning pain, and are relieved with anti-acid therapies. Classic duodenal ulcer symptoms occur when acid is secreted without a food buffer, 2–5 hours after meals or on an empty stomach (such as nocturnally). Although symptoms are typically in the epigastric area, they may localize to either the left or right upper quadrants or the hypochondrium. In patients with ulcer symptoms, symptomatic periods may be followed by symptom-free periods of weeks or months. Other symptoms that have been associated with ulcers include belching, anorexia, early satiety, nausea, vomiting, and weight loss. It is important to note that only 30–40% of patients with severe bleeding from peptic ulcer disease have symptoms from their ulcers prior to the GI bleeding.

B. Laboratory Findings

The laboratory findings for bleeding peptic ulcer disease are nonspecific and include anemia with a decrease in hemoglobin (which, if acute, will be normocytic) and an elevated ratio of blood urea nitrogen to creatinine of greater than 30:1 in some patients. *Helicobacter pylori* serology may be indicative of current or prior infection. In the rare patient with Zollinger-Ellison syndrome, the serum gastrin level will be elevated, although more commonly a mildly to moderately elevated gastrin level is due to PPI use.

C. Imaging Studies

Upper endoscopy is the primary modality to detect peptic ulcers, due to its combination of both high sensitivity and specificity, as well as its capability of providing endoscopic therapy. Barium studies, although capable of detecting peptic ulcers, should be avoided in the acute setting, as barium interferes with further endoscopic treatments and other imaging modalities. In patients with ongoing upper GI bleeding without an identifiable cause on upper endoscopy, or who have recurrent bleeding uncontrolled by upper endoscopy, angiography may define the source of the bleeding and provide treatment (either with placement of a coil or embolization of the involved artery).

Differential Diagnosis

As the symptoms of peptic ulcer disease are nonspecific, other causes of upper abdominal pain should be considered, including gastroesophageal reflux disease, nonulcer dyspepsia, cholelithiasis, choledocholithiasis, pancreatic disease, and malignancy. These conditions, however, are not typically associated with GI bleeding. The differential diagnosis of lesions seen at endoscopy that appear as peptic ulcers includes NSAID-induced damage, infectious etiologies, and malignant disease, including adenocarcinoma and lymphoma. Ischemic disease as a cause of bleeding in the upper GI tract is unusual.

Complications

Complications of peptic ulcer disease include bleeding, perforation, and obstruction. However, most patients with peptic ulcers do not develop these complications. Patients with bleeding peptic ulcers may develop aspiration pneumonia or complications of endoscopic therapy, such as respiratory depression and perforation. The tissue damage associated with ulcers may worsen with endoscopic treatment, particularly with thermal methods of cautery. This is a potential advantage of endoclip use, which should not further damage an already compromised mucosa.

Treatment

The principles of treatment of peptic ulcer disease are those outlined previously for treatment of upper GI bleeding and are detailed in Figure 30–4. Patients initially must be

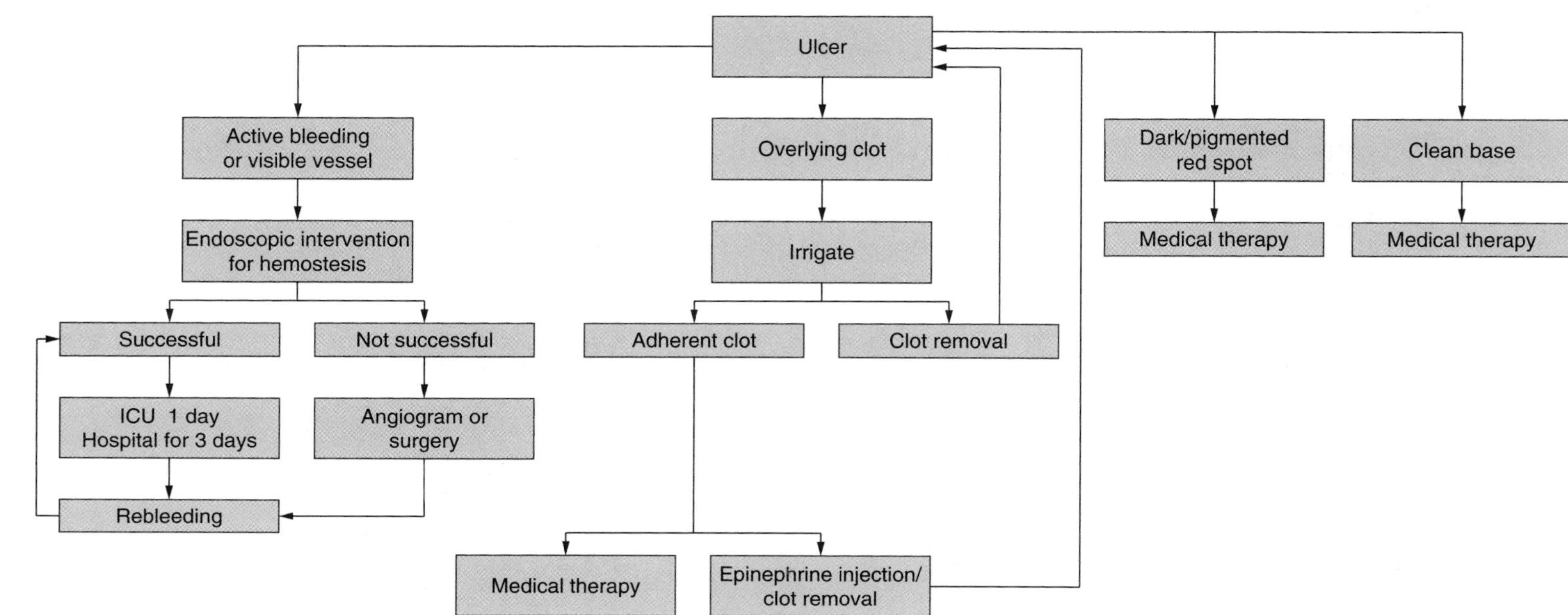

▲ **Figure 30–4.** Algorithm for the management of ulcers and acute gastrointestinal bleeding. ICU, intensive care unit. (Adapted, with permission, from Eisen GM, Dominitz JA, Faigel DO, et al; American Society for Gastroenterology. Standards of Practice Committee. An annotated algorithmic approach to upper gastrointestinal bleeding. *Gastrointest Endosc.* 2001;53:853–858.)

adequately resuscitated and stabilized. Decisions on whether to admit patients and how to optimally manage them depend on the clinical presentation and initial bleeding severity. Patients should be kept NPO and evaluated with an early upper endoscopy.

In patients requiring endoscopic therapy, use of adjuvant medical therapy with PPIs is routinely administered. In patients who do not have high-risk endoscopic stigmata of hemorrhage and who do not require endoscopic therapy, medical treatment can be initiated with H_2-receptor antagonists or PPIs, to begin the healing process. The presence of *H pylori* should be sought by endoscopic biopsy, serology, or breath testing, and patients who have *H pylori* should undergo eradication therapy to decrease the risk of recurrent bleeding and peptic ulcer disease. If other identifiable factors are present such as medications, including NSAIDS and aspirin, these should be discontinued if possible. There is some evidence that patients with bleeding peptic ulcers who do not have *H. pylori* present will have a worse prognosis.

Endoscopic therapy should be performed in patients with high-risk endoscopic stigmata of recent hemorrhage, which include active bleeding and presence of a nonbleeding visible vessel. Optimal treatment is combination therapy consisting of injection combined with a thermal coagulation method or with endoclip therapy. Although the approach is controversial, patients who have an adherent clot over an ulcer should be considered for endoscopic therapy and aggressively treated medically.

Patients who have large ulcers (>2 cm) or ulcers in locations associated with large arteries (eg, the high lesser curvature of the stomach near the left gastric artery or the posterior inferior wall of the duodenal bulb near the gastroduodenal artery) should be aggressively treated and considered for early angiographic intervention or surgery, especially with a hemodynamically significant bleed. However, angiography and surgery usually can be avoided with optimal medical and endoscopic therapy, and reserved for use in patients who have persistent or recurrent upper GI bleeding, those with large ulcers, or those with perforation. Surgery is directed at control of bleeding, such as ligation of the bleeding artery and oversewing of the ulcer. Surgery can also be performed for other complications of peptic ulcers, including perforation and nonhealing or giant ulcers. Whether surgical treatment to reduce acid production such as a vagotomy is needed is unclear due to the availability of effective antisecretory medications.

Course & Prognosis

The natural history of patients with bleeding peptic ulcers is that the majority will spontaneously stop bleeding and will not require emergency treatments. In patients who have bleeding requiring endoscopic therapy, the majority can be controlled with endoscopic measures. An angiographic intervention or surgery is needed only in a small number of patients who have ongoing or severe upper GI bleeding, not controllable by endoscopic and medical therapies. Mortality, typically from comorbid illnesses and in patients who were already hospitalized, remains significant in patients who have upper GI bleeding in peptic ulcer disease. After discharge from the hospital, it is unusual for patients to require readmission for recurrent bleeding if the previously described management measures have been instituted and if the patient does not have further need for anticoagulation. A comprehensive approach to the management of patients with bleeding peptic ulcers including a multidisciplinary team approach results in optimal outcomes.

Chan FK, Chung SC, Suen BY, et al. Preventing recurrent upper gastrointestinal bleeding in patients with *Helicobacter pylori* infection who are taking low-dose aspirin or naproxen. *N Engl J Med.* 2001;344:967–973. [PMID: 11274623]

Hawkey CJ. Risk of ulcer bleeding in patients infected with *Helicobacter pylori* taking non-steroidal anti-inflammatory drugs. *Gut.* 2000;46:310–311. [PMID: 10573289]

Lai KC, Hui WM, Wong WM, et al. Treatment of *Helicobacter pylori* in patients with duodenal ulcer hemorrhage—a long-term randomized, controlled study. *Am J Gastroenterol.* 2000;95: 2225–2232. [PMID: 1107222]

Sung JJ, Lau JY, Ching JY, et al. Continuation of low-dose aspirin therapy in peptic ulcer bleeding: a randomized trial. *Ann Intern Med.* 2010;152:1–9. [PMID: 19949136]

Wong GL, Wong VW, Chan Y, et al. High incidence of mortality and recurrent bleeding in patients with Helicobacter pylori-negative idiopathic bleeding ulcers. *Gastroenterology.* 2009;137:525–531. [PMID: 19445937]

2. Mallory-Weiss Tears

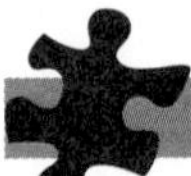

ESSENTIALS OF DIAGNOSIS

- Associated with repeated vomiting and retching
- Endoscopy is the best test for diagnosis

General Considerations

A Mallory-Weiss tear is a common cause of upper GI bleeding, accounting for approximately 5% of all cases. As the tears are relatively superficial, most heal within 24–48 hours. Mallory-Weiss tears may not be visualized on upper endoscopy, especially if the procedure is not performed promptly. Although in most patients the tears resolve spontaneously, massive bleeding can occur from Mallory-Weiss tears in patients who have portal hypertension, especially if esophageal varices are present.

Pathogenesis

Mallory-Weiss tears occur at the gastroesophageal junction in the distal esophagus or proximal stomach and may be single or multiple. Typically, these tears form after repeated and severe vomiting or retching. The tears may extend into the underlying venous or arterial plexuses.

Clinical Findings

A. Symptoms and Signs

The typical presentation of a Mallory-Weiss tear is acute upper GI bleeding in a young to middle-aged man, following repeated vomiting or retching after drinking alcohol. The antecedent history of retching and vomiting may not always be obtained. If there are other systemic signs, such as fever, chest pain, and shortness of breath, the Boerhaave syndrome (esophageal perforation) should be considered.

B. Laboratory Findings

The laboratory findings for a Mallory-Weiss tear are nonspecific and are similar to those for peptic ulcer disease.

C. Imaging Studies

Upper endoscopy, performed promptly, is the diagnostic (and therapeutic procedure) of choice. The tears can be seen as single or multiple longitudinal disruptions of the mucosa of the distal esophagus, at the gastroesophageal junction, within a hiatal hernia, or in the stomach just below the gastroesophageal junction with associated bleeding (Plate 58). As the injury of a Mallory-Weiss tear is relatively superficial and subtle, upper GI radiographs are typically nondiagnostic and not indicated.

Differential Diagnosis

The differential diagnosis of Mallory-Weiss tears includes other lesions of the gastroesophageal junction, including reflux esophagitis, infectious esophagitis, pill-induced esophagitis, Cameron lesion, and Dieulafoy lesion. Mallory-Weiss tears are focal lesions within an otherwise normal-appearing region of mucosa, which distinguishes them from reflux or infectious esophagitis. Patients with pill-induced esophagitis often have injury higher up the esophagus, and this etiology may be suspected by history. A Dieulafoy lesion is associated with a normal-appearing adjacent mucosa and the presence of a protuberant artery several centimeters below the gastroesophageal junction.

Complications

Although the natural history of Mallory-Weiss tears is that they are self-healing, patients may have ongoing bleeding or rebleeding. This is more likely with deeper tears or in anticoagulated patients. It is also possible to have a perforation (Boerhaave syndrome) either spontaneously, due to repeated vomiting, or after endoscopic therapy leading to mediastinitis.

Treatment

Endoscopic treatment of patients with Mallory-Weiss tears is indicated if there is active bleeding or a nonbleeding visible vessel at the time of endoscopy. Combination therapy with injection initially to slow or stop the bleeding followed by cautery is effective in most patients. However, because the injury is a tear of the lining (and the esophagus lacks a serosa), overinjection and overcauterization should be avoided. Endoclips have been used for this indication, are effective, and should not cause additional damage to the tissue. In cases of associated portal hypertension or esophageal varices, endoscopic therapy must be cautiously performed and cautery therapy should be avoided. These patients can be treated with sclerotherapy, band ligation, or endoclip placement. Medical therapy should be initiated in patients with Mallory-Weiss tears, but has not been shown to alter the natural history of the acute bleeding. Surgical intervention, with oversewing of a vessel, is rarely needed in patients with Mallory-Weiss tears.

Course & Prognosis

The natural history of Mallory-Weiss tears is that bleeding will stop spontaneously and healing will start to occur within 24–48 hours in the majority of patients. Rebleeding is unusual once bleeding has ceased.

Park CH, Min SW, Sohn YH, et al. A prospective, randomized trial of endoscopic band ligation vs epinephrine injection for actively bleeding Mallory-Weiss syndrome. *Gastrointest Endosc.* 2004;60:22–27.

3. Dieulafoy Lesion

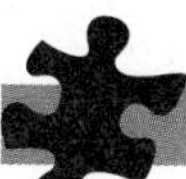

ESSENTIALS OF DIAGNOSIS

- Massive bleeding
- Most often located below the gastroesophageal junction in cardia
- May be difficult to diagnose

Pathogenesis

A Dieulafoy lesion is a dilated, aberrant submucosal vessel that erodes through otherwise normal surrounding epithelium not associated with an ulcer. Although originally described in 1884 by Gallard, the French surgeon Georges Dieulafoy 14 years later designated the lesion "exulceratio simplex." The arteries are usually 1–2 mm in size, which is approximately ten times the caliber of mucosal capillaries, although they can be larger. The typical location is in the upper stomach along the high lesser curvature, within 6 cm of the gastroesophageal junction. Dieulafoy lesions have been reported in other areas throughout the GI tract, including the esophagus, duodenum, and colon. The cause of a Dieulafoy lesion is unknown, although the lesion may be congenital. When a Dieulafoy lesion bleeds, massive arterial bleeding will occur. The typical patient with a Dieulafoy lesion is a man, with multiple comorbidities, already hospitalized for other problems.

Clinical Findings

A. Symptoms and Signs

A patient with a Dieulafoy lesion often presents with a massive acute upper GI bleed. However, the bleeding may be self-limited in nature or follow a stuttering course. In active bleeding, the diagnosis is confirmed by finding a visible vessel with active arterial pumping, without an associated ulcer or mass. The diagnosis can be difficult, as the location may be dependent within the stomach during endoscopy and as bleeding is often so massive that the area may be covered with blood and thus the source may not be visualized. In the absence of active bleeding, the lesion is even more difficult to see, as it may appear as a small and subtle raised area, such as a nipple or visible vessel without an associated ulcer. Although not widely available, the use of a Doppler probe can provide the correct diagnosis of a visible vessel in this situation. In patients with massive bleeding and no obvious cause, the lesser curvature within 6 cm of the gastroesophageal junction should be carefully inspected for evidence of a Dieulafoy lesion.

B. Imaging Studies

Upper endoscopy is the primary modality to detect a Dieulafoy lesion. If bleeding has stopped and there is doubt about the nature of the lesion, the use of a Doppler probe if available or endoscopic ultrasound with Doppler flow may be helpful to confirm the diagnosis.

Treatment

Endoscopic treatment is the primary modality for bleeding control of a Dieulafoy lesion. Combination therapy with injections of epinephrine followed by cautery may be used, or endoclips may be placed. There are also reports of band ligation over a Dieulafoy lesion. The risk of recurrent bleeding following endoscopic treatment is relatively high due to the large size of the underlying artery. It may be helpful to tattoo the area with ink or place an endoclip at or near the site to help localize the area for subsequent endoscopic therapy or future operative treatment. In patients with recurrent bleeding, an attempt to repeat endoscopic therapy is reasonable; however, surgical therapy may be necessary. Surgical treatment of a Dieulafoy lesion is typically a wedge resection, as simple oversewing has a high rebleeding rate.

Baxter M, Aly EH. Dieulafoy's lesion: current trends in diagnosis and management. *Ann R Coll Surg Engl.* 2010;92:548–554. [PMID: 20883603]

Lara LF, Sreenarasimhaiah J, Tang SJ, Afonso BB, Rockey DC. Dieulafoy lesions of the GI tract: localization and therapeutic outcomes. *Dig Dis Sci.* 2010;55:3436–3441. [PMID: 20848205]

4. Vascular Malformations

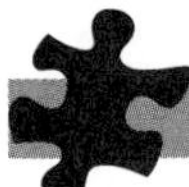

ESSENTIALS OF DIAGNOSIS

- Wide spectrum of disorders
- Can cause acute or chronic bleeding
- Variable bleeding rates

General Considerations

Various terms are used to describe vascular malformations of the upper GI tract, including arteriovenous malformations, vascular ectasia, angiodysplasia, and telangiectasia. Although these lesions can present as acute, overt upper GI bleeding, they are frequently a source of chronic occult GI bleeding and iron deficiency anemia. Vascular malformations of the upper GI tract may be associated with small bowel angioectasias (also of obscure origin).

Pathogenesis

Vascular malformations of the upper GI tract may be arterial or venous in origin. The majority are idiopathic with unknown causes. The spectrum of vascular malformations includes Dieulafoy lesions, as previously discussed, watermelon stomach (gastric antral vascular ectasia), Osler-Weber-Rendu syndrome (hereditary hemorrhagic telangiectasia), blue rubber bleb nevus syndrome, and radiation-induced telangiectasias.

Clinical Findings

Bleeding from upper GI vascular malformations is typically intermittent and low-grade in nature, although it can be acute and overt. The endoscopic appearance can be variable, but includes a superficial collection or tuft of blood vessels (Plate 59). These also can be detected by angiography, with findings including an early filling vein, a vascular tuft, and a late draining vein.

Treatment

The primary treatment of vascular malformations is endoscopic therapy. Endoscopic therapy with thermal coagulation is the treatment of choice, with cautery applied initially to the periphery and then at the center of the lesion. There should be whitening of the mucosa and ablation of all visible vascular tissue. Argon plasma coagulation is an effective treatment of vascular malformations. It is important to avoid overdistention (by the argon gas) of the stomach or small intestine during therapy, as well as to avoid contact with tissue when using argon plasma coagulation therapy. Repeated therapy should not be applied to the same location due to the risk of transmural injury and perforation, especially in the small bowel.

Various medications have been used in an attempt to treat vascular malformations in the upper GI tract. Combination estrogen–progesterone therapy has been widely used, but overall has yielded inconsistent results. Angiography and surgery can be offered for failures of endoscopic and medical therapy, but are rarely necessary.

5. Watermelon Stomach (Gastric Antral Vascular Ectasia)

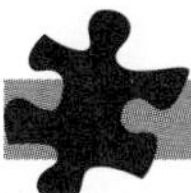

ESSENTIALS OF DIAGNOSIS

- Idiopathic or associated with portal hypertension
- Characteristic endoscopic appearance of radiating rows of vascular malformations extending outward from the pylorus

Pathogenesis

Watermelon stomach or gastric antral vascular ectasia (GAVE) is a relatively unusual cause of upper GI bleeding. This condition can occur along with, or be confused with, portal hypertensive gastropathy. In this condition vascular malformations occur in rows of reddish stripes that radiate outward from the pylorus, in a pattern that resembles the stripes on a watermelon. These stripes represent rows of vascular malformations and the entity is easy to recognize in the classic form. However, watermelon stomach may have a less organized appearance, with more scattered erythema and vascular malformations, making it more difficult to recognize.

The cause of watermelon stomach is idiopathic; however, it may be due to gastroduodenal prolapse and has been noted to occur in patients with cirrhosis, portal hypertension, and systemic sclerosis. Patients with concomitant portal hypertension have bleeding that is more difficult to control, requiring treatment of the underlying portal hypertension.

Clinical Findings

The diagnosis of watermelon stomach is based on the classic endoscopic appearance of radiating rows of vascular malformations originating from the pyloric area (Plate 60). Although the diagnosis is made by the characteristic endoscopic appearance, it can be confirmed by histology from endoscopic biopsy. Biopsies of watermelon stomach show areas of vascular ectasia associated with spindle cell proliferation and fibrohyalinosis. The bleeding that occurs is typically chronic and low grade, often associated with iron deficiency anemia and occult bleeding. It is unusual to have acute or massive upper GI bleeding from watermelon stomach.

Treatment

Endoscopic therapy is effective at treating watermelon stomach, especially in the absence of concomitant portal hypertension. This may be done with multipolar electrocoagulation or argon plasma coagulation. Several courses of treatment are required to obliterate the vascular ectasias and decrease or stop bleeding. In refractory patients with watermelon stomach, radiofrequency ablation and cryotherapy have been used with success. Although most patients respond to endoscopic therapy, surgery may be needed for patients who have persistent bleeding despite endoscopic management. Surgical management with antrectomy prevents further bleeding.

Ripoll C, Garcia-Tsao G. Treatment of gastropathy and gastric antral vascular ectasia in patients with portal hypertension. *Curr Treat Options Gastroenterol.* 2007;10:483–494. [PMID: 18221609]

Ripoll C, Garcia-Tsao G. Management of gastropathy and gastric vascular ectasia in portal hypertension. *Clin Liver Dis.* 2010;14: 281–295. [PMID: 20682235]

Sebastian S, O'Morain CA, Buckley MJ. Review article: current therapeutic options for gastric antral vascular ectasia. *Aliment Pharmacol Ther.* 2003;18:157–165. [PMID: 12869075]

LESS COMMON CAUSES OF NONVARICEAL BLEEDING

1. Aortoenteric Fistula

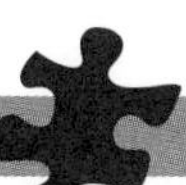

ESSENTIALS OF DIAGNOSIS

- High index of suspicion is needed for diagnosis
- Massive bleeding may cause exsanguination
- Rapid diagnosis and progression to surgery are required

Aortoenteric fistulas occur when there is a direct communication between the aorta and the GI tract. These typically occur in patients who have had a prosthetic aortic graft that erodes into the intestine. They also can occur from aortic aneurysms, after radiation therapy, or from postinfectious aortitis (eg, from syphilis or tuberculosis), trauma, or tumor invasion.

The third and fourth portion of the duodenum is the most common site of aortoenteric fistulas, followed by the jejunum and the ileum. Patients may have a "herald" bleed with initial hematemesis or hematochezia, which may spontaneously remit. This may then be followed by massive bleeding, including exsanguination, making it important to diagnose this condition as early as possible. Intermittent bleeding can occur if a blood clot temporarily seals a fistulous connection. Abdominal or back pain occurs in about half of patients. Signs of fever or infection may be present. On physical examination, a bruit may be heard or a pulsatile mass may be palpable.

A high index of suspicion is needed to properly diagnose a patient with an aortoenteric fistula while there is still time for successful management. In a patient who has a known risk factor, such as previous aortic grafting, this diagnosis should be considered early in the course. It should also be suspected in patients with bleeding from the third or fourth portion of the duodenum, particularly with massive bleeding. Aortic graft material may occasionally be seen at endoscopy protruding into the bowel lumen. The diagnosis can be confirmed by CT with angiography or angiography directly. Diagnostic tests need to be done in an expeditious manner along with surgical evaluation.

The management of an aortoenteric fistula is surgical. The mortality rate of an unrecognized fistula is 100%, whereas the mortality for a recognized fistula is 30%. Treatment consists of surgical repair of the aortoenteric fistula.

Lemos DW, Raffetto JD, Moore TC, et al. Primary aortoduodenal fistula: a case report and review of the literature. *J Vasc Surg.* 2003;37:686–689. [PMID: 12618713]

2. Hemobilia

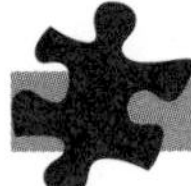

ESSENTIALS OF DIAGNOSIS

- Triad of jaundice, biliary colic, and GI bleeding
- Consider in patients after trauma or hepatic intervention

Hemobilia, bleeding that occurs from the hepatobiliary tract, is a rare cause of acute upper GI bleeding. Hemobilia should be considered in patients who have had a recent history of hepatic or biliary tract injury. This includes trauma to the area and percutaneous (or transjugular) liver biopsies, and percutaneous transhepatic cholangiograms or biopsies. Hemobilia can also occur from gallstones, cholecystitis, hepatobiliary tumors, hepatic abscesses, and aneurysms.

The classic triad of hemobilia is biliary colic, obstructive jaundice, and GI bleeding. Obstructive jaundice may be associated with biliary sepsis. Patients with this triad should be considered as potentially having hemobilia.

The diagnosis of hemobilia can be difficult by upper endoscopy. A side-viewing duodenoscope is very helpful to look at the ampulla directly or to perform endoscopic retrograde cholangiopancreatography (ERCP) (Plate 61). A tagged red blood cell scan or angiography can be done to localize the source of bleeding.

Treatment is directed at the primary cause of bleeding. Although occasionally treatment can be carried out endoscopically, it usually needs to be done angiographically (such as by arterial embolization) or surgically.

Parsi MA. Hemobilia: endoscopic, fluoroscopic, and cholangioscopic diagnosis. *Hepatology.* 2010;52:2237–2238. [PMID: 21105096]

3. Hemosuccus Pancreaticus

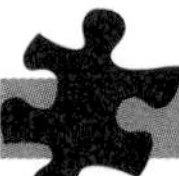

ESSENTIALS OF DIAGNOSIS

- Suspect when bleeding is associated with pancreatic disease
- Best detected with a side-viewing duodenoscope

Hemosuccus pancreaticus occurs when there is bleeding from the pancreatic duct. This is a rare cause of upper GI bleeding that can be due to chronic pancreatitis, pancreatic pseudocysts, and pancreatic tumors. Bleeding occurs when there is erosion into a vessel, forming a direct communication with the pancreatic duct. It can also occur after a therapeutic endoscopy of the pancreas, including pancreatic sphincterotomy or stone removal.

The diagnosis of hemosuccus pancreaticus should be suspected when upper GI bleeding occurs in the setting of pancreatic disease. Although it can be difficult to detect by routine endoscopy, a side-viewing duodenoscope and ERCP may reveal the source of the bleeding. The diagnosis can be confirmed by abdominal CT scan, angiography, or intra-abdominal exploration. Mesenteric angiography is an important adjunct for diagnosis and treatment, often with coil embolization to control the acute bleeding. For persistent or massive bleeding, surgery with resection of the bleeding area or ligation of the bleeding vessel may be required.

Etienne S, Pessaux P, Tuech JJ, et al. Hemosuccus pancreaticus: a rare cause of gastrointestinal bleeding. *Gastroenterol Clin Biol.* 2005;29(3):237–242. [PMID: 15864172]

4. Cameron Lesion

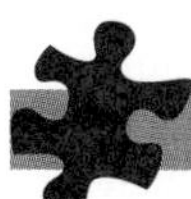

ESSENTIALS OF DIAGNOSIS

- ▶ Close inspection of hiatal hernia during endoscopy is needed
- ▶ Acute or chronic GI bleeding

Cameron lesions are erosions or ulcers that occur in the distal aspect of a hiatal hernia. Although this may be an incidental finding, a Cameron lesion can be responsible for acute or chronic upper GI bleeding and iron deficiency anemia. The mechanism of formation of a Cameron lesion is incompletely understood, although potential causative factors include gastroesophageal reflux and mechanical trauma of the area.

Management of a Cameron lesion depends on the clinical situation. Patients with acute bleeding can usually be treated by endoscopic methods. Patients who do not have acute bleeding, but have chronic blood loss may be treated with medical therapy, such as PPI therapy and iron repletion. Surgical repair of the hiatal hernia is curative, but rarely needed.

Maganty K, Smith RL. Cameron lesions: unusual cause of gastrointestinal bleeding and anemia. *Digestion.* 2008;77:214–217.

5. Upper Gastrointestinal Tumors

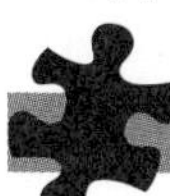

ESSENTIALS OF DIAGNOSIS

- ▶ Benign and malignant tumors can bleed
- ▶ Bleeding may be slow or massive

Neoplasms of the upper GI tract account for less than 3% of cases of upper GI bleeding. These tumors may be malignant tumors (primary or metastatic) such as adenocarcinomas, lymphomas, and melanomas, or can be benign, such as leiomyomas or GI stromal tumors.

The symptoms that suggest bleeding may be from a GI tumor include those that may be attributable to the primary tumor, such as dysphagia from esophageal cancer or gastric outlet obstruction due to carcinoma of the stomach. Other symptoms are nonspecific, including cachexia, weight loss, and early satiety.

Bleeding from an upper GI tumor can be from diffuse mucosal erosions or ulcerations, or from erosion of the tumor into an underlying vessel (Plates 62 and 63). The bleeding may be slow or may be massive. If the diagnosis of a tumor is not previously known, it may be detected at the time of endoscopy and confirmed by brushings or biopsies. Endoscopic ultrasound may be needed to evaluate submucosal masses.

Endoscopic treatment of patients with upper GI bleeding can be offered, but is less effective in the setting of tumors. Typically endoscopic treatments, although they may be effective, should be used as a temporizing measure prior to more definitive measures such as surgery, because rebleeding will frequently occur after endoscopic control of bleeding, thus requiring a more durable approach. Recent attempts at endoscopically treating bleeding tumors include the use of argon plasma coagulation at high power settings and the application of glue. Medical therapy is ineffective in this setting, although palliative measures may be provided, including chemotherapy and radiation of the primary tumor.

Patients who have bleeding due to an upper GI malignancy have a very poor prognosis. The majority of patients will die within 3 months. However, patients who have a benign upper GI tumor that bleeds should be cured by surgical resection.

Heller SJ, Tokar JL, Nguyen MT, Haluszka O, Weinberg DS. Management of bleeding GI tumors. *Gastrointest Endosc.* 2010; 72:817–824. [PMID: 20883861]

VARICEAL BLEEDING

1. Gastroesophageal Varices

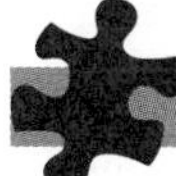

ESSENTIALS OF DIAGNOSIS

- ▶ Sign of advanced liver disease
- ▶ Larger varices bleed more often
- ▶ Associated with a high rate of bacterial infections
- ▶ May involve the esophagus, stomach, or both

General Considerations

Esophageal and gastric varices may occur without any clinical symptoms. In patients with cirrhosis, particularly in more advanced stages, screening measures are performed to detect varices in an attempt to decrease the risk of initial bleeding. Acute variceal bleeding is different from nonvariceal bleeding in many respects. Only 50% of patients with a variceal hemorrhage stop bleeding spontaneously (compared with approximately 80–90% of patients with nonvariceal upper GI bleeding). Following cessation of active variceal bleeding, there is a high risk of recurrent bleeding within 6 weeks. The time of greatest risk is within the first 48–72 hours, and over 50% of all rebleeding episodes occur within the first 10 days. Recurrent variceal bleeding may occur in up to 70% of patients within 6 weeks of the index bleed. Survival during the 6 weeks following the index bleed is directly related to rebleeding. Risk factors for rebleeding include age greater than 60 years, large varices, severe initial bleed (hemoglobin <8 g/dL on admission), and renal failure. Mortality is between

15% and 50% for each bleeding episode, and 70–80% in those with continuous bleeding. In recent years there has been a decrease in the mortality due to the prevention of rebleeding by the use of earlier, more effective endoscopic therapy along with effective vasoactive medications as well as the prevention of infection due to the use of prophylactic antibiotics. Variceal hemorrhage is responsible for one third of all deaths due to cirrhosis.

Pathogenesis

Esophageal and gastric varices develop as a result of portal hypertension. Portal hypertension can be from prehepatic causes (eg, portal vein thrombosis and schistosomiasis), from hepatic disease (cirrhosis most commonly), and from posthepatic disease (eg, hepatic vein thrombosis, cardiac failure, and constrictive pericarditis). Varices are dilated venous collaterals with a weak wall that have a tendency to rupture and can bleed massively. Varices may be isolated to the stomach if they are due to splenic vein thrombosis, acute pancreatitis, or a pancreatic tumor.

Clinical Findings

A. Symptoms and Signs

The symptoms of variceal bleeding are nonspecific and include hematemesis, melena, and hematochezia. Patients may feel lightheaded and dizzy, and those with severe liver disease may have hepatic encephalopathy. Other associated signs and symptoms are manifestations of cirrhosis, including jaundice, spider telangiectasia, palmar erythema, ascites, and Dupuytren contractures.

B. Laboratory Findings

Abnormalities of the liver enzymes (alanine aminotransferase and aspartate aminotransferase) are seen in patients with active hepatocellular damage. Patients may have hyperbilirubinemia and poor synthetic function, with hypoalbuminemia and an elevated INR. Patients with bone marrow suppression from alcohol may have pancytopenia; those with hypersplenism may have low platelets. In patients with liver failure, hypoglycemia may occur, and in those with hepatorenal syndrome, blood urea nitrogen and creatinine are elevated.

C. Imaging Studies

Upper endoscopy is the primary diagnostic modality and allows for endoscopic therapy. The Japanese Research Society for Portal Hypertension criteria includes a size (or form) classification. Small straight varices are classified as F1, enlarged tortuous varices occupying less than one third of the esophageal lumen are F2, and large coil-shaped varices that occupy more than one third of the esophageal lumen are F3. Barium radiographs may be suggestive of large varices; however, they are not sensitive to small varices, and the use of barium impedes further diagnostic or therapeutic attempts. Abdominal CT or abdominal ultrasound may show the presence of collateral vessels. Portal vein angiography may also demonstrate the presence of collaterals or recanalization of the umbilical vein. Hepatic venous pressure gradients of more than 12 mm Hg are a predictor of bleeding.

Differential Diagnosis

The differential diagnosis includes all the nonvariceal causes of upper GI bleeding. Patients with cirrhosis and upper GI bleeding are found to have a variceal source of bleeding in 50–90% of cases. Patients with cirrhosis can also bleed from esophagitis, peptic ulcer disease, Mallory-Weiss tears, and other nonvariceal sources.

Complications

Bleeding from esophageal or gastric varices may be massive and uncontrollable, resulting in severe hemorrhage and death. Acute variceal bleeding in a patient with cirrhosis may precipitate further worsening of liver disease, with increasing hepatic encephalopathy and development of the hepatorenal syndrome. Bacterial infections are present in up to 20% of cirrhotic patients with GI bleeding, and subsequently develop in an additional 50% of patients during hospitalization for variceal bleeds. The use of prophylactic antibiotics in patients with acute variceal bleeding has been shown to decrease the rates of subsequent infection, spontaneous bacterial peritonitis, bacteremia, and death.

Treatment

Patients with acute variceal bleeding are typically treated with multiple modalities simultaneously, including medical therapies and endoscopic management. Over-resuscitation should be avoided, as over vigorous volume repletion has been associated with precipitation of further bleeding. In addition radiologic and surgical treatments may be needed.

A. Medical Therapy

In patients with suspected variceal bleeding, medical therapy to reduce bleeding should be initiated prior to endoscopic evaluation. The use of prophylactic antibiotics given before endoscopy in cirrhotic patients reduces infectious complications and decreases mortality.

Medications have been shown to decrease active variceal bleeding. In the past, intravenous vasopressin was given to constrict the mesenteric vasculature and decrease portal venous blood flow. A systemic vasodilator, such as intravenous nitroglycerin, was concurrently administered to reduce the adverse effects related to the systemic vasoconstriction, which include myocardial, cerebral, bowel, and extremity ischemia. However, this combination of vasopressin and nitroglycerin is rarely used now because of the availability of other medications with fewer side effects.

Terlipressin is a synthetic analog of vasopressin that is released in a sustained and slow manner. It appears to have a similar ability to control bleeding and reduce mortality as vasopressin, without many of the systemic side effects. Terlipressin is not currently available in the United States, but is used in other countries.

Somatostatin and its analog, octreotide, have been extensively studied in patients with bleeding esophageal and gastric varices. These drugs indirectly cause vasoconstriction and decrease portal blood flow. Octreotide is given as a bolus injection of 25–50 mcg followed by a continuous infusion of 25–50 mcg/h intravenously. Octreotide and somatostatin have been found to be useful in achieving hemostasis and preventing early rebleeding. Once patients are stabilized from the acute variceal bleeding episode, β-blockers are given to prevent rebleeding. (See Chapter 47 for additional discussion of portal hypertension.)

B. Endoscopic Therapy

The treatment of choice for bleeding esophageal varices is endoscopic hemostasis (Plates 64 and 65). The objective of endoscopic therapy is to find the source of the bleeding and to treat it. Varices are evaluated for signs of either active bleeding or markers of recent bleeding. These markers include large tortuous varices with red wale marks (longitudinal red streaks on varices that resemble red, corduroy wales), cherry red spots (discrete cherry red spots that are flat on a varix), and hemocystic spots (raised discrete red spots that overlie varices that appear as "blood blisters"). Platelet or fibrin plugs are white nipple-like projections that project from a varix indicative of a site with recent bleeding and with a very high risk of bleeding.

Endoscopic therapies are initially applied to the distal esophagus at the gastroesophageal junction and then extended proximally. Most variceal bleeding is from the distal 5–10 cm of the esophagus. Gastric varices are poorly responsive to traditional endoscopic therapies and do not respond to typical endoscopic banding and injection treatments (Plate 66). Recent reports of the use of cyanoacrylate injections for bleeding gastric varices are promising, although not approved for use in the United States.

Endoscopic injection sclerotherapy is an established method of injecting esophageal varices directly using a freehand technique with 1–3 mL of a sclerosing agent (sodium morrhuate or ethanolamine) at each site. Numerous techniques and agents have been used to sclerose varices. Although this technique is effective, esophageal variceal band ligation is more effective, associated with less rebleeding, fewer complications, and a lower mortality rate, and requiring fewer treatment sessions to obliterate the varices.

Endoscopic esophageal variceal band ligation therapy is a method of placing elastic bands over varices, similar to the technique of banding hemorrhoids. This is typically performed within the distal 5 cm of the esophagus. Varices are suctioned into a banding device, and the bands are released around the base of the varices. Esophageal variceal band ligation controls acute bleeding in 90% of patients, with a rebleeding rate of 30%. Endoscopic variceal ligation is the treatment of choice for controlling acute esophageal variceal hemorrhage. A drawback of the banding technique is that it can be difficult to perform in the setting of active bleeding; it may be hard to localize the exact source of bleeding with the restricted endoscopic view afforded by the banding device, and blood may pool within the banding mechanism. In addition, it is not feasible to perform banding in the retroflexed position in the stomach due to the nature of the device.

C. Balloon Tamponade

Balloon tamponade is an effective way to achieve short-term hemostasis but should be reserved for patients whose variceal bleeding cannot be controlled by endoscopic therapy or who are having massive bleeding that prohibits an endoscopic attempt. A commonly used device is the Sengstaken-Blakemore tube, which has a large 250-mL gastric balloon and an esophageal balloon, as well as a gastric suctioning port. In patients with massive bleeding uncontrollable by other measures, this tube can be placed with the gastric balloon first inflated after radiographic confirmation of proper position. If necessary, the esophageal balloon can be carefully inflated. However, the use of the esophageal balloon is associated with esophageal wall necrosis and rupture, a lethal complication. If definitive therapy is not performed, recurrent bleeding likely will occur when the balloon is deflated. In general, balloon tamponade should be used in an effort to temporarily stabilize a patient prior to the performance of a more definitive treatment.

D. Radiologic Therapy

The main radiologic therapy is transjugular intrahepatic portosystemic shunt (TIPS). TIPS is a radiologic procedure that creates a portosystemic shunt via a transjugular approach. In this procedure, a connection is made between the portal and hepatic veins and a stent is placed between the two veins. Complications include encephalopathy due to the shunting, shunt occlusion with rebleeding, and shunt migration. Although TIPS is very effective at controlling bleeding (immediate hemostasis in 93% and rebleeding in 12% of patients), in general TIPS is reserved for patients who have persistent variceal bleeding despite endoscopic and medical attempts to control. One recent randomized multi-center trial that compared TIPS (using a stent covered with polytetrafluoroethylene (e-PTFE)) with optimal medical and endoscopic therapies in patients at a high risk of rebleeding found improved rates of rebleeding and mortality with TIPS treatment. In consideration of this study, Child-Pugh B or C disease patients who are at very high risk of rebleeding should be considered for possible TIPS treatment early in their hospital course.

E. Surgical Therapy

Various surgical therapies can be performed to control esophageal and gastric variceal bleeding. These include creation of a portosystemic shunt, which may be a portal caval shunt (nonselective) or a distal splenorenal shunt (selective). Alternately, esophageal transection can be performed, in which the distal esophagus is transected and then stapled back together after ligation of varices, with devascularization of the gastroesophageal junction (Sugiura procedure). The ultimate operation to control variceal bleeding is liver transplantation. This is an option in patients who already are planned to have a liver transplantation due to poor liver function. In general, the patients who have the best outcomes with surgical shunt therapy have relatively well-preserved liver function (Child-Turcotte-Pugh class A), but have failed endoscopic treatment.

Course & Prognosis

Variceal bleeding is a significant cause of rebleeding and mortality. Variceal bleeding will stop in approximately 50% of patients, but those who have continued bleeding have a mortality that approaches 80%. Patients have a high risk of rebleeding (up to 70%) until gastroesophageal varices are obliterated. If a patient survives the initial bleeding episode, repeated courses of band ligation are performed approximately every 2 weeks until the varices are obliterated. This technique is combined with medical therapy using β-blockade. The prognosis for patients with bleeding gastroesophageal varices is poor, even with control of bleeding varices, as this is indicative of progressive liver disease. Patients die from hepatic decompensation, rebleeding, infections, renal failure, and other complications.

2. Portal Hypertensive Gastropathy

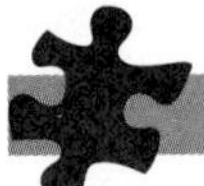

ESSENTIALS OF DIAGNOSIS

- Characteristic "snakeskin" endoscopic appearance
- Rare cause of acute bleeding

Clinical Findings

Portal hypertensive gastropathy, also called congestive gastropathy, occurs with edema and capillary venous dilation in the submucosa and mucosa of the stomach. This causes friability and can result in bleeding with rupture of the ectatic vessels. Endoscopically, the appearance is a reticular, mosaic-like pattern of pink mucosa, with a characteristic "snakeskin" appearance. In patients with cirrhosis and portal hypertension, gastric mucosal blood flow is increased, leading to congestion and hyperemia of the stomach.

Portal hypertensive gastropathy may develop after treatment of esophageal varices by either endoscopic sclerotherapy or band ligation therapy. It is postulated that treatment of the esophageal varices increases backpressure into the stomach, leading to the development of gastric congestion. Overall this is a relatively rare cause of acute upper GI bleeding, although it may be a source of chronic blood loss in cirrhotic patients.

Treatment

The goal of treatment of portal hypertensive gastropathy is to decrease portal pressures and therefore stop bleeding. Endoscopic treatments are not effective in this disorder. The affected area is diffuse, and pharmacologic agents that decrease blood flow, such as octreotide, can be used acutely. Low-dose propranolol (20–40 mg/day) is often given initially, with the dose then increased and adjusted until bleeding stops or side effects occur. Patients with uncontrolled bleeding may need TIPS therapy or shunt surgery. In patients with decompensated liver disease, liver transplantation is indicated.

Abid S, Jafri W, Hamid S, et al. Terlipressin vs octreotide in bleeding esophageal varices as an adjuvant therapy with endoscopic band ligation: a randomized double-blind placebo-controlled trial. *Am J Gastroenterol.* 2009 Mar104:617–623. [PMID: 19223890]

Bañares R, Albillos A, Rincón D, et al. Endoscopic treatment versus Endoscopic plus pharmacologic treatment for acute variceal bleeding: a meta-analysis. *Hepatology.* 2002;35: 609–615. [PMID: 11870374]

Bernard B, Grangé JD, Khac EN, et al. Antibiotic prophylaxis for the prevention of bacterial infection in cirrhotic patients with gastrointestinal bleeding. *Hepatology.* 1999;29:1655–1661. [PMID: 10347104]

Carey W. Portal hypertension: diagnosis and management with particular reference to variceal hemorrhage. *J Dig Dis.* 2010;12:25–32 [PMID: 21091935]

Chavez-Tapia NC, Barrientos-Gutierrez T, Tellez-Avila FI, Soares-Weiser K, Uribe M. Antibiotic prophylaxis for cirrhotic patients with upper gastrointestinal bleeding. *Cochrane Database Syst Rev.* 2010;8:CD002907. [PMID: 20824832]

Corley DA, Cello JP, Adkisson W, et al. Octreotide for acute Esophageal variceal bleeding: a meta-analysis. *Gastroenterology.* 2001;120:946–954. [PMID: 11231948]

D'Amico G, De Franchis R. Cooperative Study Group. Upper digestive bleeding in cirrhosis. Post-therapeutic outcome and Prognostic indicators. *Hepatology.* 2003;38:599–612. [PMID: 12939586]

García-Pagán JC, Caca K, Bureau C, et al; Early TIPS (Transjugular Intrahepatic Portosystemic Shunt) Cooperative Study Group. Early use of TIPS in patients with cirrhosis and variceal bleeding. *N Engl J Med.* 2010;362:2370–2379.

Greenspoon J, Barkun A. The pharmacological therapy of non-variceal upper gastrointestinal bleeding. *Gastroenterol Clin North Am.* 2010;39:419–432. [PMID: 20951910]

Kumar A, Singh S, Madan K, Garg PK, Acharya SK. Undiluted N-butyl cyanoacrylate is safe and effective for gastric variceal bleeding. *Gastrointest Endosc.* 2010;72:721–727. [PMID: 20883849]

Mishra SR, Chander Sharma B, Kumar A, Sarin SK. Endoscopic cyanoacrylate injection versus beta-blocker for secondary prophylaxis of gastric variceal bleed: a randomized controlled trial. *Gut.* 2010;59:729–735. [PMID: 20551457]

Monescillo A, Martínez-Lagares F, Ruiz-del-Arbol L, et al. Influence of portal hypertension and its early decompression by TIPS placement on the outcome of variceal bleeding. *Hepatology.* 2004;40:793–801. [PMID: 15382120]

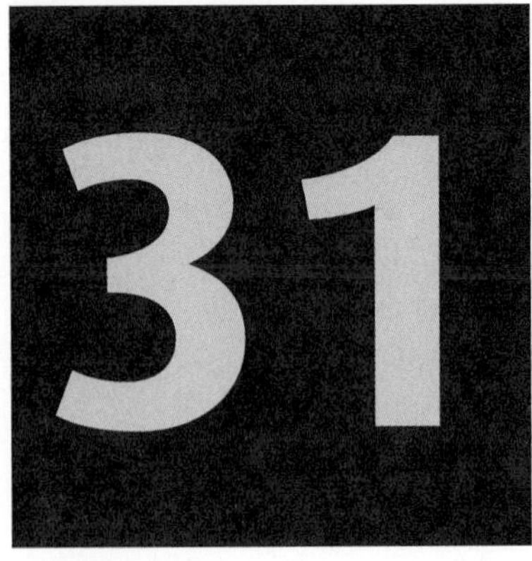

Acute Lower Gastrointestinal Bleeding

Linda S. Lee, MD
John R. Saltzman, MD

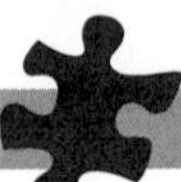

ESSENTIALS OF DIAGNOSIS

- Diverticulosis, arteriovenous malformations, and ischemic colitis are the most common causes of lower GI bleeding.
- Clinical presentation ranges from occult to overt bleeding.
- Endoscopic and radiologic tests can provide both diagnosis and therapy.
- Urgent colonoscopy may have increased diagnostic yield but does not clearly lead to decreased rates of rebleeding.

General Considerations

Lower gastrointestinal (GI) bleeding is defined as bleeding that occurs from a source distal to the ligament of Treitz. This chapter discusses only colonic sources of bleeding; upper GI bleeding and obscure (small bowel) GI bleeding are explored elsewhere (see Chapters 30 and 33).

Lower GI bleeding accounts for about 20% of major GI bleeding and is less common and generally less severe than upper GI bleeding. There are 20–27 hospitalizations per 100,000 adults in the United States due to lower GI bleeding. It generally occurs in older adults with a mean age between 63 and 77 years old. Nearly 80% of lower GI bleeding stops spontaneously, similar to upper GI bleeding. The overall mortality rate of lower GI bleeding is 2–4%. Similar to upper GI bleeding, patients who begin lower GI bleeding as outpatients have a significantly lower mortality rate (3.6%) than those who develop lower GI bleeding as inpatients (23%).

Barnert J, Messmann H. Diagnosis and management of lower gastrointestinal bleeding. *Nat Rev Gastroenterol Hepatol.* 2009;6:637–646. [PMID: 19881516]

Longstreth G. Epidemiology and outcome of patients hospitalized with acute lower gastrointestinal hemorrhage: a population-based study. *Am J Gastroenterol.* 1997;92:419–424. [PMID: 9068461]

EVALUATION OF LOWER GI BLEEDING

Definition of Bleeding

Hematochezia is defined as bright red blood per rectum and usually implies a left colonic source, although it can be caused by a more brisk, proximal source of bleeding. Maroon stools are maroon-colored blood mixed with stool and are often associated with a right colonic source of bleeding; however, they also can result from a more brisk, proximal source of bleeding. Melena refers to black, tarry, foul-smelling stool that results from the bacterial degradation of hemoglobin over a period of at least 14 hours. It usually implies an upper GI source of bleeding although it may be associated with right colonic bleeding in cases of slow motility. Ingestion of iron, bismuth, charcoal, and licorice should be excluded since they all can turn stool black. Occult blood refers to the presence of small quantities of blood in the stool that does not change its color and can only be detected by performing a stool guaiac card test. Blood loss of at least 5–10 mL/day can be detected by stool guaiac card tests. The GI tract normally loses about 0.5–1.5 mL of blood per day, which is not usually detected by guaiac tests.

Diagnostic Approach

When patients initially present with lower GI bleeding, they should be triaged and managed based on the severity of the hemorrhage (Figure 31–1).

Patients who have minor bleeding with scant hematochezia represent 75–90% of all patients with lower GI bleeding and may be evaluated as outpatients. For patients over the age of 50 years, colonoscopy should be performed to evaluate the source and to screen for colon cancer. In younger patients with rectal bleeding, there is debate regarding the necessity of a colonoscopy versus flexible sigmoidoscopy. Several studies demonstrate that 10–30% of patients with rectal bleeding had proximal lesions, which would have been missed by

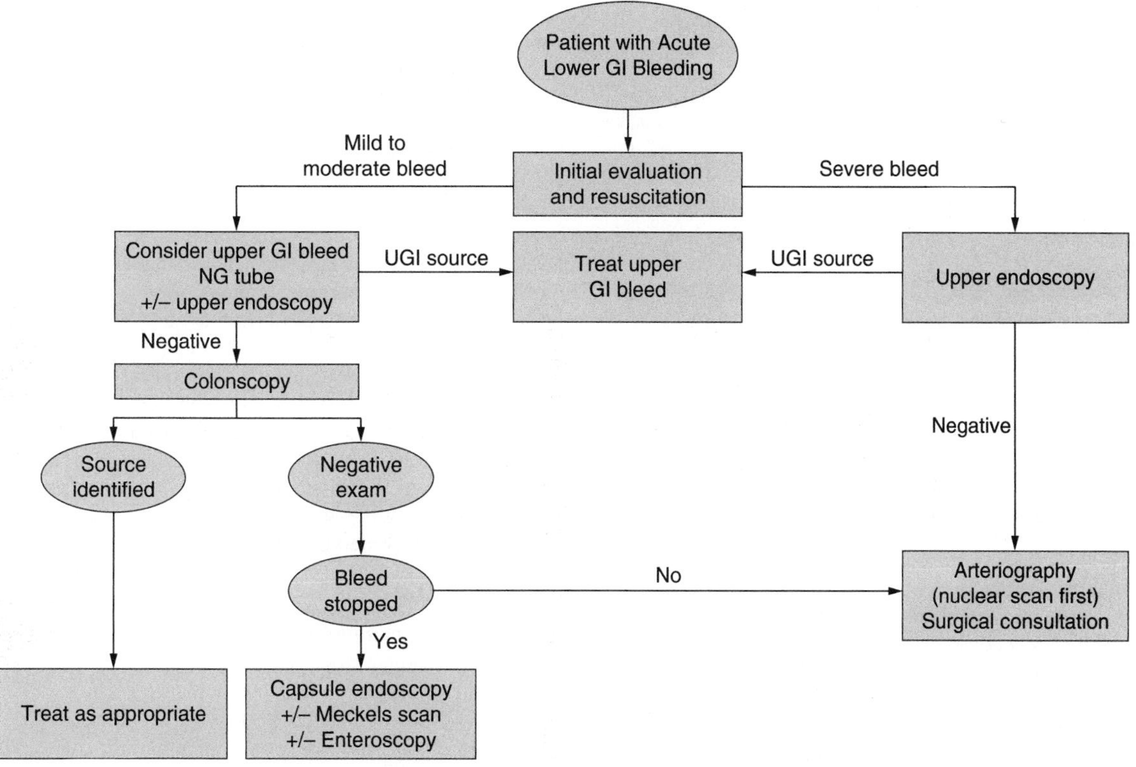

▲ **Figure 31–1.** Algorithm for the management of patients with suspected lower gastrointestinal (GI) bleeding. NG, nasogastric; UGI, upper gastrointestinal.

flexible sigmoidoscopy. Other studies found that no cancers and only a very few polyps would have been missed by flexible sigmoidoscopy in patients with "outlet-type bleeding," defined as blood seen during or after defecation on the toilet paper or in the toilet bowl without symptoms or special risk factors for colorectal neoplasia.

Physicians are unable to reliably predict based on history alone, which patients with rectal bleeding will have significant pathology. As patients grow older, it becomes cost-effective to perform a full colonoscopy. Patients in their mid-30s or older should likely be evaluated with a colonoscopy, whereas patients in their 20s with outlet-type bleeding may undergo flexible sigmoidoscopy. If no lesion is discovered to explain the hematochezia, those patients should then undergo a full colonoscopy.

Another category of patients presents with chronic intermittent bleeding that manifests as guaiac-positive stool or iron deficiency anemia, or both. Evaluation of these patients can usually occur in the outpatient setting; however, if the patients are severely anemic with cardiopulmonary symptoms or disease, inpatient admission should be considered for further monitoring, evaluation, and management. All of these patients must be evaluated with colonoscopy. About 25–41% of these patients will have abnormalities on upper endoscopy. Therefore, if no source is identified on colonoscopy or if the patient has upper gastrointestinal symptoms, an upper endoscopy should be performed. Asymptomatic patients may also harbor upper GI abnormalities, and those with iron deficiency anemia should undergo an upper endoscopy.

Other patients with lower GI bleeding include those with episodic severe bleeding and continuous active bleeding who must be evaluated in the hospital. It is important to be aware that about 10–15% of cases initially thought to represent lower GI bleeding ultimately have an upper gastrointestinal source. Clues to the presence of a possible upper GI source include hematochezia with hemodynamic instability, melena, and a history of upper GI bleeding. Placement of a nasogastric tube or obtaining a prompt upper endoscopy examination should be done to rule out an upper GI source in patients with severe lower GI bleeding.

Davila RE, Rajan E, Adler DG, et al. Standards of Practice Committee. ASGE Guideline: the role of endoscopy in the patient with lower-GI bleeding. *Gastrointest Endosc.* 2005;62: 656–660. [PMID: 16246674]

Lewis JD, Brown A, Localio AR, et al. Initial evaluation of rectal bleeding in young persons: a cost-effectiveness analysis. *Ann Intern Med.* 2002;136:99–110. [PMID: 11790061]

Song LWK, Baron TH. Endoscopic management of acute lower gastrointestinal bleeding. *Am J Gastroenterol.* 2008;103: 1881–1887. [PMID: 18796089]

Strate LL, Naumann CR. The role of colonoscopy and radiological procedures in the management of acute lower intestinal bleeding. *Clin Gastroenterol Hepatol.* 2010;8:333–343. [PMID: 20036757]

Initial Clinical Evaluation

During the initial clinical evaluation of patients with suspected acute lower GI bleeding, resuscitation should proceed simultaneously with the placement of two large-bore peripheral catheters or a central line followed by administration of intravenous fluids (normal saline or lactated Ringer's solution) or packed red blood cells (RBCs), or both.

A. Symptoms and Signs

1. History—The history in these patients should focus on factors that could be associated with potential causes: blood coating the stool suggests hemorrhoidal bleeding while blood mixed in the stool implies a more proximal source; bloody diarrhea and tenesmus is associated with inflammatory bowel disease while bloody diarrhea with fever and abdominal pain especially with recent travel history suggests infectious colitis; pain with defecation occurs with hemorrhoids and anal fissure; change in stool caliber and weight loss is concerning for colon cancer; abdominal pain can be associated with inflammatory bowel disease, infectious colitis, or ischemic colitis; painless bleeding is characteristic of diverticular bleeding, arteriovenous malformation (AVM), and radiation proctitis; nonsteroidal anti-inflammatory drug (NSAID) use is a risk factor for diverticular bleeding and NSAID-induced colonic ulcer; and recent colonoscopy with polypectomy suggests postpolypectomy bleeding.

Patients should be asked about symptoms of hemodynamic compromise, including dyspnea, chest pain, lightheadedness, and fatigue.

2. Physical findings—The physical examination should focus on the following areas:

A. Vital signs—Orthostatic hypotension implies at least a 15% loss of blood volume.

B. Abdominal examination—Evaluate for tenderness, masses, liver span, and splenomegaly.

C. Rectal examination—Key elements include inspection of the anus, palpation for masses, characterization of the stool color, and stool guaiac card test.

B. Laboratory Findings

Among the blood tests that should be performed are a complete blood count, prothrombin time/INR, partial thromboplastin time, electrolytes, and typing and cross-matching for blood products.

Coagulopathy and thrombocytopenia should be immediately corrected if possible. Platelets should be maintained above 50,000/mL and coagulopathy should be corrected with vitamin K or fresh frozen plasma. Vitamin K should be taken orally unless the patient has cirrhosis or biliary obstruction, in which case it should be administered subcutaneously. The full effect of vitamin K is not obtained for 12–24 hours, unlike fresh frozen plasma, which immediately reverses coagulopathy. The intravenous formulation of vitamin K reverses coagulopathy more quickly and may be used in cases of severe bleeding, however, patients should be monitored for anaphylaxis. The effects of fresh frozen plasma last about 3–5 hours and large volumes (>2–3 L) may be required to completely reverse coagulopathy, depending on the initial prothrombin time. Recombinant activated factor VII has been approved for use in patients with hemophilia A and B with factor VIII and IX inhibitors. Evidence of possible benefit in patients with cirrhosis and GI bleeding has been demonstrated, although the optimal dose is unclear and recombinant activated factor VII is very expensive.

C. Diagnostic Tests

Diagnostic evaluation must be performed after patients have been adequately resuscitated. If an upper GI source is suspected, an upper endoscopy should be performed first. Lower GI evaluation can be performed with anoscopy, flexible sigmoidoscopy, colonoscopy, rarely barium enema, and various radiologic studies.

1. Anoscopy—Anoscopy is useful only for diagnosing bleeding sources from the anorectal junction and anal canal, including internal hemorrhoids and anal fissures. It is superior to flexible sigmoidoscopy for detecting hemorrhoids in an outpatient setting and can be performed quickly in the office or at the bedside as an adjunct to flexible sigmoidoscopy and colonoscopy.

2. Flexible sigmoidoscopy—Flexible sigmoidoscopy uses a 65-cm long sigmoidoscope that visualizes the left colon. It can be performed without sedation and only minimal preparation with enemas. However, the diagnostic yield of flexible sigmoidoscopy in acute lower GI bleeding is only 9%. The role of anoscopy and flexible sigmoidoscopy in inpatients with acute lower GI bleeding is limited, since most patients should undergo colonoscopy.

3. Colonoscopy—Colonoscopy is the test of choice in the majority of patients with acute lower GI bleeding since it can be both diagnostic and therapeutic. The diagnostic accuracy of colonoscopy in lower GI bleeding ranges from 48% to 90%, and urgent colonoscopy appears to increase diagnostic yield. This wide range in yield is partially explained by different criteria for diagnosis, as often if no active bleeding, non-bleeding visible vessel, or adherent clot is found, bleeding is attributed to a lesion if blood is present in the area. The presence of fresh blood in the terminal ileum is presumed to indicate a noncolonic source of bleeding.

The overall complication rate of colonoscopy in acute lower GI bleeding is 1.3%. Bowel preparation is safe and well-tolerated in most patients. The complication rate of colonoscopy in an unprepped colon may be higher. About 2–6% of colonoscopy preparations in acute lower GI bleeding are poor. Between 4 and 8 L of a polyethylene glycol (PEG) prep solution should be administered orally or via nasogastric tube until the effluence is clear. Antiemetics and prokinetics such as metoclopramide 10 mg should be given as needed during the preparation, especially if a rapid and large volume of a PEG prep solution is needed. In patients at risk of aspiration or fluid overload the preparation must be cautiously administered.

4. Urgent colonoscopy—Multiple validated scoring systems exist to predict the probability of rebleeding, surgery, and mortality in upper GI bleeding. This enables appropriate triage and aggressive management of high-risk patients and potentially early discharge of low-risk patients. Few studies have stratified patients by severity of lower GI bleeding. The strongest risk factors identified for mortality in lower GI bleeding are advanced age, intestinal ischemia, and the presence of two or more comorbidities.

It is not clear that aggressive treatment with urgent colonoscopy improves the outcome in patients with severe lower GI bleeding. There are two prospective randomized trials to date of patients with significant lower GI bleeding who were randomized to standard care or urgent colonoscopy. Patients in the standard care arm underwent elective colonoscopy within 4 days of admission while patients undergoing urgent colonoscopy were administered 4–6 L of a PEG prep solution orally or via a nasogastric tube over 3–4 hours and underwent colonoscopy within 8 to 12 hours of hospitalization or diagnosis of hematochezia. More sources of bleeding were identified in the urgent colonoscopy group in one study, but there was no difference in early or late rebleeding, length of hospital stay, surgery, mortality, or complications in either study. Therefore, it is unclear if urgent colonoscopy influences patient outcome despite the increased identification and treatment of a source of bleeding, and further larger studies are needed.

Green BT, Rockey DC, Portwood G, et al. Urgent colonoscopy for evaluation and management of acute lower gastrointestinal hemorrhage: a randomized controlled trial. *Am J Gastroenterol.* 2005;100:2395–2402. [PMID: 16279891]

Laine L, Shah A. Randomized trial of urgent vs. elective colonoscopy in patients hospitalized with lower GI bleeding. *Am J Gastroenterol.* 2010;105:2636–2641. [PMID: 20648004]

Strate LL, Ayanian JZ, Kotler G, Syngal S. Risk factors for mortality in lower intestinal bleeding. *Clin Gastroenterol Hepatol.* 2008; 6:1004–1010. [PMID: 18558513]

Velayos FS, Williamson A, Sousa KH, et al. Early predictors of severe lower gastrointestinal bleeding and adverse outcomes: a prospective study. *Clin Gastroenterol Hepatol.* 2004;2:485–490. [PMID: 15181617]

5. Barium enema—There is no role for barium enema in the evaluation of acute lower GI bleeding. It may impede the performance of a colonoscopy or subsequent angiography due to the presence of barium in the colon. In young patients with minor hematochezia who have a negative flexible sigmoidoscopy, barium enema can be an alternative to colonoscopy.

6. Tagged red blood cell scan—Tagged RBC scan and angiography may be the tests of choice in patients with massive lower GI bleeding that prevents colonoscopy, in those with ongoing bleeding and a negative colonoscopy, or in patients who have not yet been prepared for a colonoscopy. Although tagged RBC scan is solely a diagnostic examination, angiography, like colonoscopy, can be both diagnostic and therapeutic.

A bleeding rate of at least 0.1–0.5 mL/min is required for detection by tagged RBC scan. An injected radiotracer circulates in the blood and extravasation of blood into the GI lumen can be identified on a series of static images captured after injection or on multiple sequential dynamic images obtained at 15- or 30-second intervals (Figures 31–2A and 31–2B). Two radiotracers have been used for tagged RBC scan: technetium 99m (^{99m}Tc) sulfur colloid and ^{99m}Tc-labeled RBC, which involves labeling the patient's RBCs in vitro and then reinjecting them into the patient. Sulfur colloid is rapidly cleared by the reticuloendothelial system and, therefore, leaves the blood pool within minutes, which provides approximately a 10-minute window to detect extravasation. RBC labeling is superior because the red cells persist for at least 24 hours in the circulation. This allows for longer and repeated imaging if the patient rebleeds during this time window. Typically a 90-minute imaging period is used as the diagnostic yield plateaus at this time.

About 45% of tagged RBC scans for lower GI bleeding are positive. Accuracy of localization of the bleeding site ranges from 24% to 91%. Scans that are positive within 2 hours were 95–100% accurate in localizing the bleeding site compared with 57–67% accurate for scans positive after 2 hours. Because of the relatively high rate of false localization, confirmatory studies are required before proceeding to surgery.

Tagged RBC scan is most useful before angiography because it selects patients who are bleeding sufficiently for an angiogram and it may allow more targeted angiography with decreased contrast load. A positive tagged RBC scan increases the diagnostic yield of angiography 2.4 times by selecting out patients who are not actively bleeding at the time of tagged RBC scan. It is important that following a positive tagged RBC scan, urgent angiography be performed within 1 hour if feasible. Delaying angiography may lead to increased negative results because lower GI bleeding is often episodic and intermittent.

7. Angiography—A more rapid rate of bleeding of at least 0.5–1.5 mL/min is necessary for detection during angiography (Figure 31–3) compared with tagged RBC scan. Patients who

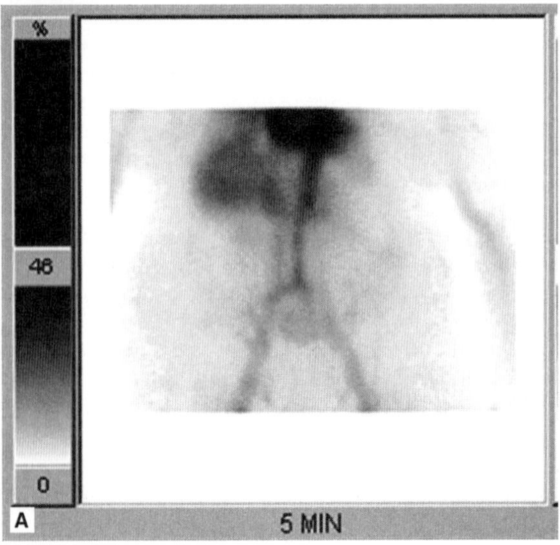

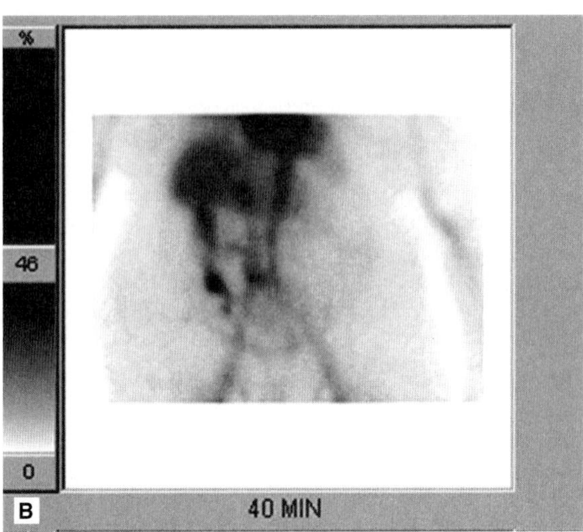

▲ **Figure 31–2.** **A.** Baseline tagged red blood cell scan. **B.** Tagged red blood cell scan with active bleeding from the right colon.

are massively bleeding and hemodynamically unstable should be resuscitated and proceed directly to angiography without tagged RBC scan. The diagnostic yield of angiography ranges from 27% to 77% with a mean of 47%; sensitivity and specificity are 47% and 100%, respectively. Complications of angiography occur in 10–20% of patients and include renal failure, hematoma, ischemia, and infarction. Provocative testing using anticoagulants (eg, intravenous heparin and intra-arterial tissue plasminogen activator) and vasodilators (intra-arterial tolazoline) can increase diagnostic yield although concern for significant complications exist. Further studies are necessary to optimize the efficacy and prove the safety of this approach.

▲ **Figure 31–3.** Angiography with active bleeding from the right colon.

Maleux G, Roeflaer F, Heye S, et al. Long-term outcome of transcatheter embolotherapy for acute lower gastrointestinal hemorrhage. *Am J Gastroenterol* 2009;104:2042–2046. [PMID: 19455109]

8. Multidetector-row computed tomography—Recent advances in the technology of computed tomography (CT) may lead to a future role for CT scan in lower GI bleeding. Multidetector-row CT (MDCT) incorporates several improvements, which allow enhanced delineation of mesenteric vessels: faster scanning time, more accurate acquisition of images in arterial and venous phases, and improved three-dimensional display. Patients do not ingest any water or contrast material orally and, after an initial unenhanced CT scan, images are obtained during the arterial phase to identify extravasation of contrast into the bowel lumen. Preliminary studies using angiography as the gold standard demonstrate sensitivity and specificity of 90.9% and 99% for detecting acute GI bleeding with MDCT and 100% accuracy in localization of bleeding site. Single-detector CT scan can detect bleeding rates of 0.3 mL/min, and MDCT may approach the detection ability of tagged RBC scans.

Table 31–1. Common sources and prevalence of lower gastrointestinal bleeding.

Source	Prevalence (%)
Diverticulosis	17-44
Colonic angiodysplasia	2-30
Ischemia	9-21
Malignancy	4-14
Hemorrhoids/anorectal	4-11
Postpolypectomy	6
Unknown	8-12

Data from Longstreth GF. Epidemiology and outcome of patients hospitalized with acute lower gastrointestinal hemorrhage: a population-based study. *Am J Gastroenterol.* 1997;92:419; Strate LL, Orav EJ, Syngal S. Early predictors of severity in acute lower intestinal tract bleeding. *Arch Intern Med.* 2003;163:838; and Zuccaro G Jr. Management of the adult patient with acute lower gastrointestinal bleeding. American College of Gastroenterology Practice Parameters Committee. *Am J Gastroenterol.* 1998;93:1202.

Copland A, Munroe CA, Friedland S, Triadafilopoulos G. Integrating urgent multidetector CT scanning in the diagnostic algorithm of active lower GI bleeding. *Gastrointest Endosc.* 2010; 72:402–405. [PMID: 20674629]

Frattaroli FM, Casciani E, Spoletini D, et al. Prospective study comparing multi-detector row CT and endoscopy in acute gastrointestinal bleeding. *World J Surg.* 2009;33:2209–2217. [PMID: 19653032]

9. Magnetic resonance angiography—Magnetic resonance angiography is not typically used in acute lower GI bleeding because it lacks the resolution to detect hemorrhage from small blood vessels. A new blood pool contrast agent may help localize the bleeding to a bowel segment. This contrast agent remains in the intravascular space for many hours, and subsequent imaging could identify extravascular contrast.

Differential Diagnosis

The differential diagnosis of acute lower GI bleeding is broad, although the vast majority of such bleeding is due to diverticulosis, ischemic colitis, AVMs, neoplasia, and hemorrhoids (Table 31–1). Following evaluation, the cause of lower GI bleeding remains uncertain in about 12% of cases.

SPECIFIC CAUSES OF ACUTE LOWER GI BLEEDING

1. Diverticulosis

Diverticulosis is the most common cause of lower GI bleeding. It is more prevalent in developed countries and older patients. Although 5–10% of people under the age of 40 have diverticulosis, nearly two-thirds of people older than 80 years are affected. A detailed discussion of diverticular disease appears in Chapter 21.

About 75–80% of people with diverticulosis are asymptomatic; however, 3–20% experience diverticular bleeding. Massive bleeding occurs in 3–5% of patients. Risk factors for diverticular bleeding include the use of NSAIDs, advanced age, and right colon location. Bleeding occurs at the site of penetration of the vasa recta, with the vasa recta stretched over the dome of the diverticula, resulting in segmental wall weakness and predisposing to rupture. Abrupt painless bleeding characterizes diverticular bleeding; mild lower abdominal cramping may occur before passage of bright red or maroon blood due to the cathartic nature of blood in the intestines. Melena is unusual for arterial bleeding from diverticulosis. Guaiac-positive stool alone and iron deficiency anemia are not consistent with diverticular bleeding.

Over 75% of diverticula are located in the left colon. Bleeding diverticula detected during angiography usually occur in the right colon whereas 60% of bleeding diverticula diagnosed at colonoscopy are located in the left colon. The vast majority of diverticular bleeding stops spontaneously. Colonoscopy is often the initial diagnostic procedure performed to rule out other lesions and determine the bleeding site, which is found in less than 22% of cases. Urgent colonoscopy increases the chance of detecting a bleeding site. If bleeding without a clear source persists or recurs, tagged RBC scan can be performed followed by immediate angiography, if positive, or by possible repeat colonoscopy, if negative. An algorithm for management of diverticular bleeding is included in Chapter 21 (see Figure 21–5).

There are multiple endoscopic options if a bleeding diverticulum is identified, including epinephrine injection, bipolar coagulation, combination therapy, and mechanical therapy. Epinephrine injection in four quadrants can control bleeding or close the mouth of the diverticulum by tamponade. The majority of bleeding vessels or nonbleeding visible vessels identified during endoscopy are located on the neck of the diverticulum. Once a site of a bleeding diverticulum is identified, the location should first be marked with a submucosal injection of ink or application of a endoclip. This allows for precise localization of the bleeding area if further endoscopic, angiographic or surgical therapy is needed. Thermal therapy should be avoided at the dome of the diverticulum. Bipolar coagulation should be performed with 10–15 watts of power, moderate pressure, and short 1-second pulses. Clots can be removed using the cold guillotine technique (similar to the technique for upper GI bleeding) and any underlying lesion should be treated appropriately. A small study suggested that endoscopic treatment is successful long term: none of the patients treated endoscopically had recurrent bleeding over a median of 30 months compared with 53% of patients treated medically who rebled. There are case reports of successful treatment of bleeding diverticula using mechanical therapy with endoclips or endoscopic band ligation (Plates 67 and 68).

Angiography offers another treatment option. Continuous, selective intra-arterial vasopressin infusion stops bleeding in about 90% of cases, with up to 50% rebleeding after discontinuing the infusion. Despite this temporary effect in many patients, vasopressin infusion can be helpful to allow bowel preparation before a semi-elective definitive surgical procedure. However, it can cause abdominal pain and should be avoided in patients with known coronary artery disease.

Superselective embolization with microcatheters uses 2.5–3 French microcatheters, which are advanced through conventional 5 French catheters to access smaller, more distal vessels. Various embolic agents are used, including gel foam, polyvinyl alcohol, and microcoils. Treatment success ranges from 44% to 91%, with rates of rebleeding from 6% to 34%. Recurrent bleeding 1 month after embolization occurs in less than 15% of patients with diverticular hemorrhage compared with over 40% with nondiverticular causes such as AVM. Major ischemic complications requiring surgery appear to occur in less than 6% of cases.

Persistent massive hemorrhage, transfusion requirement over 4 units in 24 hours, and recurrent diverticular bleeding are potential indications for surgery, which is needed in 18–25% of people requiring transfusions. Mortality rate is still relatively high at 10% even with directed segmental resection, and the rebleeding rate is 14% at 1-year follow-up. Blind segmental resection should be avoided due to rebleeding rates as high as 33% and mortality rates ranging from 20% to 57%. Rebleeding rates as low as 0% but mortality rates ranging from 0% to 33% have been reported for blind subtotal colectomy. Therefore, aggressive efforts should be made to localize a bleeding site preoperatively.

Repeat diverticular bleeding occurs in 25–35% of patients, and 50% of these people experience a third episode of diverticular hemorrhage. NSAID use is a potential risk factor; however, whether avoiding NSAIDs reduces the chance of rebleeding is unclear.

Funaki B. Superselective embolization of lower gastrointestinal hemorrhage: a new paradigm. *Abdom Imaging.* 2004;29: 434–438. [PMID: 15024510]

Jensen DM, Machicado GA, Jutabha R, et al. Urgent colonoscopy for the diagnosis and treatment of severe diverticular hemorrhage. *N Engl J Med.* 2000;342:78–82. [PMID: 10631275]

Song LWK, Baron TH. Endoscopic management of acute lower gastrointestinal bleeding. *Am J Gastroenterol.* 2008;103:1881–1887. [PMID: 18796089]

2. Arteriovenous Malformation

AVMs are the reported source of lower GI bleeding in 3–40% of patients. They are usually congenital and occur in 1–2% of colon autopsy specimens. AVMs are ectatic mucosal and submucosal blood vessels that have a direct communication between the arteries and veins without intervening capillaries. Over half are located in the right colon, and 47% of patients experience painless hematochezia similar to diverticular hemorrhage. Patients with bleeding AVMs can present with chronic, intermittent bleeding. Risk factors for bleeding include advanced age (older than 60 years), right-sided location, and possibly certain conditions (aortic stenosis and chronic renal failure).

Angiography is considered the gold standard in diagnosing AVMs. Findings include ectatic slowly emptying veins, vascular tufts, or early filling veins. The diagnostic sensitivity of colonoscopy is 80–90% with the characteristic finding of a 2- to 10-mm, red, fernlike flat lesion with ectatic vessels radiating from a central vessel. Poor bowel preparation and use of meperidine, which transiently decreases mucosal blood flow, could potentially hinder the identification of AVMs. Use of naloxone may enhance colonic vasculature and AVM identification.

Bleeding AVMs discovered during colonoscopy can be treated with a variety of thermal therapies. Contact electrocautery should begin with the outer feeder vessels and progress toward the central vessel (Plates 69 and 70). Argon plasma coagulation has become a popular noncontact method, with a reported 77–83% success rate. Nonbleeding AVMs without evidence of GI bleeding should not be treated. However, if there is a history of guaiac-positive stool or iron deficiency anemia, AVMs should be treated even if not actively bleeding.

There is a potential role for medical treatment of AVMs. Only case series and reports have suggested the benefit of octreotide administered subcutaneously in doses ranging from 100 mcg to 500 mcg two times a day by decreasing the need for transfusions. Long-term estrogen–progesterone treatment for 1 year did not decrease rebleeding from AVMs in a randomized trial. Another study that suggested benefit from hormone therapy had a study population containing 50% of patients with Osler-Weber-Rendu disease. Therefore, this subset of patients may experience decreased bleeding from AVMs with hormone therapy.

Junquera F, Feu F, Papo M, et al. A multicenter, randomized, clinical trial of hormonal therapy in the prevention of rebleeding from gastrointestinal angiodysplasia. *Gastroenterology.* 2001;121: 1073–1079. [PMID: 11677198]

Kwan V, Bourke MJ, Williams SJ, et al. Argon plasma coagulation in the management of symptomatic gastrointestinal vascular lesions: experience in 100 consecutive patients with long-term follow-up. *Am J Gastroenterol.* 2006;101:58–63. [PMID: 16405534]

Szilagyi A, Ghali MP. Pharmacological therapy of vascular malformations of the gastrointestinal tract. *Can J Gastroenterol.* 2006;20:171–178. [PMID: 16550261]

3. Ischemic Colitis

The diagnosis of colonic ischemia is established by a combination of clinical setting, physical diagnosis, and diagnostic studies. The differential diagnosis includes infectious colitis, inflammatory bowel disease, diverticulitis, radiation enteritis, and colon cancer. In hospitalized patients *Clostridium difficile* infection must be excluded. Although there are no specific blood tests for colonic ischemia, elevations may be noted in the white blood cell count and in amylase, creatine phosphokinase, and serum lactate levels. Most plain radiographs in colonic ischemia have nonspecific findings, although thumbprinting due to submucosal edema and pneumatosis may be seen typically in patients with more advanced disease.

Diagnostic testing with CT scans may reveal segmental thickening of the involved colon. Endoscopic evaluation with sigmoidoscopy or colonoscopy may be used to confirm the diagnosis in patients whose diagnosis is unclear and who do not have signs of peritonitis or perforation. Care must be taken to avoid overdistention with air during the examination to prevent worsening of ischemic damage. Endoscopic findings typically occur in a segmental distribution and vary depending on the degree of damage, ranging from pale mucosa with petechial bleeding to cyanotic, necrotic bowel. Angiography is usually not indicated in colonic ischemia as the blood flow to the colon returns to normal by the time of clinical presentation.

4. Neoplasm

Neoplasms of the colon may present with GI bleeding. In patients over the age of 50 years, rectal bleeding is due to a neoplasm in about 10% of cases; however, neoplasms are an uncommon source of rectal bleeding in persons younger than age 50. Although most bleeding from colonic neoplasms tends to be low grade and occult, bleeding may be brisk and overt at times. Bleeding occurs due to erosion or ulceration of the lesion. Distal lesions (left side and rectum) are more likely to present with bright red blood per rectum whereas more proximal lesions tend to present with maroon stool, melena, or occult blood.

The diagnosis of a neoplasm as the source of lower GI bleeding is typically done by colonoscopy, with biopsies performed to confirm the diagnosis. Larger neoplasms may be detected on CT scans. The therapeutic options for those patients with bleeding neoplasms are limited. Standard endoscopic therapies have marginal effectiveness. The use of fibrin glue has been reported to be effective in small studies (Plates 71 and 72). The treatment for most patients with bleeding colonic neoplasms is surgical resection.

5. Hemorrhoids

Hemorrhoids and other anorectal disorders (solitary rectal ulcers and anal fissures) are an important source of lower GI bleeding. Hemorrhoids are dilated submucosal vessels in the anus, which are considered internal if above the dentate line (Plate73) and external if below. Hemorrhoids are extremely common and usually asymptomatic but can present with pruritus, thrombosis, or hematochezia. Bleeding from hemorrhoids occurs when there is rupture of a blood vessel.

The clinical manifestations of bleeding hemorrhoids include painless hematochezia with the stool being coated with bright red blood. Further bleeding may occur, with blood dripping into the toilet bowl or staining underwear. Although bleeding from hemorrhoids is usually low grade, high volume or massive bleeding may occur rarely. Severe bleeding from hemorrhoids may occur in patients with a coagulopathy. Acute treatment for most patients with bleeding hemorrhoids is not needed, since most episodes are mild and resolve spontaneously. Topical medical treatments help decrease inflammation, and surgery is rarely needed for those with persistent or massive bleeding.

6. Postpolypectomy Bleeding

Postpolypectomy bleeding occurs after 1–6% of polypectomies and is the leading major complication following colonoscopy with polypectomy. Acute hemorrhage occurring at the time of polypectomy accounts for less than 50% of cases. Therapeutic options include resnaring the stalk of the polypectomy site to apply pressure, injection therapy with epinephrine, contact or noncontact thermal treatment with bipolar coagulation or argon plasma coagulation, and endoclip application (Plates 74 and75). Although bleeding usually occurs within 7 days, delayed bleeding can occur up to 29 days following polypectomy when the eschar falls off the site. Polypectomy bleeding is usually self-limited and over 70% of cases resolve with supportive care.

Risk factors for postpolypectomy bleeding include removal of large polyps (greater than 1 cm in diameter), age over 65 years, cardiovascular or chronic renal disease, platelet dysfunction, and coagulopathy. Multiple studies have tried to identify techniques to reduce the risk of postpolypectomy bleeding. Only submucosal injection of saline has proven useful in large polyps, and it is unclear whether the type of electrical current (blended vs cutting), placement of prophylactic endoclips, or use of an endoloop decreases the risk of bleeding.

Rabeneck L, Paszat LF, Hilsden RJ, et al. Bleeding and perforation after outpatient colonoscopy and their risk factors in usual clinical practice. *Gastroenterology.* 2008;135(6):1899–1906. [PMID: 18938166]

7. NSAID-Induced Bleeding

While it is well known that NSAIDs are among the most common causes of peptic ulcer disease, it is less appreciated that NSAIDs can damage the large intestine and cause lower GI bleeding. Characteristic endoscopic findings include single or multiple well-defined ulcers with normal intervening mucosa that are classically found in the terminal ileum and proximal colon and a single or multiple diaphragm-like strictures with normal intervening mucosa. Only 21% of patients with colonic ulcers have simultaneous gastric ulcers. Clinical presentation is variable and includes guaiac-positive stool, iron deficiency anemia, hematochezia, crampy abdominal pain, weight loss, and change in bowel habits. NSAID-induced colonic ulcers may also be an incidental finding in asymptomatic patients. Because pathology from NSAID-induced colonic ulcers is nonspecific, diagnosis is made after excluding other potential causes of colonic ulcers including infectious, ischemic, and inflammatory. Symptomatic patients usually respond within a few days after cessation of NSAIDs. If NSAIDs cannot be discontinued, concomitant therapy with misoprostol, sulfasalazine, or metronidazole may protect the mucosa from damage and help heal ulcers.

Kurahara K, Matsumoto T, Iida M, et al. Clinical and endoscopic features of nonsteroidal anti-inflammatory drug-induced colonic ulcerations. *Am J Gastroenterol.* 2001;96: 473–480. [PMID: 11232693]

8. Radiation Proctitis

Pelvic radiation can cause both acute and chronic radiation proctitis. Acute damage presents within 3 months of radiation therapy with diarrhea, tenesmus, and, rarely, bleeding. Chronic radiation proctitis typically occurs 9–14 months following radiation in up to 20% of patients but can occur years later (Plate 76). Bleeding is a prominent symptom caused by mucosal atrophy and fibrosis, which result in chronic mucosal ischemia.

There are no standardized recommendations for treatment of bleeding from radiation proctitis. Endoscopic therapy appears superior to medical treatment in reducing severe bleeding, with nearly 75% success following endoscopic treatment compared with 33% for medical therapy. Multiple oral and topical therapies have been investigated (mainly in small clinical trials or case series), and a few may be effective, including sucralfate enema, short-chain fatty acid enema, and topical formalin therapy.

Endoscopic management with heater probe and bipolar coagulation has proved effective in controlling bleeding during a mean of four treatment sessions performed every 4–6 weeks. Argon plasma coagulation has received more attention recently, with 85–100% success in reducing or stopping bleeding over a mean of two to three treatments every 1–2 months. All visible telangiectasias are obliterated at each session, while rectal ulcers resulting from previous treatments are avoided. Short-term complications occur in 7% of patients and include rectal pain and fever. Rare major complications include rectovaginal fistula, anal or rectal stricture, and perforation, presumed secondary to accumulation of combustible gas. A full bowel preparation is safest since there have been rare reports of explosions of gas during argon plasma coagulation when an enema preparation was used. During long-term follow-up over 1–5 years, recurrent bleeding occurred in 0–8% of patients.

Hyperbaric oxygen may represent another therapeutic option and is believed to promote angiogenesis and collagen formation, leading to reepithelialization. The few recent case series selected patients who had failed previous medical or endoscopic therapy for hyperbaric oxygen treatment, and report a 75–100% decrease or cessation of bleeding. The treatment regimen is rigorous; for example, one study placed patients in a hyperbaric chamber at a pressure of 2.4 atmospheres with 100% oxygen for 90 minutes 5–7 days per week for an average of 36 sessions. Hyperbaric oxygen therapy may be considered before proceeding to surgery in patients who are refractory to standard medical and endoscopic treatment.

Karamanolis G, Triantafyllou K, Tsiamoulos Z, et al. Argon plasma coagulation has a long-lasting therapeutic effect in patients with chronic radiation proctitis. *Endoscopy.* 2009;41:529–531. [PMID: 19440956]

Endoscopic Management of Acute Biliary & Pancreatic Conditions

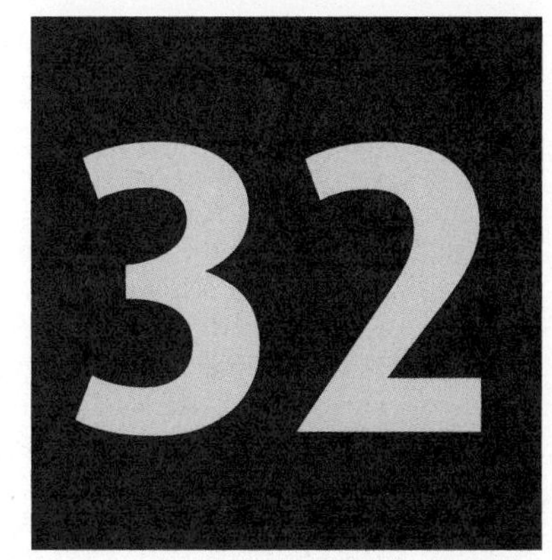

Christopher C. Thompson, MD, MSc, FACG, FASGE

General Considerations

Since the introduction of endoscopic retrograde cholangiopancreatoscopy (ERCP) in 1968 and endoscopic sphincterotomy in 1974, the management of various biliary and pancreatic illnesses has evolved from surgical to endoscopic methods with substantial improvements in patient outcomes. Additionally, development of custom accessories has improved procedural efficiency and success rates; these include balloons and baskets for stone extraction, lithotripsy devices, stents, drains, and duodenoscope-assisted cholangiopancreatoscopy. In expert centers success rates for many endoscopic interventions exceed 90%.

Several acute biliary and pancreatic conditions are amenable to endoscopic diagnosis and therapy. ERCP has been shown to have better outcomes than surgery when dealing with most ductal obstructions and leaks. Additionally, ERCP may have a limited role in the diagnosis of bleeding conditions and the treatment of associated complications. This chapter details endoscopic treatment options for these conditions.

ACUTE CHOLANGITIS

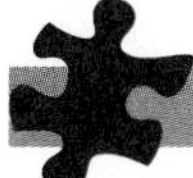

ESSENTIALS OF DIAGNOSIS

- Diagnosis of acute biliary obstruction with cholangitis relies on clinical findings, blood counts, blood chemistries, biochemical profile, and imaging studies such as MRI with MRCP.
- Endoscopic biliary drainage is the standard of care, with emergent drainage for patients not responding to antibiotics and supportive measures or showing signs of clinical deterioration (ie, hypotension, altered mental states, and signs of continuing infection such as persistent fever).

Acute cholangitis is characterized by biliary stasis and infection of the bile ducts. In 1877, Charcot defined the clinical triad of fever, right upper quadrant pain, and jaundice that is present in up to 70% of patients with acute cholangitis. The spectrum of clinical presentation ranges from mild pain and low-grade fever, to a fulminate course with hypotensive sepsis. In 1959, the Charcot triad was modified to include hypotension and mental status changes, subsequently known as the Reynolds pentad. Clinical presentation is, however, not useful in differentiating between suppurative and nonsuppurative cholangitis, which can only be determined at the time of therapy. In the latter form, bacteria are still present in bile, but without the formation of pus. Suppurative cholangitis has a more acute course and is less likely to respond to antibiotics; however, either form is potentially life threatening, and when acute cholangitis is suspected urgent diagnosis and treatment are critical.

Pathogenesis

Bile duct obstruction and infection are requisite for the development of cholangitis. Over 90% of cases are attributed to common bile duct stones. Other causes of obstruction include iatrogenic biliary instrumentation and endoprostheses. Less common causes include malignant biliary obstruction, benign bile duct strictures, ampullary adenomas, periductal adenopathy, choledochal cysts, parasites, and blood clots.

Following bile duct obstruction and biliary stasis, infection may occur either by direct ascent from the bowel, or via the lymphatics or portal vein. The latter assumes translocation of bacteria from the bowel into the portal circulation and subsequent clearance of bacteria by the reticuloendothelial system with excretion into bile. Although the origin of infecting organisms is questionable, the most common organisms are enteric and often polymicrobial. *Escherichia coli, Klebsiella, Enterobacter,* and *Proteus* are most common, while enterococcus and anaerobes are less frequent. Positive bile cultures are seen in approximately one third of patients with bacteremia.

Clinical Findings

Initial studies include blood cultures, a complete blood count, and a full biochemical profile. Several noninvasive imaging studies are available to diagnose biliary obstruction. Abdominal ultrasound is sensitive for intrahepatic biliary dilation; however, it is poor at identifying choledocholithiasis, with a sensitivity of less than 30%. Additionally, up to one third of patients with choledocholithiasis do not have evidence of biliary dilation, and cholangitis can occur before the bile duct becomes dilated. Nuclear hepatobiliary imaging can detect biliary obstruction earlier than ultrasound, with higher sensitivity. However, magnetic resonance imaging (MRI) with magnetic resonance cholangiopancreatography (MRCP) is most accurate, with a sensitivity of 97%. ERCP is no longer viewed as an initial diagnostic option and is reserved for therapy.

Treatment

A. Supportive Care

Supportive care with restoration of fluid and electrolyte balance and broad-spectrum antibiotics, including gram-negative coverage, should be promptly instituted. Additionally, anaerobic coverage should be included if there is a history of prior instrumentation. Up to 85% of patients will respond to these conservative measures allowing for semi-elective biliary drainage within 48 hours. Emergent drainage is indicated in those patients who do not respond to conservative measures or when clinical deterioration occurs, particularly with the development of hypotension or alteration of mental status.

B. Endoscopic Biliary Drainage

Endoscopic biliary drainage is the standard of care for most causes of cholangitis. Definitive therapy typically involves endoscopic sphincterotomy with removal of stones or other obstructions. This has proven to be safer than surgical options. Complete clearance of gallstones is possible in up to 90% of cases on the initial procedure, with morbidity and mortality rates of 6% and near 0%, respectively.

It is important to avoid excess contrast injection, since this may precipitate cholangiovenous reflux and sepsis. Bile should initially be aspirated to decompress the collecting system, with samples sent for culture. The amount of contrast injected should be half that of the bile removed.

If the patient is particularly ill or on anticoagulation, a two-step approach may be preferred, consisting of ERCP with stent placement alone followed by definitive endoscopic sphincterotomy and stone removal when the patient is more appropriately prepared. Additionally, when stones are too large to remove, stents may be placed as a temporizing measure to ensure adequate drainage.

Mechanical or electrohydraulic lithotripsy may be necessary for the complete removal of large common duct stones. This should not be attempted during the initial treatment of acute cholangitis.

C. Percutaneous Transhepatic Cholangiography and Rendezvous Procedures

When endoscopic drainage is not possible, percutaneous transhepatic cholangiography (PTC) with drainage is indicated. The degree of urgency similarly depends on the clinical situation; however, emergent drainage should be performed if partial injection occurred on attempted ERCP. Since its introduction in 1974, PTC has evolved into numerous therapeutic interventions including stenting, stone removal, and in rare cases, even sphincterotomy. In the setting of acute cholangitis, the initial procedure is limited to drainage of the obstructed system. Definitive therapy with stone removal can be achieved on subsequent procedures. A wire may be placed through the transhepatic access and into the duodenum allowing for endoscopic stone removal; this is referred to as a rendezvous procedure. If endoscopic access to the biliary system is not possible, a series of procedures is typically required involving upsizing of drains and various methods of lithotripsy.

Endoscopic ultrasound (EUS) may also be used to access the biliary system and perform a rendezvous procedure. Although only small case series have been reported, early results are encouraging. In this procedure a 19-gauge EUS needle is used for fine needle aspiration of the bile duct via a transduodenal or transgastric route. Following drainage, contrast may be injected and a wire passed. If the wire is placed successfully through the papilla and into the duodenum, it may be used to guide retrograde access and perform a rendezvous procedure. If the wire is unable to pass from the duct and into the duodenum, a stent may be placed antegrade into the bile duct as a temporary measure.

Gupta K, Mallery S, Hunter D, et al. Endoscopic ultrasound and percutaneous access for endoscopic biliary and pancreatic drainage after initially failed ERCP. *Rev Gastroenterol Disord.* 2007;7:22–37. [PMID: 17392627]

Mallery S, Matlock J, Freeman ML. EUS-guided rendezvous drainage of obstructed biliary and pancreatic ducts: report of 6 cases. *Gastrointest Endosc.* 2004;59:100–107. [PMID: 14722561]

Shami VM, Kahaleh M. Endoscopic ultrasound (EUS)-guided access and therapy of pancreatico-biliary disorders: EUS-guided cholangio and pancreatic drainage. *Gastointest Endosc Clin N Am.* 2007;27:581–593. [PMID: 17640584]

Surgical Drainage

Surgical biliary drainage carries significant risk of morbidity and a mortality rate as high as 40%. This is reserved for cases in which endoscopic and percutaneous methods fail.

Lipsett PA, Pitt HA. Cholangitis. In: Blumgart LH, Fong Y (eds). *Surgery of the Liver and Biliary Tract.* Saunders, 2000; 917–926.

GALLSTONE PANCREATITIS

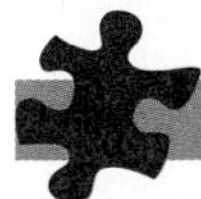

ESSENTIALS OF DIAGNOSIS

- ▶ Diagnosis is guided by clinical picture and imaging studies (eg, MRCP).
- ▶ Endoscopic drainage and papillotomy is reserved for suspected ascending cholangitis, established choledocholithiasis, or deteriorating course.

Gallstone pancreatitis is defined as acute pancreatitis with clinical evidence of gallstones, in the absence of other causes of pancreatitis. A clinical definition is needed for this condition, since calculi are often challenging to demonstrate by abdominal imaging during an acute attack, and frequently pass spontaneously into the bowel. Although this is the most common cause of acute pancreatitis, the exact pathogenesis remains unclear, and in up to 30% of patients with acute pancreatitis, the cause is considered idiopathic.

Pathogenesis

Several theories have been proposed to explain the development of gallstone pancreatitis.

Gallstones can be identified in the stool of up to 94% of patients with acute gallstone pancreatitis compared with only 10% in patients with symptomatic cholelithiasis and no history of pancreatitis. The bile reflux theory, first postulated by Lancereaux in 1899, suggests that as stones pass through the ampulla it is disrupted allowing reflux of bile, and other duodenal contents, into the pancreatic duct with subsequent intraglandular pancreatic enzyme activation.

The association of an impacted gallstone at the ampulla of Vater and fatal acute pancreatitis, first described by Opie in 1901, prompted the development of the common channel theory. This theory suggests that impaction of a stone at the ampulla of Vater leads to increased biliary pressures that exceed pancreatic duct pressure, with secondary reflux of bile into the pancreatic duct. This theory is weakened by the fact that some patients do not have common channels, and by studies that have shown sterile bile does not activate proteolytic enzymes. Nevertheless, infected bile is a potent stimulator of these enzymes due to the presence of bacterial amidase and the theory remains popular.

A third theory, the obstructive theory, suggests an increase in pancreatic duct pressure alone due to complete pancreatic duct obstruction is sufficient to trigger gallstone pancreatitis. This has been suggested by various animal models and remains a favored concept.

The exact pathogenesis is likely multifactorial, and depending on patient anatomy and stone size any one of these theories may be more applicable.

Clinical Findings

A. Symptoms and Signs

Although the diagnosis of acute gallstone pancreatitis is a clinical one, there are no signs or symptoms that are specific for the condition. A thorough history excluding other potential causes of pancreatitis is essential. Alcohol, lipid levels, infectious agents, and medications should be considered.

B. Laboratory Findings

Once other etiologies have been excluded, the likelihood of gallstone pancreatitis must be determined. Several biochemical parameters have been evaluated with conflicting results.

Various studies have shown aspartate aminotransferase (AST), bilirubin, alkaline phosphatase, or γ-glutamyl transpeptidase (GGTP) to be most sensitive at predicting gallstone pancreatitis; however, there is no consensus and none of these parameters is specific.

C. Imaging Studies

Several abdominal imaging modalities are available and some are more useful than others at helping make the diagnosis.

Abdominal ultrasound is good at identifying gallstones, with 92% accuracy, and has the advantages of being widely available, inexpensive, and noninvasive. However, as 10% of the adult population have gallstones, this is not adequate for the diagnosis of gallstone pancreatitis. Ultrasonography has a sensitivity between 55% and 91% for identifying bile duct dilation, which is associated with a higher prevalence of choledocholithiasis; however, this is highly operator dependant and is not sensitive at detecting common duct stones.

CT is good at identifying cholelithiasis and can be used to measure common bile duct diameter. Additionally, helical CT cholangiography is an evolving technique that has sensitivities as high as 95% in diagnosing choledocholithiasis; however, the contrast agents required cause significant nausea, and the technique is not highly utilized.

MRCP is an accurate and noninvasive modality, with a sensitivity and specificity for detecting choledocholithiasis of 81–100% and 92–100%, respectively. Although MRCP is expensive and may miss stones smaller than 5 mm, the technique is comparable to diagnostic ERCP and intraoperative cholangiography and has emerged as the noninvasive diagnostic modality of choice.

EUS also has sensitivity and specificity of 88–97% and 96–100%, respectively; however, the technique is invasive and requires sedation. Thus, the role of EUS is not well established in most centers where MRCP is available.

ERCP was historically the diagnostic procedure of choice with accuracy similar to MRCP; however, it is associated with complication rates as high as 15% that include cholangitis, pancreatitis, perforation, and bleeding. With improved accuracy and increased availability of less invasive modalities, ERCP is no longer considered to be a first-line diagnostic procedure.

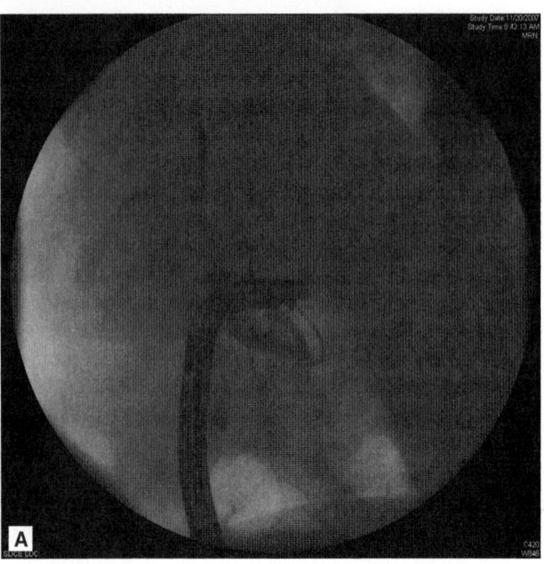

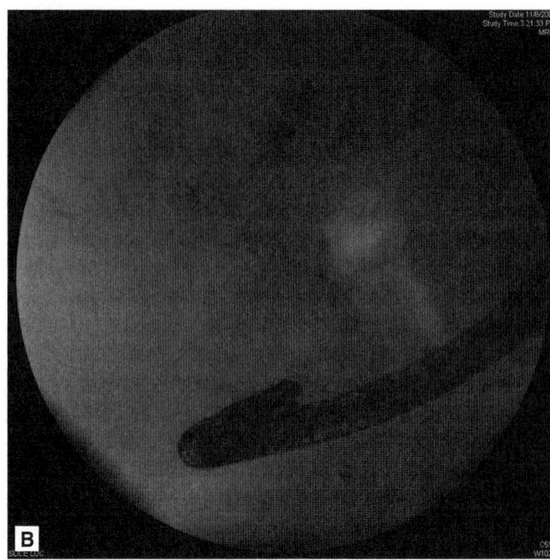

▲ **Figure 32–1. A:** Common bile duct stones in a patient with cholangitis. **B:** Stent placement adjacent to stones for temporary drainage.

Treatment

The management of acute gallstone pancreatitis has been controversial. Supportive care with aggressive intravenous hydration, nothing by mouth, and pain control is similar to the management of pancreatitis due to other etiologies; however, timing and method of common bile duct exploration for possible gallstone removal have been the focus of many studies. It is clear that ERCP is favored over surgery due to significantly better patient outcomes, with lower morbidity and mortality (Figure 32–1). The exact timing of ERCP has been more difficult to establish and depends on severity of illness. What appears to be consistent is that in patients with biliary pancreatitis and associated cholangitis, early drainage is indicated, typically within 48 hours of onset and after initial stabilization. Additionally, patients with clinical deterioration, as indicated by fever, increasing pain, and confusion, are likely to benefit from urgent ERCP. In patients without obstructive jaundice, early ERCP does not appear to be beneficial. Also, in patients with a mild course of biliary pancreatitis, up to 80% will have already passed the culprit stone and urgent ERCP is not recommended. A recent meta-analysis also looked at this question, and specifically assessed the role of early ERCP in patients with predicted severe acute pancreatitis, without cholangitis. Three randomized trials, consisting of a total 450 patients, qualified for inclusion in the meta-analysis. Subgroup analysis showed that early ERCP was not associated with improvement in overall complications or mortality from acute pancreatitis, regardless of predicted severity of pancreatitis.

Additionally, although endoscopic sphincterotomy has been shown to be protective regarding future episodes of gallstone pancreatitis, cholecystectomy remains the standard of care. More than 25% of patients who do not undergo cholecystectomy will have a recurrent episode, or related biliary complication, in the following 6 weeks. Early cholecystectomy is safe, and the preferred timing is upon resolution of pancreatitis and prior to hospital discharge.

Acosta JM, Katkhouda N, Debian KA. Early ductal decompression versus conservative management for gallstone pancreatitis with ampullary obstruction. *Ann Surg.* 2006;243:33–40. [PMID: 16371734]

Freitas ML, Bell RL, Duffy AJ. Choledocholithiasis: evolving standards for diagnosis and management. *World J Gastroenterol.* 2006;12:3162–3167. [PMID: 16718834]

Hernandez V, Pascual I, Almela P, et al. Recurrence of acute gallstone pancreatitis and relationship with cholecystectomy or endoscopic sphincterotomy. *Am J Gastroenterol.* 2004;99: 2417–2423. [PMID: 15571590]

Petrov MS, van Santvoort HC, Besselink MG, et al. Early endoscopic retrograde cholangiopancreatography versus conservative management in acute biliary pancreatitis without cholangitis a meta-analysis of randomized trials. *Ann Surg.* 2008;247: 250–257. [PMID: 18216529]

BILE DUCT INJURIES

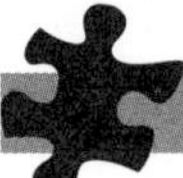

ESSENTIALS OF DIAGNOSIS

- Bile duct leaks, transection, and occlusion from ligature or strictures occur most often after cholecystectomy.
- Diagnosis can be established by imaging, including ultrasound to identify fluid accumulations and HIDA scan to detect occlusion or active leakage.

Types of bile duct injuries include leaks, transection, occlusion (ligation or stricture), or a combination. The majority of bile duct injuries are iatrogenic, most commonly following laparoscopic cholecystectomy, with an incidence of 0.3–2%. Common reasons for injury include aberrant anatomy, inadequate exposure, and otherwise difficult cases. Additional causes of bile duct injury include other biliary surgery, liver biopsy, penetrating or blunt abdominal trauma, and, rarely, spontaneous perforation.

Clinical Findings

Patients usually present with abdominal pain that may be diffused or localized. Nausea, anorexia, and abdominal distention due to ileus may also be seen. Clinically apparent ascites and bile peritonitis are less common. Fever is often absent, and laboratory evaluation typically reveals leukocytosis and nonspecific liver function test abnormalities. Initial imaging studies should involve abdominal ultrasound to assess for fluid collections or abnormalities in the biliary tree such as focal dilation, and radionuclide biliary scintigraphy to assess for ongoing leakage. Technetium-99m–labeled hepatoiminodiacetic acid derivative (HIDA) scanning is most accurate, approaching 100%.

Treatment

Bile duct injuries were historically managed surgically, but with significant morbidity and mortality. Endoscopic intervention has replaced surgery in the majority of cases. The flow of bile is pressure dependent, and it will follow the path of least resistance. The objective of endoscopic therapy is to make the path to the duodenum that of lowest resistance. This requires stenting the sphincter of Oddi or sphincterotomy. The procedure reduces the leakage of bile and allows healing of the defect. Additionally, drainage of large fluid collections either surgically or percutaneously is important for prompt resolution of pain and prevention of infection.

The Bergman classification system is useful for grading severity and prognosticating response to therapy. Type A injuries are leaks from the cystic duct or the ducts of Luschka. They are typically mild and have a near-100% response rate to ERCP with sphincterotomy or stent placement (Figure 32–2). Type B lesions are high-grade leaks of the common bile duct or main hepatic ducts with or without stricturing. These may be amenable to endoscopic therapy, with a 71% response rate to stenting. Bridging the defect with the stent is important for resolution of type B defects. Type C injuries consist of strictures without leak. Endoscopic stent placement is now considered the standard of care for these lesions. Costamagna and others have shown that upsizing and the use of multiple stents are critical to success. Type D injuries are complete transections of the biliary system. Diagnosis is best made by MRCP, and surgical hepaticojejunostomy is standard of care.

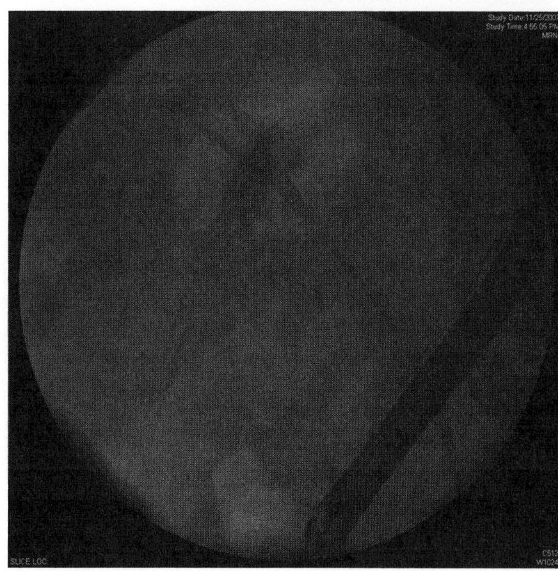

▲ **Figure 32–2.** Type A bile duct injury with extravasation of contrast from the cystic duct.

Aduna M, Larena JA, Martin D, et al. Bile duct leaks after laparoscopic cholecystectomy: value of contrast-enhanced MRCP. *Abdom Imaging.* 2005;30:480–487. [PMID: 15688109]

Bridges A, Wilcox CM, Varadarajulu S. Endoscopic management of traumatic bile leaks. *Gastrointest Endosc.* 2007;65:1081–1085. [PMID: 17531646]

Costamagna G, Shah SK, Tringali A. Current management of postoperative complications and benign biliary strictures. *Gastrointest Endosc Clin N Am.* 2003;13:635-648. [PMID: 14986791]

Demetriades D, Salim A, Berne TV. Liver and bile duct injury. In: Blugmart LH, Fong Y (eds). *Surgery of the Liver and Biliary Tract.* Saunders, 2000;1035–1056.

Sandha GS, Bourke MJ, Haber GB. Endoscopic therapy for bile leak based on a new classification: results in 207 patients. *Gastrointest Endosc.* 2004;60:567–574. [PMID: 15472680]

Shah JN. Endoscopic treatment of bile leaks: current standards and recent innovations. *Gastrointest Endosc.* 2007;65:1069–1072. [PMID: 17531644]

Zyromski NJ, Lillemoe KD. Current management of biliary leaks. *Adv Surg.* 2006;40:21–46. [PMID: 17163093]

PANCREATIC DUCT INJURIES

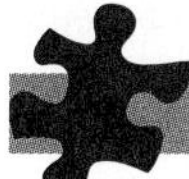

ESSENTIALS OF DIAGNOSIS

- Pancreatic duct injuries may be iatrogenic or occur after trauma or necrotizing pancreatitis.
- Diagnosis may be suspected on computed tomographic (CT) examination; however, MRCP is more specific.

The reported incidence of pancreatic injury is relatively low, ranging from 0.2% to 6% following abdominal trauma. However, the exact incidence is difficult to determine as many patients with significant abdominal trauma never have a laparotomy. Additionally, while the retroperitoneal location affords some degree of protection to the gland, it can also mask signs of significant injury.

The majority of affected patients are men under 40 years of age. Penetrating trauma is responsible for over 70% of traumatic injuries, with gunshot wounds and stabbings being most common. Location of injury following penetrating trauma is uniform among head and neck, body, and tail, with less than 5% having an injury at multiple sites. Blunt trauma is responsible for roughly 20% of injuries, with motor vehicle accidents accounting for the majority of cases. The distribution is similar to that of penetrating trauma, with a slight preponderance for pancreatic body injuries due to compression of the gland against the underlying spine at this location. Iatrogenic causes are also notable and are more commonly seen after pancreatic surgery, splenectomy, and ERCP.

Irrespective of the method of injury, the degree of injury ranges from simple contusion to complete transection, and typically results in local inflammation and fluid collections. Additionally, associated injury is typical and varies depending on location of injury. Penetrating injuries to the head are associated with major vascular injury in over 50% of cases. Hollow viscus injuries are also common, occurring nearly in 40% of cases, with liver and spleen injuries in less than 20% of cases. Overall mortality rates are between 10% and 31%, with over 50% of deaths occurring within 48 hours of presentation. Early mortality is typically due to associated injuries, with less than 10% due to pancreatic injury.

The majority of patients managed nonoperatively will develop a complication related to the pancreatic injury. Pseudocysts occur in up to 75% of patients who survive beyond 48 hours. Pancreatic fistula, pancreatitis, and peripancreatic abscess are also seen in roughly 30%. Although several organ injury grading systems exist, the most important factor in predicting clinical course and guiding therapy is the integrity of the main pancreatic duct. This is a key element of the diagnostic and management strategy.

Clinical Findings

Presenting symptoms vary from minimal pain or nausea to frank peritonitis and hemodynamic instability. With severe presentations and penetrating wounds, imaging or laparotomy is requisite and diagnosis is relatively straightforward. Diagnosis is more challenging and often delayed with more subtle presentations or when other injuries serve as confounders.

A. Symptoms and Signs

Epigastric pain is the most common symptom following blunt pancreatic trauma, with a pattern of initial abatement followed by escalation over the subsequent 6–8 hours. Physical examination is neither sensitive nor specific, and even profound pancreatic injury may not be detected on initial examination. If pain is present, it is often out of proportion to tenderness, and guarding is unusual.

B. Laboratory Findings

No single laboratory test is adequate for early detection. Serum amylase at time of admission is unreliable. Elevation of serum amylase may be seen due to causes other than pancreatic trauma, including bowel injury, head trauma, alcohol ingestion, profound hypotension, and salivary gland damage. Early reports showed that only 8% of patients with elevated serum amylase at the time of admission were found to have pancreatic injury. In other series, only 14% of patients with confirmed pancreatic gland injury had elevated amylase at the time of admission. Additionally, isoenzymes were not found to significantly improve diagnostic accuracy in this setting. Serial amylase levels have, however, been found to be useful in identifying pancreatic injury and guiding management. As such, consistently normal serum amylase levels have a negative predictive value of 93–98%, and persistently abnormal or rising levels have sensitivity as high as 89%. Nevertheless, additional diagnostic modalities are typically needed.

C. Imaging Studies

Plain film radiographs and ultrasound are of limited value. Loss of a distinct psoas margin or a halo of air surrounding the kidney or psoas may suggest a retroperitoneal process, however, this is nonspecific.

Abdominal CT scan is useful and may have findings specific to the diagnosis, including pancreatic transaction, local hematoma, fluid separating the pancreas and splenic vein, pancreatic enlargement, and increased attenuation of the peripancreatic fat. In lieu of these, the admission CT scan may hold signs suggestive of pancreatic injury, including fluid in the lesser sac, thickening of the anterior renal fascia, and associated injuries to local structures. CT rarely shows ductal disruption. Sensitivity for detecting pancreatic injury by initial CT scan alone ranges from 60% to 80%, and repeat imaging may be helpful. Specificity is high, ranging from 80% to 100%, although CT tends to underestimate degree of injury.

MRCP is particularly good at identifying pancreatic injury and at characterizing type and degree of damage. Complete visualization of normal size main ducts occurs in 97% of patients. MRCP is excellent at clarifying ductal status and at detailing parenchymal injury. ERCP is no longer considered a first-line diagnostic option, due to its invasive nature.

Treatment

Management is dependant on type and degree of injury. Severe cases with associated injury to local structures usually require emergent surgery. In such cases, the first priority is control of hemorrhage followed by complete pancreatic evaluation. This requires significant tissue dissection and mobilization.

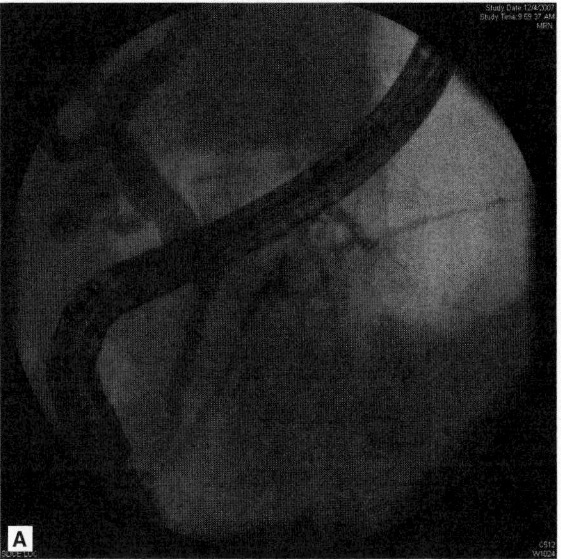

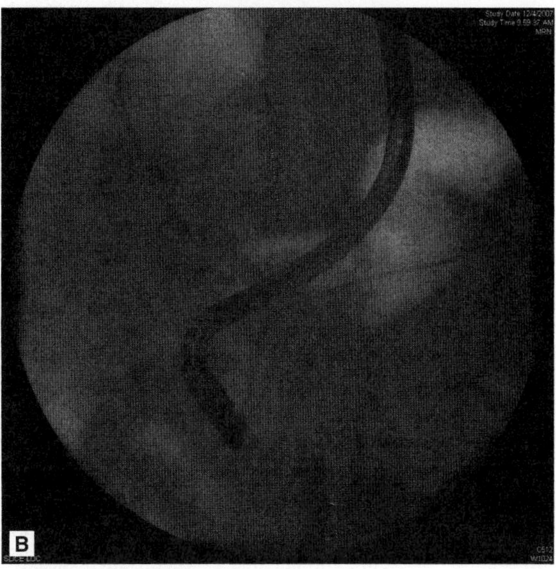

▲ **Figure 32–3. A:** Pancreatic duct disruption at genu. **B:** Stent bridging disruption.

If parenchymal damage is seen, the integrity of the main pancreatic duct must be assessed. Intraoperative pancreatography may be performed in a variety of ways and is effective at identifying ductal disruption. If ductal injury is not present, typical management involves debridement and wide external drainage. If ductal injury is identified, choice of procedure depends on location of the injury. For distal injuries, distal pancreatectomy is preferred. The surgical approach to proximal ductal injuries is more varied and duodenal diversion may be necessary.

ERCP with pancreatic stent placement is a less invasive alternative that should be considered when emergent surgery is not required and when disruption is suggested on imaging (Figure 32–3). Stent insertion is technically possible in 95% of cases, and outcomes appear to vary depending on the degree and location of disruption. Partial disruptions in the body and head appear to have the highest response rates. Additionally, placement of a stent that bridges the disruption is associated with better outcomes. In a recent series of 43 patients described by Telford and colleagues, multivariable analysis found that only bridging stent position was correlated with successful outcome. In this series bridging position was associated with a 92% success rate, compared with a 44% success rate for stents that merely cross the papilla. This is unlike the treatment of bile duct leaks, where elimination of the biliary duodenal pressure gradient by stenting across the papilla is sufficient. Patients with complete duct disruptions do not fare as well with endoscopic treatment; however, data are limited. Pancreatic duct stent placement is relatively safe and complications are well defined, including occlusion, migration, stricture formation, infection, and duodenal erosion. In a study by Varadarajulu and associates, a complication rate of 7.1% was seen for stent placement in the treatment of pancreatic duct disruption. Finally, pancreatic cyst drainage may be required and may be performed via a transgastric approach; however, fluid collection encapsulation takes several weeks and must occur before it is safe to proceed with endoscopic therapy.

Telford JJ, Farrell JJ, Saltzman JR, et al. Pancreatic stent placement for duct disruption. *Gastrointest Endosc.* 2002;56:18–24. [PMID: 12085030]

Varadarajulu S, Noone TC, Tutuian R, et al. Predictors of outcome in pancreatic duct disruption managed by endoscopic transpapillary stent placement. *Gastrointest Endosc.* 2005;61: 568–575. [PMID: 15812410]

HEMORRHAGIC BILIARY & PANCREATIC CONDITIONS

Hemobilia and hemosuccus pancreaticus are rare and potentially life-threatening conditions that are typically considered late in the diagnostic evaluation of the bleeding patient. Each condition has specific etiologies, requiring a unique approach to diagnosis and management.

1. Hemobilia

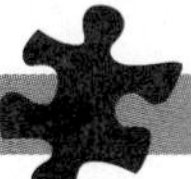

ESSENTIALS OF DIAGNOSIS

- Hemobilia can occur after trauma, gallstones, tumor, and vascular disorders and should be suspected in patients with hemorrhage, biliary colic, and jaundice.
- Diagnosis may be suggested by MRI with MRCP; however, selective arteriography is most accurate.

Hemobilia is an abnormal communication between blood vessels and bile ducts either within the liver or the extrahepatic biliary tree. Clinical manifestations are due to blood loss and biliary obstruction due to blood clots. Symptoms include melena in 90% and hematemesis in 60%, biliary colic in 70%, and jaundice in 60%. These three cardinal symptoms when together are known as the Quincke triad. The spectrum of hemobilia spans massive exsanguination causing shock and minor recurrent hemobilia resulting in chronic anemia. Whenever biliary symptoms are present in the setting of gastrointestinal bleeding or anemia, the diagnosis should be considered.

Pathogenesis

Common causes of biliary-vascular fistula that lead to hemobilia include blunt or penetrating trauma, iatrogenic etiologies, gallstones, tumors, and vascular disorders. Presentation may be immediate or several months after the inciting event. Additionally, parasites, choledochal cysts, portal hypertension, and blood coagulation defects may be implicated. Of these, iatrogenic causes are most common, with liver biopsy and PTC the most frequent.

When a communication is formed by one of these mechanisms, blood follows the path of least resistance and results in hemobilia. Blood clots may form leading to symptoms of biliary obstruction; however, bile has fibrinolytic properties that serve to dissolve clots and clear the duct of fibrin deposits. Clots are more likely to cause obstruction when they are sheltered from the bile stream as is the case with T-tubes or other biliary drains. Additionally, continuous hemorrhage with clot formation may exceed the rate of fibrinolysis leading to jaundice. The clots typically take the form of a luminal cast, and the consistency may vary from soft to well defined and firm.

In rare cases where the pressure in the biliary tree is greater than that of the vascular system, bilhemia occurs. This is typically seen with distal bile duct obstruction and low hepatic vein pressure. Symptoms include rapidly worsening jaundice and elevated direct bilirubin without increase in liver transaminases. Mortality rates in this rare condition are as high as 50%. ERCP with drainage is the initial therapy of choice, with surgery reserved for failed cases.

Clinical Findings

The diagnosis of hemobilia is typically easy to make if it is considered in the differential. Upper endoscopy is essential to rule out other sources of bleeding, and use of a side-viewing duodenoscope for proper evaluation of the papilla is recommended. Biliary imaging to evaluate for clotted blood is also helpful. Ultrasonography has been used with success; however, MRI with MRCP is more sensitive and can show active bleeding. Selective arteriography is most accurate for verifying suspected hemobilia and specifically identifying the source. Blood clots may be seen at ERCP; however, endoscopic therapy is not a long-term solution for hemostasis.

Treatment

Treatment of hemobilia is dependant on the cause. Transarterial embolization is the preferred method for hepatic artery sources. Surgical ligature or resection is reserved for embolization failure and hemorrhage from the gallbladder. Liver resection may also be required for central liver rupture and some tumors. At the present time, ERCP is not an accepted therapeutic option for the treatment of hemobilia; however, ERCP is the preferred alternative for restoring biliary patency when the bile duct is obstructed with clots (Figure 32–4). If bleeding stops spontaneously and treatment of obstruction is required prior definitive bleeding therapy, stent placement may be preferable to sphincterotomy and clot extraction as the latter may lead to recurrent hemorrhage.

Sandblom JP. Hemobilia and bilhemia. In: Blumgart LH, Fong Y (eds). *Surgery of the Liver and Biliary Tract.* Saunders, 2000; 1319–1342.

2. Hemosuccus Pancreaticus

Hemosuccus pancreaticus, or hemorrhage from the pancreatic duct, is also rare and management depends on the underlying cause. Episodic bleeding and sharp epigastric pain are the most common presenting symptoms. Anemia may be

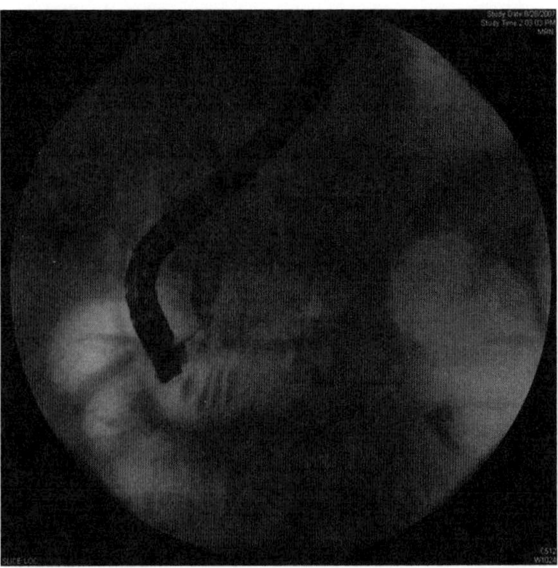

▲ **Figure 32–4.** Blood clot in bile duct seen in a patient with hemobilia.

the only sign in up to 10% of patients. Endoscopy to look for a clot at the papilla is unreliable for diagnosis, and there is no endoscopic therapeutic option. Common etiologies include splenic artery aneurysm and chronic pancreatitis with pseudoaneurysm. Other less common causes include malignancy, acute pancreatitis, and pseudocyst. CT angiography is the diagnostic modality of choice and can make the diagnosis with high accuracy even in patients without active bleeding. Data on MRCP are limited. Transarterial embolization is the suggested treatment for primary splenic artery aneurysms, whereas surgical arterial ligation and targeted pancreatectomy is preferred in the setting of chronic pancreatitis.

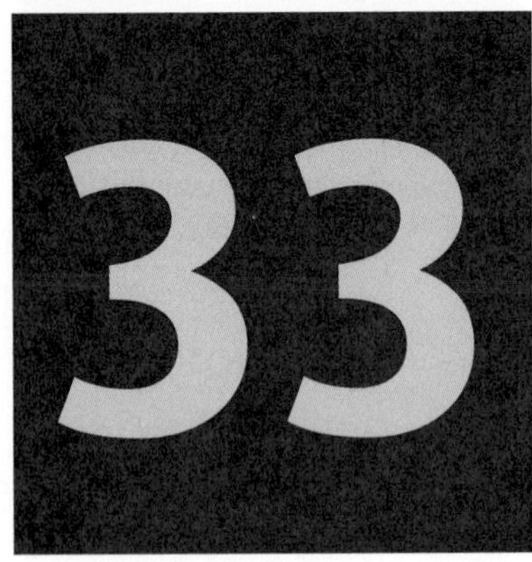

Wireless Capsule Endoscopy & Deep Small Bowel Enteroscopy

Anne C. Travis, MD, MSc, FACG
John R. Saltzman, MD

CAPSULE ENDOSCOPY

General Considerations

The first human ingestion of a video capsule endoscope occurred in 1999, and high-quality images from healthy human volunteers were described in 2000. A commercially available capsule was approved by the U.S. Food and Drug Administration (FDA) for use in the United States in August 2001, having been approved for use in Europe earlier that year. Between 2001 and 2007, more than a half million capsule endoscopy studies were performed.

Currently, three video capsules are available for use in the United States. Two are made by Given Imaging (Yoqneam, Israel). One capsule, the PillCam SB2, images the small bowel, while the other, the PillCam ESO2, is designed for imaging of the esophagus. Olympus Medical Systems Corporation (Tokyo, Japan) has also released a small bowel capsule, the EndoCapsule. Two other capsules have been developed and are being studied in clinical trials. The first is a colon capsule for colorectal cancer screening (Given Imaging), and the second is the MiRo capsule (Intro-Medic Co, Ltd, Seoul, South Korea), which uses electric field propagation to transmit the images.

The PillCam SB2 is composed of a complementary metal oxide silicon (CMOS) chip camera, a short focal length lens, six white light-emitting diode (LED) illumination sources, two silver oxide batteries, and a UHF band radio telemetry transmitter. Improvements in the design of CMOS image sensors, application-specific integrated circuits (ASICS) and white LED illumination, along with the development of nontoxic batteries made from silver oxide, allowed for the development of video capsules. The PillCam SB2 and the PillCam ESO2 capsules are 11 × 26 mm and weigh 3.7 g. The images acquired by the capsules have a field of view of 156 degrees, with eightfold magnification and a 1–30 mm depth of view. The capsules have a resolution of 0.1 mm that allows for the visualization of individual villi. The small bowel capsule transmits two 256 × 256 pixel color images per second for a total of 8 hours (~55,000 images), and the esophageal capsule transmits nine images per second from each of its two lenses, for a total of 18 images per second over the course of 20 minutes (~22,000 images). The EndoCapsule is similar to the PillCam SB2, but instead of a CMOS chip it has a charge-coupled device.

Arnott ID, Lo SK. The clinical utility of wireless capsule endoscopy. *Dig Dis Sci.* 2004;49:893–901. [PMID: 15309874]

Cave DR. Technology insight: current status of video capsule endoscopy. *Nat Clin Pract Gastroenterol Hepatol.* 2006;3: 158–164. [PMID: 16511550]

Mishkin DS, Chuttani R, Croffie J, et al; Technology Assessment Committee, American Society for Gastrointestinal Endoscopy. ASGE Technology Status Evaluation Report: wireless capsule endoscopy. *Gastrointest Endosc.* 2006;63:539–545. [PMID: 16564850]

Swain P. Wireless capsule endoscopy. *Gut.* 2003;52(Suppl IV): iv48–iv50. [PMID: 12746269]

Indications

The indications for small bowel and esophageal capsule endoscopy are summarized in Table 33–1.

A. Obscure Gastrointestinal Bleeding

Obscure gastrointestinal bleeding refers to bleeding that persists or recurs, without a source identified after standard endoscopic evaluation with upper endoscopy and colonoscopy. Obscure gastrointestinal hemorrhage can be subdivided into obscure-overt and obscure-occult gastrointestinal bleeding. Patients with obscure-overt gastrointestinal bleeding present with visual evidence of bleeding, such as hematemesis, melena, or hematochezia. Obscure-occult bleeding is manifested by stool that is positive for occult blood, frequently with iron deficiency anemia. Obscure bleeding accounts for approximately 5% of patients with gastrointestinal bleeding, and the source

Table 33–1. Indications for small bowel and esophageal capsule endoscopy.

Indications for small bowel capsule endoscopy
Obscure gastrointestinal bleeding
Diagnosis of Crohn disease
Evaluation of disease activity in established Crohn disease
Small bowel tumors
Diagnosis of celiac disease
Evaluation of refractory celiac disease
Polyp surveillance in polyposis syndromes
Surveillance for graft rejection after small bowel transplant
Detection of graft-versus-host disease
Evaluation of unexplained abdominal pain
Evaluation of unexplained diarrhea
Indications for esophageal capsule endoscopy
Screening for esophageal varices
Screening for Barrett esophagus
Detection of esophagitis

of bleeding is frequently from the small bowel, between the ligament of Treitz and the ileocecal valve.

Common causes of small bowel bleeding include vascular ectasias, small bowel tumors, Crohn disease, and nonsteroidal anti-inflammatory drug (NSAID) enteropathy (Table 33–2; see also Plates 77 and 78). Vascular ectasias are the most common cause of obscure gastrointestinal bleeding, accounting for 30–40% overall, and are responsible for the majority of obscure gastrointestinal bleeds in older patients. Patients between the ages of 30 and 50 years are more likely to have a small bowel tumor as the source of their bleeding. Finally, young patients often are found to have an ulcerated Meckel diverticulum as the source, although it should be remembered that bleeding from a Meckel diverticulum may occur at any age.

Table 33–2. Sources of small bowel bleeding.

Vascular ectasias, often associated with:
Advanced age
Chronic renal failure
Valvular heart disease
Von Willebrand disease
Scleroderma with CREST syndrome (calcinosis cutis, Raynaud phenomenon, esophageal dysmotility, sclerodactyly, telangiectasias)
Hereditary hemorrhagic telangiectasia syndrome (Osler-Weber-Rendu syndrome)
Small bowel tumors
Small bowel gastrointestinal stromal tumors (eg, leiomyoma, leiomyosarcoma)
Adenocarcinoma
Lymphoma
Carcinoid
Kaposi sarcoma
Metastatic cancer (eg, melanoma)
Crohn disease
NSAID enteropathy
Pelvic radiotherapy
Dieulafoy lesions
Aortoenteric fistulas
Meckel diverticula
Small bowel polyps
Small bowel varices
Hemosuccus pancreaticus
Strongyloides stercoralis
Pseudoxanthoma elasticum

NSAID, nonsteroidal anti-inflammatory drug.

Gralnek IM. Obscure-overt gastrointestinal bleeding. *Gastroenterology.* 2005;128:1424–1430. [PMID: 15887123]

Leighton JA, Goldstein J, Hirota W, et al. Obscure gastrointestinal bleeding. *Gastrointest Endosc.* 2003;58:650–655. [PMID: 14595294]

B. Crohn Disease

In patients with Crohn disease limited to the small bowel, or in those with indeterminate colitis, arriving at a correct diagnosis can be difficult. Capsule endoscopy can help diagnose small bowel Crohn disease by providing mucosal detail that is not available radiologically (Plate 79). It also provides the opportunity to visualize areas of the bowel not accessible by standard endoscopy. Because capsule endoscopy has a resolution of 0.1 mm, it is able to detect small, superficial defects, such as aphthoid ulcers. It is important to note, however, that not all mucosal ulcerations occur as a result of Crohn disease (Table 33–3). Ten to 23% of normal volunteers who are not taking NSAIDs will have mucosal breaks and other lesions seen on capsule endoscopy, and 50–71% of NSAID users will have evidence of small bowel injury (red spots, erosions, and ulcerations). Therefore, it is important to use capsule endoscopy findings in combination with other clinical information to arrive at the correct diagnosis.

C. Small Bowel Tumors and Polyposis Syndromes

Benign and malignant small bowel tumors are found in approximately 6–8% of people and can be seen on capsule endoscopy (Plate 80). Capsule endoscopy may be able to detect tumors years before they would be detected by other imaging modalities, potentially increasing the chance to remove them while still localized.

Capsule endoscopy can also detect small bowel polyps in patients with hereditary polyposis syndromes. Peutz-Jeghers syndrome and familial adenomatous polyposis (FAP) are two of the hereditary polyposis syndromes that are associated with small bowel polyps and malignancies. Patients with Peutz-Jeghers syndrome form hamartomatous polyps within the gastrointestinal tract, along with mucocutaneous pigmentation. The polyps have a predilection for the small bowel and will develop in more than 90% of patients (Plate 81). Complications from the polyps include gastrointestinal bleeding, anemia, intestinal obstruction, intussusception, and development of cancer. Patients with Peutz-Jeghers syndrome have

Table 33–3. Differential diagnosis of small bowel erosions and ulcerations.

Inflammatory
Crohn disease
Sarcoidosis
Behçet syndrome
Drugs and medications
Antibiotics
Aspirin
Cocaine
Chemotherapy
NSAIDs
Potassium supplements
Methamphetamine
Infections
Bacterial
Mycobacterium tuberculosis
Mycobacterium avium-intracellulare complex
Yersinia enterocolitica
Yersinia pseudotuberculosis
Typhlitis
Salmonella
Actinomycosis israelii
Viral
Cytomegalovirus
Fungal and yeast
Histoplasma capsulatum
Cryptococcosis
Parasitic
Protozoan
Helminthic
Anisakiasis
Neoplastic
Adenocarcinoma
Carcinoid tumor
Lymphoma
Lymphosarcoma
Metastatic disease
Collagen vascular disease
Churg-Strauss syndrome
Dermatomyositis
Giant cell arteritis
Henoch-Schönlein purpura
Lymphomatoid granulomatosis
Mixed connective tissue disease
Polyarteritis nodosum
Polymyositis
Rheumatoid arthritis vasculitis
Systemic lupus erythematosus
Takayasu arteritis
Thromboangiitis obliterans
Thrombotic thrombocytopenic purpura
Wegener granulomatosis
Trauma
Intussusception
Foreign body
Incarcerated hernia
Celiac disease
Chronic idiopathic enterocolitis
Eosinophilic gastroenteritis
Food allergies
Graft-versus-host disease
Heavy metal poisoning
Hypogammaglobulinemia
Ischemia
Lymphocytic enteritis
Malnutrition
Meckel diverticulum with heterotopic gastric mucosa
Radiation
Uremia
Zollinger-Ellison syndrome

NSAID, nonsteroidal anti-inflammatory drug.

a 13% lifetime risk of developing small bowel cancer, so surveillance of the small intestine is recommended. Traditionally, patients have undergone radiographic imaging with a small bowel series or enteroclysis every 2 years, starting at age 10. This approach exposes a patient to significant amounts of ionizing radiation. In addition, radiologic evaluation with small bowel follow-through, computed tomography (CT) enteroclysis, or magnetic resonance enteroclysis lacks sensitivity for detecting small polyps. Push enteroscopy has also been employed, but is only able to visualize a portion of the upper small bowel. Capsule endoscopy on the other hand, is capable of detecting small polyps throughout the small bowel.

D. Celiac Disease

Celiac disease affects up to 0.3–1% of Caucasians. Celiac disease has traditionally been diagnosed by detection of antibodies (eg, antiendomysial and tissue transglutaminase antibodies), followed by endoscopy with biopsies of the small bowel to confirm the diagnosis. Capsule endoscopy has been proposed as a possible alternative to endoscopy for the diagnosis of celiac disease. Capsule endoscopy findings of celiac disease include scalloping, a mosaic mucosal pattern, loss of mucosal folds, visible vessels, and micronodularity (Plates 82 and 83). An advantage of capsule endoscopy is that it allows for visualization of the entire small bowel, and symptom severity in celiac disease is more closely related to the length of small bowel involved and not to the severity of the villous atrophy seen on biopsy.

Capsule endoscopy may have an even more important role in the evaluation of refractory celiac disease. Celiac disease can be complicated by small bowel adenocarcinoma, lymphoma (including enteropathy-associated T-cell lymphoma), and ulcerative jejunitis. In patients who fail to respond to a gluten-free diet or who have a recurrence of symptoms while on a gluten-free diet, further evaluation is needed to differentiate between refractory celiac disease (ie, celiac disease that does not respond to a gluten-free diet), ongoing gluten ingestion (intentional or unintentional), or a complication of celiac disease.

E. Other Applications

Capsule endoscopy has also been used to evaluate for evidence of small bowel graft-versus-host disease in patients following bone marrow transplantation, to look for evidence of rejection following small intestinal transplantation, and to evaluate for radiation enteritis. However, in the case of suspected radiation enteritis, the risk for capsule retention is increased. In addition, capsule endoscopy may detect small intestinal varices or portal hypertensive enteropathy in patients with portal hypertension.

The PillCam ESO2 was designed to visualize the esophagus and can be used to detect findings such as esophageal varices, erosive esophagitis, and Barrett esophagus.

Contraindications

Capsule endoscopy is contraindicated in some patients. Because cooperation is required, demented patients are not good candidates for capsule endoscopy. Capsule endoscopy is also contraindicated in patients with cardiac pacemakers or defibrillators (due to concerns that the capsule could interfere with the cardiac device) and in pregnant women (due to a lack of data on the effects of capsule endoscopy in pregnancy). Many centers, however, perform capsule endoscopy in patients with pacemakers or defibrillators, and studies have suggested that the capsules may not interfere with the devices. In addition, the cardiac devices have not been shown to disrupt the capsule study (with the exception of one instance of images being lost as a capsule passed the pulse generator of an abdominally implanted pacemaker). Finally, there have been no reports of a cardiac device malfunctioning due to a capsule study. Patients should be instructed not to undergo magnetic resonance imaging until passage of the capsule has been confirmed, which can be done with a plain abdominal radiograph if the capsule was not noted to pass naturally.

Patients with gastrointestinal tract obstructions, strictures, or fistulas (either suspected or demonstrated on imaging studies) should not undergo capsule endoscopy because of an increased risk of capsule retention or obstruction. A patency capsule (Agile Patency Capsule, Given Imaging) is available to establish small bowel patency in patients with suspected strictures or obstructions. The capsule is a dummy capsule with a transmitter. The patient swallows the capsule, and then after 30 hours a hand-held scanner or a plain abdominal film is used to determine if the capsule is still present in the small bowel. If it is not, then it is safe to proceed with the capsule endoscopy study. If the capsule is retained due to a stricture or obstruction it will begin to dissolve after 30 hours.

In patients with swallowing disorders, such as achalasia, esophageal strictures, esophageal diverticula, or gastroparesis, the capsule may need to be delivered using a special delivery device to ensure that it enters and traverses the small bowel during its recording time. Two devices are currently available, the AdvanCE device (US Endoscopy, Mentor, Ohio) and the PillCam Express (Given Imaging). Both devices are composed of a catheter that is passed through the channel of a gastroscope. A cap that holds the capsule is then screwed onto the end of the catheter. The scope is then advanced blindly into the esophagus (the cap obscures visualization). Once in the esophagus, the catheter can be advanced slightly to allow for limited visualization. The scope is then advanced to the small bowel, where the capsule is deployed. A standard upper endoscopy examination should be carried out before using the devices to detect any abnormalities that could complicate capsule delivery. Alternative delivery methods include placing the capsule in the stomach by inserting it through an over-tube and then advancing it to the small bowel using snares or nets.

Procedure

A. Small Bowel Examination

1. Patient preparation—Studies can be performed on both inpatients and outpatients. For a small bowel study, a patient fasts for 8–12 hours before the examination. Some centers also have the patient consume only clear liquids for up to 24 hours prior to the examination. Data are conflicting, but some studies suggest that preparing the small bowel with 2–4 L of a polyethylene glycol solution may improve visualization (oral phospho soda should not be used, as it has been shown to increase gastric emptying time). A consensus panel at the 2005 International Conference on Capsule Endoscopy (ICCE), however, did not recommend a bowel preparation other than fasting prior to the study. In cases where there is concern for slowed gastric transit, such as in diabetic patients, a prokinetic agent such as metoclopramide or erythromycin is given approximately 30–60 minutes prior to the study. The ICCE consensus panel, however, did not recommend routine use of prokinetic agents. Some centers give patients simethicone prior to the study in an attempt to decrease air bubbles that can obscure the view of the mucosa, although this, too, was not recommended by the ICCE consensus panel.

2. Techniques—Prior to capsule ingestion, an eight-element sensor array is attached to the patient's abdomen, or a sensor belt is placed around the patient's abdomen. Removing the magnet that is packaged with the capsule activates the capsule. The patient then swallows the capsule in an upright position, or the capsule is placed endoscopically (see preceding text), and images are transmitted to a recording device worn about the patient's waist. During the study, patients are instructed to avoid activities that could lead to sensor detachment, such as exercise. After 2 hours, the patient is allowed to have clear liquids, and a light meal can be consumed after 4 hours. At the end of the study, the images are downloaded to a computer workstation equipped with proprietary software (either the RAPID Application, Given Imaging, Norcross,

GA, or the Endo Capsule Software, Olympus, Tokyo, Japan). A physician can then read the study and generate a report, a process that takes on average 40–60 minutes. To aid in reading the study, the software has features such as a blood indicator that marks areas with suspected bleeding.

To allow real-time viewing of the images, hand-held devices have been developed. A possible disadvantage is that reading a study in real time takes significantly longer than reviewing downloaded images (the average small bowel transit time is ~4 hours). However, in certain situations, real-time imaging may have a role. For example, the capsule could be administered in the emergency department with immediate viewing to help guide further evaluation and management.

B. Esophageal Examination

1. Patient preparation—For the esophageal examination, patients need to fast for 2 hours prior to ingesting the capsule.

2. Techniques—A three-element sensor array is attached to the patient's chest, and the patient consumes 100 mL of water with simethicone while standing. The patient then lies supine and the capsule is swallowed with a 10-mL sip of water. The patient remains supine for 2 minutes, and then progressively moves into an upright position (30 degrees for 2 minutes, 60 degrees for 1 minute, then upright for the remainder of the study). The images are then downloaded to the workstation and reviewed.

Due to difficulty with adherence to the ingestion protocol, an alternative simplified ingestion protocol has been developed for the esophageal examination. The patient lies in the right lateral decubitus position with his or her head on a pillow. The patient then swallows the capsule with a sip (approximately 15 mL) of water. The patient remains on the right side and takes an additional sip of water every 30 seconds for a total of 7 minutes. After 7 minutes, the patient sits upright and takes an additional sip of water. The patient may then get up and walk for the remainder of the study. The images are then downloaded to the computer workstation for review.

Outcomes

A. Obscure Gastrointestinal Bleeding

Obscure gastrointestinal bleeding is the most common indication for performing a capsule endoscopy. The overall yield of capsule endoscopy is 55–70%, and leads to alterations in management in approximately one third of patients (range, 25–71%). However, the yield is highly dependent on the indication for the study. In a 2004 study of 100 patients, if active bleeding was suspected, the yield was 92%, but the yield dropped to only 13% for patients with a previous overt gastrointestinal bleed (time between the bleed and capsule endoscopy ranged from 10 days to 1 year). For patients with occult gastrointestinal hemorrhage, the yield was intermediate at 44%. A second study of 47 patients from 2005, however, showed a yield of 100% for patients with ongoing bleeding, 67% for patients with prior overt bleeding (time between the bleed and capsule endoscopy ranged from 7 to 90 days), and 67% for occult gastrointestinal bleeding.

The difference in these two studies when it comes to patients with previous overt gastrointestinal bleeding may relate to the amount of time elapsed between the bleed and the capsule endoscopy. In the first study, 25 of the 31 patients had their capsule endoscopy studies at least 2 months after the bleeding episode, and the study found that the yield for capsule endoscopy dropped off in parallel with the length of time between the bleed and the capsule endoscopy. In patients who had an interval of 10–14 days, the yield was 67%, compared with 6% for those with an interval of 4–12 months. In the second study, the average time between the bleed and the capsule endoscopy was only 16 days, which may explain the much higher yield in this group. In the second study, when capsule endoscopy was compared with the gold standard of intraoperative enteroscopy, capsule endoscopy had a sensitivity of 95%, a specificity of 75%, a positive predictive value of 95%, and a negative predictive value of 86% for detecting a bleeding source.

Capsule endoscopy has also been compared with push enteroscopy, small bowel barium radiography (small bowel follow-through or enteroclysis), CT angiography, and mesenteric angiography in the evaluation of obscure gastrointestinal bleeding. A pooled analysis of seven prospective studies that compared capsule endoscopy with push enteroscopy demonstrated that capsule endoscopy had a yield of 71%, compared with 29% for push enteroscopy (although other studies have estimated the yield of push enteroscopy to be higher, at 40–65%). In a meta-analysis of 14 studies, the yield of capsule endoscopy in detecting clinically significant findings for obscure gastrointestinal bleeding was 56%, compared with 26% for push enteroscopy ($P < .001$). In that same meta-analysis, three studies that compared capsule endoscopy with small bowel barium radiography were analyzed. Capsule endoscopy had a 42% yield for detecting clinically significant lesions, compared with 6% for small bowel barium radiography ($P < .001$). A prospective study that compared capsule endoscopy with both CT angiography and mesenteric angiography in 25 patients who were able to complete all three studies found that capsule endoscopy was superior to CT angiography, detecting a bleeding source in 72% of patients compared with CT angiography, which detected a bleeding source in only 24% ($P = .005$). Capsule endoscopy also had a higher yield than mesenteric angiography, which had a yield of 56%, although the difference between the two studies did not reach statistical significance ($P = .29$).

Whether capsule endoscopy should be repeated in a patient with a negative examination has been examined. One small study found that 18 of 24 patients (75%) undergoing repeat capsule endoscopy for the evaluation of obscure-overt or obscure-occult gastrointestinal bleeding had new findings, and in 15 patients (62.5%), the findings resulted in a change in management. However, a second study with a median follow-up of 19 months found that in 18 patients with obscure-overt gastrointestinal bleeding who had negative capsule endoscopies, only one rebled (5.6%), compared with 15 of 31 patients (48.4%) who had positive capsule studies. Therefore, it is reasonable to wait for evidence of rebleeding before repeating a capsule endoscopy, since a large percentage of patients with a negative capsule endoscopy will not have further bleeding.

Capsule endoscopy has also been used in the evaluation of acute gastrointestinal bleeding in the emergency department. A study of 24 patients presenting with nonhematemesis gastrointestinal bleeding found that if capsule endoscopy was performed within 24 hours of presentation, the yield for identifying a bleeding source was 63% (10/16). In addition, capsule endoscopy demonstrated active bleeding in 54% (13/24) of the study patients.

Cave DR. Obscure gastrointestinal bleeding: the role of the tagged red blood cell scan, enteroscopy and capsule endoscopy. *Clin Gastroenterol Hepatol.* 2005;3:959–963. [PMID: 16234039]

Hartmann D, Schmidt H, Bolz G, et al. A prospective two-center study comparing wireless capsule endoscopy with intraoperative enteroscopy in patients with obscure GI bleeding. *Gastrointest Endosc.* 2005;61:826–832. [PMID: 15933683]

Pennazio M, Santucci R, Rondonotti E, et al. Outcome of patients with obscure gastrointestinal bleeding after capsule endoscopy: report of 100 consecutive cases. *Gastroenterology.* 2004;126: 643–653. [PMID: 14988816]

Sachdev RM, Hibbert PL, Pearlmutter M, et al. Capsule endoscopy in the emergency room for acute non hematemesis gastrointestinal bleeding. *Am J Gastroenterol.* 2004;99:S295–296

Saperas E, Dot J, Videla S, et al. Capsule endoscopy versus computed tomographic or standard angiography for the diagnosis of obscure gastrointestinal bleeding. *Am J Gastroenterol.* 2007;102:731–737. [PMID: 17397406]

Triester SL, Leighton JA, Leontiadis GI, et al. A meta-analysis of the yield of capsule endoscopy compared to other diagnostic modalities in patients with obscure gastrointestinal bleeding. *Am J Gastroenterol.* 2005;100:2407–2418. [PMID: 16279893]

B. Crohn Disease

Capsule endoscopy is superior to other diagnostic modalities in detecting small bowel disease when the suspicion for Crohn disease is high (Table 33–4). A meta-analysis demonstrated that capsule endoscopy is superior to small bowel radiography, colonoscopy with ileoscopy, CT enterography or enteroclysis, and push enteroscopy for the detection of nonstricturing small bowel Crohn disease (incremental yields of 40%, 15%, 38%, and 38%, respectively). Overall, capsule endoscopy had a yield of 46–72% for detecting small bowel Crohn disease. It had a yield of 33–70% in patients with suspected Crohn disease, and a yield of 68–86% in patients with established Crohn disease. It is possible, however, that the yield of capsule endoscopy for suspected Crohn disease is significantly lower in practice because patients being evaluated for possible Crohn disease do not always fulfill the selection criteria used in studies. In a study of patients being evaluated for abdominal pain who had undergone previous endoscopic or radiographic evaluations, a cause was detected by capsule endoscopy in only 6% of those with abdominal pain alone, and in 13% of those with abdominal pain and diarrhea. Capsule endoscopy can also help in the evaluation of indeterminate colitis. In patients with indeterminate colitis, two retrospective studies of capsule endoscopy have demonstrated small bowel ulcerations in 33–49% of patients, suggesting (but not proving) a diagnosis of Crohn disease.

Table 33–4. Factors associated with positive capsule endoscopy studies in patients with suspected small bowel Crohn disease.

Abdominal pain
Diarrhea
Weight loss
Nonspecific abnormalities on small bowel imaging
Elevated erythrocyte sedimentation rate
Anemia
Low serum albumin

In addition to detecting small bowel Crohn disease, capsule endoscopy can help in defining the extent of disease, diagnosing a Crohn flare, or detecting a postoperative recurrence in patients with established disease. In one study, patients who were suspected of having a Crohn flare underwent capsule endoscopy. In 20% there was no active disease, suggesting that the symptoms may have been due to other causes, such as a superimposed functional disorder.

Kornbluth A, Legnani P, Lewis BS. Video capsule endoscopy in inflammatory bowel disease: past, present, and future. *Inflamm Bowel Dis.* 2004;10:278–285. [PMID: 15290925]

C. Small Bowel Tumors and Polyposis Syndromes

Capsule endoscopy is capable of detecting tumors and polyps of all sizes throughout the small bowel; however, because many of the tumors are submucosal, it can be difficult at times to differentiate a tumor from the transient bulges that are frequently seen during capsule endoscopy. In addition, a tumor may only be seen tangentially on one frame of the study, making characterization of the mass difficult, especially when it comes to size. Because capsule endoscopy lacks biopsy capability, arriving at a definitive diagnosis is rarely possible using capsule endoscopy alone. However, a presumptive diagnosis can be made in some cases, such as in a patient with a small bowel mass and known metastatic melanoma (see Plate 80).

In a study of patients with polyposis syndromes, capsule endoscopy detected polyps in 10 of 11 patients (91%) with Peutz-Jeghers syndrome. That study also examined patients with FAP. It found that 24% of FAP patients (5 of 12 patients) with duodenal adenomas had distal jejunal or ileal polyps detected on capsule endoscopy. In patients without duodenal adenomas, however, more distal polyps occurred in only 12%. Of note, capsule endoscopy often failed to achieve adequate visualization of the ampulla of Vater, an area of frequent polyp and adenocarcinoma development in patients with FAP. Therefore, capsule endoscopy is not a substitute for standard surveillance using a side-viewing duodenoscope with ampullary biopsies.

Schulmann K, Hollerbach S, Kraus K, et al. Feasibility and diagnostic utility of video capsule endoscopy for the detection of small bowel polyps in patients with hereditary polyposis syndromes. *Am J Gastroenterol.* 2005;100:27–37. [PMID: 15654777]

D. Celiac Disease

In a small, blinded study of 20 patients (10 with celiac disease and 10 with controls), capsule endoscopy had a sensitivity of 70%, a specificity of 100%, a positive predictive value of 100%, and a negative predictive value of 77% for the diagnosis of celiac disease. Interobserver agreement for experienced capsule endoscopists was perfect ($\kappa = 1.0$). Patients with extensive small bowel involvement were more likely to have classic celiac disease symptoms, including diarrhea and weight loss, whereas those with only proximal involvement had mild, nonspecific symptoms.

Studies have also looked at using capsule endoscopy in patients with refractory celiac disease. In a study of 47 celiac disease patients with persistent abdominal pain, occult blood loss, or refractory iron deficiency anemia, capsule endoscopy identified lesions in 87% (41 of 47 patients). The capsule endoscopy studies detected findings consistent with celiac disease in a majority of patients (32 with villous atrophy, 29 with scalloping and fissuring, and 9 with a mosaic pattern). Additional findings included ulcerations (21 patients), nodularity (6 patients), an adenocarcinoma (1 patient), a polyp (1 patient), a stricture (1 patient), an intussusception (1 patient), and a submucosal mass (1 patient). This study suggests that in patients with ongoing symptoms, despite the report of adherence to a gluten-free diet, capsule endoscopy has a high yield for identifying abnormalities.

Culliford A, Daly J, Diamond B, et al. The value of wireless capsule endoscopy in patients with complicated celiac disease. *Gastrointest Endosc.* 2005;62:55–61. [PMID: 15990820]

Petroniene R, Dubcenco E, Baker JP, et al. Given capsule endoscopy in celiac disease: evaluation of diagnostic accuracy and interobserver agreement. *Am J Gastroenterol.* 2005;100: 685–694. [PMID: 15743369]

E. Esophageal Capsule Endoscopy

The PillCam ESO2 was designed to visualize the esophagus and can be used to detect findings such as esophageal varices, erosive esophagitis, and Barrett esophagus. In a study of 32 patients, there was 97% concordance between capsule endoscopy and upper endoscopy for the detection of varices, and 91% concordance for the diagnosis of portal hypertensive gastropathy.

Limitations

An advantage of capsule endoscopy is that it has the potential to image the entire length of the small bowel. However, in many instances there is poor visualization of areas of mucosa due to quick passage, inability to insufflate, tangential views, and debris. Additionally, in approximately 15% of cases, the capsule does not reach the colon prior to the battery running out (currently about 8 hours). A significant limitation is that capsule endoscopy lacks biopsy capability. This can be a problem because findings such as erythema, aphthous ulcerations, or frank ulcerations are seen in multiple disorders (see Table 33–3). In addition, nodules cannot be biopsied to determine if there is an underlying malignancy. Some of these limitations can now be addressed using deep small bowel enteroscopy if an abnormality is found on capsule endoscopy (see "Deep Small Bowel Enteroscopy," later in this chapter).

Complications

The most important complication related to capsule endoscopy is capsule retention. Overall, the risk of retention is 1–2%. Many of the disorders for which capsule endoscopy is being employed, such as Crohn disease or radiation enteritis, can increase the risk of retention. Patients with Crohn disease are at increased risk because of possible small bowel strictures (which may be missed on conventional imaging). In the setting of established Crohn disease, the risk or retention increases to 4–13%. In patients with established Crohn disease, small bowel radiographic imaging (small bowel follow-through or CT enteroclysis) should be performed prior to capsule endoscopy to decrease the risk of retention. The use of a patency capsule (Agile Patency System, Given Imaging Ltd, Yoqneam, Israel) can also decrease the risk of retention (see "Contraindications" discussed earlier).

Capsule retention is often associated with the identification of significant pathologic findings that often require further surgical or endoscopic intervention. In a study of 733 cases, capsule retention occurred in 1.9% (14 patients). Of these, all occurred at a site of pathology (Crohn disease [5], small bowel stenosis [5], small bowel neoplasm [3], and mesenteric ischemia [1]). Eleven patients underwent surgery for capsule removal, two had the capsule removed endoscopically, and one (with mesenteric ischemia) did not have the capsule removed. Deep small bowel enteroscopy is one option for retrieving capsules that are retained in the mid or distal small bowel and are thus out of reach of a standard enteroscopy (see the later section on "Deep Small Bowel Enteroscopy").

Uncommon complications of capsule endoscopy include aspiration of the capsule, impaction at the cricopharyngeus, or retention in a Zenker or Meckel diverticulum. A case of aspiration was noted in a patient who was part of the study of 733 capsule endoscopy examinations. In that case, the patient was able to expel the capsule by coughing. These complications reinforce the need to evaluate patients carefully for swallowing disorders prior to performing a capsule endoscopy study.

Cheifetz AS, Kornbluth AA, Legnani P, et al. The risk of retention of the capsule endoscope in patients with known or suspected Crohn's disease. *Am J Gastroenterol.* 2006;101:2218–2222. [PMID: 16848804]

Rondonotti E, Herrerias JM, Pennazio M, et al. Complications, limitations, and failures of capsule endoscopy: a review of 733 cases. *Gastrointest Endosc.* 2005;62:712–716. [PMID: 16246685]

DEEP SMALL BOWEL ENTEROSCOPY

General Considerations

The small bowel is on average 430 cm (14 ft) long. Push enteroscopy with an over-tube, however, can at most be advanced to 160 cm beyond the ligament of Treitz. With the advent of wireless capsule endoscopy, it is now possible to visualize the entire length of the small bowel, but capsule endoscopy lacks biopsy and therapeutic capability. Lesions detected by capsule endoscopy that are beyond the reach of a push enteroscope can now be evaluated using deep small bowel enteroscopy. Total enteroscopy is possible with balloon- or spiral-assisted enteroscopy and has the advantage of allowing for biopsies and for therapeutic interventions. Yamamoto and colleagues first described double balloon enteroscopy in 2001, and it was FDA approved for use in the United States in the fall of 2004 (Double Balloon Technology, Fujinon, Wayne, NJ). Since then, two additional systems using single balloon enteroscopy (Single Balloon Enteroscope System, Olympus, Tokyo, Japan) and spiral enteroscopy (Spirus Endo-Ease Discover SB System, Spirus Medical, Stoughton, MA) have become available.

Jonnalagadda S. Double balloon enteroscopy: wired technology meets wireless. *Gastroenterology.* 2006;131:327–329. [PMID: 16831620]

Yamamoto H, Sekine Y, Sato Y, et al. Total enteroscopy with a nonsurgical steerable double balloon method. *Gastrointest Endosc.* 2001;53:216–220. [PMID: 1174299]

Indications

Deep small bowel enteroscopy is used most often for the evaluation of obscure gastrointestinal bleeding, small bowel radiographic abnormalities, abnormalities identified on capsule endoscopy, chronic diarrhea and malabsorption, and in polyposis syndromes to detect and remove polyps (Table 33–5). It has also been used to biopsy and dilate small bowel strictures, to screen for disease recurrence in patients with a history of small bowel malignancies, and to evaluate patients with refractory celiac disease. In patients who have undergone roux-en-Y gastric bypass, it can visualize the defunctionalized stomach and gain access to the bile and pancreatic ducts.

Table 33–5. Indications for deep small bowel enteroscopy.

Obscure gastrointestinal bleeding
Small bowel radiographic abnormalities
Abnormalities seen on capsule endoscopy
Chronic diarrhea and malabsorption
Detection and removal of polyps in polyposis syndromes
Dilation and biopsy of small bowel strictures
Screening for recurrence of small bowel malignancy
Refractory celiac disease
Visualization of the defunctionalized stomach after Roux-en-Y gastric bypass
Access to the bile and pancreatic ducts after Roux-en-Y gastric bypass or Roux-en-Y hepaticojejunostomy

Di Caro S, May A, Heine DG, et al. DBE European Study Group. The European experience with double balloon enteroscopy: indications, methodology, safety and clinical impact. *Gastrointest Endosc.* 2005;62:545–550. [PMID: 16185969]

Gerson LB. Double balloon enteroscopy: the new gold standard for small-bowel imaging? *Gastrointest Endosc.* 2005;62:71–75. [PMID: 15990822]

Procedure

A. Patient Preparation

Patients who are undergoing an antegrade (per os) study, fast for 8–12 hours prior to the study. For a retrograde (per anus) study, a standard colonoscopy preparation is employed.

B. Techniques

1. Double balloon enteroscopy—The double balloon enteroscopy system is composed of an enteroscope, an over-tube, and a balloon pump controller. The system uses two latex balloons, one on the end of the enteroscope and one on the end of the over-tube (Figure 33–1). Through a combination of antegrade and retrograde approaches, the entire small bowel can be examined in 42–86% of patients.

The examination can be carried out using conscious sedation or propofol, although some centers prefer general anesthesia due to the length of the study and the potential for patient discomfort. During an antegrade study, the scope and over-tube are advanced until both are within the duodenum. The balloon on the end of the over-tube is then inflated to anchor the small bowel. The scope is then advanced. When the scope can no longer be advanced, the balloon at the tip

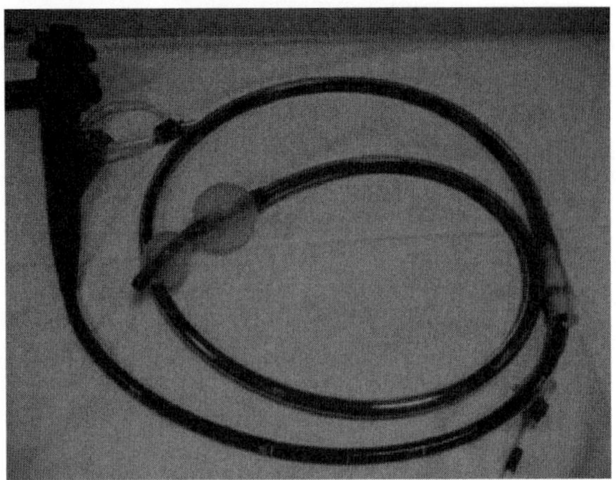

▲ **Figure 33–1.** Double balloon enteroscope.

of the scope is inflated, again anchoring the small bowel. The balloon on the over-tube is then deflated and the over-tube is advanced until it reaches the end of the scope. At this point, the balloon on the end of the over-tube is again inflated. With both balloons inflated, the scope and the over-tube are gently withdrawn until resistance is met. In so doing, the small bowel is pleated onto the over-tube and loops are reduced. The balloon on the scope is then deflated and the scope is again advanced. This sequence is repeated until the lesion of interest is reached or until the scope can no longer be advanced. Fluoroscopic guidance may be used to aid with scope advancement and reductions. When a retrograde approach is employed, the scope and over-tube are advanced until they are both within the terminal ileum, and the same sequence is carried out.

Using the antegrade approach, an average of 240–270 cm of small bowel can be examined. With the retrograde approach, an average of 140–150 cm of small bowel can be visualized. The reported rates of complete small bowel visualization (often through a combination of antegrade and retrograde examinations) vary widely (4–86%), with higher rates being reported in Japan and lower rates in Europe and the United States.

The current therapeutic double balloon enteroscope (Fujinon EN-450T5; Fujinon Inc, Saitama, Japan) has 140-degree field of view and a working length of 200 cm. It has a forceps channel diameter of 2.8 mm, which will accommodate biopsy forceps, argon plasma coagulation probes, bipolar hemostasis probes, cytology brushes, Roth nets, snares, and injection needles. The over-tube is 135 cm with an outer diameter of 13.2 mm.

2. Single balloon enteroscopy—The single balloon enteroscopy system is similar to the double balloon system except that instead of having a balloon on the end of the enteroscope, the tip of the enteroscope can be angulated sharply to anchor the scope. Average depths of small bowel insertion are 133 to 270 cm for antegrade studies and 73 to 199 cm for retrograde studies.

3. Spiral enteroscopy—Spiral enteroscopy uses an enteroscope designed for double or single balloon enteroscopy and an overtube with a soft, raised helical spiral. The enteroscope is advanced into the small bowel along with the overtube. As the overtube is rotated, the small bowel is pulled onto the overtube. The system was developed as an alternative to balloon-assisted enteroscopy in the hope that it would be a simpler and faster method. Currently it is only performed from an antegrade (per os) approach. Reported insertion depths are similar to those seen with antegrade studies performed using balloon-assisted enteroscopy.

Outcomes

The majority of data available on outcomes comes from research on double balloon enteroscopy, although early results reported for single balloon and spiral enteroscopy appear similar. The diagnostic yield for double balloon enteroscopy ranges from 43% to 80%, with a therapeutic yield of 18–55%. In a 2005 study of 137 patients by May and colleagues, double balloon enteroscopy had a diagnostic yield of 80%. The majority of the patients were being evaluated for obscure gastrointestinal bleeding (67%). Other indications included polyposis syndromes (10%), abdominal pain (8%), subileus or severe abdominal pain in the setting of Crohn disease (4%), chronic diarrhea or malabsorption (2%), non-Hodgkin lymphoma of the small bowel (2%), and intestinal obstruction by a foreign body (2%). A new diagnosis was made in 34% of patients and a diagnosis was confirmed in 30%. In 12% of the patients, the study determined the extent of a previously known diagnosis, and in 10% of the patients a previously made diagnosis was excluded. Findings included ulcerations, polyps, tumors, angiodysplasias, small bowel diverticula, foreign bodies (video capsules and dentures), hypertensive enteropathy, and bleeding sources outside of the small bowel. Endoscopic therapy was employed in 41.5% of the patients (argon plasma coagulation, polypectomy, foreign body extraction, dilation, and injection of dilute epinephrine). Medical treatments were started or changed in 17% (mainly in patients with Crohn disease of the small bowel). Surgical therapy was recommended as a result of the study in 17.5% of patients. Double balloon enteroscopy had no treatment implications in only 14.5% of the patients studied.

In a second study of 353 patients from 2007, May and associates found a similar diagnostic yield of 75% for small bowel lesions. Sixty percent of the patients were being evaluated for suspected small bowel bleeding, 10% had chronic abdominal pain, 9% had a polyposis syndrome, 8% had Crohn disease, and 13% underwent the study for other indications, including foreign body extraction. The findings influenced subsequent therapy in 67%. Endoscopic therapy was performed in 59%, and medical therapy was initiated or changed in 19%. Twenty-two percent of the patients required surgery. Not surprisingly, the majority of patients who received endoscopic therapy suffered from small bowel bleeding (74%).

Khashab MA, Lennon AM, Dunbar KB, et al. A comparative evaluation of single balloon enteroscopy and spiral enteroscopy for patients with mid-gut disorders. *Gastrointest Endosc.* 2010;71:766–772. [PMID: 20619404]

May A, Nachbar L, Ell C. Double balloon enteroscopy (push-and-pull enteroscopy) of the small bowel: feasibility and diagnostic and therapeutic yield in patients with suspected small bowel disease. *Gastrointest Endosc.* 2005;62:62–70. [PMID: 15990821]

May A, Nachbar L, Pohl J, et al. Endoscopic interventions in the small bowel using double balloon enteroscopy: feasibility and limitations. *Am J Gastroenterol.* 2007;102:527–535. [PMID: 17222315]

Tsujikawa T, Saitoh Y, Andoh A, et al. Novel single balloon enteroscopy for the diagnosis and treatment of the small intestine: preliminary experiences. *Endoscopy.* 2008;40:11–15. [PMID: 18058613]

Limitations

The primary limitation of deep small bowel enteroscopy is incomplete mucosal visualization. As noted above, the small bowel can be examined in 4–86% of patients using a combined antegrade and retrograde approach with double balloon enteroscopy, leaving a significant percentage of patients with incomplete small bowel visualization. Most commonly this occurs due to inability to advance the scope through the entire length of small bowel. Deep small bowel enteroscopy is also limited by the fact that it typically requires two operators (at least one of whom is a physician), and it is very time consuming, with an average procedure time of 73–115 minutes for balloon-assisted enteroscopy, though the time required for spiral-assisted enteroscopy may be less. In addition, because of potential patient discomfort, some centers use general anesthesia, which can make procedures logistically more difficult to arrange and expensive.

Complications

The most common adverse event is abdominal pain, the day of or the day after the procedure. This occurs in up to 20% of patients. Patients also may report a sore throat. Perforations have been reported, including multiple perforations following chemotherapy for lymphoma and following small bowel polypectomy. Post-procedure paralytic ileus and pancreatitis have also been reported. Bleeding has been seen following polypectomies.

The overall major complication rate in May's study of 353 patients, cited earlier, was 3.4%. Bleeding occurred in 1.1%, perforation in 1.7%, and enteritis in 0.6%. This, however, underestimates the risk associated with individual interventions. Of the 46 patients who underwent polypectomies, 5 (10.8%) suffered complications. Bleeding occurred in 2 (4.3%), and perforation occurred in 3 (6.5%). All of the complications in patients undergoing polypectomy occurred after the removal of polyps that were larger than 3 cm. Argon plasma coagulation had a lower complication rate of 1 in 108 (0.9%).

Thus, while the overall rate of complications is low, patients undergoing polypectomy should be advised that there is a significant complication rate associated with the removal of large polyps, as are often seen in Peutz-Jeghers syndrome. However, given that the alternative in these patients is intraoperative enteroscopy, which has a morbidity rate up to 30% and a mortality rate of 2%, deep small bowel enteroscopy is still an attractive option.

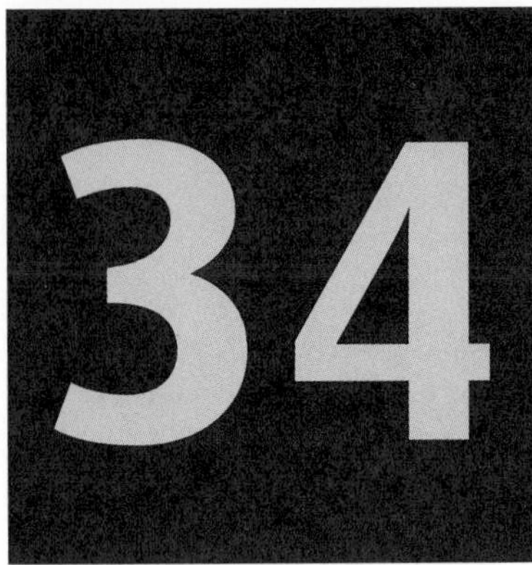

Gastrointestinal Foreign Bodies

Christopher C. Thompson, MD, MSc, FACG, FASGE

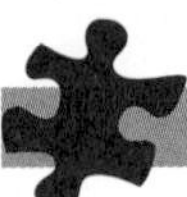

ESSENTIALS OF DIAGNOSIS

- Plain films should be the initial diagnostic study; obtain both lateral and posteroanterior films of the neck, chest, and abdomen as indicated.
- Avoid oral contrast.
- Endoscopic evaluation may be required for objects that are potentially radiolucent in patients with a compelling history but negative imaging findings.
- Impacted meat is typically radiolucent and is the most common esophageal foreign body in adults; perform endoscopy promptly in all cases with clinical evidence of obstruction and failure to pass on initial medical management.
- Many foreign bodies pass spontaneously, but certain objects (eg, sharp objects and batteries) need urgent intervention.

General Considerations

Gastrointestinal foreign bodies occur in all age groups and are commonly seen by the gastroenterologist, as well as by those in various surgical disciplines. The endoscopic removal of foreign bodies dates back to the early 1900s, with more widespread adoption following the advent of the fiberscope in 1957. Methods of diagnosis and treatment have continued to evolve since that time with the development of specialized accessories and improved procedural efficacy.

Foreign body ingestion, including dietary foreign bodies or food bolus impaction, currently represents the second most common indication for emergent gastrointestinal endoscopy, after gastrointestinal hemorrhage. Patients with foreign body ingestion typically present to their primary care physician or the emergency department, and the majority of foreign bodies pass spontaneously. Nevertheless, significant complications may arise resulting in approximately 1500–1600 deaths in the United States annually. Therefore, it is essential for the endoscopist to efficiently determine which patients require therapeutic intervention, and to be comfortable with proper methods of extraction. This chapter reviews indications for foreign body removal, the typical diagnostic evaluation, and endoscopic techniques for foreign body management.

Clinical Findings

A. Symptoms and Signs

Following foreign body ingestion patients may present in a variety of ways, ranging from asymptomatic to having signs and symptoms of complete esophageal obstruction or frank perforation. In the majority of cases a careful clinical history provides the correct diagnosis. Clinical history may be less reliable in children younger than age 5 years, the mentally ill, and in otherwise uncooperative patients. In such populations, symptoms and diagnostic studies are more critical to clarifying the diagnosis.

Most true foreign body ingestions are seen in children between the ages of 1 and 5 years who swallow small household items or toys. Fortunately, most of these objects are small and blunt, and they typically pass spontaneously. Adults who ingest true foreign bodies often have psychiatric disturbance, mental retardation, alcoholism, or identifiable reasons for secondary gain, such as prisoners. Dietary foreign bodies and food bolus impactions typically occur in older adults, denture wearers, and those with underlying esophageal disorders.

Presenting symptoms are determined by the type of foreign body ingested and its location.

1. Esophageal foreign bodies—Esophageal foreign bodies may result in symptoms of dysphagia, odynophagia, or signs of complete esophageal obstruction, including inability to swallow secretions, drooling, and regurgitation. Sudden onset of odynophagia following eating suggests impaction of a bone, sharp food fragment, toothpick, or similar objects in the esophagus. Respiratory symptoms such as coughing and stridor are common in younger children as their compliant tracheal rings are more easily compressed by an adjacent esophageal foreign body. Upper airway obstruction is a rare presentation for adults with an esophageal foreign body; however, meat bolus impaction at the level of the cricopharyngeus can result in respiratory obstruction, which has been referred to as "steak house syndrome." Subcutaneous emphysema in the supraclavicular area or the neck suggests perforation of the esophagus or hypopharynx. Esophageal perforation by sharp objects at the level of the aortic arch may also result in an aortoesophageal fistula. This typically presents with a herald bleed, followed by massive hemorrhage. Fortunately these presentations are rare.

2. Gastric foreign bodies—Gastric foreign bodies are generally asymptomatic, except when they are large enough to be associated with postprandial emesis and early satiety. Longstanding foreign bodies or those that are sharp and pointed may become impacted in the gastric wall and result in inflammation, ulceration, hemorrhage, or perforation. These patients often present with pain or bleeding.

3. Small bowel foreign bodies—Foreign bodies that have made their way to the small bowel typically remain asymptomatic. Symptoms of small bowel foreign bodies are typically those of perforation or obstruction.

B. Physical Findings

Physical examination may yield important clues to identifying complications due to ingested foreign bodies. Crepitus in the supraclavicular and cervical areas suggests perforation of the hypopharynx or esophagus. Large gastric foreign bodies may occasionally be palpable on abdominal examination. Peritoneal signs often suggest gastric or intestinal perforation, and physical findings typical of bowel obstruction may occur with small bowel foreign bodies.

C. Imaging Studies

The plain film radiograph should be the initial diagnostic study. Both lateral and posteroanterior films should be obtained of the neck, chest, and abdomen. This is important in identifying small or flat objects that may overlie the spine, and in determining the exact location of a foreign body. The lateral film is often essential in differentiating between tracheobronchial and esophageal locations. Perforation may also be identified if the object is seen extending beyond the lumen wall, or if a soft tissue mass is seen adjacent to the object. Plain films should also be obtained to evaluate food bolus impactions, as the presence of bone fragments may alter the endoscopic management.

Objects that are relatively radiolucent, such as plastic, wood, most glass, and small bones, may not be seen on plain film, in which case xeroradiography or computed tomography may be helpful in making the diagnosis.

Contrast studies should be avoided. Gastrografin is contraindicated as it is very hypertonic and can result in a severe chemical pneumonitis if aspirated, and barium can obscure endoscopic visualization, thereby complicating therapy.

Endoscopic evaluation may also be required, even in the absence of imaging findings, for a possible radiolucent object and compelling history. Additionally, endoscopy is often the therapeutic method of choice.

Treatment

Although the majority of foreign bodies pass spontaneously, certain objects need urgent intervention. The type of foreign body and its location determine management. In general, all esophageal foreign bodies, elongated and sharp gastric foreign bodies, and blunt objects should be removed from the stomach after persisting 2 weeks. Endoscopic removal may be technically challenging depending on the object shape and material, and several accessories are available to enhance procedural success. Details of management follow.

A. Foreign Body Classification and Management

A wide variety of ingested foreign bodies may be encountered by the gastrointestinal endoscopist. Roughly 75% of all foreign bodies pass spontaneously, with 1% resulting in serious complication or surgery.

Foreign bodies may be broadly classified as true foreign bodies or dietary foreign bodies. They may be further categorized as dull or sharp, blunt or pointed, long or short, toxic or nontoxic, and as food bolus impactions. These features are associated with prognosis, and depending on anatomic location may indicate when urgent removal is necessary.

1. Sharp and pointed objects—The most common sharp objects include fish or chicken bones and toothpicks; however, razor blades, hat pins, nails, and fragments of glass may also be seen (Figure 34–1 and Plate 84). Although the majority of such objects can pass safely through the gastrointestinal tract, perforation rates are as high as 35%. Thus, endoscopic removal is necessary if the object is within reach of the endoscope. When the object is above the cricopharyngeus, referral to an otolaryngologist for direct laryngoscopy is indicated. Otherwise, urgent flexible endoscopy should be considered. If the object has passed beyond the duodenum, daily radiographs should be obtained to determine its location and detect free air or other evidence of complications. If the object fails to progress for 3 consecutive days, then surgical intervention should be considered.

2. Long objects—Long and narrow foreign bodies such as toothbrushes and stiff wires are associated with a high incidence of perforation as they have difficulty passing the fixed curves of the duodenum. Objects 6 cm in length or longer are particularly problematic, and early endoscopic intervention is recommended.

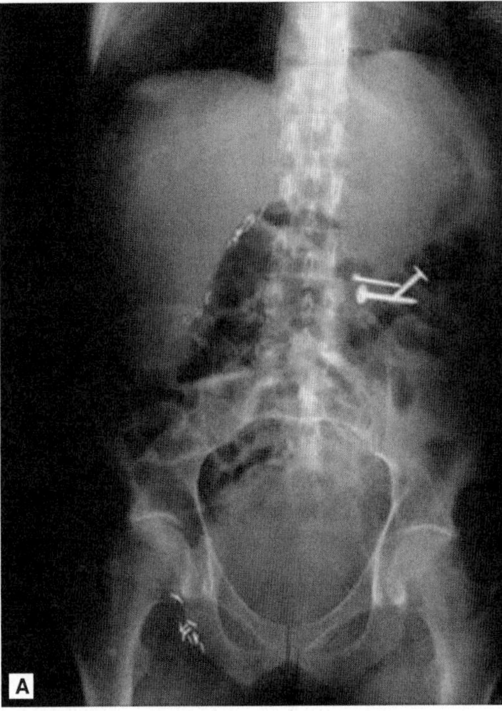

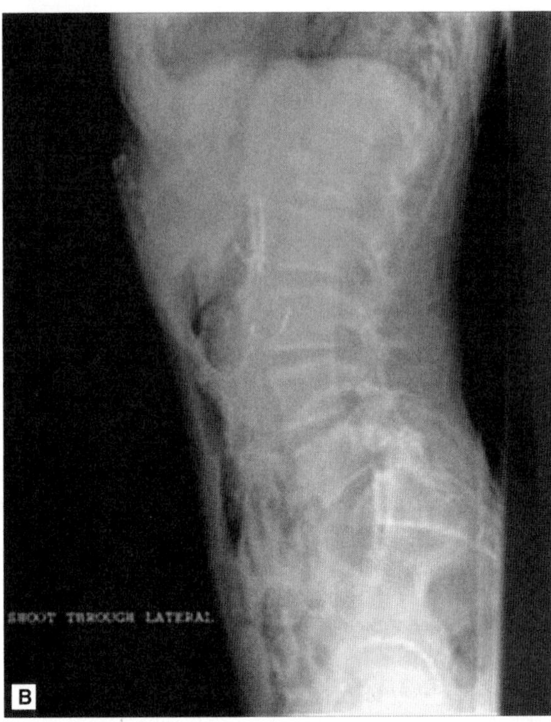

▲ **Figure 34–1.** Plain film radiographs. **A:** Posteroanterior film showing nails. **B:** Lateral film showing a razor blade.

3. Blunt foreign bodies—This is perhaps the most diverse class of ingested foreign bodies and is the most common in the pediatric population. In a review describing the management of 242 foreign bodies, coins were the most common foreign body ingested by children. Other objects in this class include marbles, small toys, and disc batteries. Conservative outpatient management is indicated for the vast majority of blunt foreign bodies that have passed into the stomach. Rounded objects larger than 2.5 cm are less likely to pass the pylorus, and endoscopic removal should be considered if the object fails to pass the stomach within 2–3 weeks. If the object successfully passes through the stomach, a radiograph should be obtained every 3–4 days to assess passage. Surgical removal should be considered if the object remains in the same location for more than 1 week.

Button batteries or disc batteries require special consideration. The most common disc battery systems include silver oxide, manganese dioxide, and mercuric oxide. These typically contain alkaline solutions of either sodium hydroxide or potassium, which can cause direct corrosive effects or low-voltage burns. Liquefaction necrosis of the esophagus and perforation can also occur. Urgent endoscopic evaluation with battery removal is thus indicated. If battery disruption is noted, heavy metal levels should be monitored in the blood and urine. Mercury poisoning is a rare complication of battery disruption. Copper, nickel, and lead poisoning have also been reported after prolonged retention of various metallic foreign objects. If a disc battery successfully passes into the stomach, it will typically pass the gastrointestinal tract without consequence. Forceps should be avoided if endoscopic removal is attempted as they can lead to battery disruption. Cathartics and acid suppression have no proven role and should also be avoided.

4. Toxic foreign bodies—Internal concealment of illicit drugs wrapped in plastic or latex packages, also known as "body packing," is seen with higher frequency in regions of drug trafficking. Package rupture or leakage can be fatal, and such foreign bodies require special consideration. Endoscopic removal should not be attempted.

Drug packages can be subdivided into three types. Type 1 includes condoms and balloons. These typically appear as a density with surrounding halo of gas on radiography. Each condom can contain 3–5 g of cocaine, and ingestion of 1–3 g may be lethal. As these packages are very susceptible to breakage, surgical removal should be considered early.

Type 2 and type 3 packages consist of layers of tubular latex or plastic, with or without aluminum foil. Type 2 packages may appear similar to type 1 on radiography. Type 3 packages are typically smaller and may not be seen on radiographs. These packages are less susceptible to breakage and, if identified, they may be followed with daily radiographs. Indications for surgery include failure of the package to progress on the daily radiograph, evidence of intestinal obstruction, visualization of broken packages on radiograph, passage of broken packages, or development of consequential symptoms.

5. Food bolus impaction—Impacted meat is the most common esophageal foreign body in adults. Total esophageal obstruction is implied by drooling and inability to swallow secretions. This is an indication for urgent endoscopic intervention. Ideally all meat boluses should be extracted or advanced into the stomach urgently (within a few hours of ingestion) as patients are at risk for aspiration. Additionally, with prolonged bolus impaction there is risk for local esophageal ischemia and pressure ulceration, and with time the bolus may be partially digested, requiring piecemeal removal. The administration of glucagon (1.0 mg intravenously) may also be attempted prior to endoscopy to encourage spontaneous passage. This may be repeated at 10 minutes, however, if this is not effective further doses are not recommended. Glucagon has little effect on the proximal esophagus but causes substantial relaxation of the smooth muscle of the lower esophageal sphincter, allowing spontaneous passage of the bolus in up to 50% of cases. Patients with structural abnormalities are less likely to respond to this form of medical therapy. Glucagon is contraindicated in patients with underlying pheochromocytoma, insulinoma, and Zollinger-Ellison syndrome. Papain and other meat tenderizers should be avoided. Many impactions occur in the proximal esophagus and careful attention must be paid to this area on initial esophageal intubation. Additionally, many patients with food bolus impactions have underlying esophageal disease, such as peptic stricture, Schatzki ring, or eosinophilic esophagitis. Local trauma and edema often preclude an accurate diagnosis of such conditions at the initial endoscopic evaluation, and subsequent studies are typically required. This may include repeat upper endoscopy with biopsy several weeks after resolution of the food bolus impaction.

6. Rectal foreign bodies—Numerous objects, including bottles, vibrators, various fruits and vegetables, flash lights, light bulbs, and a propane tank, have been reported in the literature. Because of this wide variety of objects and the varying degree of trauma that may be seen, it is important to have a systematic approach to the diagnosis and management of retained rectal foreign bodies. Additionally, delayed presentations are common, due to embarrassment and reluctance to seek medical attention, and patients are often not entirely truthful regarding important details, further complicating management. Manual or surgical removal is commonly required, and colorectal surgeons are typically asked to manage these cases. It is important to exclude perforation in all patients with abdominal imaging/CT scan, prior to considering endoscopy. Surgery is indicated in all cases of perforation. In addition, objects that are 10 cm in diameter, have been in place for more than 2 days, and that are proximal to the rectum, typically require surgical removal. If a transanal approach is feasible, anal sphincter relaxation is critical. Perianal nerve block, and/or spinal anesthetic, should be considered in addition to intravenous conscious sedation. Perforation may only be noticed after extraction, and imaging after foreign body removal is also important.

B. Methods of Removal

The removal of esophageal foreign bodies dates back to the early 1900s with Chevalier Jackson, who published a series of over 3000 cases in 1936; however, foreign body extraction using the flexible fiberoptic endoscope was not reported until 1972. Throughout the 1980s and 1990s endoscopes evolved and several accessories were developed to assist in the removal of ingested foreign bodies. Methods of removal in current use are detailed in this section.

Prior to removal, a complete history and physical examination are essential to determine the need for removal and to assess the safety of the procedure. This will also help in selection of the correct instruments based on the type of foreign body and its location.

1. Sedation—When planning foreign body extraction, the first decision involves determining the type of sedation that is most appropriate for the patient. Many patients who have ingested foreign material are poor candidates for conscious sedation. History of alcoholism, drug abuse, or certain psychiatric conditions may render them difficult to sedate and increase associated procedural risk. General anesthesia with endotracheal intubation provides deeper sedation and additional airway protection that may be desirable in certain circumstances.

2. Choice of endoscope—The second decision involves which type of endoscope to use. Forward-viewing (single-channel or double-channel) or side-viewing endoscopes may each have a role, and selection should not be arbitrary. The forward-viewing endoscopes have an advantage over side-viewing endoscopes in visualizing the esophagus and most parts of the stomach and small bowel. Double-channel endoscopes are also particularly useful for removing elongated objects as accessories may be passed through both channels, which may be helpful in positioning the object for capture or holding it in a straight position for extraction. The double-channel endoscope, however, is larger in diameter than the single-channel endoscope and may not be useable with all accessories, such as a hood or some overtubes. Additionally, the double-channel endoscope may be too large for use in infants or small children due to concern for tracheal compression. The side-viewing endoscope provides better visualization of the medial aspect of the lesser curve and the periampullary area in the small bowel, and may be useful in addressing foreign bodies lodged in these areas.

3. Choice of accessories—Several accessories may facilitate the endoscopic management of foreign bodies. Various devices are available to protect the gastrointestinal tract or airway during extraction, and to grasp objects of different sizes and shapes.

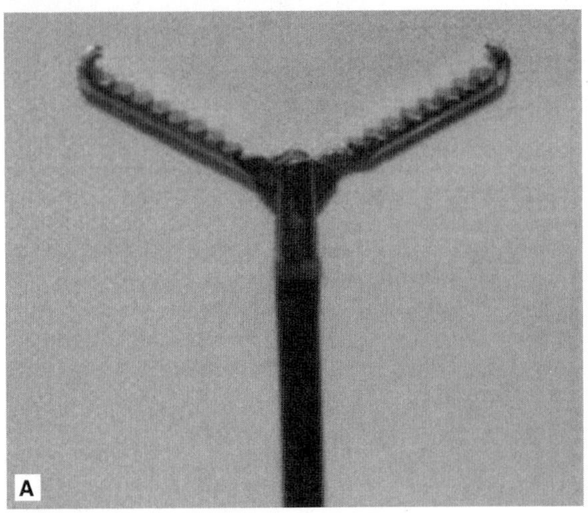

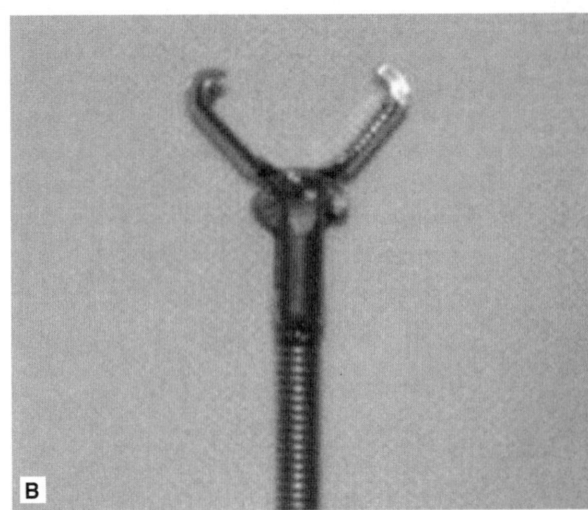

▲ **Figure 34–2.** Graspers. **A:** Alligator forceps **B:** Rat-toothed forceps.

A. Forceps and snares—Different types of forceps or graspers are available, and certain varieties may be more or less useful for specific materials. Rat-toothed forceps and alligator forceps are more effective than standard biopsy forceps at grasping various foreign materials, including plastics and metal (Figure 34–2). Snares, biliary stone retrieval baskets, and snares fitted with netting may also be useful for contending with certain objects. Netted snares are particularly useful for dealing with objects that are prone to crumbling and button batteries.

The way the objects are grasped is also important. For elongated objects it is important to grasp them at one end and keep the long axis in line with the esophagus. For sharp objects it is critical to grasp the object such that the sharp end is trailing. Additionally, when planning a procedure it is recommended that various instruments be tested on a similar object, as this will reduce procedure time and could lead to improved outcomes.

B. Overtubes—An overtube is a plastic sheath with an inner diameter large enough to accommodate an endoscope, and several varieties are available (Figure 34–3). Use of an over-tube should be considered if multiple intubations are anticipated, additional if airway protection is desired, or sharp objects have been ingested.

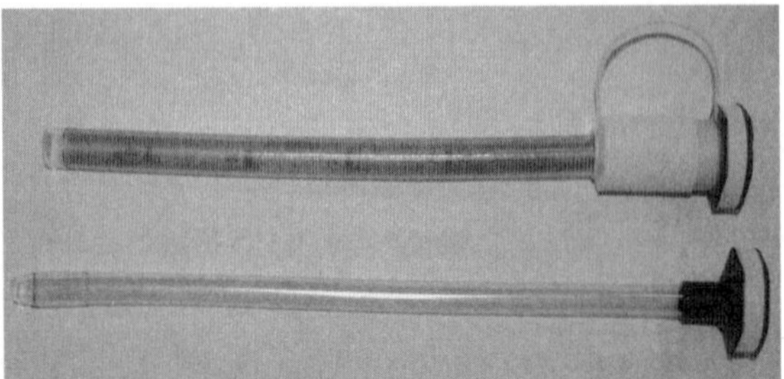

▲ **Figure 34–3.** Overtube and internal introducer with tapered tip.

Overtubes come in various lengths and may extend to the midesophagus or into the proximal stomach. There are two methods for placing overtubes. Reusable overtubes may be introduced over a snug fitting wire-guided Savary dilator, and single-use overtubes may be preloaded over the endoscope with the matching tapered-tip introducer. It is not acceptable to place a reusable overtube by preloading it over an endoscope as the resulting gap between the endoscope and the overtube could result in perforation of the hypopharynx. The inner diameter of the overtube varies depending on the specific product but is typically less than 14 mm in diameter. This feature can be limiting when dealing with large objects.

C. Hoods—The foreign body hood is an alternative to the overtube and is particularly useful when dealing with sharp foreign objects (Figure 34–4). The protective hood is attached to the bending segment of the endoscope and is folded back to avoid compromising endoscopic visualization. After the object is grasped using the appropriate endoscopic accessories, the endoscope is withdrawn. As the hood passes through the lower esophageal sphincter it is folded forward, covering the object and protecting the gastric cardia and esophagus from contact with the object. Unlike the overtube, the hood does not provide additional airway protection.

C. Alternatives to Removal

For food bolus impactions, it may be safer to push the object into the stomach rather than attempt removal. This must be done with care. It is essential to first evaluate the area beyond the foreign body, to make certain there is no stricture, or other anatomic defect. Gentle pressure may then be applied to the object to facilitate passage. This is typically not acceptable for large true foreign bodies.

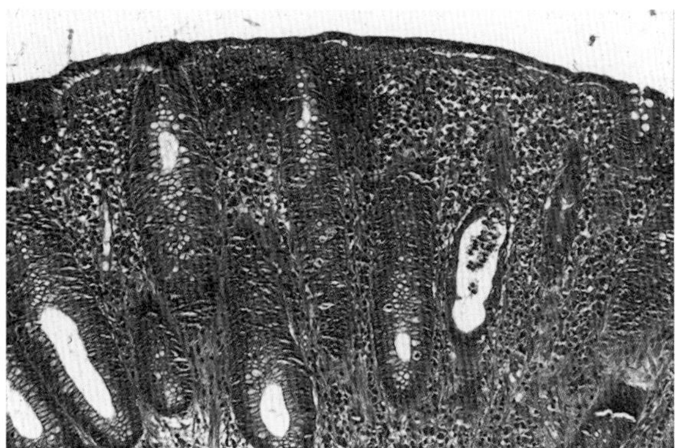

▲ **Plate 1.** Rectal mucosal biopsy specimen from a patient with dysentery caused by shigellosis. There is considerable mucosal inflammation caused by infiltration with polymorphonuclear leukocytes and mononuclear cells, as well as substantial damage to surface epithelial cells. However, mucosal architecture is generally preserved with straight, closely adjacent crypts. A crypt microabscess is seen on the right.

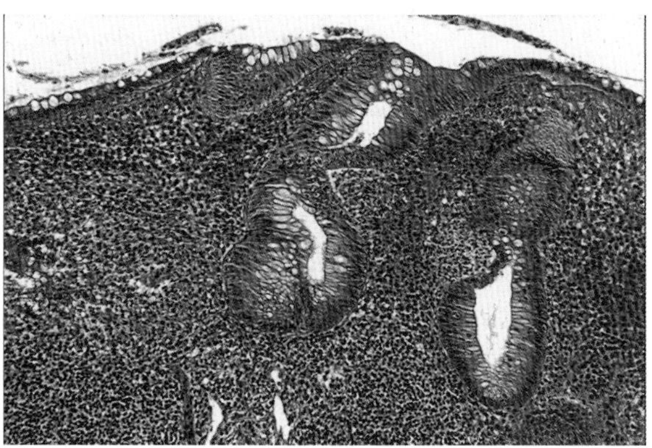

▲ **Plate 2.** Rectal mucosal biopsy specimen from a patient with dysenteric stools caused by a flare of chronic ulcerative colitis. The mucosa is heavily infiltrated with polymorphonuclear leukocytes and mononuclear cells. In contrast to Plate 1, mucosal architecture is markedly distorted, with substantial reduction in crypts and distortion of those that remain.

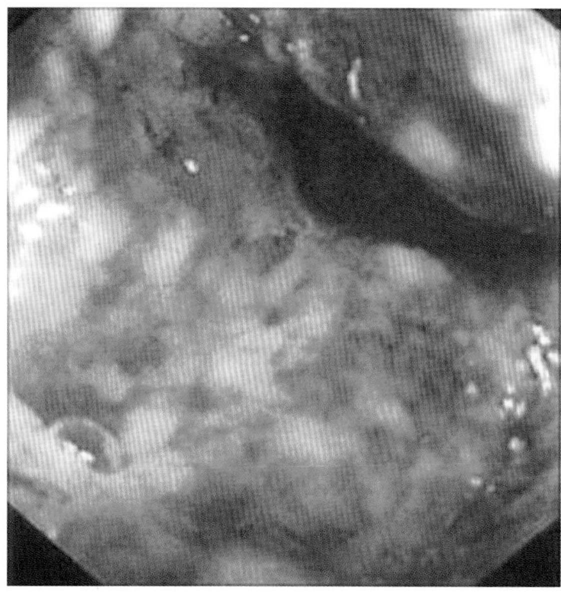

▲ **Plate 3.** Endoscopic appearance of colonic ischemia. (Used with permission from David Stockwell, MD.)

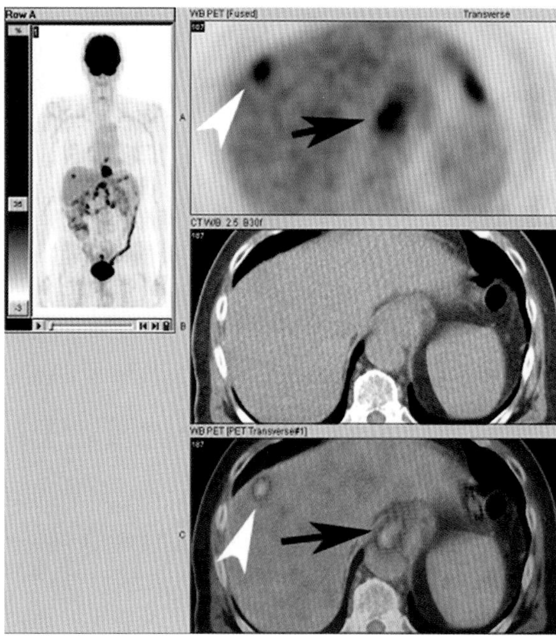

▲ **Plate 4.** Esophageal carcinoma. Fused PET-CT image shows a "hot spot" (*black arrow*) at the level of the distal esophagus corresponding to squamous cell carcinoma. Note the hepatic metastasis (*white arrowhead*).

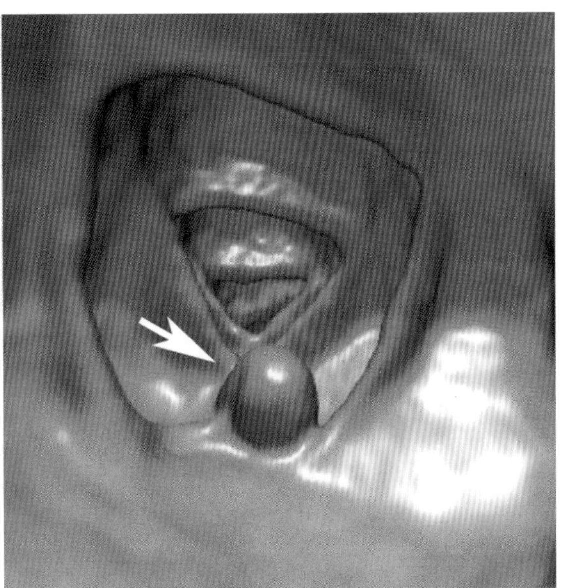

▲**Plate 5.** Colonic polyp. Three-dimensional endoluminal reconstructed image confirms the presence of a colonic polyp (*arrow*). (For corresponding axial MDCT image, see Figure 9–17 in the text.)

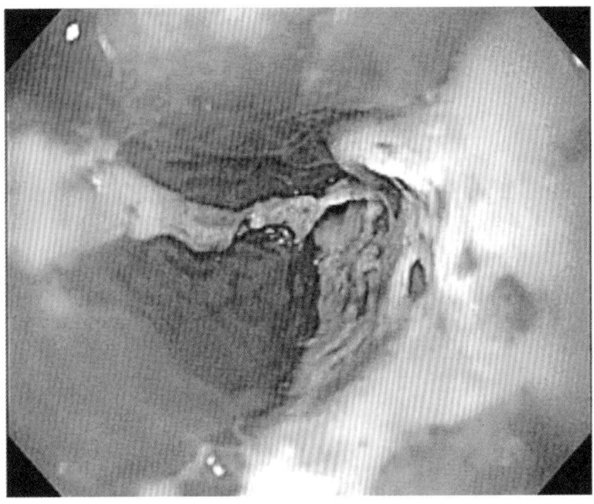

▲**Plate 6.** Severe erosive esophagitis with peptic stricture.

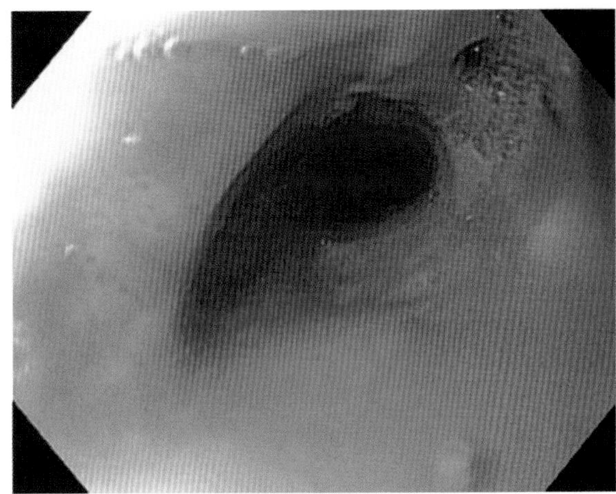

▲**Plate 7.** Esophageal stricture prior to dilation.

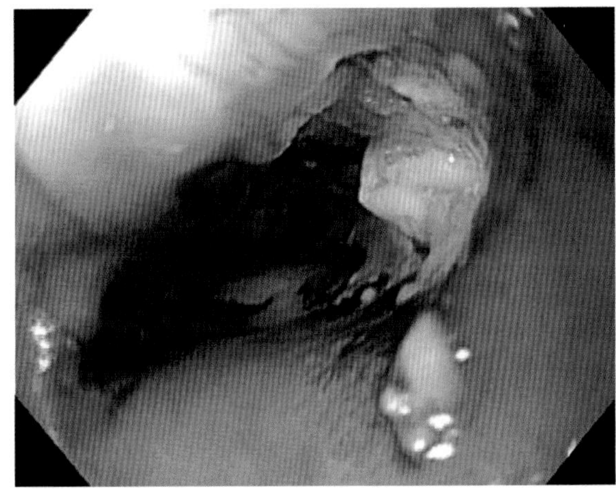

▲**Plate 8.** Postdilation appearance of esophageal stricture shown in Plate 7.

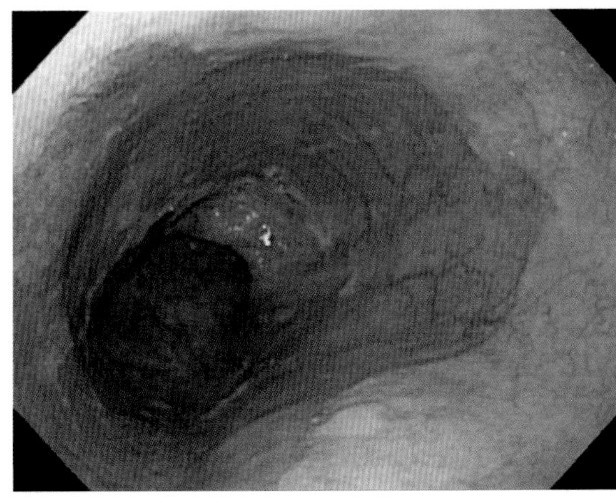

▲**Plate 9.** Endoscopic appearance of Barrett esophagus.

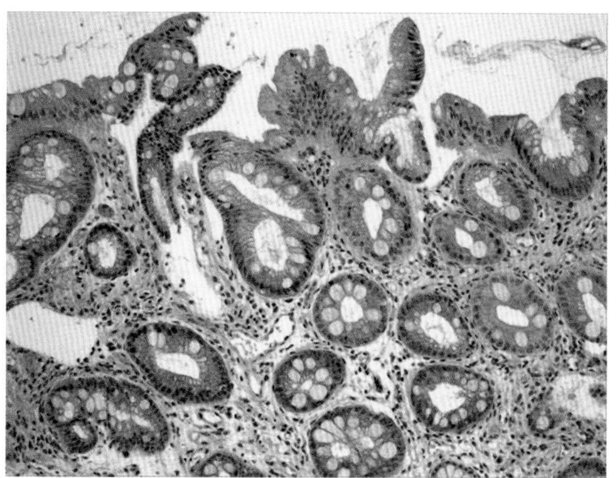

▲ **Plate 10.** Histopathologic findings in nondysplastic Barrett esophagus. Note the glandular epithelium containing goblet cells. (Used with permission from Jason Hornick, MD, PhD, Brigham and Women's Hospital.)

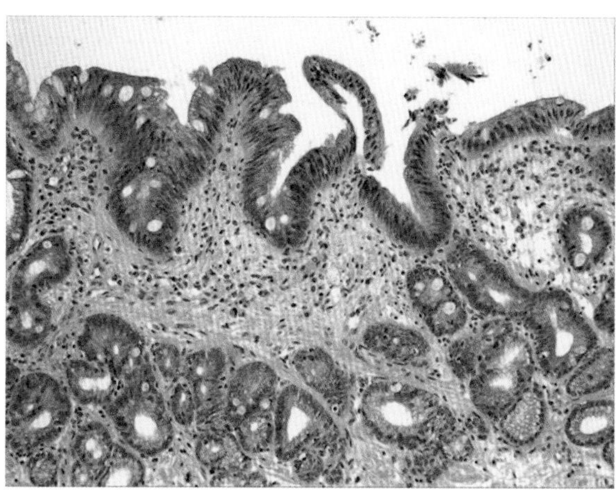

▲ **Plate 11.** Histopathologic findings of low-grade dysplasia in Barrett esophagus. The surface epithelium displays nuclear stratification, limited to the lower half of the cytoplasm. (Used with permission from Jason Hornick, MD, PhD, Brigham and Women's Hospital.)

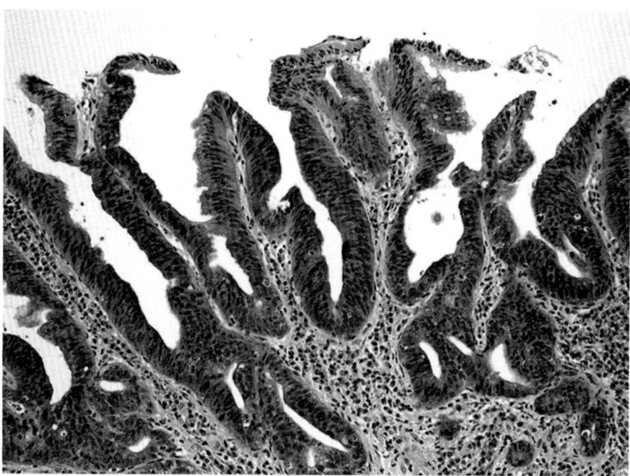

▲ **Plate 12.** Histopathologic findings of high-grade dysplasia in Barrett esophagus. There is full-thickness nuclear stratification and the mucosa has a villous appearance. (Used with permission from Jason Hornick, MD, PhD, Brigham and Women's Hospital.)

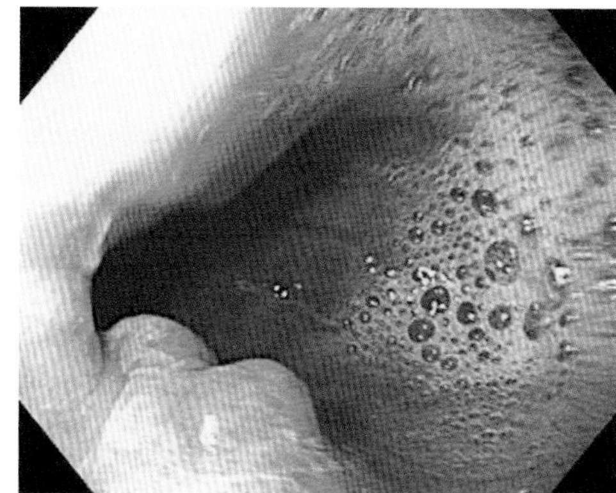

▲ **Plate 13.** Nodule of high-grade dysplasia in Barrett esophagus.

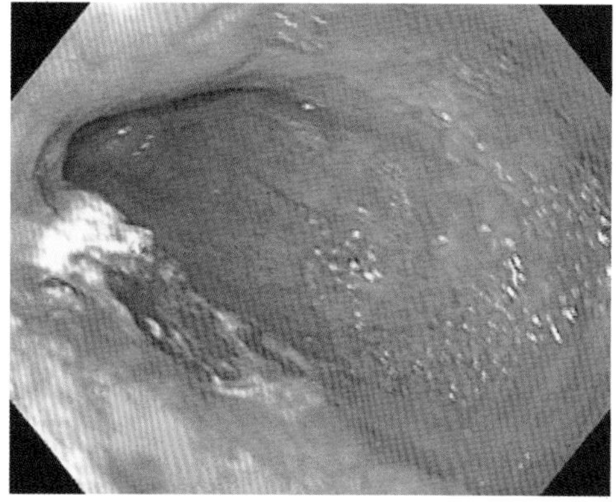

▲ **Plate 14.** Same area shown in Plate 13 after endoscopic mucosal resection.

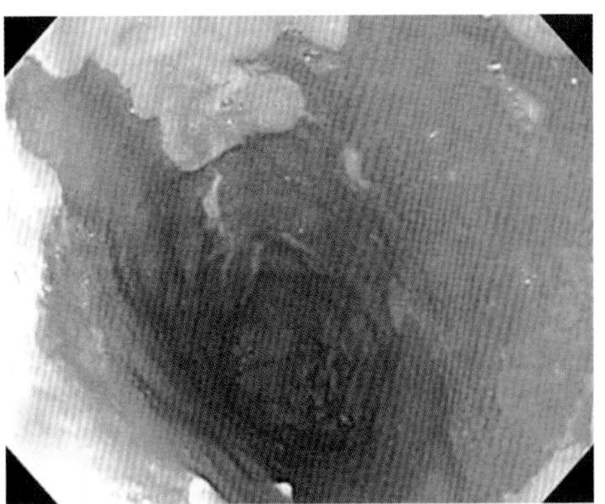

▲ **Plate 15.** Barrett esophagus with high-grade dysplasia and intramucosal adenocarcinoma.

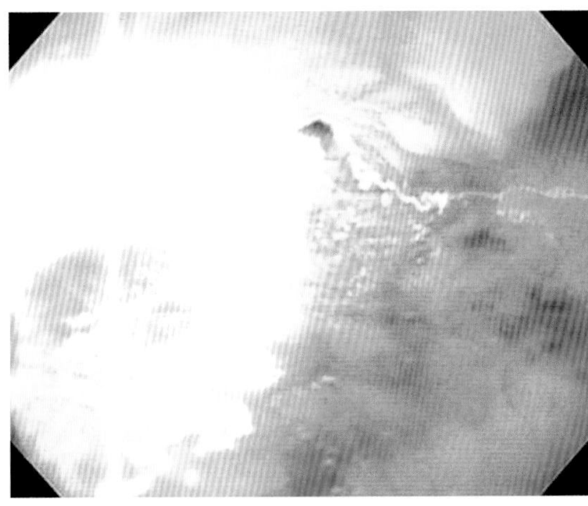

▲ **Plate 16.** Barrett esophagus. Same area as in Plate 15 showing illumination with laser light during photodynamic therapy.

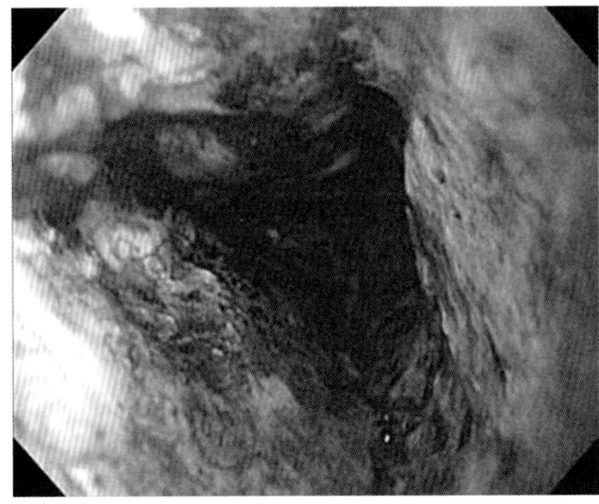

▲ **Plate 17.** Barrett esophagus segment 48 hours after illumination; same area as in Plates 15 and 16.

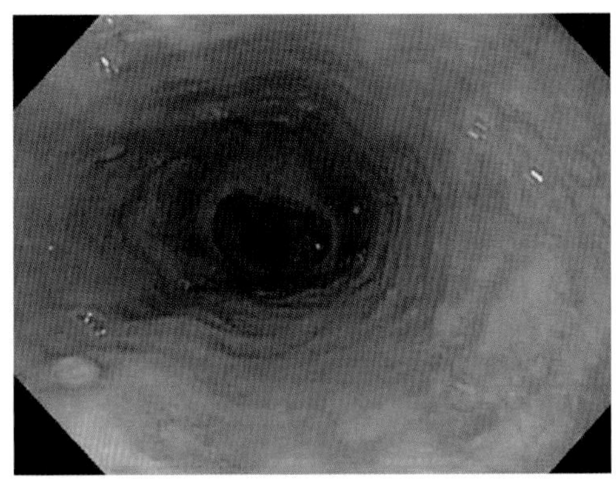

▲ **Plate 18.** Endoscopic findings in eosinophilic esophagitis. Note trachea-like mucosal rings.

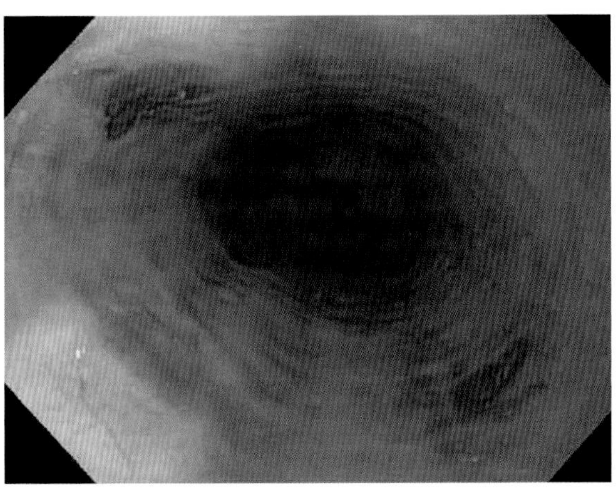

▲ **Plate 19.** Eosinophilic esophagitis. Note mucosal lacerations.

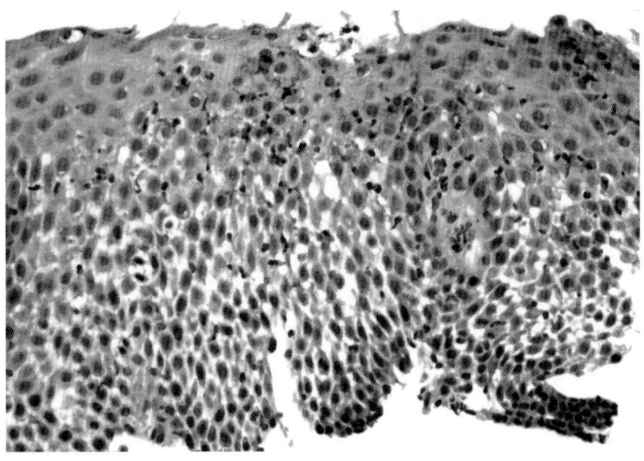

▲ **Plate 20.** Histologic findings in eosinophilic esophagitis. Note increased eosinophils in the squamous mucosa.

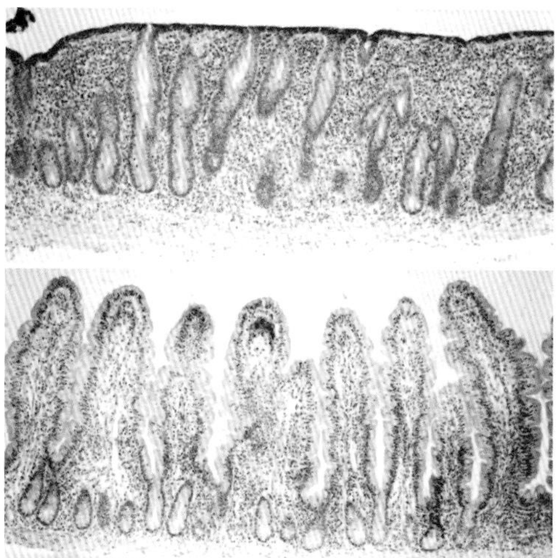

▲ **Plate 21.** The upper panel shows a characteristic severe lesion from a patient with untreated celiac sprue. Villi are absent, crypts are hyperplastic, and the lamina propria is infiltrated with many mononuclear cells. For comparison, the lower panel shows a biopsy sample from a normal volunteer showing normal mucosal architecture with tall villi and shallow crypts and just a few mononuclear cells in the lamina propria.

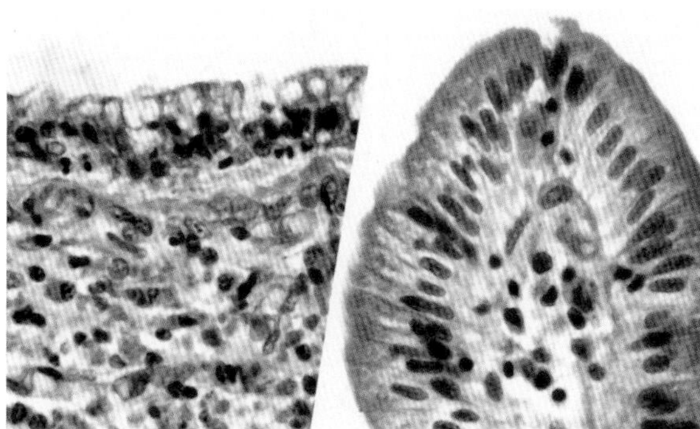

▲ **Plate 22.** The left panel shows at higher magnification the absorptive surface of the biopsy sample from the patient with celiac sprue shown in the upper panel of Plate 21. The surface absorptive cells are decreased in height and vacuolated, and the nuclei have lost their polarity. Numerous intraepithelial lymphocytes (IELs) can be seen between adjacent epithelial cells. The underlying lamina propria is heavily infiltrated with lymphocytes and plasma cells. For comparison, in the panel on the right is the tip of a villus from the biopsy sample shown in lower panel of Plate 23 from a normal individual. In contrast to the panel on the left, the absorptive cells are tall and have a well-developed brush border, with only occasional IELs evident between epithelial cells.

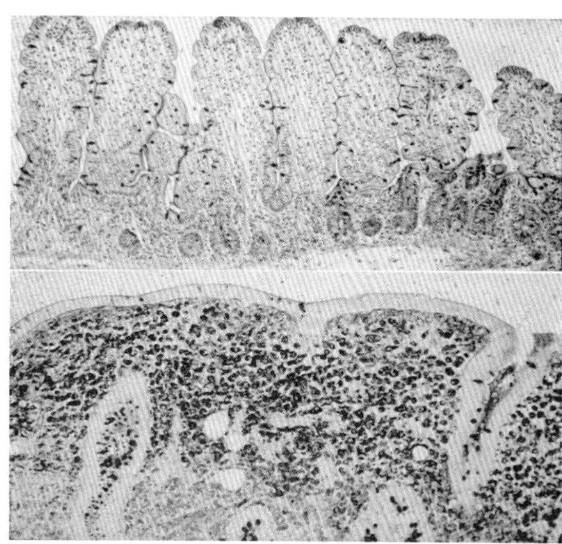

▲ **Plate 23.** Upper panel shows a biopsy sample obtained from a normal volunteer and stained with periodic acid–Schiff (PAS) stain. The glycoprotein-rich epithelial cell brush border and the goblet cell mucous are PAS-positive. The biopsy sample in the lower panel was obtained from a patient with untreated Whipple disease. The villus architecture is markedly distorted and the lamina propria is packed with large PAS-positive macrophages that virtually replace the lymphocytes and plasma cells that would normally be seen. Additionally, profiles of dilated lymphatics are evident in the lamina propria.

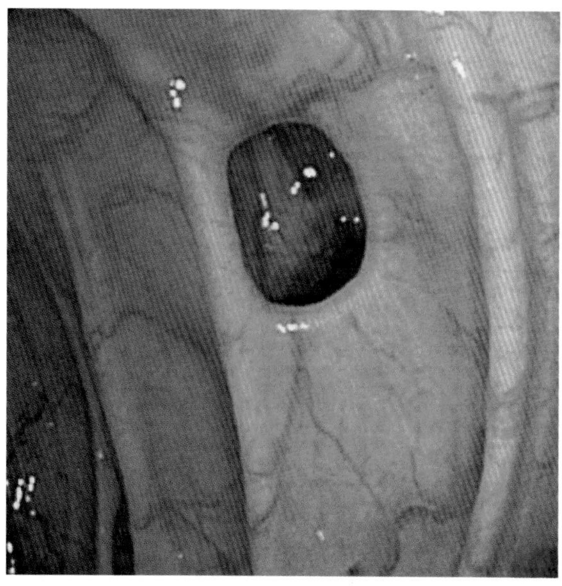

▲ **Plate 24.** Diverticulum.

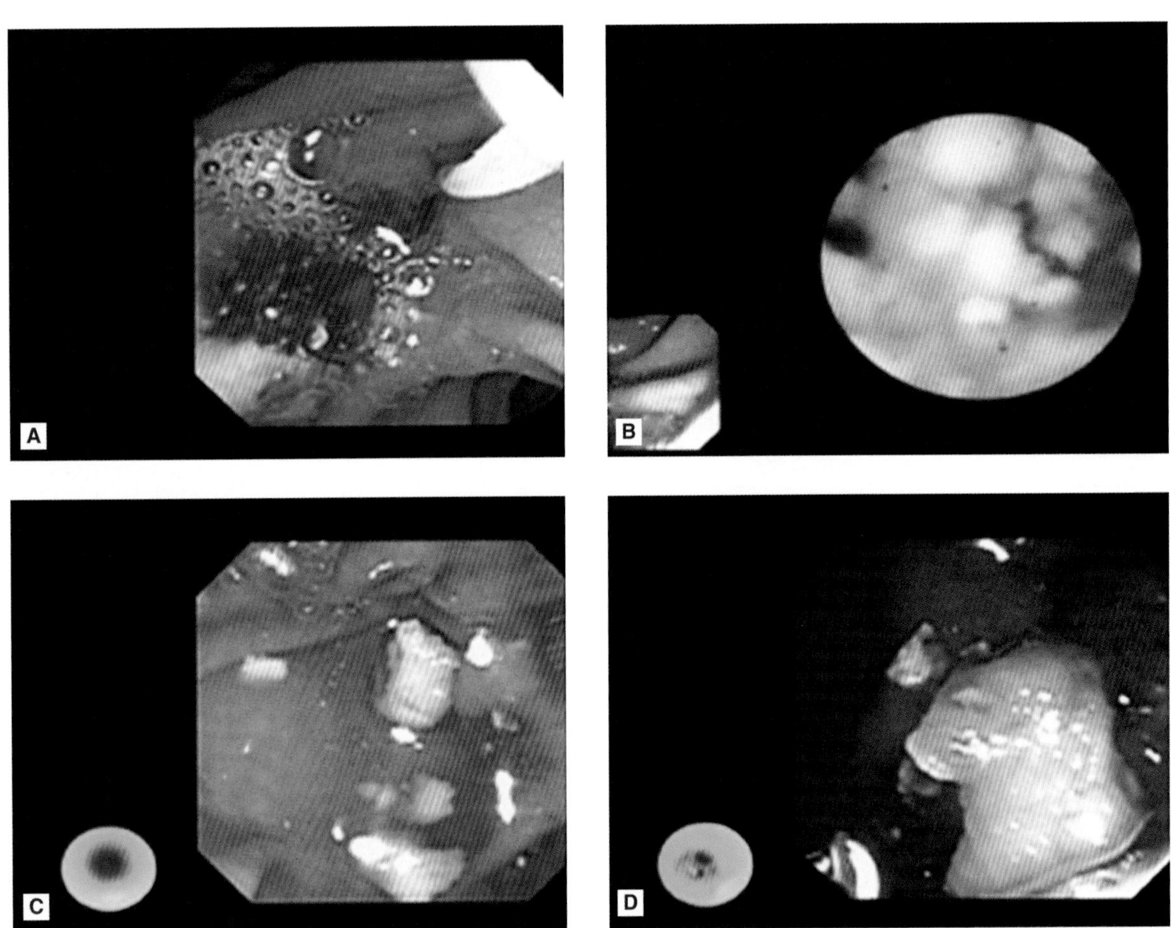

▲ **Plate 25.** ERCP + ESWL: Symptomatic Pancreatic Duct Stones. **A.** area of papilla in the duodenum, **B-D.** stones. (Used with permission from David Leslie Carr-Locke, MD.)

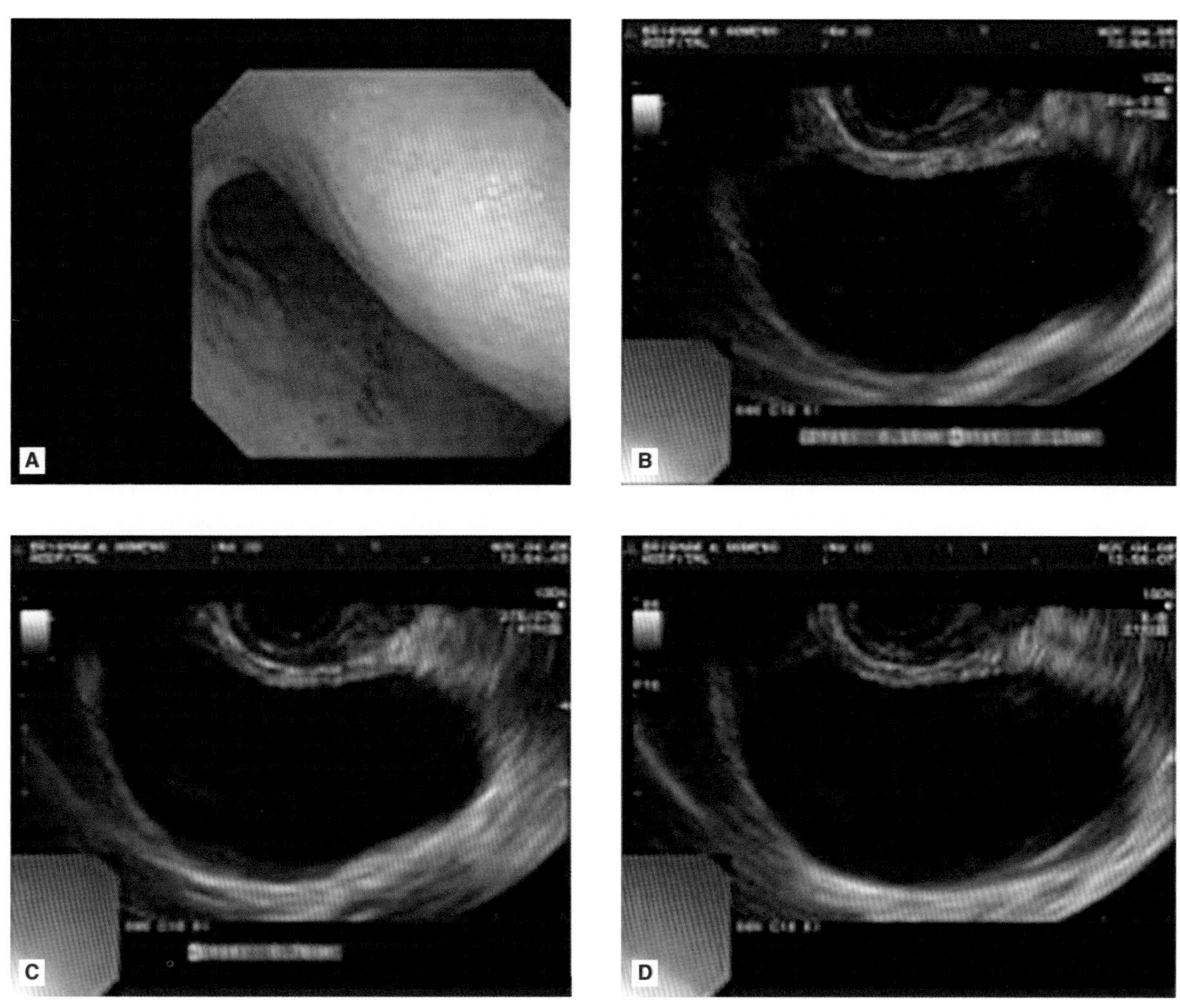

▲ **Plate 26. A.** gastric bulge, **B-D.** EUS of pseudocyst. (Used with permission from Christopher Thompson, MD.)

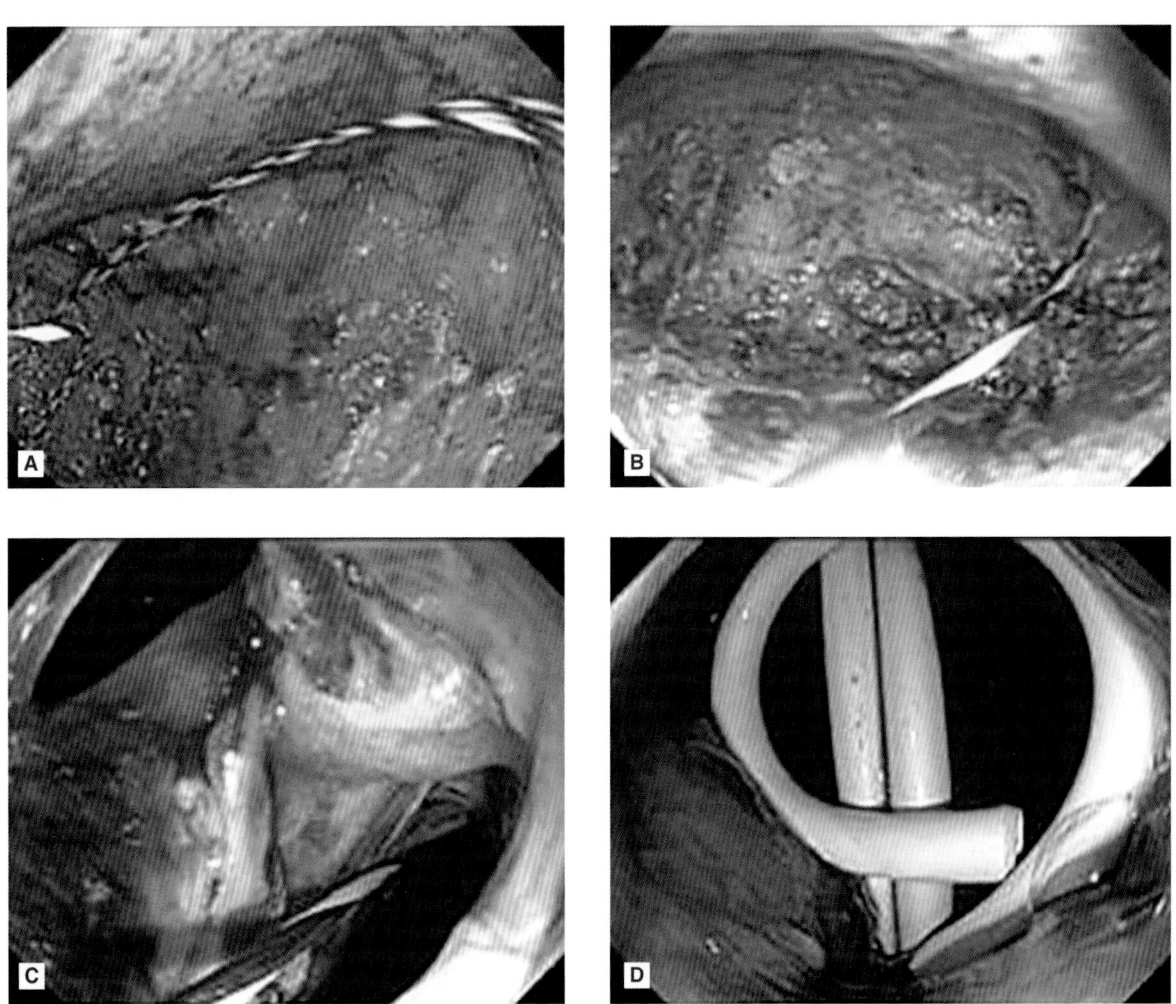

▲ **Plate 27.** Step-Wise Images (Plates 26, A-D and 27 A-D) of Endoscopic Drainage of Symptomatic Pancreas.
A. pseudocyst, **B.** wire in cyst cavity, **C.** cystogastrostomy site with wire, **D.** residual pigtail catheters.
(Used with permission from Christopher Thompson, MD.)

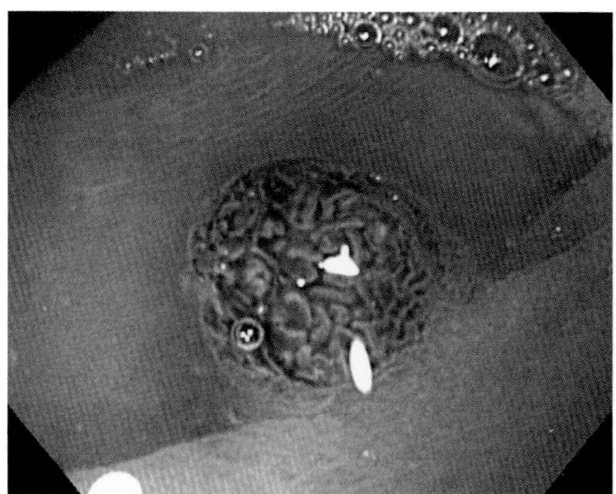

▲ **Plate 28.** Endoscopic view of a diminutive adenomatous polyp before cold snare excision (narrow band imaging mode).

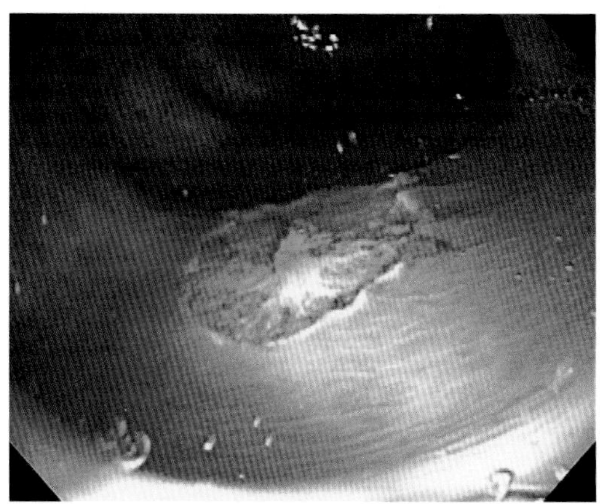

▲ **Plate 29.** Diminutive adenomatous polyp after cold snare excision. Same patient as in Plate 28.

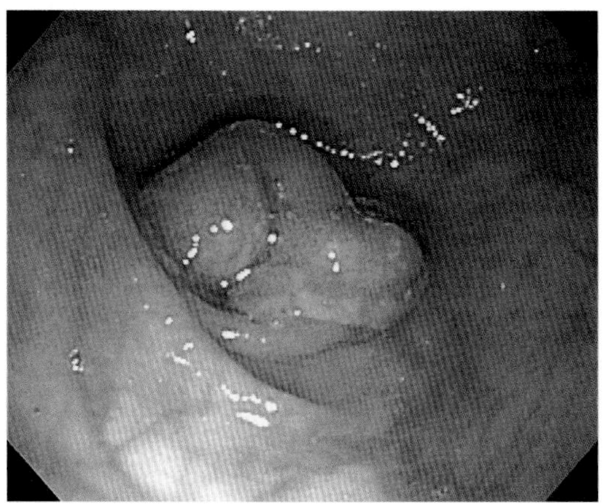

▲ **Plate 30.** Sessile adenomatous polyp.

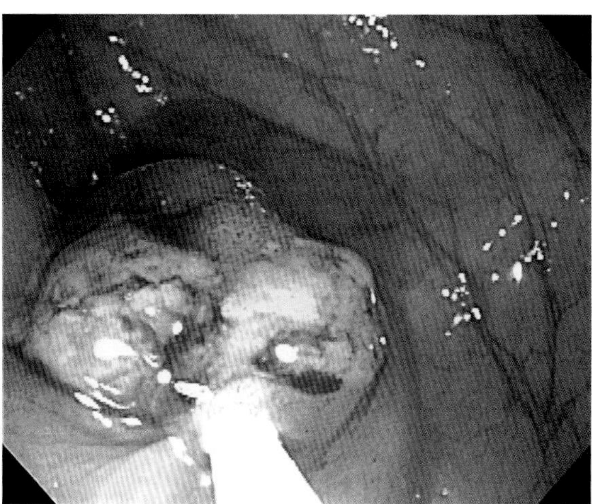

▲ **Plate 31.** Sessile adenomatous polyp undergoing hot snare polypectomy without mucosal injection. Same patient as in Plate 30.

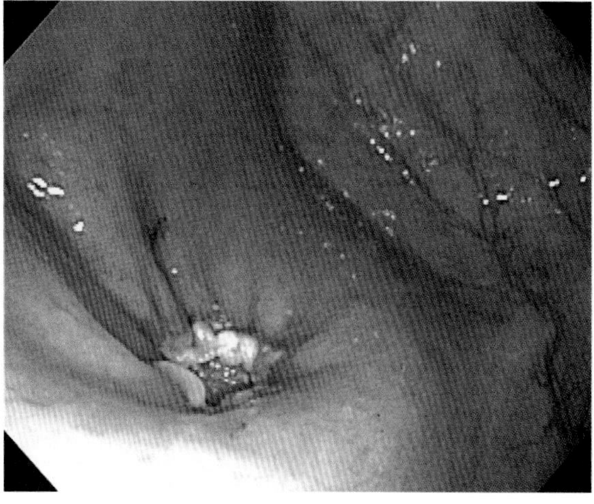

▲ **Plate 32.** Appearance immediately after polypectomy. Same patient as in Plate 30.

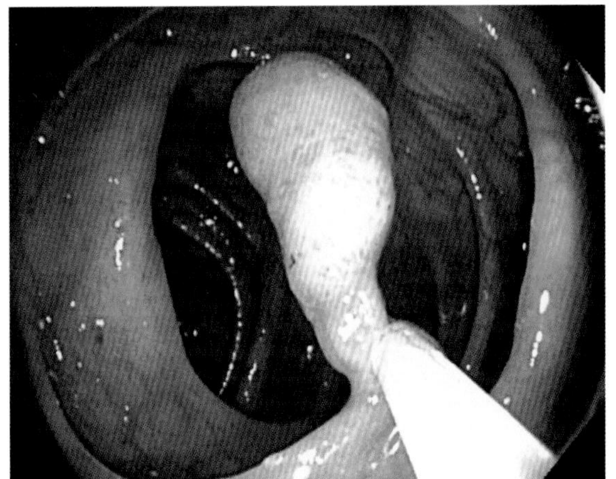

▲ **Plate 33.** Endoscopic view of a standard snare polypectomy for a pedunculated polyp.

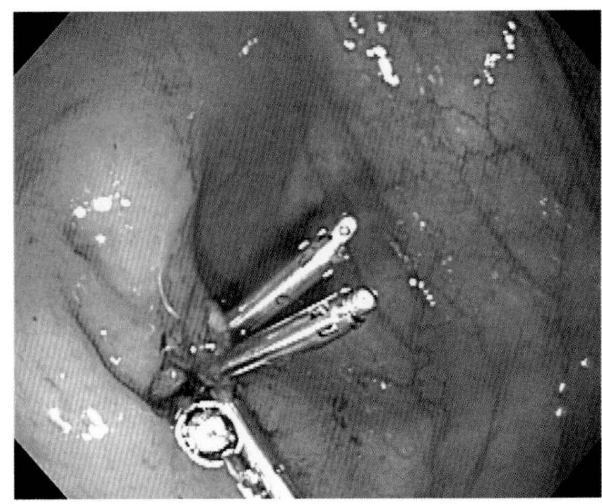

▲ **Plate 35.** Hemostatic clips applied after polypectomy for hemostasis and suspected perforation. Same patient as in Plate 30.

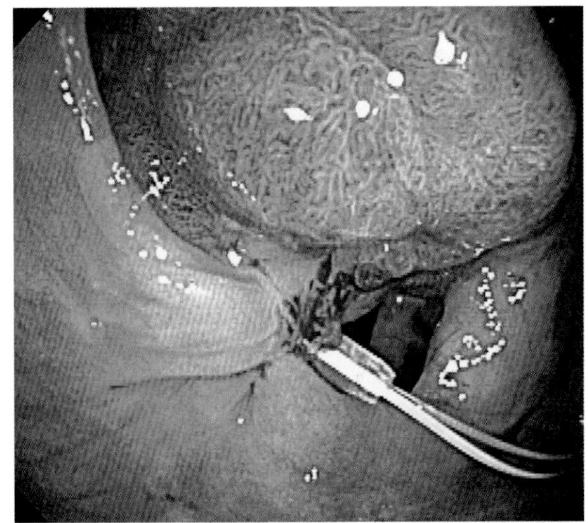

▲ **Plate 34.** Snare polypectomy for a large pedunculated polyp, with endoloop in place prior to snare resection.

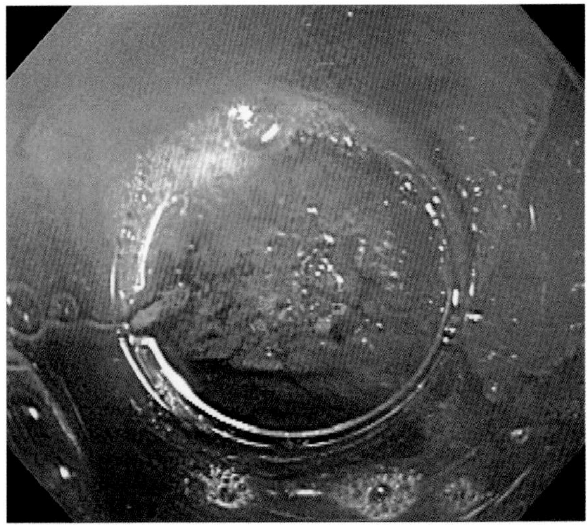

▲ **Plate 36.** Endoscopic mucosal resection: cap method with transparent cap positioned over irregular nodule in Barrett mucosa.

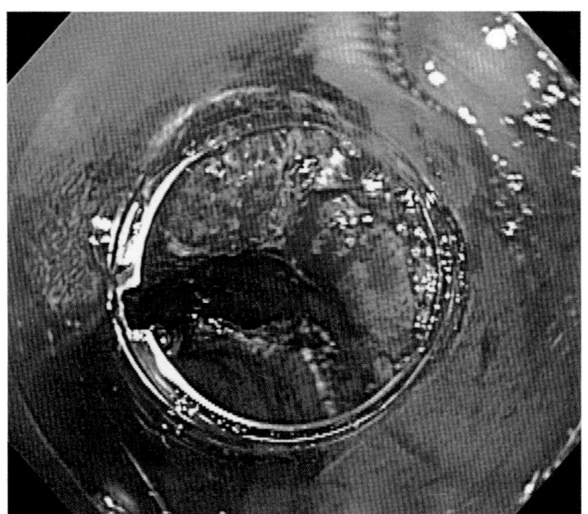

▲ **Plate 37.** Barrett nodule after suction and snare resection (snare not shown). Same patient as in Plate 36.

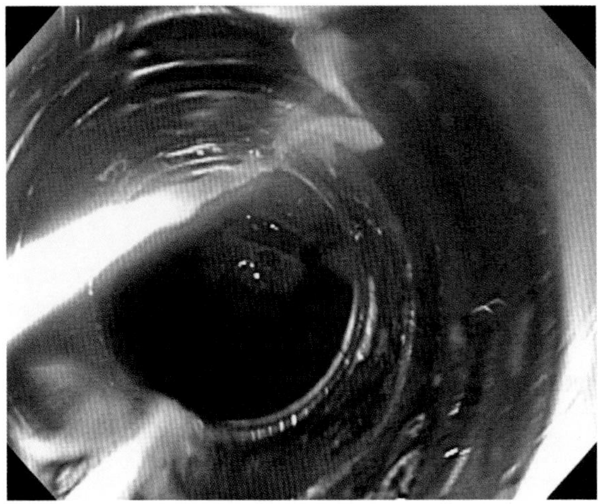

▲ **Plate 38.** Endoscopic mucosal resection: band ligation method with Barrett nodule ligated.

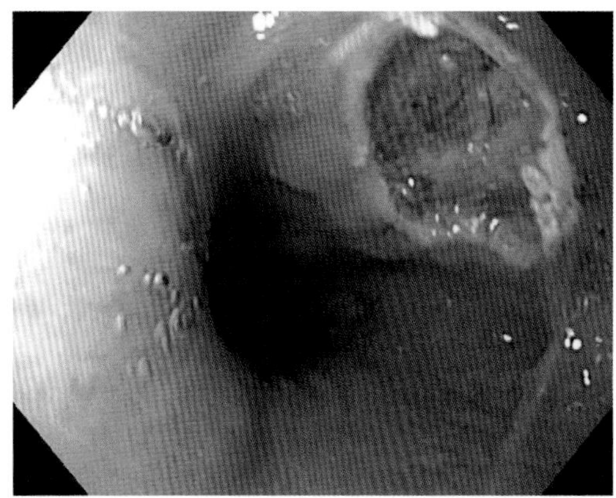

▲ **Plate 39.** Barrett nodule after snare resection. Same patient as in Plate 38. (Courtesy of Dr John R. Saltzman, Brigham and Women's Hospital.)

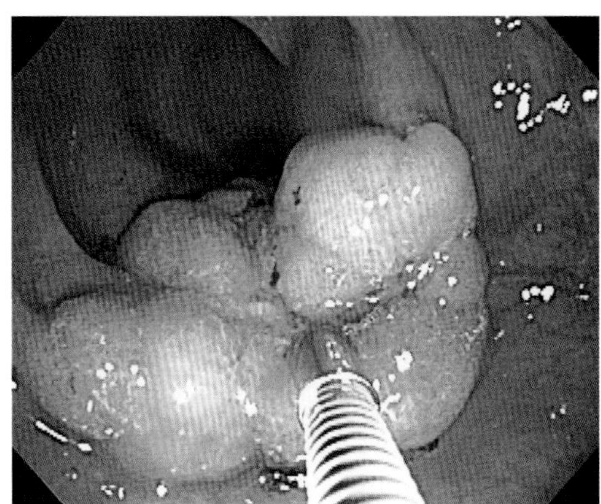

▲ **Plate 40.** Endoscopic mucosal resection: needle injection method.

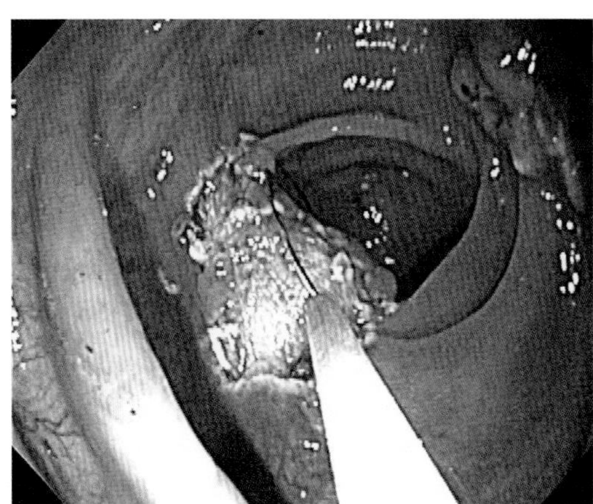

▲ **Plate 41.** Endoscopic mucosal resection: piecemeal snare polypectomy.

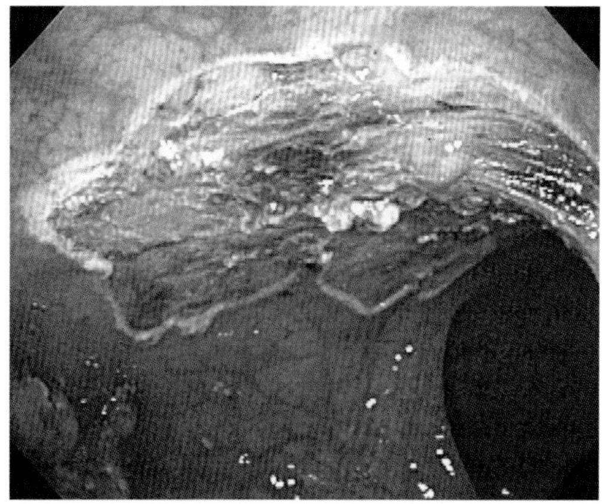

▲ **Plate 42.** Appearance after snare resection. Same patient as in Plate 41.

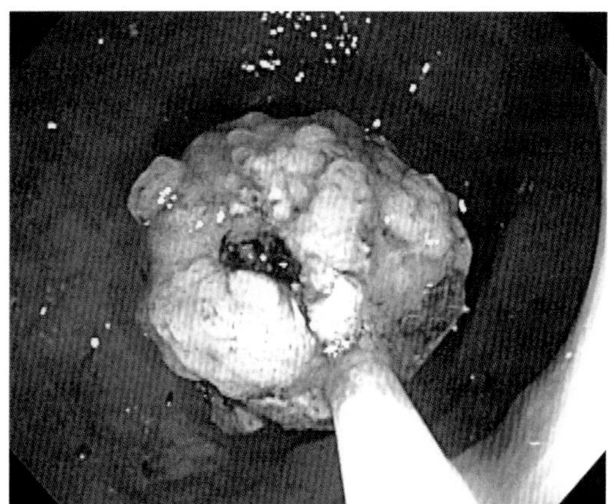

▲ **Plate 43.** Endoscopic mucosal resection: net retrieval of specimens.

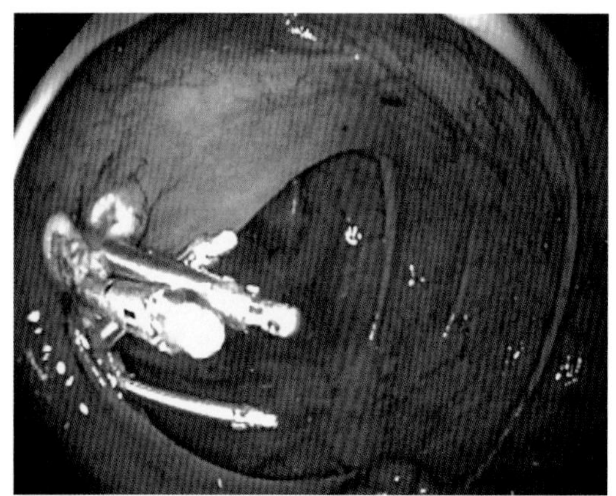

▲ **Plate 44.** Endoscopic mucosal resection: closure of the mucosal defect with clips.

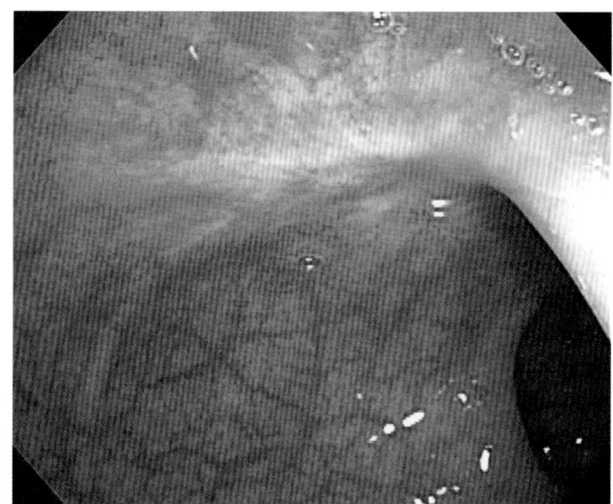

▲ **Plate 45.** Endoscopic mucosal resection: scar after 3 months.

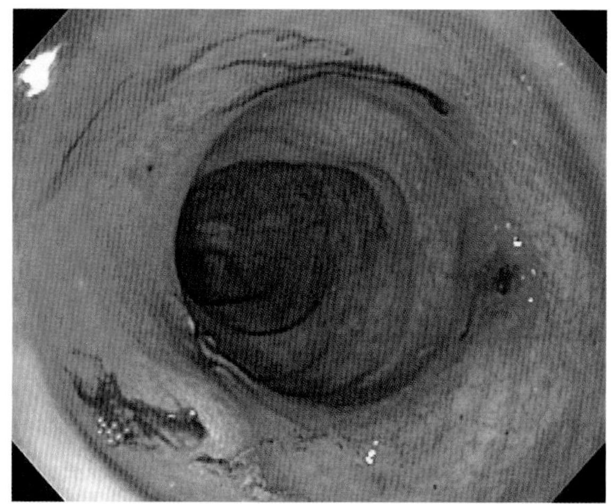

▲ **Plate 46.** Ink marking a polypectomy site.

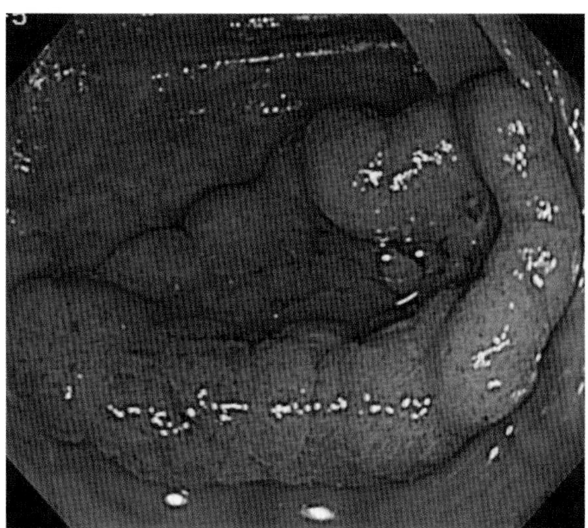

▲ **Plate 47.** Endoscopic submucosal dissection: large sessile polyp. (Used with permission from Professor Yutaka Saito, National Cancer Center Hospital, Tokyo, Japan.)

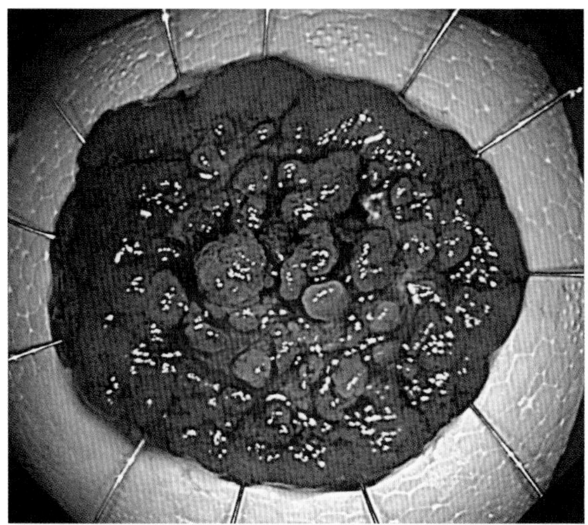

▲ **Plate 48.** Resected specimen in one piece. Same patient as in Plate 44. (Used with permission from Professor Yutaka Saito, National Cancer Center Hospital, Tokyo, Japan.)

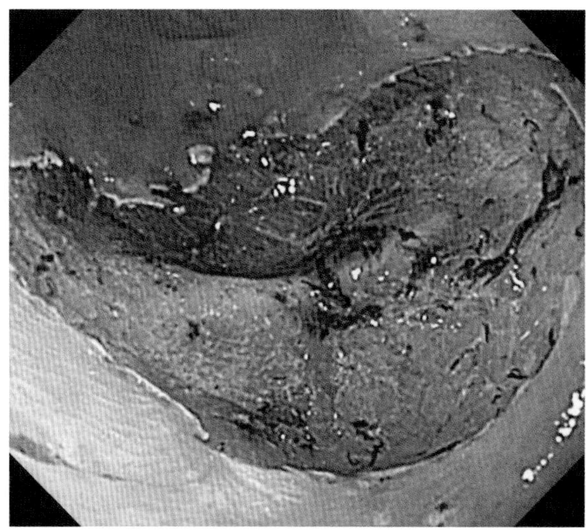

▲ **Plate 49.** Mucosal defect after endoscopic submucosal dissection. Same patient as in Plate 44. (Used with permission from Professor Yutaka Saito, National Cancer Center Hospital, Tokyo, Japan.)

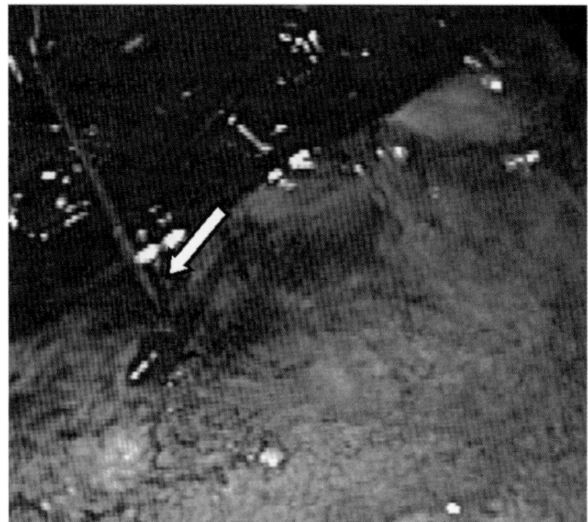

▲ **Plate 50.** Actively bleeding gastric ulcer.

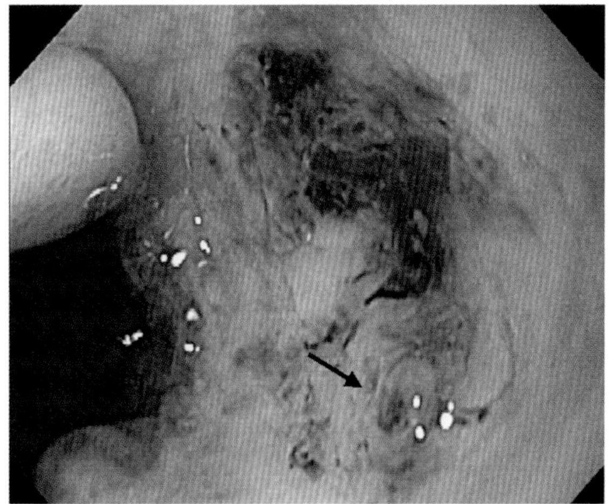

▲ **Plate 51.** Nonbleeding visible vessels. Giant duodenal ulcer occupying the entire duodenal bulb, with a nonbleeding visible vessel at bottom right (*arrow*).

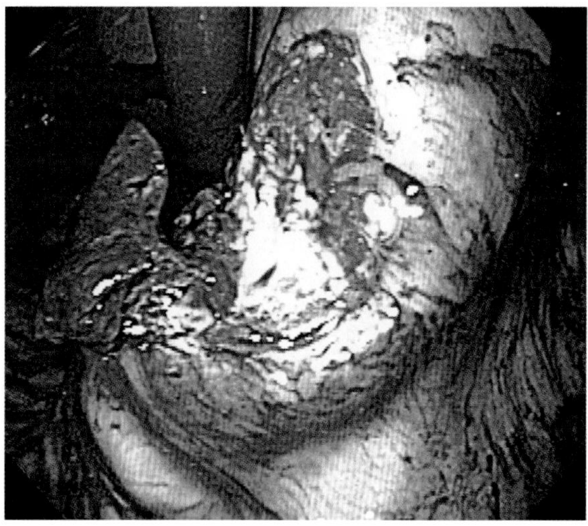

▲ **Plate 53.** Adherent clot on a gastric ulcer.

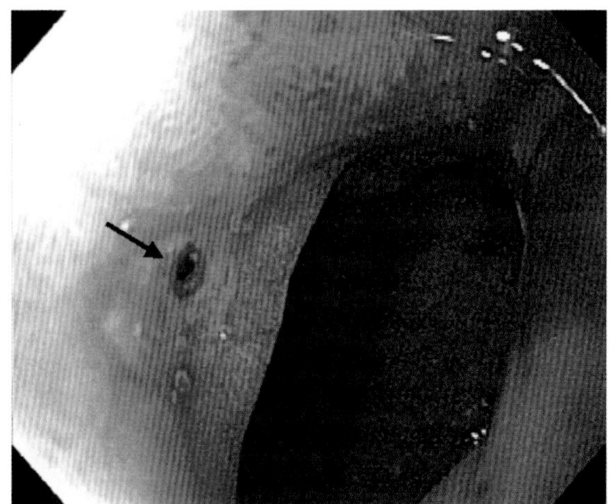

▲ **Plate 52.** Nonbleeding visible vessels. A pyloric channel ulcer with a pigmented, nonbleeding visible vessel (*arrow*).

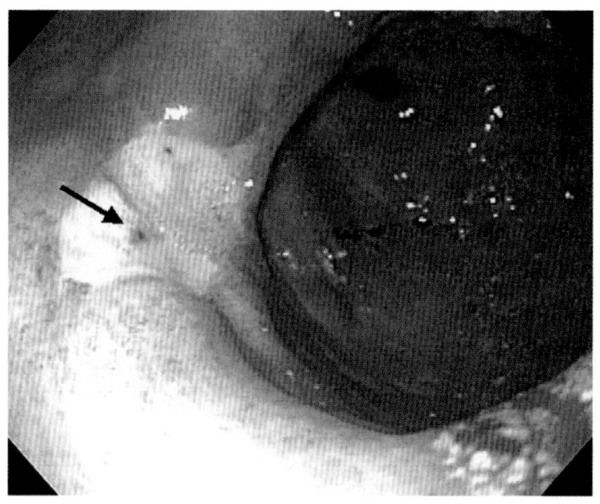

▲ **Plate 54.** Flat spot on a gastric ulcer (*arrow*).

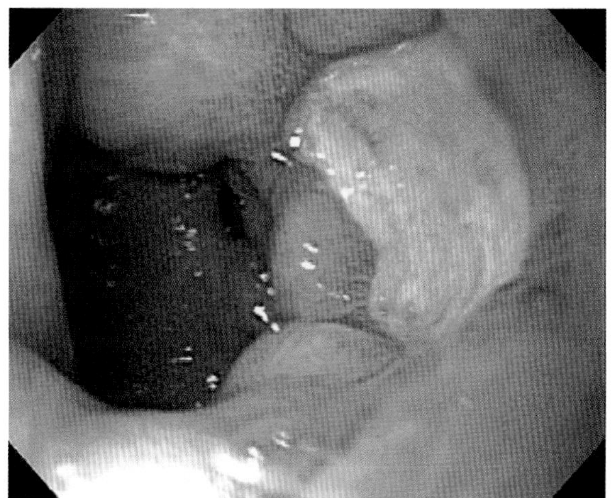

▲ **Plate 55.** Clean based prepyloric ulcer.

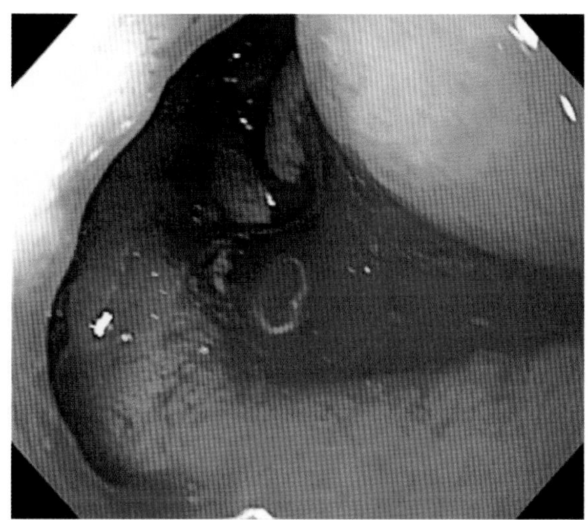

▲ **Plate 56.** Duodenal ulcer with active bleeding.

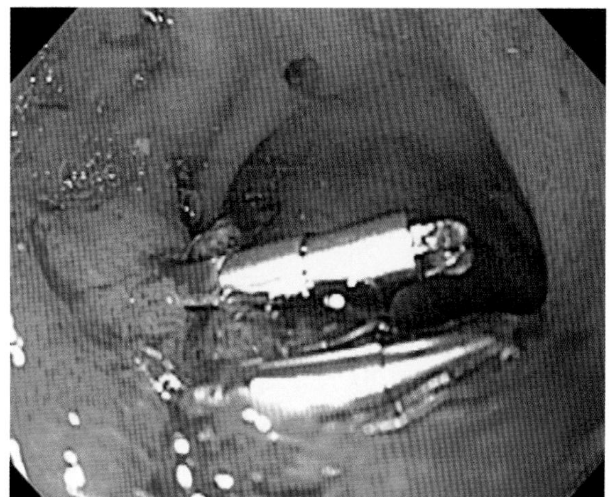

▲ **Plate 57.** Duodenal ulcer controlled by placement of two hemoclips.

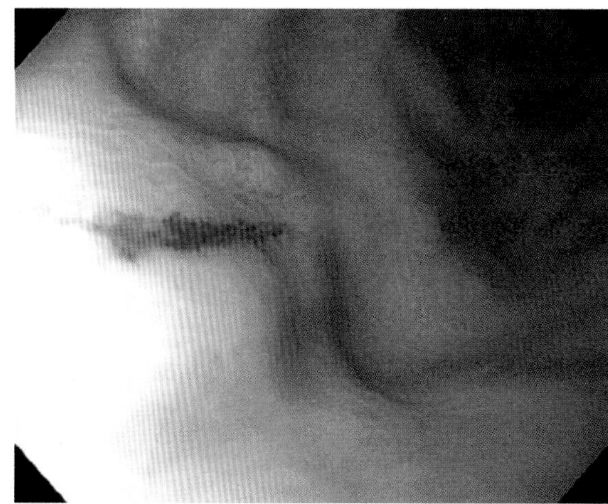

▲ **Plate 58.** Linear Mallory-Weiss tear just below the gastroesophageal junction.

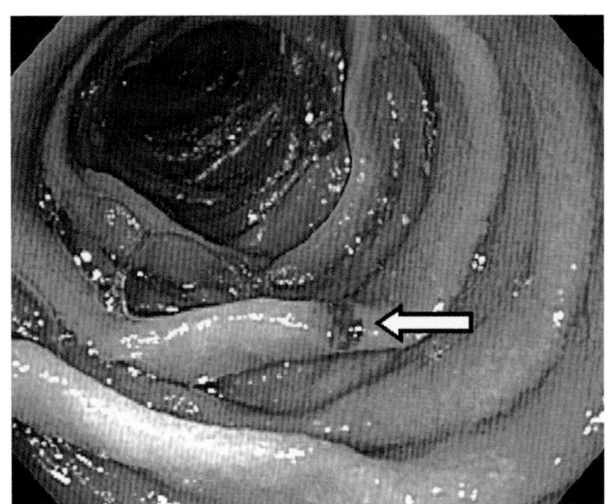

▲ **Plate 59.** Vascular malformation in the duodenum (*arrow*).

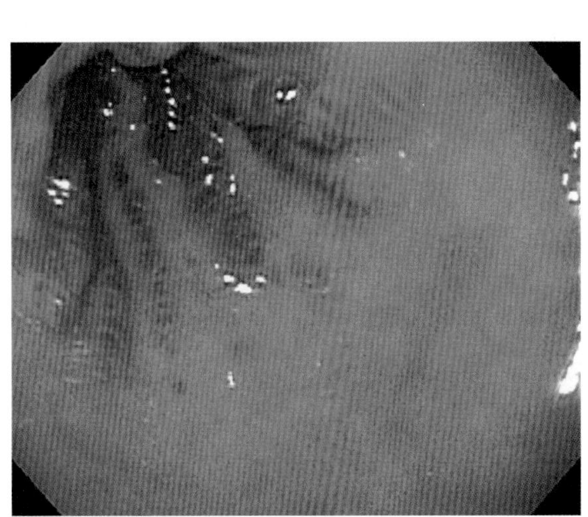

▲ **Plate 60.** Watermelon stomach.

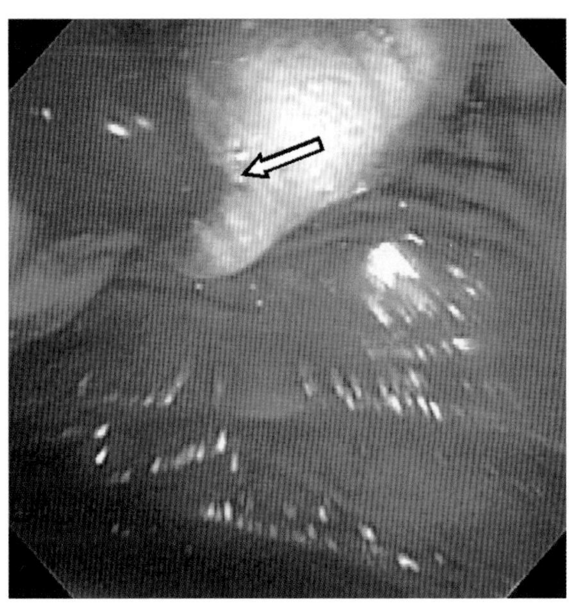

▲ **Plate 61.** Hemobilia with active bleeding and clots coming from ampullary orifice (*arrow*).

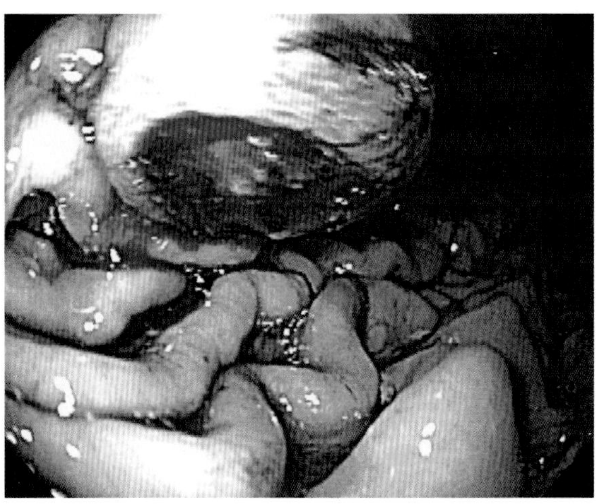

▲ **Plate 62.** Metastatic sarcoma to the stomach with active bleeding.

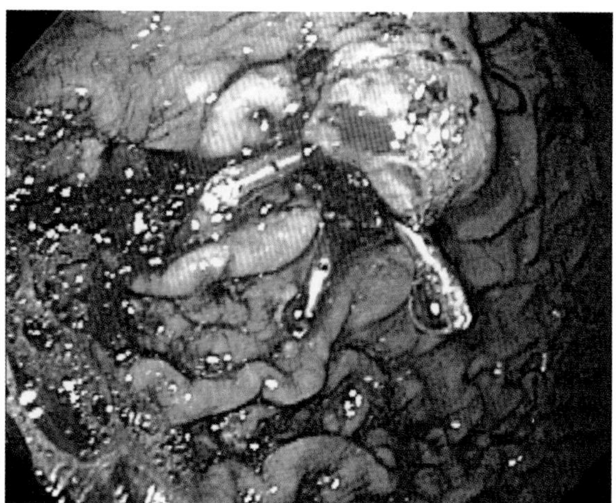

▲ **Plate 63.** Metastatic sarcoma treated by placement of hemoclips.

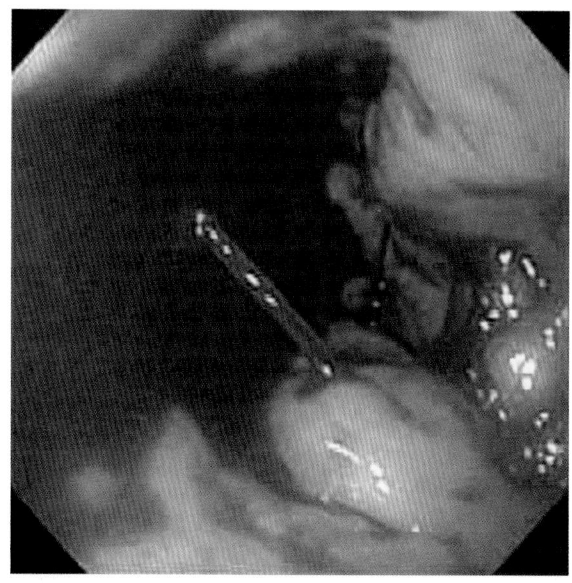

▲ **Plate 64.** Esophageal varices. Actively bleeding esophageal varix.

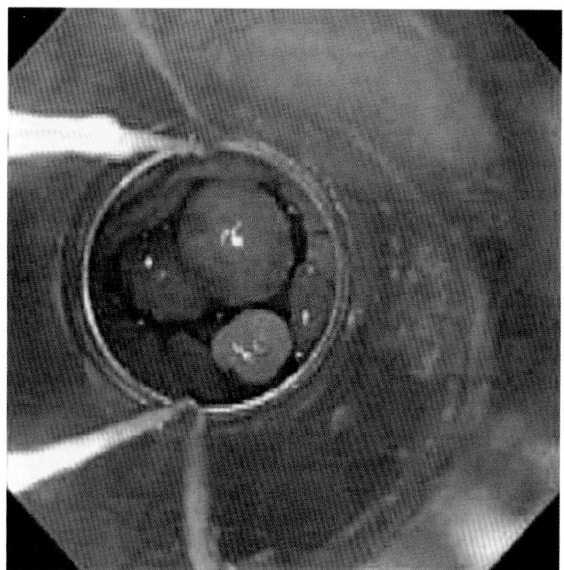

▲ **Plate 65.** Esophageal varices post-band ligation therapy.

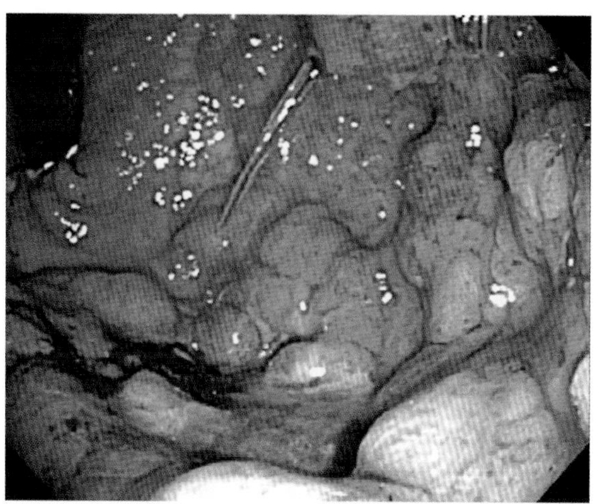

▲ **Plate 66.** Gastric varices in the body and fundus.

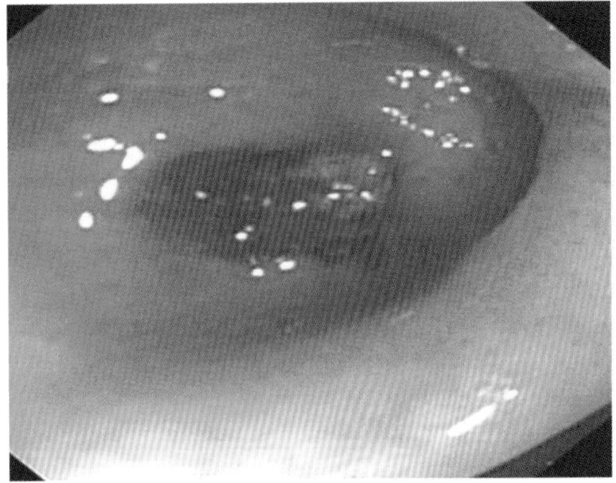

▲ Plate 67. Diverticulum with a large, oozing visible vessel.

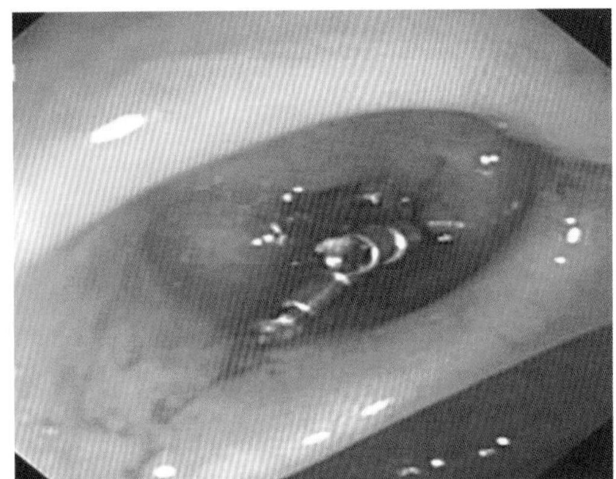

▲ Plate 68. Post-treatment of diverticulum with two endoclips.

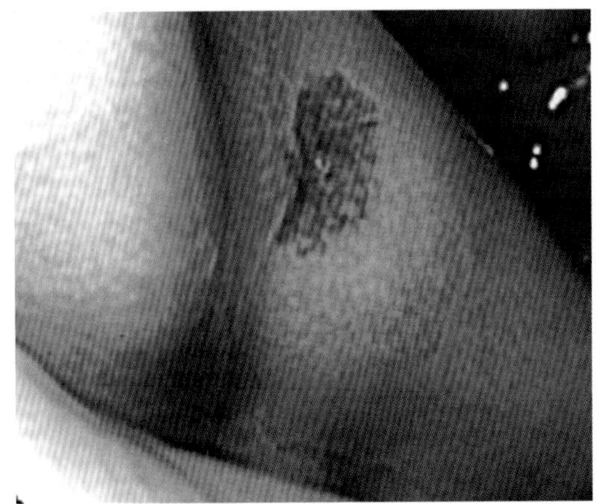

▲ Plate 69. Arteriovenous malformation in a patient with lower gastrointestinal bleeding.

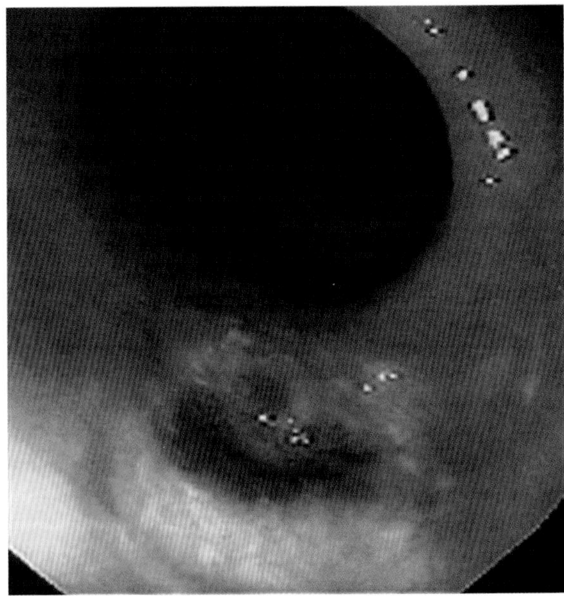

▲ Plate 70. Post-treatment of arteriovenous malformation with bipolar cautery.

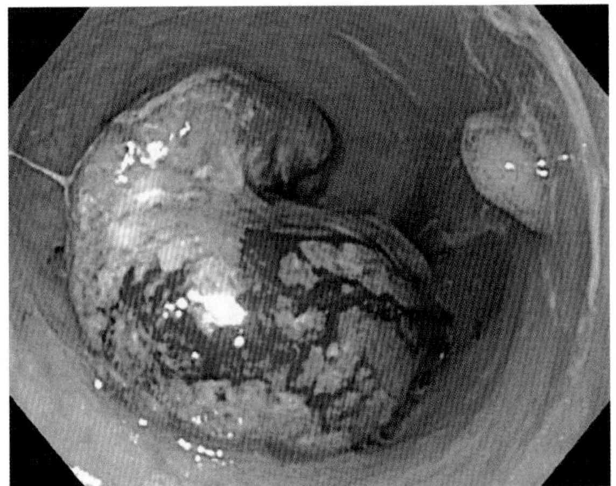

▲ Plate 71. Colon cancer.

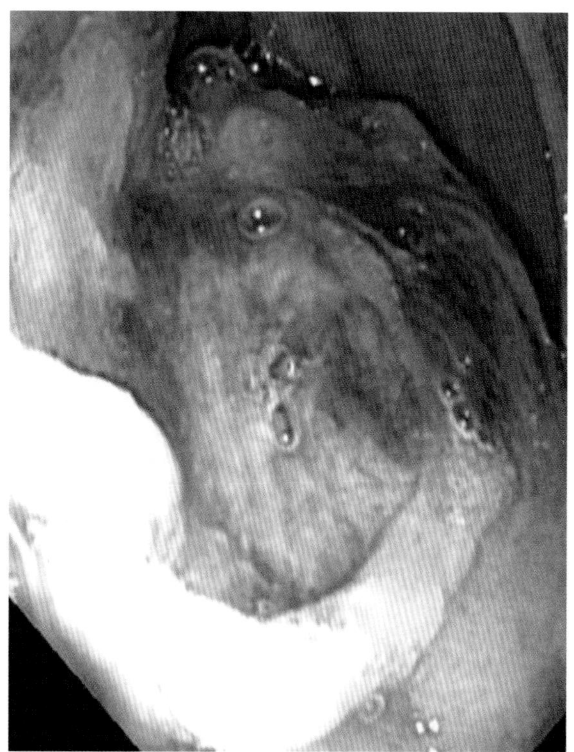

▲ **Plate 72.** Post-treatment with Tisseel fibrin glue.

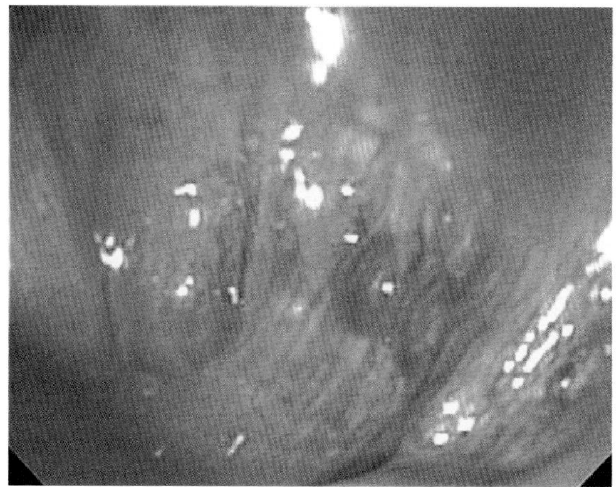

▲ **Plate 73.** Multiple internal hemorrhoids.

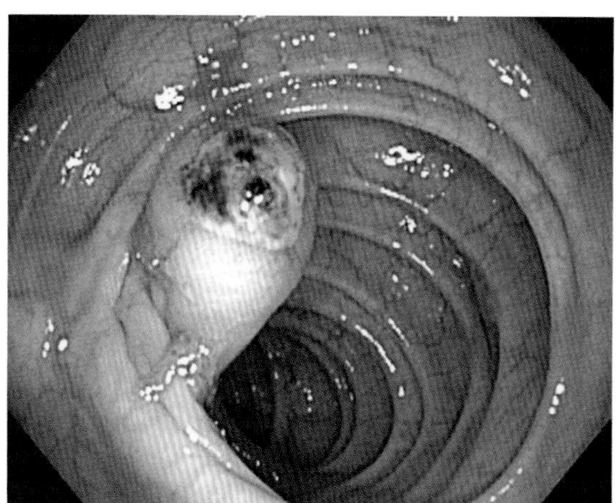

▲ **Plate 74.** Visible vessels at polypectomy site.

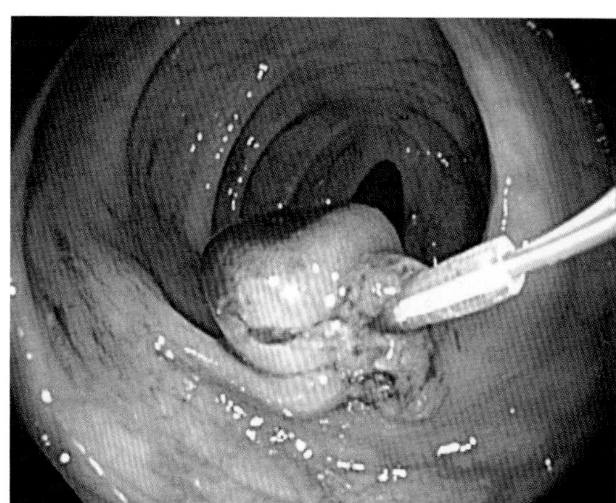

▲ **Plate 75.** Bleeding controlled with placement of an endoloop.

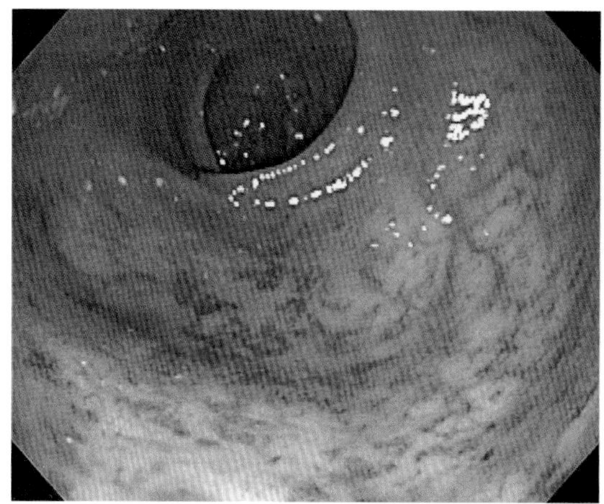

▲ **Plate 76.** Chronic radiation proctitis.

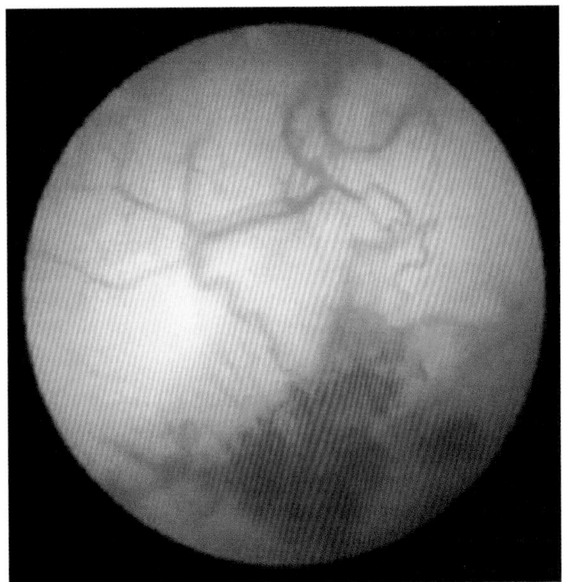

▲ **Plate 77.** Small bowel angioectasia.

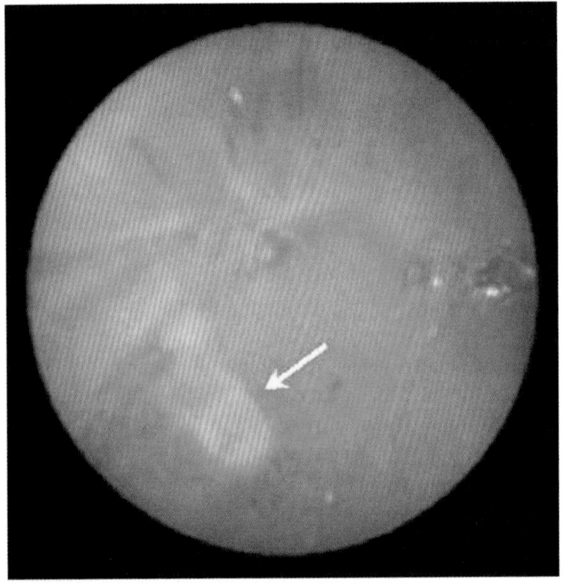

▲ **Plate 78.** Small bowel ulcer (NSAID associated).

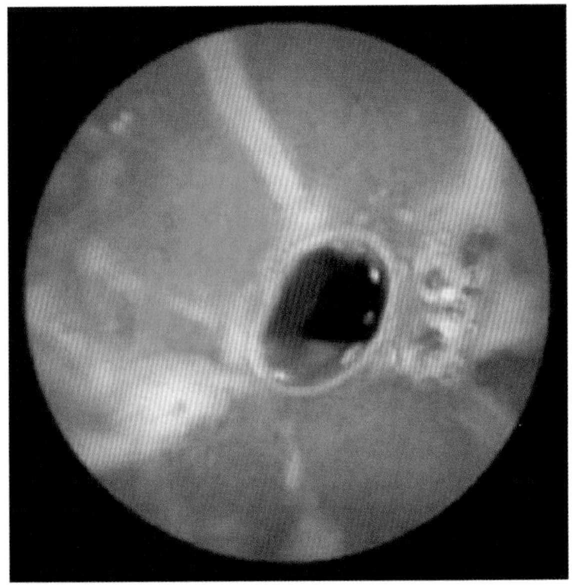

▲ **Plate 79.** Small bowel Crohn disease.

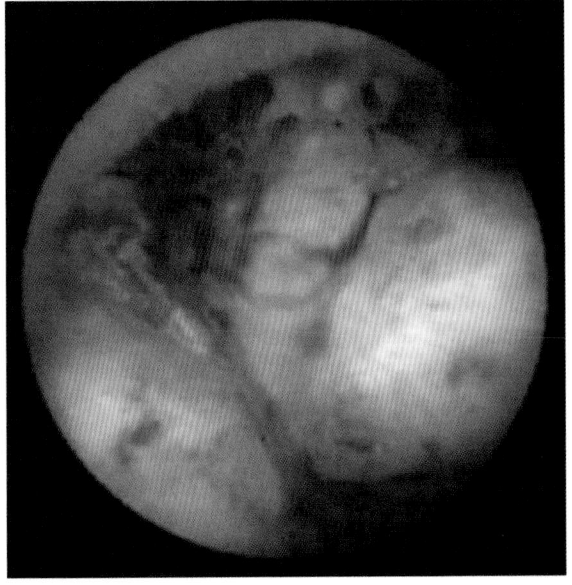

▲ **Plate 80.** Metastatic melanoma.

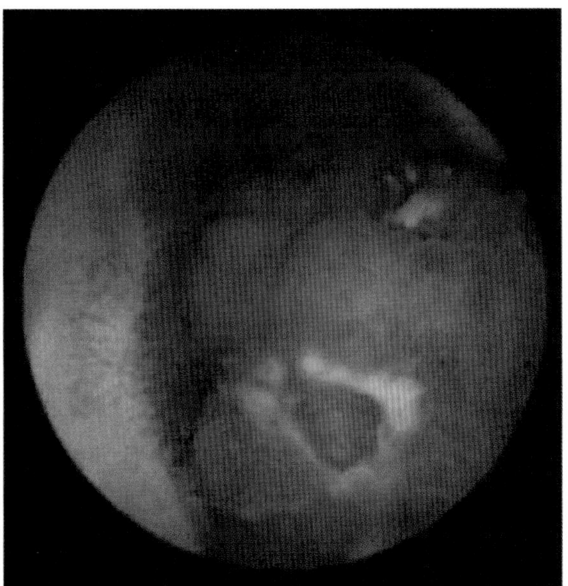

▲ **Plate 81.** Peutz-Jeghers polyp.

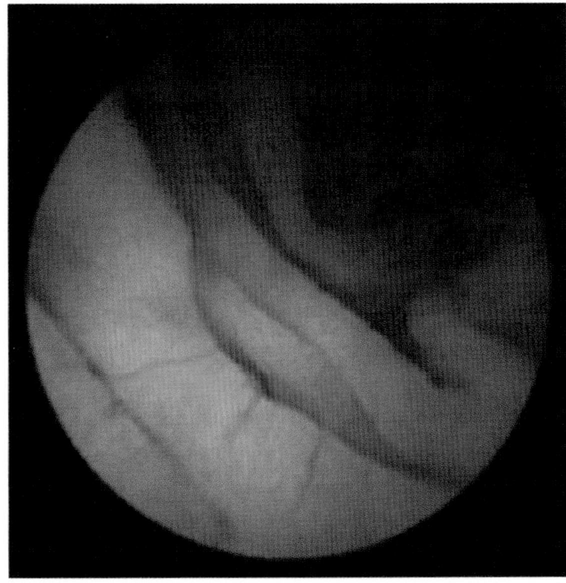

▲ **Plate 82.** Scalloping and mucosal fissures in celiac disease.

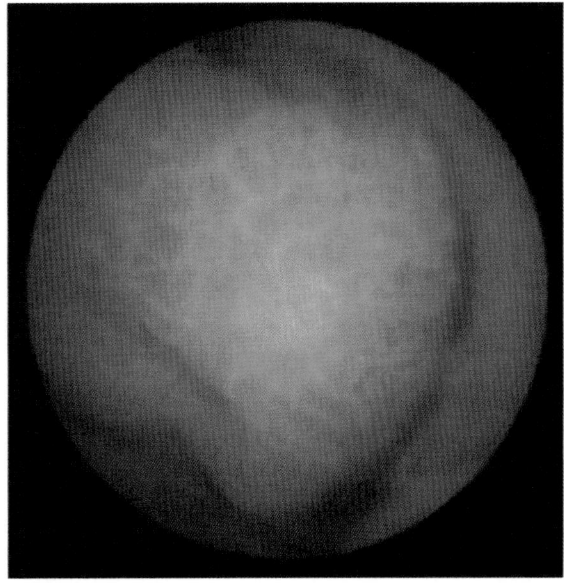

▲ **Plate 83.** Mosaic pattern of mucosa in celiac disease.

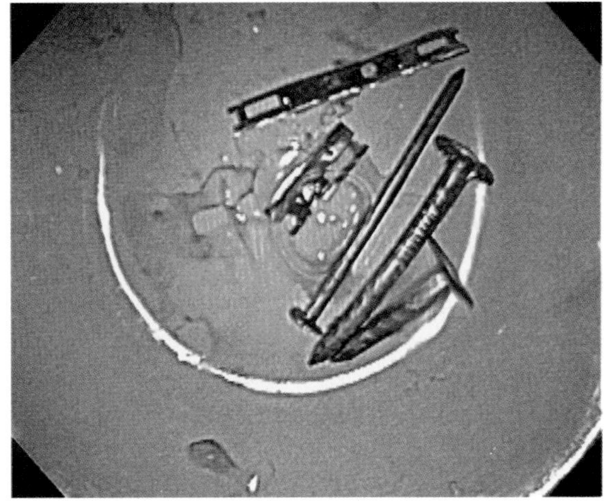

▲ **Plate 84.** Nails and razor blades in the stomach.

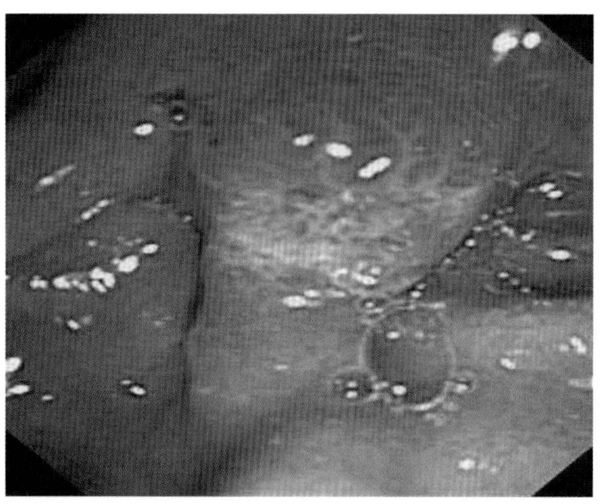

▲ **Plate 85.** Adenoma of the papilla.

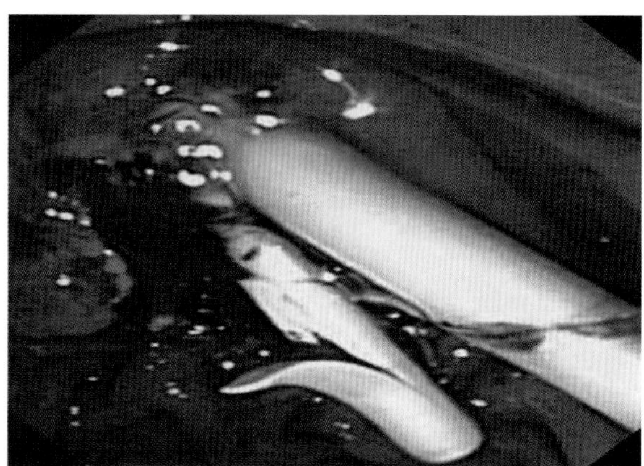

▲ **Plate 87.** Biliary and pancreatic stents in place.

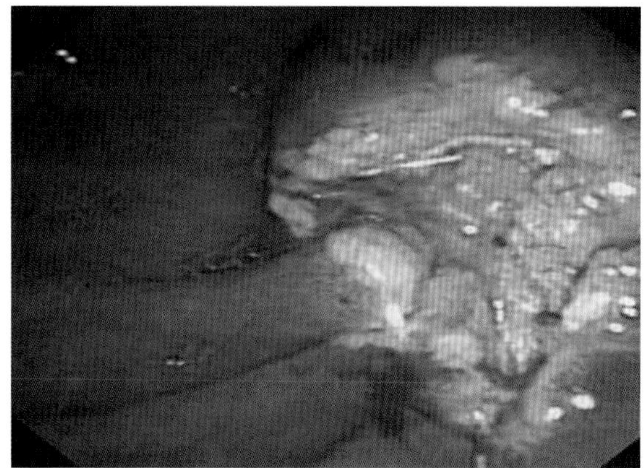

▲ **Plate 86.** Appearance immediately after papillectomy.

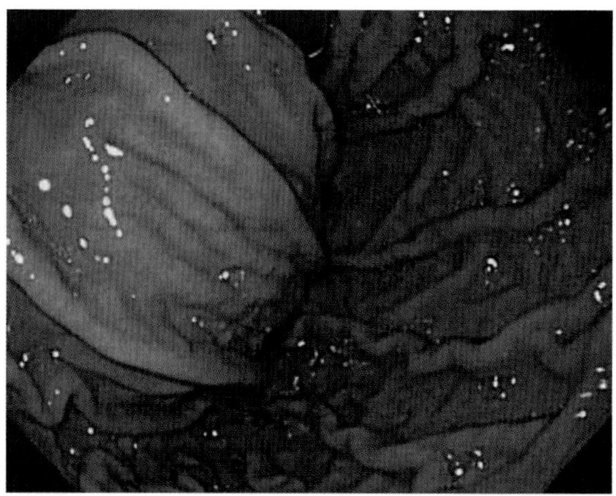

▲ **Plate 88.** Bulge along the proximal posterior gastric wall.

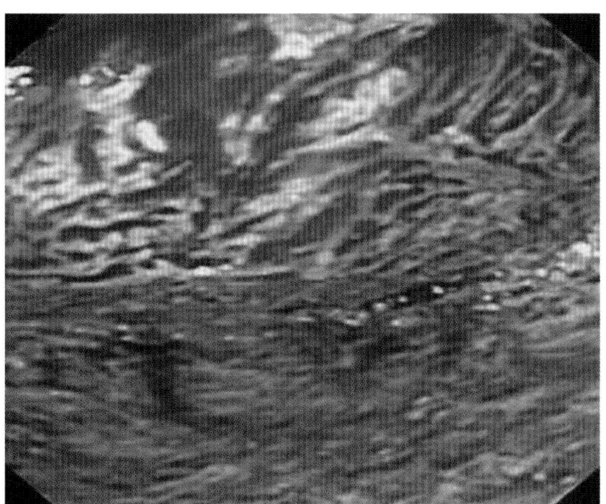

▲**Plate 89.** View inside a pseudocyst.

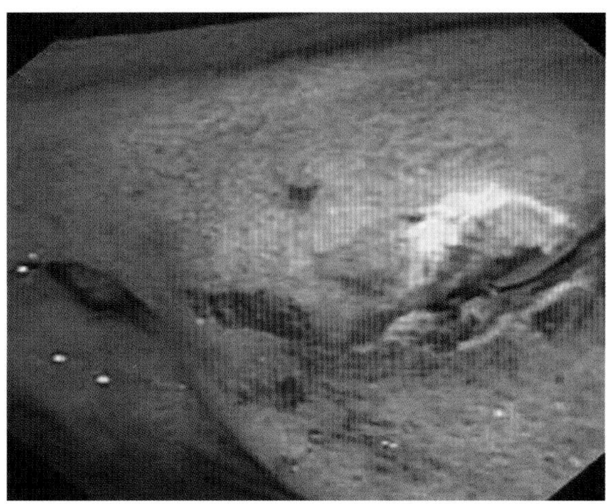

▲**Plate 91.** Endoscopic therapy for pancreas divisum showing minor papillotomy.

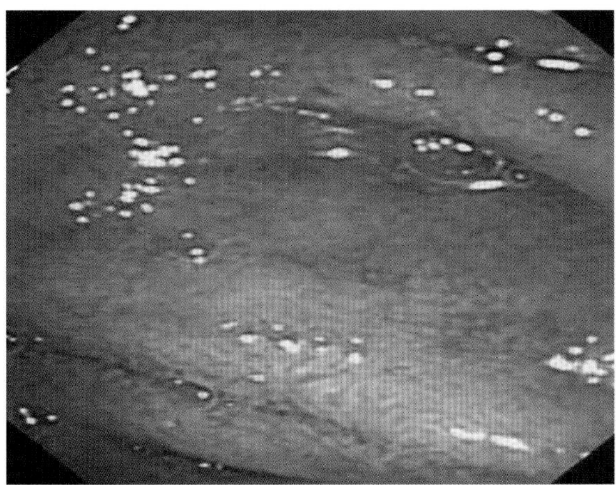

▲**Plate 90.** Endoscopic therapy for pancreas divisum showing minor papilla.

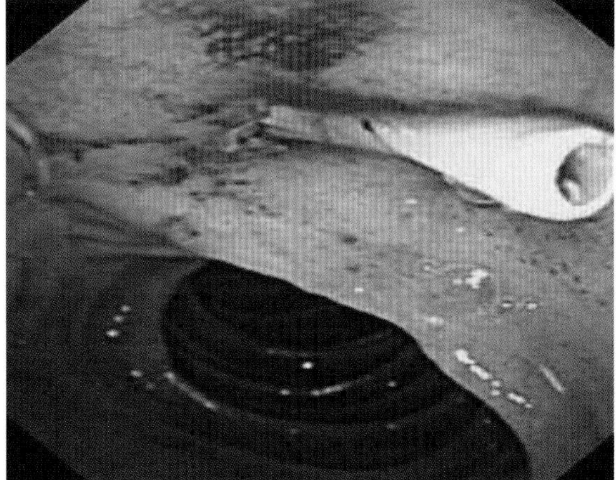

▲**Plate 92.** Endoscopic therapy for pancreas divisum showing stent placed across papillotomy.

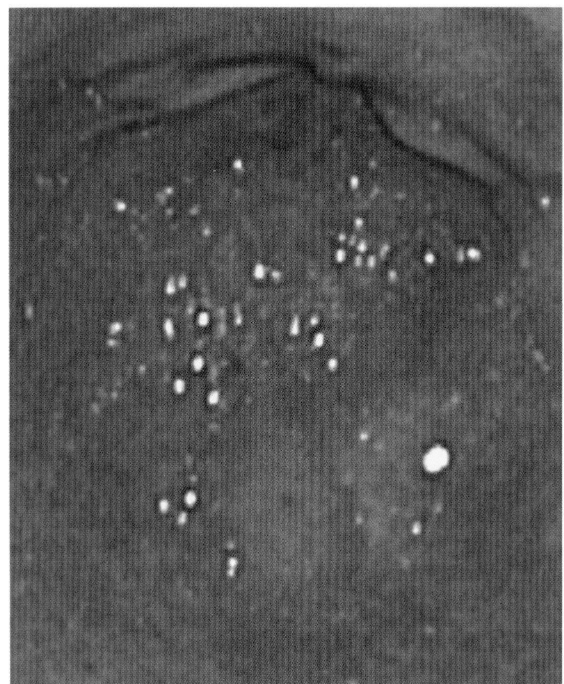

▲ **Plate 93.** Lipoma.

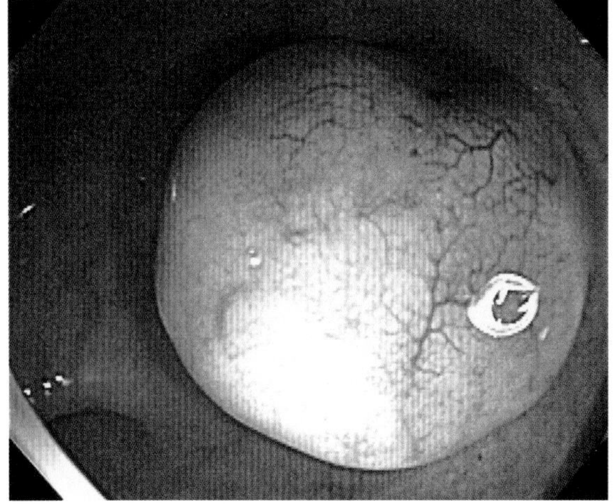

▲ **Plate 94.** Rectal carcinoid.

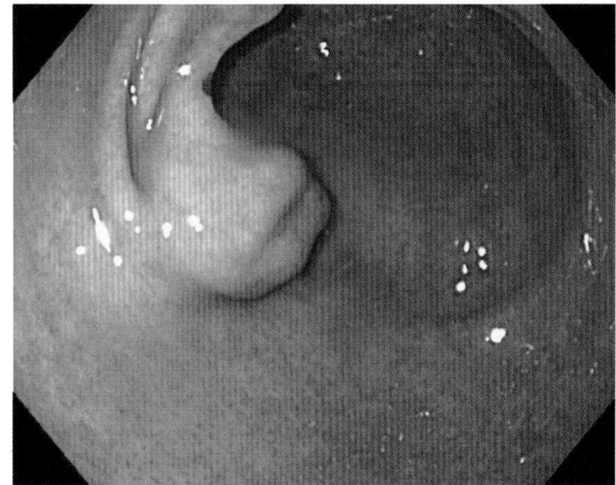

▲ **Plate 95.** Pancreatic rest.

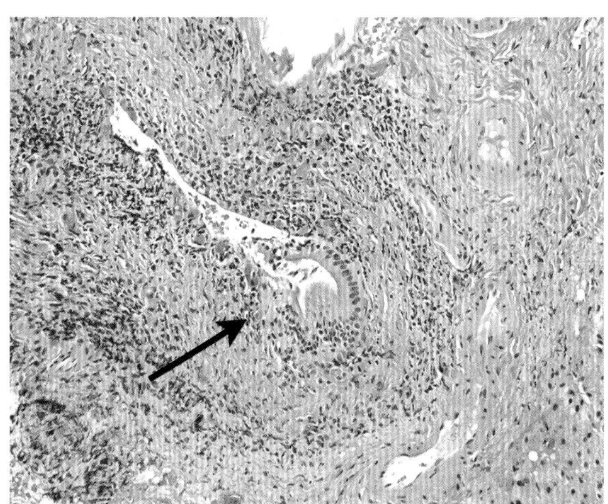

▲ **Plate 96.** Nonsuppurative destructive cholangitis. A large bile duct (*arrow*) shows lymphocytic inflammation and periductal ("onion-skin") fibrosis. (Used with permission from Jason L. Hornick, M.D., Ph.D., Brigham and Women's Hospital.)

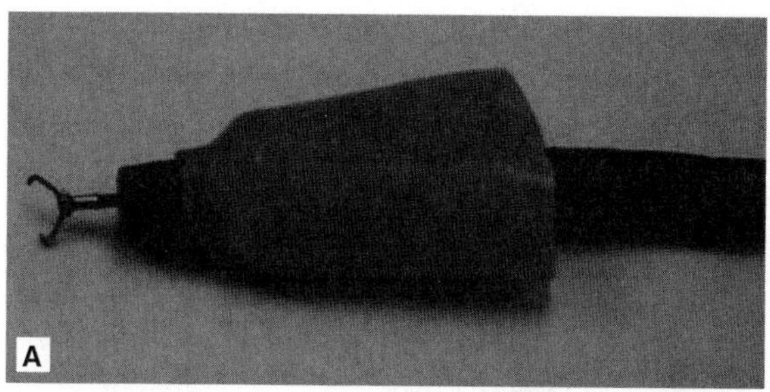

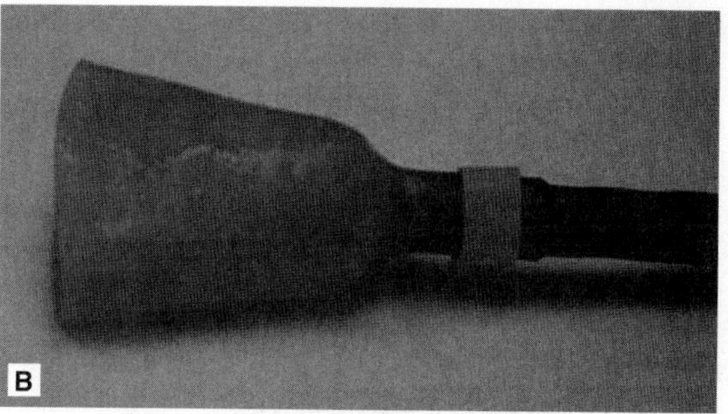

▲ **Figure 34–4.** Foreign body hood protector. **A:** Open configuration. **B:** Closed hood, following acquisition of a foreign body and withdrawal of the endoscope.

Athanassiadi K, Gerazounis M, Metaxas E, et al. Management of esophageal foreign bodies: a retrospective review of 400 cases. *Eur J Cardiothorac Surg.* 2002;21:653–656. [PMID: 11932163]

Ciriza C, García L, Suárez P, et al. What predictive parameters best indicate the need for emergent gastrointestinal endoscopy after foreign body ingestion? *J Clin Gastroenterol.* 2000;31:23–28. [PMID: 10914771]

Lin HH, Lee SC, Chu HC, et al. Emergency endoscopic management of dietary foreign bodies in the esophagus. *Am J Emerg Med.* 2007;25:662–665. [PMID: 17606092]

Yong PT, Teh CH, Look M, et al. Removal of a dinner fork from the stomach by double-snare endoscopic extraction. *Hong Kong Med J.* 2000;6:319–21. [PMID: 11025854]

Endoscopic Retrograde Cholangiopancreatography (ERCP)

Linda S. Lee, MD
David L. Carr-Locke, MA, MD, DRCOG, FRCP, FASGE

General Considerations

Endoscopic retrograde cholangiopancreatography (ERCP) (Figure 35–1) is a combined endoscopic and fluoroscopic procedure that was introduced in the early 1970s to allow access to the biliary and pancreatic ductal systems and their openings at the major and minor duodenal papillae. ERCP has evolved from a purely diagnostic technique, performed by a few, into a complex set of procedures integrating diagnosis and therapy for a wide variety of pancreatobiliary disorders offered in all major medical centers. ERCP requires dedicated training in order to acquire the range of techniques that include endoscopic papillectomy, sphincter of Oddi manometry, biliary sphincterotomy, pancreatic sphincterotomy, stone removal, tissue sampling, placement of plastic and metallic stents, and drainage of pancreatic fluid collections. Although it has become a highly successful therapeutic modality, ERCP also carries an overall morbidity of 7% that includes pancreatitis (4%), hemorrhage (1%), cholangitis (1%), perforation (0.5%), and death (0.1%). With the advent of magnetic resonance cholangiopancreatography (MRCP) (Figure 35–2) which safely and noninvasively images the pancreatic and biliary tracts, the need for purely diagnostic ERCP has appropriately diminished considerably while the demands for therapy have grown.

Baron T, Kozarek RA, Carr-Locke DL. *ERCP*. Elsevier Saunders, 2007.

DISORDERS OF THE MAJOR DUODENAL PAPILLA

1. Adenoma & Carcinoma

Small intestinal tumors represent 2.4% of all gastrointestinal malignancies and over half of these are found in the duodenum. Duodenal adenomas may occur sporadically or in 50–100% of patients with familial adenomatous polyposis (FAP) and are most commonly in the periampullary location. Papillary adenomas may be detected as an incidental finding during upper endoscopy performed for another indication or may manifest with recurrent pancreatitis, weight loss, or biliary obstruction. The frequency of carcinoma in papillary adenomas ranges from 30% to 65%.

Adenomas of the papilla follow the adenoma–carcinoma sequence similar to that seen in the colon; thus, resection of these lesions is recommended. Traditionally, the approach was surgical resection by pancreaticoduodenectomy because the presence of malignancy could not be completely excluded based on preoperative biopsies. Due to significant morbidity, even with improvements in surgery, endoscopic resection is currently the treatment of choice. Since the first reports of endoscopic resection of the papilla in the early 1990s, endoscopic papillectomy or ampullectomy has gained wider acceptance as a less invasive therapy.

Accurate preoperative diagnosis and staging of papillary lesions is essential. ERCP with biopsies and endoscopic ultrasound are the current accepted approach for diagnosis and staging of local invasion and assessment of lymph node status. Invasive cancer is a contraindication to endoscopic resection. Inoperable ampullary cancer causing biliary obstruction is best treated by sphincterotomy if feasible or by placement of a self-expanding metal stent.

The technique of ampullectomy involves inspection of the papilla with a side-viewing duodenoscope, and ERCP to define any intraductal tumor extension and to opacify the ducts with contrast to aid in identifying the ductal orifices after the procedure is completed. Most experts resect the papilla and some surrounding normal mucosa en bloc with an electrocautery polypectomy snare and retrieve the specimen for histopathologic examination. Residual adenomatous tissue at the margins of the resection site can be ablated with contact thermal or noncontact argon plasma coagulation. After resection, a short polyethylene pancreatic stent is placed to minimize the risk of post-procedural pancreatitis,

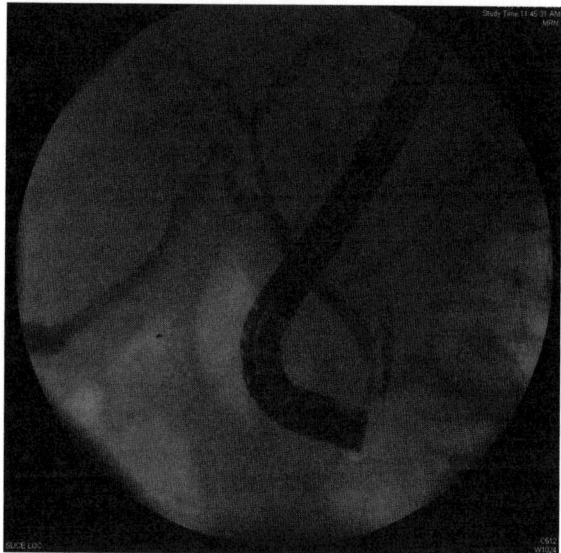

▲ **Figure 35–1.** ERCP radiograph showing standard endoscope position and normal biliary and pancreatic ductal systems.

and many endoscopists also place a biliary stent if a sphincterotomy has not been performed (Plates 85, 86, and 87). The stents are endoscopically removed about 1 month later, and the site is inspected for residual adenoma. Surveillance endoscopy with a duodenoscope is offered every 6–12 months.

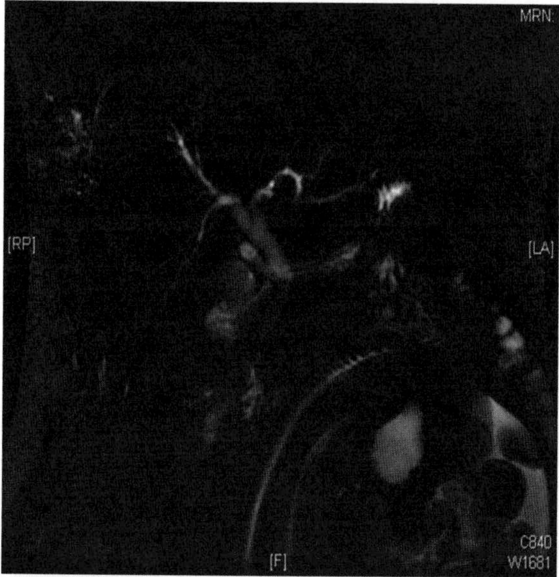

▲ **Figure 35–2.** MRCP image showing small distal common bile duct stones during late pregnancy.

Kahaleh M, Shami VM, Brock A, et al. Factors predictive of malignancy and endoscopic resectability in ampullary neoplasia. *Am J Gastroenterol.* 2004;99:2335–2339. [PMID: 15571579]

2. Sphincter of Oddi Dysfunction

The sphincter of Oddi is a complex muscular structure that surrounds the distal pancreatic duct, bile duct, and ampulla of Vater. This sphincter mechanism lies mostly within the duodenal wall and measures 6–10 mm in length. Functionally, the sphincter of Oddi is independent from the duodenal smooth muscle system. It serves to prevent reflux of duodenal contents into the ductal system and controls the flow of bile and pancreatic juice into the duodenum.

Sphincter of Oddi dysfunction (SOD) describes an abnormality within the sphincter, either motility related (dyskinesia or spasm) or structural (stenosis), and can involve the biliary sphincter, the pancreatic sphincter, or both. In pancreatic-type SOD, patients typically present with episodic pancreatic-type epigastric pain radiating to the back with pancreatic enzyme abnormalities or frank acute pancreatitis. The more common biliary-type SOD occurs postcholecystectomy and patients experience abdominal pain similar to the preoperative pain of suspected biliary origin. Each type of SOD has three subtypes:

- Biliary-I patients have biliary-type pain, abnormal liver enzyme values greater than twice normal, documented on two or more occasions with normalization in between attacks, and dilated common bile duct greater than 8 mm diameter.
- Biliary-II patients have biliary-type pain but only one or two of the preceding criteria.
- Biliary-III patients have only biliary-type pain and no other abnormalities.
- Pancreatic-I patients have recurrent pancreatitis or typical pancreatic pain, elevated pancreatic enzymes 1.5–2 times the upper limit, and dilated pancreatic duct greater than 5 mm.
- Pancreatic-II patients have pancreatic pain and one or two of the above criteria.
- Pancreatic-III patients have only pancreatic-type pain.

Sphincter function can be evaluated by noninvasive methods that include hepatobiliary scintigraphy, ultrasound assessment of pancreatic and bile duct after secretin or cholecystokinin stimulation, and secretin-stimulated MRCP. The gold standard diagnostic test for SOD, however, is manometric assessment of basal sphincter pressure by sphincter of Oddi manometry (SOM), which involves the use of solid state or perfusion low-compliance catheters that can measure the biliary and pancreatic sphincter pressures through ports located at the distal end. Multiple station pull-throughs are performed and graphic recording of the pressures are displayed on a dedicated workstation. The patient must be sedated for the procedure, but narcotics and smooth muscle relaxants are usually avoided as they may interfere with the recordings. A basal sphincter pressure greater than 40 mm Hg above duodenal pressure is considered to be abnormal, and sphincterotomy (incision of the intraduodenal portion of the common bile duct or pancreatic duct sphincter muscle) is the current standard treatment of choice for SOD in the appropriate clinical setting.

Symptomatic patients with type I SOD benefit from sphincterotomy (90–100%) regardless of manometry findings. Thus, manometry is not required for this group of patients. In type II SOD, 50–70% of patients with elevated basal sphincter pressure on manometry will benefit from sphincterotomy while only 20–40% of patients with type III SOD and elevated basal sphincter pressure on SOM benefit from sphincter ablation.

The rate of complications is high in patients with suspected SOD undergoing ERCP with pancreatitis being most common and occurring up to 20–40%. The risk of pancreatitis is reduced by temporary stenting of the pancreatic duct.

Behar J, Corazziari E, Guelrud M, Hogan W, Sherman S, Toouli J. Functional gallbladder and sphincter of oddi dysfunction. *Gastroenterology*. 2006;130:1498–1509. [PMID: 16678563]

Sgouros SN, Pereira SP. Systematic review: sphincter of oddi dysfunction—non-invasive diagnostic methods and long-term outcome after endoscopic sphincterotomy. *Aliment Pharmacol Ther*. 2006;24:237–246. [PMID: 16842450]

BILIARY SYSTEM

1. Bile Duct Stones

Bile duct stones occur in up to 15% of symptomatic patients with cholelithiasis and in up to 2% of cholecystectomies performed for acalculous biliary disease. Patients may present with abdominal pain of biliary origin, cholangitis (see Chapter 32 on Biliary Emergencies), jaundice, pancreatitis, transient elevation of transaminases, or filling defect with or without biliary ductal dilation on imaging studies such as transabdominal ultrasound, computed tomography (CT), and MRCP. When choledocholithiasis is suspected, therapy is directed toward extraction of the stones from the biliary tree to minimize serious complications such as severe pancreatitis, sepsis, and death. Stone extraction can be achieved endoscopically, surgically, or by the transhepatic approach radiologically.

Endoscopic removal of bile duct stones is the treatment of choice in centers with expertise in this technique (Figure 35–3). Since the first descriptions of endoscopic sphincterotomy in 1974, the role of ERCP in the management of bile duct stones has undergone tremendous growth. The standard techniques of stone extraction require access to the bile duct by deep cannulation. Once stones are identified on a cholangiogram, a biliary sphincterotomy is usually performed under direct endoscopic guidance to the maximum extent of endoscopic landmarks using a bow-type sphincterotome, a catheter carrying a cutting electrosurgical wire at its distal end.

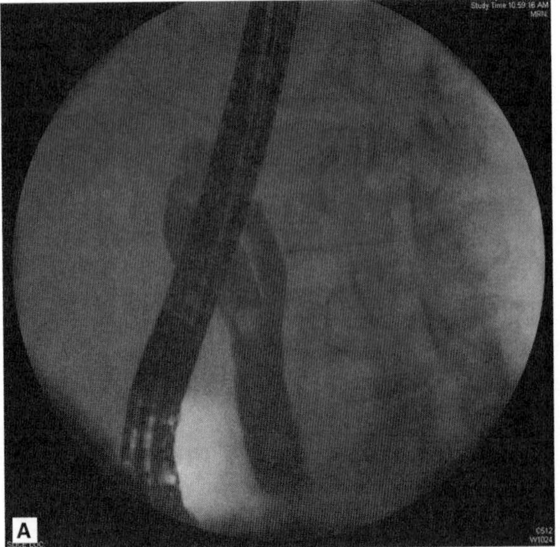

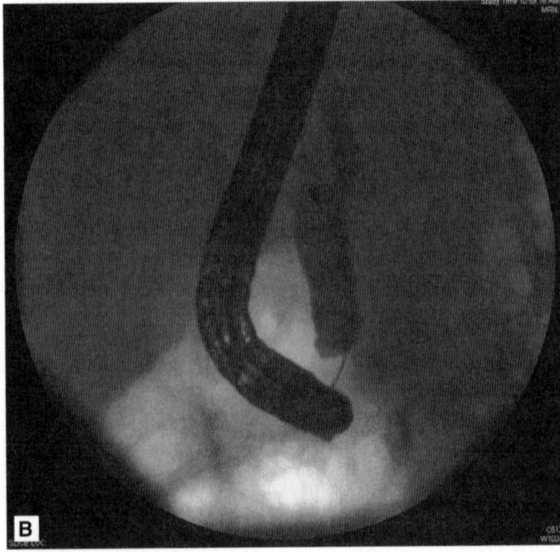

▲ **Figure 35–3.** ERCP images showing (**A**) bile duct stones being extracted by (**B**) basket.

An attempt at stone extraction should always be made after biliary sphincterotomy except in urgent, unstable situations. The most commonly used accessories for this purpose are balloon catheters and metal wire baskets (see Figure 35–3). These standard techniques can achieve success in up to 90% of bile duct stones while the remaining 10% of cases require more advanced techniques. In particular, stones larger than 15 mm present a challenge and often require additional endoscopic techniques such as mechanical, electrohydraulic, or laser lithotripsy. When complete stone removal fails, insertion of a biliary stent provides temporary drainage, minimizing the risk of biliary sepsis, before further endoscopic attempts at duct clearance can be made. This stenting approach can lead to over 90% success at stone clearance following two ERCP attempts.

Multivariate analysis of large series of sphincterotomies has shown that five risk factors for complications are significant: suspected SOD, cirrhosis, difficult bile duct cannulation, precut (access) papillotomy, and use of a combined percutaneous-endoscopic procedure. The rate of complications was highest when the indication for the procedure was suspected SOD (22%) and lowest when the indication was removal of bile duct stones within 30 days of laparoscopic cholecystectomy (5%). Endoscopists who performed more than one sphincterotomy per week had lower rates of all complications (8.4% vs 11.1%, $P = 0.03$) and severe complications (0.9% vs 2.3%, $P = 0.01$) than those who did less then one per week.

As an alternative to sphincterotomy, endoscopic balloon dilation of the papilla was introduced in the 1980s. This involves the use of a hydrostatic balloon positioned across the papilla and inflated under high pressure while dilation is monitored fluoroscopically. Endoscopic balloon dilation alone in the treatment of bile duct stones is associated with higher rates of pancreatitis (7.4%) compared to sphincterotomy (4.3%) and need for mechanical lithotripsy (20.9% vs 14.8%). This technique is used regularly in Southeast Asia without high morbidity, but due to increased incidence of pancreatitis in Western populations, balloon dilation of papilla is not recommended as a routine first-line option in the management of bile duct stones.

Large balloon dilation (LBD) of a prior sphincterotomy, however, appears safe and effective especially for large bile duct stones. Two randomized trials reported similar success in removing large bile duct stones with this technique compared to sphincterotomy alone or with mechanical lithotripsy. The latter study suggests lower overall complications, especially cholangitis, with LBD and sphincterotomy.

Hepatolithiasis, the presence of stones in the intrahepatic biliary tree above the hepatic duct confluence, is difficult to treat and poses a major challenge to the endoscopist in countries where is this is common. Surgery is often required but rarely solves the problem, since stone recurrence is high.

Attam R and Freeman ML. Endoscopic papillary large balloon dilation for large common bile duct stones. *J Hepatobiliary Pancreat Surg.* 2009;16:618–623.

2. Cholelithiasis with Choledocholithiasis

When patients present with the combined problem of gallstones in the gallbladder and bile duct simultaneously, there are two questions to answer: (1) what is the best method for clearing the bile duct, and (2) what should be done with the gallbladder? The sequential options are (1) laparoscopic cholecystectomy with laparoscopic bile duct exploration, (2) laparoscopic or open cholecystectomy followed by postoperative ERCP, (3) preoperative ERCP followed by cholecystectomy (laparoscopic or open), (4) open cholecystectomy with open exploration of the bile duct, (5) ERCP and no cholecystectomy, and, in special circumstances, (6) a range of additional and much less commonly used surgical and nonsurgical techniques such as percutaneous cholecystostomy, percutaneous access to the bile duct (including percutaneous cholangioscopy), techniques for Mirizzi syndrome, management of hepatolithiasis, and approaches to recurrent stones after biliary and nonbiliary upper gastrointestinal surgery. It is unlikely that one option will be appropriate for all clinical circumstances in all centers in all countries because the variables of disease states, patient demographics, and risk stratifications; available endoscopic, radiologic, and surgical expertise; patient preferences; and health care economics will all have significant influences on practice.

In patients with contemporaneous cholelithiasis and choledocholithiasis, it is usually the latter that dominates the acute clinical presentation and leads to intervention for pain, obstructive jaundice, cholangitis, pancreatitis, or any combination thereof. Less commonly, asymptomatic bile duct stones are discovered incidentally on noninvasive imaging for nonbiliary indications, during evaluation of symptomatic cholelithiasis, or intraoperatively during cholecystectomy. Since the universal adoption of laparoscopic cholecystectomy as the primary method for treating cholelithiasis in the early 1990s, only a minority of surgeons have mastered the techniques required for laparoscopic transcystic or direct choledochal exploration to treat choledocholithiasis and there has been reluctance to convert to open bile duct exploration for this indication. ERCP has become the standard approach for acute presentations of choledocholithiasis and with the overall success of endoscopic bile duct clearance, surgical management of choledocholithiasis is rarely necessary.

Following endoscopic bile duct clearance, the decision to leave the gallbladder in situ and follow the patient expectantly (option 5, earlier) compared with routine laparoscopic cholecystectomy has been questioned as there is an unacceptably high incidence of cholecystitis unless the gallbladder is empty. Where the expertise is available, elective management of cholelithiasis and choledocholithiasis by the laparoscopic approach is optimal.

Carr-Locke DL. Cholelithiasis plus choledocholithiasis: ERCP first, what next? *Gastroenterology.* 2006;130:270–272. [PMID: 16401489]

3. Mirizzi Syndrome

First described by Mirizzi in 1948, this syndrome is a rare complication of gallstone disease and refers to stone impaction in the neck of the gallbladder or the cystic duct, with subsequent inflammation and extrinsic compression of the main bile duct leading to obstructive jaundice and cholangitis (Figure 35–4). Type I refers to extrinsic compression of the main bile duct secondary to a stone in the cystic duct or gallbladder, and type II occurs when there is cholecystocholedochal fistula.

Treatment of Mirizzi syndrome has traditionally been surgical. Endoscopic management consists of drainage and decompression of the bile duct or gallbladder, or both, prior to surgical intervention but can be definitive if the impacted stone can be fragmented and removed.

4. Benign Bile Duct Strictures

Benign biliary strictures have many causes, with the most common being anastomosis, operative injury, and chronic pancreatitis. Patients present with cholestasis, cholangitis, or, rarely, secondary biliary cirrhosis. In the past, surgical management was the standard approach, with an associated morbidity and mortality, but currently endoscopic therapy with dilation and stenting offers a less invasive and effective line of therapy (Figure 35–5). The insertion of multiple plastic biliary stents, to achieve maximum dilation of the bile duct, has gained acceptance and carries an 80% long-term success rate over mean 14-year follow-up with a less than 10% complication rate. The use of self-expanding metal stents in benign bile duct strictures has not been advocated until the recent availability of fully covered stents, which are potentially removable.

Primary sclerosing cholangitis remains one of the rare diagnostic indications for ERCP despite the advancement of MRCP, it has reduced sensitivity for PSC limited to peripheral intrahepatic ducts. In the presence of a dominant stricture in PSC, balloon dilation with or preferably without short-term stenting is the treatment of choice.

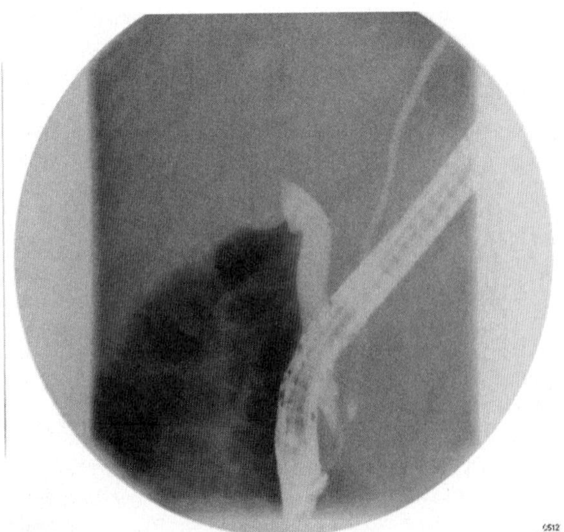

▲ **Figure 35–4.** ERCP image of Mirizzi syndrome.

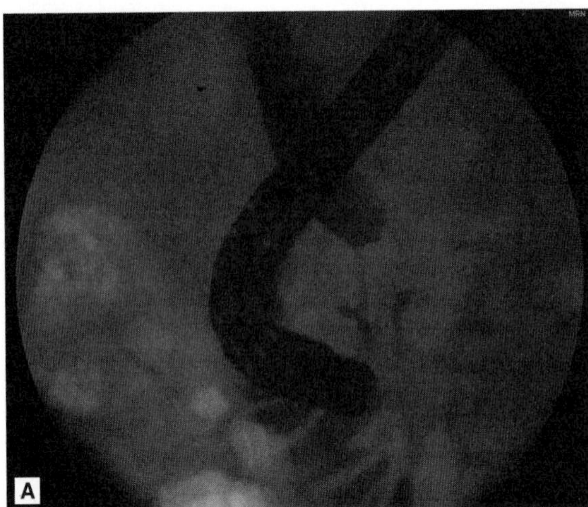

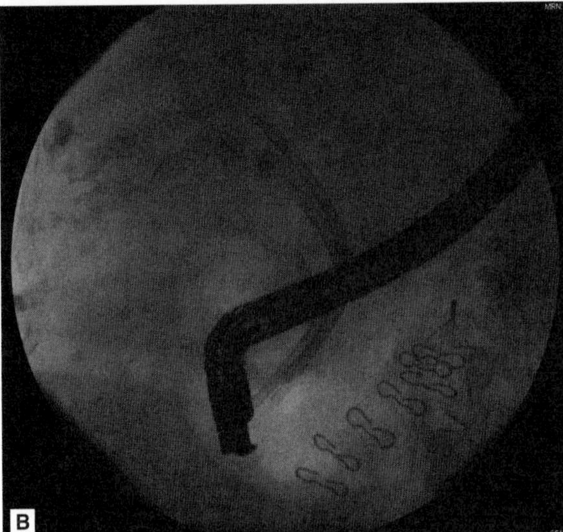

▲ **Figure 35–5.** ERCP sequence showing **(A)** benign biliary stricture and **(B)** placement of multiple plastic stents.

Catalano MF, Linder JD, George S, et al. Treatment of symptomatic distal common bile duct stenosis secondary to chronic pancreatitis: comparison of single vs. multiple simultaneous stents. *Gastrointest Endosc.* 2004;60:945–952. [PMID: 15605010]

Costamagna G, Tringali A, Mutignani M, et al. Endotherapy of postoperative biliary strictures with multiple stents: results after more than 10 years of follow up. *Gastrointest Endosc.* 2010;72:551–557. [PMID: 11474384]

5. Malignant Bile Duct Strictures

Biliary obstruction secondary to malignant bile duct stricture of pancreatic, biliary, or metastatic origin is now usually palliated by stent placement. Polyethylene plastic or self-expandable metal stents (SEMS) may be used, although a recent randomized study suggested that use of plastic stents before surgical resection of pancreatic cancer led to increased complications due to stent occlusion and cholangitis. Short uncovered SEMS and the newly available fully covered metal stents may be more appropriate for tumors that may be surgically resectable, and both the efficacy and cost-effectiveness of this approach certainly warrant study. SEMS are commonly used for their ease of deployment, high patency rate, and cost-effectiveness in patients who survive for more than 6 months following stent placement because the reintervention rate is drastically reduced compared with plastic stents (Figure 35–6). Metal stents remain patent twice as long as polyethylene stents, a median of about 270 days versus 125 days. Unlike plastic stents, SEMS occlude not from a bacterial biofilm but from tumor ingrowth or over-growth, tissue hyperplasia at the ends of the stent, and migration. Uncovered and partially covered SEMS appear to have similar rates of patency with a higher migration rate in partially covered stents based on recent randomized trials.

Tissue sampling of bile duct strictures is important in defining their nature (benign vs malignant) and can be achieved by forceps biopsy, brush cytology, and needle aspiration. Biliary brush cytology is the most common method of sampling and has low sensitivity of 30–60% but a specificity over 90%. The sensitivity for brush cytology is higher for primary bile duct tumors (80–86%) and when combined with biopsies of the stricture (63%). Additional molecular techniques such as fluorescence in situ hybridization, digital image analysis, and flow cytometry may improve accuracy.

Baron TH, Harewood GC, Rumalla A, et al. A prospective comparison of digital image analysis and routine cytology for the identification of malignancy in biliary tract strictures. *Clin Gastroenterol Hepatol.* 2004;2:214–219. [PMID: 15017605]

Baron TH, Kozarek RA. Preoperative biliary stents in pancreatic cancer—proceed with caution. *N Engl J Med.* 2010;362:170–172. [PMID: 20071708]

6. Bile Leak

Injury to the bile duct is a well-recognized complication of cholecystectomy. Postoperative bile leak occurs in up to 0.5% of patients after open cholecystectomy and up to 2% after laparoscopic cholecystectomy, and cystic duct leaks are the most common type. Patients may present with

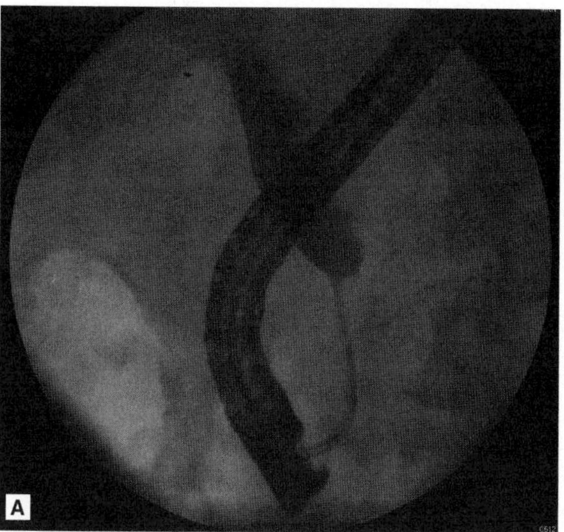

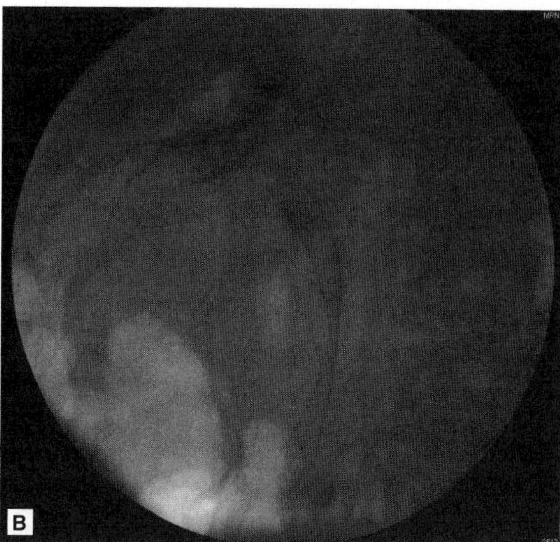

▲ **Figure 35–6.** ERCP images showing **(A)** malignant biliary obstruction and **(B)** placement of a self-expanding metallic stent.

abdominal pain, abdominal tenderness, fever, and bilious drainage through a drain when present. ERCP is the most accurate technique in defining the biliary anatomy, delineating the site of the leak, and providing definitive therapy (Figure 35–7), which is highly successful. Endoscopic therapy is most commonly achieved by stent placement to decrease the pressure gradient between the bile duct and duodenum, allowing preferential flow of bile through the transpapillary route and sealing of the leak site. The stent does not have to cross the leak site unless there is a major bile duct injury.

7. Bile Duct Cysts

Choledochal cysts are congenital anomalies typically seen in children and young adults but can be diagnosed at any age. They may affect the intrahepatic biliary tree, extrahepatic biliary tree, or both. They occur in 1 in 13,000 to 1 in 2,000,000 live births and are three times more common in females than in males.

The cysts are commonly classified into five types, with type I the most common and type V the least. Type I (80–90%) involves the extrahepatic bile duct and is subclassified into IA (common type), IB (segmental dilation), and IC (diffuse dilation). Type II (2%) is a diverticulum in the main bile duct. Type III cysts (1.4–5%) involve the intraduodenal portion of the bile duct and are also referred to as choledochoceles. Type IV (13%) is the second most common type and more frequently seen in adults. It is subclassified into IVA (multiple intrahepatic and extrahepatic cysts) and IVB (multiple extrahepatic cysts). Type V (<1%), or Caroli disease, refers to single or multiple dilations of intrahepatic bile ducts (Figure 35–8).

Anomalous pancreatobiliary union (APBU) is frequently associated with a long common channel (>15 mm). The risk of biliary malignancy (gallbladder and bile duct) is increased when APBU is present, with an overall risk of 14% in patients with choledochal cysts and 50% in those without. The classic presenting symptoms and signs of jaundice, abdominal mass, and pain are more common in children than adults (82% vs 25%, respectively). Adults often present with vague abdominal pain, cholecystitis, cholangitis, and pancreatitis.

Many choledochal cysts are detected on imaging studies such as abdominal ultrasonography and CT scan done for other reasons. ERCP usually establishes the diagnosis, classifies bile duct cysts, and detects the presence of APBU, but MRCP is increasingly being used as a noninvasive imaging modality since it has an accuracy rate of 96% for choledochal cyst detection.

Surgical management (cyst excision and biliary reconstruction) is the recommended approach for all except type III cysts to avoid the risk of biliary tract malignancy. Management of choledochocele by biliary sphincterotomy has been recommended and complete excision is not necessary due to the exceedingly low risk of malignancy.

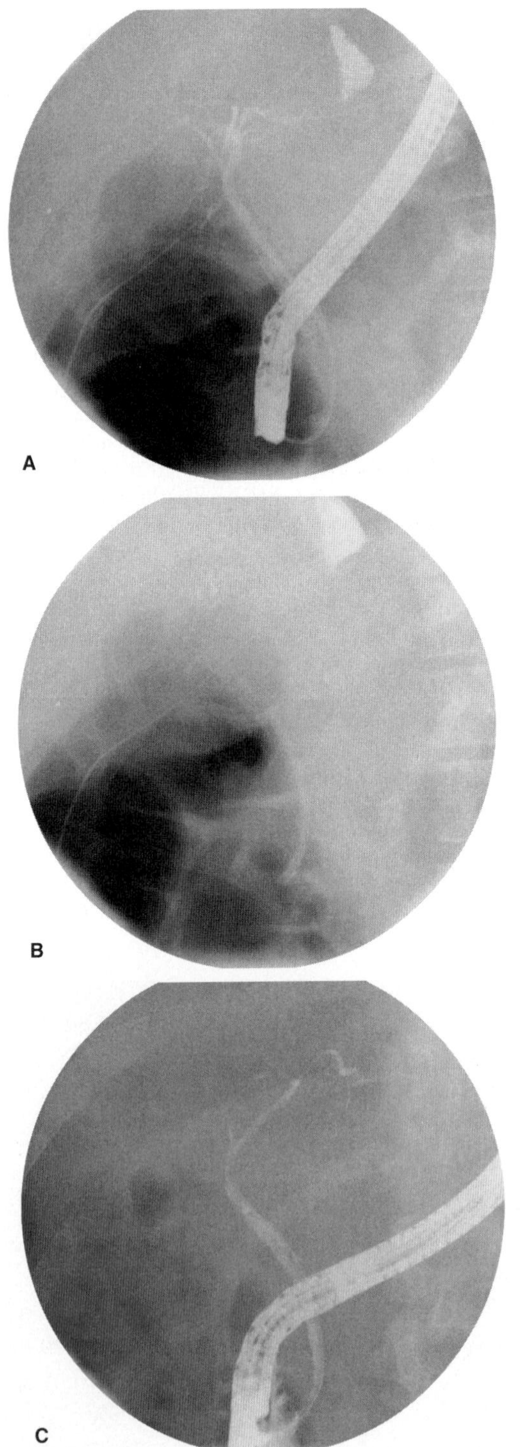

▲ **Figure 35–7.** ERCP images showing (**A**) bile leak after partial left hepatectomy, (**B**) treatment by a short 10-French plastic stent, and (**C**) no leak present at the time of stent removal.

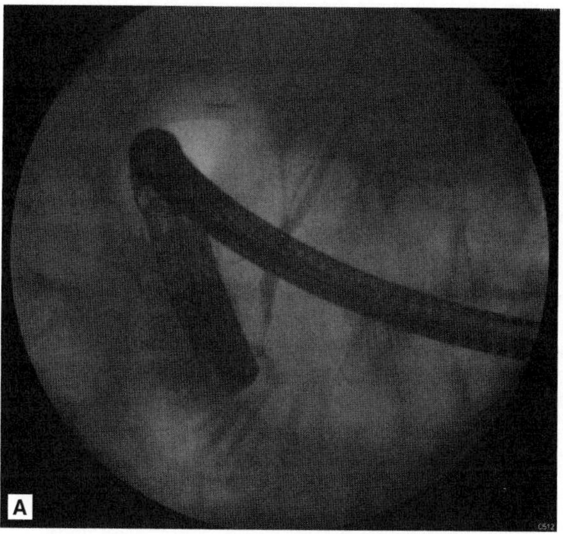

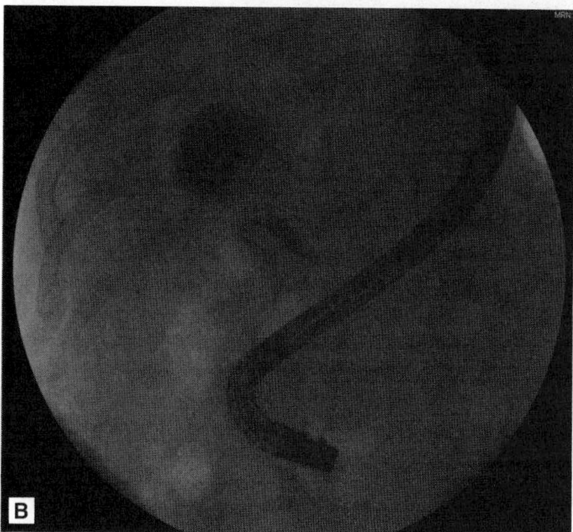

▲ **Figure 35–8.** ERCP images of choledochal cysts. **A:** Type 1 with anomalous union of the bile and pancreatic ducts. **B:** Type 5 with a single large intrahepatic cyst.

PANCREAS

1. Gallstone Pancreatitis

The goal of therapeutic ERCP in the setting of acute gallstone pancreatitis is to clear the bile duct of stones that, if left in place, may worsen the severity of pancreatitis and increase the risk of further attacks. The role of urgent ERCP and sphincterotomy in gallstone pancreatitis has been shown to improve morbidity and mortality in select patients with severe attacks, but has little or no benefit in patients with mild pancreatitis, since the majority of these patients pass the stones spontaneously and recover with supportive care. Tables 35–1 and 35–2 summarize the results. A more recent randomized trial excluding patients with cholangitis confirmed the lack of benefit of early ERCP in gallstone pancreatitis. Cholecystectomy should be planned for the same admission, if possible, but can be delayed after sphincterotomy since this confers a degree of protection from further pancreatitis.

Table 35–1. ERCP in mild biliary pancreatitis.

Country	N	Morbidity (%)		Mortality (%)	
		ERCP	Conventional	ERCP	Conventional
United Kingdom[a]	68	11.8	11.8	0	0
Hong Kong[b]	69	17.6	17.1	0	0
Poland[c]	155	10.0[e]	25.3	0	5.3
Germany[d]	160	41.7	47.4	2.4	0

[a]Data from Neoptolemos JP, Carr-Locke DL, London NJ, et al. Controlled trial of urgent endoscopic retrograde cholangiopancreatography and endoscopic sphincterotomy versus conservative treatment for acute pancreatitis due to gallstones. *Lancet*. 1988;2:979–983. [PMID: 2902491]
[b]Data from Fan ST, Lai EC, Mok FP, et al. Early treatment of acute biliary pancreatitis by endoscopic papillotomy. *N Engl J Med*. 1993;328:228–232. [PMID: 8418402]
[c]Data from Nowak A, Marek TA, Nowakowska-Dulawa E, et al. Biliary pancreatitis needs endoscopic retrograde cholangiopancreatography with endoscopic sphincterotomy for cure. *Endoscopy*. 1998;30:A256–A259. [PMID: 9932792]
[d]Data from Folsch UR, Nitsche R, Ludtke R, et al. Early ERCP and papillotomy compared with conventional treatment for acute biliary pancreatitis. The German Study Group on Acute Biliary Pancreatitis. *N Engl J Med*. 1997;336:237–242. [PMID: 8995085]
[e]$P < .05$ compared with conventional treatment.

Table 35–2. ERCP in severe biliary pancreatitis.

Country	n	Morbidity (%)		Mortality (%)	
		ERCP	Conventional	ERCP	Conventional
United Kingdom[a]	53	24.0[e]	60.7	4.0	17.9
Hong Kong[b]	58	13.3	53.6	0	17.9
Poland[c]	50	39.1[e]	74.0	4.3[a]	33.3
Germany[d]	46	65.4	70.0	23.1	14.3

[a]Data from Neoptolemos JP, Carr-Locke DL, London NJ, et al. Controlled trial of urgent endoscopic retrograde cholangiopancreatography and endoscopic sphincterotomy versus conservative treatment for acute pancreatitis due to gallstones. *Lancet.* 1988;2:979–983. [PMID: 2902491]
[b]Data from Fan ST, Lai EC, Mok FP, et al. Early treatment of acute biliary pancreatitis by endoscopic papillotomy. *N Engl J Med.* 1993;328: 228–232. [PMID: 8418402]
[c]Data from Nowak A, Marek TA, Nowakowska-Dulawa E, et al. Biliary pancreatitis needs endoscopic retrograde cholangiopancreatography with endoscopic sphincterotomy for cure. *Endoscopy.* 1998;30:A256–A259. [PMID: 9932792]
[d]Data from Folsch UR, Nitsche R, Ludtke R, et al. Early ERCP and papillotomy compared with conservative treatment for acute biliary pancreatitis. The German Study Group on Acute Biliary Pancreatitis. *N Engl J Med.* 1997;336:237–242. [PMID: 8995085]
[e]$P < .05$ compared with conventional treatment.

Oria A, Cimmino D, Ocampo C, et al. Management in patients with acute gallstone pancreatitis and biliopancreatic obstruction: a randomized clinical trial. *Ann Surg.* 2007;245:10–17. [PMID: 17197959]

2. Nonbiliary Acute Pancreatitis

ERCP plays a role in delineating and treating those patients with pancreatic-type SOD presenting with unexplained pancreatitis and other rarer causes of pancreatitis, such as ampullary adenoma, pancreas divisum, autoimmune disease, rare tumors, and helminths if not detected by noninvasive imaging.

3. Chronic Pancreatitis

Chronic pancreatitis is a progressive disease that is characterized by persistent inflammation, fibrosis, atrophy of the gland, and ductal abnormalities. Chronic pancreatitis causes significant morbidity related to chronic abdominal pain, loss of exocrine and endocrine function, and complications such as pancreatic stones, strictures, and fluid collections.

Pancreatic duct pressure may be elevated secondary to strictures, stones, or outflow obstruction at the level of the major papilla. The goal of therapeutic ERCP is to decompress the pancreatic ductal system and relieve the obstruction with the hope of minimizing attacks of recurrent pancreatitis and alleviating chronic abdominal pain.

Benign strictures and stone disease of the main pancreatic duct (Figure 35–9) can result in ductal hypertension, which may be the basis of relapsing pain and recurrent pancreatitis. Strictures are treated by balloon or catheter dilation and insertion of one or more plastic stents that are exchanged every 2–4 months for up to 1 year. Stone extraction is technically feasible if the stones are small, few in number, located in the head of the pancreas, and not impacted. A pancreatic sphincterotomy is usually required, and the stones are removed with a basket or balloon similar to bile duct stones. Stones located in the upstream duct proximal to a stricture require stricture dilation prior to extraction. Direct pancreatoscopy and electrohydraulic lithotripsy of

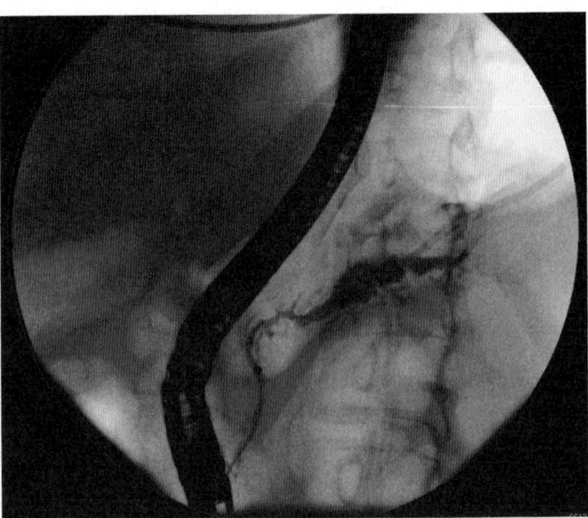

▲ **Figure 35–9.** ERCP showing chronic pancreatitis with narrowed main duct in the head, ectatic side branches, and an irregular dilated main pancreatic duct in the body and tail. A transgastric stent is in place.

pancreatic duct stones offers an additional option, although extracorporeal shock wave lithotripsy alone appears to be as effective as combined therapy with ERCP for pancreatic duct stones. While most studies have shown an overall long-term pain relief in about 67% of patients who undergo endoscopic therapy, surgery seems to offer more durable pain relief with fewer procedures.

Dumonceau JM, Costamagna G, Tringali A, et al. Treatment for painful calcified chronic pancreatitis extracorporeal shock wave lithotripsy versus endoscopic treatment: a randomized controlled trial. *Gut.* 2007;56:545–552. [PMID: 17047101]

Rosch T, Daniel S, Scholz M, et al. Endoscopic treatment of chronic pancreatitis: a multicenter study of 1000 patients with long-term follow-up. *Endoscopy.* 2002;34:765–771. [PMID: 12244496]

4. Pancreatic Ductal Disruption & Fluid Collection

Pancreatic duct disruption and fluid collections can be the result of acute or chronic pancreatitis. Ongoing pancreatic duct disruption can be healed in 78–92% of cases with stent placement across the disruption; success rates plummet to 23–44% with transpapillary stents that do not bridge the leak. A pseudocyst is a collection of amylase-rich pancreatic juice enclosed by a wall of nonepithelialized, fibrous, or granulation tissue. Symptomatic pseudocysts may be drained percutaneously (radiologically), surgically, or endoscopically. Endoscopic drainage of pancreatic pseudocysts can be performed by using transpapillary or transmural (transgastric, transduodenal) placement of endoprostheses. The transpapillary approach is utilized for pseudocysts communicating with the main pancreatic duct, with the tip of the stent positioned in the cyst cavity after a pancreatic sphincterotomy. Fluid collections not clearly communicating with the pancreatic duct are drained using the transmural approach. The goal is to establish a communication between the cyst cavity and gastric or duodenal lumen for continuous drainage of pancreatic juice. The major prerequisite for such a procedure is a distance between the cyst and gastrointestinal tract of 10 mm or less best determined during endoscopic ultrasound (EUS), and recent studies suggest that technical success is improved with EUS-guided drainage compared to the non-EUS guided approach (Figure 35–10, Plates 88 and 89).

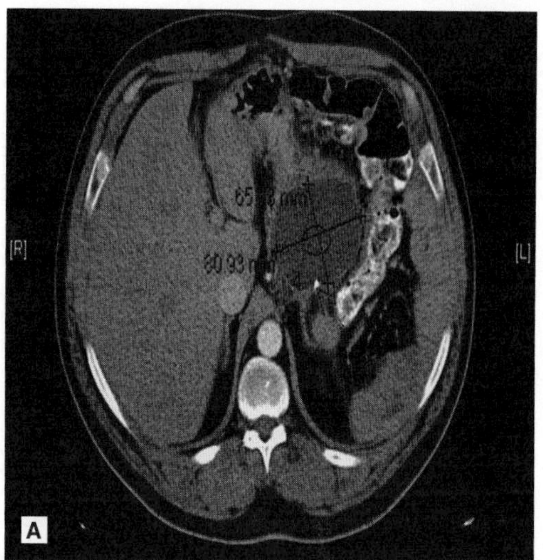

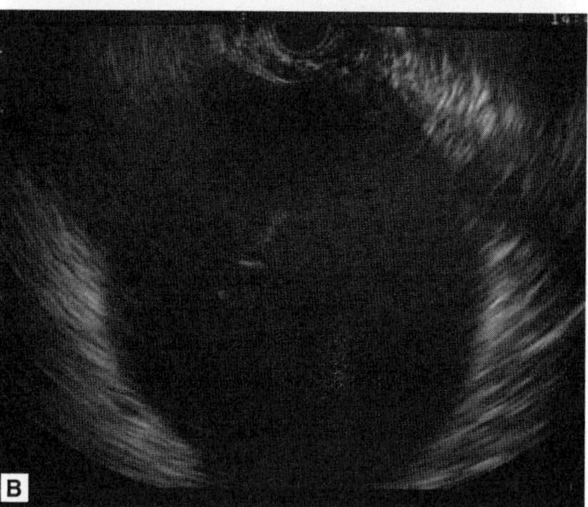

▲ **Figure 35–10.** Sequence of pseudocyst drainage: (**A**) computed tomographic (CT) scan showing retrogastric pseudocyst, (**B**) endoscopic ultrasound image with needle inside cyst, (**C**) balloon dilation of the cystgastrostomy track, (**D**) double pigtail stents across cystgastrostomy stoma, and (**E**) follow-up CT scan showing resolution. See also Plates 88 and 89.

Park DH, Lee SS, Moon SH, et al. Endoscopic ultrasound-guided versus conventional transmural drainage for pancreatic pseudocysts: a prospective randomized trial. *Endoscopy.* 2009;41:842–848. [PMID: 19798610]

5. Pancreas Divisum

Pancreas divisum, the failure of fusion of dorsal and ventral pancreatic ductal systems during embryogenesis, is the most common variant of pancreatic ductal anatomy and occurs in about 10% of individuals (Plates 90, 91, and 92). The relationship between pancreas divisum and pancreatitis remains controversial, but endoscopic therapy in patients with recurrent pancreatitis and a normal dorsal duct aims at decompressing the dorsal pancreatic duct by minor papillotomy and temporary stent insertion with greater than 80% long-term success. These patients were the first group shown to develop ductal changes resulting from stent therapy, and care must be taken to avoid this complication by not leaving stents in place longer than necessary.

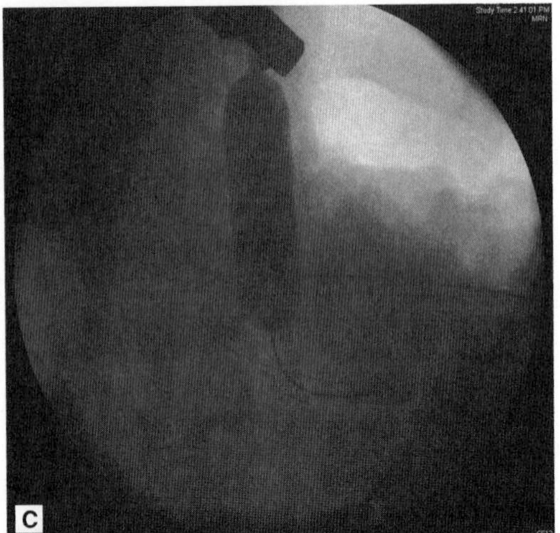

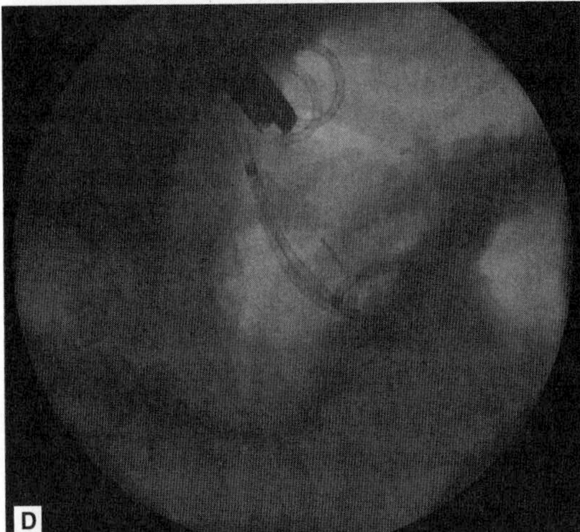

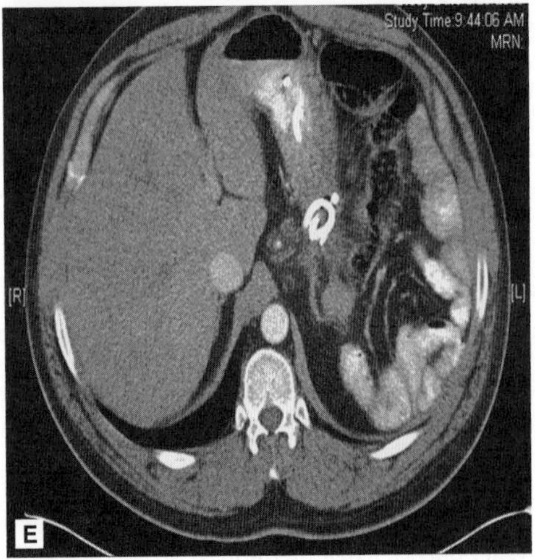

▲ **Figure 35–10.** *(Continued)*

Gerke H, Byrne MF, Stiffler HL, et al. Outcome of endoscopic minor papillotomy in patients with symptomatic pancreas divisum. *JOP*. 2004;5:122–131. [PMID: 15138333]

6. Autoimmune Pancreatitis

The first case of chronic inflammatory sclerosis of the pancreas with possible underlying autoimmune mechanism was reported in 1961, but the terminology of "autoimmune pancreatitis" (AIP) was not proposed until 1995. The epidemiology of AIP is not well known but a prevalence of 5% has been reported among patients with chronic pancreatitis (see Chapter 27). Diagnostic criteria include (1) pancreatic imaging studies showing diffuse narrowing of the main pancreatic duct with irregular walls and diffuse enlargement of the pancreas, (2) laboratory data demonstrating abnormally elevated levels of serum γ-globulin, or immunoglobulin G, or the presence of autoantibodies, (3) histopathologic examination of the pancreas showing fibrotic changes with lymphocyte and plasma cell infiltration, and (4) response to steroid therapy in select patients. For diagnosis of AIP, various combinations of the above criteria are used in the Mayo Clinic, Japan Pancreas Society, and Korean criteria. Although ERCP is part of the diagnostic criteria of the Japan Pancreas Society, MRCP is most commonly used in the Western countries. There is currently no therapeutic role for ERCP in this condition unless there is concomitant biliary obstruction.

Park DH, Kim MH, Chari ST. Recent advances in autoimmune pancreatitis. *Gut*. 2009;58:1680–1689. [PMID: 19240063]

7. Intraductal Papillary Mucinous Neoplasm

Intraductal papillary mucinous neoplasm (IPMN) is a cystic neoplasm of the pancreas that involves the main pancreatic duct, side branches, or both. It is characterized by intraductal growth of mucin-producing epithelium, segmental or diffuse ductal dilation, and, when the tumor is in the head of the pancreas, a gaping or "fish-mouth" papilla from which large amounts of mucus flow (Figure 35–11). IPMN occurs more commonly in elderly men who may present with recurrent pancreatitis and/or diabetes. Jaundice and weight loss can be the presenting symptoms in cases with malignant transformation.

Several imaging modalities are used to diagnose IPMN, including CT, EUS, magnetic resonance imaging, and ERCP. A pancreatogram is usually remarkable for dilated pancreatic ducts, intraluminal filling defects, and mural nodules. During ERCP, pancreatic juice can be aspirated for cytology, and transpapillary brushings and biopsies can be obtained from suspicious lesions seen on pancreatography. Direct pancreatoscopy involves the use of an ultrathin endoscope of 10-French diameter or less introduced through the working channel of a duodenoscope and advanced into the pancreatic

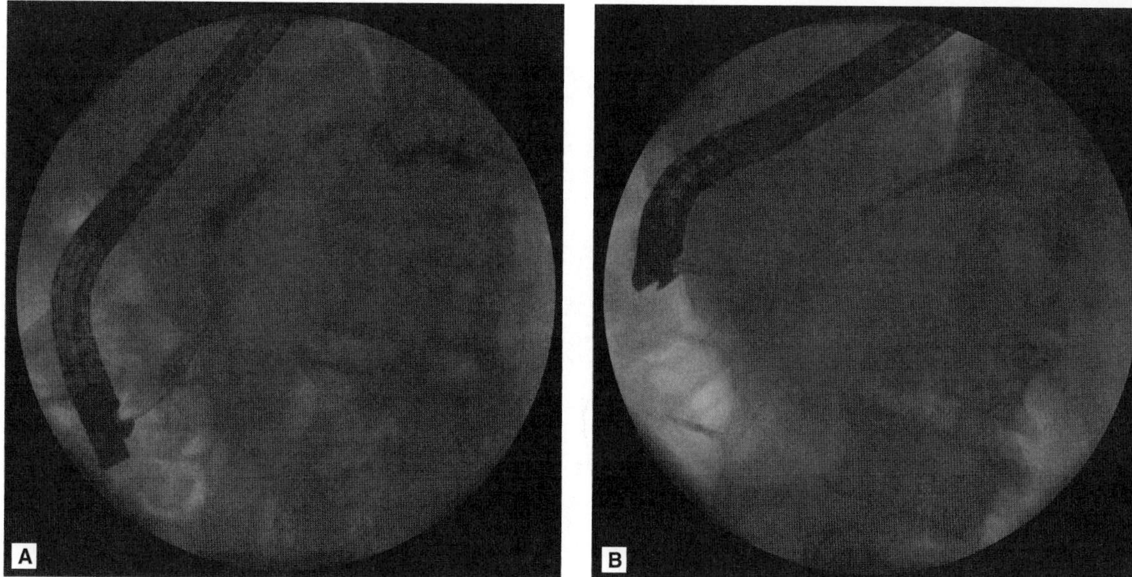

▲ **Figure 35–11.** ERCP in a patient with IPMN showing (**A**) a dilated main pancreatic duct with a mucus filling defect, and (**B**) direct pancreatoscopy, which demonstrated the ductal tumor.

duct through the major papilla. The ductal epithelium can be examined, and directed biopsies of suspicious mural nodules or masses can be performed. Pancreatoscopy has been increasingly used as an adjunct to other imaging modalities for diagnosis and determining the extent of IPMN, because the tumor is easily seen as a "cluster of eggs" appearance when it affects the main duct and surgical resection currently aims to be as conservative as possible. A recent study suggests that intraductal ultrasound during ERCP may also prove useful at defining the extent of IPMN preoperatively.

Yasuda K, Sakata M, Ueda M, et al. The use of pancreatoscopy in the diagnosis of intraductal papillary mucinous tumor lesions of the pancreas. *Clin Gastroenterol Hepatol.* 2005;3:S53–S57. [PMID: 16012998]

Endoscopic Ultrasound

Linda S. Lee, MD

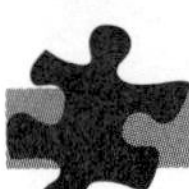

ESSENTIALS OF DIAGNOSIS

- Endoscopic ultrasound (EUS) is a critical tool in cancer staging and is superior to computed tomography (CT) and positron emission tomography (PET) in esophageal cancer staging.
- EUS-guided fine needle aspiration (EUS-FNA) is the most sensitive method for diagnosing pancreatic cancer; accuracy of EUS is similar to CT for assessing vascular invasion.
- EUS helps evaluate submucosal lesions, although the yield of EUS-FNA is lower for submucosal than for extraluminal lesions.
- EUS is emerging as an important tool in diagnosing chronic pancreatitis.
- Diagnostic yield for EUS is similar to MRCP in detecting choledocholithiasis, but initial EUS has the greatest cost-utility.

General Considerations

Endoscopic ultrasound (EUS) has emerged as the premier tool for staging cancers and has revolutionized the role of gastrointestinal endoscopy in diagnostic imaging inside and outside the gastrointestinal tract. EUS merges endoscopy, which is limited to visualizing the lumen of the gastrointestinal tract, with ultrasonography, which allows imaging of the layers of the gastrointestinal wall and surrounding structures. Tissue diagnosis can be obtained with EUS-guided fine needle aspiration (EUS-FNA), which uses a catheter with a retractable needle that can be advanced into visualized tissue. Exciting advances in the therapeutic application of EUS have begun with this technique, including the well-established endoscopic pseudocyst drainage and more recent rendezvous techniques with endoscopic retrograde cholangiopancreatography (ERCP) as well as possibilities of EUS-guided fine needle injection (EUS-FNI) therapy.

A. Equipment

Radial scanning echoendoscopes were the first instruments used with the advent of EUS in the 1980s (Figure 36–1). The ultrasound transducer is mounted on the tip of the endoscope and rotates 360 degrees to provide cross-sectional images perpendicular to the long axis of the endoscope (Figure 36–2). The endoscopic viewing optic is mounted proximal to the ultrasound transducer and provides an oblique view of the lumen. A new forward-viewing echoendoscope has been developed. To overcome the problem of ultrasound waves traveling through an air-filled lumen, a balloon that can be filled with water surrounds the ultrasound transducer. Various ultrasonic frequencies between 5 and 20 MHz are used.

Linear array echoendoscopes provide ultrasound images along the long axis of the endoscope usually in an 80- to 105-degree arc (Figures 36–2 and 36–3). This is critical to allow simultaneous imaging of the needle and target lesion during EUS-FNA. A variety of needles, including 19-, 22-, and 25-gauge, can be passed through the endoscopic working channel.

In high-frequency ultrasound probe sonography, a catheter with a tiny mechanically rotating ultrasound transducer at the tip is inserted through the endoscopic working channel (Figure 36–4). The probe images with frequencies between 12 and 30 MHz, and higher resolution allows for more detailed imaging but with decreased depth of penetration. Newer generation probes include wire-guided probes that can be introduced into the biliary and pancreatic ducts to perform intraductal ultrasound.

B. Technique

Typically a standard upper endoscopy or flexible sigmoidoscopy for a rectal EUS is performed before the EUS to identify the area of interest and to ensure the echoendoscope can be passed safely in the gastrointestinal tract. The echoendoscope is passed in a "blind" manner similar to the duodenoscope.

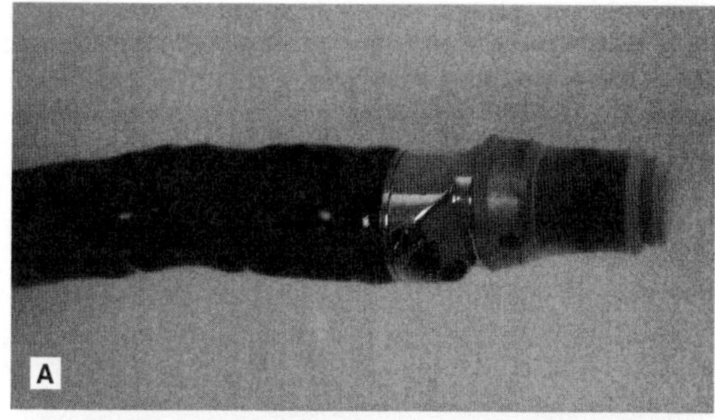

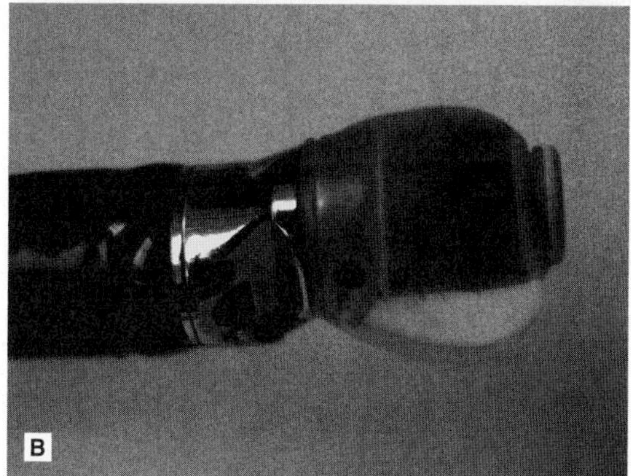

▲ **Figure 36–1. A:** Radial echoendoscope. **B:** Radial echoendoscope with balloon inflated.

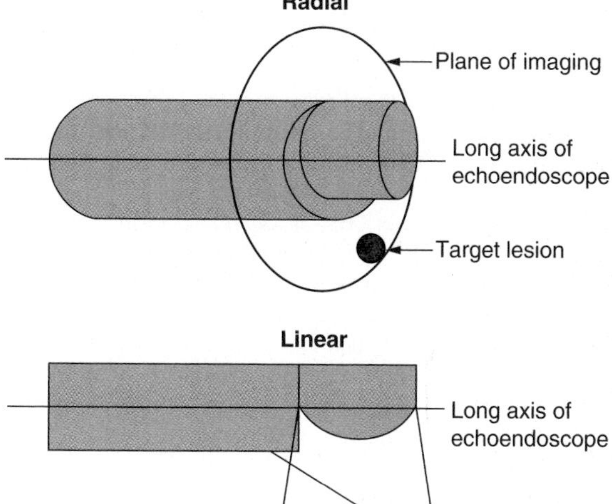

▲ **Figure 36–2.** Imaging planes for radial and linear echoendoscopes. The radial echoendoscope provides images in a plane perpendicular to the long axis. The linear echoendoscope provides images along the long axis in an 80–105-degree arc with fine needle aspiration capability.

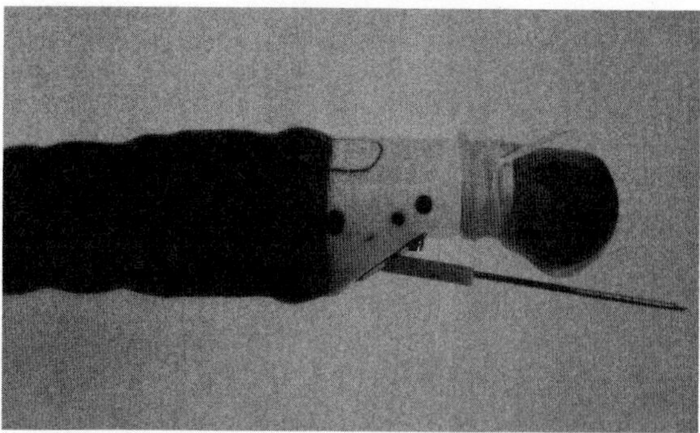

▲ **Figure 36–3.** Linear echoendoscope.

Once the echoendoscope has been advanced to the area to be imaged, a water interface is established between the ultrasound transducer and the gastrointestinal wall. This can be done by inflating the balloon on the tip of the transducer or by filling the gastrointestinal lumen with water, or both. Once a sufficient water interface has been established, EUS images should be obtained perpendicular to the lesion of interest because oblique images commonly distort the gastrointestinal wall and lead to false interpretations.

EUS-FNA is performed with the linear echoendoscope. The needle is advanced under endosonographic guidance into the lesion of interest, the stylet is withdrawn, and suction may be applied using a 10- to 25-cc syringe while advancing the needle back and forth within the lesion.

C. Normal EUS Anatomy

EUS imaging of the gastrointestinal wall layer typically reveals five layers alternating in bright and dark bands (Figure 36–5). The first bright or hyperechoic layer closest to the probe represents the superficial mucosa; the second

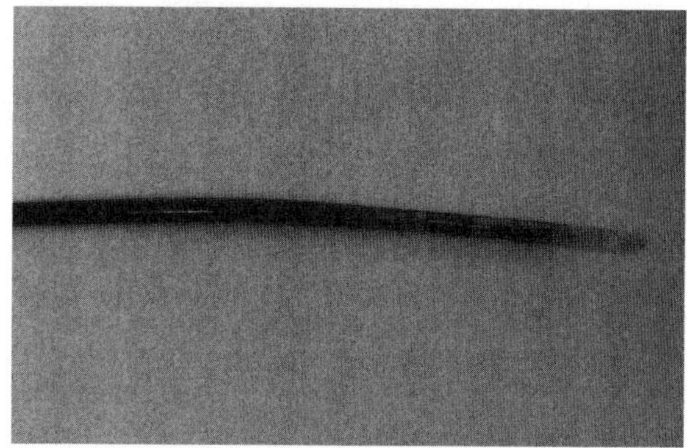

▲ **Figure 36–4.** High-frequency ultrasound probe.

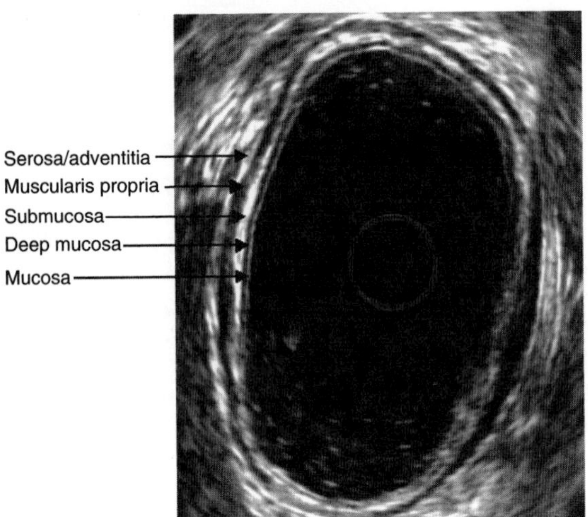

▲ **Figure 36–5.** EUS image of normal gastrointestinal wall layers.

Table 36–1. Accuracy of imaging modalities for T and N staging of gastrointestinal cancers.

Modality	T Stage	N Stage
Esophageal Cancer		
CT	50%	50-60%
PET	—	60%
EUS	61-90%	75%
EUS-FNA	—	87%
Gastric Cancer		
Multidetector-row CT	77-89%	50-75%
MRI	71-83%	52%
EUS	65-92%	50-87%
Rectal Cancer		
CT	52-76%	54-70%
Endorectal coil MRI	75-91%	65-76%
EUS	63-95%	70-75%

CT, computed tomography; EUS, endoscopic ultrasound; FNA, fine needle aspiration; MRI, magnetic resonance imaging; PET, positron emission tomograph.

dark or hypoechoic layer corresponds to the deep mucosa or muscularis mucosa; the third hyperechoic layer is the submucosa; the fourth hypoechoic layer is the muscularis propria; and the fifth hyperechoic layer represents the serosa or adventitia. The normal thickness of the gastrointestinal wall varies from 2 to 4 mm.

CANCER STAGING

Most cancers are staged according to the TNM system of the American Joint Commission on Cancer. Depth or extent of tumor invasion (T), presence or absence of locoregional lymph nodes (N), and presence or absence of distant metastases (M) are captured by the TNM system. The stages of tumor invasion are defined as Tis, limited to mucosa, lamina propria intact; T1, invades lamina propria or submucosa; T2, invades muscularis propria; T3, invades adventitia and serosa; and T4, invades surrounding structures.

1. Esophageal Cancer

As with many cancers, the prognosis of esophageal cancer correlates with stage at diagnosis. Recent changes to staging esophageal cancer include the following: subdividing N stage based on number of lymph nodes; separating T4 into T4a for resectable tumor invading the pleura, pericardium, or diaphragm and T4b for unresectable tumor invading other adjacent structures such as the aorta, trachea, etc; and classifying celiac lymph nodes as regional lymphadenopathy. Although the optimal management of patients with locally advanced esophageal cancer remains controversial, preoperative chemoradiation appears to improve survival compared with surgery alone in patients with stage IIb or stage III cancer and possibly stage IIa. Thus, accurate staging is important to select the appropriate patients for preoperative treatment. The TNM staging includes tumors at the gastroesophageal (GE) junction and the proximal 5 cm of the stomach extending into the GE junction or esophagus. Multiple studies have confirmed the superiority of EUS over CT in T and N staging of esophageal cancer (Table 36–1). Both CT and fluorodeoxyglucose–positron emission tomography (FDG-PET) identify more distant metastases than EUS, and FDG-PET appears superior to CT.

Carcinoma in situ (Tis) is often not visible on EUS. With the high-frequency ultrasound probes, T1 stage can be separated into T1m (tumor confined to mucosa) and T1sm (tumor invading submucosa). About 8–35% of T1sm tumors have local lymph node metastases. Patients with stage T1sm cancer have a lower 5-year overall survival rate of 58% compared with 91% for T1m; therefore, local endoscopic therapy should not be performed for T1sm lesions.

For each T stage (Figure 36-6), positive nodes increase the overall tumor stage and predict a worse prognosis. EUS characteristics suggestive of a malignant lymph node include size greater than 1 cm, round, well defined, and hypoechoic. Presence of all four features predicts malignancy in 80–100% of cases, but only 20–40% of all malignant lymph nodes have all four findings. FNA of lymph nodes improves accuracy of nodal staging compared with EUS alone. If FNA is not possible, the number of lymph nodes correlates with 5-year survival, and the recent change to the staging system now

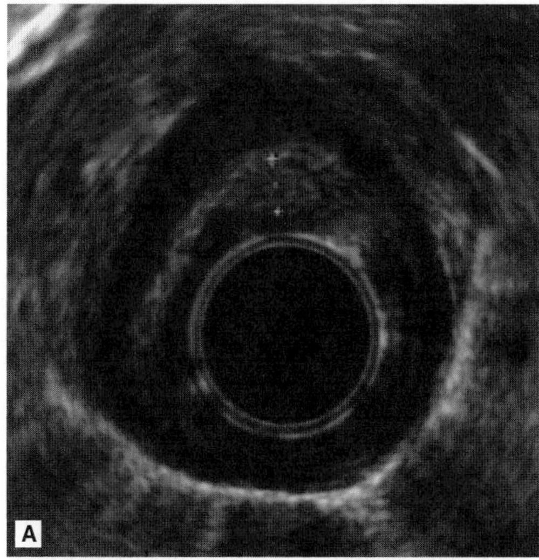

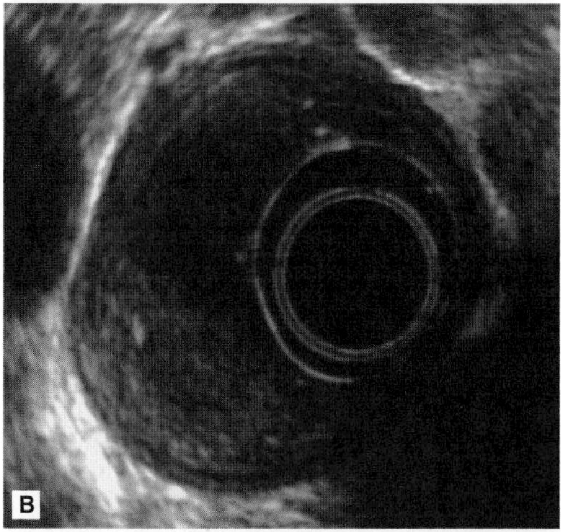

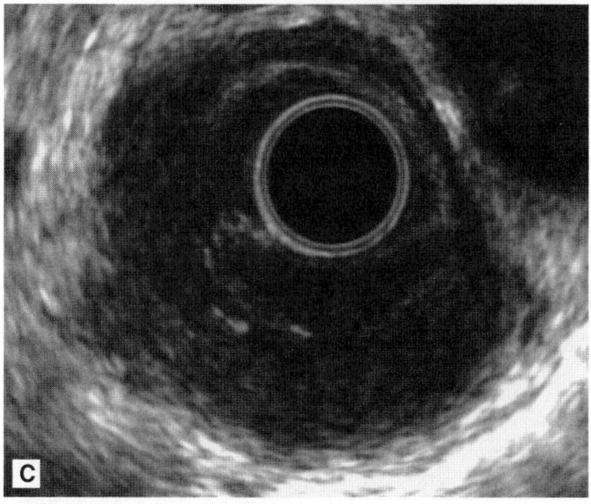

▲ **Figure 36–6.** EUS images of esophageal cancer. **A:** Stage T1. **B:** Stage T2. **C:** Stage T3.

incorporates number of metastatic regional lymph nodes in nodal staging. Restaging of esophageal cancer following chemoradiation with EUS is significantly less accurate than pretreatment staging. Accuracy of T staging is about 37–60%, and the majority of tumors are overstaged presumably due to peritumor inflammation and fibrosis being mistaken for tumor. Reduction in the cross-sectional area or thickness of the tumor by more than 50% has been associated with response to treatment and possibly improved survival.

The clinical impact of EUS on management of esophageal cancer has been demonstrated in several studies. Treatment strategy was changed in about 75% of patients following EUS-FNA, and performance of EUS was associated with increased recurrence-free survival and overall survival. This was attributed to greater use of chemoradiation following more accurate preoperative staging with EUS.

Jost C, Binek J, Schuller JC, et al. Endosonographic radial tumor thickness after neoadjuvant chemoradiation therapy to predict response and survival in patients with locally advanced esophageal cancer: a prospective multicenter phase II study by the Swiss Group for Clinical Cancer Research (SAKK 75/02). *Gastrointest Endosc.* 2010;71:1114–1121.

Liu L, Hofstetter WL, Rashid A, et al. Significance of the depth of tumor invasion and lymph node metastasis in superficially invasive (T1) esophageal adenocarcinoma. *Am J Surg Pathol.* 2005;29:1079–1085. [PMID: 16006804]

Pfau PR, Perlman SB, Stanko P, et al. The role and clinical value of EUS in a multimodality esophageal carcinoma staging program with CT and positron emission tomography. *Gastrointest Endosc.* 2007;65:377–384. [PMID: 17321235]

Shimpi RA, George J, Jowell P, Gress FG. Staging of esophageal cancer by EUS: staging accuracy revisited. *Gastrointest Endosc.* 2007;66:475–482. [PMID: 17725937]

2. Gastric Cancer

With a study demonstrating improved survival in patients who underwent perioperative chemotherapy with at least stage II operable gastric adenocarcinoma, preoperative staging for gastric adenocarcinoma assumes more importance (see stages under esophageal cancer). EUS appears similar to multidetector-row CT and magnetic resonance imaging (MRI) for T and N staging. EUS-FNA of lymph nodes should increase accuracy for N staging. As with esophageal cancer, EUS can identify superficial mucosal tumors, which may be amenable to endoscopic mucosal resection. Limitations in accuracy of EUS staging in gastric cancer include early cancers, large or ulcerated lesions, and lesions at the cardia or incisura.

EUS-staging of gastric mucosa–associated lymphoid tissue (MALT) lymphomas is 95% accurate for T staging and seems to predict response to *Helicobacter pylori* treatment. Complete remission occurs in 78% of patients with T1m disease compared with 12.5% of patients with T1sm tumor. Therefore, EUS may allow early selection of patients with higher T stage disease for consideration of other treatments.

Caletti G, Fusaroli P, Togliani T. EUS in MALT lymphoma. *Gastrointest Endosc.* 2002;56(Suppl 4):21–26. [PMID: 12269963]

Hwang SW, Lee DH, Lee SH, et al. Preoperative staging of gastric cancer by endoscopic ultrasonography and multidetector-row computed tomography. *J Gastroenterol Hep.* 2010;25:512–518. [PMID: 20370729]

3. Rectal Cancer

Local recurrence of rectal cancer occurs in 10–40% of cases despite surgical excision. Preoperative chemoradiation followed by radical resection for tumors that have extended into the perirectal fat or have local lymph nodes (T3/T4, N1, or both) decreases local recurrence by about half and possibly improves survival. There are limited data on the benefits of adjuvant chemoradiation in patients with unfavorable T1 or T2 tumors. Tumor size greater than 3 cm, poorly differentiated histology, and lymphovascular invasion are associated with increased risk of lymph node metastases. Local recurrence can be as high as 11–29% for T1 tumors and 25–62% for T2 tumors, which most likely reflects lymph node involvement occurring in 0–12% of T1 and 12–28% of T2 tumors. Therefore, local excision, which does not remove the mesorectum containing lymph nodes, rather than radical resection should be performed in only select patients with favorable T1 tumors.

Accurate staging of rectal cancer is again critical for correct patient selection for the appropriate preoperative and operative treatment. EUS remains superior to CT for both T and N staging; however, the accuracy of EUS appears comparable to endorectal coil MRI for both T and N staging.

The modest accuracy of EUS for staging rectal cancer is attributed to several factors, including inflammation surrounding the tumor, leading to overstaging; operator experience; and level of tumor in the rectum, with distal lesions being staged less accurately. In contrast to its utility for esophageal cancer, EUS-FNA of regional lymph nodes in rectal cancer does not appear to significantly improve accuracy of N staging. The greatest impact of EUS-FNA may reside in early T-stage tumors which, if node positive, would necessitate preoperative treatment. A recent study suggested that antibiotics are not necessary for transrectal EUS-FNA procedures due to low rates of bacteremia.

EUS-FNA may offer a powerful method to survey for local recurrence of rectal cancer, which often occurs extraluminally following surgical resection. Standard endoscopy is inadequate for detecting these recurrences, and CT scan is limited due to artifacts from surgical metal clips and the inability to differentiate between postoperative changes and recurrence. Sensitivity of EUS for detecting recurrence is 91–100% compared with 82–85% for CT scan, with limited specificity for EUS of 57% that improves to 93% with EUS-FNA. There is no standard recommendation for surveillance with EUS following surgical resection; however, the patients who may benefit most include those with more advanced stage tumors at diagnosis. The greatest risk of recurrence occurs in the first 2 years following surgery; therefore, EUS may be performed every 3–6 months during this time.

Bianchi P, Ceriani C, Palmisano A, et al. A prospective comparison of endorectal ultrasound and pelvic magnetic resonance in the preoperative staging of rectal cancer. *Ann Ital Chir.* 2006;77: 41–46. [PMID: 15910358]

Mutusamy VR, Chang KJ. Optimal methods for staging rectal cancer. *Clin Cancer Res.* 2007;13:6877s–6884s. [PMID: 18006793]

4. Pancreatic Cancer

The role of EUS in pancreatic cancer includes diagnosis (Figure 36–7) and staging. Tissue diagnosis is important to confirm malignancy and rule out metastatic lesions to the pancreas, which comprised 11% of masses referred for EUS-FNA in one study. EUS-FNA is the most accurate diagnostic modality, with 80–95% sensitivity and near 100% specificity compared with CT- or ultrasound-guided FNA, which have sensitivity ranging from 62% to 81%. Diagnostic sensitivity diminishes to 73% in the setting of chronic pancreatitis. Presence of an onsite cytopathologist increases diagnostic accuracy while reducing procedure time, number of needles used, and overall procedure cost. EUS-FNA is favored because of its accurate detection of small lesions less than 1.5 cm, and because the needle tract along which seeding can theoretically occur is resected for lesions in the pancreatic head. Tumor spread along the needle tract was suspected in one case report of a patient who developed recurrent cancer within the gastric wall 16 months after complete resection of a T1N0M0 pancreatic tumor located in the pancreatic tail. Therefore, for potentially resectable tumors located in the pancreatic body or tail, the options of proceeding directly to surgery without a tissue diagnosis versus EUS-FNA should be carefully considered.

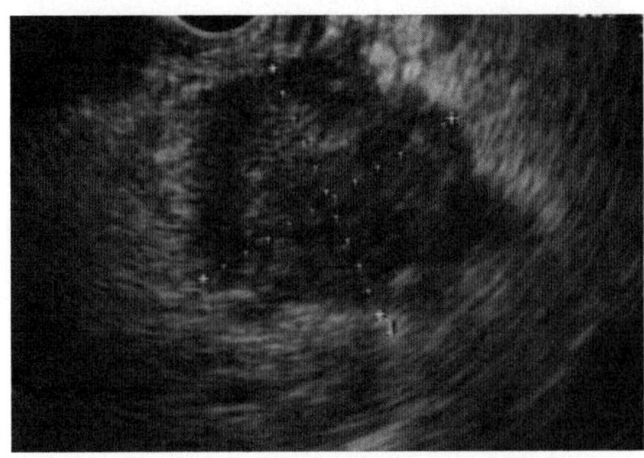

▲ **Figure 36–7.** EUS image of a pancreatic mass.

The best outcome in pancreatic cancer occurs in patients without nodal, vascular, or systemic metastases (5-year survival up to 25%). More accurate patient selection could reduce unnecessary surgeries in patients with unresectable tumors. A recent review of studies comparing EUS and CT for preoperative staging of pancreatic cancer concluded that it is unclear which modality is superior for both tumor and nodal staging.

EUS criteria for vascular invasion include abnormal vessel contour, loss of hyperechoic interface between the tumor and blood vessel, tumor in the vessel lumen, and presence of collateral vessels in the absence of a main vascular structure. Presence of any one of these criteria indicates vascular invasion. A recent meta-analysis examining the accuracy of these EUS criteria for assessing vascular invasion demonstrated 73% sensitivity and 90% specificity. EUS is more reliable for evaluating invasion into the portal vein and splenic confluence than the superior mesenteric artery or vein. With recent advances in helical CT and MRI, these modalities will most likely surpass EUS for vascular staging. Initial staging should be performed with pancreatic protocol CT scan. EUS will still have a potentially important impact on staging through identifying and sampling lymph nodes, ascites, and hepatic lesions.

Pancreatic neuroendocrine tumors are notoriously difficult to diagnose, and EUS is particularly helpful in evaluating these tumors (Figure 36–8). Because most insulinomas occur in the pancreas, sensitivity of EUS is highest for these neuroendocrine tumors at 83%. Gastrinomas and glucagonomas more commonly occur in extrapancreatic sites leading to decreased diagnostic sensitivity for EUS and a more important role in diagnosis for somatostatin receptor scintigraphy, CT, and MRI.

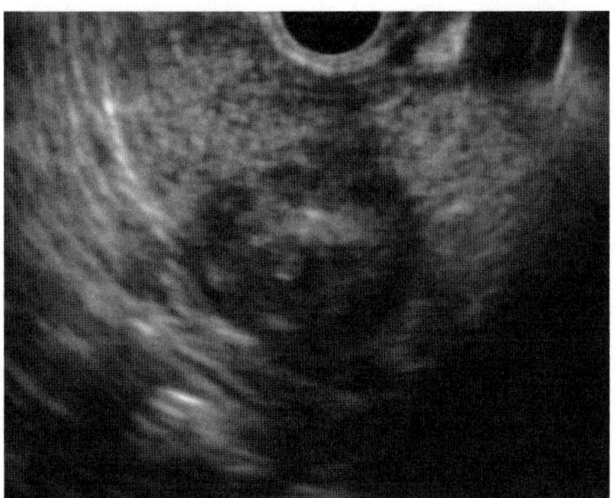

▲ **Figure 36–8.** EUS image of a pancreatic neuroendocrine tumor.

Horwhat JD, Paulson EK, McGrath K, et al. A randomized comparison of EUS-guided FNA versus CT or US-guided FNA for the evaluation of pancreatic mass lesions. *Gastrointest Endosc.* 2006;63:966–975. [PMID: 16733111]

5. Other Gastrointestinal Malignancies

Early detection of small hepatocellular carcinomas remains problematic, with over 70% of lesions smaller than 1 cm missed by MRI. Preliminary study of EUS in detecting early hepatocellular carcinoma reports promising results. In one study, patients with cirrhosis and at high risk for hepatocellular carcinoma because of elevated α-fetoprotein levels or abnormal radiologic findings underwent ultrasound, CT, MRI, and EUS or EUS-FNA; diagnostic accuracy was 38%, 69%, 92%, and 94%, respectively. EUS alone had a lower accuracy of 65% mainly due to poor specificity. Complications following EUS-FNA of hepatic lesions occurred in about 4% of patients and included bleeding, fever, and abdominal pain, and death in one patient with obstructive jaundice who developed cholangitis. Further studies are necessary to define the role and safety of EUS-FNA in hepatocellular carcinoma.

Cholangiocarcinoma also remains a difficult diagnostic dilemma. Several small studies suggest EUS-FNA is safe and useful in diagnosing biliary strictures following negative ERCP brush cytology, with sensitivity ranging from 43% to 86% and 100% specificity based on surgical pathology. EUS finding of bile duct wall thickness of 3 mm or greater was found to have 79% sensitivity and specificity. Intraductal ultrasound (IDUS) offers data about depth of tumor invasion and invasion into the pancreas and portal vein, with accuracies greater than 85%. Therefore, EUS, EUS-FNA, and probably IDUS should be included in the armamentarium for evaluating potentially malignant biliary strictures.

DeWitt J, Misra VL, LeBlanc JK, et al. EUS-guided FNA of proximal biliary strictures after negative ERCP brush cytology results. *Gastrointest Endosc.* 2006;64:325–333. [PMID: 16923477]

Inui K, Miyoshi H, Yoshino J. Bile duct cancers: what can EUS offer? Intraductal US, 3D-IDUS? FNA—is it possible? *Endoscopy.* 2006;38(Suppl 1):47–49. [PMID: 16802223]

Thuluvath PJ. EUS-guided FNA could be another important tool for the early diagnosis of hepatocellular carcinoma. *Gastrointest Endosc.* 2007;66:274–276. [PMID: 17643699]

6. Lung Cancer

The scope of EUS is not limited to the gastrointestinal tract, and it can have a major impact on staging in lung cancer, which remains the leading cause of cancer-related mortality in the United States. As with gastrointestinal cancers, accurate staging is critical in determining prognosis and appropriate treatment for patients with lung cancer. Standard staging methods include CT, PET, transbronchial FNA, mediastinoscopy, and thoracoscopy. EUS-FNA can access areas complementary to the other techniques, and approximately 14% of thoracotomies can be avoided by performing EUS-FNA in addition to mediastinoscopy.

Annema JT, van Meerbeeck JP, Rintoul RC, et al. Mediastinoscopy vs endosonography for mediastinal nodal staging of lung cancer. *JAMA.* 2010;304:2245–2252.

NONMALIGNANT LESIONS

1. Submucosal Lesions

For submucosal lesions, accurate preoperative diagnosis can prevent unnecessary surgical resection of benign lesions. Before EUS, this was difficult because submucosal lesions grow underneath the mucosa and cannot be readily diagnosed by endoscopy and biopsy. EUS appears most useful for differentiating submucosal lesions from extrinsic compression and for characterizing the submucosal lesion. Extrinsic compression from adjacent organs or blood vessels is correctly differentiated from a submucosal lesion in 94% of cases. Using EUS, the size, layer of origin, margins, and echo-pattern of the submucosal lesion are determined; the layer of origin and echotexture are most useful in suggesting a diagnosis (Table 36–2) although imaging alone is only 45.5% accurate for diagnosis. Malignancy can be inferred from larger lesions (>3 cm) with irregular margins. EUS-guided FNA has limited diagnostic yield with definitive diagnosis possible in only 34–43% of cases although a recent study suggests a higher yield up to 68%.

The most common submucosal lesion is a gastrointestinal stromal tumor (GIST), which has a mesenchymal cell of origin. On EUS, GISTs are hypoechoic and typically arise from the fourth muscularis propria layer (Figure 36–9). Presence

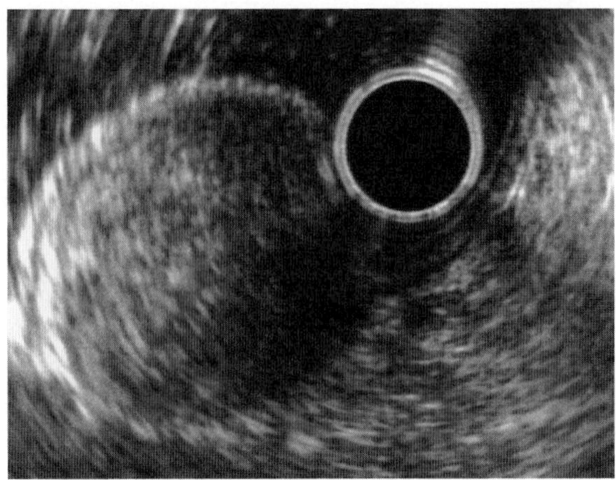

▲ **Figure 36–9.** EUS image of a gastrointestinal stromal tumor.

of an irregular border, cystic spaces, echogenic foci, and size greater than 3 cm are suggestive of malignancy. Lipoma is the second most common submucosal lesion and may be readily diagnosed during endoscopy by its yellowish hue and soft texture. If the diagnosis is unclear, EUS should be performed; it will reveal a hyperechoic lesion arising from the third submucosal layer (Figure 36–10 and Plate 93). Cysts are also easily diagnosed by EUS as anechoic structures lying within the second or third layer.

Table 36–2. Endoscopic ultrasound (EUS) characteristics of submucosal lesions.

Lesion	EUS Characteristic
GIST	Hypoechoic, 4th layer
Lipoma	Hyperechoic, 3rd layer
Carcinoid	Mildly hypoechoic; 1st, 2nd, or 3rd layer
Cyst	Anechoic, 2nd or 3rd layer
Pancreatic rest	Hypoechoic or heterogeneous; 2nd, 3rd, 4th layer; ductal structures
Granular cell tumor	Heterogeneous, 3rd layer

GIST, gastrointestinal stromal tumor.

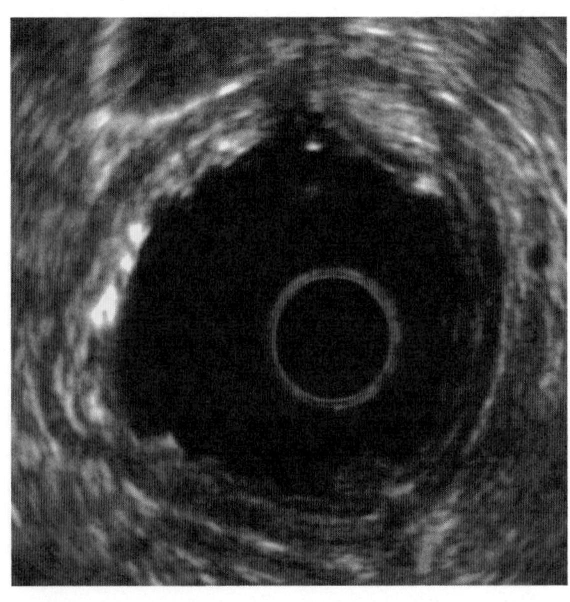

▲ **Figure 36–10.** EUS image of a lipoma. (For an endoscopic view, see Plate 93.)

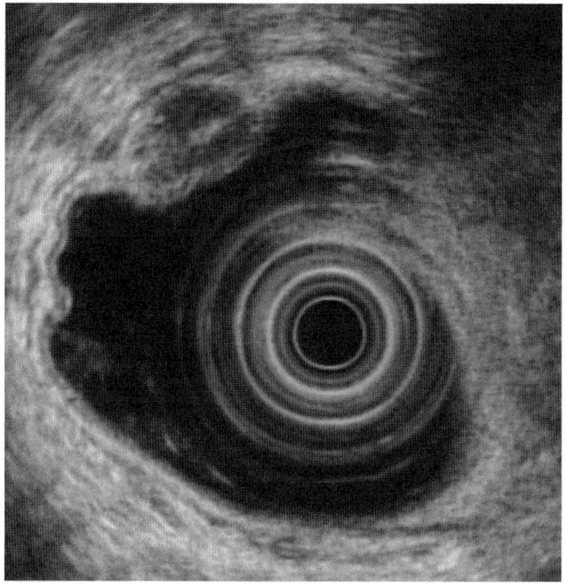

▲ **Figure 36–11.** EUS image of a rectal carcinoid. (For an endoscopic view, see Plate 94.)

Carcinoids are mildly hypoechoic, homogeneous and typically arise from the first, second, or third layer (Figure 36–11 and Plate 94). Size is usually predictive of malignancy, and they are usually benign if less than 2 cm. Other malignant submucosal tumors include metastases, which are rare, and lymphomas, which may appear as hypoechoic heterogeneous masses within the gastrointestinal wall.

A few other benign submucosal lesions include pancreatic rests and granular cell tumors. Pancreatic rests are submucosal deposits of ectopic pancreatic tissue that typically occur in the antrum and have a characteristic umbilicated appearance on endoscopy. On EUS, they appear hypoechoic or heterogeneous, arise from the second, third, or fourth layer and may contain anechoic ductal structures (Figure 36–12 and Plate 95). Granular cell tumors are believed to arise from neural tissue and appear heterogeneous within the third submucosal layer.

Management of these submucosal lesions is guided by their diagnosis, size, location, and potential for malignancy. GISTs with several EUS features raising concern for malignancy should be removed surgically. Smaller benign-appearing GISTs may be observed, although the appropriate follow-up interval is unknown. Lipomas should only be removed if symptomatic. Carcinoids smaller than 2 cm confined to the first three layers can be removed endoscopically, whereas larger lesions involving the fourth muscularis propria layer should be surgically resected.

Mekky MA, Yamao K, Sawaki A, Mizuno N, Hara K, Nafeh MA, Osman AM, Koshikawa T, Yatabe Y, Bhatia V. Diagnostic utility of EUS-guided FNA in patients with gastric submucosal tumors. *Gastrointest Endosc.* 2010;71:913–919. [PMID: 20226456]

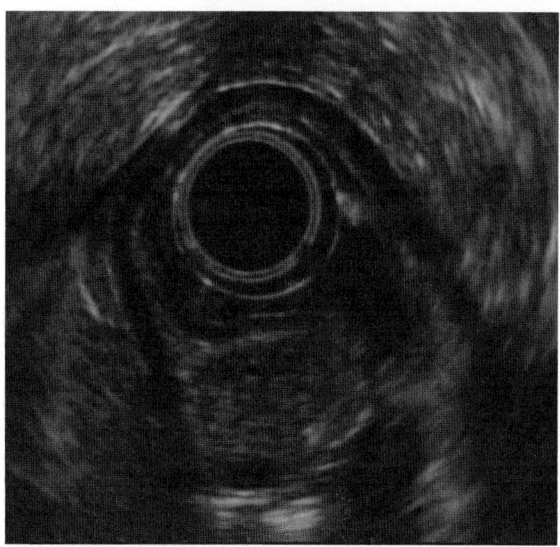

▲ **Figure 36–12.** EUS image of a pancreatic rest. (For an endoscopic view, see Plate 95.)

Philipper M, Hollerbach S, Gabbert HE, et al. Prospective comparison of endoscopic ultrasound-guided fine-needle aspiration and surgical histology in upper gastrointestinal submucosal tumors. *Endoscopy.* 2010;42:300–305. [PMID: 20306384]

2. Thickened Gastric Folds

Large gastric folds present a diagnostic dilemma that often necessitates multiple diagnostic studies. The differential diagnosis is broad and includes malignant and benign conditions (Table 36–3). Endoscopic appearance does not usually enable differentiation between malignant and benign conditions, and superficial mucosal biopsies may miss a malignancy. Snare resection or cap-assisted endoscopic mucosal resection increases diagnostic yield from 17% to 87% but carries an increased risk of complications from bleeding and potentially perforation.

Table 36–3. Causes of thickened gastric folds.

Malignant	Benign
Adenocarcinoma Lymphoma	Hypertrophic gastritis Ménétrier disease Lymphoid hyperplasia Zollinger-Ellison syndrome Gastric varices Benign hyperrugosity Granulomatous disease (Crohn, sarcoidosis, secondary syphilis) Eosinophilic gastritis Acute *Helicobacter pylori* gastritis

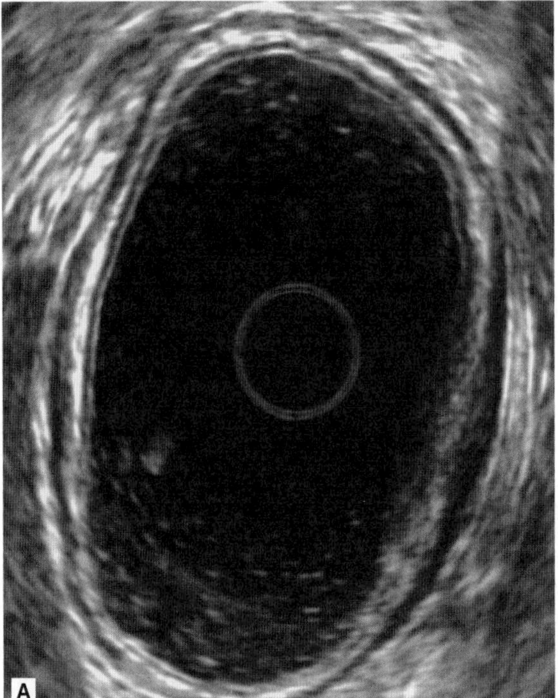

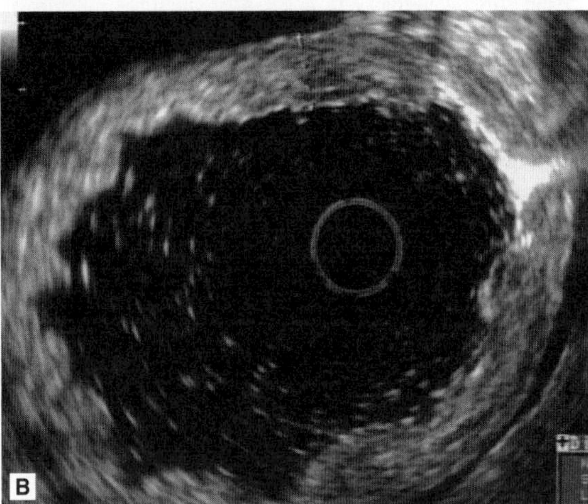

▲ **Figure 36–13.** EUS images of the gastric wall. **A:** Normal gastric wall. **B:** Thickened gastric wall.

Few studies exist examining the utility of EUS in evaluating a thickened gastric wall (Figure 36–13). The main predictor of malignancy is thickening of the deep gastric layers, including submucosa, muscularis propria, and serosa, whereas enlargement of the superficial mucosal layers is associated with benign conditions or MALT lymphoma, which is usually readily diagnosed with biopsies. Ascites and lymph nodes are present in over 60% of patients with gastric wall thickening from malignancy.

Ginès A, Pellise M, Fernández-Esparrach G, et al. Endoscopic ultrasonography in patients with large gastric folds at endoscopy and biopsies negative for malignancy: predictors of malignant disease and clinical impact. *Am J Gastroenterol.* 2006;101:64–69. [PMID: 16405535]

3. Pancreatic Cysts

Pancreatic cysts are increasingly discovered, since abdominal imaging studies have improved in quality and have become more frequently utilized. These lesions are often of unclear clinical significance and pose a diagnostic dilemma. Pseudocysts account for the majority of pancreatic cysts while an increasing minority is pancreatic cystic neoplasms, which may be benign serous cystadenomas or premalignant or malignant mucinous lesions that include mucinous cystic neoplasms or intrapapillary mucinous neoplasm (IPMN). Therefore, it is important to differentiate among these different cysts.

Serous cystadenomas occur anywhere throughout the pancreas typically in women over the age of 60 years. On radiology or EUS imaging, they usually appear microcystic and less commonly macrocystic or solid due to the presence of numerous microcysts that give the appearance of a homogeneous hypoechoic mass. A central calcification is pathognomonic but is only seen in about 10% of serous cystadenomas. Malignant transformation is very rare, and these cysts can typically be followed.

Mucinous cystic neoplasms are premalignant lesions that generally occur in women between 40 and 50 years old. They typically appear macrocystic in the body and tail of the pancreas with a rare, but pathognomonic, peripheral eccentric calcification. IPMN is also a mucinous cystic neoplasm that arises from the pancreatic ductal epithelium and communicates with the main duct, side branches, or both (Figure 36–14).

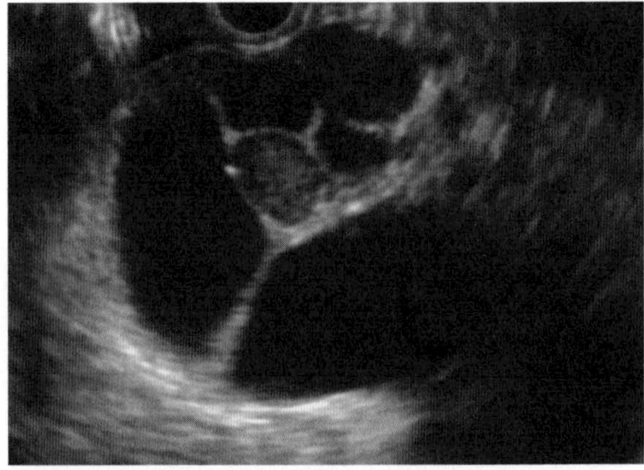

▲ **Figure 36–14.** EUS image of intraductal papillary mucinous neoplasm.

Table 36–4. Diagnostic markers for pancreatic cysts.

Marker	Sensitivity	Specificity
CEA <5 ng/mL (serous vs other lesions)	100%	86–93%
CEA >400 ng/mL (mucinous vs other lesions)	57%	100%
Cytology (mucinous vs other lesions)	27%	100%
Amylase >5000 units/mL (pseudocyst vs other lesions)	61–94%	58–74%
k-ras mutation (mucinous vs other lesions)	11–45%	45%
Allelic loss amplitude	67%	66%

CEA, carcinoembryonic antigen.

It occurs more commonly in men between the ages of 50 and 60 years. About 40% of main-duct IPMNs contain malignancy at the time of diagnosis. Features suggestive of malignancy in side-branch IPMNs include presence of a mass, mural nodules, dilated main pancreatic duct, and cyst size greater than 3 cm, although a recent study demonstrated presence of malignancy in smaller cysts.

Accurate preoperative diagnosis of serous cystadenoma, mucinous cystadenoma, and mucinous cystadenocarcinoma using CT scanning occurs in about 20–30% of cases. MRCP may be more helpful than endoscopic retrograde pancreatography (ERP) in diagnosing IPMN by delineating the main pancreatic duct, side branches, and communicating cystic lesions. EUS imaging alone is not sufficient to diagnose pancreatic cystic lesions. EUS-FNA probably improves diagnostic yield for pancreatic cystic lesions; however, the optimal cyst fluid markers remain unknown. Current evidence suggests that carcinoembryonic antigen (CEA) may be most useful while cytology has poor sensitivity and accuracy in differentiating mucinous from nonmucinous lesions as well as benign from malignant or premalignant lesions (Table 36–4). Molecular analysis of pancreatic cyst DNA for mutations, including early *k-ras* mutation followed by allelic loss, has been similarly disappointing in differentiating mucinous from non-mucinous cystic lesions.

Further work is necessary to discover new and more accurate markers of malignancy and mucinous cystic lesions as pancreatic cystic lesions are increasingly uncovered on incidental imaging studies.

Noh KW, Pungpapong S, Raimondo M. Role of endosonography in non-malignant pancreatic diseases. *World J Gastroenterol.* 2007;13:165–169. [PMID: 17226895]

4. Chronic Pancreatitis

Diagnosis of chronic pancreatitis remains challenging, especially because there is no defined gold standard. Histology may be considered the true gold standard; however, it is available in a minority of patients, sampling error may occur if only a core biopsy specimen is obtained, and there is no consensus on a histologic grading scale for severity of chronic pancreatitis. ERP is less attractive as a diagnostic modality due to its potential complications and decreased sensitivity for early-stage chronic pancreatitis. In addition, the Cambridge classification for ERP changes in chronic pancreatitis was based on expert consensus and has not been validated. Only one study has compared secretin-stimulated functional studies with histology; it found accuracy of the functional test to be 81%.

EUS is an attractive alternative diagnostic possibility due to its relatively low morbidity and ability to assess both parenchymal and ductal features. EUS criteria for chronic pancreatitis include the following parenchymal and ductal changes: hyperechoic foci, hyperechoic strands, lobulation, cysts, calcifications, main duct dilation, main duct irregularity, hyperechoic walls of the main duct, and visible side branches (Figure 36–15). Retrospective studies have noted that the presence of four or more EUS criteria had 84–91% sensitivity and 86–100% specificity for diagnosing chronic pancreatitis using histology as the gold standard. The threshold for diagnosing chronic pancreatitis can be varied depending on whether one is trying to establish or exclude the diagnosis. In the previous study, presence of five or more criteria had 100% specificity. In a population at low to moderate risk of chronic pancreatitis, EUS is most accurate when unambiguously normal with two or fewer criteria or abnormal with five or more criteria present. This is especially true in elderly patients, in whom up to three EUS criteria

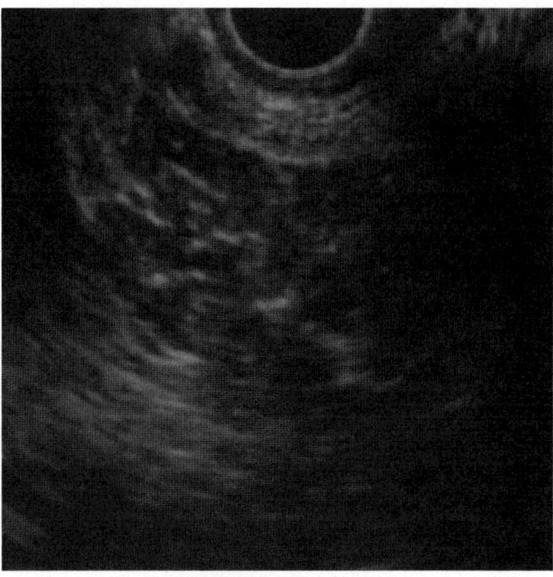

▲ **Figure 36–15.** EUS image of chronic pancreatitis demonstrating lobularity.

for chronic pancreatitis may be present without actual pancreatic disease. Certain features including calcification and lobulation are more indicative of chronic pancreatitis, and recently a weighted scoring system accounting for these factors has been proposed.

The clinical significance of the presence of three or four EUS criteria for chronic pancreatitis is unclear. The addition of FNA does not appear to increase diagnostic yield for chronic pancreatitis. A study comparing EUS and MRCP using the gold standards of ERP, histology, or long-term clinical follow-up of median 15 months demonstrated higher sensitivity of 93% for EUS compared with 65% sensitivity for MRCP, and similar specificity of 90–93%. The combination of both studies yielded higher sensitivity and specificity of 98% and 83%. Therefore, the less invasive modalities of EUS and MRCP have largely supplanted ERCP in the diagnosis of chronic pancreatitis. The expert consensus Rosemont EUS criteria for chronic pancreatitis has been proposed, however, has not been validated and interobserver variability for diagnosing chronic pancreatitis was no better using the Rosemont classification than the standard EUS criteria. More recent studies suggest that the addition of endoscopic pancreatic function testing, which can be performed during routine endoscopy or endoscopic ultrasound, may enable earlier diagnosis of chronic pancreatitis.

Wallace MB. Chronic pancreatitis. *Gastrointest Endosc.* 2009; 69:S117–S120. [PMID: 19179134]

5. Autoimmune Pancreatitis

Autoimmune pancreatitis (AIP) can be extremely difficult to diagnose and often mimics pancreatic cancer in presentation with a pancreatic mass. EUS-FNA findings are often nonspecific. Use of a 19-gauge trucut needle has been reported in small case series to yield histologic diagnosis of AIP. In addition, a small Japanese study has proposed novel EUS criteria for AIP, which remains to be validated. Certainly appreciation of a diffusely hypoechoic, enlarged pancreas with chronic inflammatory cells on cytology should raise the concern for AIP.

Mizuno N, Bhatia V, Hosoda W, et al. Histological diagnosis of autoimmune pancreatitis using EUS-guided trucut biopsy: a comparison study with EUS-FNA. *J Gastroenterol.* 2009;44: 742–750. [PMID: 19434362]

6. Bile Duct Stones

EUS has similarly proven to be a powerfully accurate and safe method for detecting choledocholithiasis. A meta-analysis of randomized controlled blinded trials comparing EUS and MRCP with the gold standard of ERCP or intraoperative cholangiography in patients with suspected bile duct stones demonstrated sensitivity for EUS and MRCP of 93% and 85%, with similar specificities of 96% and 93%, respectively. A cost-analysis study indicated that initial EUS rather than MRCP had the greatest cost-utility by reducing unnecessary ERCP procedures.

Arguedas MR, Dupont AW, Wilcox CM. Where do ERCP, endoscopic ultrasound, magnetic resonance cholangiopancreatography, and intraoperative cholangiography fit in the management of acute biliary pancreatitis? A decision analysis model. *Am J Gastroenterol.* 2001;96:2892–2899. [PMID: 11693323]

Verma D, Kapadia A, Eisen G, Adler D. EUS vs. MRCP for detection of choledocholithiasis. *Gastrointest Endosc.* 2006;64:248–254. [PMID: 16860077]

THERAPEUTIC ENDOSCOPIC ULTRASOUND

With the advent of EUS-FNA, a new realm of diagnostic possibilities was discovered, followed more recently by various innovative therapeutic techniques. The following sections discuss both well-established and more experimental therapeutic uses of EUS-FNA.

1. Celiac Plexus Neurolysis & Block

Celiac plexus neurolysis (CPN) refers to the permanent destruction of the celiac plexus using absolute ethanol. Temporary block of the plexus with corticosteroid injection is termed celiac plexus block (CPB). Pancreatic pain is predominantly controlled by the celiac plexus. CPN using surgical and transcutaneous approaches has been used for many years; however, major complications including paralysis occur in about 1% of cases, which makes the endoscopic approach a potentially more attractive option.

The EUS technique involves first flushing a 22-gauge needle with normal saline to clear the needle of air followed by insertion of the needle 1 cm cranial and anterior to the take-off of the celiac artery and aspiration to ensure no blood returns. There has been recent interest in injecting the celiac ganglia visible during EUS, however, further research is necessary to validate this approach. For CPN, 10 mL of 0.25% bupivacaine is injected followed by 20 mL of 98% absolute ethanol. For CPB, 20 mL of 0.25% bupivacaine is injected followed by 80 mg of triamcinolone. This is a safe technique without reported incidences of paralysis. Minor complications include transient diarrhea in 4–15% of patients, transient increase in pain in 9%, and transient orthostasis in 1%. Normal saline is administered during the procedure, and patients should be monitored for 2 hours post-procedure for orthostasis. Major complications include retroperitoneal bleed and peripancreatic abscess.

A recent meta-analysis suggests that EUS-CPN offers safe and effective pain relief for patients with pancreatic cancer and chronic pancreatitis. Nearly 80% of patients with pancreatic cancer experience pain relief while the response rate and durability are lower in chronic pancreatitis, with initial 55% response rate that decreases to 10% at 24 weeks.

Pain reduction lasts about 20 weeks following EUS-CPN in pancreatic cancer compared with 2 weeks for chronic pancreatitis with EUS-CPB.

Penman ID. Coeliac plexus neurolysis. Best Practice and Research Clinical. *Gastroenterology.* 2009;23:761–766. [PMID: 19744638]

Puli SR, Reddy JBK, Bechtold ML, Antillon MR, Brugge WR. EUS-guided celiac plexus neurolysis for pain due to chronic pancreatitis or pancreatic cancer pain: a meta-analysis and systematic review. *Dig Dis Sci.* 2009;54:2330–2337. [PMID: 19137428]

2. Pseudocyst Drainage

Pancreatic pseudocysts are the most common cyst in the pancreas, and studies suggest that even large pseudocysts greater than 6 cm can be followed conservatively until symptoms develop or the cyst increases in size. Surgical drainage had been the standard of care but carries a 10% morbidity rate and a 1% mortality rate; therefore, radiologic and endoscopic drainage have replaced surgical drainage as initial treatment. Complications of endoscopic pseudocyst drainage include early bleeding, perforation of adjacent structures, and infection. Traditionally, endoscopic pseudocyst drainage was performed by piercing the endoscopically visible bulge. Access to the pseudocyst can be achieved by using a needle-knife with electrocautery or the Seldinger technique, which advances a guidewire through a 19-gauge needle. Retrospective studies suggest that the rate of bleeding is reduced to 4.6% using the Seldinger technique compared with 15.7% using the needle-knife. After establishing access to the cavity, the opening is dilated with a balloon followed by placement of several pigtail stents.

EUS allows drainage of pseudocysts that do not create a visible bulge and has changed the management of about 25% of patients undergoing endoscopic pseudocyst drainage. EUS is helpful for several reasons, including detecting blood vessels in the wall of the pseudocyst or path of drainage, confirming that the distance between the wall of the pseudocyst and the gastric wall is less than 1 cm, and characterizing the pseudocyst and its contents. Presence of necrotic debris within the pseudocyst necessitates either surgical debridement or endoscopic necrosectomy, which involves entering the cavity with the endoscope and removing necrotic debris with a variety of accessories. This technique is still evolving and needs to be compared with surgical management. Two randomized trials comparing EUS-guided pseudocyst drainage with non–EUS-guided techniques both suggest that the technical success rate is higher for EUS-guided drainage although complication rates were similar.

Park DH, Lee SS, Moon SH, et al. Endoscopic ultrasound-guided versus conventional transmural drainage for pancreatic pseudocysts: a prospective randomized trial. *Endoscopy.* 2009;41:842–848. [PMID: 19798610]

Varadarajulu S, Christein JD, Tamhane A, Drelichman ER, Wilcox CM. Prospective randomized trial comparing EUS and EGD for transmural drainage of pancreatic pseudocysts. *Gastrointest Endosc.* 2008;68:1102–1111. [PMID: 18640677]

3. Rendezvous Procedure & EUS-Guided Transluminal Drainage

Endoscopic decompression of biliary and pancreatic obstruction has been traditionally performed via ERCP, with greater than 90% success in biliary drainage by skilled endoscopists. Unsuccessful endoscopic drainage results from surgically altered anatomy, tumor invasion, periampullary diverticulum, endoscopist inexperience, or other causes. Alternative therapeutic options include percutaneous transhepatic drainage or surgery. Morbidity from percutaneous transhepatic drainage is not insignificant, ranging from 4% to 32% with a mortality rate up to 5.6%. Therefore, EUS-guided decompression offers a potentially attractive endoscopic alternative for failed ERCP procedures.

To date there have been only small case series detailing the technique of EUS-guided biliary and pancreatic drainage, which involves either a rendezvous procedure with ERCP or the creation of an EUS-guided enterobiliary or enteropancreatic fistula. During a rendezvous procedure, a 19- or 22-gauge needle is used to access the pancreatic duct or the bile duct via an intrahepatic or extrahepatic approach under EUS guidance. A guidewire is then advanced into the duodenum, followed by exchange of the echoendoscope for a duodenoscope to complete the procedure. One study suggested that puncture of the bile duct closest to the point of obstruction may increase technical success whereas another suggested that entering the extrahepatic bile duct may lead to greater complications.

Another EUS-guided technique involves creating an enterobiliary or enteropancreatic fistula. The intrahepatic bile duct or pancreatic duct is punctured with a 19-gauge needle followed by guidewire placement, dilation of the puncture tract to 4–6 mm, and placement of metal or plastic pigtail stents. Small studies have reported a 90% success rate with the EUS-approach and complications in 10–17%, including cholangitis, bile leak, and self-limited pneumoperitoneum.

Barkay O, Sherman S, McHenry L, et al. Therapeutic EUS-assisted endoscopic retrograde pancreatography after failed pancreatic duct cannulation at ERCP. *Gastrointest Endosc.* 2010;71:1166–1173. [PMID: 20303489]

Kim YS, Gupta K, Mallery S, Li R, Kinney T, Freeman ML. Endoscopic ultrasound rendezvous for bile duct access using a transduodenal approach: a cumulative experience at a single center. A case series. *Endoscopy.* 2010;42:496–502. [PMID: 20419625]

4. EUS-Guided Fine Needle Injection

EUS-FNI encompasses injection of any material through the needle. Biweekly EUS-guided injection of cyanoacrylate into gastric varices until they are obliterated may reduce rebleeding rates compared with non–EUS-guided injections administered only during episodes of bleeding. Additional larger studies are necessary to determine the efficacy and complications of this technique.

EUS has revolutionized staging of many cancers, and it may allow more directed and potentially more efficacious anticancer treatments such as brachytherapy and local injection of antitumor therapy. A few small case series have demonstrated the feasibility of placing radioactive seeds into head and neck cancer, lymph nodes, and pancreatic cancer. The technique involves withdrawing the stylet about 1 cm and backloading the radioactive seed into a 19-gauge needle. Similarly, inactive radiographic markers, termed fiducials, which serve as targets for CyberKnife radiation therapy, can be placed under EUS guidance. The CyberKnife system delivers high doses of precisely targeted, small beams of radiation using real-time image guidance. This revolutionary technique reduces radiation exposure of surrounding organs, the total time of radiation treatment, and side effects compared with conventional radiotherapy. Fiducials have traditionally been placed surgically or percutaneously; however, safe EUS-guided delivery of fiducials into abdominal (predominantly pancreatic cancer) and mediastinal tumors has recently been demonstrated in several studies.

Targeted local injection of anti-tumor therapy under EUS-guidance is feasible. EUS has been used to deliver allogenic mixed lymphocyte culture (cytoimplant), antitumor viral therapy, and dendritic cells into pancreatic adenocarcinoma and a novel gene therapy agent, TNFerade, which is a replication-deficient adenovector containing human tumor necrosis factor-α gene, into pancreatic and esophageal adenocarcinoma. A phase I trial using cytoimplant in patients with pancreatic cancer was halted early because patients in the control arm receiving gemcitabine therapy had better outcomes. Another trial using the antitumor viral therapy was also stopped early due to poor response and a high rate of complications, including sepsis and duodenal perforation. Early trials of TNFerade in pancreatic and esophageal cancer suggest possibly improved rates of remission and survival and warrant further studies.

Chang KJ, Irisawa A. EUS 2008 working group document: evaluation of EUS-guided injection therapy for tumors. *Gastrointest Endosc.* 2009;69:S54–S58. [PMID: 19179171]

FUTURE DIRECTIONS

EUS continues to grow as a diagnostic and therapeutic modality. In the future, EUS will be coupled with other imaging modalities to allow more accurate diagnosis of both benign and malignant lesions. The realm of therapeutic EUS will require the development of innovative devices and accessories and perhaps new echoendoscopes to allow many potential procedures to become a reality.

1. New Diagnostic Uses of EUS

Recent development of three-dimensional (3D) software to allow rendering of two-dimensional (2D) EUS images into 3D images may allow more accurate tumor staging. A study of rectal cancer staging using 2D and 3D radial EUS demonstrated no difference in staging for T1 and T2 tumors. However, 40% of patients with tumors identified as T3N0 by 2D EUS were upstaged to T3N1 using 3D EUS. Overall accuracy of staging for 2D and 3D EUS was 71.4% and 88.6%, respectively.

Combining EUS with CT images and a real-time guidance system called the image-registered gastroscopic ultrasound (IRGUS) system may improve the diagnostic capability of EUS. The system uses a miniaturized tracking sensor that is attached to the tip of an echoendoscope and allows real-time displays of the position of the echoendoscope within a previously obtained CT scan. In a porcine model, endosonographers were more efficient and effective, identifying 25% more basic structures in a timed trial using the IRGUS system compared with standard EUS, and 90% of the users preferred the IRGUS system.

Techniques using contrast agents, elastography, and digital image analysis (DIA) with fluorescence in situ hybridization (FISH) appear promising in their ability to detect malignancies (Table 36–5). Several different contrast agents have been used, including Levovist, Albunex, Optison, and Sonovue. Following contrast injection, benign lesions such as inflammatory changes from chronic pancreatitis enhance and appear hyperechoic whereas malignant tumors are underperfused and hypoechoic.

Elastography is based on the principle that cancer changes the elastic properties or the hardness of tissue. Slight compression of tissue by an ultrasound transducer displaces the tissue, and the elasticity distribution of the tissue before and after compression can be compared. In addition to enhancing the different tissue properties of malignant compared

Table 36–5. New diagnostic techniques for detecting malignancies.

Diagnostic Technique	Sensitivity	Specificity
Contrast agents	94%	89-100%
Elastography (pancreatic mass)	80.6–100%	92.9%
DIA/FISH (various malignancies)	97%	100%
Standard cytology	87%	100%

DIA, digital image analysis; FISH, fluorescence in situ hybridization.

with normal tissue, the search for new molecular markers of malignancy continues. The techniques of DIA and FISH assess the nuclear DNA content and presence of aneuploidy to diagnose malignancy.

Finally, the horizons of EUS may be expanding with a study exploring the application of EUS-FNA and the heart. Six animals survived for 2 weeks following introduction of an EUS needle into the left atrium and coronary artery. In a separate study in humans, three patients underwent successful aspiration of pericardial fluid and puncture of a left atrial mass using EUS-FNA.

Giovannini M. Contrast-enhanced endoscopic ultrasound and elastosonoendoscopy. *Best Prac Res Clin Gastroenterol.* 2009;23: 767–779. [PMID: 19744639]

2. Future Therapeutic Uses of EUS

The realm of therapeutic EUS is in its infancy and may be slow to develop given a relatively limited number of endosonographers and the lack of incentive for instrument manufacturers to invest time and resources in this area. There have been a few animal studies using a new EUS-guided suturing system to create gastrojejunal anastomoses, perform posterior gastropexy for gastroesophageal reflux, and remove lymph nodes.

Expanding on the premise of EUS-FNI, experimental pig models have demonstrated the feasibility of EUS-guided radiofrequency ablation, photodynamic therapy, and embolization of the portal vein using ethylene vinyl alcohol co-polymer (Enteryx). There are a few case reports of successful treatment of splenic and superior mesenteric artery pseudoaneurysms using thrombin injected into the vessels under EUS guidance. In a recent randomized study of EUS-guided ethanol versus saline injection of pancreatic cysts, the technique appears safe and potentially effective at decreasing the size of the cyst although only 33% of cysts had completely resolved on short-term follow-up. In addition, EUS has been used to drain a variety of intra-abdominal collections including pelvic and intra-abdominal abscesses, bilomas, and hematomas.

Hawes RH, VanDam J, Varadarajulu S. EUS 2008 working group document: interventional EUS—a road map for the future. *Gastrointest Endosc.* 2009;69:S1–S2. [PMID: 19179130]

Kaul V, Adler DG, Conway JD, et al. Interventional EUS. *Gastrointest Endosc.* 2010;72:1–4. [PMID: 20381044]

Approach to the Patient with Jaundice & Abnormal Liver Tests

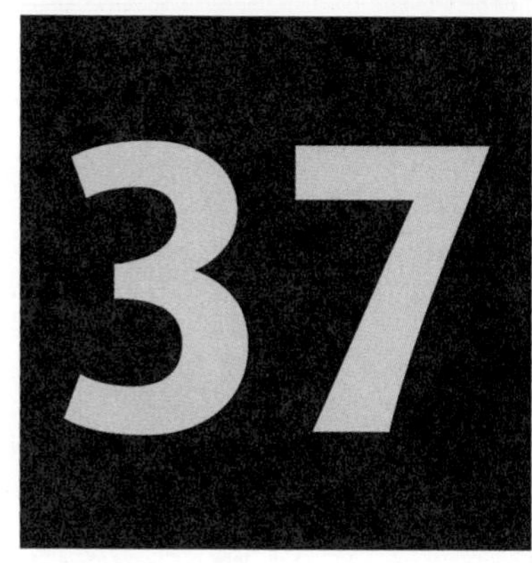

Norton J. Greenberger, MD

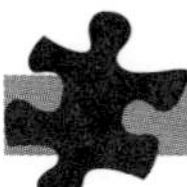

ESSENTIALS OF DIAGNOSIS

- Jaundice is most often caused by decompensation of preexisting chronic liver disease, alcoholic hepatitis, and gallstone disease.
- Careful history, physical examination, and routine laboratory tests lead to accurate diagnosis in 85% of patients with jaundice.
- Cirrhosis can be diagnosed on the basis of two physical findings (asterixis, ascites) and two laboratory findings (decreased serum albumin [<2.8 g/dL], prolonged prothrombin time [INR >1.6]).
- Dilated intrahepatic bile ducts indicate obstruction from extrahepatic causes (stone, structure, tumor).
- Absence of dilated ducts in jaundiced patients with serum bilirubin >10 mg/dL suggests intrahepatic cholestasis.
- Sepsis, drugs, sickle cell disease, and chronic hepatitis are the most common causes of intrahepatic cholestasis.

General Considerations

Jaundice refers to the yellowish discoloration of tissue resulting from the deposition of bilirubin in tissues; this indicates that the serum bilirubin is likely 3.0 mg/dL or higher. Jaundice most often is the result of acute or chronic liver disease, or biliary tract disease, and less commonly the result of hemolytic disorders. The differential diagnosis of jaundice has changed significantly in the past decade due largely to a sharp decline in the incidence of viral hepatitis types A and B as a result of immunization. The most common causes of jaundice in the adult population now are decompensation of preexisting chronic liver disease, alcoholic hepatitis, sepsis and abnormal hemodynamic conditions, and gallstone disease.

Pathogenesis

Jaundice can occur as a result of acute or chronic parenchymal liver disease, extrahepatic biliary tract obstruction (due to stone, stricture, or tumor), intrahepatic cholestasis (having several causes, as detailed below), and hemolytic anemia. Serum bilirubin derives from the degradation of senescent red cells in the reticuloendothelial system. Each day a normal individual destroys 50 mL of red blood cells, which gives rise to 7.5 g of hemoglobin. Each gram of hemoglobin that is degraded results in production of 35 mg of bilirubin. Unconjugated bilirubin is liquid soluble, water insoluble, and hence circulates bound to albumin. The hepatic processing of bilirubin involves uptake of unconjugated bilirubin, conjugation with uridine diphosphate glucuronyl transferase, transfer to the bile canaliculus, and excretion into the intrahepatic biliary tree (Figure 37–1). Bilirubin is excreted in the bile primarily as bilirubin diglucuronide (80%), bilirubin monoglucuronide (20%), and unconjugated bilirubin (<1%). Any disease process that results in an increased load of unconjugated bilirubin presented to the liver, impaired conjugation, or impaired excretion of conjugated bilirubin, either intrahepatic or extrahepatic, can lead to accumulation of bilirubin in the blood, resulting in jaundice.

Clinical Findings

A. Symptoms and Signs

On the basis of a detailed history and a carefully conducted physical examination, along with the routine liver tests summarized below, the examiner should be able to formulate a differential diagnosis and be correct in over 85% of the patients who present with jaundice and evidence of liver disease. The importance of a careful history and physical examination along with critical evaluation of the standard liver tests cannot be overemphasized.

Table 37–1 summarizes the specific information to be obtained from patients with jaundice or liver disease.

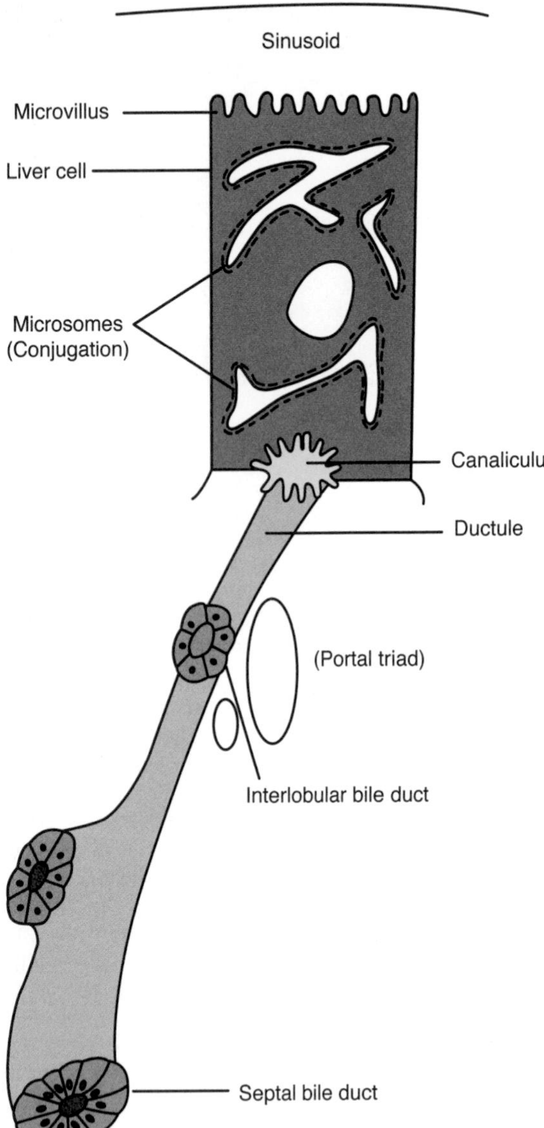

▲ **Figure 37–1.** Anatomy of the intrahepatic biliary system. (Reproduced, with permission, from Sherlock S, Dooley J. *Diseases of the Liver and Biliary System*, 10th ed. London: Blackwell Science, 1997:218.)

The information is grouped into that relating to viral hepatitis, medications, alcohol use, and miscellaneous relevant information.

Table 37–2 summarizes characteristic findings on physical examination in patients with jaundice. Attention should be paid to the peripheral stigmata of liver disease, including spider angioma, which characteristically occurs above the clavicles in the distribution of the superior vena cava.

Table 37–1. Specific information to obtain from patients with jaundice or liver disease.

Viral hepatitis
Ask about:
Blood transfusion (especially if before 1990)
Intravenous drug use
Sexual practices:
• Anal-receptive intercourse
• Sex with a prostitute
• History of sexually transmitted disease
• Multiple sexual partners (>5/y)
• Intercourse with persons infected with hepatitis B or C
Contact with persons with jaundice
Changes in taste and smell
Needlestick exposure
Work in renal dialysis units
Work in trauma units, operating rooms, or other settings in which exposure to users of IV drugs may occur
Shared razors or toothbrushes
Body piercing (ears, nose)
Tattoos
Intranasal cocaine use
Special risk factors for hepatitis A:
No immunization (older adults)
• Travel to endemic areas
• Ingestion of raw shellfish (harvested from contaminated waters)
• Exposure in settings where clusters of hepatitis may occur (eg, institutions)
Medication use
Review:
All prescription medications
Ask specifically about:
All over-the-counter drugs
Vitamins (especially vitamin A)
Any foods, herbal preparations, or home remedies purchased in a health food store
Alcohol use
Obtain detailed *quantitative* history of both recent and previous alcohol use from patient *and* family members
Ask whether patient has experienced withdrawal symptoms, or been cited for driving-under-the-influence
Miscellaneous information
Ask about:
Pruritus (suggests cholestasis either intrahepatic or extrahepatic)
Evaluation of jaundice (dark urine, light stools)
Recent changes in menstrual cycle (amenorrhea suggests chronic liver disease, often cirrhosis)
Review:
History of anemia, sickle cell disease, known hemoglobinopathy, artificial heart valves
Symptoms suggestive of biliary colic, chronic cholecystitis
Family history of liver disease, gallbladder disease

Adapted, with permission, from Greenberger NJ. History taking and physical examination for the patient with liver disease. In: Schiff ER, Sorrell MF, Maddrey WC (eds). *Schiff's Diseases of the Liver*, 10th ed, vol 1. Philadelphia: Lippincott Williams & Wilkins, 2007:4.

Table 37–2. Characteristic physical findings in the patient with jaundice.

General inspection
Scleral icterus
Pallor
Wasting
Needle tracts
Evidence of skin excoriations
Ecchymosis or petechiae
Muscle tenderness and weakness
Lymphadenopathy
Evidence of pneumonia
Evidence of congestive heart failure
Peripheral stigmata of liver disease
Spider angiomata
Palmar erythema
Gynecomastia
Dupuytren contracture
Parotid enlargement
Testicular atrophy
Paucity of axillary and pubic hair
Eye signs mimicking hyperthyroidism
Abdominal examination
Hepatomegaly
Splenomegaly
Ascites
Prominent abdominal collateral veins
Bruits and rubs
Abdominal masses
Palpable gallbladder
Signs of decompensated hepatocellular disease
Jaundice
Ascites
Oliguric hepatic failure
Hepatic encephalopathy
• Fetor hepaticus
• Asterixis
• Behavioral alterations (confusion, disorientation, failure to complete simple mental tasks)

Adapted, with permission, from Greenberger NJ. History taking and physical examination for the patient with liver disease. In: Schiff ER, Sorrell MF, Maddrey WC (eds). *Schiff's Diseases of the Liver*, 10th ed, vol 1. Philadelphia: Lippincott Williams & Wilkins, 2007:6.

More than 15 spider angiomata indicate the presence of significant liver disease and likely portal hypertension. The triad of gynecomastia, Dupuytren contracture, and parotid enlargement is a clear indication that alcohol is the most likely cause of the patient's liver disease. Splenomegaly, ascites, and prominent abdominal collateral veins indicate the presence of portal hypertension and in all likelihood the presence of esophageal or gastric varices, or both. Hepatic encephalopathy is suggested by the presence of asterixis and behavioral alterations.

The following point bears special emphasis. A clinician can make a firm diagnosis of cirrhosis on the basis of two physical findings and two laboratory findings. These four features—the presence of *asterixis* and *ascites*, along with *decreased serum albumin (<2.8 g/dL)* and a *prolonged prothrombin time*—clearly indicate cirrhosis. This statement is based on an older Mayo Clinic study in which over 500 patients with chronic liver disease were evaluated; the preceding compilation of clinical features was present in approximately 98% of patients with proven cirrhosis of the liver.

B. Laboratory Findings

Liver tests that are useful in the differential diagnosis of jaundice are summarized in Table 37–3. Four altered liver test findings point to a diagnosis of chronic liver disease (eg, cirrhosis): (1) decreased serum albumin, (2) elevated serum globulins, (3) prolonged prothrombin time, and (4) decreased cholesterol.

The serum bilirubin level exceeds 20 mg/dL rarely in patients with acute viral hepatitis, infrequently in patients with cirrhosis, and rarely in those with obstructive jaundice due to a common duct stone or pancreatic cancer. The highest serum bilirubin levels are seen in cirrhosis with accompanying oliguric hepatic failure (ie, hepatorenal syndrome). The reason is that if extrahepatic obstruction is present, the serum bilirubin level will rise to about 15 mg/dL but the compensatory mechanism is the kidney and the excess bilirubin will be excreted, resulting in bilirubinuria. In oliguric hepatic failure this compensatory mechanism is lost, which explains why the highest serum bilirubin levels are seen in advanced cirrhotic liver disease with hepatorenal syndrome.

Serum aminotransferases are characteristically increased to values above 400 IU/L in acute viral hepatitis and are usually less than 400 IU/L in cirrhosis and less than 400 IU/L in over 90% of patients with obstructive jaundice. Of note, in patients with choledocholithiasis with or without cholangitis, serum aminotransferases may be in the hepatitis range (ie, 800–1000 IU/L); however, within 2–3 days elevated values will fall abruptly.

Serum alkaline phosphatase is disproportionately elevated in obstructive jaundice, with values four- to tenfold or greater than normal, whereas these values usually are normal or minimally elevated in acute viral hepatitis or cirrhosis. Serum albumin and globulin levels are very helpful in that both are usually normal in acute viral hepatitis and usually normal with obstructive jaundice of brief duration. The serum albumin level is frequently decreased in cirrhosis whereas globulins are increased, and the finding of hypergammaglobulinemia and hypoalbuminemia in someone with liver disease almost always means that the patient has chronic liver disease.

The prothrombin time and partial thromboplastin time are usually both normal in acute viral hepatitis. However, in a patient with acute viral hepatitis, a prolonged prothrombin time and an international normalized ratio (INR) greater than 1.8 may be the harbinger of submassive necrosis of the liver and impending liver failure. The prothrombin time and partial thromboplastin time are prolonged in chronic

Table 37–3. Differential test results in patients with acute, chronic, and obstructive hepatobiliary disease.

	Acute Liver Disease	Chronic Liver Disease	Obstructive Liver Disease
	Viral Hepatitis	Cirrhosis	CBD Stone, Pancreatic Cancer
Serum bilirubin (mg/dL)	<20	<20[a]	<20
ALT/AST (IU/L)	>400	<400	<400[a]
Alkaline phosphatase	NL-↑2×	NL-4↑×	4-↑10×
Serum albumin/serum globulins (g/dL)	NL/NL	↓/↑	Usually NL
PT/PTT	NL/NL[a]	↑/↑	NL-may be ↑[a]
Cholesterol	NL	NL-↓	NL
Hepatitis serologies (A, B, C), EBV, CMV	May be helpful	—	—
Abdominal ultrasound	—	May be helpful	93% sensitivity and 95% specificity if bilirubin >10 mg/dL for 10 days

ALT, alanine aminotransferase; AST, aspartate aminotransferase; CBD, common bile duct; CMV, cytomegalovirus; EBV, Epstein-Barr virus; NL, normal limits; PT, prothrombin time; PTT, partial thromboplastin time; ↓ decreased; ↑ increased.
[a]Special circumstances may apply.

liver disease and cirrhosis. The prothrombin time may be prolonged in patients with prolonged obstructive jaundice because of failure to absorb vitamin K. In this setting, however, the prothrombin time will normalize with administration of vitamin K.

Serum cholesterol is frequently low in patients with chronic liver disease. The usual serologies to obtain in patients with jaundice include tests for hepatitis A, B, and C as well as Epstein-Barr virus and cytomegalovirus.

C. Imaging Studies

Abdominal ultrasound is a very helpful examination in patients with jaundice and obstructive-type chemistries. In a patient with serum bilirubin of 10 mg/dL or higher and in whom the elevation has persisted for more than 2 weeks, ultrasound has a sensitivity and specificity of approximately 95%. The presence of dilated ducts indicates that the process is extrahepatic. If dilated ducts are not demonstrated, it may indicate that the patient has a disorder causing intrahepatic cholestasis (Table 37–4).

Differential Diagnosis

A. Differential Diagnosis of Jaundice

As previously noted, the differential diagnosis of jaundice has changed significantly since the advent of immunization for hepatitis A and B. Prior to 2000, viral hepatitis was the cause of jaundice in 85–90% of patients younger than age 30 years. In patients presenting with jaundice who were between the ages of 40–60 years, alcoholic liver disease was the most common diagnosis, occurring in 50–70%. In patients 60–80 years of age without a history of blood transfusion, excessive alcoholic use, contact with a person with jaundice, or use of putative medicines, the diagnosis in over 80% was either gallstones and their complications or cancer of the pancreas.

Table 37–4. Spectrum of disorders and causes resulting in intrahepatic cholestasis.

Category (see Figure 37-1)	Cause
Hepatocellular	Viral hepatitis (especially type A) Alcoholic liver disease Chronic hepatitis α_1-Antitrypsin deficiency
Canalicular	Drug induced (phenothiazine, alkylated steroids) Postoperative Sepsis Parenteral nutrition Hodgkin disease Sickle cell disease Toxic shock syndrome Amyloidosis
Ductule	Primary biliary cirrhosis Sarcoidosis
Ducts	Primary sclerosing cholangitis Caroli disease Intrahepatic atresia
Recurrent	Recurrent cholestasis of pregnancy Dubin-Johnson syndrome Benign recurrent intrahepatic cholestasis

Table 37–5. Differential diagnosis of jaundice.[a]

Cause	Age		
	<30	40–60 y	60–80 y
Viral hepatitis	85-90%		
Alcoholic liver disease		50-70%	
Gallstones and complications			80% (bracketed with Cancer of the pancreas)
Cancer of the pancreas			
Chronic hepatitis	5%	5-10%	
Drug-induced jaundice		<5%	<5%
Sickle cell anemia	<5%	<5%	<5%
Glibert syndrome	2-7%	2-7%	
Primary biliary cirrhosis[b]		1%	1%
Primary sclerosing cholangitis[b]		1%	1%

[a]Reflects incidence of jaundice as reported between 1991 and 2000.
[b]Data on incidence are insufficient.

Chronic hepatitis was the cause of jaundice in 5% of patients across the age spectrum. Drug-induced jaundice occurred in less than 5% of individuals (Table 37–5).

Recent studies call attention to changing trends in the differential diagnose of jaundice (Table 37–6). In a review of 732 patients with serum bilirubin levels greater than 3 mg/dL, the most common cause was decompensation of chronic liver disease, occurring in 20.5% of the patients. Alcoholic hepatitis was present in 16.5%. Acute viral hepatitis was less frequently a cause of acute onset jaundice in 8.8% of the patients, a decline in incidence that is attributed to increased immunization of children and pregnant women against hepatitis A and B. Other hepatic causes of jaundice included acute autoimmune hepatitis and drug-induced jaundice. An extrahepatic etiology was evident in nearly half the patients, with sepsis, gallstone disease, hemolysis, and malignancy accounting for the bulk of cases.

Sepsis is a cause of jaundice due to intrahepatic cholestasis (see Table 37–4). Sickle cell anemia, which is common among African Americans, also may be characterized by intrahepatic cholestasis (see Table 37–4).

Gilbert syndrome, or chronic idiopathic unconjugated hyperbilirubinemia, occurs in 2–7% of the population and is associated with entirely normal liver tests and absence of bilirubinuria. The importance of making this diagnosis is that patients are so identified and unnecessary testing is avoided.

Primary biliary cirrhosis and primary sclerosing cholangitis are being increasingly recognized as important causes of jaundice, although in both of these disorders the diagnosis is being made earlier with the use of biochemical tests, liver biopsy, and imaging studies.

Table 37–6. Causes of jaundice identified in one recent survey.

Cause	Percentage of Cases
Hepatic Etiology (n = 406; 55%)	
Decompensation preexisting chronic liver disease	**20.5%**
Alcoholic hepatitis	**16.5%**
Acute viral liver disease	**8.8%**
HBV	[5.0]
HCV	[2.0]
HAV	[1.0]
EBV	[0.5]
HIV	[0.3]
Acute autoimmune hepatitis	**0.3%**
Drug-induced	**3.9%**
Acetaminophen	[3.3]
HAART	[0.4]
Valproate	[0.1]
Metabolite	[0.1]
Extrahepatic Etiology (n = 326; 45%)	
Sepsis/abnormal hemodynamic state	**22%**
Gallstone disease	**14%**
Hemolysis	**2.5%**
Malignancy	**6.2%**
Pancreatic biliary	[2.9]
Metastatic	[3.5]

EBV, Epstein-Barr virus; HAART, highly active antiretroviral therapy; HAV, hepatitis A virus; HBV, hepatitis B virus; HCV, hepatitis C virus; HIV, human immunodeficiency virus.
Adapted, with permission, from Vuppalanchi R, Liangpunsakul S, Chalasani N. New onset jaundice. *Am J Gastroenterol.* 2007;102: 558–562.

B. Differential Diagnosis of Intrahepatic Cholestasis

The spectrum of disorders causing intrahepatic cholestasis is summarized in Table 37–4. At every site in the intrahepatic biliary tree, there are disorders associated with jaundice. Thus, hepatocellular causes, including viral hepatitis (especially type A), alcoholic liver disease, chronic hepatitis, and α_1-antitrypsin deficiency can be associated with intrahepatic cholestasis. Canalicular cholestasis may be drug induced (eg, caused by phenothiazines or alkylated steroids), or associated with the postoperative state, sepsis, parenteral nutrition, Hodgkin disease, sickle cell disease, toxic shock syndrome, or amyloidosis. The ductules are the source of jaundice in primary biliary cirrhosis and sarcoidosis; the larger ducts in primary sclerosing cholangitis, Caroli disease, and intrahepatic biliary atresia. Recurrent jaundice occurs with recurrent cholestasis of pregnancy, benign recurrent intrahepatic cholestasis and Dubin-Johnson syndrome. Jaundice can occur in patients with sepsis, especially gram-negative sepsis, because gram-negative bacilli elaborate toxins that interfere with canalicular function (ie, canalicular membrane ATPases). It should also be remembered that patients with intrathoracic or intra-abdominal bleeding may develop jaundice because of the large bilirubin pigment load. Every 50 mL of blood loss produces up to 250 mg of bilirubin; thus, a patient who has experienced a 5-unit intraperitoneal or intrathoracic bleed may have 2500 mg of bilirubin presented for excretion, overwhelming the body's uptake, conjugation, and excretion mechanisms for handling bilirubin.

C. Differential Diagnosis of Chronic Hepatitis

The differential diagnosis of chronic hepatitis is depicted using a mnemonic device in Table 37–7. The letters in the left-hand column—A, B, C, D1, D2, E1, E2, F, and H—correspond to the categories of possible causes of chronic hepatitis.

Chronic hepatitis may be due to autoimmune disease in which the subtypes are anti–nuclear body smooth muscle positive, anti-actin positive, anti–LKM-1 positive, and anti–liver surface antigen positive. The most common entity in the United States is anti–nuclear and smooth muscle (F-actin)–positive disease. Approximately 5% of patients with acute hepatitis B develop chronic hepatitis. Approximately 70% of patients with acute hepatitis C develop chronic hepatitis. Hepatitis D occurs only with hepatitis B. Various drugs, including α-methyldopa, isoniazid, Augmentin®, and nitrofurantoin, are associated with jaundice. In the United States, the drug most frequently associated with jaundice is amoxicillin and its various derivatives. Wilson disease is a rare cause of jaundice but needs to be considered because it is eminently treatable. α_1-Antitrypsin deficiency also needs to be considered. Nonalcoholic fatty liver disease (NAFLD) is the most common cause of liver test abnormalities and is discussed in detail in Chapter 43. Hemochromatosis is another important cause of liver disease and is detailed in Chapter 41.

Table 37–7. Differential diagnosis of chronic hepatitis.

A	Autoimmune • ANA-SMA positive • Anti-actin positive • Anti-LKM-1 positive • Anti-SLA positive
B	Hepatitis B
C	Hepatitis C
$D_{(1)}$	Hepatitis D (only with hepatitis B)
$D_{(2)}$	Drugs (α-methyldopa, isoniazid, nitrofurantoin)
$E_{(1)}$	Wilson disease
$E_{(2)}$	α_1-Antitrypsin
F	Nonalcoholic fatty liver disease (NAFLD)
H	Hemochromatosis

ANA, antinuclear antibody; SLA, soluble liver antigen.

Diagnostic Considerations in Patients with Elevated Serum Aminotransferases

An elevation in aminotransferase in asymptomatic individuals is common, occurring in over 8% of the U.S. population. Recent surveys by the National Health and Nutrition Examination Survey (NHANES) have provided important information on aminotransferase elevations in asymptomatic individuals in the United States. The third annual NHANES survey reported on 15,676 adults over the age of 17 years. Aminotransferase elevation was defined by an aspartate aminotransferase (AST) value greater than 37, and an alanine aminotransferase (ALT) value greater than 42 and was classified as explained if there was (1) evidence of hepatitis B, (2) hepatitis C, (3) iron overload (ie, transferrin saturation >50%), or (4) alcohol consumption greater than two drinks per day for men and greater than one drink per day for women. Aminotransferase elevation was classified as unexplained if any of the preceding four factors were absent.

Prevalence of aminotransferase elevation in the United States was 7.9%. Aminotransferase elevations were more common in men (9.3%) compared with women (6.6%), and in Mexican Americans (14.9%) and non-Hispanic blacks 8.1% compared with non-Hispanic whites (7.1%). Known causes occurred in 31% of the patients, with the most common causes being alcohol, hepatitis C virus, hemochromatosis, and hepatitis B virus. The cause was unexplained in two thirds of cases but was associated with higher body mass index, dyslipidemia, diabetes, hypertension, and insulin resistance. Among patients with a body mass index greater than 40, over half had NAFLD. Many patients with these findings have the metabolic syndrome. Fifteen percent of such patients may already have cirrhosis.

Uncommon but important causes of asymptomatic amino-transferase elevations included chronic acetaminophen use greater than 4 g/day, celiac sprue, and use of statins. Elevations in aminotransferase values in statin users ranged from 0.5% to 3% and were dependent in large part on the dose of statin. It bears emphasizing that despite the aminotransferase elevations noted in users of statins, only rare cases of significant liver disease have been reported in such patients, and in those cases another cause was usually identified.

Clark JM, Brancati FL, Diehl AM. The prevalence and etiology of elevated aminotransferase levels in the United States. *Am J Gastroenterol.* 2003;98:960–967. [PMID: 12809815]

Greenberger NJ. History taking and physical examination for the patient with liver disease. In: Schiff ER, Sorrell MF, Maddrey WC (eds). *Schiff's Diseases of the Liver,* 10th ed. Philadelphia: Lippincott Williams & Wilkins, 2007:3–18.

Vuppalanchi R, Liangpunsakul S, Chalasani N. New onset jaundice: how often is it caused by idiosyncratic drug-induced liver injury in the United States. *Am J Gastroenterol.* 2007; 102:558–562. [PMID: 17156142]

Acute Liver Failure

Sonal Kumar, MD
Amir A. Qamar, MD

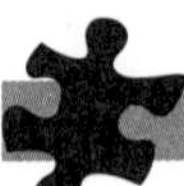

ESSENTIALS OF DIAGNOSIS

- Drugs, toxins, viral hepatitis, and hypoperfusion are the most common causes of acute liver failure (ALF).
- Laboratory findings may confirm the cause and severity of presentation.
- Consider acetaminophen toxicity in all patients, even without a history of toxic ingestion, particularly when serum aminotransferase levels are very high (>1000 units).
- Depending on timing of ingestion, acetaminophen levels may not be elevated even in cases of overdose.
- Rapid diagnostic and psychiatric evaluation is required at presentation.

General Considerations

Acute liver failure (ALF) affects approximately 2000 people in the United States each year. The most widely accepted definition of ALF includes evidence of coagulation abnormality (international normalized ratio [INR] ≥ 1.5), and encephalopathy in a patient without preexisting cirrhosis and with a hepatic illness manifested by hyperbilirubinemia of less than 26 weeks' duration.

The U.S. Acute Liver Failure Study Group (ALFSG) was formed in 1997 as a consortium of centers aimed at capturing nationwide data on ALF. Results of 1147 patients enrolled from 1998 to 2007 found that the most common causes of ALF were acetaminophen overdose (46%), indeterminate (14%), idiosyncratic drug reactions (11%), and viral hepatitis A or B (10%).

Currently in the United States, spontaneous survival occurs in approximately 45% without liver transplantation. The outcome of ALF, however, varies by etiology with favorable prognoses being found with acetaminophen overdose, hepatitis A, and ischemia, and poor prognoses with drug-induced ALF, hepatitis B, and indeterminate cases.

Larson AM, Polson J, Fontana RJ, et al. Acute Liver Failure Study Group. Acetaminophen–induced acute liver failure: results of a United States multicenter, prospective study. *Hepatology.* 2005;42:1364–1372. [PMID: 16317692]

Lee WM. Acute liver failure in the United States. *Semin Liver Dis.* 2003;23:217–226. [PMID: 14624381]

Lee WM, Squires RH, Jr, Nyberg SL, et al. Acute liver failure: Summary of a workshop. *Hepatology.* 2008;47:1401–1415. [PMID: 18318440]

Ostapowicz G, Fontana RJ, Schiødt FV, et al. Results of a prospective study of acute liver failure at 17 tertiary care centers in the United States. *Ann Intern Med.* 2002;137:947–954. [PMID: 12484709]

Clinical Findings

The constellation of clinical findings in ALF includes jaundice in a previously healthy person, often preceded by malaise or nausea, and the rapid onset of altered mental status and coma accompanied by laboratory evidence of coagulopathy and acute hepatic injury.

A. Symptoms and Signs

History-taking should include a review of all possible exposures to viral infection, drugs, and toxic ingestions, as well as risk factors for underlying chronic liver disease. If the patient shows evidence of severe encephalopathy, a history should be obtained from family members.

Jaundice and right upper quadrant tenderness may or may not be present. An enlarged liver may be seen early in viral hepatitis, malignant infiltration, congestive heart failure, or acute Budd-Chiari syndrome. Alternatively, there may be decreased hepatic dullness to percussion, indicating diminished hepatic mass. The most critical part of the physical examination is the periodic assessment of mental status.

B. Laboratory Findings

Initial laboratory analysis should aim to determine the cause of ALF, the severity of presentation, and the need for treatment of associated complications (Table 38–1).

Table 38–1. Initial laboratory analysis in acute liver failure.

Prothrombin time/INR
Chemistries
• Sodium, potassium, chloride, bicarbonate, calcium, magnesium, phosphate
• Glucose
• AST, ALT, alkaline phosphatase, GGT, total bilirubin, albumin
• Creatinine, blood urea nitrogen
Arterial blood gas
Arterial lactate
Complete blood count
Blood type and screen
Acetaminophen level
Toxicology screen
Viral hepatitis serologies
• Anti-HAV IgM
• HBsAg
• Anti-HBc IgM
• Anti-HEV
• Anti-HCV[a]
Ceruloplasmin level[b]
Pregnancy test (females)
Ammonia (arterial if possible)
Autoimmune markers
• ANA
• ASMA
Immunoglobulin levels
HIV status
Amylase and lipase

ANA, antinuclear antibody; ASMA, anti-smooth muscle antibody; ALT, alanine aminotransferase; AST, aspartate aminotransferase; GGT, γ-glutamyl transferase; HAV, hepatitis A virus; HBc, hepatitis core antigen; HCV, hepatitis C virus; HEV, hepatitis E virus; HBsAg, hepatitis B surface antigen; IgM, immunoglobulin M; INR, international normalized ratio.

[a]Done to recognize potential underlying infection.

[b]Done only if Wilson disease is a consideration (eg, in patients younger than 40 years without another obvious explanation for acute liver failure); in this case uric acid level and bilirubin to alkaline phosphatase ratio may be helpful as well.

Reproduced, with permission, from Polson J, Lee WM; American Association for the Study of Liver Diseases. AASLD position paper: the management of acute liver failure. *Hepatology*. 2005;41:1179–1197. [PMID: 15841455]

Liver biopsy, usually done via the transjugular route because of coagulopathy, may be indicated when certain conditions such as autoimmune hepatitis, metastatic liver disease, lymphoma, or herpes simplex virus are suspected.

Complications

Significant neurologic, cardiopulmonary, and renal sequelae are associated with ALF. Cerebral edema and intracranial hypertension are the most serious of these complications. Mortality is related to neurologic status and infection, which require careful monitoring (see next section). Acute renal failure complicates ALF in approximately 30–50% of patients and can be a sign of poor prognosis.

Treatment

A. General Management Concerns

Because ALF often involves the rapid deterioration of mental status and the potential for multiorgan failure, patients should be managed in the intensive care unit. Table 38–2 outlines general treatment recommendations for intensive care management of patients with ALF. For patients not at a transplant center, the possibility of rapid progression of ALF makes early consultation with a transplant facility critical. Accordingly, plans for transfer to a transplant center should begin in patients with any abnormal mentation.

Early institution of antidotes or specific therapy may prevent the need for liver transplantation and reduce the likelihood of poor outcome. *N*-acetylcysteine (NAC) is the antidote for acetaminophen-induced acute liver failure, but some data suggests intravenous NAC improves transplant-free survival in non–acetaminophen-induced liver failure, particularly in those patients in early stage. Other measures appropriate for specific causes of ALF are described in detail later in this chapter.

Jalan R. Acute liver failure: current management and future prospects. *J Hepatol.* 2005;42(Suppl):S115–S123. [PMID: 15777566]

Lee WM, Hynan LS, Rossaro L, et al. Intravenous *N*-acetylcysteine improves transplant-free survival in early stage non-acetaminophen acute liver failure. *Gastroenterology.* 2009;137:856–864. [PMID: 19524577]

Polson J, Lee WM. American Association for the Study of Liver Diseases. AASLD position paper: the management of acute liver failure. *Hepatology.* 2005;41:1179–1197. [PMID: 15841455]

B. Management of Common Complications

1. Neurologic complications—Patients with grade I–II encephalopathy (Table 38–3) should be transferred to a liver transplant facility and listed for transplantation. Sepsis, gastrointestinal bleeding, hypoglycemia, hypoxemia and electrolyte abnormalities can worsen encephalopathy. Consider a brain-computed tomography (CT) scan to rule out other causes of decreased mental status. Stimulation and overhydration can cause elevations in intracranial pressure (ICP) and should be avoided. Unmanageable agitation may be treated with short-acting benzodiazepines in small doses, but may mask the severity of encephalopathy, limiting its prognostic value. Lactulose can be considered at this stage, but abdominal distention should be assessed at regular intervals, and the dose of lactulose should be titrated to avoid intravascular depletion. A report from the ALFSG on 117 patients suggests that use of lactulose in the first 7 days

Table 38–2. Intensive care of acute liver failure.

Complication	Treatment Measures
Cerebral edema and intracranial hypertension	Grade I/II encephalopathy: • Consider transfer to liver transplant facility and listing for transplantation • Brain CT—rule out other causes of decreased mental status; little utility to identify cerebral edema • Avoid stimulation, avoid sedation if possible • Antibiotics—surveillance and treatment of infection required; prophylaxis possible helpful • Lactulose—possible helpful Grade III/IV encephalopathy: • Continue management strategies listed above • Intubate trachea (may require sedation) • Elevate head of bed • Consider placement of ICP monitoring device • Immediate treatment of seizures required; prophylaxis of unclear value • Mannitol—use for severe elevation of ICP or first clinical signs of herniation • Hyperventilation—effects short-lived; may use for impending herniation
Infection	Surveillance for and prompt antimicrobial treatment of infection required Antibiotic prophylaxis possibly helpful but not proven
Coagulopathy	Vitamin K—give at least 1 dose FFP—give only for invasive procedures or active bleeding Platelets—give for platelet counts <10,000/mm³ or invasive procedures Recombinant activated factor VII—possibly effective for invasive procedures Prophylaxis for stress ulceration—give H_2-blocker or PPI
Altered hemodynamics and renal failure	Pulmonary artery catheterization Volume replacement Pressor support (dopamine, epinephrine, norepinephrine) as needed to maintain adequate mean arterial pressure Avoid nephrotoxic agents Continuous modes of hemodialysis if needed NAC, prostacyclin—effectiveness unknown Vasopressin—not helpful in ALF; potentially harmful
Metabolic concerns	Follow closely—glucose, potassium, magnesium, phosphate Consider nutrition—enteral feedings if possible or total parenteral nutrition

ALF, acute liver failure; CT, computed tomography; FFP, fresh frozen plasma; ICP, intracranial pressure; NAC, *N*-acetylcysteine; PPI, proton pump inhibitor.
Adapted, with permission, from Polson J, Lee WM; American Association for the Study of Liver Diseases. AASLD position paper: the management of acute liver failure. *Hepatology*. 2005;41:1179–1197. [PMID: 15841455]

Table 38–3. Grades of encephalopathy.

Grade	Description
I	Changes in behavior with minimal change in level of consciousness
II	Gross disorientation, drowsiness, possibly asterixis, inappropriate behavior
III	Marked confusion, incoherent speech, sleeping most of the time but arousable to vocal stimuli
IV	Comatose, unresponsive to pain, decorticate or decerebrate posturing

Reproduced, with permission, from Polson J, Lee WM; American Association for the Study of Liver Diseases. AASLD position paper: the management of acute liver failure. *Hepatology*. 2005;41:1179–1197. [PMID: 15841455]

after diagnosis is associated with a small increase in survival time, but with no difference in severity of encephalopathy or in overall outcome.

For patients who progress to grade III–IV encephalopathy, intubation for airway protection is generally required. Many centers use propofol for sedation because it may reduce cerebral blood. The head of the bed should be elevated to 30 degrees, and electrolytes, blood gases, glucose, and neurologic status monitored frequently.

The cause of intracranial hypertension in ALF is probably multifactorial, combining cytotoxic brain edema due to an increase in cerebral blood volume and cerebral blood flow due to inflammation and toxic products of the diseased liver. Cerebral edema inside the cranial vault raises ICP and decreases cerebral perfusion assessed by cerebral perfusion pressure (CPP; defined as mean arterial pressure minus intracranial pressure).

Factors that increase ICP need to be avoided, including high positive end-expiratory pressure, frequent movements, neck vein compression, fever, arterial hypertension, hypoxia, coughing, sneezing, seizures, head-low position, and respiratory suctioning.

Evidence of increased ICP includes unequal pupil size and lack of pupillary reaction to light. Patients with cerebral edema may have systemic hypertension and bradycardia (Cushing reflex), increased muscle tone followed by decerebrate rigidity and posturing, abnormal papillary reflexes (usually dilation), and finally brainstem respiratory patterns and apnea. Brain herniation from elevated ICP is the immediate cause of death in 35% of patients with ALF, and 15–20% of patients listed for transplantation die from increased ICP. Cerebral edema is rarely seen in patients with grade I–II encephalopathy but increases to 65–75% in patients with grade IV coma and is the leading cause of death in these patients.

Seizure is common in patients with ALF, although presentation is often subclinical and likely due to use of sedatives and paralytics in intubated patients. Seizures aggravate intracranial hypertension and should therefore be promptly controlled with phenytoin. Small clinical trials using prophylactic phenytoin have shown no mortality benefit and unclear impact on cerebral edema or prevention of seizures.

The use of ICP monitoring in patients with ALF is common but not universal. Clinical signs of elevated ICP are not always present, and neurologic changes such as papillary dilation or decerebrate posturing are often present only late in the course. The risks of ICP monitoring in ALF patients include bleeding and infection, with subdural and intraparenchymal monitors demonstrating greater reliability but increased rates of complications when compared with epidural catheters. A survival benefit with the use of ICP monitoring has not been shown.

The goal is to maintain ICP below 20 mm Hg and CPP above 70 mm Hg. Evidence of elevated ICP such as pupillary abnormalities, decerebrate posturing, or monitoring suggesting ICP above 20–25 mm Hg and CPP below 50–60 mm Hg, should prompt intervention.

Interventions may include support of systemic blood pressure to maintain adequate CPP or the use of mannitol, which in doses of 0.5–1 g/kg has been demonstrated to decrease cerebral edema in the short term and improve survival. The efficacy of mannitol in patients with ICP may be affected by acute renal failure and oliguria. The dose may be repeated as needed as long as serum osmolality has not exceeded 320 mOsm/L. In order to be able to use mannitol repeatedly, fluid can be taken off with hemofiltration, which by itself reduces ICP. Prophylactic administration of mannitol is not indicated.

Hyperventilation has also been shown to cause quick reductions in ICP, but the effect is short-lived and therefore may be of therapeutic benefit only in situations of life-threatening intracranial hypertension to prevent herniation.

Barbiturate agents such as thiopental or pentobarbital may be considered when severe intracranial hypertension does not respond to other measures.

Other therapies are being explored but currently lack adequate supporting data to recommend use, including indomethacin, hypothermia, and hypertonic saline.

Detry O, De Roover A, Honore P, et al. Brain edema and intracranial hypertension in fulminant hepatic failure: pathophysiology and management. *World J Gastroenterol.* 2006;12:7405–7412. [PMID: 17167826]

Jalan R. Intracranial hypertension in acute liver failure: pathophysiological basis of rational management. *Semin Liver Dis.* 2003; 23:271–282. [PMID: 14523680]

Jalan R, Olde Daminck SW, Deutz NE, et al. Moderate hypothermia prevents cerebral hyperemia and increase in intracranial pressure in patients undergoing liver transplantation for acute liver failure. *Transplantation.* 2003;75:2034–2039. [PMID: 12829907]

Jalan R, Olde Daminck SW, Deutz NE, et al. Moderate hypothermia in patients with acute liver failure and uncontrolled intracranial hypertension. *Gastroenterology.* 2004;127:1338–1346. [PMID: 15521003]

Murphy N, Auzinger G, Bernal W, et al. The effect of hypertonic sodium chloride on intracranial pressure in patients with acute liver failure. *Hepatology.* 2002;39:464–470. [PMID: 14767999]

Wijdicks EF, Nyberg SL. Propofol to control intracranial pressure in fulminant hepatic failure. *Transplant Proc.* 2002;34:1220–1222. [PMID: 12072321]

2. Cardiovascular complications—Increased cardiac output and low systemic vascular resistance are characteristic of ALF. Pulmonary artery catheterization should be considered to monitor volume status. Hypotension should be treated preferentially with fluids, but systemic vasopressor support with agents such as epinephrine, norepinephrine, or dopamine should be used if fluid replacement fails to maintain mean arterial pressure of 50–60 mm Hg. Vasoconstrictive agents (especially vasopressin) should be avoided. Relative adrenal insufficiency occurs frequently in patients with ALF, and may contribute to cardiovascular collapse. Moderate doses (200–300 mg/day) of hydrocortisone have been shown to improve the vasopressor response to norepinephrine in hypotensive patients with sepsis and ALF.

Stravitz RT, Kramer AH, Davern T, et al. Intensive care of patients with acute liver failure: recommendations of the U.S. Acute Liver Failure Study Group. *Crit Care Med.* 2007; 35:2498–2508. [PMID: 17901832]

3. Pulmonary complications—Pulmonary edema and pulmonary infections are commonly seen in patients with ALF. Mechanical ventilation may be required. However, positive end-expiratory pressure can worsen cerebral edema and decrease hepatic blood flow.

4. Coagulopathy and gastrointestinal bleeding—Impaired hepatic synthesis of clotting factors, increased consumption of factors, low-grade fibrinolysis, and intravascular coagulation are typical of ALF. Thrombocytopenia is common and may also be dysfunctional. The prophylactic correction of INR with fresh frozen plasma is not recommended, and replacement therapy is recommended only in the setting of hemorrhage or prior to invasive procedure. Vitamin K (5–10 mg subcutaneously) should be given to treat an abnormal prothrombin time, regardless of whether there is poor nutritional status. Administration of recombinant factor VIIa has shown promise; however, this treatment approach requires further study. The use of gastrointestinal hemorrhage prophylaxis with a proton pump inhibitor is recommended.

Munoz SJ, Reddy KR, Lee WM and the Acute Liver Failure Study Group. The coagulopathy of acute liver failure and implications for intracranial pressure monitoring. *Neurocrit Care.* 2008;9: 103–107. [PMID: 18379899]

Shami VM, Caldwell SH, Hespenheide EE, et al. Recombinant activated factor VII for coagulopathy in fulminant hepatic failure compared with conventional therapy. *Liver Transpl.* 2003;9: 138–143. [PMID: 12548507]

5. Renal failure—Prevention of renal failure by ensuring adequate systemic blood pressure, treating infections, and avoiding nephrotoxic agents is important. Intravascular volume deficits are often present on admission and volume replacement is required. Acute renal failure may occur due to dehydration, hepatorenal syndrome, or acute tubular necrosis. Renal failure may be even more common with acetaminophen overdose or other toxic ingestions due to direct nephrotoxicity causing acid-base disturbances and lactic acidosis. Prompt fluid resuscitation with crystalloids for low arterial pressure, or colloids in pre-hepatorenal syndrome along with midodrine and octreotide, have been suggested. If renal dysfunction, fluid balance, and metabolic derangements necessitate renal replacement, continuous therapies such as continuous venovenous or arteriovenous hemofiltration should be used as they cause less fluctuation in hemodynamics and ICP than intermittent hemodialysis.

6. Nutrition, electrolytes, and metabolic derangements—ALF is a high catabolic state, and adequate nutrition is essential. Caloric goal for patients should be approximately 25–30 kcal/kg/d. In patients with grade I or II encephalopathy, enteral feeding should be initiated early. Parenteral nutrition should be used only if enteral feeding is contraindicated as it increases the risk of infection. Severe restriction of protein is not beneficial; 60 g/day of protein is generally reasonable. Fluid replacement with colloid (eg, albumin) is preferred rather than crystalloid (eg, saline); all solutions should contain dextrose to maintain euglycemia.

Multiple electrolyte abnormalities are common in ALF. Correction of hypokalemia is essential as hypokalemia increases renal ammonia production, potentially exacerbating encephalopathy. Hyponatremia is a poor prognostic indicator, and the desirable levels are above 125 mEq/L. Hypophosphatemia is especially common in patients with acetaminophen-induced ALF and in those with intact renal function. Hypoglycemia occurs in many patients with ALF and is often due to depletion of hepatic glycogen stores and impaired gluconeogenesis. Plasma glucose concentration should be monitored and hypertonic glucose administered as needed.

Pathikonda M, Munoz SJ. Acute liver failure. *Ann Hepatol.* 2010; 9:7–14. [PMID: 20308717]

Schilsky ML, Honiden S, Arnott L, Emre S. ICU management of acute liver failure. *Clin Chest Med.* 2009;30(1):71–87. [PMID: 19186281]

7. Infection—Bacterial and fungal infections are common in ALF, with one study demonstrating culture-proven infection in 80% of ALF patients. Infection remains one of the leading causes of mortality in patients with ALF. Defective cellular and humoral immunity as well as presence of indwelling catheters, coma, broad-spectrum antibiotics, and medications that suppress immunity all predispose to infection. Localizing symptoms of infection such as fever and sputum production are frequently absent, and the only clues to an underlying infectious process may be worsening of encephalopathy or renal function. There must be a low threshold for obtaining frequent cultures (blood, urine, and sputum), chest radiographs, and paracentesis. Bacteria that enter through the skin, such as streptococci and staphylococci, tend to predominate, and therefore broad spectrum antibiotics (quinolones or third-generation cephalosporin) are generally used. Fungal infections, particularly in the setting of broad-spectrum antibiotics, are also common, and disseminated fungemia is a poor prognostic sign. Aggressive surveillance is essential, as prophylactic antibiotics have shown little benefit, though empiric antibiotic administration can be considered where infection or the likelihood of impending sepsis is high.

Table 38–2 summarizes these and other strategies in the ICU management of ALF patients.

C. Liver Transplantation

The advent of transplantation has changed survival from as low as 15% in the pre transplant era to more than 60% today. Liver transplantation is indicated for many patients with ALF, and survival rates of 56–90% can be achieved. In addition to transplantation, better critical care and the trend toward more benign causes, such as acetaminophen, all contribute to improved survival rates. Spontaneous survival is now around 45%.

The application of transplantation among patients with ALF remains low, suggesting that the full potential of this modality may not be realized. Timely availability of an allograft is one of the major factors determining transplant outcomes. In the largest U.S. study, only 29% of patients received a liver graft, while 10% of the overall group (one fourth of patients listed for transplantation) died on the waiting list. Other series have reported death rates of those listed for transplant as high as 40%.

Current United Network for Organ Sharing (UNOS) criteria for priority (Status 1) listing are (1) onset of any degree of hepatic encephalopathy within 8 weeks of onset of acute liver injury; (2) absence of preexisting liver disease; (3) life expectancy of less than 7 days; and (4) in the intensive care unit (ICU) requiring either mechanical ventilation, renal dialysis, or with severe coagulopathy (INR 2.0).

In the ALFSG, the transplantation rate was higher in the groups with lower short-term spontaneous survival, making overall survival similar in all groups: acetaminophen, 73%; drug induced, 70%; indeterminate group, 64%; and other causes, 61%. Causes of death for the 101 patients who died within the 3-week period included cerebral edema, multiorgan failure, sepsis, cardiac arrhythmia or arrest, and respiratory failure. The median time to death after admission was 5 days.

Brown RS Jr, Russo MW, Lai M, et al. A survey of liver transplantation from living adult donors in the United States. *N Engl J Med.* 2003;348:818–825. [PMID: 12606737]

Farmer DG, Anselmo DM, Ghobrial RM, et al. Liver transplantation for fulminant hepatic failure: experience with more than 200 patients over a 17-year period. *Ann Surg.* 2003;237:666–675. [PMID: 12724633]

Lee WM, Squires RH, Jr, Nyberg SL, et al: Acute liver failure: Summary of a workshop. *Hepatology.* 2008; 47:1401–1415. [PMID: 18318440]

D. Liver Support Systems

Clinical experience with bioartificial systems is mostly confined to small numbers of patients in uncontrolled trials. One systematic review of 12 randomized trials (with a total 483 patients) assessing artificial and bioartificial support systems for acute or acute-on-chronic liver failure as a "bridge" to transplantation showed no significant effect on mortality compared with standard medical therapy. Currently, available liver support systems are not recommended for the treatment of ALF.

Prognosis

Due to the scarcity of organs and the importance of the timing and decision regarding transplantation, the ability to assess prognosis in ALF is critical. The most important determinant of short-term (3 week) outcome appears to be the cause of the ALF. In the ALFSG patients with acetaminophen overdose, hepatitis A virus infection, shock liver, or pregnancy-related ALF, short-term survival without transplantation was 50% or greater. Patients with other etiologies had a survival rate of less than 25% without transplantation. Age and length of time between onset of illness and onset of encephalopathy, previously reported as prognostic, were not prognostic in the AFLSG.

Table 38–4. Potentially helpful indicators[a] of poor (transplant-free) prognosis in patients with acute liver failure.

Etiology	Idiosyncratic drug injury Acute hepatitis B (and other non-hepatitis A viral infections) Autoimmune hepatitis Mushroom poisoning Budd-Chiari syndrome Indeterminate cause
Coma grade on admission	III IV
King's College criteria	**Acetaminophen-induced ALF:** • Arterial pH < 7.3 (following adequate volume resuscitation) irrespective of coma grade OR • PT >100 seconds (INR 6.5) + serum creatinine >300 mol/L (93.4 mg/dL) in patients in grade III/IV coma **Non-acetaminophen-induced ALF:** • PT >100 seconds irrespective of coma grade OR • Any 3 of the following, irrespective of coma grade: –Drug toxicity, indeterminate cause of ALF –Age <10 years or >40 years –Jaundice to coma interval >7 days –PT >50 seconds (INR 3.5) –Serum bilirubin >300 mol/L (17.5 mg/dL)

ALF, acute liver failure; INR, international normalized ratio; PT, prothrombin time.
[a]None of these factors, with the exception of Wilson disease and possibly mushroom poisoning, are either necessary or sufficient to indicate the need for immediate liver transplantation.
Adapted, with permission, from Polson J, Lee WM; American Association for the Study of Liver Diseases. AASLD position paper: the management of acute liver failure. *Hepatology.* 2005;41: 1179–1197. [PMID: 15841455]

The traditional King's College Hospital criteria (Table 38–4) have been the most commonly used and most frequently tested of the numerous proposed criteria for determining prognosis in ALF. Several studies evaluating these criteria have shown positive predictive values ranging from 70% to nearly 100% and negative predictive values from 25% to 94%. Fulfillment of these criteria suggests that without transplantation, the patient has a very high mortality risk. The model for end-stage liver disease (MELD) has not shown the same conclusive benefits in ALF patients.

Alternative criteria based on decreased levels of factor V in patients with encephalopathy was shown to have improved sensitivity in determining a poor prognosis in acute viral hepatitis.

Shakil AO. Predicting the outcome of fulminant hepatic failure. *Liver Transpl.* 2005;11:1028–1030. [PMID: 16123964]

SPECIFIC CAUSES OF ACUTE LIVER FAILURE

1. Acetaminophen

The ALFSG reports a rise in the annual percentage of acetaminophen-related ALF from 28% in 1998 to 39% in 2003, with subsequent studies reporting acetaminophen overdose to account for up to 46% of all cases. These numbers may underestimate the contribution of acetaminophen to ALF. In one study using a new acetaminophen detection assay, 20% of ALF patients with indeterminate etiology were found to have acetaminophen-containing protein adducts released from dying hepatocytes, suggesting that unrecognized acetaminophen poisoning may have contributed to ALF. Acetaminophen may also contribute to ALF due to viral hepatitis, as patients may be taking acetaminophen products for relief of viral symptoms. A report from France showed ALF in acute hepatitis A patients was significantly associated with acetaminophen use.

Alcohol use, starvation, and acute illness may deplete glutathione, predisposing to liver injury from acetaminophen. In the ALFSG, participants who developed acetaminophen-induced ALF after ingesting less than 4 g acetaminophen per day before presentation more often used alcohol (65% vs 37%), more often reported unintentional overdose (74% vs 40%), and were older (median, 46 years vs 34 years) than other study participants.

Clinical Findings

Clinical signs and symptoms are dependent on the time since ingestion, which is defined into different phases. Phase 1 (first 24 hours) symptoms include anorexia, nausea/vomiting, lethargy, and diaphoresis. During phase 2 (24–72 hours), symptoms may improve, but laboratory abnormalities exist. In phase 3 (72–96 hours), nausea and vomiting can recur and be more severe. It can be accompanied by jaundice, malaise, and central nervous system symptoms. Liver test abnormalities peak during this stage. In phase 4 (4–14 days), liver damage resolves.

Acetaminophen toxicity should be considered in all patients with ALF even without a history of toxic ingestion, particularly in patients with very high aminotransferase values (ie, >1000 units/mL). Acetaminophen levels should be drawn on initial evaluation; however, keep in mind that depending on the timing of ingestion, acetaminophen levels may not be elevated even in overdose.

Treatment

If ingestion is suspected within a few hours of presentation, activated charcoal (1 g/kg orally) may be useful up to 3–4 hours after ingestion and does not reduce the effectiveness of oral *N*-acetylcysteine (NAC). The administration of NAC, which replenishes glutathione stores, is recommended in any patient with ALF in whom acetaminophen overdose is suspected. Although early administration enhances efficacy, some benefit has been shown even when NAC is given as late as 36 hours, and possibly even 48 hours, after ingestion. A 20-hour intravenous dosing regimen may be the therapy of choice when oral administration is not possible. No studies have shown any difference between oral and intravenous routes of administration. Allergic reactions to NAC may be treated with antihistamines and epinephrine for bronchospasm or discontinuation if necessary.

Prognosis

In the ALFSG, among 275 patients with acetaminophen-induced ALF, 65% survived, 27% died without transplantation, and 8% underwent transplantation. However, nearly one-third of those reaching the threshold of encephalopathy died. Extended acetaminophen dosing, delay in seeking medical attention, and failure to institute NAC therapy are associated with greater morbidity and mortality. Suicidal intent, a history of previous suicide attempts, or evidence of substance abuse may preclude transplant consideration. Outcomes appear to be similar between patients with suicidal intent and unintentional overdose once the patient develops ALF.

Chun LJ, Tong MJ, Busuttil RW. Acetaminophen toxicity and acute liver failure. *J Clin Gastroenterol.* 2009;43:342–349. [PMID: 19169150]

Lee WM. Acetaminophen and the US Acute Liver Failure Study Group: lowering the risks of hepatic failure. *Hepatology.* 2004;40:6–9. [PMID: 15239078]

Sato RL, Wong JJ, Sumida SM, et al. Efficacy of superactivated charcoal administration late (3 hours) after acetaminophen overdose. *Am J Emerg Med.* 2003;21:189–191. [PMID: 12811710]

Schmidt LE, Dalhoff K. Serum phosphate is an early predictor of outcome in severe acetaminophen-induced hepatotoxicity. *Hepatology.* 2002;36:659–665. [PMID: 12198658]

2. Viral Hepatitis

A. Hepatitis A

ALF is rare in hepatitis A (0.35%), but some studies suggest that women, the elderly, and patients with underlying liver disease may be at greater risk of morbidity and mortality with acute hepatitis A infection. Since the introduction of hepatitis A vaccines in 1995, reported cases of hepatitis A in the United States have declined by more than 85%, and with it, the incidence of hepatitis A–associated liver failure has also declined. Patients with hepatitis A infection in whom liver failure develops have a good prognosis (>60% survival), although some require liver transplantation. Recommendations for routine early childhood immunization beginning at age 12–23 months have further reduced the number of ALF cases due to hepatitis A.

Eisenbach C, Longerich T, Fickensher H, et al. Recurrence of clinically significant hepatitis A following liver transplantation for fulminant hepatitis A. *J Clin Virol.* 2006;35:109–112. [PMID: 16185915]

Rezende G, Roque-Afonso AM, Samuel D, et al. Viral and clinical factors associated with the fulminant course of hepatitis A infection. *Hepatology.* 2003;38:613–618. [PMID: 12939587]

Taylor RM, Davern T, Munoz S, et al. Fulminant hepatitis A virus infection in the United States: incidence, prognosis, outcomes. *Hepatology.* 2006;44:1589–1597. [PMID: 17133489]

B. Hepatitis B and D

Acute hepatitis B infection is the most common viral cause of ALF, accounting for 8% of cases in the ALFSG. Besides in the United States and United Kingdom, it is one of the most important causes of ALF. The incidence of ALF caused by hepatitis B may be underestimated, as some studies have shown evidence of hepatitis B infection by polymerase chain reaction (PCR) in patients who underwent transplantation for what was classified non-A, non-B hepatitis. Precore or pre-S mutant hepatitis B viruses cause infection but do not produce hepatitis B e antigen and may be difficult to diagnose by routine serology. Because rapid destruction of hepatocytes occurs in patients with fulminant hepatitis, some patients have no detectable hepatitis B surface antigen and lower hepatitis B virus DNA levels; however, high-titered immunoglobulin M anti–hepatitis B core antigen is required for diagnosis of acute hepatitis B.

A study in the United States comparing two separate cohorts of patients with hepatitis B–associated ALF versus chronic infection demonstrated that patients with ALF were more likely to be non-Asians and more likely to have genotype D than patients with chronic hepatitis B. In general, the care of patients with viral hepatitis B is supportive as liver transplant is the only effective treatment option. Lamivudine, entecavir, and adefovir, used to treat chronic hepatitis B, have also been used in ALF, but the data is conflicting.

Lee HC. Acute liver failure related to hepatitis B virus. *Hepatol.* 2008;38:S9–S13. [PMID: 19125959]

Ozasa A, Tanaka Y, Orito E, et al. Influence of genotypes and pre-core mutations on fulminant or chronic outcome of acute hepatitis B virus infection. *Hepatology.* 2006;44:326–334. [PMID: 16871568]

Wai CT, Fontana RJ, Polson J, et al. Clinical outcome and virological characteristics of hepatitis B related acute liver failure in the United States. *J Viral Hepatol.* 2005;12:192–198. [PMID: 15720535]

C. Hepatitis C

The role of hepatitis C infection in ALF is controversial. Studies from Japan and India report the presence of anti-hepatitis C virus antibody or hepatitis C virus RNA among patients with ALF, but studies in France, the United States, and the United Kingdom have not shown hepatitis C to be a significant cause of ALF.

D. Hepatitis D

In the United States, infection with hepatitis D virus accounts for fewer than 10% of all cases of acute hepatitis related to hepatitis B virus. It has been suggested that a majority of cases of ALF in patients positive for hepatitis B are due to delta virus rather than to hepatitis B alone.

E. Hepatitis E

Hepatitis E occurs in epidemics in which a high incidence of ALF is seen, particularly in pregnant women. In pregnancy, the fatality rate approaches 40%. Hepatitis E has only rarely been identified in the United States but should be considered in anyone with recent travel to endemic areas such as Russia, Pakistan, Mexico, or India.

Chau TN, Lai ST, Tse C, et al. Epidemiology and clinical features of sporadic hepatitis E as compared with hepatitis A. *Am J Gastroenterol.* 2006;101:292–296. [PMID: 16454833]

F. Atypical Viral Hepatitides

Adenovirus-induced ALF is rare, but multiple cases have been reported after allogeneic stem cell transplantation, liver transplantation, chemotherapy, and renal transplantation. It has an aggressive clinical course and poor prognosis.

Similarly, cytomegalovirus, Epstein-Barr virus, and herpesviruses 1, 2, and 6 are occasionally implicated as causes of ALF. ALF related to herpesvirus infection is usually associated with immunosuppressive therapy or pregnancy, although occurrences of herpes virus–induced ALF have been reported in healthy individuals. Skin lesions are present in only about 50% of cases, and liver biopsy is often helpful in establishing the diagnosis. Treatment should be initiated with acyclovir for suspected or documented cases. Varicella virus has been rarely implicated in hepatic failure and can also be treated with acyclovir.

Nakazawa H, Ito T, Makishima H, et al. Adenovirus fulminant hepatic failure: disseminated adenovirus disease after unrelated allogeneic stem cell transplantation for acute lymphoblastic leukemia. *Intern Med.* 2006;45:975–980. [PMID: 16974062]

3. Non-Acetaminophen Drug Toxicity

Many drugs produce idiosyncratic liver failure (Table 38–5), including halothane, sulfonamides, phenytoin, and isoniazid. In the ALFSG, 13% of ALF cases were attributed to idiosyncratic drug-induced hepatotoxicity.

Drugs most frequently associated with idiosyncratic ALF, as reported by the ALFSG, were antibiotics (especially isoniazid), nonsteroidal analgesics, antiepileptics, statins, and herbal preparations. Two drugs prominently implicated in this study, bromfenac and troglitazone, have been withdrawn by the U.S. Food and Drug Administration.

Table 38–5. Drugs that may cause idiosyncratic liver injury leading to acute liver failure.

Single Agents Associated with Hepatotoxicity	
Allopurinol	Labetalol
Amiodarone	Lisinopril
Amphetamines/ecstasy	Metformin
Dapsone	Methyldopa
Diclofenac	Nefazodone
Didanosine	Nicotinic acid
Disulfiram	Ofloxacin
Efavirenz	Phenytoin
Etoposide	Propylthiouracil
Flutamide	PZA
Gemtuzumab	Quetiapine
Halothane	Statins
Imipramine	Sulfonamides
Isoflurane	Tolcapone
Isoniazid	Troglitazone
Ketoconazole	Valproic acid
Combination Agents with Enhanced Toxicity	
Amoxicillin-clavulanate	
Rifampin-isoniazid	
Trimethoprim-sulfamethoxazole	
Herbal Products/Dietary Supplements Associated with Hepatotoxicity	
Bai Fang herbs	Jin Bu Huan
Chaparral	Kava kava
Comfrey	Lipo Kinetix
Germander	Ma Huang
Greater celandine	Pennyroyal
Gum Thistle	Rattleweed
He Shan Wu	Senecio
Heliotrope	Skullcap
Impila	Sunnhemp

Adapted, with permission, from Polson J, Lee WM; American Association for the Study of Liver Diseases. AASLD position paper: the management of acute liver failure. *Hepatology*. 2005;41:1179–1197. [PMID: 15841455]

Amoxicillin–clavulanate was the most common drug implicated in another registry that included 461 patients with drug-induced liver injury. The fluorinated hydrocarbons trichloroethylene and tetrachloroethane also produce ALF, often with associated renal failure, in people who sniff glue or those exposed to industrial cleaning solvents.

Clinical Findings

Identification of drug-induced ALF requires careful history taking, including all medications, over-the-counter preparations, vitamin supplements, herbal supplements, and health foods. Peripheral eosinophilia, skin rash, and fever may be seen when associated with hypersensitivity; however, many cases of drug-induced hepatotoxicity are nonallergic and idiosyncratic. Aminotransferase levels are often only moderately elevated (in contrast with acetaminophen-induced liver failure, and most other causes of ALF).

Treatment

Initial treatment of drug-induced liver disease includes supportive care, exclusion of other causes of liver injury, and withdrawal of the offending agent. Corticosteroids are not indicated unless there is evidence of a hypersensitivity reaction.

Patients with non–acetaminophen drug-induced ALF have a poor outcome overall, with only 25% recovering spontaneously, and a 60–80% mortality rate without liver transplantation. The outcome of drug-induced acute liver failure is predicted by the degree of liver dysfunction, but not by the class of drugs, drug injury pattern, age, gender, obesity, or timing of cessation of drug use. Hyman Zimmerman, in an observation known as "Hy's rule," noted that if both drug-induced hepatocellular injury and jaundice were present simultaneously without biliary obstruction (or hemolysis), a mortality rate of at least 10% could be expected.

Andrade RJ, Lucena MI, Fernández MC, et al. Drug-induced liver injury: an analysis of 461 incidences submitted to the Spanish registry over a 10-year period. *Gastroenterology*. 2005;129:512–521. [PMID: 16083708]

Andrade RJ, Robles M, Fernández-Castañer A, et al. Assessment of drug-induced hepatotoxicity in clinical practice: a challenge for gastroenterologists. *World J Gastroenterol*. 2007;13:329–340. [PMID: 17230599]

Bernal W, Donaldson N, Wyncoll D, et al. Blood lactate as an early predictor of outcome in paracetamol-induced acute liver failure: a cohort study. *Lancet*. 2002;359:558–563. [PMID: 11867109]

Björnsson E, Olsson R. Outcome and prognostic markers in severe drug-induced liver disease. *Hepatology*. 2005;42:481–489. [PMID: 16025496]

Ohmori S, Shiraki K, Inoue H, et al. Clinical characteristics and prognostic indicators of drug-induced fulminant hepatic failure. *Hepatogastroenterology*. 2003;50:1531–1534. [PMID: 14571779]

Ranganathan SS, Sathiades MJ, Sumanasena S, et al. Fulminant hepatic failure and paracetamol overuse with therapeutic intent in febrile children. *Indian J Pediatr*. 2006;73:871–875. [PMID: 17090896]

Reuben A, Koch DG, Lee WM. Drug-induced acute liver failure: results of a U.S. multicenter, prospective study. *Hepatology*. 2010;52:2065–2076. [PMID: 20949552]

4. Mushroom Poisoning

Mushroom poisoning is common in Western Europe, with 50–100 fatal cases reported yearly. *Amanita phalloides* is the most common species implicated. Hepatic failure is preceded by muscarinic effects such as profuse sweating, vomiting, and diarrhea. Diagnosis should be suspected in patients with a history of severe vomiting, diarrhea, and abdominal cramping within hours to a day of ingesting wild mushrooms. Gastric lavage and activated charcoal via nasogastric tube to remove stomach contents and to decrease the toxin in the enterohepatic circulation has been used although there are no definitive studies of usefulness. The cholera-type diarrhea seen most commonly as an effect of phalloidin during the first 24 hours of illness can produce a profound metabolic alkalosis requiring vigorous fluid resuscitation and electrolyte replacement. Penicillin G, in doses of 250,000–1,000,000 units/kg/day, is used as treatment and is believed to work by displacing amanitin from plasma protein-binding sites and allowing for increased renal excretion. Sibilin (milk thistle) also has cytoprotective abilities against amatoxin. Both antidotes are used commonly despite no controlled trial demonstrating benefit. Patients should be considered for transplantation as very low rates of survival have been reported without it. Of note, encephalopathy is not always present in severe cases and should not be an absolute prerequisite for deciding on transplantation. One study of 27 cases showed that an interval between ingestion and diarrhea of less than 8 hours was a very early predictor of fatal outcome. Later on, prothrombin index and non acetaminophen and acetaminophen King's College criteria were more reliable indicators of prognosis.

Escudié L, Francoz C, Vinel JP, et al. Amanita phalloides poisoning: reassessment of prognostic factors and indications for emergency liver transplantation. *J Hepatol.* 2007;46:466–473. [PMID: 17188393]

Soysal D, Cevik C, Saklamaz A, et al. Coagulation disorders secondary to acute liver failure in Amanita phalloides poisoning: a case report. *Turk J Gastroenterol.* 2006;17:198–202. [PMID: 16941253]

5. Autoimmune Hepatitis

Most patients with autoimmune hepatitis exhibit clinical features of chronic hepatitis, but some present with ALF or an acute-on-chronic presentation. Diagnosis of ALF due to autoimmune hepatitis can be difficult, and other causes need to be ruled out. Autoantibodies may be absent, and liver biopsy is often needed to obtain a diagnosis. Corticosteroids should be initiated (prednisone, 40–60 mg/day), but many patients do not respond even to larger, pulsed doses of steroids. Transplantation listing should therefore be considered in all patients with this presentation.

Czaja AJ. Treatment of autoimmune hepatitis. *Semin Liver Dis.* 2002;22:365–378. [PMID: 12447708]

Kotoh K, Enjoji M, Nakamuta M, et al. Arterial steroid injection therapy can inhibit the progression of severe acute hepatic failure toward fulminant liver failure. *World J Gastroenterol.* 2006;12:6678–6682. [PMID: 17075983]

6. Wilson Disease

ALF is rare in Wilson disease and appears to be more common in women. It is frequently associated with hemolytic anemia as hepatocyte necrosis results in the massive release of copper ions into the circulation. Clinical signs include jaundice, hemoglobinuria, and renal failure. Diagnosis can be difficult because ceruloplasmin, serum copper, urinary copper, and even liver biopsy with copper staining can be unreliable. As with autoimmune hepatitis, patients may have evidence of cirrhosis and still present with signs of ALF when rapid deterioration occurs. Kayser-Fleischer rings are present in 50% of patients presenting with ALF due to Wilson disease. Findings suggestive of the disease include very high bilirubin level (>20 mg/dL), markedly decreased serum albumin and cholesterol levels, decreased serum alkaline phosphatase, decreased uric acid, and a serum AST that runs higher than ALT (over 4:1) due to hemolysis. A high bilirubin (mg/dL) to alkaline phosphatase (IU/L) ratio (>2) is a reliable indicator of Wilson disease in this setting.

ALF due to Wilson disease is nearly always fatal without transplantation, making early identification and immediate listing for transplant critical. Treatment to acutely lower serum copper and limit further hemolysis should include continuous hemofiltration, plasmapheresis, or plasma exchange. Penicillamine is not recommended in ALF as there is a risk of hypersensitivity.

Roberts EA, Schilsky ML. American Association for the Study of Liver Diseases. Diagnosis and treatment of Wilson disease: an update. *Hepatology.* 2008;47:2089–2111. [PMID: 18506894]

7. Malignancy & Vascular Causes

Vascular causes of ALF include portal vein thrombosis, hepatic vein thrombosis, veno-occlusive disease, and ischemic hepatitis. Ischemic liver injury produces marked aminotransferase elevations, centrilobular necrosis, and ALF often with concurrent renal failure, myocardial infarction, cardiac arrest, cardiomyopathy, congestive heart failure, hypovolemia, and pulmonary embolism. Drug-induced hypotension or hypoperfusion causing ALF can be observed with long-acting niacin, cocaine, or methamphetamine.

Budd-Chiari syndrome or acute hepatic vein thrombosis can also present as ALF and often is due to an underlying prothrombotic problem. Abdominal pain, ascites, and hepatomegaly are often present as well as lactic acidosis. The diagnosis should be confirmed by imaging. Transjugular intrahepatic portosystemic shunt, surgical decompression, portocaval shunt, or thrombolysis may be beneficial in patients with acute Budd-Chiari syndrome. Transplantation may be required in patients who do not respond to venous decompression or in whom significant liver failure has occurred. It is important to rule out underlying cancer prior to transplantation.

Malignant infiltration may cause ALF. Massive hepatic enlargement may be seen. Diagnosis should be made by imaging and biopsy, and treatment for the underlying disease is indicated. Common causes include breast cancer, small cell lung cancer, lymphoma, and melanoma. Transplantation is not an option in these patients.

Kavanagh PM, Roberts J, Gibney R, et al. Acute Budd-Chiari syndrome with liver failure: the experience of a policy of initial interventional radiological treatment using transjugular intrahepatic portosystemic shunt. *J Gastroenterol Hepatol.* 2004;19: 1135–1139. [PMID: 15377290]

Murad SD, Valla DC, de Groen PC, et al. Determinants of survival and the effect of portosystemic shunting in patients with Budd-Chiari syndrome. *Hepatology.* 2004;39:500–508. [PMID: 14768004]

8. Pregnancy

Viral hepatitis is the most common cause of ALF in pregnancy and accounts for 40% of jaundice. The outcome of acute fulminant hepatitis E virus infection in pregnancy is poor. Supportive care is advocated, and termination, caesarean, or discouragement of breast feeding are not indicated. Pregnancy can also increase the risk of ALF due to herpesvirus infection, which should be treated with acyclovir. Acute fatty liver of pregnancy (AFLP) occurs during the third trimester and rarely presents as ALF. It is characterized by sudden onset of jaundice and coagulopathy, altered mental status, hypoglycemia, and elevated transaminases but not to the extent seen in acute viral or drug-related hepatitis. Steatosis documented by imaging or biopsy supports the diagnosis of AFLP. Rapid delivery is the treatment, but in 40% of cases the fetus dies before delivery. Fatty liver of pregnancy can be treated with transplantation if prompt recovery does not follow delivery. Alternatively, HELLP syndrome, which involves very high aminotransferase levels, hemolysis, thrombocytopenia, hypertension, proteinuria, and preeclampsia, occurs in 0.1–0.6% of all pregnancies and in 4–12% of women with severe preeclampsia. The only definitive treatment is emergent delivery along with antepartum stabilization of hypertension and DIC, seizure prophylaxis and fetal monitoring.

Pathikonda M, Munoz SJ. Acute Liver Failure. *Ann Hepatol.* 2010; 9:7–14. [PMID: 20308717]

9. Indeterminate Cause

Other rare causes of ALF include giant cell hepatitis or arteritis, amebic abscesses, disseminated tuberculosis, sepsis, heat stroke, and bone marrow transplantation. The cause of ALF is indeterminate in nearly 20% of adult patients in the United States. Indeterminate ALF carries a poor prognosis, with a spontaneous survival rate of 20% or less. Several reports have implicated a variety of viruses in indeterminate, ALF including togaviruses, paramyxoviruses, herpes simplex virus, SEN virus, and hepatitis C virus. The presence of many of these viruses has been discovered later by PCR, after results of routine serologic testing were negative.

This chapter is a revised version of the chapter by Dr. Jaya R. Agrawal and Dr. Amir A. Qamar that was in the previous edition of Current Diagnosis & Treatment: Gastroenterology, Hepatology, & Endoscopy.

Viral Hepatitis

39

Anna Rutherford, MD, MPH
Jules L. Dienstag, MD

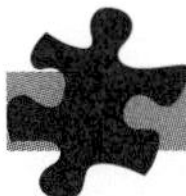

ESSENTIALS OF DIAGNOSIS

- Hepatitis A–E cause most recognized cases of acute viral hepatitis; hepatitis B, C, and D cause most recognized cases of chronic viral hepatitis.
- Hepatitis A and E are transmitted by the fecal-oral route; neither causes chronic infection.
- Hepatitis B, C, and D are acquired percutaneously; all can result in chronic infection.
- Hepatitis D can occur only in a host already infected with hepatitis B.
- All five forms can cause fulminant hepatitis, but B, D, and E are common causes, whereas A and C are very rare causes.
- Diagnostic tests appropriate to different clinical situations detect specific viral antigens and antibodies in serum by sensitive enzyme immunoassay or radioimmunoassay and viral DNA/RNA by sensitive amplification assays (eg, polymerase chain reaction).

General Considerations

Although the hepatitis viruses have been characterized extensively, the pathogenesis, diagnosis, and treatment of chronic viral hepatitis continue to be the focus of research. Sensitive and specific assays are available for all five forms (A to E) of viral hepatitis (Table 39–1). Nevertheless, at least approximately 5–10% of cases of acute and chronic hepatitis cannot be attributed to any of the known forms of viral hepatitis and do not appear to result from toxic, metabolic, or genetic conditions. A specific cause cannot be identified for approximately 50% of cases of fulminant hepatitis. Whether additional unidentified viruses cause acute or chronic liver disease remains an unanswered question; to date, despite intense investigation, no other hepatitis viruses have been identified. This chapter focuses on clinical features of the five known viruses that cause almost all recognized cases of acute and chronic hepatitis (Table 39–2).

Clinical Findings

A. Acute Viral Hepatitis

1. Symptoms and signs—Symptoms of acute viral hepatitis are usually nonspecific and include malaise, fatigue, nausea, anorexia, and arthralgias. Fever, if present, is usually low grade. With disease progression, pruritus, dark urine, scleral icterus, and jaundice may occur.

2. Laboratory findings—In any acute viral hepatitis, serum aminotransferase levels typically exceed 500 units/L and often 1000 units/L, with the alanine aminotransferase (ALT) characteristically higher than the aspartate aminotransferase (AST). Elevation of aminotransferase levels begins in the prodromal phase and precedes the rise in bilirubin level in patients with icteric hepatitis. Serum alkaline phosphatase may be normal or only mildly elevated. Serum bilirubin may be normal (anicteric cases) or elevated (icteric cases), but albumin and prothrombin time are generally normal unless the acute hepatitis is sufficiently severe to impair hepatic synthetic function. In most instances, bilirubin is divided equally between conjugated and unconjugated fractions; values above 20 mg/dL that persist late into the course of viral hepatitis are more likely to be associated with severe disease. Prolongation of the prothrombin time (>3 seconds above the control value or international normalized ratio [INR] >1.7) should raise concern and prompt close monitoring of the patient for worsening hepatic function and impending hepatic failure. Neutropenia and lymphopenia are transient and followed by a relative lymphocytosis. Hypoglycemia occurs occasionally in severe acute hepatitis. A mild and diffuse elevation of the γ-globulin fraction is common, especially in patients with acute hepatitis A.

Table 39–1. Serologic diagnosis of viral hepatitis.

	IgM Anti-HAV	HBsAg	HBeAg	IgM Anti-HBc	IgG Anti-HBc	Anti-HBs	Anti-HBe	Anti-HCV	Anti-HDV	IgM Anti-HEV
Acute hepatitis A	+	–	–	–	–	–	–	–	–	–
Acute hepatitis B	–	+	+	+	–	–	–	–	–	–
HBeAg-reactive chronic hepatitis B	–	+	+	–	+	–	–	–	–	–
HBeAg-negative chronic hepatitis B	–	+	–	–	+	–	+	–	–	–
Inactive hepatitis B carrier	–	+	–	–	+	–	+	–	–	–
Resolved hepatitis B	–	–	–	–	+	+	+	–	–	–
Post–hepatitis B vaccine	–	–	–	–	–	+	–	–	–	–
Acute or chronic hepatitis C	–	–	–	–	–	–	–	+	–	–
Acute or chronic hepatitis D	–	+	±	–	–	–	±	–	+	–
Acute hepatitis E	–	–	–	–	–	–	–	–	–	+

Anti-HAV, antibody to hepatitis A virus; anti-HBc, antibody to hepatitis B core antigen; anti-HBe, antibody to hepatitis B e antigen; anti-HBs, antibody to hepatitis B surface antigen; anti-HCV, antibody to hepatitis C virus; anti-HDV, antibody to hepatitis D virus; anti-HEV, antibody to hepatitis E virus; HBeAg, hepatitis B e antigen; HBsAg, hepatitis B surface antigen; IgG, immunoglobulin G; IgM, immunoglobulin M.

Table 39–2. Properties and clinical characteristics of viruses.

	Hepatitis A	Hepatitis B	Hepatitis C	Hepatitis D	Hepatitis E
Size	27 nm	42 nm	32 nm	36 nm	32–34 nm
Length	7.5 kb	3.2 kb	10 kb	1.7 kb	7.6 kb
Genome	RNA	DNA	RNA	RNA	RNA
Incubation	14–49 days	30–180 days	14–160 days	21–42 days	21–63 days
Transmission	Fecal-oral	Percutaneous, sexual, perinatal	Percutaneous, (especially injection drug use), sexual (rare), perinatal (rare)	Percutaneous, intrafamily	Fecal-oral
Vaccine	Available	Available	None	None (but hepatitis B vaccine protects against acute hepatitis D)	Available outside United States
Severity of acute illness	Usually mild, particularly in children	Adults: 70% subclinical, 30% clinical, <1% severe Newborn: subclinical	Usually subclinical, 1% severe	May be severe	May be severe; 20% mortality in pregnancy
Chronic infection	None	90% neonatal, 50% infants, 20% children, <1% healthy adults	>85%	5% with HBV coinfection, >90% with HBV superinfection	None

HBV, hepatitis B virus.

3. Imaging findings—Radiologic imaging studies are rarely necessary unless biliary tract disease is suspected. For example, for patients with profound cholestasis (such as occurs in hepatitis A and even more commonly in hepatitis E), ultrasonography may be helpful in excluding extrahepatic biliary tract obstruction.

4. Histologic evaluation—Liver biopsy is rarely necessary in acute viral hepatitis except when the diagnosis is questionable or when chronic hepatitis is suspected.

B. Chronic Viral Hepatitis

1. Symptoms and signs—Chronic viral hepatitis may be and is often asymptomatic; many patients are unaware of their condition until the diagnosis is made incidentally or until progression to advanced liver disease results in systemic symptoms and clinical features of hepatic dysfunction.

2. Laboratory findings—The most telling laboratory markers are the aminotransferase levels, which may be elevated continuously or may fluctuate; typically, ALT levels are higher than AST levels until cirrhosis develops, when AST levels tend to be higher. Otherwise, laboratory values that reflect hepatic function (bilirubin, albumin, prothrombin time) may be normal.

3. Imaging findings—Ultrasound, computed tomography (CT), or magnetic resonance imaging (MRI) are useful to evaluate liver parenchyma and to assess for the existence of varices, reversal of portal hepatic flow, ascites, splenomegaly, and other signs of portal hypertension; hepatic vein occlusion and other vascular abnormalities; and focal mass lesions.

4. Histologic evaluation—Although its role is evolving, liver biopsy is useful for grading the activity and for staging the progression of disease, for identifying clinically relevant histologic features (eg, steatosis, iron deposition, pathognomonic features of autoimmune liver injury, granulomatous inflammation, etc), or for adding helpful information in diagnostically challenging cases.

Differential Diagnosis

A. Acute Viral Hepatitis

Infections with other viruses, such as cytomegalovirus, Epstein-Barr virus, herpes simplex or zoster, and coxsackieviruses, can result in an acute viral hepatitis syndrome and elevated serum aminotransferase levels. Toxoplasmosis and leptospirosis may also share clinical features with acute hepatitis. If the results of serologic tests for the known hepatitis viruses (discussed later) are negative, and if clinical features are suggestive, serologic tests for these agents should be considered.

Several drugs and anesthetic agents can produce a picture similar to that of acute hepatitis; therefore, taking a careful drug history is important. A past history of unexplained and repeated episodes of hepatitis raises the possibility of underlying chronic hepatitis.

Alcoholic hepatitis is associated with a history of ethanol abuse and usually with clinical stigmata of alcoholism. In patients with alcoholic liver disease, serum aminotransferase levels rarely rise above 300 units/L, and, typically, serum AST levels exceed serum ALT levels.

When abdominal pain is prominent, acute viral hepatitis may be confused with acute cholecystitis, choledocholithiasis, ascending cholangitis, pancreatitis, or other abdominal disorders. Careful clinical and radiologic evaluation will assist in making the correct diagnosis and thereby avoiding unnecessary surgery. Cholestatic viral hepatitis may be confused with obstructive jaundice resulting from pancreatic carcinoma, common bile duct stone, other disorders that obstruct the biliary tree, or hepatic infiltrative disorders (eg, fatty infiltration, primary or metastatic tumor infiltration, extramedullary hematopoiesis, granulomatous disorders).

Clinical features help to distinguish acute hepatitis from congestive hepatopathy and acute ischemic injury, which tend to be associated primarily with aminotransferase, not alkaline phosphatase, elevations. Uncommonly, inherited metabolic disorders, such as Wilson disease, mimic acute viral hepatitis.

B. Chronic Viral Hepatitis

In the differential diagnosis of chronic viral hepatitis are autoimmune hepatitis, primary biliary cirrhosis, sclerosing cholangitis, genetic disorders such as Wilson disease, hemochromatosis, α_1-antitrypsin deficiency, alcoholic liver disease, nonalcoholic fatty liver disease, and chronic drug hepatotoxicity. Serology, biochemical testing, and liver histopathology help in arriving at the correct diagnosis in most instances.

HEPATITIS A

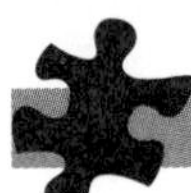

ESSENTIALS OF DIAGNOSIS

- Diagnosis of acute infection depends on the detection of immunoglobulin M (IgM) antibodies to hepatitis A virus (IgM anti-HAV).
- IgM anti-HAV, the primary immune response, is replaced by immunoglobulin G (IgG) anti-HAV, correlating with subsequent lifelong immunity.
- Presence of IgG anti-HAV in a patient with acute hepatitis indicates that the illness is not caused by HAV.

General Considerations

Hepatitis A virus (HAV) is a 27-nm nonenveloped RNA virus (genus *Hepatovirus*) that is transmitted by the fecal-oral route through ingestion of contaminated food (eg, shellfish, strawberries, onions) or water. The incubation period is 2–6 weeks, the duration of viremia is short (5–7 days), and chronic infection does not occur; therefore, percutaneous transmission is exceedingly rare.

Infection is more prevalent in areas of low socioeconomic status characterized by insufficient sanitation and poor hygienic practices, which facilitate the spread of enteric infections. In developing countries, hepatitis A is endemic, infecting most children before the age of 5–10 years. In developed countries, improved socioeconomic conditions and sanitation have led to an increase in the mean age of infection and a reduction in the prevalence of HAV exposure, as reflected by serum antibodies to HAV (anti-HAV) in the population.

Pathogenesis

As is true for all hepatitis viruses, viral replication of HAV occurs primarily within hepatocytes. Except in extraordinary circumstances, hepatitis viruses are not cytopathic; instead, liver cell damage results from host cell-mediated cytotoxicity. In hepatitis A, the necroinflammatory changes and mononuclear cell infiltrates are prominent in periportal areas, but lobular focal necrosis, ballooning hepatocytes, and apoptosis are regular features as well. In some cases, centrilobular cholestasis may be severe, particularly in adults. Serum neutralizing antibodies protect against HAV infection. HAV antigen can be demonstrated by immunohistochemical staining as fine granules in the cytoplasm of hepatocytes and Kupffer cells.

Clinical Findings

A. Acute HAV Infection

Although more than 70% of adults infected with HAV have symptoms, approximately 70% of infections in young children are asymptomatic. When hepatitis A is clinically apparent, patients present with fatigue, malaise, right upper quadrant and epigastric discomfort, loss of appetite, and, in icteric cases, dark urine and jaundice. Less commonly, HAV infection may be profoundly cholestatic and accompanied clinically by marked jaundice, acholic stools, and pruritus.

Hepatitis A results very rarely in fulminant hepatitis and does not cause chronic liver disease, although extraordinarily rare reports suggest that acute hepatitis A can trigger autoimmune hepatitis in susceptible persons. Approximately 10% of patients can have a relapsing course lasting several months (resumption of fecal viral excretion and aminotransferase elevation after initial, apparent resolution) and invariably culminating in eventual recovery. Systemic manifestations are uncommon and include arthritis and, very rarely, transverse myelitis, aplastic anemia, and leukocytoclastic vasculitis, although reports of these complications are not linked reliably to hepatitis A. Concomitant meningoencephalitis has been reported rarely. Cholestatic hepatitis with protracted, albeit ultimately self-limited, cholestatic jaundice and pruritus can occur as a variant of acute hepatitis A.

B. Serologic Assays

The diagnosis of acute HAV infection depends on the detection of IgM antibodies to HAV (IgM anti-HAV). IgM anti-HAV occurs as a primary immune response and persists for approximately 3 months, sometimes extending to 6 months after acute HAV infection. It is replaced by immunoglobulin G (IgG) anti-HAV, which correlates with subsequent lifelong immunity. Thus, if a patient who presents with acute hepatitis has IgG anti-HAV, the acute illness is not caused by HAV.

Prevention

General measures to prevent the spread of HAV infection include a safe water supply and proper environmental hygiene (eg, sewage disposal, elimination of overcrowded housing, etc). Killed HAV vaccines have a protective efficacy of 94–100% after two doses, with negligible side effects. Two such vaccines were licensed in the United States in 1995–1996 and are available worldwide. Their introduction in the United States coincided with a decline in new, reported cases of hepatitis A in the United States from an annual average of 12 cases per 100,000 population in 1995 to 1 case per 100,000 in 2007. In 2006, because of residual clusters of hepatitis A cases, including severe and even fatal instances in otherwise healthy adults, the Advisory Committee on Immunization Practices recommended routine hepatitis A vaccination of children at 1 year of age. Recommendations for vaccination of other persons in groups at increased risk for hepatitis A are listed in Table 39–3.

Immunoglobulin has also been shown to be safe and effective as both preexposure and postexposure prophylaxis against HAV infection. For preexposure prophylaxis, if immediate protection is required, travelers should receive passive immunization with immunoglobulin and begin a course of active immunization with vaccine; in this setting, preexposure passive immunization requires a single intramuscular dose of immunoglobulin (0.02 mL/kg). For postexposure prophylaxis, the same dose, given within 10–14 days of exposure, has an efficacy of approximately 85% and usually aborts or reduces the severity of, and renders clinically inapparent, HAV infection (yielding a combination of passive immunization and the durable immunity that follows acute infection). In the absence of such concomitant active immunization, the passive protection offered by immunoglobulin lasts only a few months.

Table 39–3. Indications for vaccination against hepatitis A and B.

Hepatitis A
- Travelers to countries with high or intermediate endemicity of infection, including Africa, Asia (not Japan), the Mediterranean basin, eastern Europe, the Middle East, Mexico, Central and South America, and parts of the Caribbean
- All children at age 1 year (12-23 months) as part of routine vaccinations
- Men who have sex with men and others with high-risk sexual behaviors
- Users of injection and noninjection drugs of abuse
- Persons with occupational risk for infection (eg, food handlers, child care workers, or people working with nonhuman primates)
- Persons with chronic liver disease including chronic viral hepatitis, particularly hepatitis C, in whom hepatitis A may be severe
- Susceptible persons who receive clotting factor concentrates, especially solvent-detergent treated preparations

Hepatitis B
- All children at birth (before discharge from hospital) and continued thereafter as part of routine childhood vaccinations
- Unvaccinated children <19 years of age
- At birth (along with simultaneous hepatitis B immune globulin) for babies born to HBsAg-positive mothers
- Health care workers and emergency personnel
- Public safety workers with exposure to blood in the workplace
- Clients and staff of institutions for the developmentally disabled, day care centers, and schools
- Patients undergoing hemodialysis
- Persons who have clotting factor disorders and who receive clotting factor concentrates
- Household contacts and sexual partners of persons with chronic hepatitis B
- Adoptees from countries where HBV infection is endemic
- Children who are Alaskan natives or Pacific islanders or residents in households of 1st-generation immigrants from countries in which hepatitis B is endemic
- International travelers spending >6 months in endemic areas and who may have close contact with local population or who are likely to have blood exposure from or sexual exposure with the local population
- Men who have sex with men
- HIV-infected persons
- Sexually active heterosexual men or women who have recently acquired other sexually transmitted diseases, who are sex workers, or who have multiple sexual partners
- Residents and staff of correctional facilities and residential group homes
- Persons with chronic liver disease, including chronic hepatitis C

Treatment

Treatment is largely supportive and consists of discontinuation of potentially hepatotoxic medications and restriction of alcohol intake. Neither bed rest nor dietary restrictions are effective. Most cases do not require hospitalization, which is recommended for patients with advanced age, serious underlying medical conditions, chronic liver disease, malnutrition, pregnancy, immunosuppressive therapy, hepatotoxic medications, severe vomiting that prevents adequate oral intake, and clinical and laboratory findings that suggest fulminant hepatitis. The occasional patient with fulminant hepatic failure, defined as the onset of encephalopathy within 8 weeks of the onset of symptoms, should be referred for consideration of liver transplantation.

Course & Prognosis

The overall case fatality rate for HAV infection is very low (~0.3–0.8%), although higher in adults older than age 60 years (2.6%). In some reports, morbidity and mortality were increased in the presence of a hepatitis A superinfection in patients with underlying chronic liver disease.

Advisory Committee on Immunization Practices (ACIP), Fiore AE, Wasley A, Bell B. Prevention of hepatitis A through active or passive immunization: recommendations of the Advisory Committee on Immunization Practices (ACIP). *MMWR Recomm Rep.* 2006;55:1–23. [PMID: 16708058]

Craig AS, Schaffner W. Prevention of hepatitis A with the hepatitis A vaccine. *N Engl J Med.* 2004;350:476–481. [PMID: 14749456]

Daniels D, Grytdal S, Wasley A. Surveillance for acute viral hepatitis—United States, 2007. *MMWR Surveill Summ.* 2009; 58:1–27. [PMID: 17363893]

Martin A, Lemon SM. Hepatitis A virus: from discovery to vaccines. *Hepatology.* 2006;43:S164–172. [PMID: 16447259]

Taylor RM, Davern T, Munoz S, et al. Fulminant hepatitis A virus infection in the United States: incidence, prognosis and outcomes. *Hepatology.* 2006;44:1589–1597. [PMID: 17133489]

HEPATITIS B

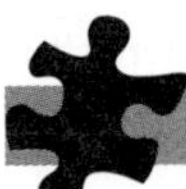

ESSENTIALS OF DIAGNOSIS

- Diagnosis relies on the presence of hepatitis B surface antigen (HBsAg).
- Presence of IgM versus IgG antibodies to hepatitis B core antigen (anti-HBc) distinguishes acute from chronic infection, and IgM anti-HBc indicates recent infection (previous 6 months).
- Hepatitis B e antigen (HBeAg) appears early in the course of infection and in self-limited cases is replaced within 2–3 months by antibody to HBeAg (anti-HBe).
- During chronic hepatitis B in patients with wild-type HBV infection, viral replication is high, infectivity is substantial, and liver injury is pronounced; this phase gives way to one of lower viral replication, infectivity, and liver injury in which patients become inactive carriers.
- In patients with precore mutations (HBeAg-negative chronic hepatitis B), HBV DNA levels fluctuate, and anti-HBe is detectable in serum.
- Presence of isolated antibodies to HBsAg (anti-HBs) is consistent with vaccine-induced immunity.
- Antibodies to both surface and core proteins (anti-HBs, anti-HBc, and anti-HBe) indicate prior HBV infection.
- Interpretation of isolated IgG anti-HBc positivity is difficult and may represent ongoing, low-level HBV infection, prior HBV infection, or a false-positive test.

General Considerations

More than 350 million people worldwide—5% of the world's population—are currently HBsAg-reactive, indicating that they are currently infected with hepatitis B virus (HBV), and as many as 50% of the world's population have had HBV infection, as reflected by the presence of anti-HBs. HBV is endemic in areas containing 45% of the world's population. In endemic areas, rates of current infection range from 8% to 25%, and exposure rates (based on the presence of anti-HBs) range from 60% to 85%. In low prevalence areas such as the United States, the prevalence of chronic HBV infection is 0.1–0.2% (1.25 million), and the annual incidence of new HBV infections is 200,000–300,000.

HBV is transmitted primarily by perinatal, percutaneous, and sexual routes. The virus can also be transmitted by inapparent percutaneous routes and close person-to-person contact, presumably via open cuts and sores, especially among children in endemic areas (eg, sub-Saharan Africa, which has a prevalence of chronic HBV infection of just under 10%). In the United States, most HBV infections occur in adolescence and early adulthood, and the most common modes of transmission are sexual and percutaneous (exposure to contaminated instruments and needles, eg, via injection drug use). In contrast, in Asia, the most common mode is perinatal transmission to infants of mothers with chronic HBV infection; in sub-Saharan African countries, in addition to perinatal spread, another common mode of transmission is horizontal spread between young children. Injection drug users are at high risk of acquiring not only HBV infection but also other blood-borne hepatitis agents, hepatitis C and D (see later sections).

Pathogenesis

HBV is a partially double-stranded, partially single-stranded DNA virus (*hepadnavirus type 1*) that replicates via reverse transcription through an RNA intermediate. Although HBV is strongly hepatotropic, viral sequences, including HBV replicative intermediates, are present in extrahepatic tissues (lymph nodes, peripheral blood mononuclear cells); however, the vast bulk of—and the only pathophysiologically relevant—HBV replication is confined to the liver. The HBV genome contains four open reading frames that encode four major proteins: (1) the S gene, which codes for the envelope protein, hepatitis B surface antigen (HBsAg); (2) the C gene, which codes for the nucleocapsid proteins hepatitis B core antigen (HBcAg) and hepatitis B e antigen (HBeAg); (3) the P (or pol) gene, which codes for the DNA polymerase, which, in turn, catalyzes transcription and reverse transcription steps involved in viral replication; and (4) the X gene, which codes for the X protein, a protein of limited clinical relevance but which upregulates the transcription of host cellular and viral genes, including those of other viruses such as HIV.

The envelope protein of the virus, HBsAg, in serum is the primary marker of HBV infection. In the hepatocyte, HBsAg is expressed in the cytoplasm and can be recognized histologically by the presence of ground-glass hepatocytes. Eight HBV genotypes (A to H) have been identified; the prevalence of HBV genotype varies depending on geographic location. In the United States the prevalences of genotypes A, B, C, D, and others are 35%, 22%, 31%, 10%, and 2%, respectively. Recent data suggest that HBV genotypes may play an important role in progression of HBV-related liver disease as well as in response to interferon therapy. Similar associations have not been clarified definitively in patients treated with oral agents (nucleoside and nucleotide analogs); therefore, the testing of HBV genotype has not yet been adopted routinely as a prelude to antiviral therapy (see later discussion).

The C region has two initiation codons and therefore two gene transcripts (precore and core), the translation of which result in two protein products (HBeAg and HBcAg). HBcAg, the protein expressed on the 27-nm nucleocapsid core particles, is not secreted into serum but is localized predominantly to the hepatocyte nucleus and is expressed also in smaller quantities on the hepatocyte surface membrane. As such, HBcAg is the target of the host immune response to infection, playing an important role in the pathogenesis of HBV-induced liver damage. The other nucleocapsid protein, HBeAg, a low-molecular-weight nonparticulate protein, is encoded by the precore plus core region of the C gene, enters the secretory apparatus of the hepatocyte, and circulates in serum; the presence of HBeAg is indicative of active viral replication and correlates with increased infectivity and liver injury. The products of the same gene, HBcAg and HBeAg, have considerable amino acid homology and immune cross-reactivity at the T-cell level. Antibody to HBcAg (anti-HBc) appears at the onset of clinical hepatitis, shortly after the appearance of HBsAg, and may be the only marker detectable between the disappearance of HBsAg and the appearance of anti-HBs (less likely to be encountered now that the sensitivity of assays for HBsAg and anti-HBs are so high). During acute hepatitis B, anti-HBe appears as clinical symptoms, and aminotransferase levels are waning; its appearance marks a transition to lower viral replication, infectivity, and liver injury.

HBeAg-negative variants result from mutations in the precore region of the C gene, with failure of HBeAg synthesis (the serologic marker linked to active virus replication) yet with continued high-level viral replication and liver injury. "HBeAg-negative" mutant HBV has been associated with fulminant hepatitis (rarely) and chronic hepatitis (commonly).

Liver injury associated with HBV infection is the product of a combination of innate and adaptive immune responses, the latter of which are effected by cytotoxic T cells directed at liver membrane complexes of host histocompatibility antigens and HBcAg. The clinical outcome of HBV infection depends on the balance between viral activity and the host immune response, as reflected by the robustness of the $CD8^+$ cytotoxic T-cell response and the release of antiviral T-cell cytokines; however, other than certain clinical features (eg, age, infection at birth, immunocompetence), what distinguishes those who recover from those who progress to chronic infection remains poorly defined. In perinatally acquired infection, immaturity of the neonatal immune system and the presence of HBV on hepatocytes shortly after birth combine to produce a level of immunologic tolerance to HBV that limits the adequacy of the host immune response to HBV. This state of immunologic tolerance can persist indefinitely. No robust cytotoxic T-cell response occurs against HBV, no clinical illness ensues, but chronic infection is almost invariable (>90%). In contrast, among young adults with acute hepatitis B, the cytotoxic T-cell response to HBV expressed on hepatocyte membranes is substantial and efficient, leading to an acute hepatitis illness and, typically, recovery; chronicity after clinically apparent acute hepatitis B in healthy, immunocompetent young adults occurs in fewer than 1% of cases.

A. Hepatocellular Carcinoma

Epidemiologically and clinically, chronic HBV infection is linked strongly to the development of hepatocellular carcinoma (HCC), which can occur in up to 50% of patients with HBV-induced cirrhosis following life-long infection acquired perinatally (see Chapter 49). The mechanism of viral oncogenesis has been studied extensively; viral integration into the host genome is required, but no consistent sites of integration have been identified (eg, adjacent to a host tumor promotor or suppressor gene). Cell turnover associated with chronic inflammation likely contributes to the pathogenesis of HCC, as do such cofactors such as alcohol use and environmental aflatoxin exposure.

B. Hepatitis B Virus Variants

1. Precore mutants or HBeAg-negative chronic HBV—A precore nucleotide mutation or core-promoter mutation can lead to premature termination of the precore protein, preventing production of HBeAg. HBeAg-negative HBV is found more frequently in HBV genotypes other than genotype A, and its prevalence was concentrated initially in Mediterranean countries. Currently, HBeAg-negative chronic hepatitis B is the predominant form of chronic hepatitis B in Europe and represents a growing proportion (~40%) of chronic hepatitis B infections in the United States. Wild-type (HBeAg-positive) chronic hepatitis B is associated with higher levels of HBV replication ($\geq 10^6$ virions/mL) than HBeAg-negative chronic hepatitis B ($\leq 10^5$ virions/mL), whereas HBeAg-negative chronic hepatitis B is more likely to be associated with fluctuating levels of HBV DNA and aminotransferase activity. In addition, in HBeAg-negative chronic hepatitis B, patients treated with antiviral therapy (see later discussion) cannot experience treatment-induced HBeAg seroconversion, which, in HBeAg-positive chronic hepatitis B, can be used as a treatment end point. Therefore, the ideal duration of therapy remains undefined in HBeAg-negative chronic hepatitis B.

2. S mutants—A mutation in the S gene has been reported in infants who are born to HBV-infected mothers but acquire HBV infection after vaccination and in liver transplant recipients who acquire breakthrough HBV reinfection despite treatment with hepatitis B immunoglobulin (HBIG). These mutations alter the antigenicity of the HBV envelope, evading neutralizing anti-HBs. Fortunately, the frequency of such mutations is limited.

3. P mutants—Mutations in the polymerase gene are associated with resistance to HBV antiviral agents such as lamivudine, adefovir, and telbivudine (see later discussion).

Clinical Findings

A. Acute Hepatitis B

The incubation period of acute hepatitis B is between 4 weeks and 6 months. Clinical symptoms are similar to those described earlier for acute hepatitis A (eg, fatigue, anorexia, jaundice), and aminotransferase elevations are the biochemical hallmark of illness. In 5–10% of patients with acute hepatitis B, a serum sickness-like syndrome with arthralgias, rash, angioedema, and, rarely, proteinuria and hematuria may develop in the prodromal phase. In children, hepatitis B may present rarely as anicteric hepatitis associated with a nonpruritic papular rash on the face, buttocks, and limbs (papular acrodermatitis of childhood).

B. Chronic Hepatitis B

Progression from acute to chronic hepatitis may be suggested by the persistence of anorexia, weight loss, and fatigue, although most patients with chronic hepatitis B are asymptomatic. Physical findings may include hepatomegaly and splenomegaly. Laboratory findings include persistence of HBsAg, detectable HBeAg in HBeAg-positive hepatitis, and elevations of aminotransferase, bilirubin, and globulin levels. Histologic features include the presence of portal inflammation, bridging or, in severe cases, multilobular hepatic necrosis, and the presence of fibrosis.

Many patients with chronic HBV infection are inactive carriers who have no symptoms, normal serum aminotransferase activity, low-level HBV DNA ($\leq 10^3$ virions/mL), circulating anti-HBe, and normal or near-normal liver histology.

Extrahepatic manifestations, when they occur, may include arthralgias, arthritis, Henoch-Schönlein purpura, generalized vasculitis (polyarteritis nodosa), glomerulonephritis, pleural effusions, pericarditis, and aplastic anemia (the latter not definitively linked to HBV infection, however). Uncommon complications of HBV infection include pancreatitis, myocarditis, atypical pneumonia, transverse myelitis, and peripheral neuropathy.

C. Serologic Assays

The diagnosis of HBV infection relies on the presence of HBsAg. Acute and chronic infections are distinguished by the presence of IgM versus IgG antibodies to HBcAg (anti-HBc). The presence of IgM anti-HBc indicates recent infection, generally within the previous 6 months. HBeAg appears early during acute hepatitis B, while viral replication is at peak levels, and in self-limited cases is replaced within 2–3 months by antibody to HBeAg (anti-HBe).

During chronic hepatitis B, in patients with wild-type HBV infection, the presence of HBeAg corresponds to a relatively highly replicative period, during which levels of HBV DNA exceed 10^6 virions/mL, infectivity is substantial, and liver injury is pronounced. Over time, this highly replicative phase gives way to a relatively low replicative phase, characterized by low-level HBV DNA ($\leq 10^3$ virions/mL) and negligible infectivity and liver injury. Patients in this phase are considered inactive carriers.

In patients with precore mutations (HBeAg-negative chronic hepatitis B), HBV DNA levels fluctuate between undetectable and approximately 10^5 virions/mL, and anti-HBe is detectable in serum. In chronic hepatitis B, anti-HBc is of the IgG class (except, rarely, during reactivation of chronic hepatitis B [eg, sero-reversion from anti-HBe-reactive back to HBeAg-reactive or during reactivation of clinically quiescent HBeAg-negative chronic hepatitis B], when IgM anti-HBc may reappear transiently). The presence of isolated anti-HBs is consistent with vaccine-induced immunity. Antibodies to both surface and core proteins (anti-HBs, anti-HBc, and anti-HBe) indicate prior HBV infection.

Interpretation of isolated IgG anti-HBc positivity is difficult and may represent ongoing, low-level HBV infection, prior HBV infection, or a false-positive test. Isolated anti-HBc with ongoing low-level HBV infection is more common in persons from high-prevalence areas, in persons with a history of injection drug use, and in patients with HIV infection.

Prevention

Hepatitis B vaccine is protective in over 90% of normal adults and in almost 100% of newborns. Recombinant vaccines have largely supplanted the original plasma-derived vaccine in most parts of the world. Common adverse effects are local reactions at the injection site (soreness, tenderness, pruritus, and swelling). The immunogenicity of hepatitis B vaccines is reduced in adults older than 40 years; among younger healthy adults, approximately 2.5–5% do not acquire protective antibodies, and such nonresponsiveness has been shown to be genetically determined.

Despite the availability of highly effective vaccines for 30 years, targeted vaccination programs for those at highest risk of infection have failed to reduce the frequency of HBV infection in the U.S. population. Currently, the U.S. Public Health Service recommends universal vaccination of all neonates and prepubertal teenagers. In addition, HBV vaccination is currently recommended for immunocompromised patients; hemodialysis patients; patients with coexisting chronic liver disease of other causes, including chronic hepatitis C; health care workers; injection drug users; and those with high-risk sexual exposures (see Table 39–3). Currently, booster immunization is not recommended routinely, although it may be useful in immunosuppressed persons who have lost detectable anti-HBs or in immunocompetent persons who sustain HBsAg inoculation after losing detectable antibody (although this subgroup appears to be protected even after loss of detectable anti-HBs).

Treatment

A. Fulminant Hepatitis B

In fulminant hepatitis B, intensive care in a specialized unit and early consideration for orthotopic liver transplantation likely reduces mortality. Only 25% of patients who have fulminant hepatitis B will survive without liver transplantation. Patients should be supported by maintaining fluid and electrolyte balance and cardiorespiratory function, controlling bleeding, treating prophylactically with broad-spectrum antibiotics, monitoring for cerebral edema, and managing other complications. Although antiviral treatment with interferon has not been shown to be of benefit in fulminant hepatitis B, treatment with oral nucleoside or nucleotide agents (described later) may be of benefit and would be recommended in most specialized treatment centers.

Corticosteroid therapy is not only ineffective but harmful, as demonstrated in clinical trials. Similarly, exchange transfusions, plasma perfusion, human cross-circulation, porcine liver cross-perfusion, and extracorporeal liver-assist devices have not been proven to be effective.

Orthotopic liver transplantation is being performed with increasing frequency, with excellent long-term results. Thus, patients should be supported maximally until spontaneous recovery or until prognostic factors indicate worsening outcome necessitating transplantation; the threshold for referring to a liver transplantation center should be very low. During and after transplantation, measures should be taken to prevent HBV infection of the graft (see later discussion).

B. Chronic Hepatitis B

The objectives of treatment for chronic hepatitis B are to suppress HBV replication and reduce liver injury. Among the end points of therapy are (1) profound reduction in circulating HBV DNA, preferably to levels undetectable by highly sensitive amplification assays; (2) in HBeAg-positive chronic hepatitis B, HBeAg seroconversion (loss of HBeAg and acquisition of anti-HBe); (3) normalization of ALT levels; (4) improvement in liver histology (reduction in the grade of necroinflammatory activity and limiting progression of, or even improving, the stage of fibrosis). Although not proven conclusively, data suggest that successful antiviral therapy has the potential to prevent or delay progression to cirrhosis, hepatic decompensation, and even HCC. Recommendations for patients with chronic hepatitis B who are candidates for treatment are summarized in Table 39–4; seven therapies are approved and currently available for treatment of chronic hepatitis B (Table 39–5).

Table 39–4. Recommendations for treatment of chronic hepatitis B.

HBe Ag	HBV DNA	ALT	Treatment Strategy
Positive	>20,000 IU/mL	≤2 × ULN	Low efficacy of treatment If ALT <ULN, observe If ALT 1-2 × ULN: • Consider biopsy for age >40 y, family history of HCC • Treat if biopsy shows substantial inflammation or any fibrosis
	>20,000 IU/mL	>2 × ULN	Treat with any of recommended agents Of the oral antiviral agents, entecavir and tenofovir are favored over earlier-generation drugs with lower barriers to resistance; PEG IFN has supplanted standard IFN Liver biopsy optional
Negative	>20,000 IU/mL	>2 × ULN	Treat with any of recommended agents (Of the oral antiviral agents, entecavir and tenofovir are favored over earlier-generation drugs with lower barriers to resistance; PEG IFN has supplanted standard IFN) Liver biopsy optional
	>2000 IU/mL	1-2 × ULN	Consider biopsy Treat if substantial inflammation or any fibrosis
	<2000 IU/mL +	<ULN	No treatment Observe (inactive carrier)

ALT, alanine aminotransferase; HBeAg, hepatitis B e antigen; HBV, hepatitis B virus; HCC, hepatocellular carcinoma; IFN, interferon; PEG IFN, pegylated interferon; ULN, upper limit of normal.

Table 39–5. Approved antiviral therapy among treatment-naïve patients with HBeAg-positive chronic hepatitis B

	IFNa	PEG IFNa	Lamivudine	Adefovir	Entecavir	Telbivudine	Tenofovir
HBV DNA Negative	37%	25%	44%	13-21%	67%	60%	76%
HBV DNA Log_{10} Reduction		–4.5	–5.5	–3.5	–6.9	–6.5	–6.2
HBeAg Loss	30%	30%	17-32%	24%	22%	26%	NA
HBeAg seroconversion		30%	16-21%	12%	21%	22%	21%
ALT normalization	23%	39%	50%	48%	68%	77%	68%
Histology improvement	NA	38%	49-56%	53%	72%	65%	74%
HBsAg loss (1 year)	8%	3%	<1%	0%	2%	0%	3%
Resistance	None	None	~14-32% year 1, ~60-70% year 5	0% year 1, 29% year 5	0% year 1, 1.2% through year 5	5% year 1, 25% year 2	0% year 3, NA beyond year 3

ALT, alanine aminotransferase; HBeAg, hepatitis B e antigen; IFN-α, interferon α; NA, not available; PEG IFN-α, pegylated interferon α.

1. Interferon-α2b—The first antiviral drug for hepatitis B, interferon-α2b (IFN-α), was approved by the U.S. Food and Drug Administration (FDA) in 1992. In patients with compensated chronic hepatitis B (including those with early cirrhosis), detectable HBeAg, and elevated aminotransferase activity, subcutaneous IFN-α injections of 10 million units three times per week or 5 million units daily for 16–24 weeks resulted in HBeAg loss in approximately 30% (along with suppression of HBV DNA to levels undetectable by relatively insensitive hybridization assays) and HBeAg seroconversion in approximately 18–20%. Patients with HBeAg-negative chronic hepatitis B should be treated for at least 12–24 months. In this early experience with interferon, almost 10% of HBeAg-reactive patients cleared HBsAg after their initial course of therapy; however, such high rates of HBsAg seroconversion have not been observed in more recent experiences. The strongest predictor of response to IFN-α in HBeAg-positive patients is a high pretreatment ALT level, but other factors favoring a response include a high histologic activity index, low HBV DNA level, and HBV genotypes A and B. Retreatment of nonresponders with a second course of IFN-α is unlikely to be of any clinical benefit.

In patients with HBeAg-negative hepatitis B, short courses of IFN-α are of little benefit and do not yield durable suppression of HBV DNA and ALT; in this patient group, long-term treatment (eg, 12–18 months) is preferable, but the durability of treatment effect is degraded over time to less than 20%, 5 years after therapy. Compensated cirrhotic patients respond as do patients with precirrhotic chronic hepatitis B; however, in decompensated cirrhosis, IFN-α may precipitate hepatic failure or be complicated by life-threatening infection or psychiatric effects and, therefore, is not recommended.

Side effects of interferon, which, in addition to the need for injection, are the major limitation to its use, include (1) flulike symptoms of fever, myalgias, fatigue, and headache; (2) marrow suppression (leukopenia, neutropenia, and thrombocytopenia); (3) anxiety, emotional lability, or depression; and (4) autoimmune disorders, primarily of the thyroid. IFN-α is accompanied by a flare in ALT in 30–40% of patients, and although flares are considered to be predictive of a favorable response, in patients with advanced or marginally compensated cirrhosis, an acute flare can precipitate decompensation.

Contraindications to IFN-α therapy include immune suppression or autoimmune disease, and severe, uncontrolled psychiatric disease or depression.

Before the availability of newer antiviral agents, IFN-α was considered a good therapeutic choice for patients with mild liver disease, low levels of HBV replication, and high serum aminotransferase levels. Some authorities recommend interferon-based therapy for young persons, based on the assumption that an approximately 30% chance of HBeAg loss with a time-confined course of therapy might be preferable for a young person to indefinite therapy with an oral agent (see later discussion). An equally compelling argument might be made to spare a young person the inconvenience and side effects of IFN-α therapy in favor of a side effect–free oral agent, which might require an extra half year to a year to achieve the same benefit as a course of IFN-α.

For all practical purposes, IFN-α as been supplanted by long-acting, once-weekly pegylated interferon for those favoring interferon therapy and by the several highly potent polymerase inhibitors for those who favor oral agents. What early studies of IFN-α have shown is that successful antiviral therapy can improve the natural history of chronic hepatitis B, improving survival and complication-free survival.

2. Pegylated interferon alfa (PEG IFN-α)—Pegylated interferons are produced by binding of a large, inert polyethylene glycol moiety to the interferon molecule, thus increasing the molecular weight of the compound, decreasing its renal clearance, altering its metabolic degradation, and increasing its half-life. Therefore, pegylated interferons can be administered by subcutaneous injection once weekly.

PEG IFN-α2a is the only pegylated interferon approved for the treatment of chronic hepatitis B in the United States. Clinical trials have demonstrated that the efficacy of PEG IFN-α2a is similar to or slightly better than that of standard IFN-α, in addition to its more convenient administration. For HBeAg-positive patients, the most definitive trial represented a comparison of 48 weeks of PEG IFN-α2a alone, versus lamivudine alone, versus combination therapy. During the 48 weeks of therapy, the level of HBV DNA suppression was highest in the combination-treatment arm, and HBeAg seroconversion occurred in a similar percentage of the three groups: 27%, 20%, and 24%, respectively. Twenty-four weeks after treatment was stopped, however, seroconversion was maintained in 32%, 19%, and 27% of the three groups, respectively, indicating that 48 weeks of PEG IFN-α2a monotherapy was superior to 48 weeks of lamivudine monotherapy as well as 48 weeks of combination therapy. In a study of HBeAg-negative patients, PEG IFN-α2a monotherapy was compared with lamivudine monotherapy versus combination therapy for 48 weeks; a sustained response, defined as suppression of HBV DNA to below 10^5 copies/mL or to undetectable by polymerase chain reaction (PCR) amplification (10^2 copies/mL) and a return to normal of ALT, was comparable in patients who received PEG IFN-α2a alone or in combination with lamivudine (100 mg), which were both better than lamivudine alone. In both HBeAg-reactive and HBeAg-negative studies, a small proportion of PEG IFN-α2a-treated study subjects experienced HBsAg seroconversion during (in the HBeAg-negative trial) or after (in the HBeAg-positive trial) therapy. Side effects and predictors of treatment response are similar to those of standard IFN-α therapy, but PEG IFN-α2a is better tolerated by most subjects.

Although some patients may choose a year of PEG IFN-α2a therapy, such therapy requires a year of weekly injections and clinically intense monitoring as well as willingness to accept interferon side effects. In these trials of PEG IFN-α2a, treatment was confined to a finite, 48-week period, which is typical of the way PEG IFN-α2a is used but not the way oral agents are used. Instead, oral agents, very well tolerated, are administered for longer periods (eg, until after HBeAg seroconversion or to maintain responsiveness in HBeAg-negative patients). In fact, the same HBeAg seroconversion rates achieved with 48 weeks of PEG IFN-α2a injection therapy occur when oral agent therapy is extended to 18–24 months. In addition, suppression of HBV DNA and ALT after interferon-based therapy in HBeAg-negative patients is lost gradually over time in the vast majority of patients. Therefore, the advantages of a year of PEG IFN-α2a therapy may be outweighed by the advantages of slightly longer treatment with substantially better tolerated oral agents. The recommended dose of PEG IFN-α2a is 180 mcg weekly for 48 weeks.

3. Lamivudine—Lamivudine, an oral nucleoside analog that inhibits viral DNA synthesis by blocking reverse transcriptase and that is cleared renally, was approved by the FDA originally for the treatment of HIV (150 mg daily) in 1995 and then for the treatment of hepatitis B (100 mg daily) in 1998.

Several large, randomized controlled trials of HBeAg-positive patients treated for 1 year documented HBeAg seroconversion (with suppression of HBV DNA to undetectable levels as determined by insensitive hybridization assays) in 16–20% of treated patients (HBeAg loss in up to a third) compared with 4–6% spontaneous seroconversion in control subjects. Furthermore, loss of detectable HBV DNA occurs in the majority of patients, normalization of ALT in ≥50% of patients, and improvement in necroinflammatory histology scores in 49–56% of patients compared with 23–25% of control subjects. Recent studies in which lamivudine was the comparator arm for new oral nucleoside analogs, demonstrated that lamivudine suppresses HBV DNA by approximately 5.5 $\log_{10}$ copies/mL. Reductions in the progression of fibrosis and progression to cirrhosis have also been demonstrated. After HBeAg seroconversion, this serologic status is maintained in approximately 80% of patients as long as a period of consolidation therapy follows the seroconversion (at least 6 months in Western patients, longer in Asian patients). For patients who do not achieve HBeAg seroconversion during the first year of therapy, HBeAg seroconversion rates increase with extended courses of therapy, but the optimal duration of treatment with lamivudine, as with other oral agents, remains to be defined.

In HBeAg-negative patients, lamivudine suppresses HBV DNA by approximately 4.5 $\log_{10}$ copies/mL, suppresses HBV DNA to undetectable levels (as determined by sensitive amplification assays) in approximately 70%, and reduces ALT to normal in approximately 75%. When therapy is discontinued, however, generally, the therapeutic effect is lost as HBV DNA and ALT return to baseline levels. Therefore, almost all HBeAg-negative patients and the majority of HBeAg-positive patients require extension of therapy indefinitely beyond the first year.

Lamivudine is safe to use in patients with cirrhosis. Clinical trials have demonstrated that lamivudine therapy for several years can reverse cirrhosis and that, unlike interferon, this drug can be used in patients with hepatic decompensation, salvaging them from a further decline and leading to reversal of decompensation. In addition, a prospective trial of lamivudine versus placebo in compensated patients with advanced fibrosis and cirrhosis demonstrated the principle that such antiviral therapy can prevent the incidence over time of hepatic decompensation; in this important study, a trend was apparent in the prevention of, or delay in, the development of HCC.

Selection of lamivudine-resistant mutations is the main concern with lamivudine monotherapy. Genotypic resistance can be detected in 14–32% of patients after 1 year of lamivudine treatment and increases to 60–70% after 5 years of treatment. The most common mutation involves substitution of methionine for valine or isoleucine in the tyrosine-methionine-aspartate-aspartate (YMDD) motif of the HBV DNA polymerase. Factors associated with resistance include long duration of treatment, high pretreatment serum HBV DNA, and, most importantly, high levels of residual virus (>10^3–10^4 virions/mL) after initiation of treatment. Although in vitro the YMDD mutation actually decreases replication fitness of HBV, compensatory mutations restore the fitness of mutant HBV, and clinical benefit is lost eventually after lamivudine resistance emerges. Lamivudine resistance is usually detected by virologic breakthrough followed by biochemical breakthrough and, in some patients, can be associated with an acute exacerbation of hepatitis or, in marginally compensated cirrhotics, with hepatic decompensation.

Most patients with confirmed lamivudine resistance should receive rescue therapy with antiviral agents, such as adefovir or the now favored tenofovir, that are effective against lamivudine-resistant HBV mutants. When adefovir or tenofovir is used to treat patients with lamivudine resistance, the new drug should be added to lamivudine therapy; for example, switching to adefovir monotherapy renders the patient susceptible ultimately to adefovir resistance.

Because of the need for long lamivudine treatment courses in most patients, because of its low barrier to resistance, and because its efficacy is inferior to that of later-generation antivirals, lamivudine is no longer a first-line treatment for chronic HBV; now that more potent, less resistance-prone antiviral agents are available, lamivudine, despite its established safety, has been supplanted as an antiviral agent for hepatitis B.

4. Adefovir dipivoxil—Adefovir is a nucleotide analog of adenosine monophosphate that can inhibit both reverse transcriptase and DNA polymerase activity and is incorporated into HBV DNA, resulting in chain termination. Adefovir is effective in suppressing wild-type HBV as well as lamivudine-resistant HBV. The recommended dose for adults with normal renal function is 10 mg orally daily. Adefovir has been shown to produce a histologic response in 53% of HBeAg-positive patients versus 25% of placebo recipients after 48 weeks of therapy, HBeAg seroconversion in 12% of patients versus 6% of placebo recipients, a 3.5 $\log_{10}$ copies/mL decrease in HBV DNA in patients versus 0.6 $\log_{10}$ copies/mL in placebo recipients, and normalization of ALT levels in 48% of patients versus 16% of placebo recipients. Approximately 30% of patients with no prior nucleotide analog treatment have a primary nonresponse to adefovir (<2 $\log_{10}$ drop in HBV DNA after 6 months of treatment), and in approximately half of adefovir-treated patients, the antiviral response is slow. This suboptimal profile, which reduced the appeal of adefovir initially, led to its replacement by tenofovir (see below) when the newer agent became available.

In HBeAg-negative patients, suppression of HBV DNA, normalization of ALT, and histologic improvement occur as well, but the therapeutic effect is lost once the drug is stopped. Thus, as is the case for therapy with other oral agents, in HBeAg-negative patients, continued treatment is needed to maintain the antiviral response. In HBeAg-negative patients who have completed 5 years of adefovir treatment, HBV DNA was undetectable in 67% and ALT was normal in 69%.

Adefovir has been shown to be effective in liver allograft recipients and in HIV-HBV coinfected patients as well as in lamivudine-resistant HBV. Adefovir resistance occurs at a slower rate than with lamivudine treatment; the cumulative probabilities of genotypic resistance to adefovir at 1, 2, 3, 4, and 5 years have been reported to be 0%, 3%, 11%, 18%, and 29%, respectively, in HBeAg-negative patients (data in HBeAg-reactive patients are not available). As previously mentioned, in patients with lamivudine-resistant HBV, if adefovir is used, lamivudine should not be *switched* to adefovir; instead, adefovir should be *added* to lamivudine therapy.

5. Entecavir—Entecavir, a carbocyclic analog of 2′-deoxyguanosine, inhibits HBV replication at three steps: priming of the HBV polymerase, reverse transcription of the negative-strand HBV DNA from the pregenomic RNA, and synthesis of the positive-strand HBV DNA. Entecavir, which suppresses HBV DNA by almost 7 $\log_{10}$ copies/mL in HBeAg-positive patients (5.2 $\log_{10}$ copies/mL in HBeAg-negative patients), is more potent than lamivudine and adefovir and, although cross-resistance occurs between entecavir and other L-nucleosides, has such a low median effective concentration in vitro that in vivo levels of drug are sufficient to be effective against lamivudine-resistant HBV. Like other L-nucleosides, entecavir is effective against adefovir-resistant HBV mutants as well. The approved oral daily dose of entecavir is 0.5 mg for treatment-naïve patients but 1.0 mg for lamivudine-resistant patients.

In HBeAg-positive patients, after 48 weeks of treatment, when compared with lamivudine, entecavir had significantly higher rates of histologic (72% vs 62%), virologic (67% vs 36% undetectable HBV DNA by highly sensitive amplification assay), and biochemical (68% vs 60% with normal ALT) responses. Among HBeAg-positive patients who underwent HBeAg seroconversion during the first year (21%) and who stopped treatment at 48 weeks, 70% remained HBeAg negative. In HBeAg-negative patients, similar rates of histologic, virologic, and biochemical improvement have been seen; however, the majority of patients relapse if treatment is stopped after 1 year.

Entecavir has a very high barrier to resistance; in nucleoside-naïve patients, entecavir resistance has not been encountered during the first year of therapy and has emerged in 1.2% of patients through year 5. In lamivudine-resistant patients, however, entecavir resistance was observed in 7% of patients at 1 year, 16% of patients at 2 years, and 51% of patients after 5 years. Therefore, although entecavir is favored above other L-nucleosides for treatment of previously untreated patients, entecavir is not recommended and should not be used as replacement therapy for lamivudine-resistant hepatitis B, FDA approval for this indication notwithstanding.

6. L-deoxythymidine (telbivudine)—Telbivudine is an L-nucleoside analog that was shown in clinical trials to be more potent than lamivudine in suppressing HBV replication. The approved dosage of telbivudine is 600 mg orally daily.

In HBeAg-positive patients, HBV DNA was undetectable in 60% of telbivudine recipients versus 40% of lamivudine recipients after 1 year and in 54% versus 8% after 2 years. Patients taking telbivudine also had significantly higher rates of normal ALT after 1 and 2 years of treatment compared with those taking lamivudine; however, as was true for entecavir, despite the substantially higher potency of telbivudine over lamivudine in suppressing HBV DNA, no difference was observed between telbivudine and lamivudine recipients in the rate of HBeAg seroconversion at the end of 1 and 2 years of treatment. In HBeAg-negative patients, telbivudine was superior to lamivudine in treatment measures by the same degree that entecavir exceeded lamivudine.

Unfortunately, telbivudine is associated with substantial resistance, and telbivudine-resistant mutations are cross-resistant with lamivudine. Like lamivudine, telbivudine selects for YMDD mutations, and genotypic resistance was observed in 5% and 25%% of HBeAg-positive patients after 1 and 2 years of therapy, respectively, and in 2.3% and 10.8% of HBeAg-negative patients after 1 and 2 years. Although one of the more (albeit not the most) potent HBV DNA inhibitors, telbivudine has a disappointing resistance profile and, therefore, does not have a role in monotherapy for HBV infection; it is not favored as first-line therapy.

7. Tenofovir disoproxil fumarate—Tenofovir is a nucleotide analogue, structurally similar to adefovir that was first approved for the treatment of HIV infection either alone or in combination with emtricitabine as a single pill. Tenofovir was approved for treatment of chronic hepatitis B in 2008. The approved oral dose of tenofovir for chronic hepatitis B treatment is 300 mg daily, although adjustments must be made for creatinine clearance <50 mL/min (as is true for other oral antiviral agents for hepatitis B).

In HBeAg-positive chronic hepatitis B, after 48 weeks of treatment, patients on tenofovir, when compared to patients treated with adefovir, had significantly higher rates of virologic (76% versus 13% undetectable HBV DNA), biochemical (74% versus 68% ALT normalization), and HBsAg loss (3% versus 0%), with similar rates of histologic response (74% versus 68%) and HBeAg seroconversion (21% versus 18%). In HBeAg-negative chronic hepatitis B, after 48 weeks of treatment, patients treated with tenofovir, when compared to those treated with adefovir, were more likely to experience suppression of HBV DNA to undetectable levels (93% versus 63%); however, biochemical and histologic reponses were similar in the two groups. Three percent of HBeAg-reactive patients treated with tenofovir for 1 year lost HBsAg; in HBeAg-negative patients, none lost HBsAg

Adefovir and tenofovir are cross-resistant. In the two principal phase-III clinical trials of tenofovir, 7 patients had virologic breakthrough during the first 2 year of treatment but had no detectable tenofovir-resistant mutations. In these large tenofovir trials, anyone who had persistent detection of serum HBV DNA at week 72 received additional treatment with emtricitabine; therefore data on resistance to tenofovir monotherapy beyond 72 weeks are limited; still, in the original cohorts followed after phase-III trials, resistance has not been encountered through year 3 of monitoring. Given its potency and limited resistance profile, the approval of tenofovir in 2008 provided a welcome, equally potent alternative to entecavir, particularly as first-line treatment of chronic hepatitis B in patients with lamivudine resistance. Currently, both entecavir and tenofovir are considered first-line oral treatments for chronic hepatitis B.

8. Other therapies—Other therapies currently being considered for approval for the treatment of HBV infection include emtricitabine (very similar to lamivudine in structure, potency/efficacy, and resistance profile) and combination therapies. A combination of emtricitabine and tenofovir, licensed for treatment of HIV infection, has the potential advantage of combination, non-cross-resistant L-nucleoside and nucleotide analog therapy. As patients begin to appear—in minuscule numbers to date—with mutations to both classes of these oral antiviral agents, interest in this combination and other combinations that can preempt the emergence of antiviral resistance will attract attention and be studied in clinical trials. To date, no advantage has been found for combinations of IFN-α or PEG IFN-α and oral agents.

C. Special Groups

1. HBV—HIV coinfection—Response rates to standard IFN-α are lower in patients with HBV-HIV coinfection. Lamivudine, emtricitabine (available currently only as a combination pill with tenofovir), and tenofovir are all nucleoside analogs with activity against both HIV and HBV; however, the rate of HBV resistance to lamivudine in HBV-HIV coinfected patients approaches 90% at 4 years. Given that antiretroviral regimens may include drugs with activity against HBV and that almost any oral regimen selected will include an agent with activity against HIV, clinicians should choose a combination antiviral regimen for HBV infection, regardless of whether or not HIV treatment is ongoing or planned. Entecavir was thought initially to have no anti-HIV activity and was considered a potential monotherapy for HBV-HIV coinfected patients not receiving HAART; however, eventually, entecavir was found to have modest activity against HIV, contraindicating its use (because of the potential for early emergence of HIV resistance) as monotherapy in patients with HIV-HBV coinfection who are not receiving HAART. To reiterate, then, in HBV-HIV coinfected patients combination antiviral therapy is the recommended choice for treating hepatitis B.

2. HBV-HDV coinfection—Refer to the later discussion of hepatitis D.

3. HBV-HCV coinfection—Limited information is available to guide treatment in this setting. Often, such patients have relatively nonreplicative chronic hepatitis B and need to be treated for hepatitis C. When both viruses need to be treated, PEG IFN-α (with ribavirin for hepatitis C) can be used to address both infections; alternatively, both diseases can be treated independently with PEG IFN-α plus ribavirin for hepatitis C and one of the oral agents for hepatitis B. Generally, antiviral therapy for hepatitis C in HCV-HBV coinfected patients yields sustained virologic responses similar to those achieved in patients being treated for HCV alone; however, suppression of HCV replication has been reported, rarely, to result in rebound replication of HBV.

4. Immunosuppressive, cytotoxic, or immunomodulatory chemotherapy—Approximately 20–50% of patients with chronic hepatitis B, including inactive carriers, have been reported to have reactivation of HBV replication associated with immunosuppressive, cytotoxic (especially if the regimen includes high-dose corticosteroids), or immunomodulatory (anticytokine) chemotherapy. This event occurs primarily as chemotherapy is withdrawn and cytolytic immune responsiveness recovers. Subclinical as well as clinically severe, even fatal, reactivations can occur, reflected initially by increases in serum HBV DNA and ALT. Prophylactic antiviral therapy should be administered to such patients with chronic hepatitis B at the onset of chemotherapy and should be maintained for at least 6 months afterward; in fact, the duration of treatment is not known, and, in some cases, discontinuing therapy proves difficult. Most of the reported experience in this setting involves lamivudine, but entecavir, similar to lamivudine in its rapid onset of action and freedom from nephrotoxicity, has also been reported to be effective as preemptive therapy to prevent chemotherapy-associated reactivation of hepatitis B and represents an appealing alternative.

D. Liver Transplantation

Liver transplantation is currently a successful therapy for end-stage chronic HBV-associated liver disease. Even with the 30% reduction in patients placed on the liver-transplantation waiting list in the decade following the introduction of oral antiviral therapy for hepatitis B, hepatitis B remains the seventh-most-common indication for liver transplantation in the United States, comprising about 4–5% of cases. Until the early 1990s, transplantation resulted in an 80% rate of reinfection in the absence of prophylaxis. The resulting hepatitis could be severe and was almost invariably chronic. The risk of reinfection was higher in patients with chronic liver disease versus fulminant disease and lower in those with HBV-HDV coinfection than in those with HBV infection alone. The introduction in 1993 of high-dose hepatitis B immunoglobulin (HBIG) perioperatively and postoperatively, combined with approval of lamivudine in 1998 for treatment of hepatitis B, has reduced graft infection rates to less than 5% in patients who receive both HBIG and a nucleoside analog posttransplantation. Given the need for long-term therapy and both the risk and consequences of lamivudine resistance in organ allograft recipients, newer drugs with higher barriers to resistance (eg, entecavir or tenofovir) and especially those with potent antiviral activity and limited nephrotoxicity (eg, entecavir) are favored first-line treatment to prevent recurrent HBV infection posttransplantation.

Disadvantages of prolonged HBIG use include cost, patient inconvenience, and intolerability. In some centers, switching from intravenous HBIG to intramuscular HBIG has been successful and associated with enhanced convenience and tolerability. No clear guideline exists for the duration of HBIG treatment post-transplantation; however, the risk of HBV reinfection was found to be negligible when HBIG was discontinued after 2 years and followed with continued use of a maintenance nucleoside or nucleotide analog treatment.

Patients who have undergone liver transplantation for HBV or HBV-HDV coinfection should have HBV DNA or HDV RNA, or both, followed every 3 months. Studies of combination nucleoside-nucleotide therapy after liver transplantation continue.

E. Postexposure Prophylaxis

For neonates born to infected mothers and any person with a percutaneous or sexual exposure, HBIG is available and is helpful to achieve immediate high-level circulating anti-HBs (passive immunization). Simultaneously, active immunization with hepatitis B vaccine should be administered as well.

Course & Prognosis

Ninety-five to 99% of healthy, immunocompetent young adult patients with clinically apparent acute HBV infection have a favorable course and recover completely. The case fatality rate is low (0.1%) but increases with age and associated comorbid systemic illnesses (eg, diabetes mellitus, congestive heart failure). The risk of chronicity is related to the age of acquisition (>90% in newborns, ~50% in young children, and 1–5% in immunocompetent adults). In addition, chronicity is more likely (>50%) in immunocompromised adults such as transplant-organ recipients, HIV-positive persons, and patients undergoing cytotoxic chemotherapy. Chronically infected patients may be inactive carriers or may have chronic hepatitis with or without cirrhosis.

Hepatitis B accounts for approximately half of all cases of fulminant viral hepatitis (see Chapter 38). The diagnosis is suggested by rising bilirubin, an increasing prothrombin time (INR), and signs of encephalopathy. Cerebral edema is common, and death usually results from a combination of brainstem compression, gastrointestinal bleeding, sepsis, respiratory failure, cardiovascular collapse, and renal failure. Survivors have complete biochemical and histologic recovery.

Patients with chronic hepatitis B, with or without HBeAg, who have highly replicative HBV infection are likely to experience the negative consequences of chronic infection, cirrhosis, hepatic decompensation, and HCC; indeed, patients with high-level HBV DNA are more likely to progress to cirrhosis and HCC than those with low-level HBV DNA, while relatively nonreplicative inactive carriers are less likely to progress to cirrhosis or to have HCC. In turn, patients with high-level HBV replication tend to progress histologically, and those with more advanced histologic stage have a worse prognosis. In one natural-history study, patients with cirrhosis had a 5-year survival of only 55% and a 15-year survival of only 40%.

Hepatitis B is a major risk factor for HCC. In HBV-endemic regions, HCC is the leading cause of cancer-related death. Cirrhosis is present in 70–80% of HBV-related HCC, and the chronic inflammation and regenerative cellular proliferation associated with cirrhosis may predispose to cellular transformation and malignancy. A proportion of patients with HBV-associated HCC, up to 20–30% in some series, do not have cirrhosis, contrasting with hepatitis C-associated HCC, almost all of which occurs in cirrhotic patients. In otherwise healthy, inactive hepatitis B carriers, the HCC incidence is 0.06–0.3% per year; in patients with chronic hepatitis, the annual incidence is 0.5–0.8%; and in those with cirrhosis, the rate of HCC is 1.5–6.6% per year. The cumulative risk of HCC almost doubles over 15 years in patients with high-level HBV DNA compared with those who have low-level HBV DNA. Furthermore, the risk of HCC is also significantly higher among men and older patients as well as in patients with a family history of HCC, a history of serologic reversion from anti-HBe to HBeAg, HBV genotype C, and coinfection with HCV. Population- and clinic-based screening programs that rely on serum α-fetoprotein (AFP) and liver imaging (primarily ultrasound) have led to identification of patients with small and potentially resectable tumors. Despite achieving earlier detection of HCC, however, such screening programs have not been shown to reduce mortality resulting from HCC (see Chapter 49). Furthermore, because of the nonspecificity of AFP elevations in chronic viral hepatitis, AFP screening is no longer recommended as part of HCC surveillance.

Dienstag JL. Hepatitis B virus infection. *N Engl J Med.* 2008;359: 1486–1500. [PMID: 18832247]

EASL clinical practice guidelines: management of chronic hepatitis B. *J Hepatol.* 2009;50:227–242. [PMID: 19054588]

Farrell G. Hepatitis B e antigen seroconversion: effects of lamivudine alone or in combination with interferon alpha. *J Med Virol.* 2000;61:374–379. [PMID: 10861649]

Lau DT, Khokhar MF, Doo E, et al. Long-term therapy of chronic hepatitis B with lamivudine. *Hepatology.* 2000;32:828–834. [PMID: 11003630]

Lau GK, Piratvisuth T, Luo KX, et al. Peginterferon alfa-2a, lamivudine and the combination for HBeAg-positive chronic hepatitis B. *N Engl J Med.* 2005;352:2682–2695. [PMID: 14987917]

Lok AS, McMahon BJ. Chronic hepatitis B. *Hepatology.* 2009;50: 661–662. [PMID: 19714720]

Marcellin P, Heathcote EJ, Buti M, et al. Tenofovir disoproxil fumarate versus adefovir dipivoxil for chronic hepatitis B. *N Engl J Med.* 2008;359:2442–2455. [PMID: 19052126]

Tan J, Lok AS. Antiviral therapy for pre- and post-liver transplantation patients with hepatitis B. *Liver Transpl.* 2007;13:323–326. [PMID: 17318864]

Wong SN, Chu CJ, Wai CT, et al. Low risk of hepatitis B virus recurrence after withdrawal of long-term hepatitis B immunoglobulin in patients receiving maintenance nucleos(t)ide analogue therapy. *Liver Transpl.* 2007;13:374–381. [PMID: 17318855]

HEPATITIS C

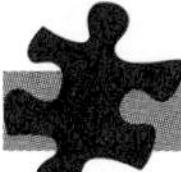

ESSENTIALS OF DIAGNOSIS

- Enzyme immunoassay (EIA) for antibody to hepatitis C virus (anti-HCV) indicates ongoing infection (rarely, past exposure).
- False-positive EIA tests occur most often in healthy blood donors and patients with rheumatoid factor; false-negative tests occur most often in immunocompromised patients (eg, hemodialysis patients, organ allograft recipients).
- Recombinant immunoblot assay (RIBA) has been supplanted by testing for HCV RNA to confirm positive tests for anti-HCV.
- HCV RNA is usually detectable in serum 7–21 days after exposure with one of the three available amplification assays (PCR, transcription-mediated amplification [TMA], and branched-chain DNA [bDNA]).
- The clinically relevant threshold between high-level and low-level HCV RNA is 800,000 IU/mL.
- Liver biopsy permits accurate assessment of the degree of inflammation and fibrosis but is not mandatory before initiating therapy.

General Considerations

Based on serologic screening (NHANES, National Health and Nutrition Examination Survey) between 1999 and 2002 of a representative cohort of the population, the U.S. Public Health Service calculated that 4.1 million people in the United States (1.6% of the population) have antibodies to hepatitis C virus (anti-HCV) and that approximately 3.2 million (1.3%) have chronic hepatitis C virus (HCV) infection. The peak prevalence observed was among persons aged 40–49 years. When a similar survey was done earlier during the 1990s, the peak prevalence of HCV infection occurred among those aged 30–39 years. In fact, this shift reflects the aging of the HCV-infected cohort who had been infected in the remote past, in the 1960s and 1970s, during an epidemic of experimentation with injection drugs. Worldwide, approximately 3% of the population (170 million people) are estimated to have chronic hepatitis C.

In the United States, HCV is the most common bloodborne infection, the leading cause of chronic liver disease, and the most common indication for liver transplantation. The Centers for Disease Control and Prevention estimates that the number of new cases of acute HCV infection has declined substantially (from 5.2 cases per 100,000 population in 1995 to 0.5 cases per 100,000 population in 2007) among persons aged 25–39, the age group that historically has highest rates of acute infection. The decline in new cases of acute hepatitis C parallels directly the decline in cases among injection drug users, which is thought to reflect the adoption of precautions in this subpopulation to minimize the risk of acquiring HIV infection. Almost all newly recognized cases of hepatitis C occur among individuals who acquired their infections several decades ago but who are just now coming to clinical recognition as they seek health care for other reasons.

Groups at risk for HCV infection include transfusion recipients (particularly those transfused before 1992, when sensitive serologic screening of donor blood began, virtually eliminating hepatitis C from the blood supply), injection drug users, hemodialysis patients, Vietnam-era veterans, and health care workers. Persons with hemophilia who received factor VIII infusions before HCV screening was initiated have a 74–90% prevalence of HCV infection. In intravenous drug users, prevalence is 72–90%. Acquisition by health care workers of hepatitis C as a result of a contaminated needlestick is inefficient, occurring in approximately 3% of those exposed and accounting for a very small proportion of HCV infections (~1%).

Sporadic HCV infection, in which the mode of transmission is unknown, is responsible for approximately 10% of cases, but in many of these, long forgotten injection drug use is the source.

Perinatal transmission is rare and inefficient, estimated to occur in only approximately 5% of infants born to HCV-infected mothers, independent of the route of delivery.

Sexual transmission of HCV can occur, but the risk is extremely low (<5% overall and closer to 1% in stable, monogamous sexual partners), and HCV is much less efficiently sexually transmitted than HBV. In the rare instance when both sexual partners are infected with HCV (0.4–3% of the sexual partners of patients with HCV infection are also infected), almost invariably, other risk factors are identified. Because of the low risk of sexual transmission of hepatitis C, the U.S. Public Health Service currently does not recommend a change in sexual practices in stable sexual partners. In the sexually promiscuous, those with sexually transmitted diseases, and sex workers, however, the risk of sexual transmission can reach 10%. In the most recent NHANES data, the risk of HCV infection was most strongly associated, independently, with injection drug use. Anti-HCV was also associated independently with Mexican-American ethnicity, birth in the United States, low family income, noninjection illicit drug use, and a lifetime total of 20 or more sexual partners.

Pathogenesis

Hepatitis C virus is a single-stranded, 9600 base-pair RNA virus (genus *Hepacivirus*). Its genome encodes core and envelope structural proteins at the 5′ end and five nonstructural proteins (including a helicase, protease, and RNA polymerase) at the 3′ end that are important in viral replication. Six major HCV genotypes have been described, designated 1–6, which are divided further into subtypes (1a, 1b, 2a, etc) of which over 50 have been described. Considerable variation exists in the geographic distribution of HCV genotypes; in the United States, approximately 70% of patients are infected with genotype 1 and the other 30% with genotypes 2 and 3. Although not predictive of the outcome of HCV infection, the genotype does predict the likelihood of treatment response and also determines the duration of treatment and the dose of ribavirin, one of the two drugs used to treat hepatitis C (see later discussion). Genotypes 1 and 4 are more refractory to interferon-based therapy compared with genotypes 2 and 3. In addition to its genotypic diversity, the heterogeneity of HCV is exaggerated by the multiple quasispecies circulating in serum, reflecting the hypervariability of regions of the HCV envelope proteins that arise as a product of evolutionary changes in the virus as it evades host immunologic containment. This viral diversity accounts for the high likelihood for HCV persistence after acute infection and the limited ability of the host to mount durable neutralizing antibodies against HCV. As a result, recovery from acute infection is unusual (<15%), and attempts to develop a protective vaccine have been frustratingly disappointing.

Levels of HCV in serum are lower (up to 10^5–10^6, rarely 10^7, virions/mL) than levels of HBV (often exceeding 10^6 and ranging to $>10^9$), and HCV antigens are not detectable in blood. The clinical features of acute and chronic hepatitis C are similar to those of hepatitis B, except that acute hepatitis C tends to be milder and progression to chronicity the rule, rather than the exception. Several histologic features are characteristic of chronic hepatitis C, including the presence of microvesicular or macrovesicular steatosis, bile duct injury, and lymphocytic follicles. As is true for the other viral hepatitides, liver injury associated with HCV infection is immunologically mediated; differences in the diversity and robustness of cytolytic T-cell responses appear to be important in distinguishing between the rare patients who recover from acute hepatitis C and the vast majority of patients who progress to chronic infection. Recently, variations in the IL28B gene were shown to affect not only responsiveness to interferon-based antiviral therapy (see below) but also likelihood of recovery from acute HCV infection; >50% of patients with the C/C haplotype at this allele experience self-limited acute HCV infection, while ~80% of patients with the T/T haplotype progress to chronic infection. A direct cytopathic effect of HCV may also contribute to the damage in some situations (eg, in immunosuppressive states, such as after liver transplantation).

Clinical Findings

A. Acute HCV Infection

Acute hepatitis C is asymptomatic in approximately 84% of cases and is usually not recognized clinically. Jaundice, fatigue, fever, nausea, vomiting, and right upper quadrant discomfort can occur, usually within 2–12 weeks of exposure and lasting from 2 to 12 weeks. The diagnosis is established by demonstration of anti-HCV, HCV RNA, or both.

B. Chronic HCV Infection

Chronic hepatitis C is also asymptomatic in most patients. ALT values fluctuate in a substantial proportion of patients. Extrahepatic manifestations, which develop in approximately 15% of patients with chronic infection, include such immune-complex disorders as essential mixed cryoglobulinemia, membranoproliferative glomerulonephritis, and leukocytoclastic vasculitis. Other extrahepatic disorders associated with chronic hepatitis C include thyroiditis, lichen planus, and porphyria cutanea tarda.

C. Serologic Assays

The first step in the diagnosis of HCV infection is the EIA for anti-HCV, which indicates past exposure (rarely) or ongoing infection (usually). The current, third-generation EIA is approximately 99% sensitive and specific. In hepatitis C, distinctions between IgM and IgG anti-HCV are not helpful; therefore, assays for IgM anti-HCV are not available. False-positive EIA tests are seen most often in populations with a low prior probability of true infection, such as healthy blood donors, and in patients with rheumatoid factor, which can result in nonspecific binding in the assay. False-negative tests are seen most often in immunocompromised patients, including hemodialysis patients and organ allograft recipients. In the past, a recombinant immunoblot assay (RIBA) was used to confirm positive tests for anti-HCV; however, RIBA has been supplanted by testing for HCV RNA.

The next step in the diagnosis of HCV infection is detection of HCV RNA in serum. HCV RNA is generally detectable 7–21 days following exposure. Currently, three types of amplification assay are available for detecting HCV RNA: PCR, transcription-mediated amplification (TMA), and branched-chain DNA (bDNA). The most sensitive PCR and TMA assays have a sensitivity of 10–50 IU/mL and a broad dynamic range; for all practical purposes, bDNA, less sensitive (10^3 copies/mL), is being supplanted by the more sensitive assays.

Quantitation of HCV RNA is based on World Health Organization–standardized international units (IU) per milliliter; the clinically relevant threshold between high-level and low-level HCV RNA is 800,000 IU/mL. The HCV genotype is not necessary for the diagnosis of HCV infection but provides valuable clinical information required for management decisions about duration of therapy and drug doses.

D. Liver Biopsy

Because the severity of liver damage cannot be determined noninvasively with adequate reliability, a liver biopsy is necessary to assess the degree of inflammation (histologic grade) and fibrosis (histologic stage) accurately. According to the current guidelines of the American Association for the Study of Liver Diseases (AASLD), a liver biopsy should be done when the results will influence whether treatment is recommended or will provide information on prognosis, but a biopsy is not mandatory in order to initiate therapy for hepatitis C.

Although some authorities have issued recommendations against performing liver biopsies prior to therapy for chronic hepatitis C, many clinicians, in weighing the risks, benefits, and costs of biopsy versus those of treatment for hepatitis C, choose to obtain a liver biopsy in patients with HCV genotype-1 infection to inform treatment decisions. For patients with genotypes 2 and 3, with a higher likelihood of response, some authorities advocate treating all patients without liver biopsy. For patients with little or no fibrosis (ie, Metavir score <2 or Ishak score <3), in whom the prognosis for progression is relatively good and for whom, therefore, treatment may be deferred, liver biopsy can be used to monitor progression of disease; however, frequency of such histologic monitoring has not been established.

Prevention

Because the injection drug-using population represents the largest reservoir of HCV infection, prevention of high-risk, drug-related behaviors is the best way to prevent the majority of new HCV infections in the United States. Even before screening of blood donors for hepatitis C began, transfusions never accounted for more than a small proportion of all cases of HCV infection in the United States. Since the advent of routine screening of the blood donor pool began in the 1990s, the annual incidence of transfusion-related infection has become negligible, and further reduction in the frequency of posttransfusion HCV infection is unlikely to have an impact on the overall prevalence of the disease.

Although success has been reported in case studies of postexposure interferon therapy, the efficacy of such an approach has not been studied systematically, and the initiation of antiviral therapy is not recommended until the diagnosis of HCV infection is established (in the setting of acute hepatitis C, antiviral therapy is nearly universally effective). Standard immunoglobulin administered after needlestick, sexual, or perinatal exposure to HCV is ineffective and is not recommended. Currently, an effective preventive vaccine is not available, and prospects for a vaccine are dim (see the discussion of pathogenesis, earlier).

Treatment

A. Interferon-α or Pegylated Interferon-α and Ribavirin

The goal of treatment in patients with hepatitis C is to prevent disease progression and the complications of infection, which is achieved by eradication of HCV infection. HCV infection is considered eradicated when a patient achieves a sustained virologic response (SVR), defined as absence of HCV RNA in serum, as demonstrated by the most sensitive amplification assay, at the end of treatment as well as 6 months later. An SVR is associated with improved histologic findings in up to 94% of patients, including both fibrosis and histologic activity index, as well as a reduced risk of progression to cirrhosis, hepatic failure, and liver-related death.

Patients who achieve an SVR almost always have a dramatic earlier reduction in the HCV RNA level, defined as a $\geq 2\text{-}\log_{10}$ drop or loss of HCV RNA at 12 weeks into therapy, referred to as an early virologic response (EVR). In one study of 453 patients who underwent 12 weeks of therapy, 86% had an EVR. Of those 86%, 65% went on to achieve an SVR. Of the 14% who did not have an EVR, only 3% achieved an SVR; in another, similar, large trial, none of the subjects who failed to achieve an EVR experienced an SVR. Furthermore, in patients with the more difficult-to-treat genotype 1, achieving a rapid virologic response (RVR), defined as a reduction in serum HCV RNA to undetectable at week 4, is associated with an SVR of ≥95%, even if treatment is confined to 24 weeks.

Currently, IFN-α and PEG IFN-α are the backbone of treatment for chronic hepatitis C. As discussed earlier, in the section on hepatitis B, IFN-α has direct antiviral activity as well as immune-modulating activity (which may or may not be involved in its activity against viral hepatitis). Pegylated interferons are produced by binding an inert polyethylene glycol moiety to interferon molecules, thereby increasing the molecular weight of the molecule, decreasing its renal clearance, and increasing its serum half-life.

In the 1990s, the sole treatment for hepatitis C was monotherapy with interferon (3 million units 3 times weekly initially for 24 weeks, then for 48 weeks), which produced low SVR rates of 10% and 20%, respectively. Later in the 1990s, ribavirin was added to interferon as combination therapy for HCV infection. Ribavirin, a synthetic guanosine analog, can inhibit several RNA and DNA viruses, including flaviruses, to which HCV is similar. Ribavirin alone has no more than a subtle antiviral effect on HCV replication; however, the combination of ribavirin with the standard interferon regimen doubled SVRs to 38–43%. Although the mechanism for ribavirin activity is not understood, ribavirin reduces the relapse rate at the conclusion of therapy, thereby increasing the SVR.

Standard interferon, administered by injection three times a week in patients with hepatitis C, has been eclipsed by PEG IFN-α. Two types of pegylated interferon, which differ in their pharmacokinetics and chemical properties, were approved by the FDA in 2001, PEG IFN-α2a and PEG IFN-α2b. In large, randomized, controlled trials, the combination of weekly injections of PEG IFN-α and twice-daily oral ribavirin yielded higher SVR rates than either three injections per week of standard IFN-α together with oral ribavirin or PEG IFN-α monotherapy. In these trials, 12-kD PEG IFN-α2b was dosed by weight (1.5 mcg/kg) and coupled with 800 mg of ribavirin; the larger, 40-kD PEG IFN-α2a was given as a fixed dose of 180 mcg with a weight-adjusted, higher dose of ribavirin (1000 mg if <75 kg and 1200 mg if ≥75 kg) for 48 weeks. In the initial two registration trials, genotype was the strongest predictor of response. In patients with genotype-1 infections, SVRs occurred in 42–46%, whereas the SVR rate in those with genotypes 2 and 3 was 76–82%. In a subsequent registration trial of PEG IFN-α2a, trial subjects were randomized to receive either 24 or 48 weeks of PEG IFN-α plus ribavirin therapy and to receive either a fixed 800-mg dose or standard 1000–1200-mg doses (based on weight <75 kg or ≥75 kg) of ribavirin. In patients with genotype 1, the SVR was highest (51%) in patients who underwent 48 weeks of treatment with PEG IFN-α and 1000–1200 mg of ribavirin; patients treated for 24 weeks or with only 800 mg of ribavirin had lower SVR rates. In contrast, among patients with HCV genotypes 2 or 3, PEG IFN-α plus a ribavirin dose of only 800 mg for 24 weeks was adequate to achieve an SVR rate of ~80%; extending therapy to 48 weeks or increasing the ribavirin dose did not increase the frequency of SVR in these genotypes. In a clinical trial, reported in 2009, weight-based daily doses of ribavirin ranging up to 1400 mg were used with PEG IFN-α2b.

Several variables are associated with an increased likelihood of achieving an SVR, among them HCV genotype other than 1, low pretreatment HCV RNA levels ($<8 \times 10^5$ IU/mL), age <40 years, body weight <75 kg, absence of bridging fibrosis or cirrhosis at baseline, non–African American ethnicity, the absence of hepatic steatosis and insulin resistance, and favorable IL28B genotype C/C (~80% SVR compared to <30% with genotype T/T or to just under 40% for T/C heterozygotes).

The presence of these poor predictors of responsiveness, however, does not preclude responsiveness absolutely and should not be a reason to deny a patient therapy.

Currently, based on the registration trials described above, a full 48 weeks of PEG IFN-α and 1000–1200 mg of ribavirin are recommended for patients with HCV genotype 1 (and 4) but only 24 weeks of PEG IFN-α and 800 mg of ribavirin for patients with HCV genotypes 2 and 3. Recognized more recently, tailoring therapy based on the rapidity of a patient's response can increase the SVR or shorten therapy, or both. The likelihood of an SVR is increased if the level of HCV RNA falls to undetectable within 4 weeks (a rapid virologic response, RVR). In patients with genotype 2 or 3 who achieve an RVR, a 12–16-week course of therapy may be as effective as one lasting 24 weeks, but only if the baseline HCV RNA level is low. Conversely, in patients with genotype 2 or 3 who have cirrhosis, some experts choose to treat a full 48 weeks; however, in most cirrhotic patients with genotype 2, and fewer with genotype 3, the recommended 24 weeks of therapy will suffice to achieve an SVR. In patients with genotype 1, among those with an RVR, especially in the subset with a low level of HCV RNA at baseline, 24 weeks of PEG IFN-α plus ribavirin therapy may suffice to yield SVRs as high as 90%. In the same vein, failure to achieve an RVR signals refractoriness to therapy; for such patients with genotype 1, extending therapy beyond 48 weeks to 72 weeks increases the likelihood of an SVR. Clinical trials have also shown that, in patients with risk factors for reduced responsiveness (eg, high level of HCV RNA, obesity), increasing PEG IFN-α (eg, to 270 mcg weekly) and ribavirin doses (eg, to 1600 mg daily) improves SVR rates.

In patients who failed to respond during therapy with, or who relapsed after, standard IFN-α and ribavirin therapy, retreatment with PEG IFN-α and ribavirin can result in an SVR in 25–40%. For relapsers or nonresponders to PEG IFN-α and ribavirin therapy, however, retreatment is unlikely to yield a successful SVR. Occasionally, retreatment with longer durations of therapy, higher doses of ribavirin, or aggressive attempts at maintaining adequate treatment doses with bone marrow support (erythropoietin) may yield an SVR in this setting, but none of these approaches has been validated or recommended.

Although eradication of HCV RNA is the primary goal for treatment of persons with chronic hepatitis C, early studies suggested that long-term, low-dose interferon treatment may reduce the progression of fibrosis or risk of hepatic decompensation, despite an absence of virologic response to treatment. Several trials were designed to evaluate the potential use of maintenance therapy in virologic nonresponders, but none demonstrated efficacy. For example, in 2008, the results of the HALT-C Trial were published; this was a large randomized controlled trial of 1050 patients with advanced fibrosis who had not responded to previous therapy with PEG IFN-α and ribavirin. These patients received either low-dose interferon or no therapy for 3.5 years, but no difference emerged between the treated and untreated-control groups in rates of death, hepatocellular carcinoma, hepatic decompensation, or ≥2-point increase in Ishak fibrosis score. Therefore, low-dose maintenance interferon is not recommended treatment in patients who do not respond to standard PEG IFN-α and ribavirin.

B. Side Effects and Monitoring

Side effects of interferon and PEG IFN-α were described earlier in relation to treatment of hepatitis B. Additional side effects are associated with combination therapy, specifically, hemolytic anemia caused by ribavirin, which reduces hemoglobin to less than 10 g/dL in 25% of patients. Red blood cell counts recover typically within 4 weeks after treatment is stopped. Because hemolytic anemia associated with ribavirin may be severe and precipitous, ribavirin is contraindicated in patients who cannot tolerate anemia, including those with unstable coronary artery, cerebrovascular, pulmonary, or renal disease as well as baseline anemia. Ribavirin can cause pruritus and rash (occasionally severe), and chest congestion or cough. In addition, ribavirin is a documented teratogen; all patients must be counseled on the danger of birth defects, and both male and female patients and their sexual partners of childbearing age should be required to use effective birth control during and for 6 months after the end of treatment.

Once a patient is started on therapy, close follow-up is essential. Monitoring of complete blood counts is necessary every 2–4 weeks during the first 2 months and then typically every 4–8 weeks during treatment. Periodic thyroid tests (thyroid-stimulating hormone levels) at the same frequency are also recommended. Virologic response should be assessed at week 4 (RVR), week 12 (EVR), end of therapy (end-treatment response), and 24 weeks after completion of therapy (SVR); many clinicians check HCV RNA levels more frequently, including at weeks 24 and 36 of therapy and at weeks 4 and 12 after completion of therapy. If an EVR is not present at 12 weeks, therapy can be stopped, especially in patients who tolerate therapy poorly. If a patient achieves an RVR, consideration may be given to shortening the duration of therapy, and if a patient has not achieved an RVR (or if HCV RNA, although reduced by ≥2 $\log_{10}$ is still detectable at week 12 [absence of a "complete" EVR]), some clinicians choose to prolong therapy beyond the recommended treatment period.

C. Special Treatment Considerations

1. Acute hepatitis C—In a small study of 60 patients with acute hepatitis C, 85% of whom presented with symptomatic disease, treatment with interferon alone or in combination with ribavirin was begun immediately upon diagnosis in 6 patients. Of the 54 who were not treated, 37 (68%) cleared HCV spontaneously within a mean of 8 weeks after diagnosis; 13 relapsed later, leaving 24 (44%) persistently HCV RNA-negative. Although the numbers are small and should be interpreted with caution, none of the nine patients with asymptomatic acute hepatitis C cleared

HCV RNA spontaneously, whereas 52% of those with symptomatic disease lost virus spontaneously, all within 12 weeks. Treatment given to those who did not recover spontaneously, beginning 3–6 months after onset of disease, led to SVR in 81%. Based on these results, the authors recommended delaying treatment 2–4 months after acute onset of acute hepatitis C to allow for spontaneous resolution. Others have presented evidence to show that earlier treatment (within 8 weeks) is superior in efficacy to treatment delayed thereafter. What is reassuring is that most studies of antiviral therapy in acute hepatitis C demonstrate a very high frequency of viral clearance when therapy is administered within the first 3 months after diagnosis; although earlier trials involved high-dose interferon, subsequent trials suggest that a 6-month course of PEG IFN-α plus ribavirin yields the same high SVR rate. Additional studies confirming these results continue to be reported.

2. Renal disease—Historically, persons with renal disease have been at increased risk of acquiring HCV infection, predominantly through blood transfusions and exposure to HCV-contaminated equipment during hemodialysis. Ribavirin is contraindicated in this population, because the drug is not removed during conventional dialysis, and its accumulation causes a dose-dependent hemolytic anemia. Treatment of patients with mild-to-moderate impairment in renal function must be individualized; however, ribavirin is not recommended in persons with creatinine clearance <50 mL/min. Consequently, therapy for patients with substantial renal impairment or on hemodialysis should be PEG IFN-α monotherapy at a reduced dose with close monitoring for interferon toxicity. As might be expected, efficacy is reduced under these circumstances.

3. Decompensated cirrhosis—Currently, interferon-based antiviral therapy is not recommended for patients with decompensated cirrhosis (ie, patients with one or more clinical complications of chronic liver disease, such as ascites, encephalopathy, variceal bleeding, or coagulopathy). Instead, liver transplantation is the treatment of choice for such patients.

In patients with decompensated cirrhosis, antiviral therapy can be complicated by an increased risk of life-threatening infections as well as accelerating hepatic decompensation. Reinfection of the donor liver allograft with HCV is almost assured, and progressive post-transplantation disease of the allograft is common. Eradication of the virus prior to transplantation is associated with a low likelihood of post-transplantation infection, providing a strong incentive to treat HCV infection before transplantation; however, treating someone with decompensated liver disease is not recommended routinely, can be associated with substantial treatment intolerability and morbidity, and should be done only in specialized centers that have experience in treating decompensated patients beginning with low drug doses that are escalated progressively, as tolerated. In addition, even in patients with such treatment-associated short-term absence of HCV RNA pretransplantation, the virus is likely to become apparent again posttransplantation after longer follow-up monitoring. If such pretransplantation antiviral therapy is initiated, low doses should be used initially and only in patients with mild degrees of hepatic compromise, with vigilant monitoring for adverse events, preferably in those who have already been accepted as candidates for liver transplantation.

Antiviral therapy for hepatitis C is indicated definitively in patients with compensated HCV-related cirrhosis who also have sufficient platelet and white blood cell counts to tolerate therapy.

4. Post-solid organ transplantation—Immunosuppression administered to prevent allograft rejection plays a role in the accelerated liver disease observed in HCV-infected patients following transplantation. Interferon has been reported to precipitate rejection of kidney grafts; thus, the absence of clear treatment benefit and the concern about precipitating rejection weigh against treating HCV infection in heart, lung, or kidney allograft recipients. The risk of precipitating rejection with interferon in liver allograft recipients appears to be low. Because, typically, HCV-related liver disease is this group is more progressive than that observed in immunologically competent persons, in most liver transplantation centers, antiviral therapy—its limitations and tolerability issues notwithstanding—is instituted once recurrent disease is established.

D. Future Treatments

Direct acting antivirals (DAAs) are currently being developed against hepatitis C viral enzymes, including the viral NS3/4A protease and NS4 polymerase, as well as other proteins critical for viral replication and assembly. Several of the DAAs, administered together with PEG IFN-α and ribavirin have been shown in phase-III clinical trials to lower HCV RNA levels rapidly and profoundly, yielding higher rates of SVR with shorter-duration therapy. The two new protease inhibitors are effective primarily in patients with genotype-1 chronic hepatitis C.

Telaprevir, an NS3/4A protease inhibitor for which phase-III clinical trials are complete, is undergoing FDA evaluation. In previously treatment-naïve subjects, when telaprevir was used in combination with PEG IFN-α and ribavirin for 12 weeks and followed by another 12–36 weeks of PEG IFN-α and ribavirin ("response-guided," ie, another 12 weeks for the ~60% whose HCV RNA was undetectable at weeks 4 and 12 [total duration of treatment 24 weeks] versus another 36 weeks for the ~40% without such an extended rapid virologic response [total treatment duration 48 weeks]), the frequency of SVR was as high as 75%, compared to only 44% with PEG IFN-α and ribavirin alone. In phase-II trials, treatment arms lacking ribavirin were found to be substantially less effective, and telaprevir combination therapy for only 12 weeks was effective but less so than 24-week regimens (12 of triple combination followed by 12 of standard-of-care PEG IFN-α and ribavirin). Data from another phase-III trial in treatment-naïve subjects showed that, for subjects managed based on "response-guided" therapy and in whom an extended RVR (HVC RNA undetectable at weeks 4 and 12) was accomplished, the SVR was ~90%; no benefit was achieved by extending standard of care PEG IFN-α and ribavirin (after 12 weeks of triple combination therapy) from 12 to 36 weeks. In treatment-experienced patients (nonresponders [who failed to clear HCV RNA during previous treatment] and relapsers [who cleared HCV RNA during treatment but who experienced a return of HCV RNA after treatment]), telaprevir combined with PEG IFN-α and ribavirin (12 weeks of triple combination therapy, followed by 36 weeks of PEG IFN-α and ribavirin) achieved SVR in 65% of subjects, compared to in only 17% treated with the former standard of care. Among these nonresponders, the frequency of SVR was 31% for prior null responders (who failed to experience a 12-week, 2-$\log_{10}$ reduction with prior standard therapy, ie, the most refractory subgroup), 67% in prior partial responders (≥2-$\log_{10}$ HCV RNA reduction at 12 weeks but virus still detectable at 24 weeks), and 86% in prior relapsers. In this trial, a 4-week lead-in phase with PEG IFN-α and ribavirin was no more effective than a treatment arm lacking a lead-in phase. The most common adverse effect of telaprevir treatment is skin rash, which occurs in a third of subjects but is sufficiently severe to result in discontinuation of triple-drug therapy in only 0.5–1.5% of patients. Anemia occurs in ~40% during telaprevir triple-drug combination therapy, which lasts only 12 weeks.

Boceprevir, another protease inhibitor that is undergoing phase-III clinical trials, is also being evaluated by the FDA. For this drug, a 4-week lead-in phase with PEG IFN-α2b and ribavirin precedes the administration of the DAA, and the triple DAA-PEG IFN-α/ribavirin regimen continues for either an additional 24 (total duration 28) or 44 (total duration 48) weeks, based on "response-guided" criteria (28 weeks if HCV RNA is undetectable at week 8 and at all time points thereafter versus 48 weeks if this criterion is not met). Triple-drug combination therapy resulted in an SVR of 65%, compared to an SVR of 38% for PEG IFN-α and ribavirin. Fewer than half of subjects qualified, based on response-guided criteria, to discontinue therapy at week 28. In experienced patients who failed to achieve an SVR during prior therapy—two-thirds relapsers, one-third partial responders, no null responders—4 weeks of PEG IFN-α and ribavirin lead-in therapy was followed by 32 weeks of triple-combination therapy (total duration of 36 weeks) or 44 weeks of triple-combination therapy (total duration 48 weeks). An SVR occurred in 59% of patients in the 36-week arm (46% of boceprevir-treated patients) and in 66% of the 48-week arm (compared to 21% of those treated with PEG IFN-α and ribavirin). The peak response to boceprevir-based triple-drug therapy in partial responders was 52% and in relapsers 75%. The most prominent adverse effect of broceprevir therapy is anemia, which occurs in half of treated patients, persists for the duration of therapy, and, in clinical trials, was treated in most cases with erythropoietin.

With FDA approval expected in 2011, the addition of a protease inhibitor to a backbone of PEG IFN-α/ribavirin will emerge as the new standard of care for patients with genotype-1 HCV infection, whether treatment-naïve or treatment-experienced (prior nonresponders and relapsers). Nucleoside polymerase inhibitors with a high barrier to resistance and with pangenotypic activity are also showing promise, and nonnucleoside polymerase inhibitors are also being studied. To date, double-combination DAA therapy without PEG IFN-α and ribavirin have been hampered by viral breakthrough. Ultimately, however, trials of potent DAA combinations with complementary mechanisms of action and a high barrier to resistance are anticipated, and the expectation is that all-oral regimens will obviate the need for IFN ± ribavirin-based therapy.

E. Ongoing Issues in Treatment

Patients inquire frequently about and use herbal medicines; however, none of the so-called complementary and alternative medications improves HCV RNA or ALT levels, and they do not improve the outcome of, or add to, standard antiviral therapy.

Despite the very important and substantial improvements in drug treatments, most patients are not benefited by these therapies. First, for many patients, treatment is contraindicated—specifically those with major, inadequately controlled depression or risk for suicide; uncontrolled, severe autoimmune disorders; marked cytopenias; active cardiopulmonary, cerebrovascular, or renal disease; or inadequately treated and active substance abuse. Second, many patients decline treatment because of their concern over side effects or they do not tolerate treatment. Third, until recent progress with DAAs, about half of all treated patients do not have a sustained response despite successful completion of therapy.

Among patients being treated for hepatitis C, those of European or Asian ancestry are more likely to respond to antiviral therapy than those of African ancestry. In 2009, a genetic polymorphism near the IL28B gene, which codes for interferon lambda, was found to be closely linked to IFN responsiveness in hepatitis C. As noted above (genetic variability at this locus is associated with both spontaneous clearance of HCV after acute infection and SVR after IFN-based antiviral therapy), patients with the C/C allele have a very high SVR, compared to those who have a T containing allele (T/T or T/C). Providing a partial explanation for differences among ethnic groups in treatment responsiveness, Europeans and Asians have far greater frequencies of the C/C allele, as compared to those of African origin, in whom T/T is predominant. This IL28B polymorphism is associated with on-treatment virologic responses as well as relapse rates and appears to be the most powerful pretreatment predictor of SVR. Although not yet introduced into routine clinical use, IL28B genotyping may become a critical tool to determine which patients are more likely to benefit from current standard-of-care, PEG IFN-based treatment regimens. Whether the association between IL28B genotypes and SVR will be maintained once new, DAA-containing regimens become the new standard of care remains to be determined.

F. Other Aspects of Disease Management

Although most patients with hepatitis C are asymptomatic, disease management goes well beyond the treatment possibilities described above. Education and counseling command attention and resources in caring for patients with hepatitis C. Because of the reported (but not universally experienced) risk of increased morbidity and mortality associated with acute hepatitis A superinfection, susceptible patients (IgG anti-HAV-negative) should be vaccinated against hepatitis A. Similarly, because of the risk of hepatitis B when superimposed on chronic hepatitis C, patients who are susceptible to HBV infection (eg, HBsAg, anti-HBs, anti-HBc-negative) should be vaccinated against hepatitis B. Excessive and frequent alcohol consumption promotes progression of chronic hepatitis C; therefore, avoidance of alcohol is recommended. Many patients inquire about diet, but no dietary restrictions or supplements have been shown to be beneficial. Finally, screening for HCC is recommended for patients with cirrhosis or advanced fibrosis. Periodic radiologic imaging (ultrasound, CT scan, or MRI) every 6–12 months is recommended. Although most clinicians still monitor α-fetoprotein (AFP) levels as part of HCC surveillance programs, AFP screening in patients with chronic hepatitis C has been shown to be highly nonspecific and is no longer recommended officially.

Course & Prognosis

In approximately 85% of persons with acute hepatitis C, chronic infection develops; the other 15% clear the virus spontaneously within the first 6 months of infection, although the rate of viral clearance appears to be less common in African Americans and those coinfected with HIV. As noted above, IL28B genetic polymorphisms are associated with likelihood of viral clearance after acute HCV infection.

In approximately 20% of patients with chronic hepatitis C, cirrhosis develops over 20–25 years of infection. By the time a patient comes to clinical attention and undergoes liver biopsy, he or she has often had chronic hepatitis C for more than two to three decades, and the biopsy provides a window on the level of liver injury during these previous decades. In addition, the levels of necroinflammatory activity and of fibrosis on such a biopsy provide prognostic information for future progression; the more severe the level of necroinflammatory activity and fibrosis found on initial biopsy, the greater the risk of progressing to cirrhosis over the ensuing 20 years. Progression to cirrhosis is more common in persons infected at older ages (particularly men), those who drink more than 50 g of alcohol daily, those who are obese or have substantial hepatic steatosis, and those with HIV coinfection. Once cirrhosis develops, the 10-year prognosis remains very good (80% survival) until signs of hepatic decompensation begin to appear (declining hepatic synthetic function, gastrointestinal bleeding associated with portal hypertension, ascites and edema, coagulopathy, hepatic encephalopathy, life-threatening bacterial infections, and hepatorenal failure); once hepatic decompensation has begun, the 10-year prognosis falls to 50% or less.

Finally, cirrhosis associated with chronic hepatitis C increases the risk of HCC dramatically. Among patients with cirrhosis and HCV infection, HCC develops at a rate estimated at between 1% and 4% annually, affecting 2–7% of cirrhotic patients over 10 years. The occurrence of HCC is confined primarily to patients who have had chronic hepatitis C for two to three decades and who have cirrhosis or, at the very least, advanced fibrosis. HCC rarely occurs in patients with chronic hepatitis C in the absence of cirrhosis or advanced fibrosis. Successful antiviral therapy in patients with chronic hepatitis C reduces, but does not eliminate, the risk of HCC; therefore, in patients with advanced fibrosis, HCC screening should be continued even after achievement of an SVR.

A. Children

Children who are infected with HCV are more likely to clear the virus spontaneously, to have milder hepatitis, and to progress less frequently to cirrhosis. In one study of German children who acquired hepatitis C genotype 1 as a result of cardiac surgery during infancy, 45% cleared the virus spontaneously, and, at a mean of 21 years after infection, only 3 of 17 had histologic evidence of advanced liver disease.

B. HCV-HIV

Coinfection with HCV and HIV is common. Approximately 25% of HIV-infected persons in the Western world have concomitant HCV infection. About 6% of HIV-infected persons fail to acquire detectable anti-HCV; therefore, HCV RNA should be tested in HIV-positive patients with risk factors for HCV infection or unexplained liver disease. Since the advent of HAART in 1996, liver disease has become an increasingly important cause of morbidity and mortality in patients with HIV/AIDS. In addition, HIV infection accelerates the course of disease associated with HCV infection. In one series, cirrhosis developed within 15 years in 25% of coinfected patients, compared with only 6.5% of those who had HCV infection alone. Finally, the likelihood of achieving an SVR after treatment for chronic hepatitis C is lower in HCV-HIV coinfection than in HCV alone: 14–29% in genotype 1 and 43–73% in genotypes 2 and 3, following 48 weeks of therapy with PEG IFN-α and ribavirin.

C. HCV-HBV

As discussed previously, coinfection with HCV and HBV increases the risk and rate of development of cirrhosis and HCC, relative to those observed in patients infected with either virus alone.

D. Hepatic Steatosis

Patients with hepatitis C and high body mass index or hepatic steatosis, or both, are at increased risk for development of fibrosis and its accelerated progression. In addition, as noted above, moderate-to-severe steatosis has been associated with advanced fibrosis and a decrease in response to interferon-based therapy.

Adinolfi LE, Gambardella M, Andreana A, et al. Steatosis accelerates the progression of liver damage of chronic hepatitis C patients and correlated with specific HCV genotype and visceral obesity. *Hepatology.* 2001;33:1358–1364. [PMID: 11391523]

Di Bisceglie AM, Shiffman ML, Everson GT, et al. Prolonged therapy of advanced hepatitis C with low-dose peginterferon. *N Eng J Med.* 2008;359:2429–2441. [PMID: 19052125]

Dienstag JL, McHutchison JG. American Gastroenterological Association medical position statement on the management of hepatitis C. *Gastroenterology.* 2006;130:225–230. [PMID: 16401485]

Dienstag JL, McHutchison JG. American Gastroenterological Association technical review on the management of hepatitis C. *Gastroenterology.* 2006;130:231–264. [PMID: 16401486]

Fried MW, Shiffman ML, Reddy R, et al. Peginterferon alfa-2a plus ribavirin for chronic hepatitis C virus infection. *N Engl J Med.* 2002;347:975–982. [PMID: 12324553]

Ge D, Fellay J, Simon JS, et al. Genetic variation in IL-28B predicts hepatitis C treatment-induced viral clearance. *Nature.* 2009;461:399–401. [PMID: 19684573]

Ghany MG, Strader DB, Thomas DL, et al. Diagnosis, management, and treatment of hepatitis C: an update. *Hepatology.* 2009;49:1335–1374. [PMID: 19330875]

Hadziyannis SJ, Sette H Jr, Morgan TR, et al. Peginterferon-alpha-2a and ribavirin combination therapy in chronic hepatitis C: a randomized study of treatment duration and ribavirin dose. *Ann Intern Med.* 2004;140:346–355. [PMID: 14996676]

Hezode C, Forestier N, Dushieko G, et al. Telaprevir and peginterferon with or without ribavirin for chronic HCV infection. *N Engl J Med.* 2009;360:1839–1850. [PMID: 19403903]

Kwo PY, Lawitz EJ, McCone J, et al. Efficacy of boceprevir, an NS3 protease inhibitor, in combination with peginterferon alfa-2b and ribavirin in treatment-naïve patients with genotype 1 hepatitis C infection (SPRINT-1): an open-label, randomized, multicentre phase 2 trial. *Lancet.* 2010;376:705–716. [PMID: 20692693]

Mangia A, Santoro R, Minerva N, et al. Peginterferon alfa-2b and Ribavirin for 12 weeks vs. 24 weeks in HCV genotype 2 or 3. *N Engl J Med.* 2005;352:2609–2617. [PMID: 15972867]

Manns MP, McHutchinson JG, Gordon SC, et al. Peginterferon alfa-2b plus ribavirin compared with interferon alfa-2b plus ribavirin for initial treatment of chronic hepatitis C: a randomised trial. *Lancet.* 2001;358:958–965. [PMID: 11583749]

McHutchinson JG, Everson GT, Gordon SC, et al. Telaprevir with peginterferon and ribavirin for chronic HCV genotype 1 infection. *N Engl J Med.* 2009;360:1827–1838. [PMID: 19403902]

McHutchinson JG, Manns MP, Muir AJ, et al. Telaprevir for previously treated chronic HCV infection. *N Engl J Med.* 2010;362:1292–1303. [PMID: 20375406]

O'Leary JG, Chung, RT. Management of hepatitis C virus coinfection in HIV-infected persons. *AIDS Read.* 2006;16:313–316. [PMID: 16795921]

Shiratori Y, Imazeki F, Moriyama M, et al. Histologic improvement of fibrosis in patients with hepatitis C who have sustained response to interferon therapy. *Ann Intern Med.* 2000;132:517–524. [PMID: 10744587]

Thomas DL, Thio CL, Martin MP, et al. Genetic variation in IL28B and spontaneous clearance of hepatitis C virus. *Nature.* 2009;461:798–801. [PMID: 19759533]

HEPATITIS D

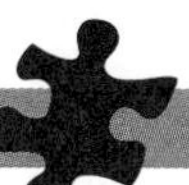

ESSENTIALS OF DIAGNOSIS

- Infection occurs only in the presence of HBV and is detected by demonstrating anti-HDV (distinctions between IgM and IgG anti-HDV are not helpful).
- HDV RNA detected in serum by molecular hybridization or PCR assays is helpful in confirming the diagnosis.
- Testing for IgM and IgG anti-HBc helps distinguish between acute, simultaneous HBV-HDV coinfection (IgM anti-HBc–positive) and HDV superinfection in patients with chronic HBV infection (IgG anti-HBc–positive).

General Considerations

Hepatitis D virus (HDV) requires the helper function of hepatitis B virus; therefore, in nature, hepatitis D occurs exclusively in patients with hepatitis B. Infection with HDV occurs worldwide, but incidence and prevalence data vary substantially from region to region and are influenced periodically by immigration patterns of patients from high endemic areas. On a worldwide basis, 15 million people with chronic hepatitis B are estimated to harbor concomitant HDV infection. Although hepatitis D was first identified and recognized in southern Europe during the 1970s, the prevalence and incidence of HDV infection declined dramatically, presumably in parallel with measures introduced to control HBV infection and with shifts in the migration patterns that amplified its spread in the 1970s. A higher prevalence of HDV infection persists in older southern European populations, representing residual infection in the cohort of patients infected several decades ago when HDV infection was endemic there.

In nonendemic areas, HDV is transmitted primarily by percutaneous routes, especially in injection drug users and their sexual contacts. In parts of the Mediterranean and other endemic areas, transmission is perpetuated by close personal contact (eg, within families).

Pathogenesis

HDV, the agent that causes hepatitis D or "delta," as named originally, is a unique hepatitis virus with the smallest known genome (1.7 kb) of any animal RNA virus. The 36-nm HDV virion comprises an RNA genome, a single HDV-encoded antigen, and a lipoprotein envelope provided by HBV.

Although under unusual circumstances (eg, associated with immunosuppression after liver transplantation) HDV can replicate autonomously, generally it is a defective virus that requires the simultaneous presence of HBV for complete virion assembly and secretion. Consequently, as noted, HDV infection and replication can occur only in a host with HBV infection. HDV infection can be acquired during (a) simultaneous acute HBV-HDV coinfection, which is limited in duration by the duration of the HBV infection; and (b) acute HDV superinfection of a person with chronic hepatitis B (including inactive carriers), in whom HDV infection almost invariably becomes chronic, lasting as long as the underlying chronic HBV infection. Because HDV "takes over" the replicative machinery of HBV, HDV infection usually results in suppression of HBV replication; thus, patients with both HBV and HDV infection tend to have markers of low-level HBV replication (HBsAg positive, HBeAg negative, anti-HBe positive) and low-level or undetectable HBV DNA.

In acute HDV infection, microvesicular steatosis and granular eosinophilic necrosis may be seen histologically. In chronic hepatitis D, necroinflammatory activity is often severe, but no specific histologic features are noted, and HDV antigen (HDVAg) is localized by immunohistochemical staining in hepatocyte nuclei. HDV genotypes (I–III) and specific clinical features of hepatitis D seem to cluster in distinct geographic areas. Genotype I is most common in the Western world and Africa, where acute hepatitis D is more likely to be fulminant, and chronic infection is more likely to progress rapidly to cirrhosis. Genotype II is predominantly an Eastern genotype and is thought to be less pathogenic than genotype I. Genotype III is seen almost exclusively in Central and South America, where HDV superinfection in persons with underlying chronic hepatitis B tends to be associated with severe, often fulminant, hepatitis.

Clinical Findings

A. Acute HBV-HDV Coinfection

Acute coinfection is characterized by hepatitis, which can be severe, with hepatocellular necrosis and inflammation. The majority of cases, however, are self-limited, with clearance of HBV and therefore HDV. Fulminant hepatitis is infrequent overall, reported in approximately 5% of outbreaks of coinfection among injection drug users and their sexual partners, but is still more than 10 times more common than in patients with acute hepatitis B alone.

B. Chronic HBV-HDV Infection

Most cases emanate from acute HDV superinfection of a patient with underlying chronic hepatitis B, including those with chronic hepatitis and inactive carriers. In chronic HBV-HDV infection, HDV viremia continues, although at lower levels than is seen during the period of acute HDV superinfection. On biopsy, necroinflammatory lesions are notable and are typically more severe than those seen in patients with chronic HBV infection alone. Episodes that resemble acute hepatitis can also mark the course in chronic coinfection. Labrea fever is an unusual form of delta hepatitis (HDV superinfection in a population with endemic HBV infection) described in the Amazon basin and in which fulminant hepatitis results in jaundice, fever, and black vomitus.

C. Serologic Assays

HDV infection is detected by demonstrating the presence of anti-HDV. Distinctions between IgM and IgG anti-HDV are not helpful. The nucleocapsid HDV protein is always encapsidated within an envelope of HBsAg; therefore, circulating levels of HDVAg are undetectable, and commercial HDVAg assays are not available. HDV RNA can be detected in serum by either molecular hybridization or PCR assays, which are helpful in confirming the diagnosis and in monitoring viremia during a course of antiviral therapy.

In patients with HDV infection, testing for IgM and IgG anti-HBc helps distinguish between acute, simultaneous HBV-HDV coinfection (IgM anti-HBc–positive) and HDV superinfection in someone already harboring chronic HBV infection (IgG anti-HBc–positive).

Prevention

Because of its requirement for chronic HBV infection, HDV infection can be prevented by vaccinating susceptible persons with hepatitis B vaccine. No effective vaccine is available for preventing HDV superinfection in persons who are already HBsAg-positive.

Treatment

Despite the reliance of HDV on concomitant HBV infection, the oral polymerase inhibitors that suppress HBV replication have not been shown to be effective in the treatment of hepatitis D. IFN-α is currently the only licensed drug for treatment of HDV. Clinical trials in the early 1990s provided evidence than IFN-α is effective in the treatment of HDV infection, but the rate of relapse is high, and efficacy is proportional to the dose and duration of treatment; high-dose, long-duration therapy lasting at least 1 year is required. More recently, PEG IFN-α monotherapy for 12 months has been shown to result in a 43% SVR; the addition of ribavirin does not offer further benefit. Patients with decompensated cirrhosis resulting from chronic hepatitis D are good candidates for liver transplantation; even before the widespread use of HBIG and polymerase inhibitors to prevent recurrent hepatitis B after liver transplantation, patients with hepatitis D were less likely to experience HDV-HBV reinfection of the allograft. Currently, with efficient antiviral therapy to prevent recurrent HBV infection posttransplantation, recurrent hepatitis D after transplantation is even less of a threat.

Targeting specific steps in the HDV life cycle have been contemplated as the basis of potential new therapies for HDV, such as prenylation inhibitors. Prenylation is a site-specific lipid modification of proteins, and viruses can also make use of this posttranslational modification provided by their host cells. Depriving a virus access to prenylation can have dramatic effects on the targeted virus's life cycle, and pharmacological inhibitors of prenylating enzymes have been developed and shown to have potent antiviral effects in both in vitro and in vivo systems. Because prenylation inhibitors target a host cell function, are available in oral form, and are surprisingly well tolerated in human trials, these compounds represent an attractive new class of antiviral agents with potential for broad-spectrum activity.

Course & Prognosis

A. Acute HBV-HDV Coinfection

Acute coinfection resolves in 80–95% of cases, following clearance of HBV, without which HDV infection cannot continue. In 2–20% of cases, however, fulminant hepatitis develops; in series from endemic areas, 30% of cases of fulminant hepatitis B represent simultaneous acute hepatitis D. In addition, 2–5% of cases of acute HBV-HDV coinfection result in chronic infection. Finally, in acute simultaneous HBV and HDV infection among injection drug users, case fatality rates approaching 5% have been reported.

B. Acute HDV Superinfection

Unlike acute coinfection, HDV superinfection results in chronic HDV-HBV in almost all cases, fostered by the persistence of HBV infection. Similar to acute coinfection, acute HDV superinfection results in fulminant hepatitis in 2–20% of cases. Hepatitis D superinfection rarely resolves unless HBV infection resolves. In some outbreaks of severe HDV superinfection in populations with a high rate of HBV infection, mortality exceeding 20% has been reported.

C. Chronic HBV-HDV Infection

Initial descriptions of chronic hepatitis D were consistent with severe liver disease; however, some patients with chronic HDV infection have very mild liver disease and may even be inactive HDV carriers. Generally, chronic hepatitis D progresses more frequently and more rapidly to cirrhosis than chronic hepatitis B, but after years of infection, severity and progression appear to lessen as the disease becomes more quiescent. Although chronic HBV infection is a well recognized risk factor for the development of HCC, a similar association has been demonstrated for chronic HDV infection. Overall, the pattern of disease progression appears to vary with geography, genotype, and mode of transmission. Slowly progressive, mild disease is more common in endemic areas. On the other hand, HDV-associated disease appears to be more severe in nonendemic areas, where injection drug use is the main form of transmission.

Bordier BB, Ohkanda J, Liu P, et al. In vivo antiviral efficacy of prenylation inhibitors against hepatitis delta virus. *J Clin Invest.* 2003;112:407–414. [PMID: 12897208]

Canbakan B, Senturk H, Tabak F, et al. Efficacy of interferon alpha 2b and lamivudine combination treatment in comparison to interferon alpha-2b alone in chronic delta hepatitis: a randomized trial. *J Gastroenterol Hepatol.* 2006;21:657–663. [PMID: 16677149]

Castelnau C, Le Gal F, Ripault MP, et al. Efficacy of peginterferon alpha-2b in chronic hepatitis delta: relevance of quantitative RT-PCR for follow-up. *Hepatology.* 2006;44:728–735. [PMID: 16941695]

Farci P. Treatment of chronic hepatitis D: new advances, old challenges. *Hepatology.* 2006;44:536–539. [PMID: 16941704]

Lau DT, Doo E, Park Y, et al. Lamivudine for chronic delta hepatitis. *Hepatology.* 1999;30:546–549. [PMID: 10421666]

Niro GA, Ciancio A, Gaeta GB, et al. Pegylated interferon alpha-2b as monotherapy or in combination with ribavirin in chronic delta hepatitis. *Hepatology.* 2006;44:713–720. [PMID: 16941685]

Rizzetto M. Hepatitis D: thirty years after. *J Hepatol.* 2009;50:1043. [PMID: 19285743]

Taylor JM. Hepatitis delta virus. *Virology.* 2006;344:71–76. [PMID: 16364738]

Wedemeyer H, Heidrich B, Manns MP. Hepatitis D virus infection—not a vanishing disease in Europe! *Hepatology.* 2007;45:1331–1333. [PMID: 17464980]

HEPATITIS E

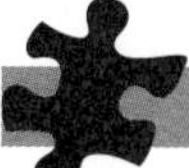

ESSENTIALS OF DIAGNOSIS

- Diagnosis is established by demonstrating the presence of serum IgM antibody to hepatitis E virus (anti-HEV) by immunoassay or HEV RNA by PCR (these assays are not available routinely in the United States).
- IgM anti-HEV is detectable for only a few months after acquisition of HEV, and IgG anti-HEV for ~1 year.
- A vaccine has been developed that is effective in preventing hepatitis E, but this vaccine is not available in the United States.

General Considerations

Outbreaks occur in the Indian subcontinent, Central America, Africa, northwest China, and the Central Asian Republics (the former Soviet Union), where hepatitis E virus (HEV) infection is endemic. HEV is transmitted predominantly through the fecal-oral route, and most reported outbreaks of infection have been related to the consumption of fecally contaminated drinking water. Unusual for an enteric virus, HEV is not readily spread via person-to-person transmission. The highest attack rate occurs in young adults, a subpopulation that, ordinarily, would be immune to enterically transmitted endemic agents. Genotypes 3 and 4, more common in the United States, are relatively nonvirulent and associated with inapparent infection, whereas genotypes 1 and 2, common in endemic areas, are relatively virulent, accounting for the clinically apparent, often severe disease in these regions.

In countries where HEV infection is not endemic, the disease has been observed in travelers returning from endemic regions; in nonendemic countries, HEV accounts for fewer than 1% of cases of acute viral hepatitis. HEV can infect pigs, suggesting that some cases of human transmission may result from contact across species. Although clinically apparent hepatitis E is uncommon in the United States, as many as 20% of the population harbor antibodies to HEV, hypothesized to be attributed to low-pathogenicity genotypes acquired via exposure to a swine reservoir.

Pathogenesis

HEV is a small, 32–34 nm, nonenveloped spherical, 7600-base-pair RNA virus (genus *Hepacivirus*) that was identified in 1983. Transmission is through the fecal-oral route, and, like other hepatitis viruses, the main target cells are hepatocytes. Various geographically distinct isolates have been classified into at least four human genotypes (plus a fifth in nonhuman hosts), but all genotypes share at least one major serologically cross-reactive epitope, despite substantial genomic variability, permitting the development of an effective vaccine.

Clinical Findings

The incubation period for hepatitis E ranges from 2 to 10 weeks; the clinical course of acute hepatitis E is similar to that of acute hepatitis A, but generally acute hepatitis E is more severe. Like acute hepatitis A, acute hepatitis E has an insidious onset, most commonly beginning with a several-day prodromal phase with flulike symptoms, fever, abdominal pain, nausea and vomiting, dark urine and clay-colored stools, diarrhea, and, in a small proportion of cases, a transient macular skin rash. The prodromal phase is followed by the development of jaundice in icteric cases, resolution of the prodromal symptoms, pronounced elevation of amino transaminase levels, elevated bilirubin levels, and, in a proportion of patients with cholestatic features, more often in hepatitis E than in the other viral hepatitides, alkaline phosphatase elevations. Histologically, cholestasis with rosette formation of hepatocytes and polymorphonuclear leukocytes may be prominent. Acute hepatitis E can be very severe in pregnant women, in whom the mortality rate can reach 15–25%.

The diagnosis of HEV infection is established by demonstrating the presence of serum IgM anti-HEV by immunoassay or HEV RNA by PCR. IgM anti-HEV is undetectable after a few months, and even IgG anti-HEV does not persist much beyond 1 year. These assays are not available routinely in the United States but can be obtained in specialized labs (eg, at the Centers for Disease Control and Prevention).

Prevention

Immunoglobulin, produced in countries where HEV is endemic, has not been shown to confer protection against HEV. Prophylactic measures to minimize the occurrence of HEV infection involve improved sanitation and sanitary handling of food and water. Boiling water appears to reduce the risk of infection. Because person-to-person transmission is rare, isolation of affected patients is not indicated.

A recombinant polypeptide vaccine was shown to be effective in a randomized, double-blind, placebo-controlled trial involving nearly 2000 mostly male members of the Nepalese army. The volunteers received three doses of the vaccine or placebo at 0, 1, and 6 months. A total of 69 cases of definite HEV infection occurred at least 14 days after the third injection, 3 in the vaccine group (0.3%) and 66 in the placebo group (7.4%). The efficacy of the vaccine was 85.7% after two doses and 95.5% after all three. The vaccine was well tolerated, with similar serious adverse events in the two groups. Studies are underway to determine the length of protective efficacy of the vaccine and its safety in different sub-population groups, including pregnant women. This vaccine is available in endemic regions but not in the United States.

Treatment

Treatment is largely supportive (see the discussion of hepatitis A treatment earlier in this chapter).

Course & Prognosis

Acute hepatitis E is self-limited; acute illness usually lasts 1–4 weeks, although some patients have a prolonged cholestatic hepatitis lasting 2–6 months. Neither persistent viremia (chronic hepatitis E) nor cirrhosis follows acute infection. Fulminant hepatitis can occur, however, with an overall case fatality rate of 0.1–4%. For unclear reasons, as previously noted, fulminant hepatitis occurs more frequently during pregnancy, resulting in an inordinately high mortality rate of 15–25%, primarily affecting women in the third trimester. In addition, acute hepatitis E can cause hepatic decompensation in patients with preexisting liver disease and in persons who are malnourished.

Chau TN, Lai ST, Tse C, et al. Epidemiology and clinical features of sporadic hepatitis E as compared with hepatitis A. *Am J Gastroenterol.* 2006;101:292–296. [PMID: 16454833]

Emerson SU, Purcell RH. Running like water—the omnipresence of hepatitis E. *N Engl J Med.* 2004;351:2367–2368. [PMID: 15575050]

Krawczynski K. Hepatitis E vaccine—ready for prime time? *N Engl J Med.* 2007;356:949–951. [PMID: 17329703]

Shrestha MP, Scott RM, Joshi DM, et al. Safety and efficacy of a recombinant hepatitis E vaccine. *N Engl J Med.* 2007;356:895–903. [PMID: 17329696]

Chronic Nonviral Hepatitis

Chinweike Ukomadu, MD, PhD

This chapter discusses a group of conditions that result in chronic inflammation of the liver, ultimately leading to fibrosis, cirrhosis, and liver failure. The epidemiology, pathogenesis, and management of autoimmune hepatitis, Wilson disease, and α_1-antitrypsin deficiency are described.

AUTOIMMUNE HEPATITIS

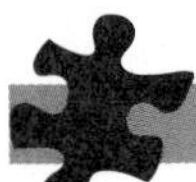

ESSENTIALS OF DIAGNOSIS

- Characterized by the presence of autoantibodies and elevated serum IgG levels.
- More common in women than in men.
- Diagnosis is made on the basis of serologic findings (abnormal liver biochemical tests, autoantibodies, elevated IgG) and histologic findings, and by ruling out other chronic liver diseases (drug-induced liver injury, viral hepatitis, inherited and metabolic liver disorders).
- Overlap syndromes include features of other chronic liver disorders (eg, primary biliary cirrhosis, primary sclerosing cholangitis).

General Considerations

Autoimmune hepatitis (AIH) is a heterogeneous group of chronic inflammatory hepatic disorders identified by the presence of circulating autoantibodies and elevated serum γ-globulins. The pathogenesis of the disease is unclear, although it is believed that genetic predisposition in susceptible individuals ultimately leads to an immunologic process directed against hepatocytes. Among the many suspected inciting factors in those genetically predisposed are toxins and infectious agents. The inflammatory disorder can result in hepatocellular necrosis and collapse or in fibrosis and cirrhosis. The disease is present in all racial groups and all age groups but is more common in women than in men, with a frequency of 3.6:1. It is responsible for approximately 5.9% of the liver transplantations performed in the United States.

Krawitt EL. Autoimmune hepatitis. *N Engl J Med.* 2006;354:54–66. [PMID: 16394302]

Manns, MP, Czaja AJ, Gorham JD, et al. Diagnosis and management of autoimmune hepatitis. *Hepatology.* 2010;51:2193–2213. [PMID: 20513004]

Pathogenesis

The mechanism of hepatic injury in AIH is not well characterized. There appear to be both genetic and environmental influences.

AIH is classified into two distinct sub-types based on the presence of autoantibodies. The clinical relevance of this classification system is, however, unclear as it is not certain that autoantibodies play a role in disease pathogenesis. Type 1 disease is present in patients who test positive for antinuclear antibody (ANA) or anti–smooth muscle antibody (ASMA), or both. This is the most common form and has been linked to HLA DRB 10301 (DR3) and DRB 10401 (DR4). Type 2 disease is present in patients who are positive for anti–liver kidney microsomal (ALKM) antibody. This form is common in Europe and is often present in younger women in the second and third decades of life. The linkage is to HLA DRB 10701. A third variant (Type 3) characterized by the presence of antibody to the soluble liver antigen (ASLA) has been abandoned because the ASLA is also present in some patients with Type 1 or Type 2 AIH. Currently, ASLA is touted as a possible prognostic marker for identifying patients who may relapse after cessation of corticosteroid therapy.

It is worth noting that in some patients, autoimmune hepatitis may be part of a larger syndromic manifestation of autoimmune polyendocrinopathy, candidiasis, and ectodermal dystrophy (APECED). This is disorder, caused by a mutation in the gene for the autoimmune regulator protein (AIRE), is inherited in an autosomal recessive fashion. In classic (nonsyndromic) AIH, genetic predisposition is inferred by associations with HLA alleles as discussed above. However, inheritance of AIH is not Mendelian in nature but polygenic. Therefore genetic screening of affected individuals and their kin for classic non-syndromic AIH is of limited clinical importance.

The frequency with which autoantibodies occur varies in the general population. For example, a positive ANA result is found in 67% of patients with AIH. It is present alone in 13% of patients but is accompanied by the ASMA in an additional 54%. It can be present in patients who have primary biliary cirrhosis, primary sclerosing cholangitis, viral hepatitis, drug-induced hepatitis, and non-alcoholic steatohepatitis (NASH). ASMA is present in 87% of patients with AIH. It is seen alone in 33% of patients and in combination with ANA in 54% of patients. The target antigen is thought to be actin and nonactin components of the smooth muscle. In fact, a serologic test for a component of actin (F-Actin) is now used in place of the ASMA assay by many laboratories in screening for AIH. The ALKM antibody is seen in 4% of patients and is often seen in the absence of ANA and ASMA. The target is thought to be the enzyme CYP2D6, which shares homology to hepatitis C. As a result, the ALKM antibody can be falsely positive in patients who are chronically infected with the hepatitis C virus. It is important to realize, however, that the presence of autoantibody by itself is not diagnostic (see later discussion of diagnostic criteria, and Table 40–1).

Finnish-German APACED consortium. An autoimmune disease, APECED, caused by mutations in a novel gene featuring two PHD-type zinc-finger domains. *Nature Genetics*. 1997; 17:399–403. [PMID: 9398840]

Manns MP, Czaja AJ, Gorham JD, et al. Diagnosis and management of autoimmune hepatitis. *Hepatology*. 2010;51:2193–3023. [PMID: 20513004]

Clinical Findings

In addition to the presence of autoantibodies and elevated γ-globulins, the patient's gender, a detailed clinical history, a multitude of diagnostic serologic tests, liver biopsy findings, and the response to a trial of steroids aid in the diagnosis of AIH. The goal of the clinical evaluation is to solidify the diagnosis of AIH while eliminating processes that may mimic AIH (Table 40–1). Thus, several other causes of hepatitis need to be excluded (see "Differential Diagnosis," later).

Historic information helps elucidate potential toxin-induced causes of hepatitis, including alcohol. Serologic evaluations help eliminate viral hepatitis and inherited liver diseases (eg, Wilson disease, hemochromatosis, α_1-antitrypsin deficiency). Additionally, primary sclerosing cholangitis and primary biliary cirrhosis need to be excluded. Personal and family history of AIH should be sought.

A. Symptoms and Signs

The most common presenting symptoms are fatigue (seen in 87% of patients), dark urine and light-colored stools (77%), right upper quadrant pain (48%), and anorexia (30%). Physical examination findings include hepatomegaly (seen in

Table 40–1. Simplified diagnostic criteria for autoimmune hepatitis (AIH)

Variable	Result	Score[a]
ANA or SMA	≥1:40	1
ANA or SMA or LKM or SLA	≥1:80 ≥1:40 Positive	2*
IgG	>upper normal limit >1.10 times upper normal limit	1 2
Liver histology (evidence of hepatitis is a necessary condition)	Compatible with AIH Typical AIH	1 2
Absence of viral hepatitis	Yes	2 ≥6: probable AIH ≥7: definite AIH

*Addition of points achieved for all autoantibodies (maximum, 2 points). For details, see reference cited below.

a. Scores from criteria above are summed. Prior to steroid therapy a definite diagnosis requires a score >7, while a probable diagnosis requires a score of 6 or higher.

AIH, autoimmune hepatitis; ANA, antinuclear antibody; SMA, smooth muscle antibody; LKM, liver kidney microsomal (antibody); SLA, soluble liver antigen; IgG, immunoglobulin G.

Adapted with permission from: Hennes EM, Zeniya M, Czaja AJ, et al. Autoimmune, cholestatic and biliary disease: simplified criteria for the diagnosis of autoimmune hepatitis. *Hepatology*. 2008;48:169–176. [PMID: 18537184]

78% of patients), spider angiomata (58%), palpable spleen (40%), scleral icterus (46%), ascites (20%), and encephalopathy (14%).

AIH is associated with several other autoimmune disorders. Among the most common are autoimmune thyroiditis, rheumatoid arthritis, and ulcerative colitis. Additional conditions, although rare, include insulin-dependent diabetes mellitus, Sjögren syndrome, Graves disease, dermatitis herpetiformis, vitiligo, myasthenia gravis, pernicious anemia, and celiac sprue.

B. Laboratory Findings

The presentation of AIH is variable. Severe AIH characterized by marked elevation in transaminases (>10 times the upper limit of normal) is the presentation in around 40% of patients. Approximately 3% of these patients have liver failure on presentation. Around 40% of those with untreated severe AIH disease die within 6 months; 40% of the survivors are cirrhotic at presentation, and 54% have varices within 2 years. The 5-year mortality is approximately 58%. In patients who have an alanine aminotransferase (ALT) level more than 10 times the upper limit of normal or serum γ-globulins three times the upper limit normal or who have bridging necrosis on histology, 82% are cirrhotic within 5 years, and mortality is 45% during this period of time.

C. Histologic Findings

Liver biopsy should be performed, and the resulting histologic evaluation should be consistent with findings known to be present in AIH. Findings consistent with interface hepatitis, and presence of a lymphoplasmacytic infiltrate in the portal area, are reliable clues and helpful histologic findings. Histologic changes suggestive of biliary tract disease (eg, granulomas), as seen in patients with primary biliary cirrhosis should not be present in the canonical form of AIH.

D. Diagnostic Criteria

Among patients whose diagnosis is not straightforward, response to corticosteroids can aid in determining if AIH is likely. As a result of discrepancies and difficulties in diagnosis, a scoring system for AIH has been designed. An original scoring system developed by Alvarez et al has been felt by many to be too cumbersome. A revised and simplified version of this scoring system is shown in Table 40–1. Prior to treatment with corticosteroids, a definite diagnosis implies a score of greater than 7; a probable diagnosis implies a score of 6 or higher.

Alvarez F, Berg PA, Bianchi FB, et al. International Autoimmune Hepatitis Group Report: review of criteria for diagnosis of autoimmune hepatitis. *J Hepatol.* 1999;31:929–938. [PMID: 10580593]

Hennes EM, Zeniya M, Czaja AJ, et al. Autoimmune, cholestatic and biliary disease: simplified criteria for the diagnosis of autoimmune hepatitis. *Hepatology.* 2008;48:169–176. [PMID: 18537184]

Differential Diagnosis

The differential diagnosis of AIH includes various forms of acute and chronic hepatitis. These include toxin-induced hepatitis, hepatotropic (hepatitis A–E viruses) and nonhepatotropic viral hepatitis (cytomegalovirus, Epstein-Barr virus, herpes simplex virus, and varicella virus) infections, metabolic liver disorders such as NASH, and inherited liver disorders such as hemochromatosis, Wilson disease, and α_1-antitrypsin deficiency.

Treatment

The cornerstone of treatment is the use of immunosuppressive agents (Table 40–2). Induction of remission should include corticosteroids. Noncorticosteroid immunomodulatory agents such as azathioprine and mycophenolate mofetil may be used for maintenance.

In three distinct randomized clinical trials on adults with severe AIH, those who received prednisone as part of the initial therapy had clinical and histologic improvement in addition to lower mortality when compared with those who did not receive the drug. Table 40–3 summarizes clinical outcomes of two published trials. Improvement in clinical indices occurs, as well, in patients who are already cirrhotic at the time of diagnosis. As a result, corticosteroids remain the standard therapy for AIH, either given alone or in combination with azathioprine.

Although therapy is effective, side effects of corticosteroid therapy include osteopenia, diabetes mellitus, hypertension, and Cushing syndrome. Budesonide (a glucocorticoid with a high hepatic first-pass clearance) and deflazacort (a derivative of prednisolone with decreased risk of osteopenia and diabetes mellitus) have been used to help limit side effects associated with prednisone. Until recently there had not been enough evidence that any of these glucocorticoids were equivalent or superior to prednisone. However a recent study showed that budesonide in combination with azathioprine was superior to a tapering regimen of prednisone and azathioprine in induction and maintenance of remission in non cirrhotic AIH patients.

Azathioprine has been used as monotherapy for the treatment of AIH, but only after remission has been induced and sustained, and then corticosteroids tapered off. Many practitioners do not use azathioprine alone unless there is some compelling reason to avoid corticosteroids, given the evidence that corticosteroids are superior to many other immunomodulators for induction of remission. Potential side effects of azathioprine include leukopenia, pancreatitis, and drug-induced hepatitis.

Table 40–2. Treatment of autoimmune hepatitis.

Agent	Dose	Adverse Effects
Prednisone	40–60 mg/day with subsequent taper	Cushingoid appearance Diabetes mellitus Hypertension Osteopenia
Budesonide	3 mg two or three times daily	As above for prednisone but markedly reduced in degree and frequency
Azathioprine	50–100 mg/day (1–2 mg/kg/day)	Leukopenia Drug-induced hepatitis Pancreatitis Gastrointestinal upset
Mycophenolate mofetil	1 g twice daily	Leukopenia Diarrhea/colitis Nausea
Cyclosporine	3–5 mg/kg/day	Hypertension Renal failure
Cyclophosphamide	1–1.5 mg/kg/day	Cystitis Pancytopenia

Cyclosporine has been used with some promising results, especially in children, as a result of concerns of the side effects of steroids. Biochemical improvement as evidenced by decreased ALT and γ-globulin levels and increased albumin often occurs. There is improvement in average growth velocity, and side effects (hypertension and renal impairment) are minimal when serum levels are kept low.

Mycophenolate has been tried as a rescue therapy in patients with AIH. It normalizes ALT and improves the ability to taper prednisone to lower doses. In addition, histology is improved, and the medicine is well tolerated except for mild leukopenia.

Cyclophosphamide, tacrolimus, and methotrexate have been used either alone or in combination with corticosteroids with limited success.

Table 40–3. Clinical outcome of prednisone use in autoimmune hepatitis.

Soloway et al[a]		
Clinical Event	**Prednisone or Prednisone plus Azathioprine (35 patients)**	**Azathioprine or Placebo (28 patients)**
Death in 6 months	1	12
Esophageal variceal hemorrhage	0	3
Resolution of ascites	5	0
Development of ascites	1	12
Murray-Lyon et al[b]		
Clinical Event	**Prednisone (22 patients)**	**Azathioprine (25 patients)**
Death in 2 years	1	6
Esophageal variceal hemorrhage	0	5

[a]Data from Soloway RD, Summerskill WH, Baggenstoss AH, et al. Clinical, biochemical, and histo-logical remission of severe chronic active liver disease: a controlled study of treatments and early prognosis. *Gastroenterology*. 1972;63:820–833. [PMID: 4538724]

[b]Data from Murray-Lyon IM, Stern RB, Williams R. Controlled trial of prednisone and azathioprine in active chronic hepatitis. *Lancet*. 1973;1:735–737. [PMID: 4121073]

Manns, MP, Czaja AJ, Gorham JD, et al. Diagnosis and management of autoimmune hepatitis. *Hepatology*. 2010;51:2193–2213. [PMID: 20513004]

Manns MP, Woynarowski M, Kreisel W, et al. Budesonide induces remission more effectively than prednisone in a controlled trial of patients with autoimmune hepatitis. *Gastroenterology*. 2010;139:1198–1206. [PMID: 20600032]

Prognosis

Response to prednisone is excellent, with 80–100% of patients responding. Even among cirrhotic patients, reversal of signs of decompensation (ascites, jaundice, coagulopathy) can occur with treatment. Failure of bilirubin to decrease to less than 15 mg after 2 weeks of corticosteroid therapy suggests a very poor prognosis.

For many patients with AIH, lifelong immunosuppressive therapy has usually been the norm. This has led investigators to ask whether remission can be maintained in some patients after complete withdrawal of therapy. Indeed, studies suggest that between 10% and 40% of persons remain in remission after therapy is withdrawn. Laboratory indices, AST, ALT, bilirubin, and g-globulin should be normal before attempted withdrawal of drug therapy.

Relapse after therapy withdrawal does not preclude attainment of sustained remission, although it usually requires the reinstitution of high-dose steroid therapy. The laboratory markers that correlate with remission are serum γ-globulin levels and stage of fibrotic disease. Patients with markedly elevated globulin levels and cirrhosis are most at risk. Many practitioners obtain a liver biopsy to ensure that there is no inflammatory activity before withdrawing therapy. For patients who fail immunosuppressive therapy, liver transplantation is an option if they are deemed suitable candidates.

Czaja AJ, Menon KV, Carpenter HA. Sustained remission after corticosteroid therapy for type 1 autoimmune hepatitis: a retrospective analysis. *Hepatology*. 2002;35:890–897. [PMID: 11915036]

Feld JJ, Dinh H, Arenovich T, Marcus VA, Wanless IR, Heathcote EJ. Autoimmune hepatitis: effect of symptoms and cirrhosis on natural history and outcome. *Hepatology*. 2005;42:53–62. [PMID: 15954109]

Overlap Syndromes of AIH

The preceding section describes AIH in its classic form. There are, however, variants of the disorder in which serologic and clinical characteristics are mixed with other forms of chronic (often immune-mediated) liver disorders. These groups of syndromes are known as overlap syndromes. The prevalence of overlap syndromes among patients with AIH, primary sclerosing cholangitis (PSC), and primary biliary cirrhosis (PBC) has been estimated at about 18%. The two most common variants are AIH-PBC and AIH-PSC overlaps.

A. AIH-PBC Overlap

In the majority of these patients, serologic evaluations show the presence of antimitochondrial antibodies (AMAs) but histologic characteristics of AIH are present. These patients are treated as classic AIH and have an excellent response to steroid therapy. A second group of patients frequently classified as AIH-PBC overlap are negative for AMA, positive for ANA or ASMA, or both, but have histologic findings consistent with PBC. This entity has been termed autoimmune cholangitis or immune cholangiopathy. Many practitioners do not regard this as an overlap syndrome but rather consider it to be an AMA-negative form of PBC. The heterogeneity of this group of disorders has prompted investigators to look for ways of improving diagnostic accuracy. One such study found that the use of the Paris criteria, which requires the presence of 2 out of 3 criteria for diagnosis PBC and AIH was effective in the diagnosis of AIH/PBC overlap. For this study, the criteria for PBC were (1) a twofold elevation in the alkaline phosphatase or five fold elevation in the gamma glutamyltransferase, (2) appositive AMA, and (3) a liver biopsy with bile duct lesions as seen in PBC. For AIH, the diagnostic criteria was (1) elevated ALT of at least fivefold the upper limit of normal, (2) at least a two fold increase in IgG level or a positive ASMA, (3) a liver biopsy with classic findings suggestive of AIH. This criteria yields sensitivity and specificity of diagnosing AIH /PBC overlap of 92% and 97%, respectively.

B. AIH-PSC Overlap

Patients with this overlap syndrome have serologic findings suggestive of AIH (presence of ANA or ASMA, or both) but radiographic findings suggestive of PSC. This entity should be suspected in patients with a clinical diagnosis of AIH who present with pruritus and have radiographic or histologic findings of PSC, known inflammatory bowel disease (specifically ulcerative colitis), and elevated alkaline phosphatase. Treatment of these patients is difficult. Corticosteroids alone or in combination with azathioprine have not been shown to be very effective. The addition of ursodiol to corticosteroids and azathioprine, however, has been shown in one small study to be helpful (see Chapter 52).

Cjaza AJ. Frequency and nature of the variant syndromes of autoimmune liver disease. *Hepatology*. 1998;28:360–365. [PMID: 9695997]

Floreani A, Rizzotto ER, Ferrara F, et al. Clinical course and outcome of autoimmune hepatitis/primary sclerosing cholangitis overlap syndrome. *Am J Gastroenterol.* 2005;100:1516–1522. [PMID: 15984974]

Talwalkar JA, Keach JC, Angulo P, et al. Overlap of autoimmune hepatitis and Primary biliary cirrhosis: an evaluation of a modified scoring system. *Am J Gastroenterol.* 2002;97:1191–1197. [PMID: 12014727]

Kuiper EM, Zondervan PE, Van Buuren HR. Paris criteria are effective in diagnosis of primary biliary cirrhosis and autoimmune hepatitis overlap syndrome. *Clin Gastroenterol Hepatol.* 2010;8:530–534. [PMID: 20304098]

WILSON DISEASE

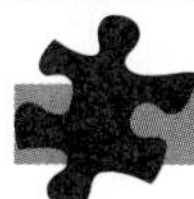

ESSENTIALS OF DIAGNOSIS

- ▶ Autosomally inherited disorder of copper metabolism.
- ▶ Genetic defect is a mutation in a P-type copper-dependent ATPase, ATP7B.
- ▶ Copper deposition in many tissues, with liver and neurologic disease the most prominent manifestations.
- ▶ Consider in any young person with chronic hepatitis or cirrhosis.
- ▶ Diagnosis is challenging and requires measurement of serum ceruloplasmin levels, measurement of urinary copper, and an ophthalmic examination; all three tests are necessary as only 40% of patients have abnormalities in all three.
- ▶ Liver biopsy is often necessary to confirm or stage disease.

General Considerations

Wilson disease is a rare disease of impaired biliary excretion of copper. It is an autosomal-recessive disorder with prevalence of approximately 1 in 30,000 persons. The defective gene is on chromosome 13 and has been identified as a copper dependent P-type ATPase. Copper is a co-factor for many proteins and is obtained through dietary consumption. On the average humans take in between 2 mg and 5 mg per day far in excess of the daily requirement of around 0.9 mg per day. Copper absorption occurs in the small intestine (duodenum and proximal jejunum), enters the portal circulation, and then is used for synthetic processes in the liver. Excess copper is secreted into bile for subsequent elimination.

Ala A, Walker AP, Ashkan K, et al. Wilson's disease. *Lancet.* 2007; 369:397–408. [PMID: 17276780]

Pathogenesis

The defective gene, *ATP7B*, encodes a transmembrane protein with two important physiologic roles: (1) transport of copper across the canalicular membrane into the biliary tract, and (2) transport of copper into the trans-Golgi network, where it complexes with an acute phase reactant and copper-binding protein, ceruloplasmin. When ATP7B is absent, copper accumulates within the lysosomes in the cell and is absent in the biliary secretions. This leads to accumulation of hepatocellular copper. Additionally, because copper is required for stability of ceruloplasmin, its serum half-life is markedly decreased in persons with Wilson disease. The low level of ceruloplasmin in patients with Wilson disease accounts for its use as a screening test (see later discussion).

Clinical Findings

Wilson disease is a disease of young people, manifesting most commonly in the second and the third decades of life. It is unusual for Wilson disease to manifest after the age of 40 and when it does, neurologic complications are often the principal presenting symptoms. Copper deposition in hepatic tissue can lead to liver disease in the form of chronic hepatitis or cirrhosis, or can present in a fulminant form known as fulminant Wilson disease.

A. Fulminant Disease

In fulminant Wilson disease there is marked transaminase elevation, with the aspartate aminotransferase (AST) level often greater than the ALT (additional AST is present as a result of accompanying Coombs-negative hemolytic anemia). Alkaline phosphatase is low, jaundice and liver failure invariably result, and survival is almost always dependent on the availability of liver transplantation.

B. Cirrhotic Disease

A more indolent form of liver disease results in cirrhosis. Patients may present with compensated disease or have significant evidence of hepatic dysfunction by the time of diagnosis. Physical signs of advanced liver disease are common, with spider angiomata, splenomegaly, and ascites.

C. Other Disease Manifestations

In addition to liver disease, patients with Wilson disease may have neurologic manifestations that represent the presenting features in 40–50% of patients. The resulting clinical manifestations occur as a result of copper deposition in many parts of the brain, including but not limited to the putamen, globus pallidus, caudate, and thalamus. Associated neurologic disorders include (1) a Parkinson-like movement disorder, (2) ataxia, (3) dystonia, and (4) tremors. Psychiatric manifestations may also occur and occasionally can dominate the presentation, with decline in performance status (eg, worsening school grades) and behavioral changes.

In addition to the liver and central nervous system, copper is deposited at other sites, leading to a range of disease manifestations. Deposition in the eye can result in Kayser-Fleischer rings and sunflower cataracts; both are visible on slit-lamp examinations. The former is a golden-brown pigment in the outside rim of the cornea, whereas the later is visualized as multicolored cataracts. Deposition of copper also occurs in the kidneys, predominantly in the proximal tubules, where a Fanconi-like syndrome may manifest. Proximal renal tubular acidosis and nephrolithiasis are possible consequences. Chondrocalcinosis, osteomalacia, and osteoarthritis are also common in patients with Wilson disease. Table 40–4 summarizes the clinical spectrum of Wilson disease.

Table 40–4. Clinical spectrum of Wilson disease.

Affected Organ	Clinical Manifestations
Liver	Chronic hepatitis Cirrhosis Fulminant liver failure
CNS	Spasticity and rigidity Ataxia Dystonia Tremors Behavioral changes Decreased performance status
Ophthalmic	Kayser-Fleischer rings Sunflower cataracts
Hematologic	Coombs-negative hemolytic anemia
Renal	Proximal renal tubular acidosis Nephrolithiasis Aminoaciduria Hypouricemia
Musculoskeletal	Chondrocalcinosis Osteoarthritis Osteomalacia Osteoporosis

D. Diagnostic Tests

The diagnosis of Wilson disease is often challenging but is based on a combination of astute clinical suspicion and laboratory data. The disease should be suspected in any young person who presents with unexplained, chronic active hepatitis or cirrhosis. Serum ceruloplasmin is an acute phase reactant and may be normal in approximately 20% of patients with Wilson disease due elevated levels in inflammatory conditions. Regardless, the initial screening test is the measurement of serum ceruloplasmin.

In patients with low ceruloplasmin or in whom there is a high clinical suspicion of Wilson disease, additional tests are needed for confirmation. These include slit-lamp examinations to look for Kayser-Fleischer rings and 24-hour urinary collection, which will show increased urinary excretion of copper (>100 mcg/24 h). Abnormalities in all three tests—ceruloplasmin, slit-lamp examination, and urinary copper measurement—are present in only about 40% of patients.

For some patients a liver biopsy is necessary and may show histologic evidence of copper deposition within the liver. In addition, measurement of the hepatic tissue content of copper can show elevated copper levels (normally ~55 mcg copper/g dry liver vs >250 mcg copper/g dry liver in Wilson disease). This is measurement is often helpful when the diagnosis is in doubt.

Although the genetic locus is known, mutational analysis is not widely used in clinical settings because of the multitude of mutations that have been identified. The most common mutation, a substitution of histidine with glutamine on amino acid 1069 of the coding sequence (H1069Q), is present in approximately 30% of patients with Wilson disease. Although widespread clinical utility of genetic testing is not common, the identification of a mutation within a family helps in screening relatives of the index case.

Ferenci P, Czlokowska A, Merle U, et al. Late-onset Wilson's disease. *Gastroenterology.* 2007;132:1294–1298. [PMID: 17433323]

Page RA, Davie CA, MacManus D, et al. Clinical correlation of brain MRI and MRS abnormalities in patients with Wilson disease. *Neurology.* 2004;63:638–643. [PMID: 15326235]

Roberts EA, Schilsky ML. Diagnosis and treatment of Wilson's disease: an update. *Hepatology.* 2008;47:2089–2111. [PMID: 18506894]

Differential Diagnosis

The differential diagnosis of Wilson disease includes acute and chronic hepatitides and depends on the form of presentation. In patients with fulminant Wilson disease, acute toxic injury, acute viral hepatitis, acute vascular hepatic injury, and AIH should be considered. For those presenting with chronic hepatitis, considerations should include toxic injury, chronic viral hepatitis, NASH, other inherited liver disorders, and AIH.

Treatment

Treatment of Wilson disease is geared toward mobilizing accumulated tissue copper (Table 40–5). At the same time, attempts should be made to prevent further copper absorption through the gastrointestinal tract. The first goal is accomplished by the use of chelating agents such as D-penicillamine and trientine. These agents bind tissue copper and then lead to elimination through the urinary tract.

D-Penicillamine is felt to be the first agent of choice, although its use is sometimes limited by side effects. These include allergic hypersensitivity reactions, proteinuria, immunosuppression, and a plethora of dermatologic changes. Penicillamine also interferes with the metabolism of pyridoxine, so it is usual to supplement for vitamin B_6, especially in children and pregnant women.

In patients who are unable to tolerate D-penicillamine, trientine should be used. Zinc, which competes with copper for intestinal absorption and therefore reduces the amount of copper that can be absorbed, is also a widely used therapeutic choice. Recent studies suggest that zinc monotherapy is not as effective as the chelating agents in preventing hepatic deterioration in patients with Wilson's disease. For those patients in whom zinc is used, many preparations are available, and gastrointestinal upset has been associated especially with the acetate form.

Lastly, dietary instructions should stress the avoidance of foods that are rich in copper, which include liver, chocolate, shellfish, and nuts.

Table 40–5. Treatment of Wilson disease.

Agent	Initial Dose	Maintenance Dose	Comment
Penicillamine	Adult: 250–500 mg/day to maximum of 1200–1500 mg/day in 2–4 divided doses Children: 20 mg/kg/day	Adult: 750–1000 mg/day in 2 divided doses	Give 1 h before or 2 h after eating Many possible acute-onset and delayed side effects Monitor: complete blood count, proteinuria Give vitamin B_6, 50 mg weekly
Trientine	Adult: 1200–800 mg/day in 2–3 divided doses Children: 20 mg/kg/day	Adult: 900–1200 mg/day in 2–3 divided doses	Give 1 h before or 2 h after eating Fewer side effects than penicillamine Safety in pregnancy unclear
Zinc	150 mg (elemental) in 3 divided doses	Same	Safe in pregnancy Some preparations may cause gastrointestinal upset

Roberts EA, Schilsky ML. Diagnosis and treatment of Wilson's disease: an update. *Hepatology.* 2008;47:2089–2111. [PMID: 18506894]

Weiss KH, Gotthardt DN, Klemm D, et al. Zinc monotherapy is not as effective as chelating agents in the treatment of Wilson's Disease. *Gastroenterology.* Dec 23,2010. epub ahead of print.

α_1-ANTITRYPSIN DEFICIENCY

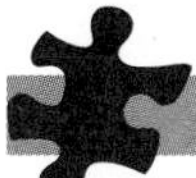

ESSENTIALS OF DIAGNOSIS

- Autosomal co-dominant disease resulting from defects in the *SERPINA1* gene.
- Produces a spectrum of disease; liver, lung, hematologic, and dermatologic complications are possible.
- Liver complications most often result from deposition of a poorly degradable mutant of α_1-antitrypsin (α_1-AT) in hepatocytes.
- Diagnosis is through measurement of serum α_1-AT levels followed by pi-typing for mutant alleles.
- Liver biopsy shows characteristic PAS-positive granules that are resistant to diastase.

General Considerations

α_1-Antitrypsin deficiency is an autosomal co-dominant disease that affects about 1 in 2000–5000 persons. It is most common in people of northern European descent.

Stoller JK, Aboussouan LS. Alpha1-antitrypsin deficiency. *Lancet.* 2005;365:2225–2236. [PMID: 15978931]

Pathogenesis

To date more than 100 mutant alleles of the culprit *SERPINA1* gene have been identified and implicated in lung, liver, or hematologic disease. The alleles are characterized phenotypically on the basis of their migration on pH gradient gels, with faster migrating variants, A (anodal), to slower migrating variants, Z. Normally migrating alleles are denoted as M; thus, individuals homozygous for the gene defect are denoted as MM. Individuals with ZZ alleles have severe deficiency of α_1-antitrypsin (α_1-AT).

Functionally, α_1-AT alleles can be categorized into four major groups:

1. Normal, with α_1-AT levels of greater than 80 mg/dL.
2. Deficiency alleles characterized by serum α_1-AT levels of less 80 mg/dL or decreased activity (eg, Z alleles). The Z allele is the most common deficiency variant, accounting for 95% of all α_1-AT deficiency. A single mutation of lysine to glutamate at position 342 is responsible.
3. Null variants in which there is a complete lack of circulating α_1-AT.
4. Dysfunctional variants in which the mutant protein results in a novel function, such as the *Pittsburgh* allele, which acts as a thrombin inhibitor.

Lomas DA, Mahadeva R. Alpha 1-antitrypsin polymerization and the serpinopathies: pathobiology and prospects for therapy. *J Clin Invest.* 2002;110:1585–1590. [PMID: 12464660]

Clinical Findings

A. Symptoms and Signs

α_1-AT deficiency causes several significant chronic clinical problems, including emphysema, which occurs mostly in the fourth and fifth decades of life as a result of unopposed activity of leukocyte elastase. This lung disease is accelerated in patients who smoke. A second clinical entity is panniculitis, which is characterized by the appearance of painful cutaneous nodules at sites of trauma. Additionally, hematologic problems can occur in persons who have the *Pittsburgh* allele, as noted earlier.

Chronic liver disease, unlike the associated lung disease, occurs due to accumulation of an insoluble and non-degraded mutant protein within hepatocytes. The spectrum of liver abnormalities includes chronic hepatitis, cirrhosis, and hepatocellular carcinoma. Among the patients with chronic hepatitis, the risk of cirrhosis has been estimated at between 12% and 50%. More than 25% of those with neonatal hepatitis die in the first decade of life.

B. Laboratory Findings

Evaluation of α_1-AT levels is usually the first step in the diagnostic workup of patients with suspected α_1-AT deficiency. For individuals with low circulating levels of α_1-AT, pi-typing is then performed to look for abnormal alleles that might lead either to lack of or for abnormal forms of α_1-AT. For patients with liver disease, histologic evaluation of the liver biopsy samples shows the presence of globules that are periodic acid-Schiff–positive and diastase-resistant.

American Thoracic Society; European Respiratory Society. American Thoracic Society/European Respiratory Society statement: standards for the diagnosis and management of individuals with alpha-1 antitrypsin deficiency. *Am J Respir Crit Care Med.* 2003;168:818–900. [PMID: 14522813]

Differential Diagnosis

The differential diagnosis is the same as for the other forms of chronic hepatitis discussed earlier.

Treatment

The only effective therapy for liver disease is transplantation in advanced cirrhosis. Recombinant α_1-antitrypsin, however, can be used in patients whose main presentation is emphysema.

Future therapies: In a mouse model of liver disease caused by aggregates of misfolded AIAT in liver, the burden of misfolded protein and the degree of liver fibrosis can be reduced by the use the autophagic enhancing drug carbamazepine. Such studies suggest that these groups of autophagy enhancing medicines may ultimately prove useful in treatment of persons with A1AT liver disease.

Hidvegi T, Ewing M, Hale P, et al. An autophagy-enhancing drug promotes degradation of mutant alpha1-antitrypsin Z and reduces hepatic fibrosis. *Science.* 2010;329:229–232. [PMID: 20522742]

Perlmutter D. Alpha-1-antitrypsin deficiency: importance of proteasomal and autophagic degradative pathways in disposal of liver disease-associated protein aggregates. *Ann Rev Med.* 2010. epub ahead of print [PMID: 20707674]

Hereditary Hemochromatosis

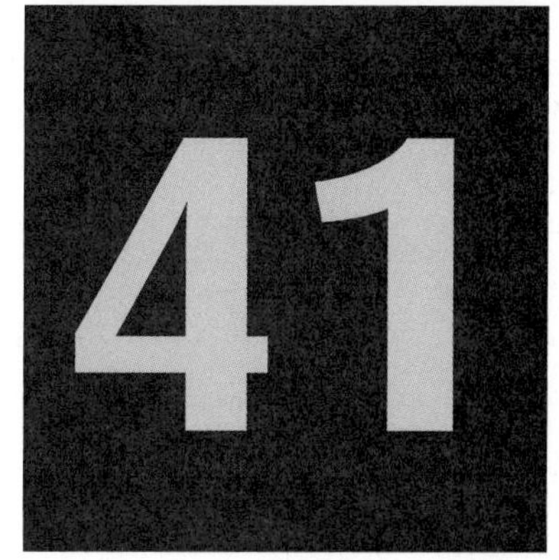

Benjamin Smith, MD
Norman D. Grace, MD

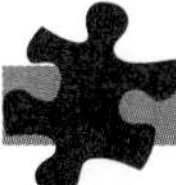

ESSENTIALS OF DIAGNOSIS

- Hemochromatosis classically refers to *HFE*-mediated genetic iron overload, but several alternatively mediated genetic iron overload syndromes have been described.
- C282Y is the major mutation and H63D the minor mutation of the *HFE* gene; individuals with two copies of C282Y or one copy of both mutations (compound heterozygote) are at risk for iron overload.
- Excess iron deposition in tissues leads to end-organ damage; advanced hemochromatosis typically involves the liver first and may also involve the pancreas, heart, pituitary gland and other organs.
- Most patients are identified by laboratory screening or family history and are asymptomatic at diagnosis.
- Symptomatic patients usually present with nonspecific complaints of fatigue, arthralgias, and abdominal pain.
- Screening studies include serum iron/total iron-binding capacity (abnormal if >45% in women, >50% in men) and serum ferritin (abnormal if >200 mcg/dL in women, >300 mcg/dL in men); if either test is positive, genetic testing should be pursued.
- Liver biopsy to assess iron concentration and hepatic iron index is indicated if serum ferritin is >1000 mcg/dL, liver tests are abnormal, or hepatomegaly is noted on physical examination.

General Considerations

Eighty percent of clinically established cases of hemochromatosis worldwide and over 90% of cases in the United States result from the autosomal-recessive inheritance of two copies of the major mutation (C282Y) of the *HFE* gene. Individuals with this genotype are described as C282Y homozygotes. Ten to 15% of Caucasian populations are heterozygotes, possessing one copy of the major mutation. This mutation is believed to have originated more than 6000 years ago amid Celtic or Viking ancestry. It has been postulated that the mutation may have had a potential selective advantage, preventing iron deficiency in the setting of scarce resources such as red meat.

Prevalence estimates of homozygosity for the C282Y mutation in populations of Northern European descent are 1 in 260 persons. Prevalence rates vary by gender and ethnicity. The disease is more common in men, which is attributed to increased dietary iron consumption as well as iron losses in women during menstruation. The disease is rarely seen in African Americans, Mexican Americans, and Asians. Approximately 90–95% of *HFE*-related hemochromatosis cases in the United States are related to homozygosity for C282Y and 80% in European populations (EASL p. 4).

One copy of the H63D mutation, the minor mutation of the *HFE* gene, may be found in 15–40% of Caucasian populations. About 4% of cases of hemochromatosis result from the inheritance of one copy of the major mutation, C282Y, and one copy of the minor mutation, H63D. These individuals are described as compound heterozygotes. However, the great majority of compound heterozygotes will not develop clinically significant iron overload. The risk has been estimated to be 200 times less than in C282Y homozygotes. H63D homozygotes typically do not develop clinically significant iron overload. Individuals with this genotype may have an elevated transferrin saturation, but an elevated ferritin should prompt a search for secondary causes of iron overload.

Phenotypic expression of these altered gene states is variable and, as a result, the proportion of patients who go on to develop clinically significant hemochromatosis remains uncertain. It has been estimated that 38–50% of C282Y homozygotes will develop iron overload, but only 10–33% will manifest hemochromatosis-related morbidity. Men are much more likely than women to develop iron overload-related disease (28% vs 1%). The majority of individuals who develop end-organ damage likely have cofactors such as significant alcohol intake or NASH. Overall, secondary causes of iron overload are still more common than primary iron overload syndromes.

Allen KJ, Gurrin LC, Constantine CC, et al. Iron-overload-related disease in HFE hereditary hemochromatosis. *N Engl J Med.* 2008;358:221–230. [PMID: 18199861]

Jackson HA, Carter K, Darke C, et al. HFE mutations, iron deficiency and overload in 10,500 blood donors. *Br J Haematol.* 2001;114:474–484. [PMID: 11529872]

Pathogenesis

A. Normal Iron Metabolism

The quantity of total body iron is closely regulated and is estimated to be approximately 3 g in women and 5 g in men. Most of this iron is incorporated into red blood cells. The remainder is stored in the liver and a small amount in skeletal muscle. Almost all iron absorption occurs in the duodenum. After iron is absorbed, it circulates bound to the carrier protein transferrin for distribution to tissues. In addition to taking up inorganic iron in this way, the duodenal enterocytes may also take up iron in the form of heme.

Most of the circulating iron is taken up within sites of erythropoiesis, where it is incorporated into hemoglobin by developing erythrons. The liver serves as a storage reservoir for iron and then releases iron back into circulation as needed. As red blood cells senesce, they are phagocytosed by macrophages which then process and release iron for recycling into newly developing cells at a controlled rate.

The amount of iron absorbed from food can be up-regulated quickly when excess iron is lost or utilized, such as through menstruation, pregnancy, or gastrointestinal bleeding. Small amounts of iron, on the order of 1–2 mg daily, are lost as cells of the gastrointestinal and urogenital tracts are shed. An Additional 1–2 mg of iron are lost daily by women during their reproductive years. However, the human body has no effective physiologic mechanism for excreting excess iron. The duodenal enterocytes must correctly sense or be signaled to absorb enough iron to replace losses but no more.

The duodenal enterocytes, hepatocytes, and macrophages all appear to play important roles in iron homeostasis. Because they function at sites distant from one another, it has been hypothesized that they communicate via a hormone or hormones. Multiple factors influence iron absorption, including both systemic and intestinal factors. Systemic factors include the level of body iron stores, erythropoietic activity, hemoglobin concentration, and oxygen saturation as well as the presence or absence of inflammatory cytokines. Intestinal factors include pancreatic insufficiency and disturbances in pH. Disorders of iron metabolism develop when disease states overwhelm the homeostatic mechanisms. For example, infections or chronic inflammation induce iron sequestration by macrophages and signal a decrease of iron absorption, leading to the anemia of chronic disease. Conversely, disorders of erythropoiesis, such as the thalassemias, release signals promoting iron absorption by developing erythrons that overwhelm the inhibitory signals generated by excessive accumulation of iron stores.

Sharma N, Butterworth J, Cooper BT, et al. The emerging role of the liver in iron metabolism. *Am J Gastroenterol.* 2005;100: 201–206. [PMID: 15654801]

B. Hereditary Hemochromatosis

In hereditary hemochromatosis, one or more genetic mutations lead to excess iron absorption relative to body iron stores. The excess iron is stored in the liver initially but, if unrecognized and untreated, the iron may deposit in multiple end organs when hepatic storage is saturated, leading to the phenotypic expression of the disease. Iron spillover has been observed once total body stores reach 4.5 g with hepatic levels in excess of 400 mcg/g of tissue.

In 1996, Feder and colleagues published the discovery of a candidate gene for hemochromatosis located on the short arm of chromosome 6, now called *HFE.* As noted earlier, two mutations are now recognized. The major mutation results from a tyrosine substitution for cysteine at the 282 amino acid position on the gene and is abbreviated Cys282Tyr or simply C282Y. The minor mutation results from an aspartate substitution for histidine at the 63rd amino acid position and is abbreviated His63Asp or simply H63D.

Feder JN, Gnirke A, Thomas W, et al. A novel MHC class I-like gene is mutated in patients with hereditary hemochromatosis. *Nat Genet.* 1996;13:399–408. [PMID: 8696333]

C. Pathophysiology of Iron Overload in Hereditary Hemochromatosis

The initial model for iron overload in *HFE*-related hemochromatosis postulated that the *HFE* mutation acted at the level of the developing duodenal crypt cell. These cells elaborate iron transporters (DMT-1), as they differentiate and migrate toward the villus tip (Figure 41–1). Within this so-called crypt-programming model, the crypt cells would correctly assess or "sense" the amount of iron in circulation through *HFE*-dependent uptake of transferrin-bound iron at their basolateral membrane and thereby program production of the appropriate number of iron transporters in the differentiating cell. The *HFE* mutation would disable normal uptake of iron by the nascent crypt cells, leading to incorrect "sensing" of an iron-deficient state and to programming of an excessive number of iron transporters (Figure 41–2).

The crypt-programming model has been challenged by recent experimental data. Changes in iron absorption occur

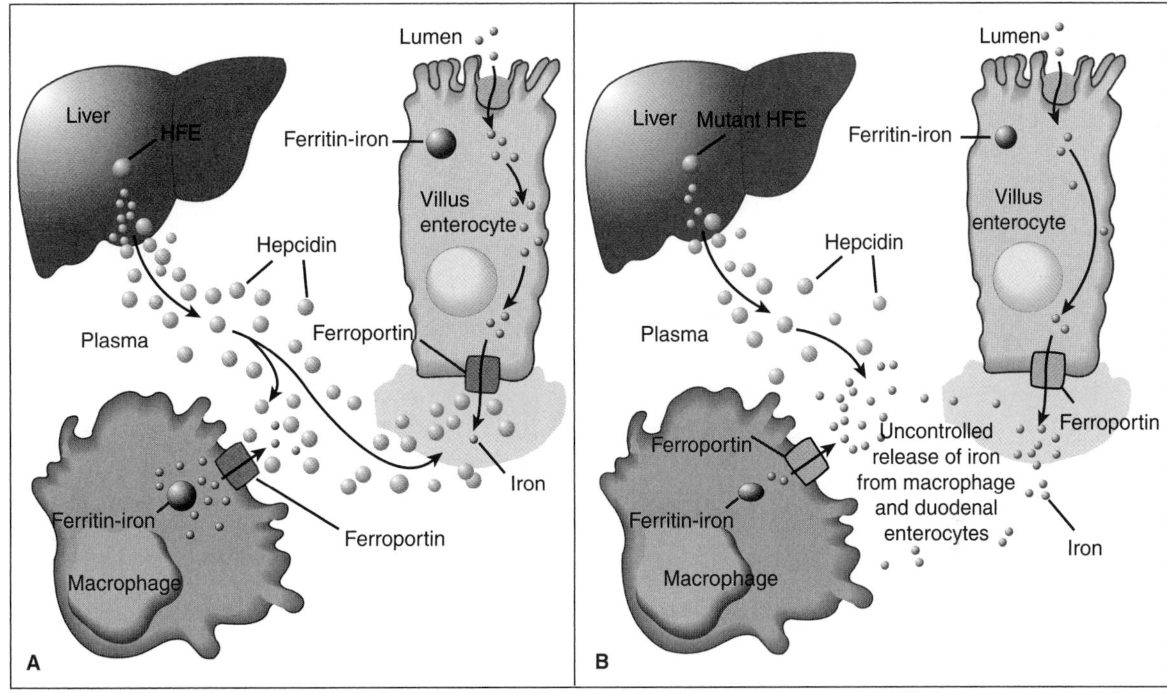

▲ **Figure 41–1.** Hepcidin model. Hepcidin normally functions as a regulatory protein, inhibiting release of iron from villus enterocytes and macrophages, which in turn inhibits iron absorption. **A:** Normal. **B:** *HFE*-related hemochromatosis. (Adapted, with permission, from Pietrangelo A. Hereditary hemochromatosis—a new look at an old disease. *N Engl J Med.* 2004;350:2389.)

within hours of a change in iron status, whereas enterocyte maturation takes days. Furthermore, other forms of iron overload, such as juvenile hemochromatosis, occur in the absence of *HFE* mutations. This suggests the existence of other factors with a more fundamental role in iron homeostasis.

Investigators have shifted their focus from the duodenum to the liver, where the protein hepcidin is now considered the key regulator of iron absorption. It was first described by Park and colleagues, who named it after its site of synthesis in the liver and its antibacterial properties. Hepcidin is a 25 amino acid peptide encoded by the *HAMP* gene. There is an inverse relationship between the level of hepcidin and iron absorption. In mouse models of hereditary hemochromatosis, decreasing hepcidin production by silencing the *HAMP* gene encoding hepcidin results in severe iron overload. In iron-deficient mice, hepcidin production is also decreased, leading to increased iron absorption. In *HFE* knockout mice with iron overload, stimulating hepcidin production successfully reverses the iron overload.

Similarly, humans with *HFE*-related hereditary hemochromatosis have low levels of hepcidin mRNA in liver biopsy specimens despite iron overload. Weinstein and colleagues reported on two patients with large hepatic adenomas overexpressing hepcidin who presented with severe microcytic anemia. Resection of the masses reversed the hematologic abnormalities.

Hepcidin appears to have several targets. The primary target is ferroportin, the main iron exporter from mammalian cells such as duodenal enterocytes. When hepcidin binds to ferroportin at the basolateral cell surface of enterocytes, this leads to ferroportin internalization and degradation. This, in turn, limits iron export from enterocytes, leading to accumulation of iron within these cells and decreased iron absorption. Reticuloendothelial macrophages also have ferroportin receptors, and the effects of hepcidin here are thought to be similar.

The mechanism by which *HFE* mutations lead to iron overload is incompletely understood. *HFE* mutations lead to low levels of hepcidin, which leads to unchecked release of iron from duodenal enterocytes and macrophages. This leads, in turn, to uncontrolled iron absorption and the hemochromatosis phenotype (see Figure 41–2). However, the pathways by which *HFE* mutations lower hepcidin levels remain to be elucidated. One theory is that *HFE* is a participant in hepatocyte sensing of body iron status, perhaps as part of a hepatocyte sensing unit together with TfR1 and TfR2. Hepatocytes elaborate TfR2 receptors on their surface which may bind to diferric transferrin (Tf) in portal blood, possibly sensing the circulating level of iron by this means.

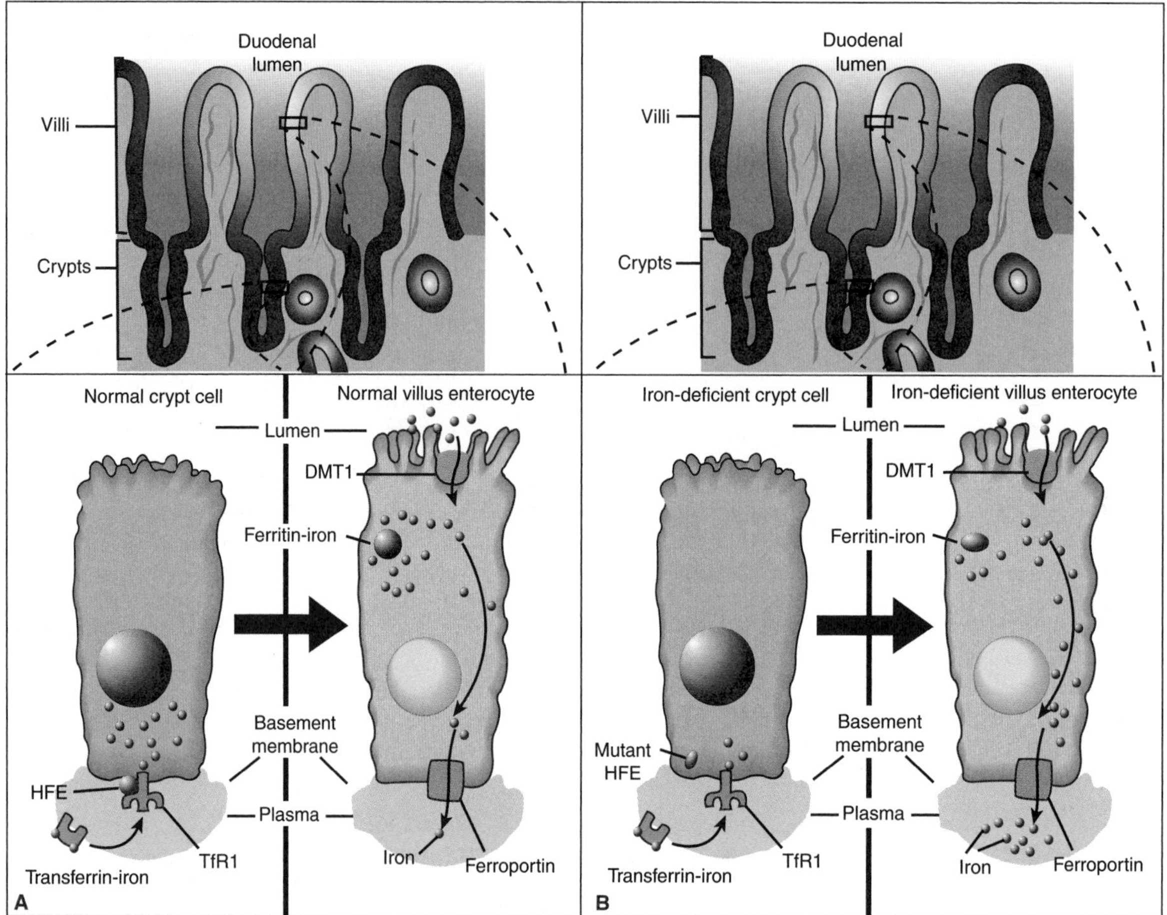

▲ **Figure 41–2.** Crypt-programming model. The *HFE* mutation interferes with duodenal uptake of iron. **A:** Normal. **B:** *HFE*-related hemochromatosis. (Adapted, with permission, from Pietrangelo A. Hereditary hemochromatosis—a new look at an old disease. *N Engl J Med.* 2004;350:2389.)

HFE mutations could theoretically influence the binding and thereby the sensing of diferric Tf by hepatocytes and lead to lower levels of hepcidin. Another sensing unit may include hemojuvelin (HJV) together with two other proteins, BMP6 and neogenin (see non-HFE HHC below for more on HJV). These two sensing units may work independently or together to modulate hepcidin expression in the nucleus of the hepatocyte through a common intracellular signal transduction cascade. The intermediaries in this cascade likely include a BMP ligand on the cell surface and intracellular mediators and modulators known as SMAD proteins.

Bridle KR, Frazer DM, Wilkins SJ, et al. Disrupted hepcidin regulation in HFE-associated hemochromatosis and the liver as a regulator of body iron homoeostasis. *Lancet.* 2003;361:669–673. [PMID: 12606179]

Fleming RE, Bacon BR. Orchestration of iron homeostasis. *N Engl J Med.* 2005;352:1741–1744. [PMID: 15858181]

Nemeth E, Tuttle MS, Powelson J, et al. Hepcidin regulates cellular iron efflux by binding to ferroportin and inducing its internalization. *Science.* 2004;306:2090–2093. [PMID: 15514116]

Park CH, Valore EV, Waring AJ, et al. Hepcidin, a urinary antimicrobial peptide synthesized in the liver. *J Biol Chem.* 2001; 276:7806–7810. [PMID: 11113131]

Pietrangelo A. Hereditary hemochromatosis: pathogenesis, diagnosis and treatment. *Gastroenterology.* 2010;139:393–408. [PMID: 20542038]

Roy CN, Enns CA. Iron homeostasis: new tales from the crypt. *Blood.* 2000;96:4020–4027. [PMID: 11110669]

Weinstein DA, Roy CN, Fleming MD, et al. Inappropriate expression of hepcidin is associated with iron refractory anemia: implications for the anemia of chronic disease. *Blood.* 2002; 100:3776–3781. [PMID: 12393428]

D. Disease-Modifying Agents

The fact that only a small percentage of C282Y homozygotes develop signs and symptoms of iron overload suggests that other genetic and environmental modifiers are present. Perhaps other proteins influencing hepcidin expression may compensate for the effects of the *HFE* mutation.

Alcohol consumption is a major environmental factor modifying disease activity. Much higher rates of cirrhosis have been observed in patients with hereditary hemochromatosis who consume more than 60 g of alcohol per day. Investigations into the mechanism of action of alcohol on exacerbating disease activity have demonstrated down-regulation of hepcidin activity as well as increased C/EBPα, DMT-1, and ferroportin expression in animal models. In addition, it is believed that alcohol and iron deposition may act synergistically to promote fibrosis through increased oxidative stress and hepatic stellate cell activation.

E. Non-*HFE* Hemochromatosis

Although *HFE* mutations are responsible for the great majority of cases of hemochromatosis worldwide, the commercial availability of testing for *HFE* mutations soon identified individuals and subpopulations with significant iron overload in the absence of these mutations. Three other gene mutations have been identified that cause autosomal-recessive iron overload with a phenotype very similar to that of *HFE*-related hemochromatosis. They are the *HJV* gene on chromosome 1, the *HAMP* gene on chromosome 19, and the *TfR2* gene on chromosome 7. All three mutations decrease hepcidin levels and lead to a primarily hepatocellular deposition of excess iron (Table 41–1).

The term *juvenile hemochromatosis* was first used in 1979 to describe an overload syndrome that resembled *HFE*-related hemochromatosis but with iron loading and end-organ damage at an early age. This form of severe hemochromatosis appears to be caused by mutations in either the *hemojuvelin* (*HJV*) or *HAMP* genes. *HJV* mutations have been identified in 12 families from France, Greece, and Canada. The possible mechanism by which hemojuvelin modulates hepcidin expression is outlined above in the pathophysiology section C. Mutations in *HJV* appear to be more common than mutations of the *HAMP* gene, which encodes hepcidin. *HAMP* mutations may lead to severe and potentially fatal iron overload before age 30, corroborating the critical role of hepcidin in iron homeostasis.

TfR2 mutations lead to a milder form of iron overload similar to *HFE*. Mutations have been identified in individuals from France and Japan. The predominant site of *TfR2* expression is in hepatocytes. The potential mechanism by which *TfR2* mutations lead to low hepcidin levels and iron overload is outlined earlier under Pathophysiology of Iron Overload, Section C.

Ferroportin is the target of hepcidin in duodenal enterocytes and macrophages. Two mutations have been identified that lead to autosomal-dominant iron overload. One mutation inactivates ferroportin and leads to retention of iron in duodenal enterocytes and macrophages, called ferroportin disease. The result is a primarily reticuloendothelial distribution of iron within the macrophage populations of the liver, spleen and bone marrow. Circulating levels of iron tend to be lower than in *HFE*-related hemochromatosis with a high serum ferritin but normal or low transferrin saturation. Since the parenchymal cells of the affected end organs do not accumulate iron in ferroportin disease, there is minimal end organ damage, and aggressive phlebotomy can actually lead to iron-restricted anemia. Ferroportin disease is the second-most-common cause of inherited hyperferritinemia after hemochromatosis caused by HFE mutations. The second ferroportin mutation partially disables the interaction between ferroportin and hepcidin, leading to hepcidin resistance. This leads to effects similar to low levels of hepcidin with a primarily hepatocellular distribution of iron similar to *HFE*-related disease.

Recognition of these different genes, and the influence of their proteins on iron metabolism, has led to a new classification of iron overload syndromes in the Online Mendelian Inheritance in Man (OMIM) database (see Table 41–1).

Table 41–1 OMIM classification of primary iron overload syndromes.

OMIM	Implicated Gene	Gene Product	Hepcidin Level	Pattern of Inheritance	Potential for Organ Damage	Hepatic Iron Deposition
Type 1	*HFE*, 6p21.3	HFE	Low	AR	Variable	Parenchymal
Type 2A	*HJV*, 1q21	Hemojuvelin	Low	AR	High	Parenchymal
Type 2B	*HAMP*, 19q13.1	Hepcidin	Absent	AR	High	Parenchymal
Type 3	*TfR2*, 7q22	Transferrin receptor 2	Low	AR	Variable	Parenchymal
Type 4	*SLC40A1*, 2q32	Ferroportin	High	AD	Low	Reticuloendothelial

AD, autosomal dominant; AR, autosomal recessive; OMIM, Online Mendelian Inheritance in Man database.
Data from the OMIM database, available at: http://www.ncbi.nlm.nih.gov/omim/online, and from Pietrangelo A. Hereditary hemochromatosis—a new look at an old disease. *N Engl J Med*. 2004;350:2383.

As noted in the Pathophysiology of Iron Overload, Section C, it is likely that the constitutive expression of hepcidin or up-regulation in response to iron depends on the hepcidin-regulating activities of the proteins noted in the OMIM, including HFE, TfR2, and HJV. These may function independently or interdependently. The relative importance of the different proteins on hepcidin expression and therefore iron metabolism is reflected by the severity of iron overload that develops in their absence: Mutations in the *HJV* (or *HAMP*) gene lead to an early development of severe iron overload, whereas either *HFE* or *TfR2* mutations alone lead to a milder phenotype that develops later in life, if at all.

It is now apparent not only that mutations in multiple genes may lead to the hemochromatosis phenotype but also that various combinations of mutations may be responsible for the variable presentation of the disease. Merryweather-Clarke and colleagues, for example, described two families of C282 heterozygotes with different mutations of the *HAMP* gene. Family members inheriting one copy of C282Y and one allele with the *HAMP* mutation develop significant iron overload. Pietrangelo and colleagues described patients with "juvenile hemochromatosis" but without either the *HAMP* or *HJV* mutations. The severe phenotype in their cases developed from inheritance of both *HFE* and *TfR2* mutations and their additive effects on iron metabolism.

The rate at which iron accumulates in the different types of hemochromatosis affects the phenotype. Mutations in the hemojuvelin and HAMP genes typically leads to overtly symptomatic disease before age twenty affecting the heart and endocrine organs. The liver is relatively spared. On the other hand, the gradual accumulation of iron that typically occurs with HFE and TfR2 mutations, leads to minimally symptomatic disease that affects the liver first and uncommonly affects the other end organs. Intermediate phenotypes may occur with other combinations of mutations.

Merryweather-Clarke AT, Cadet E, Bomfor A, et al. Digenic inheritance of mutations in HAMP and HFE results in different types of hemochromatosis. *Hum Mol Genet.* 2003;12:2241–2247. [PMID: 12915468]

Pietrangelo A. Hereditary hemochromatosis—a new look at an old disease. *N Engl J Med.* 2004;350:2383–2397. [PMID: 15175440]

Clinical Findings

A. Symptoms and Signs

Iron overload is typically an insidious process. Patients are commonly asymptomatic until 10–20 g of iron stores have accumulated in parenchymal tissues. Diagnosis is typically made earlier in men, as iron overload is often delayed by menstrual losses and decreased dietary intake in women. As a result, while men are typically diagnosed in the fourth to fifth decade of life, women are diagnosed on average a decade later. As the use of screening laboratory measures has increased, more patients are now being diagnosed in an asymptomatic stage.

1. Presentation—Clinical manifestations of iron overload include unexplained fatigue, arthralgias, weight loss, abdominal pain, and reduced libido. Identification of the most common genetic abnormalities associated with hereditary hemochromatosis has led increasingly to diagnosis in asymptomatic individuals.

Hereditary hemochromatosis can lead to iron deposition within multiple organ sites. Complications by organ system are reviewed below.

2. Liver—Elevated liver enzymes, hepatomegaly, or cirrhosis is present in greater than 95% of patients with clinically advanced hereditary hemochromatosis. Liver manifestations usually do not begin until liver stores become saturated (6–7 g). The majority of deaths related to hereditary hemochromatosis (89%) are attributable to complications of cirrhosis. Overall, the risk of hepatocellular carcinoma in patients with hereditary hemochromatosis who develop cirrhosis is 200 times that of the general population (5% annual risk after the development of cirrhosis). Pathologically, the presence of "iron-free" nodules on histologic examination has correlated with onset of hepatocellular carcinoma.

With treatment, elevations in liver function tests and hepatomegaly are reversible. No strong evidence currently exists with respect to the reversibility of portal hypertension with treatment.

3. Cardiac—Iron deposition within cardiac tissue can lead to either dilated cardiomyopathy or a mixed dilated-restrictive picture. Conduction disturbances such as atrial fibrillation or sick-sinus syndrome have also been linked with hereditary hemochromatosis. The extent of cardiac involvement is highly variable and does not necessarily correlate with the extent of other organ involvement. Dysrhythmias and cardiomyopathy are the leading cause of sudden death in patients with iron overload.

With phlebotomy, both the cardiomyopathy and dysrhythmias associated with iron deposition can be reversed, albeit to a variable extent.

4. Endocrine—Diabetes mellitus and hypogonadism are the most commonly described endocrinopathies associated with hereditary hemochromatosis. The prevalence is significantly increased in type 1 diabetes whereas the prevalence of the HFE gene in type 2 diabetes is similar to the general population. The onset of diabetes has been described in up to 65% of patients with symptomatic iron overload. The mechanism is believed to be twofold: both direct damage to pancreatic islet cells by iron deposition as well as increased insulin resistance due to higher circulating iron levels. The incidence of diabetes is increased in patients with a family history of diabetes, suggesting that a genetic predisposition is at least partially responsible. Unlike the cardiac disturbances, the diabetes associated with hereditary hemochromatosis is often nonreversible despite therapy for iron overload.

Reduced secretion of gonadotropin as a result of iron interference in the hypothalamic-pituitary axis can lead to hypogonadism. This is the second most common form of endocrinopathy associated with hereditary hemochromatosis and can present as impotence, amenorrhea, and reduced libido, as well as osteoporosis. Secondary hypothyroidism is a less common form of endocrinopathy seen in men with hereditary hemochromatosis. Patients who develop hypogonadism or hypothyroidism often require lifelong hormone supplementation.

5. Arthropathy—Twenty to 70% of symptomatic patients present with complaints of arthropathy. Classically, the second and third metacarpophalangeal and proximal interphalangeal joints of the hands are involved. In addition, the wrists, shoulders, knees, and ankles can be affected. Radiographically, joint space narrowing is accompanied by squared-off bone ends and hook-like osteophytes. These changes resemble those of calcium pyrophosphate crystal deposition disease (pseudogout). It has been difficult to tease apart the contribution of hereditary hemochromatosis to arthropathy given the relatively high prevalence of joint disease in the general population. Significant improvement in symptoms is not often observed with treatment of the underlying iron overload.

6. Pigmentation—The classically described metallic or slate-gray hue described as "bronzing" is a result of increased melanin in the dermis. In addition, direct iron deposition in the dermis contributes to the gray appearance. Although best appreciated by examining the volar (unexposed) portion of the forearms, additional sites of involvement include the face, neck, dorsum of the hands, lower legs, and genital regions. Cutaneous atrophy, flattening of the nails, and loss of body hair has also been described. Estimates of the prevalence of bronzing in symptomatic individuals range from 18% to 47%. Data is sparse with respect to changes in pigmentation with phlebotomy therapy.

B. Laboratory Findings

1. General approach—Patients suspected of iron overload, based on either symptoms or routine laboratory testing, should undergo a thorough history and review of systems. Emphasis should be placed on eliciting symptoms suggesting involvement of the gastrointestinal, cardiac, endocrine, and rheumatologic systems. Because the C282Y homozygous state does not necessarily translate into clinical disease, the diagnosis of hereditary hemochromatosis is determined by a combination of genetic, serologic, and clinical features. Current diagnostic markers include gene analysis, iron studies, liver biopsy, and response to therapy.

2. Serum iron studies—Initial evaluation usually begins with serologic testing of iron studies. All serologic testing should be conducted in the fasting state. The transferrin saturation is regarded as the single best screening test for hereditary hemochromatosis. Although widely accepted as an accurate marker of the genetic defect in *HFE*-associated hemochromatosis, there is controversy over the optimal cutoff level. Previously suggested levels include transferrin saturation of 45% or higher, 55% and higher, and 60% and higher, as thresholds. With increasing thresholds, sensitivity is sacrificed for greater specificity. However, the transferrin saturation does not reflect the extent of hepatic iron stores. The unsaturated iron-binding capacity (UIBC) has also been examined as a single test for screening patients for hereditary hemochromatosis with similar results to the transferrin saturation.

Serum ferritin has been employed as an index of the body's iron stores with a high sensitivity but a relatively low specificity. Although the ferritin level is typically greatly elevated in hereditary hemochromatosis, ferritin may also be elevated as an acute phase reactant in additional inflammatory states in the absence of the genetic disease, notably alcoholic liver disease, nonalcoholic steatohepatitis, and chronic hepatitis C. Combined measurement of the percent transferrin saturation and serum ferritin provides a simple means to exclude patients from further analysis. If either is elevated in the absence of a known inflammatory condition, further genetic testing for hereditary hemochromatosis is indicated. We generally apply a combination threshold of transferrin saturation >45% with a ferritin >200 mcg/L for women, and a transferrin saturation >50% with a ferritin >300 mcg/L for men.

C. Imaging Studies and Special Tests

1. Liver biopsy—Liver biopsy provides information relevant to the diagnosis and staging of hemochromatosis. Sampling of liver tissue provides documentation of fibrosis or cirrhosis. It also helps evaluate for additional causes of liver disease. Biopsy also allows determination of the hepatic iron index (ratio of hepatic iron concentration to age of the patient). An index greater than 1.9 is highly supportive of hereditary hemochromatosis and helps to distinguish that disease from alcoholic liver disease.

With the widespread availability of genetic testing, liver biopsy for diagnostic purposes is now reserved for cases in which either genetic testing is unavailable or non–*HFE*-related iron overload is suspected in patients with suggestive iron studies but a normal *HFE* gene analysis. Current guidelines also recommend biopsy in C282Y homozygotes or C282Y/H63D compound heterozygotes older than age 40, with a serum ferritin level greater than 1000 and abnormal liver enzymes or hepatomegaly, or both. If none of these indicators of chronic liver disease is present, studies have suggested that the presence of significant fibrosis or cirrhosis is unlikely and liver biopsy may be deferred, provided treatment to deplete iron stores is initiated. The presence of abnormal liver enzymes and hepatomegaly at any age are indications to pursue a biopsy. Younger C282Y homozygotes with normal iron studies can defer biopsy with repeat testing of iron studies every 5 years. European guidelines suggest a ferritin measurement annually. The guidelines of the American

Association for the Study of Liver Diseases (AASLD) recommend biopsy for simple C282Y heterozygotes with elevated iron studies and liver enzymes.

2. Quantitative phlebotomy—Although not providing information with respect to the extent of disease, quantitative phlebotomy can be used to diagnose iron overload. The calculated iron storage can be assessed by determining the number of phlebotomies required to produce iron deficiency. Four phlebotomy sessions of 500 mL each will remove approximately 1 g of iron. Calculated iron storage greater than 5 g is considered abnormal.

3. Imaging studies—Noninvasive imaging techniques have not yet seen widespread use in the diagnosis or staging of hereditary hemochromatosis. In general, noninvasive imaging is useful for advanced disease but is not feasible for screening of early disease.

MRI studies have found a relatively high concordance between MRI and liver biopsy with respect to detection of hepatic iron levels. MRI also has the ability to distinguish parenchymal from mesenchymal iron overload and to detect iron-free neoplastic nodules.

Transient elastography has shown promise for the detection of advanced fibrosis and cirrhosis. Similarly, the superconducting quantum interference device susceptometer (SQUID) enables an in vivo measurement of hepatic iron that appears to be quantitatively equivalent to liver biopsy measurement of hepatic iron. The technique has not yet been validated for HHC patients.

Initial studies suggest that serum hyaluronic acid levels appear to correlate well with the degree of hepatic fibrosis in HHC patients with advanced disease. If these data are corroborated, it would provide another noninvasive tool for assessing fibrosis and cirrhosis.

4. Genetic testing—Discovery of the *HFE* gene, and the C282Y and H63D mutations, has revolutionized the diagnosis of hereditary hemochromatosis. Genetic testing for these mutations should be undertaken in any patient with documentation of iron overload based on the results of laboratory testing. The results of genetic testing, however, must be combined with a patient's clinical presentation as penetrance of the genetic defect is variable, in some recent estimates below 1%. Genetic testing is not recommended for the general population. However, it should be considered in patients with porphyria cutanea tarda, *chondrocalcinosis*, hepatocellular carcinoma or type 1 diabetes mellitus.

5. Screening for hereditary hemochromatosis

A. Family screening—Screening of first-degree relatives of C282Y homozygotes is universally recommended. Siblings have a 1 in 4 to 1 in 2 chance of inheriting the mutation, depending on whether the parents are homozygous or heterozygous for the mutation. Children of C282Y homozygotes have an approximately 1 in 20 chance of inheriting two copies of the C282Y mutation.

Once an individual is identified with hemochromatosis, his or her spouse should be genotyped if the couple has more than one child. If the spouse has at least one copy of the major or minor mutation, then the children should undergo *HFE* gene testing. It is more cost-effective to directly genotype an only child. Genetic screening of family members is preferred over phenotypic screening methods due to improved efficiency, as biochemical iron overload is not always present initially. Screening of first- to third-degree relatives of carriers may detect up to 40% of at-risk individuals.

B. Population-based screening—Hereditary hemochromatosis satisfies many of the criteria set forth by the U.S. Preventative Services Task Force and World Health Organization to determine diseases appropriate for population screening. Hereditary hemochromatosis has adequate prevalence with a prolonged latent phase. In addition, treatment for the disease has been shown to be widely successful in forestalling associated complications that, if untreated, can be associated with significant morbidity and mortality. Moreover, testing for hemochromatosis is relatively inexpensive, widely available, and reliable.

Issues that have hindered acceptance of widespread screening guidelines for hereditary hemochromatosis have included varying case definitions, relatively low phenotypic expression, concerns about discrimination (ie, insurance coverage) for HFE patients who do not phenotypically express, as well as disagreement over the cost-effectiveness of general population screening.

EASL clinical guidelines for HFE hemochromatosis. *J Hepatol.* 2010:53:3–22. [PMID: 20471131]

Ombiga J, Adams LA, Tang K, et al. Screening for HFE and iron overload. *Semin Liver Dis.* 2005;25:402–410. [PMID: 16315134]

Qaseem A, Aronson M, Fitterman N, et al. Screening for hereditary hemochromatosis: a clinical practice guideline from the American College of Physicians. *Ann Intern Med.* 2005;143: 517–521. [PMID: 16204164]

Treatment

Phlebotomy has been the mainstay of treatment for iron overload. Initiation of therapeutic phlebotomy has been demonstrated to have significant survival benefit in patients with and without cirrhosis. Every four phlebotomy treatments removes approximately 1 g of iron. Although an optimal regimen has not been specified, early and rapid depletion of iron stores is the goal of therapy. Weekly phlebotomy is generally instituted in the early phase of treatment, with frequent monitoring of the hemoglobin as well as ferritin levels. In most cases, the therapeutic goal is a serum ferritin level less than 50 mcg/L. After initial depletion of iron stores, maintenance phlebotomy can be performed two to four times a year with ongoing periodic monitoring of serum ferritin levels. While there are no good data to guide the endpoint of maintenance therapy regimens, one common practice is to maintain the serum ferritin between 50 and 100 mcg/L. Some patients may reaccumulate iron very slowly, perhaps due to decreased iron absorption in the setting of proton pump inhibitor therapy or iron loss from chronic NSAID use. If iron loss is suspected , appropriate investigation should be pursued, guided by the clinical circumstances. Maintaining appropriate follow-up is the key to avoiding the damaging long-term effects of iron deposition, avoiding cirrhosis, and improving overall survival.

With the general success and relatively low cost of phlebotomy, chelation therapy for hereditary hemochromatosis is only rarely employed. Subcutaneous desferrioxamine (1–2 g daily infused over 8 hours) is typically used when phlebotomy is contraindicated or in the case of specific cardiac disease that can be improved with aggressive iron depletion.

Prognosis

HFE-related hemochromatosis is the most common autosomal-recessive disorder in Caucasians with an incidence of approximately 1:260 population. It remains underdiagnosed, although early diagnosis before the development of cirrhosis is essentially curative. The discovery of *HFE* has led to a rapid evolution of our understanding and management of this disease.

It now appears that hepcidin is the key regulator of iron homeostasis, influenced by multiple proteins, including HFE, TfR2, and HJV. Mutations in multiple genes may lead to the hemochromatosis phenotype. The unifying feature is iron overload that begins with early expansion of the plasma iron compartment, resulting from inappropriate release of iron from villus enterocytes and macrophages. Progressive parenchymal iron deposition ensues with the potential for severe organ damage.

The phenotypic expression of hemochromatosis may be influenced by multiple other host and environmental factors. For example, C282Y homozygotes experience increased rates of cirrhosis and a poorer prognosis when faced with added insults to the liver such as alcohol or nonalcoholic steatohepatitis. In addition, patients with both hereditary hemochromatosis and hepatitis C have been found to be less responsive to treatment with combination interferon and ribavirin.

Areas for future investigation include further elucidation of the molecular mechanisms of action of hepcidin and the proteins that influence its production, including HFE, TfR2, HJV, and possibly others. Testing for the multiple genes implicated in the hemochromatosis phenotype may become commercially available in the foreseeable future. Potential therapeutic applications of our rapidly expanding knowledge of iron metabolism include administration of exogenous hepcidin for the treatment of iron overload and hepcidin antagonists to treat anemia associated with chronic inflammatory states.

Adams PC. Review article. The modern diagnosis and management of hemochromatosis. *Aliment Pharmacol Ther.* 2006;23:1681–1691. [PMID: 16817911]

Yen AW, Fancher TL, Bowlus CL. Revisiting hereditary hemochromatosis: current concepts and progress. *Am J Med.* 2006;119:391–399. [PMID: 16651049]

This chapter is a revised version of the chapter by Dr Bechien U. Wu, Dr Benjamin Smith, and Dr Norman D. Grace that was in the previous edition of Current Diagnosis & Treatment: Gastroenterology, Hepatology, & Endoscopy.

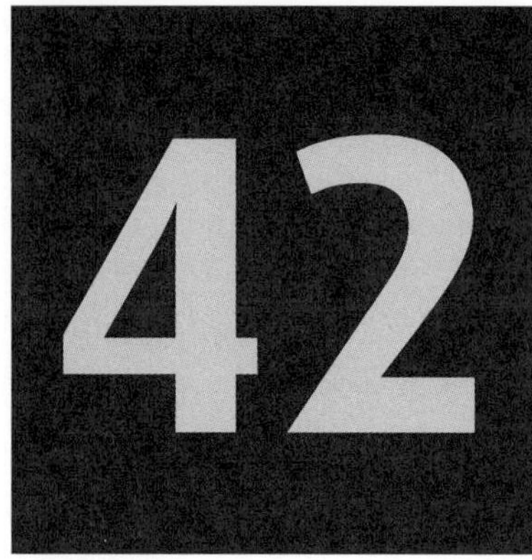

Alcoholic Liver Disease

Timothy T. Kuo, MD
Norman D. Grace, MD

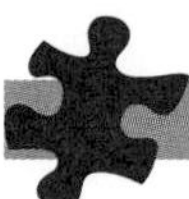

ESSENTIALS OF DIAGNOSIS

- In the United States, excessive alcohol use is defined as ingestion of >14 drinks/week in women and >21 drinks/week in men (1 drink = 12 oz beer, 1.0 oz malt liquor, 5 oz wine, or 1.5 oz 80 proof "hard liquor").
- Factors accelerating liver injury in alcoholic liver disease (ALD) include female gender, Latino and African-American ethnicity, chronic hepatitis C infection, acetaminophen overdose, and hereditary hemochromatosis.
- 75% of Asians have decreased ability to metabolize ethanol, resulting in acetaldehyde accumulation and subsequent flushing.
- Diagnosis of excessive alcohol use is suggested by increased serum ALT and AST levels, AST:ALT ratio of 2–3:1, and MCV >100.
- Accurate history of substance intake and CAGE or Alcohol Use Disorders Identification Test (AUDIT) questionnaires aid in the diagnosis of alcohol abuse.
- Liver biopsy and liver imaging cannot distinguish ALD from nonalcoholic steatohepatitis (NASH).
- Although 90–100% of heavy drinkers will develop hepatic steatosis, only 10–35% will develop alcoholic hepatitis, and 5–15% will develop cirrhosis.

General Considerations

Alcohol use in human history has played an important role in social interactions, politics, religion, medicine, and nutrition. The first use of alcohol dates back to the late stone-age Neolithic period (circa 10,000 BC) with the archeological discovery of beer jugs. Egyptian pictographs suggest wine consumption as early as 4000 BC. The use of wine and beer for medical purposes began circa 2000 BC. Sentiment toward moderation in drinking was documented in a Chinese imperial edict in the 12th century BC. The association of alcohol with liver disease appeared to have been noticed by the ancient Egyptians, who linked the use of beer with ascites, and the ancient Greeks, who described the association with jaundice and gastrointestinal bleeding.

A. Incidence and Societal Costs

Alcohol-related health problems contribute to significant health care costs worldwide. In 2003, the prevalence of alcohol-related disorders was 1.7% worldwide, and alcohol was the third leading cause of death in the United States. Data from the NIH-sponsored NESARC study suggest that 4.65% and 3.81% of American adults meet the criteria for alcohol abuse and alcohol dependence, respectively. Studies have shown that per capita alcohol consumption in both men and women is associated with mortality from liver cirrhosis.

Not all those who consume alcohol will develop Alcoholic Liver Disease (ALD) and liver cirrhosis. Among heavy drinkers, 90–100% will develop hepatic steatosis in 10 years, but only 10–35% will develop steatohepatitis and 5–15% will develop cirrhosis in the same period (Figure 42–1).

B. Definition

Epidemiologic research involving alcohol use is not without limitations. The definition of one alcohol drink varies globally and individually. In the United States, the definition used by the Centers for Disease Control and Prevention is about 0.5 oz, or 13.7 g of pure alcohol. This is equivalent to 12 oz of beer, 8 oz of malt liquor, 5 oz of wine, or 1.5 oz of 80-proof "hard liquor." In the United Kingdom and Japan, one drink equals 8 g and 19.75 g, respectively.

Lucey MR, Mathurin P, Morgan TR. Alcoholic hepatitis. *N Engl J Med.* 2009;360:2758–2769. [PMID:20347501]

Mandayam S, Jamal MM, Morgan TR. Epidemiology of alcoholic liver disease. *Semin Liver Dis.* 2004;24:217–232. [PMID: 15349801]

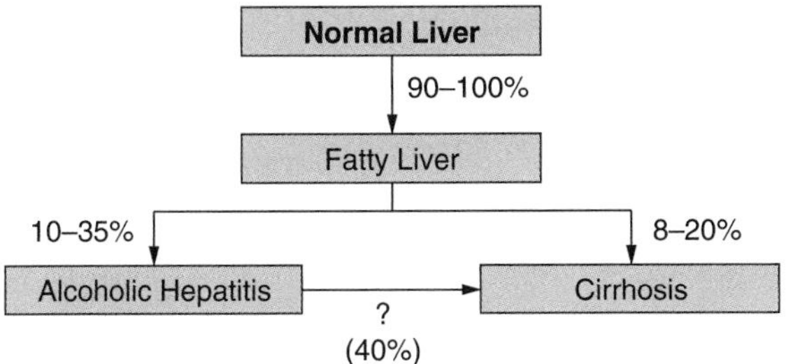

▲ **Figure 42–1.** Progression of alcoholic liver disease. (Reproduced, with permission, from McCullough AJ, O'Connor JF. Alcoholic liver disease: proposed recommendations for the American College of Gastroenterology. *Am J Gastroenterol.* 1998;93:11.)

McCullough AJ, O'Connor JF. Alcoholic liver disease: proposed recommendations for the American College of Gastroenterology. *Am J Gastroenterol.* 1998;93:2022–2036. [PMID: 9820369]

O'Shea RS, Dasarathy S, McCullough AJ. Alcoholic liver disease. *Hepatology.* 2010;51:307–328. [PMID:20034030]

Pathogenesis

A. Cofactors That Potentiate the Development of Alcoholic Liver Disease

The amount of alcohol consumption required for progression to liver cirrhosis reported by Lelback and colleagues in 1975 was 80 g of ethanol daily (equivalent to 1 L of wine, a half pint of hard liquor, or 8 beers) consumed for 10–20 years. However, as noted, not all who ingest significant amounts of alcohol will develop cirrhosis. Several cofactors are known to accelerate progression of liver disease, and the risk for ALD increases with ingestion of more than 35 drinks per week. A "safe" amount is believed to be 21 drinks per week for men and 14 drinks per week for women, in the absence of the cofactors listed below.

1. Age—Despite the legal alcohol drinking age of 21 years in the United States, a 2004 study revealed that 50% of high school students drank some amount of alcohol, and 20% of all alcohol consumption is suspected to be in individuals younger than age 21. Early alcohol use is associated with alcoholism later in life. At the opposite end of spectrum, an emergency department screening study revealed that 24.5% of subjects older than 65 years met criteria for alcohol abuse. However, the highest rate of alcohol abuse morbidity occurs among individuals aged 45–64 years, with a prevalence rate of 94.8 per 100,000.

2. Gender—The overall prevalence of alcohol abuse and related liver disease is higher among men than women. However, women are more prone than men to alcohol-related liver injury and fibrosis progression for the same amount of alcohol consumption. This may be due to different rates of alcohol metabolism, lower body mass index, effects of estrogens, or an increased intestinal permeability to endotoxin.

3. Ethnicity—Susceptibility to ALD is believed to vary among different ethnic groups. In the United States, alcoholic cirrhosis–related deaths are highest in Hispanic males, followed by black non-Hispanics, white non-Hispanics, and black Hispanics. The prevalence among females is highest in black non-Hispanics, followed by white Hispanics, white non-Hispanics, and black Hispanics. Studies in the United Kingdom suggest that South Asian men are more susceptible to alcohol-related liver injury than European men. It is unclear whether these differences are due to genetic polymorphisms, types of alcohol consumed, or access to health care.

4. Hepatitis C (HCV) infection—Between 14% and 36% of individuals with ALD also have chronic hepatitis C. The combination of HCV and ALD accelerates the progression and severity of liver disease, increases the risk for hepatocellular carcinoma, and decreases the likelihood of virologic response to interferon alfa therapy. The acceleration of liver disease has been postulated to be due to an increase in viral replication, a decrease in liver regenerative capability, and an increase in quasispecies complexity. Patients with HCV who consume excessive alcohol succumb at an earlier age. This affects the mortality in women more than men.

5. Hepatitis B (HBV) infection—In a large population study performed in Taiwan, the data suggest that chronic HBV infection and alcohol consumption increase the risk for the development of hepatocellular carcinoma.

6. Hepatocellular carcinoma—ALD and hepatitis C are the two most common causes of hepatocellular carcinoma. In a Veterans Administration study of patients between 1993 and 1998, the prevalence rate of hepatocellular carcinoma in patients with cirrhosis secondary to alcohol use was 9.1 per 100,000, whereas the rate was 7.0 per 100,000 in patients with HCV. The risk of hepatocellular carcinoma increases after consuming more than 60 g of alcohol per day for more than 10 years. Recent studies have also shown that there has been a dramatic increase in the incidence of hepatocellular carcinoma associated with hepatitis C infection, and the incidence may be comparable to that of ALD. The effect of alcohol and HCV in the development of hepatocellular carcinoma appears to be synergistic.

7. Medications—Patients with ALD appear to be at an increased risk for liver injury after ingestion of multiple or above recommended therapeutic doses of acetaminophen. This is believed to be due to rapid depletion of glutathione stores and competition with cytochrome P450 (CYP) 2E1. Although other medications may also compete with CYP450, there are limited data on increased hepatotoxicity in the setting of ALD.

8. Iron overload—The liver is able to tolerate high levels of intrahepatic iron without progression to fibrosis. However, when a cofactor, such as alcohol, is involved, liver damage is accelerated. Similar synergistic effects are also seen in nonalcoholic fatty liver disease, chronic HCV, and porphyria cutanea tarda. Both iron and alcohol generate reactive oxygen species that promote lipid peroxidation with consequent damage to cellular integrity. Alcohol has also been shown to suppress hepcidin activity in animal models. Excessive alcohol consumption (>60 g/day) in patients with hemochromatosis is associated with accelerated fibrogenesis, increased risk for hepatocellular cancer, and lower long-term survival. Because consumption of more than three drinks daily is associated with increased serum markers (ferritin) of iron overload from ALD, *HFE* genetic testing can differentiate ALD from hereditary hemochromatosis. Primary iron overload may be distinguished from secondary iron overload when the hepatic iron index is greater than 1.9 micromole per gram dry weight of liver per year of life.

9. Diet and lifestyle—There are limited data on dietary and lifestyle factors that may influence the natural history of ALD. Coffee may be protective in ALD and related cirrhosis. Studies on the effect of tobacco have been conflicting. Some studies have suggested that obesity (basal metabolic index >25 kg/m^2) for more than 10 years accelerates progression of ALD. Pork products, on the other hand, have been shown to be associated with alcoholic hepatitis and cirrhosis but not steatosis. Other lifestyle factors that may be associated with ALD progression include single status, urban dwelling, unemployment, lower socioeconomic background, daily alcohol ingestion, and variable alcoholic beverage ingestion.

Anand BS, Thornby J. Alcohol has no effect on hepatitis C virus replication: a meta-analysis. *Gut.* 2005;54:1468–1472. [PMID: 16162952]

Anand BS, Velez M. Assessment of correlation between serum titers of hepatitis C virus and severity of liver disease. *World J Gastroenterol.* 2004;10:2409–2411. [PMID: 15285030]

Chen CM, Yoon YH, Yi HY, et al. Alcohol and hepatitis C mortality among males and females in the United States: a life table analysis. *Alcohol Clin Exp Res.* 2007;31:285–292. [PMID: 17250621]

Donato F, Tagger A, Gelatti U, et al. Alcohol and hepatocellular carcinoma: the effect of lifetime intake and hepatitis virus infections in men and women. *Am J Epidemiol.* 2002;155: 323–331. [PMID: 11836196]

Douds AC, Cox MA, Iqbal TH, et al. Ethnic differences in cirrhosis of the liver in a British city: alcoholic cirrhosis in South Asian men. *Alcohol Alcohol.* 2003;38:148–150. [PMID: 12634262]

Fletcher LM, Dixon JL, Purdie DM, et al. Excess alcohol greatly increases the prevalence of cirrhosis in hereditary hemochromatosis. *Gastroenterology.* 2002;122:281–289. [PMID: 11832443]

Morgan TR, Mandayam S, Jamal MM. Alcohol and hepatocellular carcinoma. *Gastroenterology.* 2004;127(Suppl 1):S87–S96. [PMID: 15508108]

B. Alcohol Metabolism

The metabolic breakdown products of alcohol are essential in the progression of ALD. Ethanol is metabolized by alcohol dehydrogenase in the hepatic cytosol to acetaldehyde, which is subsequently metabolized in the mitochondria by acetaldehyde dehydrogenase. There are various acetaldehyde dehydrogenase isoforms. Seventy-five percent of Asians have a deficiency in acetaldehyde dehydrogenase 2, which results in accumulation of acetaldehyde, causing flushing. A similar mechanism is seen with the drug disulfiram (Antabuse), which inhibits acetaldehyde dehydrogenase, causing acetaldehyde accumulation and resultant flushing, tachycardia, nausea, vomiting, hypotension, and headache within 15–30 minutes of alcohol ingestion.

Ethanol may also be metabolized in minor hepatic pathways involving the microsomal enzyme oxidation system, via CYP2E1, and the enzyme catalase. The stomach can metabolize ethanol via gastric alcohol dehydrogenase. Women have less gastric alcohol dehydrogenase than men, offering a possible explanation for the observed increased female susceptibility to the effect of alcohol.

C. Cellular Mechanisms

Although detailed mechanisms of ethanol-induced liver injury are incompletely understood, recent scientific advances have furthered our understanding of cellular and immunologic mechanisms through the use of in vitro and in vivo models.

Animal models of alcohol ingestion have demonstrated susceptibility of the hepatic pericentral area to hypoxemia due to competitive oxygen consumption by ethanol metabolism. Decreased intestinal permeability during alcohol ingestion results in an increase in serum endotoxin (lipopolysaccharide) levels, leading, in turn, to activation of Kupffer cells, which secrete cytokines such as tumor necrosis factor α (TNFα). It is believed that TNFα can induce cytotoxicity through caspase-dependent and caspase-independent pathways, leading to increased mitochondrial permeability and ultimately cell death. Both ethanol and decreased glutathione levels can sensitize the liver to TNFα-induced cytotoxicity.

D. Immunologic Mechanisms

In alcoholic hepatitis, elevated interleukin (IL)-18 levels result in neutrophil accumulation in the liver. Subsequently, neutrophil release of reactive oxygen species results in hepatocyte injury. Acute ethanol ingestion may also result in a suppressed T-cell response, decreased monocyte function, and increased levels of IL-1 and IL-6.

Ethanol metabolites, acetaldehyde and hydroxyethyl, may potentially play a major role in alcoholic liver injury. These metabolites bind to proteins to form adducts that result in altered intracellular protein function, and these adducts may also act as a neoantigen that can stimulate immune-mediated injury. Autoantibodies to various structures of the liver, such as liver membrane antigen, liver-specific protein, and CYP450, can be found in patients with ALD.

Frezza M, di Padova C, Pozzato G, et al. High blood alcohol levels in women. The role of decreased gastric alcohol dehydrogenase activity and first-pass metabolism. *N Engl J Med.* 1990;322: 95–99. [PMID: 2248624]

Hoek JB, Pastorino JG. Cellular signaling mechanisms in alcohol induced liver damage. *Semin Liver Dis.* 2004;24:257–272. [PMID: 15349804]

Thiele GM, Freeman TL, Klassen LW. Immunologic mechanisms of alcoholic liver injury. *Semin Liver Dis.* 2004;24:273–287. [PMID: 15349805]

Clinical Findings

A. Symptoms and Signs

In the early stages, patients with ALD exhibits subtle and often no abnormal physical findings. It is usually not until development of advanced liver disease that stigmata of chronic liver disease become apparent. Early ALD is usually discovered during routine health examinations when liver enzyme levels are found to be elevated. These usually reflect alcoholic hepatosteatosis. Microvesicular and macrovesicular steatosis with inflammation are seen in liver biopsy specimens. These histologic features of ALD are indistinguishable from those of nonalcoholic fatty liver disease. The presence of cholestasis would favor the diagnosis of alcoholic hepatitis, as it is not seen in nonalcoholic steatohepatitis. Steatosis usually resolves after discontinuation of alcohol use. Continuation of alcohol use will result in a higher risk of progression of liver disease and cirrhosis.

In patients with acute alcoholic hepatitis, clinical manifestations include fever, jaundice, hepatomegaly, and possible hepatic decompensation with hepatic encephalopathy, variceal bleeding, and ascites accumulation. Tender hepatomegaly may be present, but abdominal pain is unusual. Occasionally, the patient may be asymptomatic. Table 42–1 summarizes diagnostic features of ALD.

B. Laboratory Findings

In patients with alcoholic hepatitis, the serum aspartate aminotransferase (AST) to alanine aminotransferase (ALT) ratio is greater than 2:1. AST and ALT levels are almost always less than 500. The elevated AST to ALT ratio is due to deficiency of pyridoxal-6-phosphate, which is required in the ALT enzyme synthetic pathway. Furthermore, alcohol metabolite–induced injury of hepatic mitochondria results in AST isoenzyme release. Other laboratory findings include red blood cell macrocytosis (mean corpuscular volume >100) and elevations of serum γ-glutamyl transferase, alkaline phosphatase, and bilirubin levels. Folate level is reduced in alcoholic patients due to decreased intestinal absorption, increased bone marrow requirement for folate in the presence of alcohol, and increased urinary loss. The magnitude of leukocytosis reflects severity of liver injury.

Table 42–1. Characteristic findings in alcoholic liver disease.

Hematology	Pancytopenia MCV >100
Chemistry	↑ GGT AST:ALT ≥2 ↓ or normal Albumin ↑ γ-globulin ↑ PT and PTT
Physical Findings	
Hepatobiliary	Hepatomegaly Splenomegaly
Peripheral stigmata	Palmar erythema Spider angioma Gynecomastia Parotid enlargement Dupuytren contracture Impotence Testicular atrophy Decreased body hair Peripheral muscle wasting
Imaging Studies	
Ultrasound	Enlarged or shrunken liver Increased echogenicity Nodular surface Nodules (regenerating or dysplastic) Enlarged caudate lobe Right posterior hepatic notch
CT scan	Enlarged hilar periportal space Enlarged or shrunken liver Prominent intrahepatic fissure Increased size of caudate lobe and lateral segments Nodular surface Capsular retraction Hepatic periportal lucency (due to edema)
MRI	Regenerative nodules with surrounding fibrous septa Heterogenous liver parenchyma
Liver-spleen scan	Colloid shift
Extrahepatic findings	Splenomegaly Ascites Varices

ALT, alanine aminotransferase; AST, aspartate aminotransferase; CT, computed tomography; MCV, mean corpuscular volume; MRI, magnetic resonance imaging; PT, prothrombin time; PTT, partial thromboplastin time.

Histologic features include Mallory bodies, giant mitochondria, hepatocyte necrosis, and neutrophil infiltration at the perivenular area. Mallory bodies, which are also present in other liver diseases, are condensations of cytokeratin components in the hepatocyte cytoplasm and do not contribute to liver injury. Up to 70% of patients with moderate to severe alcoholic hepatitis already have cirrhosis identifiable on biopsy examination at the time of diagnosis.

C. Imaging Studies

Radiographic imaging may show features suggestive of cirrhosis, such as a nodular liver surface, reversal of portal vein flow, splenomegaly, and gallbladder wall edema. Other findings such as enlarged caudate lobe and right posterior hepatic notch are suggestive of liver disease. Characteristic findings on ultrasound, computed tomography, and magnetic resonance imaging are summarized in Table 42–1.

D. Liver Biopsy

Liver biopsy is not mandatory for the diagnosis of ALD or acute alcoholic hepatitis, but it may be helpful when the diagnosis is uncertain. The histology may help determine prognosis and perhaps encourage alcohol cessation. In the setting of severe thrombocytopenia or a hypercoagulation state, transjugular liver biopsy is the procedure of choice. The need for liver biopsy in this situation should be decided on an individual basis, considering the risk of the procedure and potential adverse effects of corticosteroid therapy.

E. Screening for Alcohol Abuse

Screening for alcohol abuse is an important part of a routine history and physical examination. Several standard screening questionnaires have been developed. The most commonly used is the CAGE questionnaire. Nearly all alcoholic patients will have two positive responses, and 50% will have positive responses to all four questions listed below.

1. Have you felt the need to *cut* down drinking?
2. Have you ever felt *annoyed* by criticism of drinking?
3. Have you had *guilty* feelings about drinking?
4. Do you ever take a morning *eye* opener?

The World Health Organization has developed the Alcohol Use Disorders Identification Test (AUDIT) which consists of 10 questions aimed to identify heavy drinkers and those with alcohol dependency. This questionnaire has a higher sensitivity and specificity than the shorter instruments and provides more detailed information about risk.

It must be emphasized that accurate assessment of alcohol use still requires obtaining a careful history from the patient or family members. New laboratory tests have been developed to screen for recent or chronic alcohol use, but these are seldom used due to lack of commercial availability. The carbohydrate-deficient transferrin (CDT) test is based on a decreased carbohydrate moiety to transferrin caused by chronic alcohol use. However, CDT levels may be affected by serum transferrin concentrations, hypertension, primary biliary cirrhosis, liver malignancy, chronic viral hepatitis, decompensated liver disease, female sex, and age. The new turbidimetric CDT assay appears to have fewer limitations. Other experimental serologic tests for recent alcohol use include 5-hydroxytryptophol, ethyl glucuronide, phosphatidyl ethanol, sialic acid level, β-hexosaminidase, mitochondrial AST levels, and alcohol metabolites such as erythrocyte acetaldehyde and acetaldehyde adducts.

Niemelä O. Biomarkers in alcoholism. *Clin Chim Acta.* 2007;377: 39–49. [PMID: 17045579]

Differential Diagnosis

A. Nonalcoholic Steatohepatitis

Alcoholic hepatitis is usually indistinguishable by liver histology from nonalcoholic steatohepatitis (NASH). However, the ALT is usually twice that of AST in NASH, and the AST is rarely greater than 500 in alcoholic hepatitis. Careful review of the patient's history may reveal risk factors suggestive of either disease.

B. Hemochromatosis

Patients with ALD may have elevated transferrin saturation and ferritin levels similar to those seen in hemochromatosis. In murine models, alcohol causes down-regulation of hepcidin expression in the liver and a subsequent increase in the iron transporters ferroportin and DMT-1 in the duodenum. Genetic testing may reveal the *HFE* gene, but this does not rule out concurrent alcohol-related liver disease. When genetic testing is equivocal, a hepatic iron concentration (HIC) greater than 71 mcg of iron per gram of dry liver weight and a hepatic iron index greater than 1.9 (HIC divided by patient's age) may help determine the amount of total body iron overload and establish the diagnosis of hereditary hemochromatosis.

C. Acetaminophen Toxicity

Concurrent intake of alcohol can lower the toxicity threshold of acetaminophen, resulting in AST levels significantly greater than 500 IU/L. A careful history of the amount of alcohol and acetaminophen ingestion, as well as measurements of the serum acetaminophen level, can help determine therapeutic options, including need for liver transplantation referral.

Complications

Complications of ALD are similar to those for non–alcohol-related chronic liver disease. During severe acute alcoholic hepatitis, the major causes of death are liver failure, gastrointestinal bleeding, hepatorenal syndrome, and sepsis. Until the introduction of the Maddrey discriminant function (MDF), there was no method for predicting the severity of alcoholic

Table 42–2. Efficacy of various medical therapies for alcoholic liver disease.

Proven Efficacy	Further Studies Needed	Ineffective Therapy
Abstinence corticosteroid	Anti-tumor necrosis factor	Vitamin E SAMe Polyenylphosphatidylcholine Propylthiouracil Milk thistle Anabolic steroids Disulfiram

hepatitis. The MDF, which is calculated as 4.6 × [patient's prothrombin time – control prothrombin time] + total bilirubin (mg/dL), identifies patients with a high risk for early mortality. An MDF of 32 or higher is associated with spontaneous survival of 50–65%, whereas MDF below 32 is associated with survival of approximately 90%.

Treatment

Table 42–2 summarizes the efficacy of various medical therapies that have been used in the treatment of ALD.

A. Abstinence

Reversal of liver disease and improvement in survival occur with abstinence. With cessation of alcohol use, less than 20% of patients will demonstrate progression of liver disease. Five-year survival improves from 34% to 60% for those with decompensated liver disease. Six months of sobriety, along with treatment programs and support networks, is a good predictor of long-term success. Patients with chronic HCV infection should abstain from any alcohol intake, due to the risk for rapid acceleration of liver disease.

Patients with alcoholic liver disease may or may not admit to alcohol dependency. Psycho-social counseling and support groups (eg, Alcoholics Anonymous) may help maintain abstinence. The use of medications to avoid recidivism should be monitored with collaboration a psychiatrist or addiction specialist. Acamprosate, which modulates the NMDA receptor, appears to help alcohol-dependent patients to avoid relapse according to the recent Cochrane analysis. Opioid antagonist, such as disulfiram, has not been shown to enhance abstinence, and Naltrexone may be hepatotoxic.

B. Nutrition

Standard fluid, mineral, and vitamin replacement and withdrawal precautions are mandatory for patients hospitalized with decompensated liver cirrhosis. Oral as well as tube feeding has been found to be associated with decreased mortality. Continued enteral nutrition support after hospitalization also improves long-term morbidity. Dietary protein should not be restricted in alcoholic hepatitis for fear of hepatic encephalopathy. In the setting of hepatic encephalopathy, branched-chain amino acids (BCAAs) may be considered.

Patients with liver cirrhosis usually have protein malnutrition with decreased BCAAs (leucine, isoleucine, and valine). A decrease in BCAA has been associated with serum hypoalbuminemia and elevated arterial ammonia levels. Recent formulations have resolved the poor taste by incorporation of BCAA into granules. Despite some small clinical studies suggesting benefit in improving metabolite profile and hepatic encephalopathy, there is still a lack of convincing evidence to justify the use of this expensive supplement to significantly improve morbidity and mortality. In patients with alcoholic hepatitis or fulminant hepatic failure, BCAA has not been found to influence short-term or long-term survival.

Charlton M. Branched-chain amino acid enriched supplements as therapy for liver disease. *J Nutr*. 2006;136:295S–298S. [PMID: 1635102]

C. Corticosteroids

Thirteen randomized controlled trials have examined corticosteroid therapy in severe acute alcoholic hepatitis. Although five studies have shown benefit in survival, mostly in rural populations and/or in patients with concomitant hepatic encephalopathy, the remaining studies have been equivocal. Significant improvement in liver function is evident at 7 days after initiation of therapy. Overall, corticosteroid therapy is beneficial in improving 30- and 60-day mortality only in patients with severe acute alcoholic hepatitis and an MDF greater than 32, in the absence of acute gastrointestinal bleeding, renal failure, acute infection, or pancreatitis. Two-month survival with corticosteroid therapy is about 80%, but up to 40% of patients still die in 6 months. The benefit of corticosteroid therapy may be present up to 1 year. However, the benefit of corticosteroids may not extend to all those with MDF >32. In a VA cooperative study, mortality at 6 months was higher in the group with MDF >54 who received prednisolone than placebo. A recently published algorithm to determine corticosteroid use is recapitulated in Figure 42–2.

A recent study demonstrated the use of the Lille model (formula available online at http://www.lillemodel.com) in attempting to identify poor outcome at 6 months of follow-up in patients with MDF of 32 or higher treated with either prednisolone (40 g/day orally) or methylprednisolone (32 mg/day intravenously) for 28 days. Patients with a score greater than 0.45 using the Lille model had a mortality rate of 76% at 6 months. This study suggests that alternative therapies should be considered in patients with scores above 0.45 after 1 week of treatment with steroids. Recently, the Lille model has also been found to predict survival benefit at 28 days after steroid treatment.

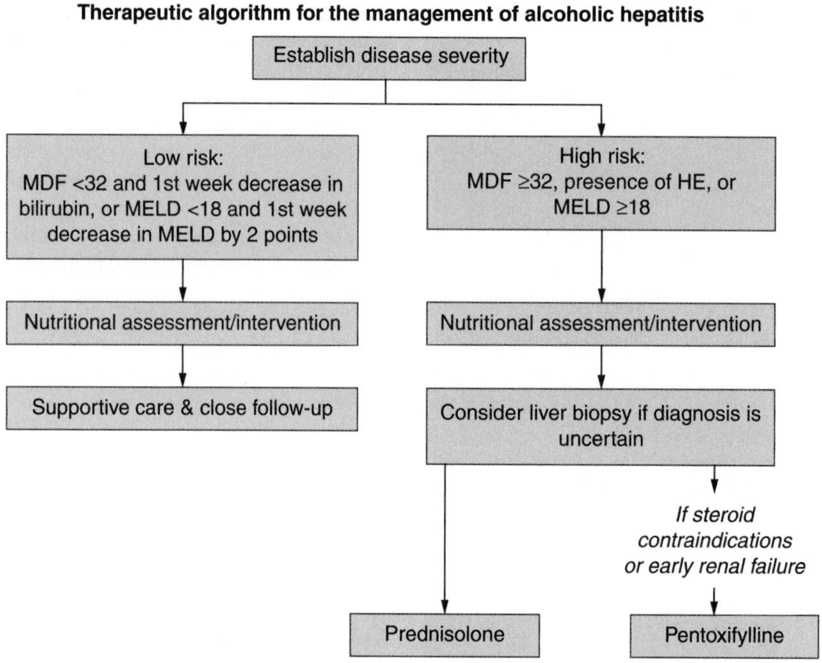

Therapeutic algorithm for the management of alcoholic hepatitis

Establish disease severity

Low risk: MDF <32 and 1st week decrease in bilirubin, or MELD <18 and 1st week decrease in MELD by 2 points

Nutritional assessment/intervention

Supportive care & close follow-up

High risk: MDF ≥32, presence of HE, or MELD ≥18

Nutritional assessment/intervention

Consider liver biopsy if diagnosis is uncertain

Prednisolone

If steroid contraindications or early renal failure

Pentoxifylline

▲ **Figure 42–2.** AASLD Practice Guidelines for the treatment of alcoholic hepatitis. (Reproduced, with permission, from O'Shea RS, Dasarathy S, McCullough AJ, Alcoholic liver disease. *Hepatology*. 2010;51:319.)

Prednisolone may have a theoretical advantage over prednisone, because it does not require hepatic metabolism for the active component. It is given at a dose of 40 mg daily for 4 weeks and can be discontinued or tapered over a 2–4 week period. Although use of corticosteroids in the treatment of ALD was recommended in a 1998 American College of Gastroenterology guideline, clinical use has been infrequent.

Maddrey WC, Boitnott JK, Bedine MS, et al. Corticosteroid therapy of alcoholic hepatitis. *Gastroenterology*. 1978;75:193–199. [PMID: 352788]

Mathurin P. Corticosteroids for alcoholic hepatitis—what's next? *J Hepatol*. 2005;43:526–533. [PMID: 16026887]

Mathurin P, O'Grady J, Carithers RL, et al. Corticosteroids improve short-term survival in patients with severe alcoholic hepatitis: meta-analysis of individual patient data. *Gut*. 2011;60:255–260. [PMID: 20940288]

D. Anti-Tumor Necrosis Factor Therapy

TNF has been implicated in the pathogenesis of ALD, and elevated levels are found in patients with alcoholic hepatitis. Anti-TNF treatment prevents liver injury in a murine model of ALD, and this therapy has also been studied in humans.

Pentoxiphylline, an inhibitor of TNF, at 400 mg orally three times per day, was shown to decrease the risk of hepatorenal syndrome in patients whose MDF is greater than 32. The 28-day mortality for the pentoxiphylline group was 24%, compared with 46% for the placebo group. Survival benefit was related to a reduction in mortality associated with the hepatorenal syndrome. The decrease in serum TNFα levels was not statistically significant when compared with placebo. Pentoxiphylline 400 mg oral daily is a reasonable alternative to corticosteroids in those with contraindications to steroid or early renal failure.

Treatment with anti-TNF monoclonal antibody (infliximab, a chimeric mouse and human antibody that neutralizes soluble TNFα) and etanercept (a p75-soluble TNF receptor Fc fusion protein) has yet to reveal survival benefit in clinical trials for ALD, which are often inadequately sized and include some patients suffering fatal complications.

Naveau S, Chollet-Martin S, Dharancy S, et al. Foie-Alcool group of the Association Française pour l'Etude du Foie. A double-blind randomized controlled trial of infliximab associated with prednisolone in acute alcoholic hepatitis. *Hepatology*. 2004;39:1390–1397. [PMID: 15122768]

E. Other Therapies

Based on the involvement of reactive oxygen species in the pathways of ALD, pilot studies using antioxidants have been performed. Vitamin E (1000 IU daily for 3 months) failed to show a benefit despite improvement in serum levels of bilirubin and the prothrombin time.

In a small study, SAMe, a precursor to glutathione, at 1200 mg orally per day improved survival in patients with alcoholic liver cirrhosis with Childs-Pugh class A or B. However, this benefit was not substantiated in a Cochrane Review. Colchicine was also determined to be ineffective in alcoholic liver cirrhosis.

Polyenylphosphatidylcholine (PPC), given to 789 patients with alcoholic liver fibrosis in a Veterans Administration Cooperative Trial, benefited those who abstained from alcohol use but not those who continued a moderate amount of alcohol consumption.

Because pericentral (zone 3) hepatocytes are relatively oxygen poor and are sensitive to hypoxic injury caused by alcohol and thyroid hormone, suppression of thyroid hormone using propylthiouracil was attempted in a clinical trial. Survival benefit was seen at 2 years when compared with placebo but only in abstinent patients. However, these findings have not been replicated in other trials.

The use of milk thistle seed has been used for 2000 years in Europe for treatment of liver diseases. The active ingredient is believed to be silymarin, which is made of silybin, silidianin, and silicristin. Silybin is believed to be the most active compound. Silymarin is believed to enhance liver regeneration and protect hepatocytes from toxicity, although the mechanism is still unclear. However, clinical trials have yet to demonstrate a clear benefit.

No benefit was seen using anabolic steroids for alcoholic hepatitis or cirrhosis. Treatment with disulfiram, which inhibits acetaldehyde dehydrogenase, is contraindicated in patients with liver disease.

Therapies related to hepatic regeneration (insulin, glucagons, and malotilate) and extracorporeal support (molecular absorbent recirculating system) have been evaluated in clinical trials, but the use of these agents remains experimental. Future therapies may include antifibrotic agents, IL-10, theophylline, and possibly thalidomide.

In summary, only steroids or pentoxifylline are currently recommended for pharmacologic treatment of alcoholic hepatitis. The combination of these two drugs has not been investigated.

F. Transplantation

Although in rare cases liver cirrhosis is reversible, the disease process remains mostly irreversible. Liver transplantation remains the only definitive therapy. Today, survival after liver transplantation is similar for patients with ALD and non-ALD. The requirements for transplant listing are the same as those for other types of liver disease, except for a 6-month sobriety prerequisite along with psychiatric evaluation and rehabilitation assistance (ie, Alcoholics Anonymous). Specific requirements vary among the transplant centers. Relapse to alcohol use after transplant listing results in delisting. Re-listing is possible in many institutions, but only after 3–6 months of sobriety.

There are limited data on transplant survival in patients transplanted for acute alcoholic hepatitis, but it is believed to be similar to that in nonacute ALD, non-ALD, and alcoholic hepatitis with MDF less than 32.

See Chapter 50 for further discussion of liver transplantation.

Neuberger J, Schulz KH, Day C, et al. Transplantation for alcoholic liver disease. *J Hepatol.* 2002;36:130–137. [PMID: 11804676].

Prognosis

The prognosis for patients with ALD depends on the liver histology as well as cofactors, such as concomitant chronic viral hepatitis. Among patients with alcoholic hepatitis, progression to liver cirrhosis occurs at 10–20% per year, and 70% will eventually develop cirrhosis. Despite cessation of alcohol use, only 10% will have normalization of histology and serum liver enzyme levels.

As previously noted, the MDF has been used to predict short-term mortality (ie, MDF ≥32 associated with spontaneous survival of 50–65% without corticosteroid therapy, and MDF <32 associated with spontaneous survival of 90%). The Model for End-Stage Liver Disease (MELD) score has also been found to have similar predictive accuracy in 30-day (MELD >11) and 90-day (MELD >21) mortality. The Glasgow alcoholic hepatitis score has also been found to be helpful in predicting survival.

Liver cirrhosis develops in 6–14% of those who consume more than 60–80 g of alcohol daily for men and more than 20 g daily for women. Even in those who drink more than 120 g daily, only 13.5% will suffer serious alcohol-related liver injury. Nevertheless, alcohol-related mortality was the third leading cause of death in 2003 in the United States. Worldwide mortality is estimated to be 150,000 per year.

Dunn W, Jamil LH, Brown LS, et al. MELD accurately predicts mortality in patients with alcoholic hepatitis. *Hepatology.* 2005;41:353–358. [PMID: 15660383].

Sheth M, Riggs M, Patel T. Utility of the Mayo End-Stage Liver Disease (MELD) score in assessing prognosis of patients with alcoholic hepatitis. *BMC Gastroenterol.* 2002;2:2. [PMID: 11835693]

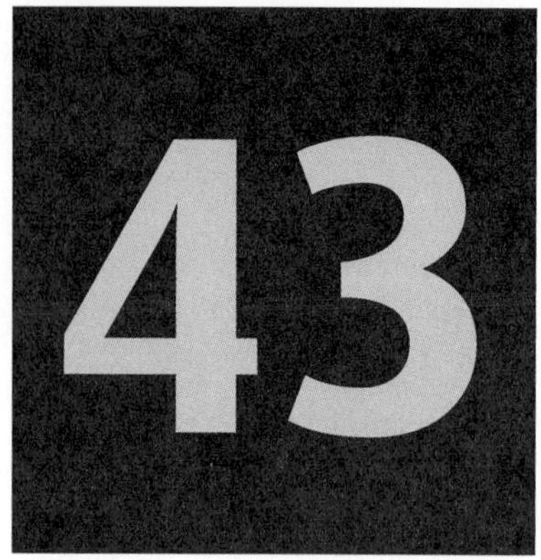

Nonalcoholic Fatty Liver Disease

David E. Cohen, MD, PhD
Frank A. Anania, MD

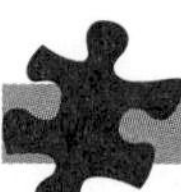

ESSENTIALS OF DIAGNOSIS

- Nonalcoholic fatty liver disease (NAFLD) is an overarching concept that includes simple steatosis and nonalcoholic steatohepatitis (NASH).
- NAFLD is commonly associated with the metabolic syndrome, obesity, diabetes, and hyperlipidemia; 80% of patients with the metabolic syndrome have NAFLD.
- Patients generally present without clinical symptoms but with mild transaminase elevations; NAFLD is the most common cause of increased serum transaminase levels.
- NAFLD is a clinical diagnosis after exclusion of other causes of liver disease.
- Ultrasound, computed tomography, and magnetic resonance imaging are useful for the detection.
- Liver biopsy is currently required to distinguish NASH from NAFLD.

General Considerations

Nonalcoholic fatty liver disease (NAFLD) is characterized by hepatic steatosis, the hepatocellular accumulation of triglycerides in the absence of significant alcohol consumption. Simple steatosis connotes fat accumulation in the absence of inflammation in the liver. By contrast, nonalcoholic steatohepatitis (NASH) indicates the presence of inflammation and fibrosis in association with hepatic steatosis. NAFLD is sometimes used as an overarching term that includes simple steatosis and NASH, but is also commonly employed to connote simple steatosis.

Whereas the histopathology of NAFLD and NASH is similar to that of alcohol-related liver disease, the etiology is quite distinct. An abundance of basic and clinical research has demonstrated that the metabolic underpinnings of NAFLD are rooted in insulin resistance. Indeed, NAFLD is commonly associated with other manifestations of insulin resistance including obesity, diabetes, and hyperlipidemia. Although early studies suggested NAFLD to be a benign condition, it is now apparent that NAFLD is a major cause of liver-related morbidity and mortality.

A. Epidemiology

The absence of signs and symptoms, combined with a lack of sensitive and specific diagnostic tests, makes estimation of the prevalence of NAFLD difficult. Elevated liver enzymes are not sensitive for detecting NAFLD and there is no current consensus that histopathology is a gold standard for diagnosis. Although likely an underestimate for these reasons, the prevalence of NAFLD is considered to be in the range of 20% in the United States and between 11.5% and 46% of the general population. By contrast, the prevalence of NASH is much lower, and in the range of 2% to 3%. As a result, the prevalences of NAFLD and NASH easily exceed chronic hepatitis C (HCV) infection, which afflicts 1.8% of the U.S. population. Recently, a common polymorphism in the gene encoding patatin-like phospholipase-3 (*PNPLA3*) (synonym adiponutrin) was shown to be strongly associated with NAFLD and its histopathologic severity.

Population-based studies have revealed that NAFLD is more common in men than women. It is more common in Hispanics compared with whites and more common in whites than blacks. It is assumed that the prevalence of NAFLD will increase over time in parallel to the epidemic of obesity and diabetes. Of particular concern is that NAFLD is increasing in the pediatric population, with prevalences estimated at around 3% of children and 20–50% of obese children.

Argo CK, Caldwell SH. Epidemiology and natural history of non-alcoholic steatohepatitis. *Clin Liver Dis.* 2009;13:511–531. [PMID: 19818302]

Browning JD, Szczepaniak LS, Dobbins R, et al. Prevalence of hepatic steatosis in an urban population in the United States: impact of ethnicity. *Hepatology*. 2004;40:1387–1395. [PMID: 15565570]

Koutsari C, Lazaridis KN. Emerging genes associated with the progression of nonalcoholic fatty liver disease. *Hepatology*. 2010;52:807–810. [PMID: 20812353]

Ruhl CE, Everhart JE. Determinants of the association of overweight with elevated serum alanine aminotransferase activity in the United States. *Gastroenterology*. 2003;124:71–79. [PMID: 12512031]

B. Association of NAFLD with the Metabolic Syndrome, Obesity, Diabetes, and Hyperlipidemia

Insulin resistance represents the most important risk factor for the development of NAFLD. Because insulin resistance is also the hallmark of the metabolic syndrome, it is not surprising that there is a close connection between NAFLD and the metabolic syndrome. Indeed, steatosis may simply characterize the hepatic manifestation of the metabolic syndrome. The metabolic syndrome is generally defined as the coexistence of three or more of the following findings: (1) increased waist circumference, (2) hypertriglyceridemia, (3) hypertension, (4) elevated fasting plasma glucose, and (5) low high-density lipoprotein (HDL) cholesterol level. Patients with metabolic syndrome have a 4- to 11-fold higher risk of developing NAFLD, and the prevalence of metabolic syndrome in patients with NAFLD ranges from 18% to 67%, depending on body weight. In NAFLD patients with the metabolic syndrome, the risk of NASH is elevated threefold.

There is also a close association of NAFLD with obesity. The prevalence of obesity in patients with NAFLD is reported to vary from 30% to 100%. In obese patients (body mass index [BMI] ≥30) the risk of NAFLD is elevated 4.6-fold. Importantly, the frequency of NASH also varies in proportion to weight. The prevalence of NASH is 3% of the lean population, but rises to 19% in obesity and to nearly 50% in morbidly obese individuals. Consistent with the close relationship of NAFLD with the metabolic syndrome, NAFLD is more common in individuals with an abdominal concentration of fat, even at lower BMI.

The prevalence of NAFLD is high in the type 2 diabetic population (50%), and the prevalence of type 2 diabetes in NAFLD patients ranges from 10% to 75%. The prevalence of NAFLD appears to increase as continuous function of fasting plasma glucose. Importantly, NASH is disproportionately represented in type 2 diabetics, with significant fibrosis and cirrhosis present in approximately 20%. In hyperlipidemic patients, the overall prevalence of fatty liver is 50%, with hypertriglyceridemia and mixed dyslipidemia conferring a fivefold risk of NAFLD. The prevalence of hyperlipidemia associated with NAFLD varies from 20% to 90%. In keeping with a strong link to the metabolic syndrome, low HDL cholesterol levels are also commonly observed in patients with NAFLD. Emerging evidence suggests that hypertension is linked to NAFLD through its relationship to insulin resistance.

Gholam PM, Flancbaum L, Machan JT, et al. Nonalcoholic fatty liver disease in severely obese subjects. *Am J Gastroenterol*. 2007; 102:399–408. [PMID: 17311652]

Hamaguchi M, Kojima T, Takeda N, et al. The metabolic syndrome as a predictor of nonalcoholic fatty liver disease. *Ann Intern Med*. 2005;143:722–728. [PMID: 16287793]

Marchesini G, Bugianesi E, Forlani G, et al. Nonalcoholic fatty liver, steatohepatitis, and the metabolic syndrome. *Hepatology*. 2003;37:917–923. [PMID: 12668987]

Parekh S, Anania FA. Abnormal lipid and glucose metabolism in obesity: implications for nonalcoholic fatty liver disease. *Gastroenterology*. 2007;132:2191–2207. [PMID: 17498512]

Pathogenesis

Current concepts indicate that insulin resistance is the primary metabolic defect leading to NAFLD (Figure 43–1). This leads to an influx into the liver of free fatty acids that are liberated from adipose tissues due to a failure of insulin to suppress hormone-sensitive lipase. In addition, elevated insulin levels associated with insulin resistance promote

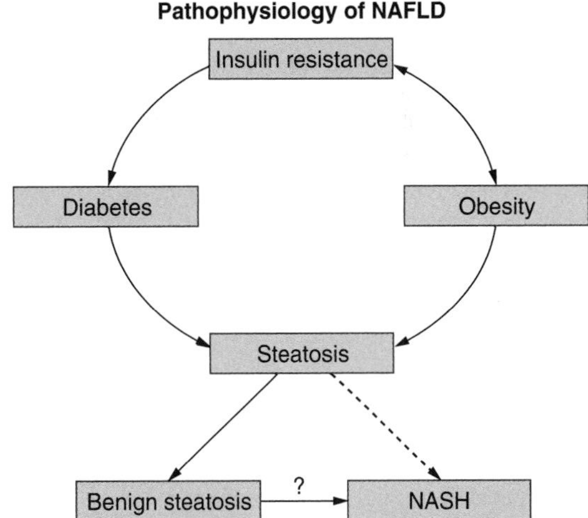

▲ **Figure 43–1.** Insulin resistance is the foundation hepatic steatosis. Type 2 diabetes is a consequence of insulin resistance, but obesity can also result in insulin resistance. As indicated by the question mark, it is not known whether there is progression of benign steatosis to nonalcoholic steatohepatitis (NASH). NAFLD, nonalcoholic fatty liver disease. (Reproduced, with permission, from Parekh S, Anania FA. Abnormal lipid and glucose metabolism in obesity: implications for nonalcoholic fatty liver disease. *Gastroenterology*. 2007;132:2191–2207. [PMID: 17498512])

continued synthesis of triglycerides in the liver. These two sources of triglycerides result in lipid-engorged hepatocytes (ie, macrovesicular hepatic steatosis alone). The presence of NAFLD appears to be a relatively innocuous occurrence, and it does not appear that progressive liver injury necessarily ensues. Although many patients with NAFLD have coexisting type 2 diabetes, this is not uniformly true. Indeed, steatosis and insulin resistance may be present in the absence of other components of the metabolic syndrome.

A prevailing hypothesis suggests that NASH evolves as a progression from NAFLD. In this regard, the presence of NALFD represents a first "hit." According to this theory, NASH develops due to a second hit whereby hepatocytes laden with triglycerides are vulnerable to additional insult. Although definitive data to support individual second hits are lacking, two categories have been described and have gained some acceptance. These are oxidative stress and specific cytokines plus lipopolysaccharides. Free fatty acids and hyperinsulinemia potentiate lipid peroxidation and the release of hydroxy free radicals, which directly injure hepatocytes by recruitment of necroinflammatory mediators. Chronic liver injury sustained over time will then lead to activation of hepatic stellate cells, creating the potential for hepatic fibrosis.

At least in certain animal models of NASH, lipopolysaccharides are released into the portal vein and are potent agonists for tumor necrosis factor α (TNFα) production, with the subsequent release of interleukins. Interestingly, the same mechanisms appear to be pathogenic in alcoholic hepatitis and produce quite similar histopathologic lesions. The combination of oxidative stress and necroinflammatory cytokines is associated with compromised mitochondrial function, which impairs electron transport and depletes adenosine triphosphate. This renders hepatocytes incapable of handling the enhanced oxidative stress. In this setting, the increased oxidative stress may overwhelm the intrinsic antioxidant capacity of the liver. Intracellular free fatty acids within the liver also promote endoplasmic reticulum stress, which leads to increase lipid synthesis and hepatocyte apoptosis via activation of c-Jun N-terminal kinase (JNK).

The majority of patients with NAFLD, but a lesser fraction of those with NASH, never progress to fibrosis, which results from a complex series of molecular events in response to all types of liver injury. However, in the setting of excess oxidative stress, stellate cells in the liver may become activated, and this results in increased deposition of extracellular matrix. Excess extracellular matrix eventually disrupts normal signal transduction between cells and the matrix on which they rest, as well as the normal flow of nutrients and blood in the liver sinusoids. The result is a wound-healing response that can compromise liver function.

Leptin is a cytokine-like hormone that circulates at increased concentrations in patients with the metabolic syndrome. Emerging evidence suggests that leptin may play an important pathogenic role in the development and progress of NASH. Leptin is synthesized by adipocytes, but also by activated hepatic stellate cells. Among its diverse activities, leptin promotes liver fibrosis, apparently as part of a wound healing response.

Adiponectin, also known as adipocyte complement–related protein (ACRP30), is a hormone produced by omental fat. Adiponectin stimulates glucose utilization and fatty acid oxidation in the liver by activating adenosine monophosphate–activated protein kinase (AMPK). Adiponectin is correlated positively with insulin sensitivity and negatively with intra-abdominal fat. Adiponectin gene expression and secretion are decreased in obesity and are lower in patients with insulin resistance, type 2 diabetes, and other conditions associated with the metabolic syndrome than in age- and sex-matched controls. Adiponectin levels measured in patients with NAFLD or NASH were found to be lower than those in age- and sex-matched controls and correlate negatively with hepatic fat. Low levels of adiponectin expression may predispose patients to the progression to NASH.

Abdelmalek MF, Diehl AM. Nonalcoholic fatty liver disease as a complication of insulin resistance. *Med Clin North Am.* 2007; 91:1125–1149. [PMID: 17964913]

Cheung O, Sanyal AJ. Recent advances in nonalcoholic fatty liver disease. *Curr Opin Gastroenterol.* 2010;26:202–208. [PMID: 20168226]

Clinical Findings

A. Symptoms and Signs

Most patients with NAFLD present because abnormal serum transaminase levels are discovered incidentally or in panels of laboratory tests sent for screening purposes. In general, patients with NAFLD are asymptomatic. If present, symptoms tend to be nonspecific and constitutional but may include right upper quadrant discomfort. On physical examination, associated findings are limited to hepatomegaly.

Because NAFLD is a diagnosis of exclusion, historical information is important. Several risk factors that increase the likelihood of NAFLD may be elicited in the history. Importantly, alcohol use must be limited to qualify as NAFLD, so that the maximum rate of alcohol intake is two standard drinks per day (140 g ethanol/week) for men, and one standard drink per day (70 g ethanol/week) for women. Other important risk factors for NAFLD include age, obesity, and type 2 diabetes. A family history of diabetes, obesity, and liver disease without a clear etiology provides important cues.

B. Laboratory Findings

Modest elevations of alanine aminotransferase (ALT) and aspartate aminotransferase (AST) are typically present at levels in the range of two- to threefold the upper limit of normal. However ALT and AST can range up to 10 times the upper limit of normal in NAFLD. The AST/ALT ratio is typically less than 1.0, and this helps to distinguish NAFLD from alcoholic liver disease (ALD). Because NAFLD is very common in the general population, it is also important to exclude other common and uncommon causes of elevated transaminase levels. These include viral hepatitis, autoimmune hepatitis, hemochromatosis, thyroid disease, drugs and, if appropriate, Wilson disease and α_1-antitrypsin deficiency. It is often useful to obtain a fasting lipid profile and plasma glucose concentration. Whereas patients with biopsy-proven NASH are more likely to also have higher levels of aspartate and alanine aminotransferases, alkaline phosphatase, gamma glutamyl transpeptidase and homeostasis model assessment of insulin resistance (HOMA-IR), currently available laboratory tests are not adequate for the predicting the presence of NASH and its severity.

Neuschwander-Tetri BA, Clark JM, Bass NM, et al. Clinical, laboratory and histological associations in adults with nonalcoholic fatty liver disease. *Hepatology.* 2010;52:913–924. [PMID: 20648476]

C. Imaging Studies

Imaging studies play key roles in the diagnosis of NAFLD. The mainstay is ultrasonography, which reveals a diffuse echogenic pattern in the setting of hepatic fat accumulation. Ultrasound is also the least invasive imaging modality and is relatively inexpensive. The sensitivity for ultrasound detection of NAFLD is in the range of 60–90%, with a specificity around 90%. These numbers depend on the degree of fat infiltration and will decline in mild cases of NAFLD. In the setting of morbid obesity, sensitivity and specificity of ultrasound are also lessened due to body habitus. Computed tomography is a reasonable but more costly imaging modality for detecting hepatic fatty infiltration, which appears as a low radiographic attenuation of the liver when compared with the attenuation of the spleen or paraspinal region. The sensitivity of computed tomography for detecting NAFLD approaches 90%. Magnetic resonance imaging allows for quantitation of hepatic fat and is the most sensitive but also the most expensive modality for detecting steatosis. These radiographic techniques share the important limitations that they cannot distinguish simple steatosis from NASH, nor can they assess the stage of disease (ie, degree of inflammation) or the presence of fibrosis.

Browning JD. New imaging techniques for non-alcoholic steatohepatitis. *Clin Liver Dis.* 2009;13:607–619. [PMID: 19818308]

D. Special Tests

The value of liver biopsy in the management of NAFLD is controversial. Histologic features that can be appreciated in NAFLD include hepatocellular steatosis and balloon degeneration, mixed inflammatory-cell infiltrates, necrosis, glycogen nuclei, and Mallory hyaline. Liver biopsy can also assess degree of fibrosis. An important limitation of liver biopsy is that sampling error can be substantial, leading to both overestimation and underestimation of degree of severity. Although liver biopsy is the only procedure that can distinguish between simple steatosis and NASH, its value in clinical practice remains uncertain. NASH accounts for a relatively small fraction of patients when compared with the high prevalence of NAFLD in the population. Therefore, most patients will have steatosis alone by biopsy, and this carries a favorable prognosis. Moreover, there are no approved therapies for NAFLD or NASH, so distinguishing between these two entities would not likely influence management. On the other hand, histopathology does provide prognostic information and, importantly, can exclude coexisting conditions. The latter consideration may become even more important as the prevalences of obesity and diabetes increase in the population. With progress in the area of surrogate markers for inflammation and fibrosis, the decision to subject patients to liver biopsy may be simplified.

Adams LA, Angulo P. Role of liver biopsy and serum markers of liver fibrosis in non-alcoholic fatty liver disease. *Clin Liver Dis.* 2007;11:25–35. [PMID: 17544970]

Angulo P, Hui JM, Marchesini G, et al. The NAFLD fibrosis score: a noninvasive system that identifies liver fibrosis in patients with NAFLD. *Hepatology.* 2007;45:846–854. [PMID: 17393509]

Treatment

Although both the prevalence and understanding of NAFLD have increased, therapies for this common condition remain very limited. At present, there are no reliable evidence-based treatments. Efforts to develop effective management strategies, including improving insulin resistance and reducing oxidant stress in the liver, are based on current understanding of NAFLD pathogenesis. Current approaches include both weight loss and pharmacotherapies.

A. Weight Loss

Considering the strong association among obesity, NAFLD, and type 2 diabetes, it is logical that improving insulin resistance would represent the cornerstone of therapy for NAFLD. Because rapid weight loss can induce or exacerbate NASH, gradual weight loss constitutes the main objective. Gradual weight loss can be achieved through therapeutic lifestyle modifications, pharmacologic treatment, and bariatric surgery.

1. Therapeutic lifestyle modifications—Lifestyle modifications are generally accepted as meritorious for the treatment for NAFLD. Because weight loss through reduced caloric intake and increased physical activity improves insulin resistance, it is logical to think it would also lead to improvements in NAFLD. A 2002 American Gastroenterology Association position paper on NAFLD advocated weight loss in the absence of randomized studies, citing the benefits of weight loss on cardiovascular risk profile. This recommendation is now supported by two randomized clinical trials of weight loss over 1 year due to intensive lifestyle intervention. In obese patients with biopsy-proven NASH, a 9% reduction in weight led to significant improvements in liver histopathology compared with controls. In patients with type 2 diabetes, an 8% reduction in weight was associated with 25% greater reduction in hepatic steatosis compared with controls as measured by MRI spectroscopy.

Lazo, M, Solga SF, Horska A, et al. Effect of a 12-month intensive lifestyle intervention on hepatic steatosis in adults with type 2 diabetes. *Diabetes Care.* 2010;33:2156–2163. [PMID: 20664019]

Promrat K, Kleiner DE, Niemeier HM, et al. Randomized controlled trial testing the effects of weight loss on nonalcoholic steatohepatitis. *Hepatology.* 2010;51:121–129. [PMID: 19827166]

2. Pharmacologic weight reduction—Appreciating that weight loss through therapeutic lifestyle modifications is not always successful, pharmacologic options are frequently sought. At present, two drugs, orlistat and sibutramine, are approved by the U.S. Food and Drug Administration for weight loss.

Orlistat reduces the absorption of dietary triglycerides by inhibiting gastric and pancreatic lipase. In randomized trials compared with dietary changes alone, orlistat reduced weight modestly over a 1-year period by 4–8 lb. This was accompanied by significant reductions in blood pressure and plasma cholesterol, with improved glucose control. Orlistat has been studied for the treatment of NAFLD in small case series and pilot studies. Significant weight reductions achieved using orlistat have been associated with improvements in liver enzymes and hepatic fat on ultrasound. Improvements in liver histology appear to require approximately 9% reductions in body weight. Limitations to the use of orlistat include dyspepsia, bloating, diarrhea, and steatorrhea; decreased absorption of fat-soluble vitamins; as well as a requirement for three times daily dosing.

Sibutramine is both a serotonergic and a noradrenergic reuptake inhibitor, which promotes satiety. Sibutramine achieves modest weight reductions in the range of 6–12 lb at 1 year. Improvements in metabolic parameters include reduced plasma insulin concentrations in type 2 diabetic patients. When used for NAFLD, sibutramine performed similarly to orlistat in promoting weight loss, reducing transaminase elevations, and decreasing hepatic steatosis as assessed by ultrasound. The safety profile of sibutramine has proved favorable, with side effects that include dry mouth, headache, insomnia, and constipation. There is also a mild increase in diastolic blood pressure (+2 mm Hg) associated with the administration of sibutramine. It is important to note that none of these pharmacotherapies is FDA approved for NAFLD and would be used as off-label if prescribed for NAFLD or NASH.

Patel AA, Torres DM, Harrison SA. Effect of weight loss on nonalcoholic fatty liver disease. *J Clin Gastroenterol.* 2009;43:970–974. [PMID: 19727004]

Sabuncu T, Nazligul Y, Karaoglanoglu M, et al. The effects of sibutramine and orlistat on the ultrasonographic findings, insulin resistance and liver enzyme levels in obese patients with nonalcoholic steatohepatitis. *Rom J Gastroenterol.* 2003; 12:189–192. [PMID: 14502318]

3. Bariatric surgery—Surgery to promote weight loss is considered for obese patients who are unable to lose weight by therapeutic lifestyle modifications. Current evidence suggests that bariatric surgery is beneficial for many morbidly obese patients with NAFLD. Bariatric surgery includes procedures that restrict caloric intake and those that promote malabsorption of nutrients. For obese patients to qualify for bariatric surgery, their BMI must generally exceed 40. Patients may also be candidates if their BMI exceeds 35 and if they suffer from a significant obesity-related disease.

Depending on the type of procedure, bariatric surgery has achieved weight loss (defined as the percentage of the pounds above ideal body weight) in the range of 48–70%, with a mean of 61%. Postoperative mortalities ranged from 0.5% to 1.1%. Importantly, metabolic parameters were markedly improved: type 2 diabetes and hypertension resolved in 77% and 62% of patients, respectively, with improvement of cholesterol and triglycerides in 70%. Resolution of the metabolic syndrome has been reported in 96% of patients at 1 year following surgery. Bariatric surgery may lower mortality rates compared with medically managed patients by as much as 89%.

NAFLD largely improves in patients who undergo bariatric surgery, with reduced steatosis, inflammation, and fibrosis all reported in several studies that utilized different surgical approaches. Whereas bariatric surgery appears to be generally safe, underlying hepatic reserve must be considered in the selection of patients in order to avoid hepatic failure in patients with cirrhosis.

Klein S, Mittendorfer B, Eagon JC, et al. Gastric bypass surgery improves metabolic and hepatic abnormalities associated with nonalcoholic fatty liver disease. *Gastroenterology.* 2006;130: 1564–1572. [PMID: 16697719]

Mathurin P, Gonzalez F, Kerdraon O, et al. The evolution of severe steatosis after bariatric surgery is related to insulin resistance. *Gastroenterology.* 2006;130:1617–1624. [PMID: 16697725]

B. Insulin-Sensitizing Agents

Because insulin resistance is central to pathogenesis, attention has been focused on antidiabetic agents that reduce insulin resistance as therapies for NAFLD and NASH. Although metformin showed initial promise in laboratory animals, results in human trials have not born this out. The thiazolidinediones (TZDs), rosiglitazone and pioglitazone, have met with more success. These drugs activate the nuclear hormone receptor peroxisome proliferator-activated receptor γ (PPARγ).

A fundamental mechanism whereby PPARγ agonists work is to increase insulin sensitivity by enhancing adiponectin production in subcutaneous and visceral fat. TZDs have proven effective in the treatment of type 2 diabetes, although weight gain is a well-recognized side effect. The PIVENS trial compared pioglitazone versus vitamin E versus placebo for the treatment of nondiabetic patients with nonalcoholic steatohepatitis. This was a phase 3, multicenter, randomized, placebo-controlled, double-blind clinical trial of pioglitazone or vitamin E (α-tocopherol) for the treatment of adults without diabetes who had biopsy-confirmed nonalcoholic steatohepatitis. It was found that pioglitazone treatment reduced hepatic steatosis and lobular inflammation but did not achieve the primary endpoint of the trial (ie, improvement in histologic features of nonalcoholic steatohepatitis, as assessed with the use of a composite of standardized scores for steatosis, lobular inflammation, hepatocellular ballooning, and fibrosis).

Sanyal AJ, Chalasani N, Kowdley KV, et al. Pioglitazone, vitamin E, or placebo for nonalcoholic steatohepatitis. *N Engl J Med.* 2010;362:1675–1685. [PMID: 20427778]

C. Medical Therapy Targeting Hepatic Oxidative Stress

Several medical therapies have sought to improve outcomes by reducing oxidant stress in the liver, which appears to play an important role in the pathogenesis of NASH. Vitamin E is an antioxidant that proved superior to placebo for the treatment of nonalcoholic steatohepatitis in adults without diabetes in the PIVENS trial. Ursodeoxycholic acid (UDCA) is a hydrophilic bile acid with hepatoprotective properties. UDCA has shown little efficacy in the treatment of NAFLD or NASH. A combination of UDCA and vitamin E has shown promise in the treatment of NASH. Betaine is a precursor of *S*-adenosyl methionine and a metabolite of choline. It has shown promise for the treatment of NASH in a limited study, which suggested that larger clinical trials are warranted, especially considering its limited side effect profile.

D. Lipid-Lowering Therapies

Based on a strong association between NAFLD and dyslipidemia, particularly elevated triglyceride and low HDL cholesterol concentrations in plasma, the use of lipid-lowering agents has been tested in pilot studies. In general, the use of statins and fibrates has led to improvements in serum transaminases. However, mixed results and limited histopathologic data preclude recommending these therapies for the treatment of NAFLD. Because patients with NAFLD are at increased risk of adverse cardiovascular events, it is important to point out that the use of statins does not appear to carry any additional risk of hepatotoxicity in these patients.

Cohen DE, Anania FA, Chalasani N. National Lipid Association Statin Safety Task Force Liver Expert Panel. An assessment of statin safety by hepatologists. *Am J Cardiol.* 2006;97:77C–81C. [PMID: 16581333]

Course & Prognosis

A challenging aspect in the care of patients with NAFLD is predicting natural history (Figure 43–2). At present, there are no agreed upon biomarkers that permit the clinician to determine prognosis accurately. Rather, histopathology is required to predict which patients with NAFLD are likely to progress to cirrhosis. Progression of liver disease is dependent on the degree of damage that is present on a liver biopsy specimen. Hepatocellular steatosis in the absence of inflammation and fibrosis suggests the NAFLD will not progress and that the clinical course will be benign. By contrast, the presence of steatohepatitis and more advanced fibrosis portend a worse prognosis, with increased likelihood of progression to cirrhosis. Whereas the overall prevalence of NAFLD approximates 20% of the population, only about 10% of these individuals (ie, 2–3% of adults in the United States) have NASH. Approximately 20% of patients with NASH will progress to cirrhosis.

Although the overall risk of cirrhosis due to NAFLD is modest, certain groups are at particular risk. Important risk factors for NASH include obesity, diabetes, and advanced

Natural History of NAFLD

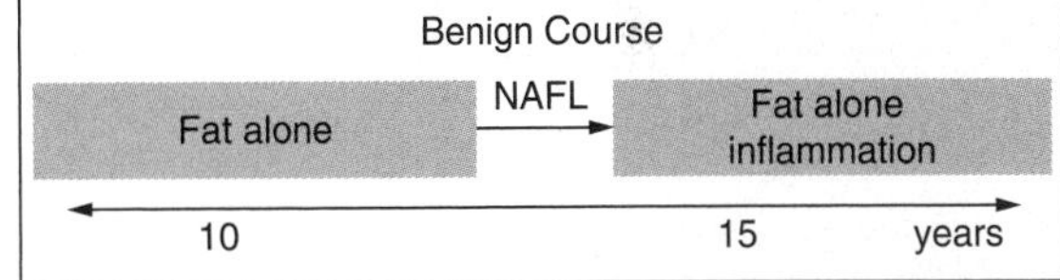

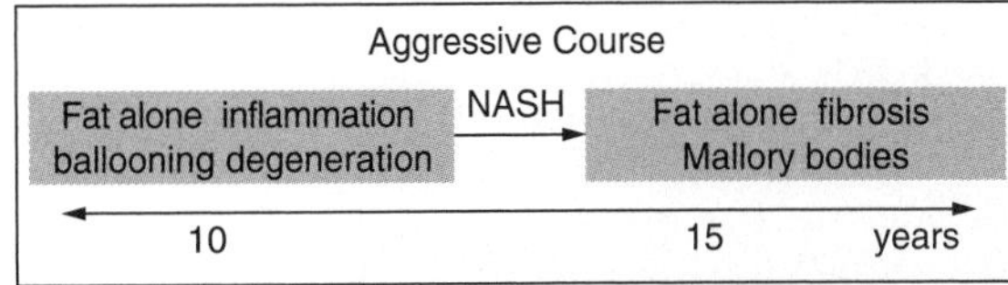

Up to 23% may progress to cirrhosis; 5% risk of hepatocellular carcinoma

▲ **Figure 43–2.** The natural history of nonalcoholic fatty liver disease depends on histopathology. Nonalcoholic fatty liver (NAFL) progresses very slowly, if at all, when fat alone is present on liver biopsy. By contrast, the presence of nonalcoholic steatohepatitis (NASH) is associated with a more accelerated progression to fibrosis. (Reproduced, with permission, from Parekh S, Anania FA. Abnormal lipid and glucose metabolism in obesity: implications for nonalcoholic fatty liver disease. *Gastroenterology*. 2007;132:2191–2207. [PMID: 17498512]) age. In the setting of morbid obesity, steatosis is present in up to 90% of patients, with NASH in up to 40% and advanced fibrosis or cirrhosis in the range of 13–14%. The prevalence of NAFLD in diabetic patients is approximately 50%, with disproportionately high representation of NASH. Fibrosis or cirrhosis is present in up to 20% of diabetic patients. Severely obese patients with diabetes have hepatic steatosis at rates of nearly 100%, of which 50% have NASH and 19% have cirrhosis. Age is also a negative prognostic indicator, with markedly increased rates of fibrosis (10-fold) in NASH patients older than 45 years (40%) compared with only 4% of NASH patients younger than 45 years.

Assessments of prognosis in NAFLD patients may also be guided by the demographics of cryptogenic cirrhosis. Prior to the appreciation of NAFLD as disease entity, the pathophysiologic basis of cirrhosis in many patients was characterized as cryptogenic. It is now considered likely that 67–75% of these individuals suffered from NASH, which led to cirrhosis and liver biopsies that had progressed beyond the point at which the etiology could be discerned. Indeed, patients with cryptogenic cirrhosis are more likely to exhibit features of the metabolic syndrome. In patients awaiting liver transplantation due to cryptogenic cirrhosis, there was increased prevalence of obesity and diabetes compared with matched controls. NASH may occur even following liver transplantation for cryptogenic cirrhosis, as has been described in patients with the diagnosis of NASH that come to transplantation.

Hepatocellular carcinoma is now recognized as a potential complication of NAFLD that progresses to NASH with cirrhosis. This risk is compounded when diabetes is present, suggesting the possibility that chronic hyperinsulinemia may provide a carcinogenic stimulus.

Overall, up to 40% of patients with cirrhosis attributable to NASH will die of liver-disease related complications or will receive a liver transplant. Of all liver transplants, approximately 10% are attributable to NASH-induced cirrhosis. Survival for patients with NAFLD is reduced compared with the general population.

Bugianesi E. Non-alcoholic steatohepatitis and cancer. *Clin Liver Dis.* 2007;11:191–207. [PMID: 17544979]

Burke A, Lucey MR. Non-alcoholic fatty liver disease, non-alcoholic steatohepatitis and orthotopic liver transplantation. *Am J Transplant.* 2004;4:686–693. [PMID: 15084161]

Fassio E, Alvarez E, Dominguez N, et al. Natural history of non-alcoholic steatohepatitis: a longitudinal study of repeat liver biopsies. *Hepatology.* 2004;40:820–826. [PMID: 15382171]

Portal Systemic Encephalopathy & Hepatic Encephalopathy

44

Norton J. Greenberger, MD

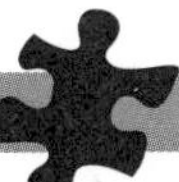

ESSENTIALS OF DIAGNOSIS

- Diagnosis can often be made during physical examination by checking for fetor hepaticus and asterixis, and evaluating mental status using serial 7's and the "A" deletion test.
- Precipitating factors include gastrointestinal bleeding, sepsis, azotemia, sedative or analgesic use, and noncompliance with medications.
- Consider other causes (eg, infections, intracranial bleeding, metabolic abnormalities), in patients with known cirrhosis and prior evidence of portal system encephalopathy who present with altered mental status.
- Mental changes in patients with subclinical or minimal hepatic encephalopathy can impair automobile handling skills; patients and their families should be advised of this risk.

General Considerations

Hepatic encephalopathy, also referred to as portal systemic encephalopathy (PSE), is a complex neuropsychiatric disorder resulting from chronic parenchymal liver disease with liver cell failure, often in conjunction with portal systemic shunts, either naturally occurring or surgically created. However, PSE can occur in individual with normal liver tests or with large spontaneous or surgically created shunts. PSE is characterized by changes in personality, level of consciousness, motor function, and cognition. Changes in cognition may be quite subtle, as pointed out below.

Hepatic encephalopathy can be characterized as being episodic or chronic resistant. The episodic form may be spontaneous, precipitated, or recurrent; in the chronic resistant form, patients have persistent mild stage 1–2 or severe stage 2–4 disease. Patients can have minimal or subclinical encephalopathy with no obvious abnormalities in cognition, personality, or behavior but with abnormal psychometric tests. Patients with advanced chronic liver disease and long-standing portal systemic shunting may also develop evidence of non-Wilsonian hepatolenticular degeneration.

Pathogenesis

Table 44–1 summarizes putative toxins that have been implicated in the pathogenesis of hepatic encephalopathy. Although the precise pathogenesis of hepatic encephalopathy is unknown, accumulation of nitrogenous products derived from the gut can have adverse effects on brain function and is believed to play a major role.

Ammonia produced by the intestine may enter the systemic circulation as a result of decreased hepatic function or portal systemic shunts. Once in brain tissue, it can block chloride channels, modulate the γ-aminobutyric acid (GABA) receptor, up-regulate peripheral benzodiazepine receptors, and increase brain glutamine. Several lines of evidence support the concept that ammonia plays a key role in the pathogenesis of hepatic encephalopathy. Ammonia levels are elevated in portal blood, peripheral blood, and cerebrospinal fluid (CSF). Factors precipitating PSE are often those that result in an increased nitrogen load and elevated blood ammonia levels. Treatment strategies are aimed at decreasing gut production of ammonia as well as decreasing blood ammonia levels. It should be pointed out, however, that there is often not a direct correlation between peripheral blood and ammonia levels and stages of hepatic encephalopathy.

Another putative gut-derived naturally occurring mediator is a benzodiazepine-like compound. Elevated benzodiazepine levels have been found in blood and CSF. Benzodiazepine antagonists can ameliorate encephalopathy, although this effect is often transient.

Other putative mediators include short-chain fatty acids, mercaptans, aromatic amino acids, and manganese. Manganese may deposit in basal ganglia and induce extrapyramidal symptoms.

Table 44–1. Putative toxins causing hepatic encephalopathy.

Toxin	Effects and Treatment Considerations
Ammonia (NH_3)	Produced by intestine; of bacterial origin Blocks chloride channels Modulates GABA receptor Up-regulates peripheral benzodiazepine receptors Increases brain glutamine Elevated in portal blood Elevated in peripheral blood and CSF Precipitating factors often increase NH_3/N_2 load Treatment strategies aim to decrease blood NH_3 levels
Naturally occurring benzodiazepines (BZDs)	Bind to benzodiazepine site of GABA receptor Elevated levels in blood and CSF BZD antagonists induce amelioration, albeit transient Unresolved issues—source and identity of actual BZDs; mechanism of increase in PSE is uncertain
Short-chain fatty acids	Synergistic effects with NH_3 causing obtundation Lactulose decreases levels Lack of correlation between plasma levels and grade of hepatic encephalopathy
Mercaptans	Synergistic effects with NH_3 Lack of correlation between plasma levels and grade of hepatic encephalopathy
Aromatic amino acids	Patients with liver failure have increased aromatic amino acids and decreased branched-chain amino acids False neurotransmitters are not found in human brain
Manganese	Probably involved in development of extrapyramidal signs Results from portal systemic shunting and reduction in biliary secretion

CSF, cerebrospinal fluid; GABA, γ-aminobutyric acid.

Clinical Findings

A. Symptoms and Signs

1. Physical findings—The diagnosis of PSE often can be made on the basis of physical examination alone. Patients may have a fetor hepaticus; this is a pungent breath odor caused by the breakdown products of sulfur-containing amino acids such as cysteine and methionine and consisting of dimethyl sulfides methanethiol and ethanethiol. Asterixis or a metabolic flapping tremor is characteristic but not pathognomonic of PSE. It can also occur in patients with chronic renal failure, pulmonary failure, and congestive heart failure.

Patients with PSE can have focal neurologic abnormalities such as increased deep tendon reflexes, unilateral or bilateral Babinski sign, and other findings such as ataxia, dysarthria, tremor, or myopathy, usually with long-standing chronic systemic shunting. These are infrequently encountered clinically.

Table 44–2. Grades of hepatic encephalopathy.

Grade	Manifestations
Subclinical (0)	Abnormal psychometric tests but no obvious abnormalities in consciousness, personality, or behavior
1	Trivial lack of awareness, short attention span, reversed day-night sleep cycle
2	Lethargy, disorientation, personality change, inappropriate behavior
3	Somnolence to semistupor, confusion, response to noxious stimuli preserved
4	Coma; no response to noxious stimuli

2. Mental status changes—The stages of hepatic encephalopathy are summarized in Table 44–2. Careful mental status testing should be performed in all patients with chronic parenchymal liver disease and cirrhosis of the liver. One approach is to ask the patient to calculate serial 7's. Patients can also be asked to write their name, and to draw a square, a star, and a spiral. Another very useful bedside test is the "A" deletion test in which the patient is asked to delete all letter A's in a paragraph of newsprint in a 1- to 2-minute period. The physician then calculates the number of A's that were not deleted.

B. Diagnostic Approach

Table 44–3 summarizes the diagnostic approach to a patient with suspected chronic PSE. The usual criteria include documented chronic parenchymal liver disease; evidence of portal systemic shunts; mental status changes, which can be subclinical; and clinical improvement with measures directed at decreasing ammonia production by the gut. The electroencephalogram (EEG) in patients with stage 2, 3, or 4 encephalopathy is usually abnormal and shows a decrease in mean cycle frequency. It is not usually necessary to perform an EEG.

1. Precipitating factors for portal systemic encephalopathy—In any patient with PSE it is important to identify precipitating factors. Table 44–4 summarizes precipitating factors and the mechanisms by which they can trigger an episode of PSE. A common problem is noncompliance with prescribed medications (eg, lactulose, because of side effects such as diarrhea).

The high prevalence of spontaneous portal systemic shunting in patients with persistent hepatic encephalopathy is not generally appreciated. A recent case-controlled study

Table 44–3. Diagnostic findings in chronic portal systemic encephalopathy (PSE).

Usual diagnostic criteria
Documented chronic parenchymal liver disease
Evidence of portal systemic shunting
• Naturally occurring (varices, venous collaterals)
• TIPS
• Surgically created shunts
Mental status changes
• Subclinical (0) → grades 1-4
Clinical improvement with measures aimed at decreasing NH_3 production/N_2 load
EEG abnormal (↓ mean cycle frequency), but test is usually not necessary
Bedside diagnosis of PSE
Fetor hepaticus grades 1-4+ (dimethyl sulfides, methanethiol, ethanethiol)
Asterixis
Mental status changes
• Serial 7's
• "A" deletion test
• Signature, star, spiral
Neurologic abnormalities
• Focal (deep tendon, Babinski reflexes)
• Non-Wilsonian hepatolenticular generations (ataxia, dysarthria, tremor)
• Myelopathy (spastic paraparesis)

EEG, electroencephalogram; TIPS, transjugular intrahepatic porto-systemic shunt.

compared prevalence of spontaneous portal systemic shunts in cirrhotic patients having recurrent or persistent PSE with that in cirrhotic patients who did not have overt signs of PSE. Fourteen patients with persistent or recurrent PSE were matched with 14 patients without evidence of PSE. The PSE evaluation included psychometric tests, EEG, mental status examination, spiral computed tomography scan, arterial and venous ammonia levels, and cerebral magnetic resonance imaging. Ten of 14 patients (71%) with recurrent PSE were found to have spontaneous shunts compared with 2 of 14 cirrhotic controls (14%). The patients with spontaneous portal systemic shunts also had a much higher incidence of abnormal results on psychometric tests (71% vs 7%). The key finding is that large spontaneous shunts might often sustain the chronicity of PSE; the presence of large shunts should therefore be sought in patients with cirrhosis and recurrent or persistent PSE. Examples are shown in Figures 44–1A and B.

Riggio O, Efrati C, Catalano O, et al. High prevalence of spontaneous portal systemic shunts in persistent hepatic encephalopathy: a case control study. *Hepatology*. 2005;42:1158–1165. [PMID: 16250033]

Table 44–4. Portal systemic encephalopathy: precipitating factors.

Precipitating Factor	Mechanism
Gastrointestinal bleeding	N_2 load, hepatic hyperfusion
Sepsis	Protein catabolism, cytokines
Azotemia	Ammonia generation (ureases)
Narcotics, benzodiazepines, antidepressants	Activation of inhibitory neurotransmission
Increased dietary protein	N_2 load
Hypokalemia	Renal ammonia generation
Diuretics	Azotemia, hypokalemia, dehydration
Constipation	NH_3 generation by colonic bacteria
Surgery	Anesthesia, hepatic hypoperfusion
Acute hepatitis	Drug, virus → liver injury, cytokines
Discontinuation of medications	Noncompliance, portal systemic shunts, TIPS, N_2 load

TIPS, transjugular intrahepatic portosystemic shunt.

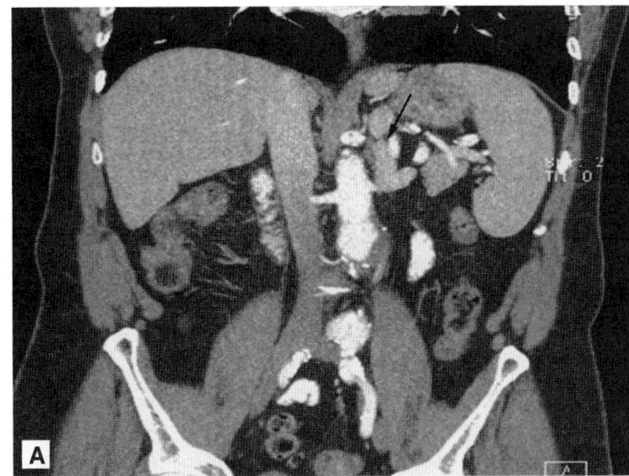

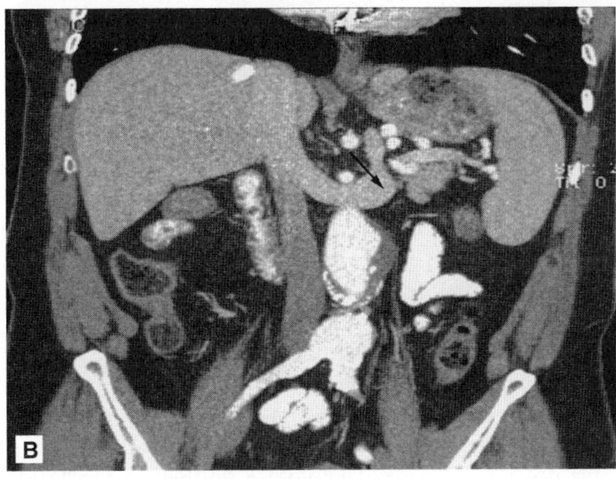

▲ **Figure 44–1. A** and **B:** Large splenic mesenteric-renal vein shunts.

2. Subclinical or minimal hepatic encephalopathy—It is important to assess all patients with established cirrhosis for the presence of minimal or subclinical encephalopathy (MHE). This is underscored by a recent study that assessed whether the ability to drive a car is impaired in cirrhotic patients with MHE. In a standardized on-road driving test covering 22 miles in 90 minutes designed for patients with brain impairment, a professional driving instructor blinded to the patients' diagnosis and test results assessed their driving performance. Four global driving categories (car handling, adaptation to lanes, overtaking, awareness of pedestrians and bike riders) and total score for driving performance were rated using a 6-point scale. Of 274 consecutive patients with liver cirrhosis, 48 fulfilled the medical and driving criteria, 14 of them with and 34 without MHE. Forty-nine individuals with gastrointestinal disease and normal liver findings served as controls. MHE was assessed by the trail-making test, digital symbol test, and complex choice reaction test. The striking findings were that MHE resulted in impaired car-handling skills and adaptation to traffic situations. Indeed, the instructor had to intervene in the driving of 5 of the 14 patients with MHE to avoid an accident. It is important to emphasize that the fitness to drive a car can clearly be impaired in patients with cirrhosis and MHE, and such patients and their families should be advised of this risk.

In patients with known cirrhosis and prior evidence of PSE who present with altered mental status, causes other than PSE may need to be considered. Patients with cirrhosis and advanced liver disease can develop intracranial hemorrhages, infections (including meningitis), sepsis, and metabolic abnormalities (including hypokalemia and hypoglycemia). In addition, patients with alcohol-related cirrhosis could present with dual problems of alcoholic withdrawal and PSE, which is a very difficult combination of disorders to treat. The only benzodiazepine that can be used for patients with both PSE and alcohol withdrawal is lorazepam because the latter drug is excreted to a greater extent by the kidneys than other benzodiazepines.

Wein C, Koch H, Popp B, et al. Minimal hepatic encephalopathy: fitness to drive. *Hepatology*. 2004;39:739–745. [PMID: 14999692]

Treatment

The management of PSE is summarized in Table 44–5. Initial treatment includes identifying and treating any precipitating factors. Attention to nutrition is also important. Rigid protein restriction is not appropriate. Patients need at least 25–35 kcal/kg and more than 200 g of carbohydrate to spare protein metabolism.

Medical treatment for PSE is based largely on efforts to control the generation of putative neuroactive toxins, most notably ammonia. Lactulose, a synthetic disaccharide consisting of galactose and fructose, is not metabolized by intestinal disaccharidases and therefore reaches the colon, where it is broken down by the fecal flora. The breakdown of lactulose to short-chain fatty acids results in a decreased fecal pH that inhibits ammonia production by urea splitting microorganisms, and traps fecal ammonia, acidifying it to ammonium chloride and resulting in an increase in fecal nitrogen excretion. Interestingly, lactose can be used in lactase-deficient patients with good results. The lactulose dose needs to be titrated so the patient is experiencing two to three loose bowel motions per day. If necessary, the fecal pH can be checked; if lactulose is, in fact, resulting in acidification of the stool, the fecal pH should be 5.0 and not the usual 7.0. Patients on lactulose should be cautioned as to the ingestion of foods that have a laxative effect (eg, excess simple sugars containing fructose, which can augment diarrhea). If diarrhea persists, the lactulose dose should be reduced.

Table 44–5. Management of chronic portal systemic encephalopathy.

Therapy	Considerations
Initial Treatment	
Precipitating factors	Identify and treat if present
Nutrition	Protein restriction (40–60 g) not appropriate to restrict protein intake to <0.75 g/kg long term (60–80 g/day) Patients need >25–35 kcal/kg and ≥200 g carbohydrate to spare protein catabolism Vegetable-based diet increases elimination of nitrogen products in stool Branched-chain amino acids are costly and data on efficacy are controversial
Nonabsorbable disaccharides	Lactulose (galactose fructose), 15–30 mL 4 times daily • Decreases fecal pH by inhibiting production of NH_3 by fecal flora • Increases fecal N_2 excretion Lactose is effective in lactase-deficient patients
Antibiotics	
Neomycin	Potential for nephrotoxicity; taper dose (1–2 g/day) for prolonged use No evidence of potentiation of response to lactulose
Metronidazole	250 mg twice daily
Rifaximin	Poorly absorbed antibiotic (550 mg 2 times daily)
Other Treatments	
Zinc	No large RCTs
Sodium benzoate	A few small trials suggest 5.0 g twice daily is beneficial; no large RCTs
Vancomycin	Small trials only

RCT, randomized controlled trial.

A controlled randomized trial of lactulose versus placebo has confirmed the efficacy of lactulose in the treatment of hepatic encephalopathy. While 12 of 61 (19.6%) patients receiving lactulose in a dosage of 30–60 mL two to three times daily developed an episode of hepatic encephalopathy, 30 of 64 (46.8%) patients receiving placebo treatment developed hepatic encephalopathy.

Rifaximin, a minimally absorbed antibiotic, has been demonstrated to be effective in treating acute episodes of hepatic encephalopathy. A recent study has established its efficacy in preventing episodes of this disease. In a randomized, double-blind, placebo-controlled trial of patients in remission from recurrent hepatic encephalopathy, 159 patients received placebo, and 140 patients received rifaximin at a dosage of 550 mg twice daily for six months. Rifaximin significantly reduced the risk of an episode of hepatic encephalopathy to 22.1% (31 of 140 patients) in the rifaximin group as compared to 45.9% in the placebo group (73 of 159 patients). Similarly, hospitalization involving hepatic encephalopathy was reported for only 19 of 140 patients in the rifaximin group (13.6%) as compared to 36 of 159 patients in the placebo group (22.6%).

Neither the study by Bass and colleagues nor the study by Sharma and colleagues addresses the effect of lactulose or combined lactulose-rifaximin therapy on gut flora and ammonia production and how changes in the flora and production correlate with the clinical efficacy of the therapy.

Antibiotics such as neomycin and metronidazole, which can alter the fecal flora, are not recommended for routine use in patients with PSE. Controlled studies have shown that neomycin in doses as high as 6 g/day is not significantly better than placebo in reducing ammonia levels. Other treatments have included zinc, sodium benzoate, and vancomycin, but no large randomized controlled trials have been performed that would permit further assessment of these treatment modalities.

Substantial rates of treatment failure remain with lactulose and/or rifaximin, highlighting the need for additional treatment strategies for this debilitating and potentially life-threatening condition.

Bass NM, Mullen KD, Sanyal A, et al. Rifaximin treatment in hepatic encephalopathy. *N Engl J Med.* 2010;362:1071–1081. [PMID: 20335583]

Prasad S, Dhiman RK, Duseja A, et al. Lactulose improves cognitive functions and health-related quality of life in patients with cirrhosis who have minimal hepatic encephalopathy. *Hepatology.* 2007;45:549–559. [PMID: 17326150]

Sharma BC, Sharma P, Agrawal A, et al. Secondary prophylaxis of hepatic encephalopathy: an open-label randomized controlled trial of lactulose versus placebo. *Gastroenterology.* 2009;137: 885–891. [PMID: 19501587]

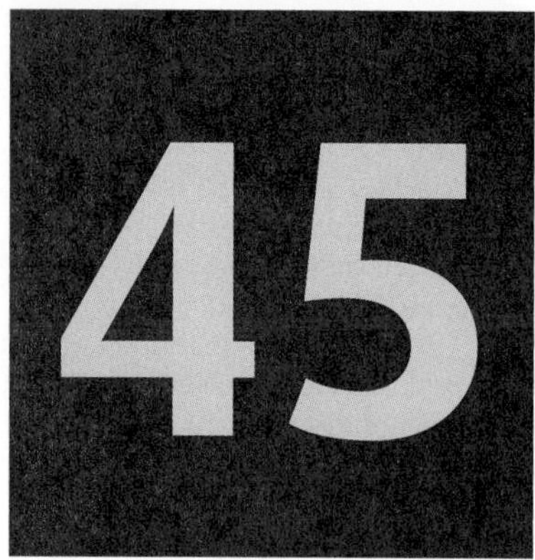

Ascites & Spontaneous Bacterial Peritonitis

Norton J. Greenberger, MD

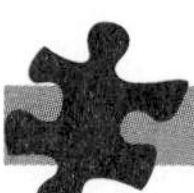

ESSENTIALS OF DIAGNOSIS

- All patients with cirrhosis and ascites on admission should undergo diagnostic paracentesis.
- Diagnosis of spontaneous bacterial peritonitis (SBP) is usually established by an elevated ascitic fluid polymorphonuclear leukocyte (PMN) count >250 cells/mL. Whereas some patients with ascites have peritoneal fluid PMN counts >250 cells/mL, *all* patients with SBP do.
- The most useful parameter for classifying ascites is the serum–albumin peritoneal fluid albumin gradient (SAAG).
- With 98% accuracy a SAAG value >1.1 g/dL is consistent with ascites secondary to portal hypertension.
- SAAG values <1.1 g/dL can occur in ascites due to infection, inflammation, or neoplasm.

ASCITES

General Considerations

The major causes of ascites are listed in Table 45–1. In North America and Europe, 90% of the cases of ascites are due to cirrhosis, malignancy, and congestive heart failure. In Europe and other countries tuberculous peritonitis is not uncommon. Ascites is a cardinal manifestation of decompensated cirrhosis of the liver. Approximately 50% of patients with cirrhosis will develop ascites within 10 years. The development of ascites in patients with cirrhosis provides important prognostic information as up to 50% of such patients will die within 5 years.

Pathogenesis

A. Development of Cirrhotogenic Ascites

Five major factors are involved in the pathogenesis of cirrhotogenic ascites: portal hypertension, hypoalbuminemia, sodium retention, water retention, and increased lymph formation.

Portal hypertension is universally present in patients with ascites secondary to cirrhosis of the liver. Two major mechanisms contribute to the development of portal hypertension: (1) distortion of the hepatic vascular architecture caused by reduction in the intrahepatic arterial bed as a result of fibrosis and nodule formation, and (2) increased production of vasodilatory substances, most importantly nitric oxide synthase.

Hypoalbuminemia results from decreased albumin synthesis that, in turn, is secondary to impaired hepatocellular synthetic function. It should be emphasized that there is no critical level of serum albumin at which ascites formation takes place. In one large series of cirrhotic patients with ascites, serum albumin levels ranged from 2.3 g% to 3.8 g%.

Increased *sodium retention* appears to be related primarily to abnormalities of proximal tubular function, and increased proximal tubular reabsorption of sodium. The latter occurs due to increased aldosterone secretion in response to changes in effective circulating blood volume. Activation of the renin-angiotensin-aldosterone system contributes to abnormal sodium retention.

It has long been appreciated that cirrhotic patients have an impaired ability to excrete a water load. A major factor in the abnormal *water retention* is abnormal delivery of sodium in the distal tubule with a consequent inability to generate free water. This is augmented by increased vasopressin secretion (antidiuretic hormone [ADH]) in response to a decreased effective circulating blood volume.

Increased *lymph formation* occurs in the liver and splanchnic circulation.

B. Hormone Alterations

Table 45–2 lists key hormone alterations in cirrhotogenic ascites. In decompensated cirrhosis, serum levels of renin, aldosterone, ADH, and norepinephrine are all increased. In patients who respond to diuretic therapy, there is normalization of these levels. However, in patients with refractory

Table 45–1. Causes of ascites.

Portal Hypertension
Cirrhosis
Alcoholic hepatitis
Fulminant and subfulminant hepatitis
Hepatic veno-occlusive disease (including Budd-Chiari syndrome)
Congestive heart failure
Constrictive pericarditis
Hypoalbuminemia
Nephrotic syndrome
Protein-losing enteropathy
Severe malnutrition
Peritoneal Diseases
Malignant ascites (carcinomatosis mesothelioma)
Ovarian disease (carcinoma, benign tumors)
Infectious peritonitis (tuberculous, fungal, etc)
Eosinophilic gastroenteritis
Starch granulomatous peritonitis
Rare in sarcoidosis and Whipple disease
Miscellaneous Disease
Myxedema
Pancreatogenous ascites (pseudocyst, disrupted duct)
Nephrogenic ascites
Chylous ascites (lymphoma, intestinal lymphangiectasia, etc)
Pseudo chylous ascites (turbid color)

ascites, despite expansion of intravascular volume, serum renin, ADH, aldosterone, and norepinephrine remain inappropriately elevated.

Circulatory dysfunction is important in cirrhotogenic ascites. Initially, plasma volume, cardiac output, and heart rate increase because the splanchnic circulation behaves functionally as a large arteriovenous fistula. With progression of liver disease, portal pressure increases further, as does splanchnic vasodilation. There is increased sodium retention and ascites formation. The renin-angiotensin-aldosterone system and sympathetic nervous system become activated in parallel with intense reduction in urinary sodium excretion to values of less than 10 mEq/24 h. Increased secretion of ADH occurs at later stages, which explains why hyponatremia is a later event in decompensated cirrhosis.

C. Decreased Effective Circulating Blood Volume

Table 45–3 contrasts changes in mean arterial pressure, plasma volume, cardiac index, plasma renin level, and norepinephrine level in cirrhotic patients with and without hepatorenal syndrome with values in healthy individuals. In patients with cirrhosis, plasma volume is increased 50% above normal; additionally, the cardiac index is increased as are plasma renin and norepinephrine levels. In patients with hepatorenal syndrome, similar changes persist despite intravascular volume repletion.

The key factors leading to the development of cirrhotogenic ascites are summarized later. Cirrhosis gives rise to portal hypertension, which results in splanchnic arterial vasodilation. Splanchnic arterial vasodilation then leads to a decreased effective arterial circulating blood volume and activation of the renin-angiotensin and sympathetic nervous systems, which, in turn, results in renal vasoconstriction and sodium retention. The splanchnic vasodilation causes increased capillary pressure and permeability that contribute to ascites. Splanchnic arterial vasodilation also results in increased venous return and increased cardiac output as it acts as an arteriovenous fistula. This, in turn, can result in pulmonary vasodilation and infrequently results in the hepatopulmonary syndrome.

Although circulating blood volume is increased in cirrhotogenic ascites, the effective blood volume (ie, the fraction present within the intrathoracic circulation that is able to influence baroreceptors, the sympathetic nervous system, and the renin-angiotensin system [ADH]) is actually reduced. This mechanism promotes sodium and water retention. A large volume of blood enters and leaves the portal venous system rapidly due to decreased splanchnic resistance. The hyperdynamic circulation leads to vasodilation of the pulmonary circulation to allow increased venous return. Increased venous return and arterial hypertension of the systemic circulation lead to increased blood volume, tachycardia, and increased cardiac output, as summarized in Table 45–3.

Clinical Findings

A. Symptoms and Signs

Patients with decompensated cirrhosis and ascites often exhibit peripheral stigmata of chronic parenchymal liver disease. These include spider angiomata, palmar erythema,

Table 45–2. Key hormone alternations in cirrhotogenic ascites.

Hormone	Decompensated Cirrhosis	Compensated Cirrhosis	Refractory Ascites
Renin	↑	NL	↑
Aldosterone	↑	NL	↑
Antidiuretic hormone	↑	NL	↑
Norepinephrine	↑	NL	↑

NL, normal limit; ↑, increased.

Table 45–3. Comparative findings in cirrhotic ascites with and without hepatorenal syndrome.

		Subjects with Cirrhosis and Ascites	
	Healthy Subjects	No HRS	HRS
Mean arterial pressure	87 ± 3	82 ± 2	69 ± 5
Plasma volume (mL/kg)	44 ± 2	66 ± 2	59 ± 4
Cardiac index (L/min/m^2)	3.0 ± 0.2	5.7 ± 0.2	5.5 ± 0.5
Plasma renin	0.5 ± 0.1	8.2 ± 2.0	31.7 ± 10.4
Norepinephrine (pg/mL)	200 ± 22	512 ± 39	1141 ± 134

HRS, hepatorenal syndrome.
Reproduced, with permission, from Arroyo V, Navasa M. Ascites and spontaneous bacterial peritonitis. In: Schiff ER (editor). *Schiff's Diseases of the Liver*, 10th ed. Lippincott Williams & Wilkins, 2007:542.

gynecomastia, parotid enlargement, Dupuytren contracture, paucity of axillary and pubic hair, and testicular atrophy, with the north-south testicular diameter being less than 3 cm. The triad of findings of *parotid enlargement, gynecomastia,* and *Dupuytren contracture* usually implies an alcoholic etiology leading to the patient's cirrhosis. The triad of findings of *hepatomegaly, ascites,* and *increased venous collateral of the anterior abdominal walls* always indicates the presence of portal hypertension.

A diagnosis of cirrhosis can be made on the basis of two physical findings and two laboratory findings. The two physical findings are asterixis and ascites; the two laboratory findings are hypoalbuminemia (serum albumin levels <2.8 g/dL) and prolongation of the prothrombin time (international normalized ratio [INR] >1.6). The presence of "classical" physical findings (eg, bulging flanks, shifting dullness, and a fluid wave), however, are only about 60–70% accurate in predicting the presence of ascites.

B. Laboratory Findings

Patients with ascites should always be evaluated with diagnostic paracentesis to determine the cause. The most useful parameter to classify ascites is the serum–ascites peritoneal fluid albumin gradient (SAAG), which is calculated by subtracting the ascites albumin concentration from the serum value. With approximately 98% accuracy a difference of greater than 1.1 g/dL is consistent with ascites secondary to portal hypertension. Conversely, gradients less than 1.1 g/dL are associated with ascites due to inflammation, infection, malignancy, and disorders such as pancreatogenous ascites, tuberculous peritonitis with ascites. Thus, the underlying cause can be readily differentiated.

In patients with cirrhotogenic ascites, measurement of urine electrolytes is important. If ascites is due to cirrhosis, urine sodium excretion will be low (eg, frequently <10 mEq/24 h) and potassium excretion increased to a value of greater than 30 mEq/24 h. This can also be used as a baseline measurement to determine the effectiveness of diuretic therapy as distal-acting agents such as spironolactone frequently cause a reversal of the abnormal sodium-potassium ratio. In addition, if patients with cirrhotogenic ascites are found to have high urine sodium excretion it would suggest another complicating factor such as malignancy.

C. Imaging Studies

In patients with ascites it is important to obtain an ultrasound examination not only to confirm the diagnosis of ascites, but also to assess the patency of the portal and hepatic veins. This is because portal or hepatic vein thrombosis can occur in the setting of cirrhosis of the liver. Ultrasonography can detect as little as 100 mL of fluid in the peritoneal cavity whereas on physical examination ascitic fluid volume usually needs to exceed 2 L to be evident. Patients with cirrhosis can develop umbilical hernias when long-standing ascites is present. Such hernias can actually increase in size if ascites persists uncontrolled.

Treatment

A. Management of Sodium Balance

Because sodium retention is a major factor in the development of ascites, a key goal of therapy is the attainment of a negative sodium balance. To achieve this, sodium output must exceed sodium input. Accordingly, appropriate sodium restriction is very important in the treatment of ascites and in maintenance of cirrhotic patients who are ascites free. In older studies severe salt restriction (22 mmol/24 h) was associated with a shorter time for resolution of ascites. More recent studies, however, have shown that there is little difference in diuretic responsiveness with sodium intakes of 50–90 mmol/day. Most authorities now believe that restriction of salt to 4 g/day is reasonable. This translates into a sodium intake of 2000 mg/day (or 20 mEq/day). Patients need detailed dietary instructions as to hidden sources of sodium in their diet.

Bed rest often facilitates diuresis because upright posture activates sodium-retaining systems and impairs renal profusion and sodium excretion. It is usually not necessary to restrict water intake unless the serum sodium is less than 125 mEq/dL. Water restriction should not be prescribed if fever, sepsis, bleeding, or azotemia are present.

Diuretics are usually required in patients with ascites, especially those with moderate to severe ascites who retain sodium avidly and for whom sodium restriction will not be sufficient to retain negative sodium balance. In such cases, it is reasonable to begin with a potassium-sparing diuretic such as spironolactone initially, given as a dosage of 100–200 mg/day. This can be increased cautiously to 400 mg/day, but one needs to watch for hyperkalemia and metabolic acidosis. The spironolactone dose need not be split and can be given once daily. An effect of spironolactone can be noted as early as 3 days after initiation of treatment. Effective therapy with spironolactone usually results in a reversal of the potassium-sodium abnormalities in the urine, with an increase of sodium excretion to more than 10 mEq/day and a decrease in potassium secretion. Other potassium-sparing diuretics include amiloride and triamterene. It is often necessary to add a loop diuretic, such as furosemide or torsemide. Furosemide is given initially at a dosage of 20–40 mg/day and can be increased to 160 mg. Torsemide is administered at a dosage of 10–20 mg/day and can be increased to 80 mg/day.

Patients with cirrhosis, ascites, and edema initially loose excess fluid from their extremities rather than abdominal fluid. It is reasonable to expect patients with cirrhosis and ascites who have been placed on a diuretic regimen and sodium restriction to lose between 0.5 and 1.0 kg/day. Losses greater than this can occur, especially with brisk diuresis, and may precipitate an episode of oliguric hepatic failure.

B. Managing Patients Who Do Not Respond to Salt and Fluid Restriction and Diuretics

The patient's fluid intake and output and urine sodium excretion should be monitored closely, especially if urine sodium excretion exceeds 50 mEq/day. This would suggest that the patient is obtaining salt-laden foods in the hospital or surreptitiously ingesting large amounts of fluid (eg, >2500 mL/24 h). In this regard, patients may also be ingesting large amounts of ice, as one pint of ice intake yields over 800 mL of fluid. Please refer to Table 45–4 for considerations in managing difficult to control ascites.

1. Definition and management of refractory ascites— Five percent of cirrhotic patients with ascites develop refractory ascites. The following criteria are usually employed to establish diagnosis of refractory ascites. Failure to respond to spironolactone, 200–400 mg/day; furosemide, 160 mg/day; restriction of dietary sodium intake to 10 mEq/day; and water restriction to 1.5–2.0 L/day, accompanied by urinary sodium excretion of less than 10 mEq/24 h.

If the patient is stable, the following options are available. Patients may respond to a large volume paracentesis. Furosemide given intravenously as a bolus results in higher initial concentrations of the drug being delivered to the renal tubule, but this may not be sustained. Accordingly, a

Table 45–4. Considerations in managing difficult to control ascites.

Problem	Suggested Approach
1. Failure to maintain a low sodium diet (≤2 gm Na^+/day)	Check urine Na^+ to see if it exceeds 50 mEq/day
2. Maximize diuretic effectiveness	Avoid split doses of furosemide
3. Maximize spironolactone use	A high urine K^+ (>30 mEq/day) and low Na^+ (<20 mEq/day) suggests too little spironolactone to not split spironolactone dosage
4. Development of hyponatremia	• Avoid excessive diuresis and hypotonic fluids • Consider a relative vasopressin V_2 receptor antagonist (see text on "Selective Vasopressin V_2 Receptor Antagonists" below)
5. Worsening renal function	• Look for NSAID or aspirin use • Avoid over-diuresis • Exclude SBP • With worsening liver disease, ie, encephalopathy, jaundice, coagulation abnormalities, consider liver transplantation
6. Refractory ascites	See below

Adapted with permission from Boyer TD. Difficult to manage ascites: causes, evaluation and management. *American Association for the Study of Liver Diseases Postgraduate Course Syllabus*, 2009:100.

Table 45–5. Outcomes in patients undergoing transjugular intrahepatic portosystemic shunt (TIPS) for refractory ascites.

	Paracentesis (N = 156)	TIPS (N = 149)
Recurrent ascites	139 (89%)	63 (42%)
Death	78 (50%)	65 (44%)
Actuarial transplant-free survival at 36 months[a]	28%	38%
Average number of PSE episodes per patient	0.63	1.13

PSE, portal systemic encephalopathy.
[a]Factors associated with transplant-free survival: age, serum bilirubin, and serum Na^+.
Data from Salerno F, Cammá C, Enea M, et al. Transjugular intrahepatic portosystemic shunt for refractory ascites: a meta-analysis of individual patient data. *Gastroenterology.* 2007;133:825–834.

furosemide drip infusing 20 mg/h can be effective in restoring diuretic responsiveness by achieving sustained elevated furosemide levels in the renal medulla.

In this setting, it is reasonable to consider adding either metolazone or hydrochlorothiazide, which act on the ascending limb, in addition to administering furosemide at 20 mg/h intravenously.

2. Large-volume paracentesis—It has been demonstrated that large-volume paracentesis (ie, removal of 4–6 L/day of fluid) with albumin replacement of 8.0 g/L of ascitic fluid removed is an effective approach in patients with refractory ascites. The rationale for including albumin is that studies have indicated that side effects occurred in 30% of patients undergoing large-volume paracentesis alone compared with 16% in patients who had paracentesis plus albumin replacement. Large-volume paracentesis is more effective than diuretics in eliminating ascites and shortening the duration of hospitalization. However, it should be emphasized that this procedure does not eliminate the need for continued diuretic therapy. Contraindications to large-volume paracentesis include sepsis, spontaneous bacterial peritonitis (SBP), recent gastrointestinal bleeding, azotemia, marked wasting, and low blood pressure.

3. Transjugular intrahepatic portosystemic shunting (TIPS)—The North American Study for the Treatment of Refractory Ascites was a multicenter randomized trial in which 109 patients with refractory ascites were randomized to medical therapy (sodium restriction, diuretics, and total paracentesis) or medical therapy plus TIPS. Although TIPS was found to be effective in 60% of patients with refractory ascites, and more effective than paracentesis, there was no difference in survival and, importantly, an increased risk of portal systemic encephalopathy and shunt problems in TIPS patients. The study authors concluded that although TIPS plus medical therapy appeared to be superior to medical therapy alone for the control of ascites, it did not improve survival, decrease hospitalization rates, or improve overall quality of life.

In contrast, a recent meta-analysis compared the effect of TIPS and large-volume paracentesis in cirrhotic patients with refractory ascites using data from four randomized controlled trials of 305 patients (149 allocated to TIPS, and 156 to paracentesis). Cumulative probabilities of transplant-free survival and of hepatic encephalopathy were estimated using Kaplan-Meyer methodology. The data are shown in Table 45–5. This meta-analysis provides evidence showing that TIPS significantly improves transplant-free survival.

4. Selective Vasopressin V_2 Receptor Antagonists—A main pathogenetic factor responsible for cirrhotogenic ascites is a nonosmotic hypersecretion of arginine vasopressin (antidiuretic hormone) related to arterial splanchnic vasodilation and arterial underfilling leading in turn to activation of baroreceptors and release of ADH. Vaptans act by antagonizing specifically the effects of ADH on the V_2 receptors located in the kidney tubules.

In two multicenter, randomized, double-blind, placebo-controlled trials, the efficacy of tolvaptan was evaluated in patients with euvolemic or hypervolemic hyponatremia. Patients received either oral placebo (223 patients) or oral tolvaptan (225) at a dose of 15 mg/daily; 63 of the patients had cirrhotic ascites. The two primary end points for all patients were the change in the average daily area under the curve for the serum sodium concentration from baseline to day 4 and the change from baseline to day 30. Serum sodium concentrations increased significantly more in the tolvaptan group than in the placebo group during the first four days and after the full 30 days of therapy with the average increase 4–6 mEq/L. During the week after discontinuation of tolvaptan on day 30, hyponatremia recurred. Side effects associated with tolvaptan included increased thirst, dry mouth, and increased urination, and an increased risk of gastrointestinal bleeding possibly related to the effect of tolvaptan on vitamin K–dependant clotting factors in platelet function.

Because of the risk of side effects it has been recommended that the use of tolvaptan be limited to the inpatient setting to correct severe hyponatremia (Na^+ <125 mEq/L). Further, a reasonable goal for treatment would be a gradual rise of serum sodium of 6–10 mEq/L to a value greater than 130 mEq/L.

C. Complications of Diuretic Therapy

Significant complications can result from inappropriate use of diuretic therapy. One should be very careful about administering diuretics to cirrhotic patients hospitalized with marked wasting, cachexia, and tense ascites, as oliguric hepatic failure can be triggered in these fragile patients. Other complications of diuretic therapy include hyponatremia, hypokalemia, metabolic acidosis, muscle cramps, and precipitation of portal systemic encephalopathy. The latter may occur if diuretic-induced hypokalemia develops.

Course & Prognosis

A recent report has helped to define the natural history of cirrhotic ascites and identify prognostic factors (Table 45–6). Two hundred sixty-three cirrhotic patients were followed for a mean of 40.9 months after onset of their first episode of ascites. The average Child-Pugh score was 8.3 and the average Model for End-Stage Liver Disease (MELD) score was 10.6. The incidence of dilutional hyponatremia was 28%. Refractory ascites occurred in 11.4%, and hepatorenal syndrome in 7.6%. Overall probability of survival at 1 year was 85%, and at 5 years was 56.5%. The 1-year probability of survival was 26.5% after dilutional hyponatremia, 31.6% after refractory ascites, and 38.5% after type 2 hepatorenal syndrome. The authors concluded that survival of cirrhotic patients with a first episode of ascites is relatively high and is minimally influenced by age, Child-Pugh score, and development of dilutional hyponatremia.

Boyer TD. Difficult to manage ascites: causes, evaluation and management. *American Association for the Study of Liver Diseases Postgraduate Course Syllabus*. 2009;99–104.

Boyer TD. Tolvaptan and hyponatremia in a patient with cirrhosis. *Hepatology*. 2010;51:699–702. [PMID: 20101750]

Planas R, Montoliu S, Ballesté B, et al. Natural history of patients hospitalized for management of cirrhotic ascites. *Clin Gastroenterol Hepatol*. 2006;4:1385–1394. [PMID: 17081806]

Salerno F, Cammà C, Enea M, et al. Transjugular intrahepatic portosystemic shunt for refractory ascites: a meta-analysis of individual patient data. *Gastroenterology*. 2007;133:825–834. [PMID: 17678653]

Sanyal AJ, Genning C, Reddy KR, et al. The North American Study for the treatment of Refractory Ascites. *Gastroenterology*. 2003;124:634–641. [PMID: 12612902]

Schrier RW, Gross P, Gheorghiade M, et al. Tolvaptan, a selective oral vasopressin V_2-receptor antagonist, for hyponatremia. *N Engl J Med*. 2006;355:2099–2112. [PMID: 17105757]

SPONTANEOUS BACTERIAL PERITONITIS

General Considerations

SBP is defined as infection of a previously sterile ascitic fluid without an apparent intra-abdominal source of infection. The prevalence of SBP in unselected hospitalized patients with cirrhosis and ascites ranges between 10% and 30%. The diagnosis is established by an elevated ascitic fluid polymorphonuclear leukocyte (PMN) count greater than 250 cells/mL. Ascitic fluid cultures are positive in 50–90% of cases, depending on the volume of the ascitic fluid culture. Inoculations of 10–20 mL of fluid into 100-mL culture bottles led to a much higher culture positivity rate versus inoculum of 1–3 mL (ie, 3% vs 53%).

The vast majority of patients with SBP have portal hypertension, ascitic fluid albumin concentration less than 1 g/dL, and SAAG greater than 1.1 g/dL. Neutrocytic ascites is defined as ascitic fluid containing greater than 250 PMNs/mL. Many patients with neutrocytic ascites, especially outpatients, have neutrocytic ascites without culture

Table 45–6. Outcomes and survival in patients hospitalized for management of cirrhotic ascites.

		Probability of Survival[a]	
	Incidence (n = 263)	1 Year	5 Years
Dilutional hyponatremia	74 (28%)	26.5%	37%
Refractory ascites	30 (4%)	31.6%	11.4%
Hepatorenal syndrome	20 (7.6%)	38.5% (type 2)[b]	11.4%

[a]Probability of survival at 1 year for all patients was 85%; at 5 years, 56.5%.
[b]For type 1 hepatorenal syndrome, survival was 7 days.
Data from Planas R, Montoliu S, Ballesté B, et al. Natural history of patients hospitalized for management of cirrhotic ascites. *Clin Gastroenterol Hepatol*. 2006;4:1385–1394. [PMID: 17081806]

positivity or evidence of SBP. In contrast, all patients with SBP have ascitic fluid PMN counts greater than 250 cells/mL and usually other findings as well. In one survey, the prevalence of SBP in a population of 427 cirrhotic outpatients (defined as PMN >250 cells/mL) was 3.5%. Of the 15 patients with neutrocytic ascites, 6 were culture positive (1.4%) and 9 were culture negative (2.1%). Eight other patients (1.9%) had bacterial ascites. The organisms cultured from the ascitic fluid in asymptomatic patients with culture-positive neutrocytic ascites and bacterial ascites were predominantly gram-positive organisms. The conclusion drawn was that SBP in outpatients with cirrhotic ascites is much less frequent, occurs in patients with less advanced liver disease, and may have a better outcome than its counterpart in hospitalized patients.

It is important to recognize the distinction between SBP and primary bacterial peritonitis (PBP). PBP develops in patients who have ascites and a perforated viscus, as in ruptured diverticulitis and appendicitis. Peritoneal fluid in PBP in cirrhotic patients with ascites who have developed a perforated viscus has the following characteristics: protein concentration greater than 1.0 g/dL and frequently greater than 3.0 g/dL; glucose concentration less than 50 g/dL; marked elevation of ascitic fluid white blood cell count often greater than 5000 PMNs/mL; ascitic fluid lactic dehydrogenase (LDH) content threefold greater than serum LDH. If PBP is suspected, computed tomography or magnetic resonance imaging should be performed to exclude a perforated viscus, and antibiotic coverage broadened against anaerobic organisms.

Pathogenesis

Bacterial translocation, which is the passage of viable microorganisms in the intestinal lumen to the mesenteric lymph nodes and other extraintestinal locations, is a major factor in the development of SBP. These are most commonly gram-negative organisms from the intestinal flora. Such translocation is facilitated by depression of the hepatic reticuloendothelial system as well as altered intestinal permeability due to edema and hypervolemia. The hepatic reticuloendothelial system is depressed in patients with cirrhosis. It is recognized that 90% of reticuloendothelial cell function resides in Kupffer cells and endothelial and sinusoidal cells. Intrahepatic shunting with portal hypertension results in decreased contact of microorganisms with reticuloendothelial cells. In addition, there is decreased phagocytic activity. Additional factors include decreased activity in ascitic fluid and decreased compliment (fibronectin), and this correlates directly with total protein level in the ascitic fluid. As previously noted, the ascitic fluid protein in SBP is characteristically less than 1.0 g/dL. Neutrophil dysfunction also results in decreased chemotaxis and decreased phagocytic and killing capacity.

Table 45–7. Clinical characteristics of spontaneous bacterial peritonitis (SBP).[a]

Clinical Features[b]	% Patients
Fever	69
Abdominal pain	59
Altered mental status	54
Abdominal tenderness	49
Diarrhea	32
Ileus	30
Hypotension	21
Hypothermia	17

[a]Clinical presentation can vary from minimally symptomatic or asymptomatic to severe abdominal pain and fever.
[b]Signs and symptoms in 489 patients with SBP.
Data from McHutchinson JG, Runyon BA. Spontaneous bacterial peritonitis. In: Surawicz CM, Owen, RL (editors). *Gastrointestinal and Hepatic Infections*. WB Saunders, 1994:17.

Clinical Findings

Clinical features of SBP are summarized in Table 45–7. It should be emphasized that SBP can occur in patients who are only minimally symptomatic and that abdominal pain is present in only about half the patients with SBP. Certain laboratory findings also predict the first episode of SBP (Table 45–8).

A recent case-control study of 70 cirrhotics with paracentesis-proven SBP and 70 matched cirrhotics without SBP demonstrated that patients with SBP have a significantly higher rate of pre-hospital use of proton pump inhibitors (69%) compared with ascitic cirrhotics hospitalized without SBP (31%). Importantly, 47% of patients receiving a proton pump inhibitor in this study had no documented indication for proton pump inhibitor treatment.

Table 45–8. Predictors of a first episode of spontaneous bacterial peritonitis (SBP).

Parameter	Value Predictive of SBP
Bilirubin	>2.5 mg/dL
Prothrombin time (INR)	>1.6
Ascitic fluid total protein	<1.0 g/dL
Serum Na	<130
Serum albumin	<2.6
Platelets	<100,000

A. Symptoms and Signs

Although SBP can occur in patients with asymptomatic cirrhotic ascites, the diagnosis should be suspected in all hospitalized cirrhotic patients with ascites, especially if abdominal pain and tenderness are present. The diagnosis should also be suspected if fever, leukocytosis, signs of sepsis, worsening renal function, worsening of encephalopathy, and a recent gastrointestinal bleed have occurred. In particular, cirrhotic patients admitted with variceal bleeding and ascites have a 40% chance of developing SBP. Accordingly, all cirrhotic patients with recent gastrointestinal bleeding should be administered antibiotic prophylaxis to prevent SBP.

B. Diagnostic Tests

A diagnostic paracentesis should be performed in all patients with cirrhosis and ascites who are admitted to the hospital, even if the admission is for other reasons. Evidence that the diagnosis of SBP is correct and that antibiotic treatment is appropriate can be obtained by doing a repeat paracentesis within 48 hours after initiation of therapy. In patients who are responding to treatment, a decrease in PMNs of at least 50% should be evident after 48 hours of treatment. If the ascites neutrophil count is greater than 250 cells/mL antibiotic therapy should be initiated, especially if any of the clinical features outlined earlier are present. Most cases of SBP are due to gut bacteria such as *E coli* and *Klebsiella,* with occasional streptococcal and, infrequently, staphylococcal infections. In these cases, broad-spectrum therapy is warranted.

Treatment

Current guidelines call for the use of a third-generation cephalosporin such as cefotaxime or ceftazidime, given at a dosage of 2 g/8 h. Other third-generation cephalosporins, such as ceftizoxime or ceftriaxone, are also suitable antibiotics. The cephalosporins have been shown to be as effective as, if not more effective than, combinations of ampicillin and an aminoglycoside.

Antibiotic therapy usually can be discontinued after 5 days. The use of intravenous albumin in the treatment of SBP is supported by randomized controlled trials that have shown that antibiotics and intravenous albumin given at a dosage of 1.5 g/kg at the time of diagnosis and then 1.0 g/kg at day 3 reduces the incidence of renal impairment and improves hospital survival compared with antibiotics given alone. This is especially important in patients with a serum bilirubin ≥4 mg/dL.

Predictors of resolution and survival in SBP include young age, absence of acidemia and renal impairment, peak serum bilirubin levels of 5 mg% or less, and community- rather than hospital-acquired SBP. The 1-year survival rate is approximately 40%.

Patients who have recovered from an episode of SBP are at a high risk of recurrence. Long-term prophylaxis with norfloxacin or trimethoprim–sulfamethoxazole is effective in preventing SBP recurrence.

Patients with cirrhosis who develop recurrent SBP in the face of norfloxacin and prophylactic therapy can be treated with cefotaxime plus metronidazole. As previously noted, patients with cirrhosis and gastrointestinal bleeding are predisposed to develop bacterial infections. Approximately 20% of these patients are already infected upon admission and an additional 50% will develop the infection during hospitalization. For these patients, a short-term, 7-day course of antibiotic prophylaxis is appropriate.

It is well established that norfloxacin is highly effective in preventing recurrent SBP in cirrhosis. A recent study by Fernández and colleagues demonstrated that primary prophylaxis with norfloxacin not only reduces the incidence of SBP, but also, importantly, delays the development of hepatorenal syndrome and improves survival. Sixty-eight patients who met the inclusion criteria were randomized to receive either norfloxacin (400 mg/day) or placebo. The results are outlined in Chapter 46, which discusses hepatorenal syndrome (see Table 46–2). Primary prophylaxis of SBP with norfloxacin was effective by causing selective intestinal decontamination and reducing bacterial translocation.

Bajaj JS, Zadvornova Y, Heuman DM, et al. Association of proton pump inhibitor therapy with spontaneous bacterial peritonitis in cirrhotic patients with ascites. *Am J Gastroenterol.* 2009;104:1130–1134. [PMID: 19337238]

Evans LT, Kim WR, Poterucha JJ, et al. Spontaneous bacterial peritonitis in asymptomatic patients with cirrhotic ascites. *Hepatology.* 2003;37:897–901. [PMID: 12668984]

Fernández J, Navasa M, Planas R, et al. Primary prophylaxis of spontaneous bacterial peritonitis delays hepatorenal syndrome and improves survival in cirrhosis. *Gastroenterology.* 2007;33:818–824. [PMID: 17854593]

Runyon BA. Ascites and spontaneous bacterial peritonitis. In: Feldman M, Friedman LS, Brandt LJ (editors). *Sleisenger and Fordtran's Gastrointestinal and Liver Disease,* 8th ed, vol 2. Saunders Elsevier, 2006;1935–1964.

Sort P, Navasa M, Arroyo V, et al. Effect of intravenous albumin on renal impairment and mortality in patients with cirrhosis and spontaneous bacterial peritonitis. *N Engl J Med.* 1999;341:403–409. [PMID: 10532325]

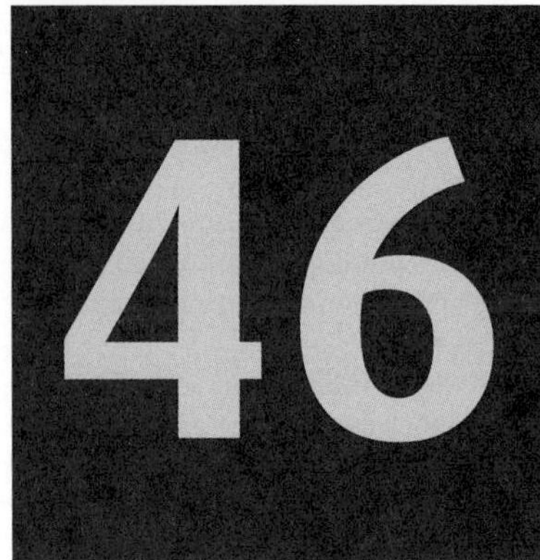

Hepatorenal Syndrome

Norton J. Greenberger, MD

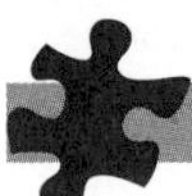

ESSENTIALS OF DIAGNOSIS

- Type 1 hepatorenal syndrome—rapid and progressive impairment of renal function defined by doubling of the initial serum creatinine level to >2.5 mg/dL or 50% reduction of the initial 24-hour creatinine clearance to <20 mL/min in less than 2 weeks.
- Type 2 hepatorenal syndrome—impairment in renal function leading to serum creatinine level >1.5 mg/dL that does not meet the criteria for type 1.
- Frequent precipitants include gastrointestinal bleeding, sepsis, spontaneous bacterial peritonitis, aggressive diuresis and paracentesis, nonsteroidal anti-inflammatory drugs (NSAIDs), and intravenous contrast agents.
- Intravenous albumin, 1.0 g/kg, should be administered on the first day of diagnosis of hepatorenal syndrome, Type 1 followed by 20–40 g/day.

General Considerations

Hepatorenal syndrome is characterized by functional kidney failure in patients with end-stage liver disease. It results in intense renal vasoconstriction without any other identifiable kidney pathology. Clinical features of hepatorenal syndrome include oliguria, dilutional hyponatremia, progressive azotemia, and hypotension. Frequent precipitants include gastrointestinal bleeding, sepsis, aggressive diuresis, and paracentesis. However, many patients develop hepatorenal syndrome as a consequence of chronic end-stage liver disease without any identifiable precipitating factors.

A. Incidence

Hepatorenal syndrome develops in 5% of patients with chronic liver disease who present with upper gastrointestinal bleeding, 30% of patients admitted with spontaneous bacterial peritonitis, 10% of patients with ascites treated with total paracentesis, and 25% of patients with severe alcoholic hepatitis. The probability of hepatorenal syndrome developing in a patient with cirrhosis and new onset of ascites is 7–10%. The 5-year probability of hepatorenal syndrome developing in a patient with cirrhosis and recurrent ascites is 40%.

B. Definition

1. Type 1 hepatorenal syndrome—Type 1 is characterized by rapid and progressive impairment of renal function defined by a doubling of the initial serum creatinine to a level higher than 2.5 mg/dL or a 50% reduction of the initial 24-hour creatinine clearance to a level lower than 20 mL/min in less than 2 weeks.

2. Type 2 hepatorenal syndrome—Type 2 is defined as impairment in renal function (serum creatinine >1.5 mg/dL) that does not meet the criteria for type 1. Prerenal failure is a preischemic state and may lead to ischemic tubular necrosis.

Salerno F, Gerbes A, Ginès P, et al. Diagnosis, prevention and treatment of hepatorenal syndrome in cirrhosis. *Gut.* 2007;56: 1310–1318. [PMID: 17389705]

Pathogenesis

In patients with cirrhosis and ascites there is activation of the renin-angiotensin and sympathetic nervous systems, resulting in elevated levels of renin, aldosterone, and norepinephrine. If cirrhotic patients undergo diuresis successfully, the levels of renin, aldosterone, norepinephrine, and antidiuretic hormone all decrease. However, in patients with end-stage liver disease complicated by hepatorenal syndrome, levels of renin, aldosterone, antidiuretic hormone, and norepinephrine are raised and remain persistently elevated despite vigorous attempts at volume expansion. This consequence occurs in part because of decreased systemic vascular resistance and splanchnic arteriolar vasodilation. The splanchnic vasodilation results from increased nitric oxide synthesis. The combination of decreased systemic vascular resistance and arterial underfilling leads to the stimulation of systemic vasoconstrictors which, in turn, causes renal vasoconstriction.

In the early stages of cirrhosis, increased systemic and local vasodilators may act to preserve renal function. The vasodilators include prostacyclin, prostaglandin E_2, nitric oxide, atrial natriuretic peptide, and the kallikrein-kinin system. Vasoconstrictors include angiotensin II, norepinephrine, neuropeptide Y, endothelin-1, adenosine, thromboxane A_2, cysteinyl leukotrienes, and F_2-isoprostanes. With the development of hepatorenal syndrome, there is decreased production of local vasodilators and increased production of vasoconstrictors. The net result is intense renal vasoconstriction affecting primarily the renal cortex. NSAIDs, and aspirin, by virtue of their inhibition of prostaglandin synthesis, may actually interfere with the production of local vasodilators in the kidney and can trigger or precipitate an episode of hepatorenal syndrome in cirrhotic patients with marginal renal function.

Planas R, Montoliu S, Ballesté B, et al. Natural history of patients hospitalized for management of cirrhotic ascites. *Clin Gastroenterol Hepatol.* 2006;4:1385–1394. [PMID: 17081806]

Clinical Findings

The major and minor criteria for diagnosis of hepatorenal syndrome are summarized in Table 46–1. Hepatorenal syndrome is characterized by oliguria (<500 mL/24 h), an unremarkable urinary sediment, a low rate of sodium secretion (<10 mEq/L), a low urine output in the absence of diuretics, and a progressive rise of plasma creatinine.

Table 46–1. Diagnostic criteria for hepatorenal syndrome.

1. Cirrhosis with ascites.
2. Serum creatinine >1.5 mg/dL.
3. Type 1 hepatorenal syndrome is characterized by a doubling of the serum creatinine to >2.5 mg/dL in less than two weeks; type 2 is characterized by a stable or less rapid course than in type 1.
4. No improvement of serum creatinine (to ≤1.5 mg/dL) after at least two days with diuretic withdrawal and volume expansion with albumin 1.0 g/kg body weight per day up to a maximum of 100 g/day.
5. Absence of shock.
6. No current or recent treatment with nephrotoxic drugs.
7. Absence of parenchymal kidney disease, i.e., no proteinuria >500 mg/day, microhematuria (>50 red blood cells per high power field), or abnormal kidneys on ultrasonography.

Modified with permission from Salerno F, Gerbes A, Ginès P, et al. Diagnosis, prevention and treatment of hepatorenal syndrome in cirrhosis. *Gut*. 2007;56:1310-1318.

Table 46–2. Types of renal failure in cirrhosis.

1. Hepatorenal syndrome—type 1 or type 2, see Table 46-1.
2. Hypovolemia–induced renal failure (gastrointestinal bleeding or fluid losses from diarrhea, or renal losses from excessive diuretic therapy).
3. Parenchymal renal disease—see Table 46-1.
4. Drug-induced renal failure—current/recent treatment with nonsteroidal anti-inflammatory drugs (NSAIDs), aminoglycosides, acetylsalicylic acid, or intravenous contrast.

Adapted with permission from Ginès P, Schrier RW. Renal failure in cirrhosis. *N Engl J Med*. 2009;361:1279–1290. [PMID: 19776409]

The onset of renal failure is typically insidious but can be precipitated by acute insults such as gastrointestinal bleeding, sepsis, spontaneous peritonitis, and overly rapid diuresis, especially in patients who have marked ascites but no peripheral edema. Although diuretics can cause azotemia and appear to trigger an episode of hepatorenal syndrome, the syndrome usually progresses even after diuretics have been discontinued and expansion has occurred with infusion of plasma expanders.

The types of renal failure in cirrhosis are summarized in Table 46–2.

The incidence and prognosis of different types of functional renal failure in cirrhotic patients with ascites has been studied in 263 consecutive cirrhotics followed for 41 ± 3 months after onset of ascites. During the follow-up period, 129 (49%) developed some type of functional renal failure. These were characterized as follows: (1) prerenal failure 72 (27%); (2) infection-induced renal failure 37 (14.1%); and (3) hepatorenal syndrome 20 (7.6%).

Montoliu S, Ballesté B, Planas R, et al. Incidence and prognosis of different types of functional renal failure in cirrhotic patients with ascites. *Clin Gastroenterol Hepatol.* 2010;8:616–622. [PMID: 20399905]

Differential Diagnosis

The differential diagnosis of hepatorenal syndrome includes acute tubular necrosis and other forms of renal disease such as glomerulonephritis and vasculitis. Patients with cirrhosis and ascites may develop acute tubular necrosis after a course of aminoglycoside therapy, the administration of a radiocontrast agent, or an episode of sepsis or bleeding. A fractional excretion of sodium above 2% and granular and epithelial cell casts in the urine sediment point to a diagnosis of acute tubular necrosis. Early in the course of hepatorenal syndrome, fractional excretion of sodium is usually below 1% and the urinary sediment is benign. It has been suggested that persistent hepatorenal syndrome with survival between 2–4 weeks or longer can result in sufficiently persistent severe renal ischemia and acute tubular necrosis, and the resultant changes in the fractional excretion of sodium.

Treatment

A. Preventive Measures

It is important to recognize incipient hepatorenal syndrome and take preventive measures. Hepatorenal syndrome develops in patients with systemic bacterial infections (ie, spontaneous bacterial peritonitis or severe alcoholic hepatitis, or both), and it is important to provide prophylactic treatment to guard against its development. This includes the administration of intravenous albumin (1.0 g/kg) on the first day of diagnosis of spontaneous bacterial peritonitis or sepsis, and another dose of albumin (1.0 g/kg) after 48 hours of antibiotic treatment. Improvement in underlying liver disease has been documented in patients with hepatorenal syndrome and severe alcoholic hepatitis who have received pentoxifylline (400 mg three times daily for 28 days).

It is well established that norfloxacin is highly effective in preventing recurrent spontaneous bacterial peritonitis in cirrhosis. A recent study by Fernández and colleagues demonstrated that primary prophylaxis with norfloxacin not only reduces the incidence of spontaneous bacterial peritonitis, but, importantly, also delays the development of hepatorenal syndrome and improves survival. Sixty-eight patients who met the inclusion criteria were randomized to receive either norfloxacin (400 mg/day) or placebo. The results are shown in Table 46–3. Note the decreased probability of spontaneous bacterial peritonitis at 1 year, decreased incidence of hepatorenal syndrome, and survival in norfloxacin recipients compared with patients receiving placebo.

Fernández J, Navasa M, Planas R, et al. Primary prophylaxis of spontaneous bacterial peritonitis delays hepatorenal syndrome and improves survival in cirrhosis. *Gastroenterology.* 2007;33: 818–824. [PMID: 17854593]

Table 46–3. Effectiveness of norfloxacin in preventing spontaneous bacterial peritonitis (SBP).[a]

	Placebo (N = 33)	Norfloxacin (N = 35)
Probability of SBP at 1 year	77%	61%
Hepatorenal syndrome	41%	28%
Probability of survival		
3 months	62%	94%
1 year	48%	60%

[a]Patients were randomized to receive norfloxacin (400 mg/day) or placebo. Main end points of the trial were 3-month and 1-year probability of survival. Secondary end points were 1-year probability of developing SBP and hepatorenal syndrome.
Data from Fernández J, Navasa M, Planas R, et al. Primary prophylaxis of spontaneous bacterial peritonitis delays hepatorenal syndrome and improves survival in cirrhosis. *Gastroenterology.* 2007;33:818–824. [PMID: 17854593]

B. Vasopressor Therapy

Accumulating data suggest that combination therapy with midodrine and octreotide may be effective and safe. The rationale for such therapy is that midodrine is a systemic vasoconstrictor and addresses the question of inappropriate vasodilation, and octreotide is an inhibitor of endogenous vasodilators. The use of terlipressin, a vasopressin, has also been studied.

Some general considerations with regard to the use of midodrine and octreotide follow. These drugs should be used for at least 7–14 days because the improvement in renal function usually occurs slowly. Therapy should be aimed at reducing the serum creatinine level to below 1.5 mg/dL (130 μmol/L). The effective doses of these drugs have varied in several studies. The recommended dosage for midodrine is usually 7.5 mg subcutaneously three times daily, and for octreotide, 200 mcg subcutaneously three times daily.

Terlipressin dosage is 0.5 or 1.0 mg intravenously every 4–6 hours and is doubled on day 4 if serum creatinine has not decreased 30% from baseline. Usual duration of therapy is 5–15 days.

The concomitant administration of albumin (1.0 g/kg on the first day, followed by 20–40 g/day) as a plasma expander appears to be necessary for the vasoconstrictor drugs to have a beneficial effect. The recurrence of hepatorenal syndrome after discontinuation of therapy in patients whose serum creatinine level normalizes is uncommon.

In one study of 13 patients with hepatorenal syndrome reported by Wong and colleagues, five patients were given midodrine (7.5–12.5 mg three times daily) and octreotide (100–200 mcg subcutaneously three times daily). The dose of midodrine was increased until a mean arterial pressure of at least 15 mm Hg was achieved.

Esrailian and colleagues compared the survival of patients with hepatorenal syndrome who received octreotide and midodrine treatment with a concurrent control group of hepatorenal syndrome patients who did not receive this treatment. Of the 81 patients, 60 were treated with octreotide plus midodrine, and 21 were controls. Mortality was significantly lower in the treatment group (43%) than in the controls (71%) ($P < 0.05$). Furthermore, 24 study patients (40%) had a sustained reduction of serum creatinine compared with only 2 controls (10%). This retrospective strongly suggests that octreotide plus midodrine treatment may improve 30-day survival. As the authors emphasize, a randomized controlled trial is needed to evaluate this treatment modality.

Two recent studies have demonstrated that terlipressin is an effective treatment to improve renal function in type 1 hepatorenal syndrome. Sanyal and colleagues studied 112 patients with type 1 hepatorenal syndrome, as defined by a doubling of serum creatinine to greater than 2.5 mg/dL in less than 2 weeks despite plasma volume expansion. Patients were randomized to receive either terlipressin (1 mg intravenously every 6 hours) plus albumin (100 g on day 1 and 25 g daily until end of treatment) or placebo plus albumin. The terlipressin dose was doubled on day 4 if serum creatinine had not decreased 30% from baseline. Treatment was continued until day 14 unless treatment success, death, dialysis, or transplantation occurred. Treatment success was defined by a decrease in serum creatinine to 1.5 mg/dL or less for at least 48 hours without dialysis, death, or relapse of hepatorenal syndrome. Treatment success at day 14 was noted in 14 of 56 terlipressin recipients (25%) versus 7 of 56 placebo recipients (12.5%). However, 6-month survival was only marginally better in the terlipressin recipients compared with those who received placebo (42.9% vs 37.5%, respectively).

Martín-Llahí and colleagues studied 46 patients with type 1 hepatorenal syndrome. Improvement in renal function occurred in 10 of 23 patients (43.5%) who received terlipressin plus albumin versus 2 of 23 patients (8.7%) who received albumin alone. Survival at 3 months was only marginally better in the terlipressin recipients compared with the placebo-treated group (27% vs 19%, respectively).

Angeli P, Volpin R, Gerunda G, et al. Reversal of type 1 hepatorenal syndrome with administration of midodrine and octreotide. *Hepatology.* 1999;29:1690–1697. [PMID: 10347109]

Esrailian E, Pantangco ER, Kyulo NL, et al. Octreotide/Midodrine therapy significantly improves renal function and 30-day survival in patients with type 1 hepatorenal syndrome. *Dig Dis Sci.* 2007;52:742–748. [PMID: 17235705]

Martín-Llahí M, Pépin MN, Guevara M, et al. Terlipressin and albumin vs albumin in patients with cirrhosis and hepatorenal syndrome: a randomized study. *Gastroenterology.* 2008;134: 1352–1359. [PMID: 18471512]

Moreau R, Durand F, Poynard T, et al. Terlipressin in patients with cirrhosis and type 1 hepatorenal syndrome: a retrospective multicenter study. *Gastroenterology.* 2002;122:923–930. [PMID: 11910344]

Sanyal AJ, Boyer T, Garcia-Tsao G, et al. A randomized, prospective, double-blind, placebo-controlled trial of terlipressin for type 1 hepatorenal syndrome. *Gastroenterology.* 2008;134:1360–1368. [PMID: 8471513]

C. Transjugular Intrahepatic Shunt (TIPS)

Wong and colleagues studied efficacy of TIPS as a treatment for type 1 hepatorenal syndrome in ascitic cirrhotic patients following improvement in systemic hemodynamics with a combination of midodrine, octreotide, and albumin. In this study, 14 ascitic cirrhotic patients with type 1 hepatorenal syndrome received medical therapy until their serum creatinine decreased to less than 1.5 mg/dL for at least 3 days followed by TIPS if there were no contraindications. Patients were assessed at 1 week and at 1, 3, 6, and 12 months post-TIPS with serial measurements. All patients received oral midodrine (2.5 mg/dL), intravenous octreotide (25 mcg/h), and intravenous albumin (50 g/day). The medical therapy with midodrine and octreotide led to improvement in 10 of the 14 patients as evidenced by a fall in serum creatinine from 2.6 mg/dL to 0.84 mg/dL post-medical treatment. The authors concluded that TIPS was an effective treatment for type 1 hepatorenal syndrome in patients with cirrhosis and ascites, following improvement of renal function with combination treatment of midodrine, octreotide, and albumin.

There is scattered additional information on the use of TIPS in patients who fulfill the criteria of hepatorenal syndrome. In two reports, one describing 16 such patients and another describing 7 patients, improvement in serum creatinine was noted over a 16-week period. However most of the patients died within 6 weeks or 6 months of the procedure.

Brensing KA, Textor J, Strunk H, et al. Transjugular intrahepatic portosystemic stent-shunt for hepatorenal syndrome. *Lancet.* 1997;349:697–698. [PMID: 9078203]

Guevara M, Gines P, Bandi JC, et al. Transjugular intrahepatic portosystemic shunt for hepatorenal syndrome: effects on renal function and vasoactive systems. *Hepatology.* 1998;28:416–422. [PMID: 9696006]

Wong F, Pantea L, Sniderman K. Midodrine, octreotide, albumin, and TIPS in selected patients with cirrhosis and type 1 hepatorenal syndrome. *Hepatology.* 2004;40:55–64. [PMID: 15239086]

D. Dialysis

Patients with hepatorenal syndrome can be treated with dialysis; this is most frequently done when a patient is waiting for liver transplantation. Although evidence suggests that improvement in liver function may result, most patients with hepatorenal syndrome who undergo dialysis do not survive in the absence of liver transplantation.

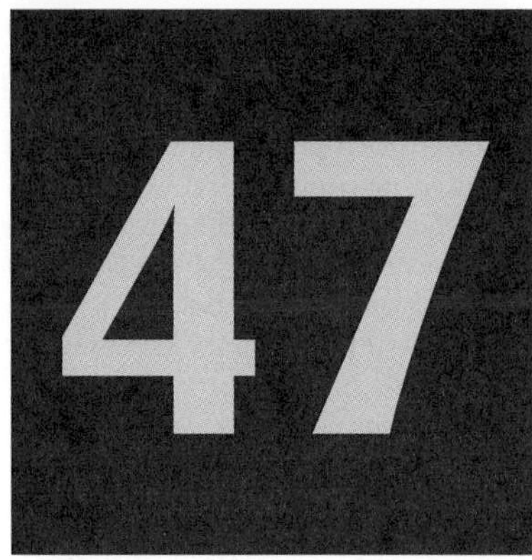

Portal Hypertension & Esophageal Variceal Hemorrhage

Norman D. Grace, MD
Melissa A. Minor, MD, MPH

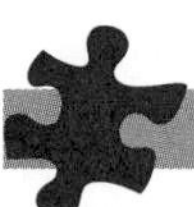

ESSENTIAL CONCEPTS

- Either nonselective β-blockers or esophageal variceal ligation can be first-line treatment for primary prophylaxis of variceal hemorrhage in patients with medium to large esophageal and high-risk small varices.
- Endoscopic variceal ligation is an alternative to pharmacologic therapy for patients intolerant to β-blockers
- Management of acute variceal hemorrhage includes resuscitation, antibiotic prophylaxis, use of vasoactive agents, and endoscopic treatment with band ligation.
- Balloon tamponade can be used as a bridge to transjugular intrahepatic portosystemic shunt (TIPS) or surgical shunt therapy.
- Hepatic venous pressure gradient (HVPG) measurements have prognostic and therapeutic value.
- TIPS, surgical shunt procedures, or liver transplantation are treatment options for patients who do not respond to medical therapy.
- Gastric varices that are contiguous with esophageal varices can be treated as esophageal varices; those below the gastroesophageal junction are best treated with endoscopic injection of glue.
- TIPS is the preferred rescue procedure for uncontrolled variceal bleeding and can be first line therapy for high risk patients.
- Portal hypertensive gastropathy is usually mild and stops spontaneously.
- Chronic bleeding from portal hypertensive gastropathy is treated with β-blockers or TIPS based on the severity of hemorrhage.

General Considerations

Chronic liver disease and cirrhosis are the 12th-leading causes of mortality in the United States. Portal hypertension and its consequences are progressively debilitating complications of cirrhosis (Table 47–1). Variceal hemorrhage, spontaneous bacterial peritonitis, and the hepatorenal syndrome are chiefly responsible for the high morbidity and mortality rates in patients with cirrhosis.

Esophageal varices develop at a rate of 5–8% per year in patients with cirrhosis and portal hypertension, and up to 80% of patients with cirrhosis will eventually develop this complication. Variceal hemorrhage occurs in 25–35% of patients with cirrhosis and large esophagogastric varices. The majority of bleeding episodes occur within the first year of diagnosis of varices. Bleeding from esophageal varices is associated with 15–20% early mortality and accounts for one-third of all deaths. If no long-term therapy is instituted after control of acute hemorrhage, 60–70% of patients will experience recurrent variceal hemorrhage. Most of these episodes occur within 6 months of the index bleed.

Pathogenesis

Portal hypertension develops as a result of two main factors: (1) an increase in intrahepatic resistance, and (2) an increase in portal blood flow. In cirrhosis, the initiating event is an increase in hepatic and portocollateral resistance. The increased resistance occurs, in part, from sinusoidal encroachment, collagen deposition, vascular tree pruning, and nodular regeneration. These elements, together with the overexpression of endogenous vasoconstrictors (eg, endothelins and leukotrienes) and the underproduction of endogenous vasodilators (primarily nitric oxide), are responsible for the increase in intrahepatic and portocollateral resistance, Systemic vasodilation follows with the increased release of neurohormonal vasodilators (eg, nitric oxide, glucagon,

Table 47–1. Causes of portal hypertension.

	Presinusoidal	Sinusoidal or Mixed
Infectious (other than hepatitis)	Schistosomiasis	—
Toxin-mediated	Azathioprine Chronic arsenic ingestion Vinyl chloride	Methotrexate Alcoholic hepatitis Hypervitaminosis A
Cirrhotic	Early biliary cirrhosis	Chronic hepatitis Alcoholic cirrhosis Cryptogenic cirrhosis Primary biliary cirrhosis
Autoimmune, oncologic, primary fibrotic	Sarcoidosis Myeloproliferative diseases Congenital hepatitic fibrosis Early primary sclerosing cholangitis	Incomplete septal fibrosis Nodular regenerative hyperplasia Primary sclerosing cholangitis
Vascular	Splenic vein thrombosis Portal vein thrombosis Cavernous transformation of the portal vein Extrinsic compression of the portal vein	—
Other	Idiopathic portal hypertension	—

Reproduced, with permission, from Wolf AT, Grace ND. Portal hypertension. In: Bayles TM, Diehl, AM (editors). *Advanced Therapy in Gastroenterology and Liver Disease*. BC Decker, 2005:675.

tumor necrosis factor, prostaglandins, and other cytokines) and results in a hyperdynamic circulatory system. This is further complicated by angiogenesis, which increases splanchnic blood flow. These factors lead to the development of ascites or hydrothorax, or both, and the formation of varices and portal hypertensive gastropathy (PHG). The goal of therapy is to interrupt the process by decreasing portal venous blood flow and/or intrahepatic and portocollateral resistance.

Bosch J, Abraldes JG, Fernandez M, et al. Hepatic endothelial dysfunction and abnormal angiogenesis: new targets in the treatment of portal hypertension. *J Hepatol.* 2010;53:558–567. [PMID: 20561700]

Clinical Findings

A. Symptoms and Signs

Patients with cirrhosis have symptoms that are nonspecific for the presence of portal hypertension. Physical findings in cirrhosis that may suggest the presence of portal hypertension include muscle wasting, spider angiomata, jaundice, splenomegaly, ascites, abdominal collateral vessels, and an altered mental status.

B. Laboratory Findings

Laboratory findings include hyperbilirubinemia, hypoalbuminemia, thrombocytopenia, and a prolonged prothrombin time. Other abnormalities that may coexist include anemia, elevated creatinine level, and hyponatremia. Although the presence of these abnormalities may indicate the presence of portal hypertension, these values often remain normal in patients with compensated or early cirrhosis.

C. Noninvasive Studies for Predicting Cirrhosis

Radiographic studies that strongly suggest cirrhosis include a small, nodular liver, ascites, splenomegaly, intra-abdominal varices, or portal and hepatic vein thrombosis; however, no test is considered a diagnostic gold standard. The current best test for diagnosing cirrhosis is liver biopsy.

1. Abdominal ultrasound—Abdominal ultrasound findings that support a diagnosis of cirrhosis include a nodular liver, with increased echogenicity. In patients with more advanced cirrhosis and portal hypertension, findings of ascites, splenomegaly and intra-abdominal varices may be detected. Unfortunately, ultrasonography is limited by interoperator variability, with a diagnostic accuracy of 85–91%. The addition of portal and hepatic vein flow Doppler images enables the assessment of hemodynamic changes that occur with cirrhosis. The reversal of portal vein flow occurs with increased hepatic resistance. This resistance results in the diversion of flow from the portal vein through portosystemic collaterals. This mechanism has been shown to be present in patients with advanced portal hypertension. Inter-observer variability, patient position, phase of respiration, cardiac output, and timing of meals limit the accuracy of Doppler ultrasound.

2. Computed tomography scan and magnetic resonance imaging—These imaging studies are limited in their ability to detect changes associated with early cirrhosis but can accurately demonstrate later changes in liver architecture, ascites, and varices. Computed tomography angiography and magnetic resonance angiography can assess portal vein patency.

3. Fibroscan—Transient elastography, known as Fibroscan, is a technique that uses pulse-echo ultrasound to measure liver stiffness as a way of detecting fibrosis. This method of measuring fibrosis is reported to have a low inter-observer variability and correlates well with the severity of fibrosis and the presence of portal hypertension.

Castera L, Le Bail B, Roudot-Thoraval F, et al. Early detection in routine clinical practice of cirrhosis and oesophageal varices in chronic hepatitis C: comparison of transient elastography (fibroscan) with standard laboratory tests and non-invasive scores. *J Hepatol.* 2009;50:59–68. [PMID: 19013661]

Ziol M, Handra-Luca A, Kettaneh A, et al. Non-invasive assessment of liver fibrosis by measurement of stiffness in patients with chronic hepatitis C. *Hepatology.* 2005;41:48–54. [PMID: 15690481]

D. Noninvasive Predictors of Esophageal Varices

Current practice guidelines recommend endoscopic screening for the presence of esophageal varices in all patients with cirrhosis. If varices are not present, screening endoscopy should be repeated within 2–3 years or sooner if there is evidence of hepatic decompensation. Several studies have recently attempted to identify noninvasive predictors of esophageal varices. A low platelet count has been associated with the presence of varices, although the discriminating threshold for the presence of varices ranges between 68,000 and 160,000/mm^2. A recent study found that patients with esophageal varices had a lower mean platelet count and a greater rate of reduction of platelets over time compared with those who did not have varices. However, several patients with cirrhosis developed varices despite having a normal (>150,000) platelet count. Non-invasive serum markers (indices combining a number of biochemical tests) have been useful in identifying cirrhotic patients in whom the risk of developing clinically significant esophageal varices is low. However, their positive or negative predictive values are insufficient to avoid screening endoscopy. Other noninvasive findings, such as splenomegaly, enlarged portal vein diameter greater than 13 mm on ultrasound imaging, and advanced Child-Pugh class, have not been reproducible predictors of esophageal varices. The predictive accuracy of suggested noninvasive markers remains low, and no markers that are currently available replace the need for endoscopic diagnosis of varices .

A promising predictor of esophageal varices is the platelet count/spleen diameter ratio as measured by abdominal ultrasound. In patients with compensated cirrhosis, the higher the ratio, the less likely it is that a patient will have varices.

Wireless capsule endoscopy has been compared with conventional upper endoscopy in identifying and characterizing esophageal varices. High sensitivity and specificity have been reported for the ability of wireless capsule endoscopy to determine the presence of esophageal varices (84–96% accuracy), the size of esophageal varices, and the presence of red wale signs. The potential benefits of capsule endoscopy include decreased study time, better patient tolerance, avoidance of intravenous conscious sedation, and possibly decreased costs. Wireless capsule endoscopy, however, is limited by inability to insufflate the esophagus, difficulty in measuring the length of varices, and image quality artifacts.

D'Amico G, De Franchis R; Cooperative Study Group. Upper digestive bleeding in cirrhosis. Post-therapeutic outcome and prognostic indicators. *Hepatology.* 2003;38:599–612. [PMID: 12939586]

D'Amico G, Garcia-Tsao G, Pagliaro L. Natural history and prognostic indicators of survival in cirrhosis. A systematic review of 118 studies. *J Hepatol.* 2006;44:217–231. [PMID: 16298014]

Lapalus MG, Ben Soussan E, Gaudric M, et al. Esophageal capsule endoscopy vs EGD for the evaluation of portal hypertension: a French prospective multicentre comparative study. *Am J Gastroenterol.* 2009;104:1112–1118. [PMID: 19337246]

Qamar AA, Grace ND, Groszmann RJ, et al; Portal Hypertension Collaborative Group. Platelet count is not a predictor of the presence of development of gastroesophageal varices in cirrhosis. *Hepatology.* 2008;47:153–159. [PMID: 18161700]

Sebastiani G, Tempesta D, Fattovich G, et al. Prediction of oesophageal varices in hepatic cirrhosis by simple serum non-invasive markers: results of a multicenter, large-scale study. *J Hepatol.* 2010;53:630–638. [PMID: 20615567]

E. Invasive Studies to Measure Portal Hypertension: Hepatic Venous Pressure Gradient

Hepatic venous pressure gradient (HVPG) measurements provide information for diagnosis, prognosis, and management of portal hypertension. The HVPG is the difference between the wedged or occluded hepatic vein pressure and the free hepatic vein pressure. Normal portal pressure (HVPG) ranges from 1 to 5 mm Hg with greater than 5 mm Hg indicating the presence of portal hypertension. In patients with sinusoidal cirrhosis, the HVPG accurately predicts the portal venous pressure gradient. An HVPG greater than 10 mm Hg identifies patients with clinically significant portal hypertension and is predictive of the development of varices. Pharmacologically reducing the HPVG more than 10% at 1 year compared with the baseline measurement significantly lowers the risk of developing varices. Similarly, a 10% increase in HPVG significantly increases the risk of developing varices.

Determining a patient's HPVG also predicts variceal bleeding, development of hepatic decompensation, development of hepatocellular carcinoma, determination of response to clinical treatment, and estimations of patient survival. Variceal bleeding can occur in patients with HVPG greater than 12 mm Hg. In patients with acute or ongoing bleeding, an HVPG greater than 20 mm Hg is associated with early

Table 47–2. Drugs used in the management of portal hypertension.

Drug	Class of Drug	Starting Dose	Maximum Dose
Propranolol	Nonselective β-blocker	40 mg twice daily	640 mg/day
Nadolol	Nonselective β-blocker	40 mg daily	320 mg/day
Timolol	Nonselective β-blocker	10 mg daily	40 mg/day
Isosorbide mononitrate	Long-acting nitrate	20 mg daily	240 mg/day
Spironolactone	Aldosterone antagonist	25 mg daily	400 mg/day
Furosemide	Loop diuretic	40 mg daily	80 mg/day
Octreotide	Splanchnic vasoconstrictor	50 mcg bolus, followed by 50 mcg/h	50 mcg/h
Norfloxacin	Quinolone antibiotic	400 mg twice daily	–

rebleeding or uncontrolled bleeding, longer intensive care unit stay, prolonged hospital stay, higher transfusion requirements, and a lower probability of survival.

Patients achieving a reduction in HVPG to less than 12 mm Hg or a reduction in HVPG of 20% after pharmacologic therapy are less likely to develop recurrent esophagogastric variceal bleeding, ascites, spontaneous bacterial peritonitis, hepatorenal syndrome, and hepatic encephalopathy. Unfortunately, only 35–45% of treated patients respond with a 20% decrease in HVPG. Patients, who do not achieve an HVPG of less than 12 mm Hg, or a 20% reduction from their baseline HVPG after pharmacologic treatment, have a high risk for recurrent variceal bleeding and a greater risk of developing complications of portal hypertension and a higher probability of death. Repeat HPVG measurements obtained 1–3 months after initiating treatment help guide therapeutic decisions.

Abraldes JG, Tarantino I, Turnes J, et al. Hemodynamic response to pharmacological treatment of portal hypertension and longterm prognosis of cirrhosis. *Hepatology.* 2003;37:902–908. [PMID: 12668985]

Ripoll C, Groszmann R, Garcia-Tsao G, et al. Hepatic venous pressure gradient predicts clinical decompensation in patients with compensated cirrhosis. *Gastroenterology.* 2007;133:481–488. [PMID: 17681169]

Treatment

A. Goal and Options

Treatment of portal hypertension includes pharmacologic management aimed at decreasing portal pressure and endoscopic therapy aimed at obliterating esophageal varices. When medical treatment fails, shunt procedures can be used to decompress high portal pressure. The goal of treatment is to interrupt the process that leads to the development of varices, refractory ascites, and hydrothorax.

De Franchis R. Revising consensus in portal hypertension: report of the Baveno V consensus workshop on methodology of diagnosis and therapy in portal hypertension. *J Hepatol.* 2010; 53:762–768. [PMID: 20638742]

Garcia-Tsao G, Bosch J. Management of varices and variceal hemorrhage in cirrhosis. *N Engl J Med.* 2010;362:823–832. [PMID: 20200386]

1. Pharmacologic therapy—Nonselective β-blockers (propranolol, nadolol, and timolol) are the cornerstones of long-term management in patients with portal hypertension (Table 47–2). β-Blockers work by decreasing cardiac output by blocking β_1-receptors and by vasoconstricting splanchnic vessels via blockade of β_2-receptors, thereby leaving unopposed α-adrenergic activity. Unfortunately, not all patients respond to maximally tolerated doses of β-blockers. In patients who fail to show a reduction in HPVG, there is often an increase in portocollateral resistance. The long-acting nitrate isosorbide mononitrate, when used in conjunction with β-blockers, has been shown to counteract this increase in portocollateral resistance. Oral nitrates may cause systemic hypotension, which limits their clinical usefulness. Carvedilol, a nonselective β-blocker with intrinsic anti-alpha-1 adrenergic activity, produces a greater reduction in the HVPG than nonselective β-blockers given as monotherapy and has been shown to be well tolerated in clinical trials.

The use of β-blockers in patients with cirrhosis is limited by their side-effect profile, which includes hypotension, fatigue, lethargy, depression, and dyspnea in patients with associated pulmonary disease. Due to concomitant diseases such as reactive airway disease, congestive heart failure, bradycardia, and heart block, 15–20% of patients are unable to take β-blockers. In patients who are candidates for β-blocker therapy, dose titration should be adjusted to patient tolerance.

Vasopressin and its analog, terlipressin, and somatostatin and its analogs, octreotide and vapreotide, have been the agents used for the management of acute variceal bleeding. These vasoconstrictive drugs act by decreasing splanchnic blood flow, resulting in a lowering of portal pressure, and by decreasing splanchnic hyperemia. Vasopressin has been demonstrated to decrease HVPG by as much as 23%. Its use is limited, however, due to significant complications, including myocardial infarction, hypertension, hyponatremia, peripheral vascular ischemia, bradycardia, and fluid retention. These side effects may be ameliorated with the concurrent use of nitroglycerin, but caution is recommended with its use, due to the risk of hypotension.

Terlipressin has a milder side-effect profile than vasopressin, and it does not appear to alter renal excretion of sodium. Its intravenous half-life is 4 hours, and its use results in a 21% decrease in HVPG. Randomized controlled trials comparing terlipressin with a placebo or no pharmacologic treatment in patients with acute variceal hemorrhage have demonstrated a significant survival benefit for terlipressin. It is safer and more effective than either vasopressin or vasopressin plus nitroglycerin.

Somatostatin has been shown to decrease portal pressure in patients with portal hypertension, but to a lesser extent than vasopressin. It works by inhibiting vasodilatory peptides from the gastrointestinal tract that have been shown to contribute to the maintenance of portal hypertension. Due to its short half-life (2 minutes), somatostatin is used as a continuous infusion after an initial bolus to treat acute variceal hemorrhage.

The somatostatin analogs, namely octreotide, lanreotide, and vapreotide, have similar pharmacologic properties to somatostatin.

Octreotide, which is used widely in the United States, is thought to act through the inhibition of the vasodilator glucagon. The intravenous half-life of octreotide, like that of somatostatin, is short; therefore, it is given as a bolus followed by a continuous infusion. Although intravenous octreotide may decrease portal pressure and bleeding from esophageal varices, its use has not been shown to improve overall survival. Similarly, vapreotide in combination with endoscopic therapy has been shown to decrease bleeding from esophageal varices more effectively than endoscopic therapy alone, but without a benefit in survival.

Together with a low-sodium diet, continuous spironolactone (100 mg/day) treatment results in a modest decrease in portal pressure. The efficacy and safety of losartan and irbesartan, angiotensin II receptor blockers, in lowering portal pressure has been established in Child Pugh class A patients but the risk of systemic hypotension and renal failure precludes their use in patients with decompensated cirrhosis. Randomized controlled trials with established clinical endpoints are needed to establish clinical efficacy.

Calés P, Masliah C, Bernard B, et al. Early administration of vapreotide for variceal bleeding in patients with cirrhosis. *N Engl J Med.* 2001;244:23–28. [PMID: 11136956]

Groszmann RJ, Garcia-Tsao G, Bosch J, et al. Portal Hypertension Collaborative Group. Beta-blockers to prevent gastroesophageal varices in patients with cirrhosis. *N Engl J Med.* 2005;353: 2254–2261. [PMID: 16306522]

2. Endoscopic variceal ligation (EVL) and sclerotherapy— EVL and sclerotherapy are local treatments for varices and do not alter the pathophysiologic processes that lead to their development. As such, even with successful EVL, varices eventually recur. EVL consists of the placement of rubber bands on variceal columns that lead to localized mucosal and submucosal necrosis and replacement of the varix by scar tissue. Band ligation carries the risk of causing esophageal ulcerations that have the potential to bleed.

Sclerotherapy involves injecting a sclerosing agent (ethanolamine oleate, sodium tetradecyl sulfate, sodium morrhuate) into or adjacent to a varix. Sclerotherapy leads to localized thrombosis and inflammation with subsequent scar formation. Both local and systemic complications of sclerotherapy occur in 20–40% of patients. Side effects include bacteremia, fever, chest pain, mediastinitis, acute esophageal ulceration (with bleeding potential), and esophageal strictures. Because of greater efficacy and fewer side effects, EVL has replaced sclerotherapy as the endoscopic treatment of choice.

Garcia-Pagán JC, Bosch J. Endoscopic band ligation in the treatment of portal hypertension. *Nat Clin Pract Gastroenterol Hepatol.* 2005;2:526–535. [PMID: 16355158]

3. Radiologic therapy—The transjugular intrahepatic portosystemic shunt (TIPS) was first introduced in the 1980s, as an alternative to surgically performed shunts. TIPS should be reserved for patients who fail pharmacologic and endoscopic management of both acute and recurrent variceal bleeding.

Placement of a TIPS bypasses the fibrosed liver and allows for unhindered blood flow between the portal and hepatic veins. A catheter is inserted into the right internal jugular vein and advanced to the hepatic venous system (usually the right hepatic vein). A needle is then used to cannulate the liver, creating a tract to the portal vein. The transhepatic tract is dilated, and a flexible metal stent is placed, resulting in a shunt between the hepatic and portal veins. Placement of TIPS is successful in greater than 90% of cases and is effective in acutely decreasing portal pressure.

Early complications of TIPS include fever, infection, renal dysfunction, intrahepatic or intraperitoneal hemorrhage, and liver failure. Furthermore, hyperbilirubinemia, secondary to hemolytic anemia, may persist until the TIPS stent is re-epithelialized. Long-term complications from TIPS placement include hepatic encephalopathy and stent occlusion. Over 20% of patients with TIPS will either develop or have worsening hepatic encephalopathy and should be prophylactically treated with lactulose, neomycin, or rifaximin. Risk factors for developing hepatic encephalopathy include older age, larger stent diameter, and prior episodes of hepatic encephalopathy. Seventy percent of patients who undergo TIPS with non-coated stents will develop stent occlusion within 1 year and 90% by 2 years. Angioplasty or additional stent placement is successful in treating stent occlusion and decreases the reocclusion rate to 10% at 2 years.

However, these complication rates are significantly reduced with the use of coated stents which have replaced non-coated stents as standard therapy. Patients treated with TIPS should have Doppler ultrasound surveillance at regular intervals to confirm stent patency, as TIPS dysfunction can result in variceal bleeding. However, angiographic assessment and measurements of portal pressure are more accurate in establishing TIPS dysfunction.

Absolute contraindications to TIPS placement include right heart failure and polycystic liver disease. Relative contraindications include systemic infection, portal vein thrombosis, biliary obstruction, and severe hepatic encephalopathy. Although TIPS can be successfully placed in most patients, placement is associated with a 30-day mortality rate of 3–15% and a procedure-related mortality rate of 2–5%.

Boyer TD, Haskal ZJ; American Association for the Study of Liver Diseases. The role of transjugular intrahepatic portosystemic shunt in the management of portal hypertension. *Hepatology.* 2005;41:386–400. [PMID: 15660434]

Bureau C, Garcia-Pagan JC, Otal P, et al. Improved clinical outcome using polytetrafluoroethylene coated stents for TIPS: results of a randomized study. *Gastroenterology.* 2004;126: 469–475. [PMID: 14762784]

4. Liver transplantation—Variceal hemorrhage is not an indication for liver transplantation. However in appropriate candidates as determined by the Model for End-Stage Liver Disease (MELD) scoring system, liver transplantation can achieve up to 95% control of variceal bleeding. Liver transplantation continues to be limited by organ availability.

5. Preprimary prophylaxis—Early treatment with β-blockers prior to the development of complications of portal hypertension may halt or delay the progression of portal hypertension. Unfortunately, the results from a large multicenter randomized controlled trial have not supported the use of nonselective β-blockers in the preprimary prophylaxis of portal hypertension. However, data from this trial show that measurements of the HVPG predict the development of esophageal varices and hepatic decompensation.

B. Primary Prophylaxis for Variceal Hemorrhage

1. Nonselective β-blockers—Because of the high morbidity and mortality in patients with cirrhosis associated with acute variceal bleeding, pharmacologic therapy aimed at preventing initial variceal bleeding is paramount (Figure 47–1). Nonselective β-blockers are the only established pharmacologic therapy for primary prophylaxis of variceal bleeding. A meta-analysis of randomized controlled trials has demonstrated their efficacy in decreasing the rates of a first variceal bleed from 24% to 15%. These studies involved primarily patients with Child-Pugh class A and B cirrhosis.

Current practice guidelines on the management of portal hypertension recommend that patients with small varices who are at increased risk of bleeding (red wale sign on endoscopy, hepatic decompensation) should be treated prophylactically with β-blockers. Patients with small varices who are not at high risk may be started on β-blockers, but their long-term efficacy has not been established. All patients with medium-to large-sized varices who are judged to be compliant and are without contraindications to or intolerance

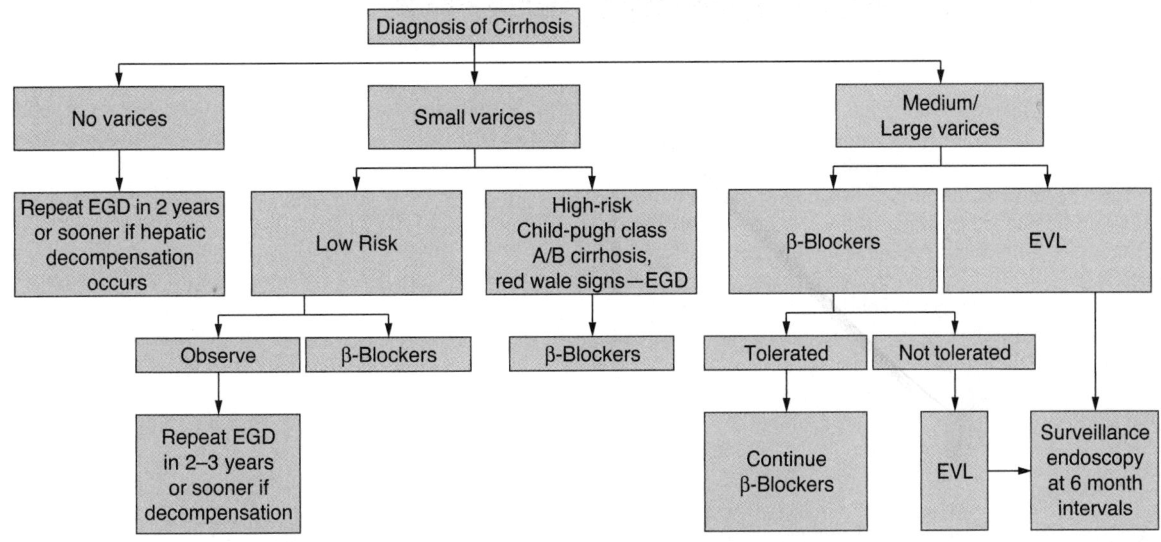

▲ **Figure 47–1.** Management algorithm for primary prophylaxis of variceal hemorrhage. EGD, esophagogastroduodenoscopy; EVL, endoscopic variceal ligation.

of nonselective β-blockers should be treated with these drugs. Therapy must be continued for a lifetime, as the risk of bleeding recurs if treatment is discontinued.

Although combining a long-acting nitrate with a nonselective β-blocker increases the number of hemodynamic responders, it has not resulted in incremental clinical benefit (ie, by preventing initial variceal hemorrhage or leading to improved survival). Similarly, combining spironolactone with β-blockers showed no benefit in decreasing rates of bleeding episodes or survival compared with treatment using β-blockers alone. Current data do not support the use of combination therapy or monotherapy with nitrates for the prevention of a first variceal bleed. A recent study suggests that carvedilol may be superior to endoscopic variceal ligation for primary prophylaxis but more data are needed to establish its clinical role.

Grace ND, Garcia-Pagan JC, Angelico M, et al. Primary prophylaxis for variceal bleeding. In: de Franchis R (editor). *Portal Hypertension IV: Proceedings from the 4th Baveno International Consensus Workshop.* Blackwell Science, 2006:168–200.

2. Esophageal variceal ligation—Nonselective β-blockers or esophageal variceal ligation are considered to be first-line therapies for the prevention of initial variceal hemorrhage. However, 15% of patients have contraindications, and an additional 15–20% are intolerant of β-blocker therapy. EVL is an excellent alternative for these patients.

For patients who undergo esophageal variceal ligation, it is recommended that the procedure be performed biweekly until the varices are obliterated. As new varices may develop after eradication treatment, it is important to continue surveillance for varices every 6 months. Endoscopic ultrasound may be used to confirm eradication of esophageal varices, but it is likely of limited utility in clinical practice.

Recent meta-analyses have shown a benefit for EVL over β-blocker therapy in preventing first variceal hemorrhage, but EVL is associated with more serious side effects and offers no survival advantage. Randomized controlled trials of EVL have been limited by a short duration of follow-up. The studies with the largest number of patients and the longest follow-up have failed to show a difference between EVL and nonselective β-blockers, either for the prevention of initial variceal bleeding or for survival. Combination therapy using β-blockers plus EVL compared with EVL alone has not been shown to decrease the risk of first variceal hemorrhage and is associated with increased side effects.

There is no role for endoscopic sclerotherapy, TIPS, surgical shunts, or liver transplantation in the primary prophylaxis of variceal hemorrhage.

dela Peña J, Brullet E, Sanchez-Hernández R, et al. Variceal ligation plus nadolol compared with ligation for prophylaxis of variceal rebleeding: a multicenter trial. *Hepatology.* 2005;41:572–578. [PMID: 15726659]

Garcia-Tsao G, Sanyal AJ, Grace ND, et al; Practice Guidelines Committee of the American Association for the Study of Liver Diseases; Practice Parameters Committee of the American College of Gastroenterology. Prevention and management of gastroesophageal varices and variceal hemorrhage in cirrhosis. *Hepatology.* 2007;46:922–938. [PMID: 17879356]

Gonzalez R, Zamora J, Gomez-Camarero J, et al. Meta-analysis: combination endoscopic and drug therapy to prevent variceal rebleeding in cirrhosis. *Ann Intern Med.* 2008;149:109–122. [PMID: 18626050]

Lo GH, Lai KH, Cheng JS, et al. Endoscopic variceal ligation plus nadolol and sucralfate compared with ligation alone for the prevention of variceal bleeding: a prospective, randomized trial. *Hepatology.* 2000;32:461–465. [PMID: 10960435]

C. Acute Variceal Hemorrhage

Patients with acute variceal bleeding may present with hematemesis, melena, or hematochezia. The initial management includes immediate resuscitation, administration of prophylactic antibiotics and vasoactive agents, and diagnostic endoscopy (Figure 47–2). It is important to consider elective intubation in patients with active bleeding to protect the airway from aspiration, especially if there is concomitant hepatic encephalopathy.

1. Resuscitation—Resuscitative measures should be aimed at replacing blood volume to a goal of a hematocrit of 25%, thereby avoiding increases in portal pressure and potential exacerbation of variceal bleeding associated with aggressive transfusion. Correcting thrombocytopenia and coagulopathy have not been shown to improve survival from an acute variceal bleed. Nonetheless, transfusing platelets in order to increase levels to greater than 50,000 and transfusing fresh frozen plasma to reverse coagulopathy may be beneficial in the acute setting. The excessive use of saline should be avoided in resuscitation, as it can worsen or precipitate the formation of ascites and volume overload.

2. Antibiotic prophylaxis—Infection in the setting of acute variceal bleeding has been associated with early rebleeding and a high mortality rate. Patients with bleeding from varices are at high risk of developing infection, including spontaneous bacterial peritonitis. Short-term antibiotics should be administered to all patients with cirrhosis and acute variceal bleeding. Norfloxacin (400 mg twice daily for 7 days) or quinolone antibiotics with a similar spectrum of activity (eg, levofloxacin, ciprofloxacin) are the preferred agents. In a recent study, intravenous ceftriaxone (1 g/day) was found to be superior to norfloxacin in patients with severely decompensated cirrhosis.

3. Vasoactive agents—As soon as variceal hemorrhage is suspected, administration of vasoactive agents should be initiated. These agents include vasopressin, vasopressin plus nitroglycerin, terlipressin, and somatostatin or its analogs. Use of vasopressin is limited by its serious side effects, which can be partially counteracted by the addition of nitroglycerin. The vasopressin analog terlipressin has fewer side effects than

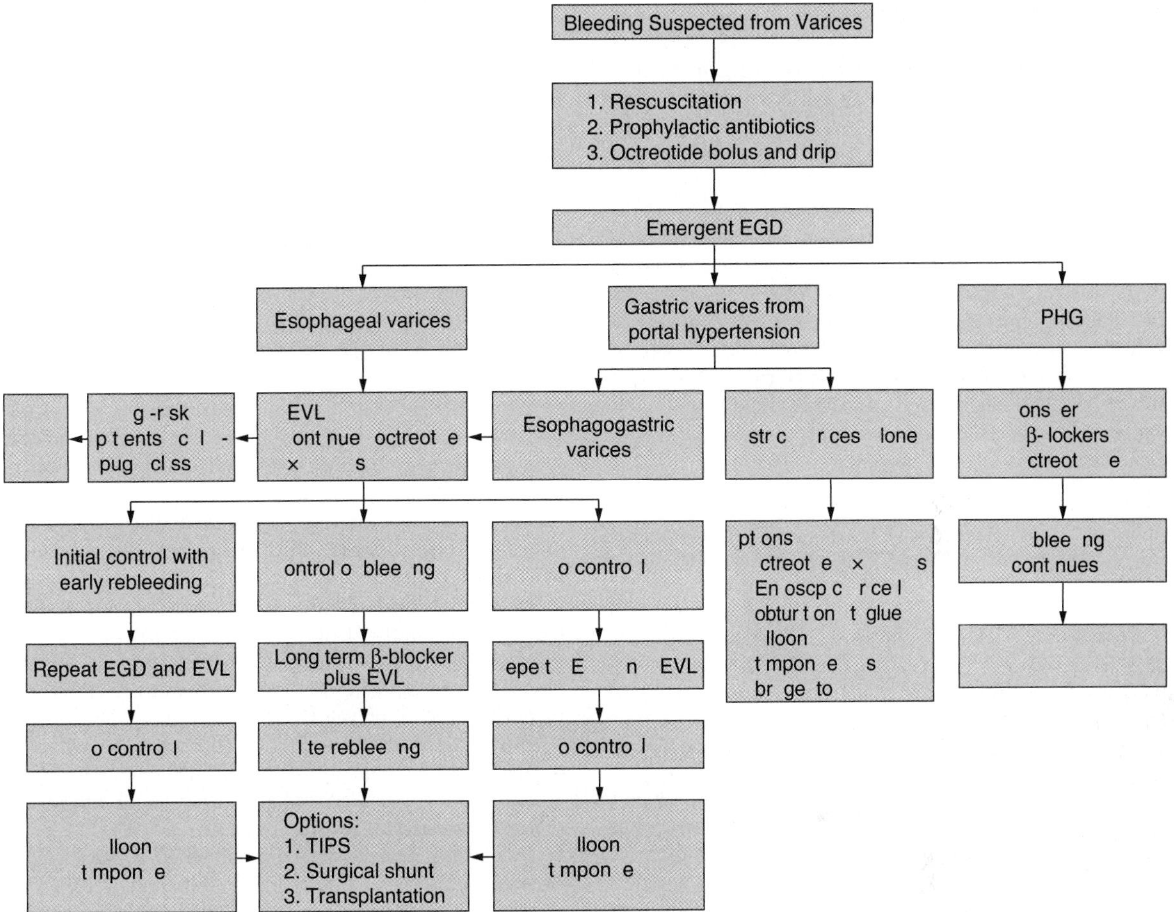

▲ **Figure 47–2.** Management algorithm for acute variceal hemorrhage. EGD, esophagogastroduodenoscopy; EVL, endoscopic variceal ligation; PHG, portal hypertensive gastropathy; TIPS, transjugular intrahepatic portosystemic shunt.

vasopressin and is the only pharmacologic agent that has a survival benefit in patients with acute variceal hemorrhage.

Octreotide has been shown to have equal efficacy to sclerotherapy in controlling bleeding. It is safe with very few side effects and can be used continuously for up to 5 days. However, its use has been associated with tachyphylaxis, and its vasoactive effects may be transient. When combined with endoscopic therapy, octreotide improves management of acute bleeding compared with EVL alone, but without a survival benefit.

β-Blockers should not be administered during an active bleed, due to the physiologic blunting of heart rate in the setting of hypotension.

4. Endoscopic therapy—Endoscopic evaluation should occur as soon as possible and within the first 12 hours of a patient presenting with an acute variceal bleed. In addition to confirming the source of bleeding, endoscopic treatments are successful in controlling hemorrhage in 90% of cases. EVL is the procedure of choice. The combination of EVL and a somatostatin analog has been shown to be more effective than either EVL or a pharmacologic agent, given as monotherapy, and is the treatment of choice.

5. Balloon tamponade—Balloon tamponade is 80% effective in immediate control of hemorrhage from esophagogastric varices. However, serious complications occur when the balloon is left inflated for more than 24 hours. The complications, which occur in 20% of cases, include aspiration, esophageal ulceration and necrosis, and esophageal perforation. Balloon tamponade is best utilized as a short-term bridge to TIPS or liver transplantation.

6. Transjugular intrahepatic portosystemic shunt (TIPS)—TIPS is used to manage variceal bleeding when endoscopic and pharmacologic treatments fail. In 90% of cases of uncontrolled bleeding, TIPS is successful in stopping bleeding. Unfortunately, mortality remains high (27–50%), probably because of the severity of illness, and rebleeding can occur in the short and long term. Predictors of early mortality include creatinine greater than 1.7 mg/dL, bilirubin greater than 5 mg/dL, a Child-Pugh score greater than 12, an APACHE II score greater than 18, and a Patch prognostic index greater than 18. TIPS is the rescue therapy of choice after two failed attempts of combined endoscopic and pharmacologic management.

The use of polytetrafluoroethylene-coated stents results in significantly less stent dysfunction and lower clinical relapse rates. Patients receiving coated stents, compared with those receiving uncoated stents, had lower rates of recurrent bleeding and hepatic encephalopathy after 2 years of follow-up. Recent studies have shown that the early use of TIPS with coated stents in patients at high risk for treatment failure (ie, Child Pugh class C patients or Child Pugh class B patients with active bleeding at endoscopy) is associated with a decrease in treatment failure and in mortality.

Bureau C, Garcia-Pagan JC, Otal P, et al. Improved clinical outcome using polytetrafluoroethylene coated stents for TIPS: results of a randomized study. *Gastroenterology.* 2004;126:469–475. [PMID: 14762784]

Garcia-Pagan JC, Caca K, Bureau C, et al. Early use of TIPS in patients with cirrhosis and variceal bleeding. *N Engl J Med.* 2010; 362:2370–2379. [PMID: 20573925]

D. Prevention of Recurrent Variceal Hemorrhage

Once the acute bleed has been controlled, secondary prevention of rebleeding is paramount. First-line therapy for prevention of recurrent variceal hemorrhage is the combination of pharmacologic therapy and EVL. For patients who fail to respond to medical therapy, TIPS, surgical shunts or liver transplantation for appropriate candidates are the options (Figure 47–3A).

Pharmacologic treatment for prevention of recurring variceal hemorrhage is initiated by administration of a nonselective β-blocker, titrated to tolerance. β-Blockers have been shown to decrease rates of rebleeding from 63% to 42% and to decrease mortality from 27% to 20%. The hemodynamic goal of β-blocker therapy is to decrease the HVPG by greater than 20% or to a level less than 12 mm Hg (Figure 47–3B). Achieving this goal has been shown to reduce rebleeding rates to less than 15%.

In patients who have an incomplete response to β-blocker monotherapy, one can consider the addition of isosorbide mononitrate. With combination therapy, the rebleeding rate appears to be lower, but at a cost of significantly greater side effects and no survival benefit.

If patients are unable to tolerate β-blockers, EVL is the preferred endoscopic treatment to prevent recurrent variceal hemorrhage. Although EVL is more effective than sclerotherapy at preventing rebleeding, the risk of rebleeding after EVL remains high, reaching 30–50% at 2 years. The combination of a nonselective β-blocker and EVL has been shown to result in a decreased rate of variceal rebleeding, a lower transfusion requirement, a lower recurrence of esophageal varices, and a trend toward improved survival. However, there are slightly increased side effects with combination therapy. Current guidelines recommend combination therapy as the treatment of choice for prevention of variceal rebleeding,.

EVL sessions should be performed every 7–14 days until complete variceal obliteration is achieved. Once varices are eradicated, continued surveillance every 6–12 months is required to screen for recurrent varices.

In patients who do not respond to pharmacologic or endoscopic therapy, alone or in combination, decompression of the portal system by use of TIPS with coated stents is the next option. Liver transplantation provides the only

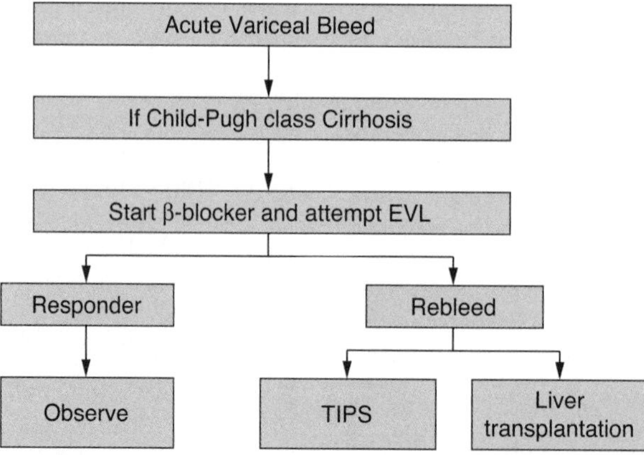

▲ **Figure 47–3A.** The role of hepatic venous pressure gradient measurements in preventing recurrent variceal hemorrhage. EVL, endoscopic variceal ligation; TIPS, transjugular intrahepatic portosystemic shunt.

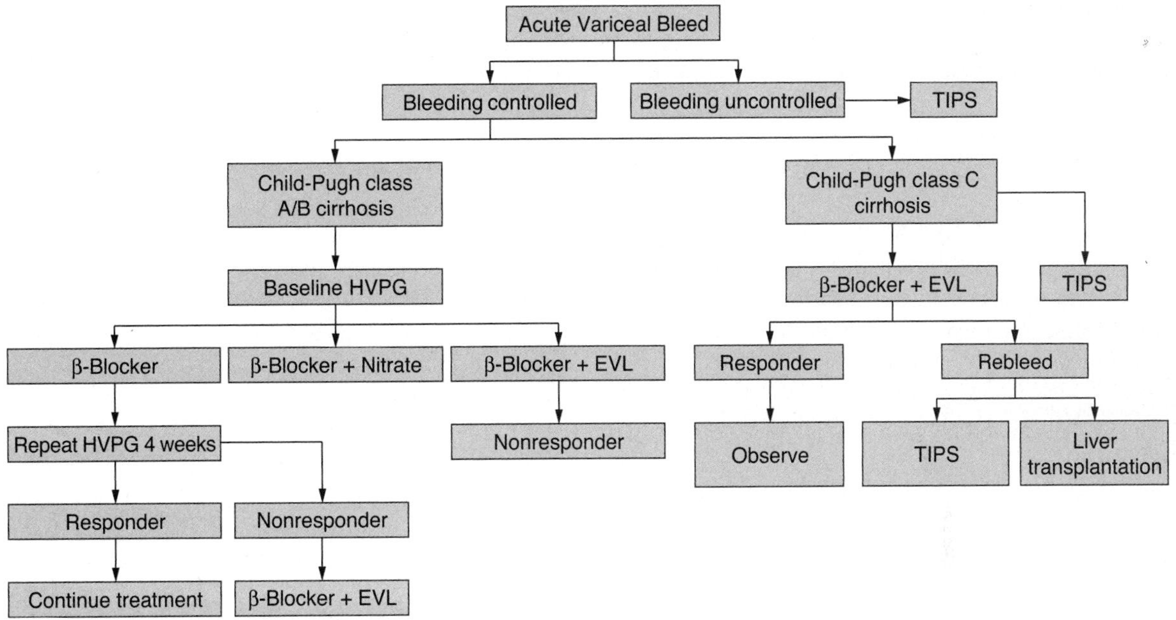

▲ **Figure 47–3B.** Prevention of recurrent variceal hemorrhage. EVL, endoscopic variceal ligation; HVPG, hepatic venous pressure gradient; TIPS, transjugular intrahepatic portosystemic shunt.

definitive treatment for rebleeding as it directly addresses the underlying liver pathology that leads to portal hypertension and the formation of varices. However, variceal bleeding is not by itself an indication for liver transplantation, which should be reserved for appropriate candidates.

Numerous meta-analyses have demonstrated that TIPS is more effective than endoscopic therapy in preventing rebleeding from varices. The drawback of TIPS is an increase in hepatic encephalopathy and the lack of a survival benefit. Endoscopic and pharmacologic therapy remains the first-line therapy for prevention of rebleeding, with TIPS reserved as a rescue therapy.

GASTRIC VARICES

General Considerations

Gastric varices are present in 20% of patients with portal hypertension and account for 10–15% of variceal bleeds. Gastric varices can occur alone or in combination with esophageal varices. Although the risk of bleeding from gastric varices is lower than that from esophageal varices, gastric variceal hemorrhages are associated with higher rates of rebleeding (between 34% and 89%) and a higher mortality rate. Gastric varices are more common in patients with extra-hepatic portal vein obstruction than in patients with cirrhosis.

A. Etiology

Management depends on the underlying etiology of the gastric varix; therefore, it is important to identify the cause of the varix before treatment. Varices that develop from portal hypertension have been treated with EVL, administration of vasoactive agents or cyanoacrylate glue, or TIPS (see Figure 47–2). Varices that develop after splenic vein thrombosis or stenosis, leading to isolated left-sided portal hypertension, are best treated with splenectomy or splenic artery embolization.

B. Classification

Gastric varices are classified according to their anatomic location in the stomach and their relationship to esophageal varices. Type 1 gastric varices, GOV1, extend from esophageal varices to the lesser curvature of the stomach. As such, they should be treated similarly to esophageal varices (ie, using EVL). Type 2 gastric varices, GOV2, extend from esophageal varices to the gastric fundus. Isolated type 1 gastric varices (IGV1) are located in the fundus, whereas isolated type 2 gastric varices (IGV2) are located elsewhere in the stomach. Risk factors for variceal bleeding include location in the fundus (GOV2, IGV1), size larger than 5 mm, presence of endoscopic red wale signs, and Child-Pugh class C cirrhosis.

Unlike esophageal varices, gastric varices can bleed with HVPG less than 12 mm Hg. This is thought to be the result of a higher prevalence of spontaneous shunting (gastrorenal shunts), which decreases portal pressure but does not decrease the reversal of flow in splenic veins that result in gastric varices.

Treatment

A. Pharmacologic Therapy

Given the high morbidity and mortality from gastric variceal bleeds, it is reasonable to treat patients empirically with vasoactive agents shown to improve bleeding outcomes in esophageal variceal hemorrhage. Similarly, nonselective β-blockers have been used for prevention of recurrent variceal bleeding.

B. Endoscopic Therapy

Endoscopy is essential for identifying gastric varices. However, because these varices can lie deep in the submucosa, standard endoscopy can underestimate their true prevalence. Most gastric varices that bleed are close to the mucosal surface and are readily identifiable.

EVL is associated with a high rate of rebleeding, and it is less successful in treating gastric variceal bleeds compared with esophageal variceal bleeds. Endoscopic variceal obturation refers to the injection of adhesive and glue agents into a varix. Tissue adhesives, including *N*-butyl-cyanoacrylate, isobutyl-2-cyanoacrylate, and thrombin, have resulted in better control of initial gastric variceal bleeding than EVL. Furthermore, gastric variceal obturation with *N*-butylcyanoacrylate has a lower rate of rebleeding and an overall survival benefit compared with EVL. Documented side effects from use of glue include fever, sepsis, retroperitoneal abscess formation, and distal embolization. Embolic complications to cerebral arteries, pulmonary arteries, coronary arteries, renal veins, and inferior vena cava have been documented. The only agent (off label) available in the United States is 2-octyl-cyanoacrylate (Dermabond). The use of thrombin injections has been reported to be effective in controlling gastric variceal bleeding but the data are limited, and more studies are needed.

If endoscopic therapy fails, placement of a Linton-Nachlas tube or Sengstaken-Blakemore tube can be lifesaving as a temporizing procedure. Balloon tamponade should only be used as a bridge to more definitive therapy (TIPS or liver transplantation), because of its associated complications.

Lo GH, Lai KH, Cheung JS, et al. A prospective, randomized trial of butyl cyanoacrylate injection versus band ligation in the management of bleeding gastric varices. *Hepatology.* 2001;33: 1060–1064. [PMID: 11343232]

Ramesh J, Limdi JK, Sharma V, et al. The use of thrombin injections in the management of bleeding gastric varices: a single-center experience. *Gastrointest Endosc.* 2008;68:877–882. [PMID: 18534583]

Tan PC, Hou MC, Lin HC, et al. A randomized trial of endoscopic treatment of acute gastric variceal hemorrhage: N-butyl-2-cyanoacrylate injection versus band ligation. *Hepatology.* 2006;43:690–697. [PMID: 16557539]

C. Transjugular Intrahepatic Portosystemic Shunt

Hemorrhage control using TIPS can be achieved in more than 90% of cases. TIPS, however, is recommended after one failed attempt of endoscopic management of gastric variceal bleeding or after early rebleeding. Unfortunately, the complication of hepatic encephalopathy and lack of survival benefit still exist. Surgical shunts are an alternative to TIPS in patients with Child-Pugh class A cirrhosis.

Ryan BM, Stockbrugger RW, Ryan JM. A pathophysiologic, gastroenterologic, and radiologic approach to the management of gastric varices. *Gastroenterology.* 2004;126:1175–1189. [PMID: 15057756]

PORTAL HYPERTENSIVE GASTROPATHY

PHG describes the endoscopic appearance of gastric erythema with a whitish mosaic-like pattern that is found in 51–98% of patients with cirrhotic and noncirrhotic portal hypertension. In part, PHG develops as a result of increased resistance to portal flow, but there is no linear correlation between the development of PHG and the level of portal pressures. The development of PHG has been correlated with the duration and severity of liver disease, presence and size of gastroesophageal varices, and previous eradication of varices by banding or sclerotherapy. The pathogenesis of PHG is not clearly understood, but it may be related to the overproduction of nitric oxide, which results in capillary dilation, or increased levels of vascular endothelial growth factor, which results in increased angiogenesis.

PHG is characterized by mucosal congestion, with dilated capillaries and venules in the mucosa and submucosa of the stomach. Endoscopically, the gastric mucosa appears erythematous and edematous, with a characteristic mosaic pattern, often described as a snakeskin appearance. In PHG, the gastric mucosa is friable and may have associated hemorrhagic spots. The gastric mucosa in patients with PHG bleeds easily on contact and is more susceptible to damage by noxious stimuli such as bile acids, aspirin, and nonsteroidal anti-inflammatory drugs. PHG is most prominent in the gastric body and fundus, but may be noted diffusely. Several endoscopic classification systems for PHG have been proposed but there is no consensus on the best system.

Patients with PHG typically present with chronic anemia and more rarely with acute blood loss. An estimated 8% of upper gastrointestinal hemorrhage in patients with cirrhosis is due to PHG bleeding, and tends to occur in patients with severe PHG. Mortality from PHG bleeding is reported to be very low.

First-line treatment for PHG includes medical therapies aimed at decreasing gastric blood flow (eg, β-blockers, octreotide, vasopressin). Small studies have shown efficacy of propranolol in decreasing rates of chronic and recurrent bleeding from PHG. If medical therapy is not tolerated or fails to reduce bleeding rates, TIPS may be beneficial.

Surgical shunts or liver transplantation are not recommended for the treatment of PHG, and endoscopic therapy has no proven benefit or safety profile. It remains to be seen how advances in argon plasma coagulation, cryotherapy, and photodynamic therapy may evolve in the future as therapeutic options for PHG.

Primignani M, Carpinelli L, Preatoni P, et al. Natural history of portal hypertensive gastropathy in patients with liver cirrhosis. The New Italian Endoscopic Club for the Study and Treatment of Esophageal Varices (NIEC). *Gastroenterology.* 2000;119: 181–187. [PMID: 10889167]

Sarin SK, Shahi HM, Jain M, et al. The natural history of portal hypertensive gastropathy: influence of variceal eradication. *Am J Gastroenterol.* 2000;95:2888–2893. [PMID: 11051364]

FUTURE TREATMENT TRENDS

Over the past 30 years, major advances in pharmacologic and endoscopic therapy for primary and secondary prophylaxis of variceal hemorrhage, together with a better understanding of resuscitative measures, have led to a marked improvement in the morbidity and mortality associated with variceal hemorrhage. Early mortality from variceal bleeding has been reduced by 50% to its present 15%. The advent of TIPS as a rescue procedure has reduced surgical shunts to a footnote. Future research will be directed toward finding alternative drugs for patients who cannot tolerate or do not benefit from the use of β-blockers. Carvedilol and simvastatin are drugs with promising futures. Moreover, the TIPS literature will have to be reassessed with the development of coated stents. Finally, a noninvasive test is needed that will give information similar to that now obtained by measurements of the HVPG for the diagnosis, prognosis, and management of patients with cirrhosis and portal hypertension.

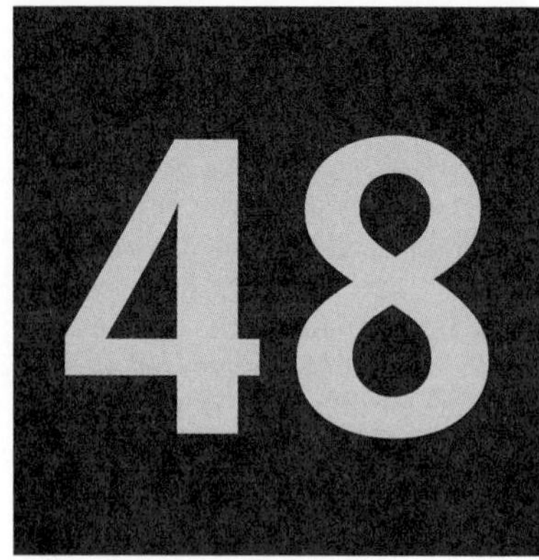

Drug-Induced Liver Disease

Willis C. Maddrey, MD, MACP, FRCP

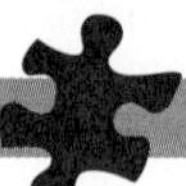

ESSENTIALS OF DIAGNOSIS

- A remarkable array of therapeutic drugs has been shown to cause hepatic injuries of many types. There are no specific diagnostic tests that establish the presence of a drug-induced liver injury; therefore, the diagnosis is often one of exclusion.
- Evidence of hepatic injury appearing days to months after adding a therapeutic drug with known or suspected potential to injure the liver suggests possible drug-induced injury.
- Improvement following discontinuation of a drug suspected to have caused liver injury (deceleration) is often helpful in diagnosis.
- In patients with few if any signs or symptoms of liver injury, hepatotoxicity may be detected only by biochemical tests showing elevated aminotransferase, bilirubin, or alkaline phosphatase levels.
- A drug-induced etiology should be considered in any patient who develops acute hepatitis with jaundice (hepatocellular injury) or jaundice associated with pruritus and elevated alkaline phosphatase levels (cholestatic or mixed injury).

General Considerations

Almost all drugs in current use have been suggested as a cause of some liver alterations, most often asymptomatic elevations of aminotransferases. Awareness of drug-induced reactions affecting the liver is receiving increased attention. A number of drugs with proven efficacy have been withdrawn from the market because of the recognition of a few cases of severe liver injury. The economic consequences after removing an approved drug from the market or markedly restricting its use are tremendous. Drug-induced injuries that lead to clinically severe liver disease garner much attention even if only a few cases are recognized (or even suggested). A challenge is to improve the methods by which the risk of drug-related hepatotoxicity with a specific drug is assessed (and hopefully predicted) so that effective plans to minimize risk can be developed.

It is well recognized that with many drugs, transient biochemical changes (usually increases in aminotransferases) occur in patients in whom there are no symptoms suggesting liver injury and that with continue use, these usually minor elevations subside as the liver adapts to the newly introduced agent. Determining the threshold of tolerance (risk-benefit factor) for mild to moderate injury caused by drugs that are effective in the treatment of serious illnesses is a difficult but important undertaking.

Hepatic injury that occurs rarely (<1 in 10,000) is designated as an idiosyncratic reaction that is defined as a response or reaction that is host dependent and dose independent. The frequency of hepatotoxicity is influenced by age, patterns of use (short courses or long-term administration), age, sex, ethnicity, and increasingly determination of genetic factors that govern metabolism of the drug and the immune responses to the drug or its metabolic products. Furthermore, transport of specific drugs into the hepatocyte from the blood and from the hepatocyte into bile is dependent on genetically influenced transporters. Evidence of clinically apparent severe events from an approved drug is rare. Significant events may not be detected in the preapproval development during which a limited (several thousand) number of patients are exposed and evidence of liver injury appears after release when large numbers of patients have been treated. The causes of these rare reactions have remained largely unknown. The challenge for further research is to identify why an agent that is well tolerated by thousands of patients may cause a devastating injury in a few. The present focus on genetic variations in drug metabolism, immune responses, and transporters is receiving much attention.

Drug-induced liver disease is usually indistinguishable (clinically and histologically) from liver injury of other causes and may only be detected through awareness of the possibility, suspicion, careful history, exclusion of other likely causes, and inquisitive persistence by the clinician.

Careful attention must be given to the time of onset, duration of therapy, and nature of the hepatic injury, as well as consideration of the roles of other drugs that may enhance production or accumulation of reactive intermediates or interfere with drug transport. Most clinicians prescribe a relatively limited panel of drugs. It is essential that the clinician become familiar with the hepatic risk profile and patterns of manifestation of the agents he or she uses. Difficulties in establishing a diagnosis are compounded by the status of the underlying disease, concomitant illnesses, and polypharmacy.

Considerable supportive evidence implicating a drug as the cause of a liver injury is found if there is resolution of manifestations of liver injury (deceleration) following withdrawal. There are problems in a patient who is receiving many drugs in deciding which agent to remove when evidence of liver injury is found.

The profile of frequency, type of reaction, and possible extent of injury for individual drugs must be considered. Minimal biochemical abnormalities, especially minor elevations of serum aminotransferases (less than three times the upper limit of normal), do not necessarily indicate that clinically important liver injury is occurring. Patients with elevated aminotransferase levels and clinical jaundice are in a group at considerable risk of an adverse outcome.

The conceptual framework of differentiating types of hepatic adverse reactions into those that are predominantly hepatocellular (elevated aminotransferase levels) and those that are predominantly cholestatic injury (elevated alkaline phosphatase levels) is useful. With some drugs, there are elements of both patterns of injury, leading to a category of a mixed reaction.

Cholestatic disorders range from mild elevations of alkaline phosphatase levels found on routine biochemical testing to symptomatic cholestatic syndromes with jaundice and pruritus that resemble primary biliary cirrhosis and primary sclerosing cholangitis. Hepatic steatosis (fatty liver) of both the microvesicular and macrovesicular types is frequently noted in liver biopsy and is a near-constant finding in obese and diabetic patients. Drugs that cause mitochondrial injury may lead to microvesicular fat accumulation. A few drugs (eg, amiodarone) lead to an acquired phospholipidosis. Several drugs are established causes of hepatic granulomatous inflammation indistinguishable from those found in a variety of infections and sarcoidosis.

Tumors induced or promoted by therapeutic drugs range from benign hepatic adenomas, associated with long-term use of oral contraceptives, to angiosarcomas, cholangiocarcinomas, and hepatocellular carcinomas.

Several helpful observations regarding drug-induced liver disease include:

1. Clinical manifestations of drug-induced hepatotoxicity are often clinically indistinguishable from those of liver disease caused by other etiologies.
2. The risk of developing serious liver injury from a drug-induced injury that is predominantly hepatocellular is considerably greater than that in patients who have cholestatic injury.
3. The appearance of clinically apparent liver disease in patients who have predominantly hepatocellular injury with clinical jaundice requires immediate attention.

Hepatic injury from a drug may have a somewhat specific "signature" as regards time of onset, type of injury, and propensity to develop severe disease. However, exceptions occur and many drugs, even those that predominantly cause hepatocellular injury, will on occasion present with a mixed hepatocellular and cholestatic injury or even predominant cholestatic injury.

It may be difficult or impossible to assess the contribution of a drug to hepatic injury in a patient who has an underlying disease or a condition that itself is known to cause liver injury (eg, disseminated carcinoma or fungal disease, chronic hepatitis or cirrhosis, HIV infection and AIDS, and multiorgan involvement from an autoimmune process). Furthermore, in settings in which many drugs are used, especially in the elderly, assigning attribution to any one agent is difficult. Additional consideration must be given to a role for herbal compounds, which may be the initiator of the hepatic findings. Obtaining an accurate history from the patient of the use of herbal products may be especially difficult. The variable timing of stopping, restarting, and substitution of drugs adds to the difficulties. Knowing the relative hepatic risks of individual agents the patient is receiving and the expected time of onset is helpful. Dilemmas are heightened when one or more of the drugs suspected to have caused hepatotoxicity are required in the treatment of a serious underlying illness.

Abboud G, Kaplowitz N. Drug-induced liver injury. *Drug Saf.* 2007;30:277–294. [PMID: 17408305]

Andrade RJ, Lucena MI, Fernandez MC, et al. Drug-induced liver injury: an analysis of 461 incidences submitted to the Spanish Registry over a 10-year period. *Gastroenterology.* 2005;129:512–521. [PMID: 16083708]

Bjornsson E, Olsson R. Outcome and prognostic markers in severe drug-induced liver disease. *Hepatology.* 2005;42:481–489. [PMID: 16025496]

Daly AK, Day CP. Genetic association studies in drug-induced liver injury. *Seminars in Liver Disease.* 2009;29(4):400–411.

Daly AK, Aithal GP, Leathart JB, et al. Basic-liver, pancreas, and biliary tract: genetic susceptibility to diclofenac-induced hepatotoxicity: contribution of UGTY2B7, CYP2C8, and ABCC2 genotypes. *Gastroenterology.* 2007;132:272–281. [PMID: 17241877]

Farrell GC. Drugs and steatohepatitis. *Seminars in Liver Disease.* 2002;22(2):185–194.

Kaplowitz N. Idiosyncratic drug hepatotoxicity. *Nat Rev Drug Discov.* 2005;4:489–499. [PMID: 15931258]

Maddrey WC. Drug-induced hepatotoxicity 2005. *J Clin Gastroenterol.* 2005;39:S83–S89. [PMID: 15758665]

Russmann S, Jetter A, Kullak-Ublick GA. Pharmacogenetics of drug-induced liver injury. *Hepatology.* 2010;52:748–761.

Stickel F, Patsenker E, Schuppan D. Herbal hepatotoxicity. *J Hepatol.* 2005;43:901–910. [PMID: 16171893]

Temple R. Hy's law: predicting serious hepatotoxicity. *Pharmacoepidemiol Drug Saf.* 2006;15:241–243. [PMID: 16552790]

Watkins PB. Idiosyncratic liver injury: challenges and approaches. *Toxicol Pathol.* 2005;33:1–5. [PMID: 15805049]

Zimmerman HJ. Drug-induced liver disease. *Clin Liver Dis.* 2000;4:73–96. [PMID: 11232192]

Clinical Findings

A. Symptoms and Signs

Early symptoms sometimes associated with drug-induced injuries are nonspecific and include loss of appetite, fatigue, lassitude, and occasionally a dull discomfort more prominent in the right upper quadrant of the abdomen. All these symptoms may be attributed to an underlying condition. There may be few clinical signs or symptoms suggesting liver injury, even in a patient who has biochemical and histologic evidence of considerable damage. These are the same symptoms that are often found in patients who have chronic viral hepatitis B or C or alcohol-induced liver disease. With a few drugs, there is the concomitant presence of fever, rash, or eosinophilia—the hallmarks of hypersensitivity reactions.

B. Genetic Testing

For several drugs that have been implicated in the pathogenesis of liver injury, there is evidence that genetically controlled metabolic or immune response pathways play important roles in determining which individuals are likely to have an adverse reaction affecting the liver (for example, flucloxacillin, isoniazid, diclofenac, and ximelagatran). The expression of genes controlling the metabolism of a drug (heightened or dampened) influences individual susceptibility to injury, and the patterns of genes affected may allow prediction of a group of individuals at increased risk. Much attention has been paid to variations in the levels of individual cytochronic p450s involved in metabolism.

Extensive evaluations of genetic polymorphisms focusing on enzymes that metabolize or transport metabolic products and those that influence the responses to injury are being undertaken as part of efforts to unravel the mystery of what causes a rare reaction designated as idiosyncratic.

One approach utilizing genetic testing is to identify a group of individuals who have experienced an adverse reaction and compare the gene profile of those patients with those who have received the drug and have not had a problem. Thus far, there is insufficient experience to fully assess the value of this approach, which is presently the focus of considerable research.

Differential Diagnosis

The development of reliable tests to detect hepatitis A–E has made the task of excluding viral hepatitis more straightforward and certain. The finding of antimitochondrial antibodies in a patient who has biochemical evidence of cholestasis and jaundice may go far to resolve whether the patient has primary biliary cirrhosis or a drug-induced syndrome that resembles the disorder. However, it must be recalled that patients with liver disorders of all types may develop superimposed drug-induced injury, which, in patients with cirrhosis and decreased hepatic reserve, is more likely to manifest as clinically significant disease.

A. Drug-Induced Chronic Hepatitis

Several drugs cause chronic hepatitis syndromes that may be largely indistinguishable from autoimmune hepatitis. Drugs that cause a pattern of chronic hepatitis include minocycline, nitrofurantoin, and methyldopa. Misdiagnosing those patients as having autoimmune hepatitis may lead to the institution of corticosteroid therapy while there is continuation of the drug. Corticosteroids serve to blunt the manifestations of the underlying ongoing injury while continued drug use leads to further damage. Generally drugs that cause chronic hepatitis are taken for extended intervals.

The majority of patients who develop drug-induced chronic hepatitis are women, and many have increased serum globulin levels as well as the presence of autoantibodies. The clinical onset of the hepatic injury may be as an acute hepatitis in a patient in whom liver biopsy changes suggest long-standing disease (acute on chronic pattern). The histologic changes may be indistinguishable from autoimmune hepatitis. In some patients chronic hepatitis may present as insidious progressive hepatic failure in a patient who develops hepatosplenomegaly and evidence of portal hypertension or ascites.

Maddrey WC. Drug-induced hepatotoxicity 2005. *J Clin Gastroenterol.* 2005;39:S83–S89. [PMID: 15758665]

Treatment

The vast majority of drug-induced elevations of serum aminotransferases occur in minimally symptomatic or asymptomatic patients who require no treatment beyond identification and withdrawal of the causation. Removal of the causative agent is generally followed by resolution of the biochemical abnormalities over several days to weeks (deceleration). Some drugs cause a hepatic reaction that closely mimics autoimmune injury. Even in these situations, withdrawal of the likely culprit is generally followed by gradual resolution. With some drugs that cause symptomatic hepatitis, especially if the increase in aminotransferases is associated with the concomitant presence of clinical jaundice, careful evaluation and often hospitalization to allow careful monitoring is required.

If drug-induced acute liver failure occurs, the patient should be viewed as a candidate for liver transplantation and referred to a transplant-capable center. Corticosteroid therapy has not definitely been established to be useful in the treatment of drug-induced liver injury. These agents have often been used in those patients with drug-induced liver injuries who also manifest hypersensitivity reactions, for example in patients with drug-induced injury caused by halothane or diphenylhydantoin.

In many patients who have drug-induced hepatocellular injury, a gradual decrease in the aminotransferase levels occurs within 1–2 weeks of removing the drug. The decrease may not occur immediately, especially with drugs whose parent compound or metabolic products accumulate in the hepatocytes. For the first several days after drug withdrawal, processes already in place may proceed, causing early concern as to whether the drug was the cause. Continued evidence of liver injury may persist for weeks to months and cause a pattern of chronic injury. The longer abnormalities persist, the greater the possibility that permanent hepatic injury is present or will develop or that the diagnosis of a drug-induced injury was not correct.

Rechallenge with a suspected drug to establish a diagnosis of drug-induced injury is seldom necessary and if the initial event has been severe (such as a presentation with clinical jaundice and marked elevations of aminotransferases), may be dangerous.

DRUGS OF SPECIAL INTEREST

1. Acetaminophen

Acetaminophen hepatotoxicity is the most frequent cause of acute liver failure in the United States and is likely the cause of (or a major contributor to) elevations of aminotransferases often found on routine evaluations. Ingestion of excessive amounts of acetaminophen (>10–15 g), used in suicidal attempts, predictably leads to liver injury ranging from elevated aminotransferases to acute liver failure and in some patients death or the need for liver transplantation. In therapeutic doses (≤4 g/day), acetaminophen is usually safe and well tolerated. The safety margin of patients who are regular users of alcohol appears to be diminished, and these individuals are at increased risk of developing acetaminophen-induced liver injury.

Factors that predispose patients to hepatic injury from acetaminophen in nonsuicidal situations include the dose ingested and are more likely to occur in a patient who has been a regular user of alcohol. First and most important is the dose of acetaminophen. Patients may have underestimated or understated the amount ingested, especially since acetaminophen is present in many widely used combination products. Ingestion of 4 g of acetaminophen given as a single agent or in combination with opioids in healthy, asymptomatic individuals was shown to elevate aminotransferase levels to greater than three times the upper limit of normal in 31–44%. Second is the role of concomitant use of alcohol. Chronic use of alcohol may induce changes in levels of CYP2E1 (the major cytochrome P450 subspecies involved in the metabolism of ethanol and in the metabolism of acetaminophen). Therefore, in this setting, the alcohol-induced increased CYP2E1 potentially leads to more acetaminophen being metabolized to yield the reactive metabolite *N*-acetyl-p-benzoquinone imine (NAPQI). In addition, the intracellular concentration of glutathione (which has the major role in binding to NAPQI, leading to its excretion as mercapturic acid) is possibly lowered in patients who regularly use alcohol, further promoting the potential for injury.

N-acetylcysteine has been shown to be effective in reducing the extent of hepatic injury from acetaminophen.

Larson AM, Polson J, Fontana RJ, et al. Acetaminophen-induced acute liver failure: results of a United States multicenter, prospective study. *Hepatology*. 2005;42:1364–1372. [PMID: 16317692]

Watkins PB, Kaplowitz N, Slattery JT, et al. Aminotransferase elevations in healthy adults receiving 4 grams of acetaminophen daily: a randomized controlled trial. *JAMA*. 2006;296:87–93. [PMID: 16820551]

2. Isoniazid

Isoniazid (INH) has been recognized as an established cause of liver injury for the past five decades. Elevations of aminotransferase levels are found in 10–20% of patients who receive the drug, with the onset of these elevations within several weeks of beginning treatment. In most patients, the elevated aminotransferase levels are not associated with symptoms suggestive of liver injury, and often the levels return to normal during continued treatment (adaptation). In patients with elevated ALT levels, discontinuation of INH is usually followed by resolution over several weeks. A few patients develop clinically evident liver disease. Many years of observation of patients receiving INH allow the following conclusions to be made:

1. Patients older than 50 years at the time of therapy are at increased risk of developing clinically important INH-induced liver injury (~1%).
2. Children younger than age 16 years seldom show evidence of hepatic injury from INH.
3. Prodromal signs and symptoms are vague and include loss of appetite. If clinically apparent jaundice develops, there is an approximately 10% mortality.
4. Continued use of INH after the appearance of nonspecific symptoms and signs of liver injury and, especially after the presence of jaundice, is associated with an increased likelihood of development of severe injury.
5. Patients who have hepatitis B, hepatitis C, and HIV are at increased risk of developing liver injury from INH.
6. Combining INH with several other drugs also used to treat tuberculosis (eg, rifampin and pyrazinamide) increases the likelihood of injury.

The principal mechanism underlying INH-induced hepatic injury stems from the effects of an intermediary metabolite. The specific toxic intermediate has not been definitely established but is likely a hydrazine derivative. Genetic polymorphisms of the genes for *N*-acetyltransferase and CYP2E1, both of which have important roles in the metabolism of INH, have been shown to influence susceptibility. Slow acetylators of INH by the enzyme *NAT2* are at higher risk of developing hepatotoxicity than are rapid acetylators and are more likely to develop severe injury. Individuals who are CYP2E1 c1/c1 (wild type) have higher levels of CYP2E1 activity than do those who are CYP2E1 c1/c2 or c2/c2 and are at increased risk.

Awareness of the risk of INH-induced liver injury and regular monitoring of aminotransferase levels in patients receiving the drug have proven effective in identifying evidence of hepatic injury early, at a time when withdrawal of the drug leads to resolution.

Huang YS, Chern HD, Su WJ, et al. Cytochrome p450 2E1 genotype and the susceptibility to antituberculosis drug-induced hepatitis. *Hepatology*. 2003;37:924–930. [PMID: 12668988]

Huang YS, Chern HD, Su WJ, et al. Polymorphism of the *N*-acetyltransferase 2 gene as a susceptibility risk factor for antituberculosis drug-induced hepatitis. *Hepatology*. 2002;35: 883–889. [PMID: 11915035]

Maddrey WC. Drug-induced hepatotoxicity 2005. *J Clin Gastroenterol*. 2005;39:S83–S89. [PMID: 15758665]

3. Minocycline

Minocycline, a tetracycline derivative used in many situations including the long-term treatment of acne, has been established to cause several types of liver damage including acute hepatitis, occasionally with features of a hypersensitivity reaction including Stevens-Johnson syndrome with fever and lymphadenopathy, chronic hepatitis closely simulating autoimmune hepatitis, and, rarely, acute liver failure. In some patients, cholestatic features may be prominent or even predominate.

Of particular interest is a minocycline-induced syndrome that simulates autoimmune hepatitis. The majority of the affected patients are women who often have taken the drug for months. Hyperglobulinemia and the presence of antinuclear antibodies and anti-DNA antibodies are found in some. The role of minocycline in the causation or unmasking of an autoimmune hepatitis is important in that misdiagnosis and treatment of presumed autoimmune hepatitis type 1 with corticosteroids may mask the minocycline-induced liver injury, which then progresses relatively unnoticed.

4. Statins & Ezetimibe

The era of the widespread, often long-term use of statin drugs to lower low-density lipoprotein and cholesterol levels through inhibition of HMG-CoA began in the 1980s. Increases of aminotransferase level to more than three times the upper limit of normal occurs in 1–3% of patients receiving statins. The extent of the elevation appears directly related to the dose.

Statin-induced aminotransferase elevations are noted within weeks to months of initiating therapy, and the increases appear to be linked in some as yet undetermined way to the changes in lipids. There have been remarkably few instances of clinically significant liver injury reliably attributable to statins. The risk of statin-induced acute liver failure is less than 1 in 1 million, and cases of statin-induced significant liver injury are infrequent in large series of patients with acute liver failure.

In asymptomatic patients receiving statins who have elevations of aminotransferases, withdrawing the statin is followed by a return of ALT to normal. In some patients, adaptation occurs during continued treatment or upon treatment with a reduced dose. Increases of bilirubin associated with the elevations of aminotransferases are extremely uncommon.

There is no convincing evidence that patients with abnormal baseline aminotransferase levels, underlying steatohepatitis, or chronic hepatitis C are at increased risk of hepatotoxicity from statins. A few reports suggesting autoimmune hepatitis may be triggered by statins have been reported.

Ezetimibe, an inhibitor of intestinal uptake of intestinal and biliary cholesterol, is another agent widely used to lower cholesterol and is often given along with a statin. There have been isolated reports of ezetimibe in individual hepatic injury. Overall, the agent has an excellent safety record.

Chalasani N, Aljadhey H, Kesterson J, et al. Patients with elevated liver enzymes are not at higher risk for statin hepatotoxicity. *Gastroenterology*. 2004;126:1287–1292. [PMID: 15131789]

Cohen DE, Anania FA, Chalasani N. An assessment of statin safety by hepatologists. *Am J Cardiol*. 2006;97:77C–81C. [PMID: 16581333]

Larson AM, Polson J, Fontana RJ, et al. Acetaminophen-induced acute liver failure: results of a United States multicenter, prospective study. *Hepatology*. 2005;42:1364–1372. [PMID: 16317692]

Stolk MF, Becx MC, Kuypers KC, et al. Severe hepatic side effects of ezetimibe. *Clin Gastroenterol Hepatol*. 2006;4:908–911. [PMID: 16797241]

Tolman KG. The liver and lovastatin. *Am J Cardiol*. 2002;89: 1374–1380. [PMID: 12062731]

Vuppalanchi RA, Teal E, Chalasani N. Patients with elevated baseline liver enzymes do not have higher frequency of hepatotoxicity from lovastatin than those with normal baseline liver enzymes. *Am J Med Sci*. 2005;329:62–65. [PMID: 15711421]

5. Amoxicillin–Clavulanate

Hepatotoxicity from the extensively used combination of amoxicillin and clavulanic acid is widely recognized and is attributed to the clavulanic acid component. Amoxicillin–clavulanate is among the most frequently identified drugs causing liver injury.

The frequency of hepatic injury from amoxicillin–clavulanate is low (~1–3 in 100,000), and the range of clinical and laboratory manifestations is broad. The drug is generally used as short duration therapy (7–10 days). The appearance of evidence of liver injury is often delayed for days to weeks after initiation of therapy; therefore, many cases of hepatic injury appear well after the course of the therapy has been completed, and the pivotal role of amoxicillin–clavulanate may be overlooked. The types of liver injury from amoxicillin–clavulanate include hepatocellular necrosis, cholestatic reactions, and, in some patients, a mixed hepatocellular-cholestatic presentation. Some patients (one to two-thirds) have signs of hypersensitivity, with rash and fever at the time hepatic injury is recognized, whereas others present with jaundice and evidence of a bland cholestasis. In general, the liver injury from amoxicillin–clavulanate is mild and self-limiting, with a gradual and complete resolution of the process over several days to weeks.

Advancing age and prolonged therapy are factors associated with the development of the cholestatic injury. Predominantly hepatocellular injury is more frequent in younger patients. A few instances of severe hepatocellular injury leading to death or the need for transplantation have been reported.

Abboud G, Kaplowitz N. Drug-induced liver injury. *Drug Saf.* 2007; 30:277–294. [PMID: 17408305]

Maddrey WC. Drug-induced hepatotoxicity. *J Clin Gastroenterol.* 2005;39:S83–S89. [PMID: 15758665]

Robles M, Toscano E, Cotta J, et al. Antibiotic-induced liver toxicity: mechanisms, clinical features and causality assessment. *Curr Drug Saf.* 2010;5:212–222. [PMID: 20210729]

6. Herbal Hazards

Hepatic injury from a variety of herbal products from around the world has been associated with hepatotoxicity. In most instances, these products have not been well characterized chemically and have not been subjected to clinical trials. For example, Pyrrolizidine alkaloids used in herbal teas in Africa and the Caribbean have been associated with the development of sinusoidal obstruction syndrome. Extracts of kava, a plant found in the South Pacific, is widely used to alleviate stress, anxiety, and sleeplessness. There are multiple reports of hepatotoxicity including instances of acute liver failure, which have been attributed to the use of kava. There is a dose relationship between kavalactones and the risk of hepatic injury.

Patients ingesting greater than 250 mg a day of kavalactones are at increased risk. The variable processes of extraction and variation in kava products exemplify the difficulties of assessing risk with herbal problems. Several herbal products for weight loss including Hydroxycut have been banned following recognition of hepatic injury.

The important lesson for the clinician is to inquire (often repeatedly) about the use of herbals and vitamins. For example, excessive use of vitamin A can lead to sinusoidal compression, fibrosis, cirrhosis, and ascites.

Fong TL, Klontz KC, Canas-Coto A, et al. Hepatotoxicity due to Hydroxycut: a case series. *Am J Gastroenterol.* 2010;105: 1561–1566. [PMID: 20104221]

Teschke R, Schulze J. Risk of kava hepatotoxicity and the FDA consumer advisory. *JAMA.* 2010;304:2174–2175. [PMID: 21081732]

Teschke R. Kava hepatotoxicity—a clinical review. *Ann Hepatol.* 2010;9:251–265. [PMID: 20720265]

Teschke R. Kava hepatotoxicity: pathogenetic aspects and prospective considerations. *Liver Int.* 2010;30:1270–1279. [PMID: 20630022]

Liver Neoplasms

Amir A. Qamar, MD
Chinweike Ukomadu, MD, PhD

General Considerations

The increased used of imaging modalities—ultrasound, computed tomography (CT), and magnetic resonance imaging (MRI)—over the past few decades has led to an increase in the detection of hepatic masses. In the noncirrhotic patient or in patients with no history of extrahepatic malignancies, most of these lesions are benign. Diagnosis is often made on the basis of radiographic appearance, and only in rare equivocal cases is histologic analysis required. In patients with cirrhosis or those with chronic hepatitis B infections, the detection of a hepatic mass often raises suspicion of a hepatocellular cancer, and frequently additional diagnostic (including histologic) and therapeutic interventions are necessary.

Liver lesions are often classified on the basis of appearance (cystic or solid) and histologic composition (hepatocellular or biliary). They can also be classified based on malignant potential (benign or malignant), and when, malignant, they can be classified based on origin of the cancerous cells (primary or metastatic). In adults, malignant tumors are more common than benign tumors and metastatic lesions account for most forms of liver neoplasms. The differential diagnosis of liver lesions includes benign lesions (eg, hemangioma, focal nodular hyperplasia, adenoma, focal regenerative hyperplasia, simple hepatic cysts, polycystic liver disease, bile ductular cystadenoma, and bile ductular hamartomas) and malignant lesions (eg, primary hepatocellular cancer, cholangiocarcinoma, metastatic tumors, lymphoma).

Shaked O, Reddy KR. Approach to a liver mass. *Clin Liver Dis.* 2009;13:193–210. [PMID: 19442914]

BENIGN LIVER TUMORS

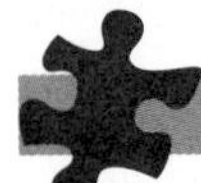

ESSENTIALS OF DIAGNOSIS

- Cavernous hemangiomas, focal nodular hyperplasia, hepatic adenomas, and nodular regenerative hyperplasia are the most common benign tumors of the liver.
- Cavernous hemangiomas are usually asymptomatic and can be identified by their classic appearance on CT and MRI.
- Focal nodular hyperplasia is common in young women and can be identified by the presence of a central stellate scar on CT or MRI.
- Hepatic adenomas are common in women of childbearing age, especially after prolonged oral contraceptive use. Because necrosis, hemorrhage, or rupture can occur, they should be surgical excised when identified.
- Nodular regenerative hyperplasia is associated with many systemic illnesses. Patients present with signs of portal hypertension. Radiographic characteristics are nonspecific, and histologic evaluation shows no fibrosis.

In clinical practice the most commonly encountered lesions are cavernous hemangiomas, focal nodular hyperplasia (FNH), hepatic adenoma, and nodular regenerative hyperplasia.

Mortele KJ, Ros P. Benign liver neoplasms. *Clin Liver Dis.* 2002; 6:119–145. [PMID: 11933585]

1. Cavernous Hemangiomas

General Considerations

This is the most common benign lesion of the liver, with a prevalence that ranges from 1% to 20% of the general population. Approximately two thirds of all cavernous hemangiomas are found in the right lobe of the liver, and more than 90% are solitary. More than 80% occur in women. Although lesions can be small (often ≤1 cm), larger lesions, especially those greater than 4 cm (giant hemangiomas), also occur; some can be as large as 25 cm (Figure 49–1).

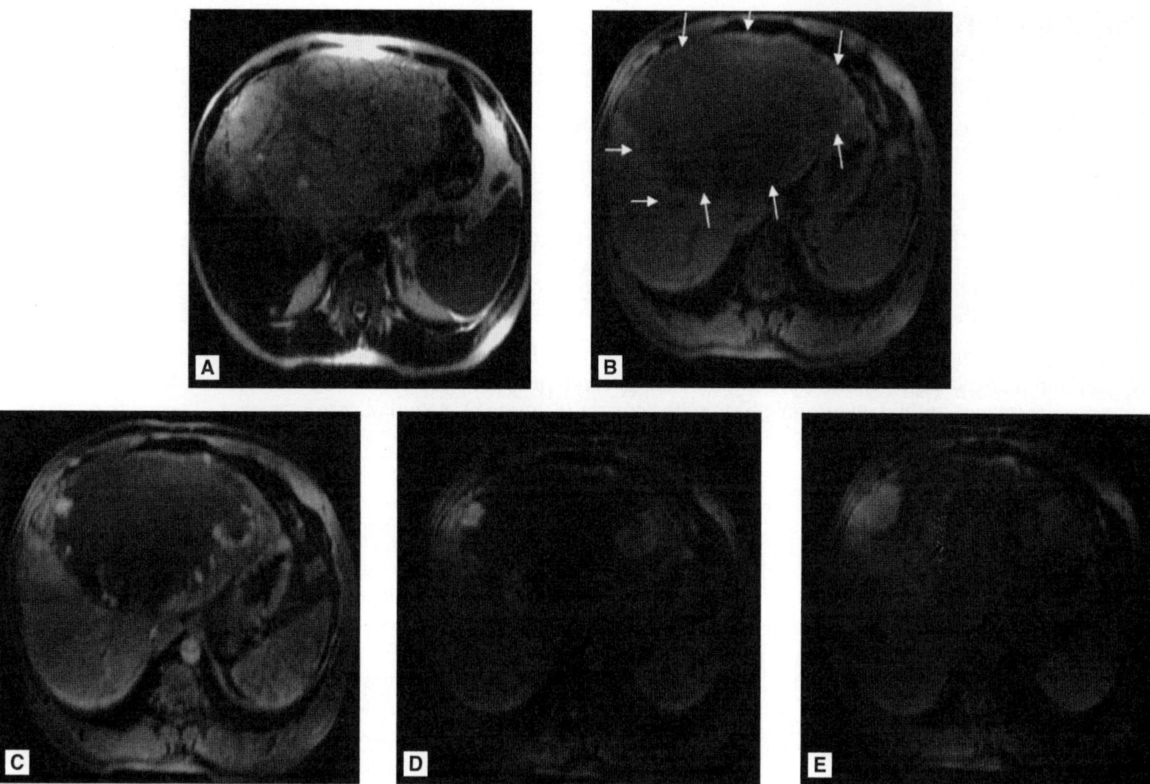

▲ **Figure 49–1.** Magnetic resonance images of a 25-cm giant hemangioma of the left hepatic lobe. The lesion is very bright on the T2-weighted image (**A**) but dark on the T1 precontrast image (**B**). Dynamic postgadolinium images show gradual nodular enhancement from the periphery to the center of the lesion on early arterial (**C**), late arterial (**D**), and delayed phase views (**E**). Arrows in B indicate the area of the hemangioma. (Used with permission from Dr Cheryl Sadow, Department of Radiology, Brigham and Women's Hospital.)

Clinical Findings

Findings on laboratory evaluation are usually normal, but signs of portal hypertension such as thrombocytopenia may be noted in patients with very large hemangiomas. The diagnostic modalities available include ultrasound, CT, and MRI. Ultrasound has sensitivity of 60–70% and specificity of 60–80% for detection of hemangiomas. Because of nonspecific findings on ultrasound, contrast-enhanced CT or MRI is often necessary for diagnosis of cavernous hemangiomas.

On CT scan, the lesions are characterized by progressive enhancement during the arterial phase that begins at the periphery of the lesion and progresses inward. The intensity of enhancement during this arterial phase resembles that of the aorta. Small hemangiomas are difficult to diagnose on contrast-enhanced CT because of inability to detect the stepwise enhancement seen in larger lesions. Because of this apparent homogenous enhancement, they may resemble hypervascular liver masses. Overall, the sensitivity of contrast-enhanced CT for diagnosis of cavernous hemangiomas is estimated at around 90%, with specificity of around 90%.

On MRI, cavernous hemangiomas appear hypodense on T1-weighted images, hyperdense on T2, and with gadolinium they show the classic peripheral enhancement with progressive inward enhancement (see Figure 49–1).

Treatment

Most cavernous hemangiomas are asymptomatic. They are usually discovered during abdominal imaging for unrelated symptoms. Treatment is usually not necessary, and there is often no need for continued surveillance. In the few instances where lesions are very large (>10 cm), symptoms such as nausea, vomiting, and early satiety can occur. In these cases, surgical resection can be performed to alleviate symptoms.

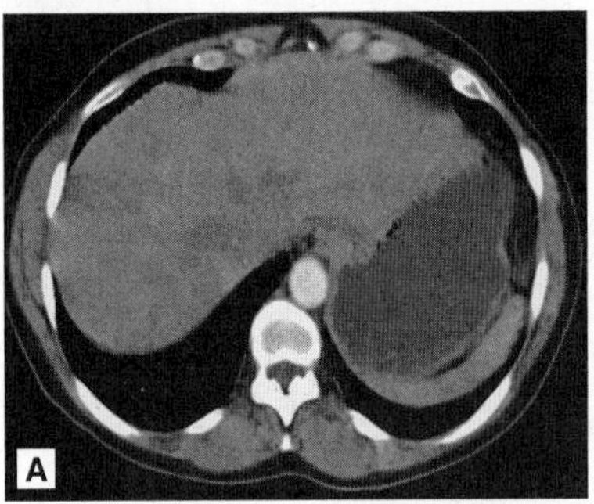

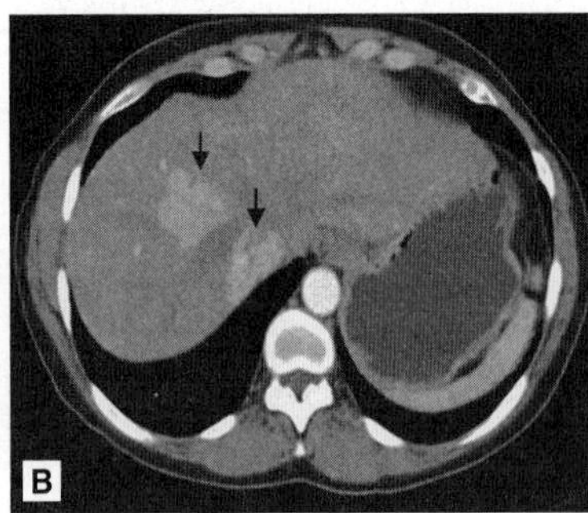

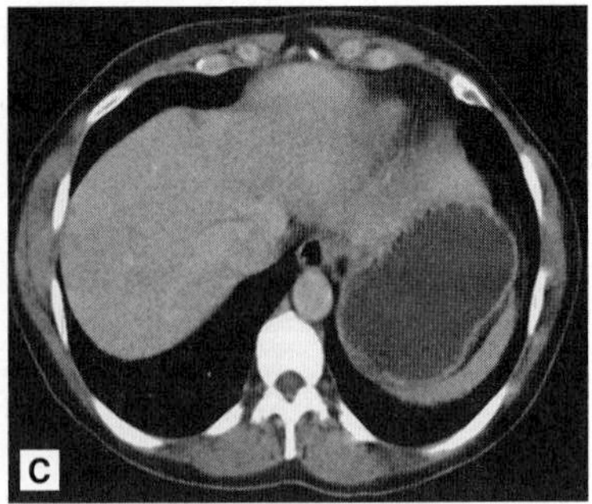

▲ **Figure 49–2.** Computed tomographic scans of focal nodular hyperplasia. The lesions are barely visible in the early arterial phase image (**A**) and not visible in the postvenous phase (**C**) but can be detected as two homogenous hypervascular images in the late arterial phase with contrast (**B**, *arrows*). A central scar is present. (Used with permission from Dr Cheryl Sadow, Department of Radiology, Brigham and Women's Hospital.)

2. Focal Nodular Hyperplasia

General Considerations

A common benign lesion of the liver, FNH is seen in 0.9% of the population. It is the second most common hepatic lesion after cavernous hemangiomas. FNH is more common in women, occurring with a frequency of 8:1. Lesions are most often solitary, but approximately 20% of patients have multiple lesions.

Pathogenesis

The mechanisms underlying development of FNH are not well understood. It has been suggested that proliferation of hepatocytes secondary to vascular malformation or vascular injury may lead to FNH. Given the higher incidence in women, a correlative link has been made to the use of oral contraceptive pills (OCPs). However, data suggesting a causative link or even the influence of OCPs on the growth of FNH are controversial. Indeed, many clinicians believe there is no link.

Clinical Findings

In more than 70% of patients with FNH, lesions are detected incidentally. In the remaining patients, symptoms (especially right upper quadrant discomfort) prompt evaluation. FNH can be classified into two broad categories: the more prevalent classic FNH, and the nonclassic FNH. Classic lesions are nodular, vascular lesions with bile duct proliferation. Radiographically, the lesions are often identified by the presence of a central scar; however, 95% of nonclassic lesions lack this feature. Histologically, the lesions are well circumscribed with proliferating hepatocytes and Kupffer cells. A central vascular scar is invariably present in the classic form of FNH.

Ultrasound can be used for the diagnosis of FNH. The central scar is seen on only 20% of ultrasounds. Doppler imaging shows increased blood flow with a pattern of abnormal blood vessels that emanate radially from a central feeding artery ("spoke-wheeling"). Because ultrasound is not considered the preferred diagnostic modality to rule out FNH, additional imaging with CT or MRI is usually the norm.

On contrast-enhanced CT, the lesion is isodense with the liver on precontrast and postcontrast images but shows homogenous enhancement during the arterial phase, along with the central scar (Figure 49–2). Figure 49–3 shows the typical MRI features of FNH. The lesion is isointense in T2-weighted images with a bright central scar (see Figure 49–3A). It is isointense or hypointense with a central dark scar on T1-weighted images (see Figure 49–3B), homogenously vascular except for the central scar in the arterial phase (see Figure 49–3C), isointense in the portal phase (see Figure 49–3D), and shows subsequent delayed enhancement of the central scar (see Figure 49–3E).

Treatment

There is no indication to treat a patient with asymptomatic FNH because malignant transformation is not felt to occur with typical FNH lesions. Symptoms caused by FNH are present in 30% of patients. These patients often present with right upper quadrant pain. Surgical resection is indicated if patients have pain that is felt to be secondary to the FNH lesions, or if there is doubt about the diagnosis of FNH.

Mathieu D, Kobeiter H, Maison P, et al. Oral contraceptive use and focal nodular hyperplasia of the liver. *Gastroenterology.* 2000; 118:560–564. [PMID: 10702207]

Nguyen BN, Fléjou JF, Terris B, et al. Focal nodular hyperplasia of the liver: a comprehensive pathology study of 305 lesions and recognition of new histologic forms. *Am J Surg Path.* 1999; 23:1441–1454. [PMID: 10584697]

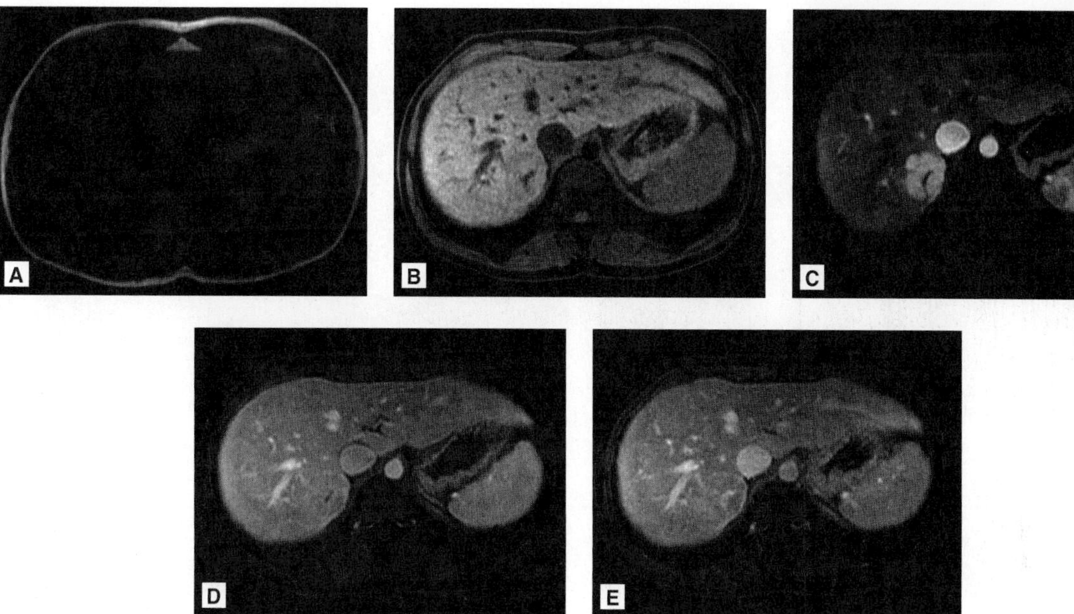

▲ **Figure 49–3.** Magnetic resonance images of focal nodular hyperplasia. The lesion is isointense with the liver on the T2-weighted image, but a bright scar is visible (**A**). On the T1-weighted precontrast image, the lesion remains isointense to slightly hypointense with liver, but a dark central scar is visible (**B**). Dynamic postgadolinium T1 image shows a homogenous hypervascular lesion except for a dark central scar (**C**). The lesion becomes isointense in the portovenous phase (**D**), with delayed enhancement of the central scar (**E**). Arrows indicate the location of the lesion. (Used with permission from Dr Cheryl Sadow, Department of Radiology, Brigham and Women's Hospital.)

Nino-Murcia M, Olcott EW, Jeffrey RB Jr, et al. Focal liver lesions: pattern-based classification scheme for enhancement at arterial phase CT. *Radiology*. 2000;215:746–751. [PMID: 10831693]

3. Hepatic Adenomas

General Considerations & Pathogenesis

This rare liver tumor is most commonly diagnosed in women aged 20–40 years. The major risk factors are OCP use, glycogen storage diseases, diabetes, and androgen use. Among patients who use OCPs there is a 30-fold increase in prevalence of hepatic adenomas. The tumors are usually solitary and increase in size during states of enhanced estrogen levels, such as pregnancy and OCP use (see Figure 9–28). Of note, hepatic Adenomatosis is a distinct entity from hepatic adenomas. Although the former syndrome is characterized by the presence of multiple hepatic adenomas, there is no association with OCP use, and it occurs equally in men and women. In addition, laboratory data usually show an elevated alkaline phosphatase level.

Clinical Findings

In approximately 20% of cases, hepatic adenomas are detected during radiographic imaging for unrelated issues in asymptomatic patients. However, many patients present with abdominal pain resulting from encroachment on neighboring tissue or overt hemorrhage of the tumor. Laboratory evaluation is usually normal in patients without hemorrhage. Histologic evaluation of hepatic adenomas often shows a circumscribed capsular tumor containing hepatocytes that appear normal but are architecturally distorted, in that bile ducts, portal venous tracts, and terminal hepatic veins are absent. The lesion often has a high fat and glycogen content, and necrosis and frank hemorrhage may be present.

Ultrasonographic evaluation can show a hyperechoic mass due to the intracellular fat, with areas that are hypoechoic as a result of hemorrhage. In the absence of contrast, CT usually shows a lesion hypodense to the liver parenchyma if there is no intramural blood. With contrast there is brisk, early enhancement as a result of the vascular nature of the tumor followed by an equally brisk washout due to arteriovenous shunting. On MRI, hepatic adenomas appear as hyperintense lesions on T2-weighted images (Figure 49–4A). On postgadolinium images, they show early arterial enhancement that rapidly washes out (Figure 49–4B and C).

Complications & Treatment

Unlike the other benign hepatic lesions, hepatic adenomas produce significant associated morbidity. The lesion can

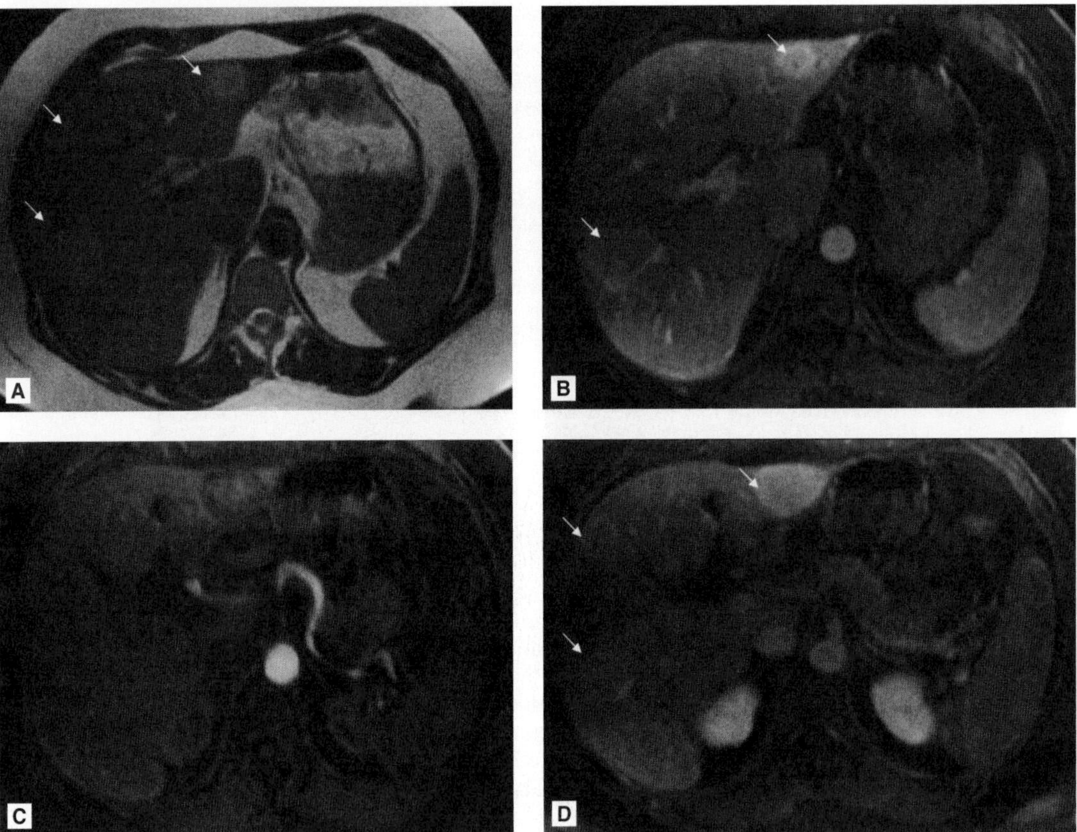

▲ **Figure 49–4.** Magnetic resonance images of hepatic adenoma: T2-weighted images (**A**) show three heterogenous masses (*arrows*). Dynamic postgadolinium T1 images shows early arterial enhancement (**B** and **C**) with washout in the delayed image (**D**). (Used with permission from Dr Koenraad Mortele, Department of Radiology, Brigham and Women's Hospital.)

lead to life-threatening hemorrhage resulting from tumor necrosis and rupture. In addition, hepatic adenomas have the potential for malignant transformation. Although adenomas may be discovered incidentally, right upper pain resulting from encroachment on neighboring tissues or from necrosis is common. Shock from hemorrhage resulting from rupture is a life-threatening emergency that requires emergent resuscitation and surgical therapy. For asymptomatic patients, surgical resection of the adenoma is the therapy of choice. OCPs can be stopped and lesions followed expectantly; however, such an approach is best in patients in whom surgical excision is not a valid option.

4. Nodular Regenerative Hyperplasia

General Considerations

This is a disorder characterized by benign proliferation of hepatocytes, resulting in nodules that range in size from 0.1 to 1 cm. It is associated with many systemic diseases, including but not limited to rheumatoid arthritis, Felty syndrome, Raynaud phenomena, myeloproliferative diseases, lupus erythematosus, polyarthritis nodosa, hereditary hemorrhagic telangiectasia, and amyloidosis, as well as with anabolic steroid use.

Clinical Findings

Patients often present with marked signs of portal hypertension, esophageal varices, upper gastrointestinal bleeding, thrombocytopenia, and ascites. Radiologic appearance is nonspecific, showing multiple nodules throughout the liver that can be confused with cirrhosis. However, histologic evaluation shows nodules that have no associated fibrosis.

Treatment

Treatment focuses on management of the complications of associated portal hypertension and hepatic dysfunction, as discussed in Chapters 44–47.

HEPATOCELLULAR CARCINOMA

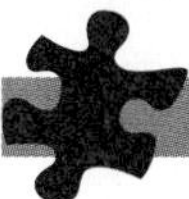

ESSENTIALS OF DIAGNOSIS

- Predisposing conditions include hepatitis B with or without cirrhosis, cirrhosis from hepatitis C, alcoholic liver disease, hemochromatosis, primary biliary cirrhosis, and possibly α_1-antitrypsin deficiency and nonalcoholic steatohepatitis.
- Screening and surveillance programs for early detection use ultrasound with or without α-fetoprotein every 6–12 months.
- CT or MRI of suspicious lesions can identify typical radiographic characteristics.
- Biopsy may be required to establish the diagnosis.

General Considerations

In the United States, hepatocellular carcinoma (HCC) has an incidence of approximately 2.4 in 100,000 persons. Globally, it is the third most common cancer, with a much greater incidence in the Middle East and Africa. Interestingly, during the past few decades the average age at occurrence of cancer has decreased. Older age, male sex, advanced compensated cirrhosis, and active liver disease predict HCC irrespective of the underlying cause of liver disease.

A. Predisposing Conditions

1. Hepatitis B—The annual incidence rate of HCC ranges between 1% and 15% depending on the presence of cirrhosis and disease activity. Even among patients without cirrhosis who are only carriers of hepatitis B virus (HBV), the incidence ranges between 0.5% and 1.0% annually. Older age groups appear to be at the highest risk of developing HCC. Asians, Africans, and patients with HBV infections acquired through vertical transmission are also at increased risk of developing HCC. In contrast, North Americans and Europeans have a lower incidence of HCC, with various cohorts reporting rates of 0–0.46% per year. The difference in HCC rates may be related to the acquisition of the HBV infection later in life among non-Asian and non-African patients. Interestingly, among Asian patients who lose the HBV surface antigen, the risk of HCC remains unchanged. Based on the increased risk of HCC among HBV-infected patients, surveillance is recommended (Table 49–1).

Table 49–1. Recommended surveillance for patients at risk for hepatocellular carcinoma (level III[a]).

Hepatitis B Carriers
Asian males >40 years
Asian females >50 years
All cirrhotic hepatitis B carriers
Family history of HCC
Africans >20 years
For noncirrhotic hepatitis B carriers not listed above, risk of HCC varies depending on severity of underlying liver disease and current and past hepatic inflammatory activity; patients with high HBV DNA concentrations and those with ongoing hepatic inflammatory activity remain at risk for HCC
Non-hepatitis B Cirrhosis
Hepatitis C
Alcoholic cirrhosis
Genetic hemochromatosis
Primary biliary cirrhosis
Although the following groups have an increased risk of HCC no recommendations for or against surveillance can be made because lack of data precludes assessment of whether surveillance would be beneficial:
• α_1-Antitypsin deficiency
• Nonalcoholic steatohepatitis
• Autoimmune hepatitis

HBV, hepatitis B virus; HCC, hepatocellular carcinoma.
[a]American Association for the Study of Liver Diseases level III: opinion of respected authorities, descriptive epidemiology.
Reproduced, with permission, from Bruix J, Sherman M; Practice Guidelines Committee; American Association for the Study of Liver Diseases. Management of hepatocellular carcinoma. *Hepatology.* 2005;42:1210.

2. Hepatitis C—Patients with hepatitis C are at the highest risk of developing HCC. The 5-year cumulative incidence has been reported to be 17–30%. Although individuals infected with hepatitis C virus (HCV) who have bridging fibrosis, but not cirrhosis, may be at risk for HCC, this risk appears to be very low. All patients with hepatitis C and cirrhosis should undergo surveillance. Whether patients with bridging fibrosis should undergo screening is currently controversial.

3. Alcoholic liver disease—The 5-year cumulative incidence of HCC in patients with alcoholic liver disease without associated Hepatitis B and C is 8%. However, infection with HBV or HCV further increases the risk of developing HCC.

4. Nonalcoholic steatohepatitis—The annual incidence of HCC in patients with nonalcoholic steatohepatitis (NASH) is 2.4%. Diabetes mellitus, a condition commonly associated with NASH, was found to be a risk factor for HCC. Whether this suggests that NASH patients are at higher risk of developing HCC is not clear, but surveillance of NASH patients with cirrhosis is recommended.

5. Genetic or inherited liver diseases—Patients with hemochromatosis who develop cirrhosis have an increased 5-year cumulative incidence of HCC that is reported to be 21%. In contrast, in Wilson disease and α_1-antitrypsin deficiency, the incidence rates of HCC are not at present very clear. HCC has been reported in patients who have α_1-antitrypsin deficiency with or without cirrhosis. In Wilson disease, the incidence of HCC is exceedingly low. Surveillance of patients with hemochromatosis and cirrhosis is recommended. For patients with α_1-antitrypsin deficiency, the American Association for the Study of Liver Diseases (AASLD) does not recommend surveillance since data are insufficient. Lastly, patients with hereditary tyrosinemia can develop HCC and in one study, primary liver cancers occurred in up to 40% of patients.

6. Autoimmune hepatitis and primary biliary cirrhosis— HCC surveillance of patients with primary biliary cirrhosis who are cirrhotic is recommended based on a study that shows an incidence similar to that of patients with HCV cirrhosis. The association between autoimmune hepatitis and HCC is not clear, but case reports have illustrated the occurrence of HCC in such patients with cirrhosis. Although surveillance of patients with autoimmune hepatitis and cirrhosis is not recommended, most practitioners do so because of a concern that cirrhosis in all forms elevates the risk of HCC.

7. Other conditions—Aflatoxin, produced by *Aspergillus flavus*, is clearly associated with HCC, particularly among patients infected with HBV.

8. Fibrolamellar hepatocellular carcinoma—This tumor, which is a distinct primary HCC, tends to occur in patients without cirrhosis who are in their 20s to 40s. The long-term prognosis is generally good with either resection or transplantation.

Degos F, Christidis C, Ganne-Carrie F, et al. Hepatitis C virus related cirrhosis: time to occurrence of hepatocellular carcinoma and death. *Gut.* 2000;47:131–136. [PMID: 10861275]

Elmberg M, Hultzcrantz R, Ekbom A, et al. Cancer risk in patients with hereditary hemochromatosis and in their first-degree relatives. *Gastroenterology.* 2003;125:1733–1741. [PMID: 14724826]

El-Serag HB, Mason AC. Rising incidence of hepatocellular carcinoma in the United States. *N Engl J Med.* 1999;340:745–750. [PMID: 10072408]

El-Serag HB, Mason AC. Risk factors for the rising rates of primary liver cancer in the United States. *Arch Intern Med.* 2000; 160:3227–3230. [PMID: 11088082]

Hassan MM, Hwang LY, Hatlen CJ, et al. Risk factors for hepatocellular carcinoma: synergism of alcohol with viral hepatitis and diabetes mellitus. *Hepatology.* 2002;36:1206–1213. [PMID: 12395331]

Sherman M. Hepatocellular carcinoma: epidemiology, risk factors, and screening. *Semin Liver Dis.* 2005;25:143–154. [PMID: 15918143]

Shibuya A, Tanaka K, Miyakawa H, et al. Hepatocellular carcinoma and survival in patients with primary biliary cirrhosis. *Hepatology.* 2002;35:1172–1178. [PMID: 11981767]

B. Screening and Surveillance

Owing to the increased risk of HCC in certain populations (ie, HCC risk >1.5% per year for non-HBV cirrhosis, >0.2% for HBV carriers), surveillance measures have been recommended, often using a combination of serologic and radiologic tests. However, despite these recommendations, a recent study reported that less than 20% of cirrhosis patients with a new diagnosis of HCC underwent regular surveillance

In the one large-scale study performed to date, from China, 18,816 patients were randomized to either surveillance with ultrasound and α-fetoprotein every 6 months or no monitoring. A 37% decrease in HCC-related mortality was noted in those who were screened compared with the unscreened cohort. The 1-, 3-, and 5-year mortality rates in the screened group were 66%, 53%, and 46% compared with rates of 31%, 7%, and 0%, respectively, in the control group. These data need further confirmatory studies. However, based on the premise that early diagnosis of HCC will lead to early treatment and reduction in mortality, surveillance measures are widely implemented in the patients groups identified in Table 49–1. Interestingly, over the past 2 decades the 2- and 4-year survival rates have doubled, suggesting that more patients are being diagnosed with localized and regional HCC thus improving prognosis.

1. Serologic screening—A persistently elevated α-fetoprotein level is a risk factor for subsequent HCC. Absolute α-fetoprotein levels have inadequate sensitivity and specificity to detect HCC. However, very high (>500 ng/mL) levels are generally associated with the presence of HCC, and if a mass is identified on subsequent imaging, biopsy is not necessarily needed to confirm the diagnosis. Other serologic studies such as des-γ-carboxy prothrombin (an abnormal prothrombin induced in patients deficient in vitamin K), glycosylated α-fetoprotein ratio, α-fucosidase, and glypican 3 need further investigation before being considered for HCC screening.

2. Radiographic imaging—Ultrasound is widely used for HCC surveillance. On ultrasonography either a hyperechoic or a hypoechoic lesion can be seen. Ultrasound has low sensitivity (~65%) but excellent specificity for the detection of liver lesions (>90%). However, there is concern that its accuracy may be limited in obese individuals and in those with multiple cirrhotic nodules.

HCC surveillance is recommended in at-risk populations, with ultrasonography performed every 6–12 months. Most hepatologists, however, use a combination of ultrasonography and α-fetoprotein every 6 months for surveillance. If a lesion greater than 1 cm is identified or a previously known nodule enlarges, further diagnostic evaluation with either contrast-enhanced CT or MRI should be performed.

Davila JA, Morgan RO, Richardson PA, et al. Use of surveillance for hepatocellular carcinoma among patients with cirrhosis in the United States. *Hepatol.* 2010;52:132–141. [PMID: 20578139]

Zhang BH, Yang BH, Tang ZY. Randomized controlled trial of screening for hepatocellular carcinoma. *J Cancer Res Clin Oncol.* 2004;130:417–422. [PMID: 15042359]

Clinical Findings

A. Symptoms and Signs

Because a significant fraction of patients with HCC are being diagnosed at early stages due to surveillance, many are asymptomatic at presentation. However, any patient with compensated cirrhosis who suddenly develops signs and symptoms of worsening hepatic function should undergo appropriate studies to exclude the development of HCC.

Among the patients who present with symptoms, weight loss, fatigue, anorexia, right upper quadrant pain, jaundice, and pruritus may be noted. Patients may also present with variceal hemorrhage, ascites, or hepatic encephalopathy. Physical examination findings often show stigmata of portal hypertension and cirrhosis. Occasionally, hepatomegaly may be present. In patients suspected of having HCC who present with peritoneal signs, hemoperitoneum should be suspected as a consequence of hemorrhage related to the tumor. Additional clinical findings may be secondary to associated paraneoplastic syndromes, including hypercholesterolemia, cryoglobulinemia, carcinoid syndrome, hypercalcemia, dysfibrinogenemia, erythrocytosis, and hypoglycemia.

B. Diagnostic Approach

With the exception of an α-fetoprotein, laboratory testing is generally not very useful and radiographic studies are required to make a diagnosis. Nevertheless, the diagnosis of HCC can be made using a combination of radiographic, laboratory, or pathologic studies. The size of the tumor influences the diagnostic evaluation.

1. Lesions larger than 1 cm—A nodule greater than 1 cm in size that has CT or MRI characteristics typical of HCC (ie, early arterial enhancement) usually is HCC; in such cases, a biopsy to confirm the diagnosis is not generally required. However, if characteristics of HCC are not seen on the initial radiographic study, then a second CT or MRI study (whichever was not performed initially) is recommended. If typical HCC characteristic are seen on the follow-up study, then the diagnosis of HCC is confirmed. If the second study still does not confirm the diagnosis of HCC, a biopsy is recommended. If a negative biopsy result is obtained in an individual with risk factors for HCC (eg, chronic HBV infection or cirrhosis), then enhanced follow-up with MRI or CT is recommended at a very short interval to ensure stability of the lesion and should be considered.

2. Lesions smaller than 1 cm—These lesions have a very low probability of being HCC. The AASLD recommends an ultrasound every 3–6 months for up to 2 years and if no growth is documented, reverting back to typical HCC surveillance guidelines thereafter. Alternatively, if the lesion enlarges, additional diagnostic testing with CT, MRI, or biopsy is recommended.

3. Metastases—Many patients with HCC have metastases to the portal and hepatic veins and inferior vena cava. Metastases to the portal, pancreatic, and para-aortic lymph nodes have also been reported. Other sites of metastasis include the lung, bone, myocardium, and adrenal gland. Imaging by Doppler ultrasound, contrast-enhanced CT, or MRI can be used to identify a thrombus in the major vessels. A contrast-enhanced CT or MRI scan is often required for nodal involvement.

Differential Diagnosis

The differential diagnosis of HCC is very broad and includes benign and malignant lesions. Among these are cholangiocarcinoma, hepatic adenoma, hemangioma, FNH, cystic neoplasms, metastatic tumors, peliosis hepatis, and lymphoma.

Treatment

Therapeutic management of HCC is influenced by the tumor size and extent, underlying liver function, and the patient's performance status. The best system of staging patients, appears to be the Barcelona Clinic Liver Cancer Proposal (Figure 49–5). Treatment options include resection, transplantation, percutaneous ablation, transarterial embolization, chemotherapy, and radiation.

Bruix J, Sherman M. Practice Guidelines Committee, American Association for the Study of Liver Diseases. Management of hepatocellular carcinoma. *Hepatology.* 2005;42:1208–1236. [PMID: 1625051]

A. Resection

Surgical resection is an option in HCC patients without cirrhosis and Child Pugh Class A cirrhosis. However, this constitutes only a small proportion of patients with HCC. The risk of hepatic decompensation after surgery is approximately 35–40%. But studies have shown that surgical resection may be a viable option for carefully chosen patients. Based on available data, it appears that patients who have compensated cirrhosis with a normal bilirubin and hepatovenous portal gradient (discussed in Chapter 47) less than 10 mm Hg may be appropriate candidates provided there is only a solitary tumor. After resection, the recurrence rate is approximately 70%. However, clinical studies have not shown any presurgical or postsurgical adjuvant therapies to be effective; thus, adjuvant therapy is not usually recommended.

Imamura H, Matsuyama Y, Tanaka E, et al. Risk factors contributing to early and late phase intrahepatic recurrence of hepatocellular carcinoma after hepatectomy. *J Hepatol.* 2003;38:200–207. [PMID: 12547409]

B. Transplantation

Both cadaveric and live donor liver transplantation have been used in patients with HCC. Based on the Milan criteria, carefully chosen patients with HCC who undergo liver transplantation have a 5-year survival rate of 70%. The patients who fulfill these criteria usually have a solitary nodule no more than 5 cm in size or three nodules each no more than

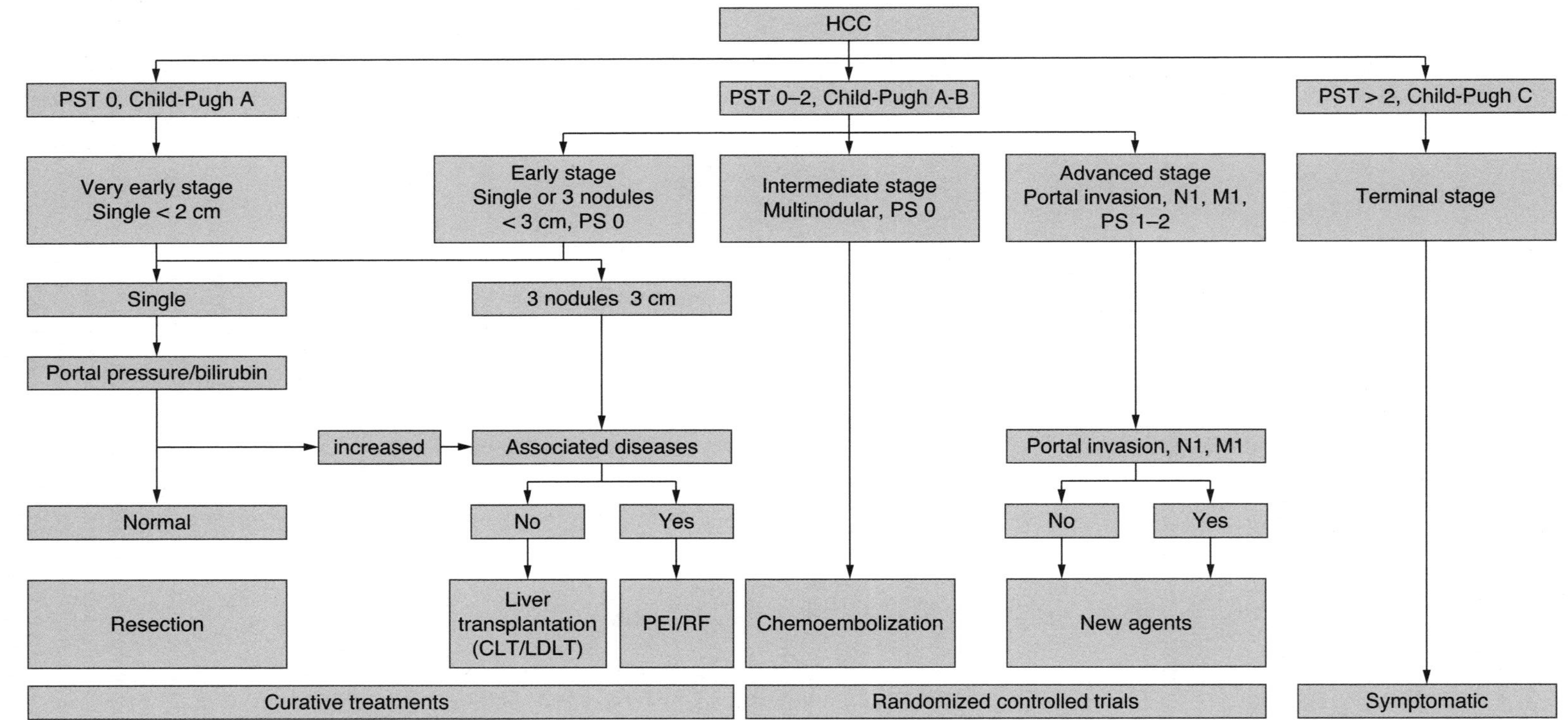

▲ **Figure 49–5.** Algorithm for staging and management of hepatocellular carcinoma (HCC). CLT, cadaver liver transplantation, LDLT living donor liver transplantation, M, metastasis, N, node, PEI, percutaneous ethanol injection, PS, performance status, PST, performance status test, RF radiofrequency (ablation) (Reproduced, with permission, from Bruix J, Sherman M; Practice Guidelines Committee; American Association for the Study of Liver Diseases. Management of hepatocellular carcinoma. *Hepatology*. 2005;42:1210.)

3 cm and no evidence of metastasis. The United Network for Organ Sharing (UNOS) has created a priority system for such patients. However, as previously noted, lesions need to be larger than 2 cm for the Model for End-Stage Liver Disease (MELD) points (the system used for prioritizing transplant necessity, discussed in Chapter 50) to be awarded. For patients who meet the criteria, a MELD score of 22 is given at the time of listing with a 10% increase in the MELD score every 3 months while on the waiting list.

In many transplant systems, the wait time can be long even with the priority MELD system, extending up to 12 months or more. Most centers with wait times greater than 6 months practice some form of preoperative therapy. For patients with small tumors, percutaneous ablative techniques using either radiofrequency ablation or ethanol can be considered. The major concerns with these techniques are hemorrhage, liver failure, and tumor seeding. For patients with multiple or larger tumors, transarterial chemoembolization can be considered. This technique is associated with a significant risk of hepatic decompensation and liver failure.

Llovet JM, Brù C, Bruix J. Prognosis of hepatocellular carcinoma: the BCLC staging classification. *Semin Liver Dis.* 1999;19: 329–338. [PMID: 10518312]

C. Percutaneous Ablation

Percutaneous ablative techniques for HCC using either ethanol or radiofrequency remain a viable option as either a bridge to transplant or for poor surgical candidates. The 5-year survival rate is satisfactory, particularly for tumors smaller than 2 cm, and can be as high as 50%. The major risks with this procedure are hemorrhage, hemoperitoneum, and seeding of the needle track.

Sala M, Llovet JM, Vilan R, et al; Barcelona Clínic Liver Cancer Group. Initial response to percutaneous ablation predicts survival in patients with hepatocellular carcinoma. *Hepatology.* 2004;40:1352–1360. [PMID: 15565564]

D. Transarterial Embolization

Transarterial embolization appears to be an effective noncurative option for a certain subset of patients with HCC. Candidates without evidence of vascular or metastatic disease or portosystemic shunting can be considered for the procedure. Liver failure after embolization is a major risk. Patients with advanced liver disease are at greater risk of morbidity and mortality with the procedure. Chemotherapeutic agents such as doxorubicin and cisplatin can be administered directly into the arterial branches supplying the tumor; in such cases, the procedure is called transarterial chemoembolization. Survival rates appear to improve 20–60% at 2 years with this intervention. Side effects related to the procedure include liver failure, chemotherapeutic side effects, and postembolization syndrome related to hepatic artery occlusion.

Bruix J, Sala M, Llovet JM. Chemoembolization for hepatocellular carcinoma. *Gastroenterology.* 2004;127(Suppl 1):S179–188. [PMID: 15508083]

E. Chemotherapy and Radiation Therapy

Generally, chemotherapy and radiation therapy have not had much of a role in the treatment of HCC. However, recent studies suggest that sorafenib may be an effective palliative option. In a recent phase III multicenter, randomized, placebo-controlled trial of 602 patients, overall survival was improved with sorafenib. Serious side effects were rare, and common side effects included diarrhea, fatigue, and hand-foot skin reaction.

Llovet JM, Ricci S, Mazzaferro V, et al; SHARP Investigators Study Group. Sorafenib in advanced hepatocellular carcinoma. *N Engl J Med.* 2008;359:378–390. [PMID: 18650514]

CHOLANGIOCARCINOMA

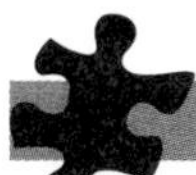

ESSENTIALS OF DIAGNOSIS

- Risk factors include biliary and liver diseases (eg, primary sclerosing cholangitis [PSC], choledocholithiasis, hepatolithiasis, hepatitis C), chronic parasitic infection, and typhoid carrier state.
- Diagnosis usually requires abdominal imaging and tissue sampling either by percutaneous biopsy or ERCP.
- Associated with a poor prognosis.

General Considerations

Although the incidence of cholangiocarcinoma is increasing globally, it remains a rare cancer with an incidence of approximately 8 per million persons.

The risk factors for cholangiocarcinoma include PSC, choledocholithiasis, hepatolithiasis, choledochal cyst, Caroli disease, bile duct adenoma, thorotrast, HCV infection, chronic parasitic infection, and typhoid carrier state. Age and smoking are also risk factors.

Shaib Y, El-Serag HB. The epidemiology of cholangiocarcinoma. *Semin Liver Dis.* 2004;24:115–125. [PMID: 15192785]

Clinical Findings

Patients may be asymptomatic, with abnormal findings that are discovered incidentally on liver biochemical or imaging tests. Alternatively, symptoms maybe present especially those suggestive of biliary obstruction or hepatic decompensation. Extrahepatic cholangiocarcinoma typically presents with obstructive symptoms.

Abdominal imaging with either CT or MRI is required. Endoscopic retrograde cholangiopancreatography (ERCP) with cytologic brushing of the biliary tree may be required. The role of serologic testing is not entirely clear, but of the many markers, CA 19-9 may be of some clinical use. Its sensitivity seems to be better in PSC than in non-PSC patients with cholangiocarcinoma when a level of 100 IU/mL is used as a cutoff.

Malhi H, Gores GJ. Cholangiocarcinoma: modern advances in understanding a deadly old disease. *J Hepatol.* 2006;45:856–867. [PMID: 17030071]

Differential Diagnosis

The differential diagnosis is similar to that of HCC (see earlier discussion).

Treatment

The best treatment option in cholangiocarcinoma is surgical resection, but even when patients are carefully selected, the 5-year survival rate is only 20–45%. The absence of positive lymph nodes, a clear resection margin (>1 cm), lack of vascular invasion, and single lesions are the predictors of good response to surgery. Patients with compromised liver function, PSC, and bilobar involvement are not candidates for surgical resection and transplantation may be considered. However, because of the high rate of disease recurrence, transplantation is generally not associated with good outcomes. A recent protocol using neoadjuvant chemotherapy and radiation followed by exploratory laparotomy to confirm down-staging of the tumor and subsequent liver transplantation is reported to be associated with a good prognosis. Further studies evaluating this approach are necessary prior to its widespread use. Otherwise, there appears to be minimal response to chemotherapy and radiation in this disease.

Most patients who present with cholangiocarcinoma are not candidates for curative therapy but require palliation. Biliary obstruction is a common complication of this disease, and decompression using endoscopic, percutaneous, or surgical approaches is often necessary. There is interest in photodynamic therapy, but further confirmatory studies are needed.

Prognosis

Overall, the prognosis is poor. Most patients develop liver failure or biliary complications, resulting in a 5-year survival rate of approximately 5%.

Jarnagin WR, Fong Y, DeMatteo RP, et al. Staging, resectability, and outcome in 225 patients with hilar cholangiocarcinoma. *Ann Surg.* 2001;234:507–517. [PMID: 11573044]

Rea DJ, Heimbach JK, Rosen CB, et al. Liver transplantation with neoadjuvant chemoradiation is more effective than resection for hilar cholangiocarcinoma. *Ann Surg.* 2005;242:451–458. [PMID: 16135931]

Silva MA, Tekin K, Aytekin F, et al. Surgery for hilar cholangiocarcinoma: a 10-year experience of a tertiary referral centre in the UK. *Eur J Surg Oncol.* 2005;31:533–539. [PMID: 15922889]

Sudan D, DeRoover A, Chinnakotla S, et al. Radiochemotherapy and transplantation allow long-term survival for nonresectable hilar cholangiocarcinoma. *Am J Transplant.* 2002;2:774–779. [PMID: 12243499]

Yeh CN, Yan YY, Yeh TS, et al. Hepatic resection of the intraductal papillary type of peripheral cholangiocarcinoma. *Ann Surg Oncol.* 2004;11:606–611. [PMID: 15172934]

Liver Transplantation

50

Amir A. Qamar, MD

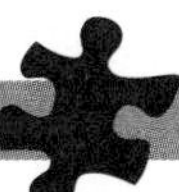

ESSENTIAL CONCEPTS

- Hepatitis C and hepatocellular carcinoma are among the leading indications for liver transplantation in the United States.
- Thorough medical, psychiatric, and social evaluation is required prior to listing patients for transplantation.
- The Model for End-Stage Liver Disease (MELD) score is widely used for prioritizing patients on the transplant waiting list.
- Liver biopsy is needed to confirm the diagnosis of acute rejection, which is common and occurs in up to 60% of patients.
- Medical and surgical complications after transplantation can occur immediately or years later.
- Biliary strictures and leaks occur in 15% of patients after transplantation.
- Long-term immunosuppression, particularly with calcineurin inhibitors, is associated with an increased risk of renal failure.

General Considerations

A. Background

Liver transplantation has radically changed the management of patients with chronic liver disease and acute liver failure. Following the first liver transplant procedure in 1963, numerous medical, surgical, and technical breakthroughs were required before transplantation became a viable therapy in liver disease. The 1-year survival rate remained low at 25% until the introduction of cyclosporine as a long-term immunosuppressant in the 1980s. Further medical developments in immunosuppression, including mycophenolate mofetil, sirolimus, tacrolimus, and azathioprine, as well as effective anti-infective treatment and prophylaxis, have resulted in 5-year survival rates of up to 85–90%.

B. Role of UNOS

The United Network for Organ Sharing (UNOS) is a nonprofit scientific organization based in Virginia that is responsible for matching donors to recipients and coordinating the organ transplantation process. UNOS has divided the United States into 11 regions to facilitate organ allocation (Figure 50–1).

INDICATIONS FOR TRANSPLANTATION

There are numerous indications for liver transplantation; common and uncommon indications are listed in Table 50–1.

1. Hepatitis C

The hepatitis C virus (HCV) infects approximately 170 million people worldwide and up to 4 million people (1–1.5%) in the United States. Based on histopathologic studies, it is believed that 5–20% of patients with hepatitis C develop cirrhosis after 20 years of infection. After the occurrence of cirrhosis, decompensation (ie, variceal hemorrhage, ascites, and hepatic encephalopathy) occurs in 25–28% of patients in a median of 3–9 years. HCV significantly contributes to the occurrence of hepatocellular carcinoma (HCC). Current studies suggest that the five-year incidence of HCC is 17–30% in HCV-induced cirrhosis per year.

Hepatitis C is one of the leading indications for liver transplantation in most countries, including the United States, accounting for up to 40% of transplant procedures performed each year. It is expected that the proportion of liver transplants resulting from HCV will increase over the next 10–15 years in response to increases in the incidence of cirrhosis and eventual decompensation or occurrence of HCC.

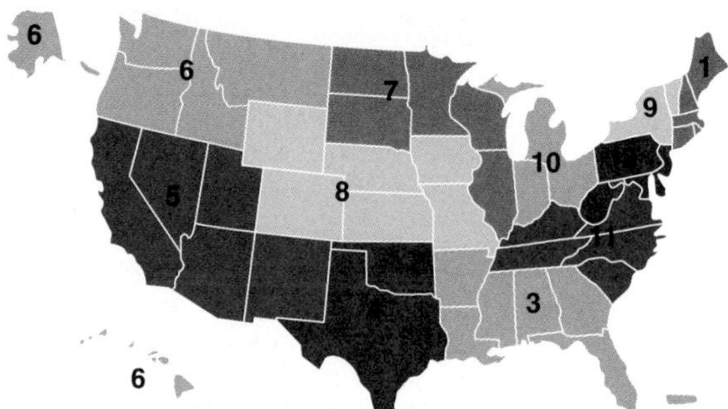

▲ **Figure 50–1.** UNOS regions. (Source: United Network for Organ Sharing.)

NOTE: *MELD score* = 9.57 × *log$_e$ creatinine mg per dL* + 3.78 × *log$_e$ bilirubin mg per dL* + 11.20 × *log$_e$ INR* + 6.43 (*constant for liver disease etiology*: 0 = *cholestatic or alcoholic*; 1 = *all other*).

Fattovich G, Pantalena M, Zagni I, et al. European Concerted Action on Viral Hepatitis (EUROHEP). Effect of hepatitis B and C virus infections on the natural history of compensated cirrhosis: a cohort study of 297 patients. *Am J Gastroenterol.* 2002;97:2886–2895. [PMID: 12425564]

Lawson A, Hagan S, Rye K, et al. Trent HCV Study Group. The natural history of hepatitis C with severe hepatic fibrosis. *J Hepatol.* 2007;47:37–45. [PMID: 17400322]

2. Hepatitis B

Until approximately 10 years ago, transplantation of patients infected with the hepatitis B virus (HBV) was controversial. The near universal recurrence of hepatitis B generally resulted in early graft loss. A major advance in the field of transplantation was the introduction of hepatitis B immunoglobulin and antiviral therapy with nucleoside and nucleotide analogs. This has resulted in a dramatic improvement in transplant outcomes, and HBV infection is now a well accepted indication with a good prognosis.

Although less prevalent than HCV in the United States, HBV remains a common cause of decompensated liver disease and HCC globally. Approximately, 350 million people globally and 730,000 people in the United States are infected with HBV. The occurrence of cirrhosis is a significant prognostic indicator, with a 50% 5-year survival among patients with hepatitis B e antigen–positive disease and cirrhosis. Both the incidence of decompensation and HCC rate are slightly lower for HBV than for HCV. Although in the United States the number of transplant procedures performed because of HBV is small, it remains an indication in a large proportion of transplants performed in many Asian and European countries.

Table 50–1. Indications for liver transplantation.

Common	Uncommon
Chronic hepatitis B	Hereditary hemochromatosis
Chronic hepatitis C	Wilson disease
Autoimmune hepatitis	α_1-Antitrypsin deficiency
Alcoholic liver disease	Glycogen storage disease
Nonalcoholic fatty liver disease	Tyrosinemia
Primary biliary cirrhosis	Urea cycle defects
Primary sclerosing cholangitis	Amyloidosis
Hepatocellular carcinoma	Hyperoxaluria
Acute liver failure	Branched-chain amino acid disorders
	Cystic fibrosis
	Alagille syndrome
	Progressive familial intrahepatic cholestasis
	Polycystic liver disease
	Budd-Chiari syndrome
	Metastatic neuroendocrine tumor

3. Alcoholic Liver Disease

Alcoholic liver disease is the most common cause of cirrhosis in the United States and results in an estimated 12,000 deaths annually. Although there is concern that patients with alcoholic liver disease are high-risk candidates for poor outcomes after liver transplantation, graft loss as a result of alcohol abuse is uncommon. In fact, the 7-year graft survival rate is very good, and better than rates reported for many other indications for liver transplantation. Presently, approximately 85% transplant centers recommend a 6-month period of abstinence from alcohol before considering a patient for liver transplantation. This stipulated period of abstinence remains unproven as there are no conclusive data to suggest that any period of abstinence is associated with a decreased risk of relapse after transplantation. The American Association for the Study of Liver Diseases (AASLD) recommends careful assessment of such patients by a health care professional experienced in the management of patients with addictive behavior.

4. Metabolic Liver Disease

Liver transplantation has been used effectively to treat several genetic and metabolic diseases associated with liver involvement (see Table 50–1).

5. Hemochromatosis

Hemochromatosis is primarily a disease of Caucasians, with a prevalence of 1 in 200–300 persons. Among patients with untreated hemochromatosis, a significant proportion can develop decompensated cirrhosis or HCC. For these patients, liver transplantation is a treatment option. The survival of patients who undergo liver transplantation for hemochromatosis is not comparable to that of patients with other genetic or metabolic liver disease treated with transplantation. This may be attributable to the presence of cardiomyopathy in patients with hemochromatosis. Among genetic and metabolic conditions, hemochromatosis is the most common reason for transplantation.

6. α_1-Antitrypsin Deficiency

This autosomal-recessive condition is a common indication for liver transplantation in children. Patients who do not develop liver disease as children can develop cirrhosis, which tends to occur in the sixth and seventh decades. The outcomes for liver transplantation in this setting are very good.

7. Wilson Disease

Wilson disease is an autosomal-recessive disease that can cause either acute or chronic liver disease. In patients with fulminant failure or decompensated cirrhosis, liver transplantation is an effective therapy with a good prognosis. Transplantation cures the defect in copper secretion, and long-term antichelating therapy is generally not required.

8. Autoimmune Liver Disease & Cholestatic Liver Disease

A significant proportion of patients with autoimmune hepatitis develop decompensated cirrhosis despite immunosuppressant therapy. In patients with decompensated disease, liver transplantation remains a viable option; excellent survival outcomes and 5-year survival of 90% are reported.

Similarly, primary biliary cirrhosis and primary sclerosing cholangitis are excellent indications for liver transplantation, and are associated with good graft survival.

9. Hepatocellular Carcinoma

Because of the increased risk of HCC in cirrhosis, most patients undergo some form of screening, which includes radiologic imaging or α-fetoprotein assessment, or both (see Chapter 49). The use of screening has resulted in the earlier detection of tumors. This has improved survival in HCC, especially in patients with small tumors. The AASLD and UNOS endorse liver transplantation as effective treatment for patients with "early HCC," defined as a solitary tumor less than 5 cm or three tumors less than 3 cm. The 5-year survival rate in this group of patients has been reported to be 70%. In 2005, UNOS also allowed patients who meet either of these criteria to receive a higher Model for End-Stage Liver Disease (MELD) score at the time of being placed on the transplant list to increase the chance of receiving a liver transplant sooner.

Sangiovanni A, Del Ninno E, Fasani P, et al. Increased survival of cirrhotic patients with a hepatocellular carcinoma detected during surveillance. *Gastroenterology*. 2004;126:1005–1014. [PMID: 15057740]

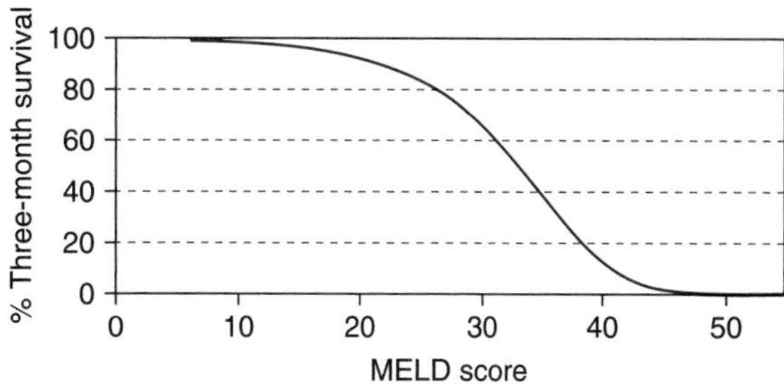

NOTE: *MELD score* = 9.57 × *log$_e$ creatinine mg per dL* + 3.78 × *log$_e$ bilirubin mg per dL* + 11.20 × *log$_e$ INR* + 6.43 (*constant for liver disease etiology:* 0 = *cholestatic or alcoholic;* 1 = *all other*).

▲ **Figure 50–2.** Estimated 3-month survival as a function of the MELD score. INR, international normalized ratio; MELD, Model for End-Stage Liver Disease. (Adapted, with permission, from Wiesner R, Edwards E, Freeman R, et al; for the United Network for Organ Sharing Liver Disease Severity Score Committee. Model for end-stage liver disease (MELD) and allocation of donor livers. *Gastroenterology*. 2003;124:94.)

10. Acute Liver Failure

Acute liver failure is a rare but life-threatening event that in many cases may result in death without a liver transplant. A detailed review of liver transplantation in acute liver failure is provided in Chapter 38.

11. Decompensating Events

Since 2002, UNOS has used the MELD score to determine the need for liver transplantation in patients with cirrhosis. As shown in Figure 50–2, the 3-month survival of patients decreases with higher MELD scores. Many transplant centers use a MELD score of 15 as a minimal listing threshold. However, there continues to be a role for the Child-Pugh score (Table 50–2). Patients with Child class B or C cirrhosis have poor survival compared with patients who have more compensated Child class A disease. In addition, patients with a history of variceal hemorrhage and spontaneous bacterial

Table 50–2. Child-Pugh scoring system.

	1	2	3
Bilirubin	<2.0	2.0-3.0	>3.0
Albumin	>3.5	3.5-2.8	<2.8
Prothrombin time	<4 seconds	4-6 seconds	>6 seconds
Ascites	Absent	Mild-moderate	Moderate-severe
Encephalopathy	Absent	Mild (grade I-II)	Severe (grade III-IV)

Score: 5–6 = Child class A; 7–9 = Child class B; >10 = Child class C.

peritonitis have decreased 1-year survival and would benefit from liver transplantation.

Kamath PS, Kim WR. Advanced Liver Disease Study Group. The model for end-stage liver disease (MELD). *Hepatology.* 2007;45:797–805. [PMID: 17326206]

12. Impaired Quality of Life

One of the major goals of liver transplantation is to improve patients' quality of life. Studies have shown that prior to transplantation, many patients experience significant impairments because of physical and emotional stress. A meta-analysis of quality of life showed that patients improved after liver transplantation.

PRETRANSPLANT EVALUATION

The evaluation of patients who are candidates for liver transplantation occurs in a multidisciplinary setting and involves hepatologists, transplant surgeons, anesthesiologists, psychiatrists, social workers, and subspecialists as needed.

Several diagnostic tests and procedures are used to evaluate patients; these are listed in Table 50–3 and described later.

1. Laboratory Evaluation

Laboratory evaluation provides information about the underlying liver disease and assessment of liver and renal function (see Table 50–3).

Importantly, evaluation of the risk of developing complications related to immunosuppression is needed. Routine studies include serologic testing for cytomegalovirus (CMV), herpes simplex virus (HSV), and Epstein-Barr virus (EBV).

Table 50–3. Liver transplant recipient evaluation.

Viral hepatitis A, B, C, D, and E serologies
HIV testing
Serologic testing for cytomegalovirus, Epstein-Barr virus, herpes simplex virus immunoglobulin G
Chest radiograph
Pulmonary function tests with arterial blood gases
Electrocardiogram
Dobutamine stress echocardiography
Magnetic resonance imaging and angiography of the liver
Esophagogastroduodenoscopy and colonoscopy
Cervical cancer screening
Mammogram
Prostate-specific antigen assay
Dental evaluation
Vaccination against hepatitis A and B, *Pneumococcus, Haemophilus influenzae*, influenza
Purified protein derivative skin test for tuberculosis
Comprehensive psychiatric and social assessment

Testing for histoplasmosis, schistosomiasis, and strongyloidiasis should be considered in patients from endemic areas. All patients should undergo skin testing for tuberculosis with purified protein derivative (PPD) and, if positive, computed tomography (CT) scan of the chest. Further testing and referral to a pulmonologist may be needed if the suspicion of tuberculosis remains.

2. Cardiopulmonary Evaluation

Cardiac and pulmonary complications of liver transplantation are the leading cause of mortality. Meticulous cardiopulmonary evaluation is required in every patient being considered for liver transplantation. Recent data have shown that maximum heart rate achieved during dobutamine stress echocardiography and MELD score adequately identify patients who would be at increased risk for cardiac mortality 4 months after transplantation. An added benefit of this test is that it can identify patients with congenital abnormalities of the heart such as a patent foramen ovale. If abnormalities are identified, they can be corrected and patients reconsidered for transplant.

Muñoz SJ, ElGenaidi H. Cardiovascular risk factors after liver transplantation. *Liver Transpl.* 2005;(Suppl 1):S52–56. [PMID: 16237716]

Tsutsui JM, Mukherjee S, Elhendy A, et al. Value of dobutamine stress myocardial contrast perfusion echocardiography in patients with advanced liver disease. *Liver Transpl.* 2006;12: 592–599. [PMID: 16555336]

3. Psychosocial Evaluation

A comprehensive psychosocial evaluation of the candidate is needed before listing. Alcohol abuse is common among liver transplant candidates. Studies have produced controversial evidence that duration of less than 6 months is associated with an increased risk of relapse after surgery. Alcohol relapse is not an ideal situation as it increases the risks of noncompliance with immunosuppressant medications and posttransplant alcoholic hepatitis.

Strong social support is needed after liver transplantation to ensure compliance with medication regimens and appointments. A comprehensive evaluation by social support services must be considered in every patient undergoing liver transplant evaluation.

Rocca P, Cocuzza E, Rasetti R, et al. Predictors of psychiatric disorders in liver transplantation candidates: logistic regression models. *Liver Transpl.* 2003;9:721–726. [PMID: 12827559]

4. Infectious Risk Workup

Given the risk of infectious complications in patients taking immunosuppressant medications, a comprehensive evaluation for infectious risk is needed. This evaluation should include serologic testing for CMV, HSV, varicella–zoster, and EBV. Patients should undergo evaluation for *Mycobacterium tuberculosis* infection using a PPD skin test and chest radiograph. Patients from regions in which strongyloidiasis, schistosomiasis, and histoplasmosis are endemic should undergo serologic evaluation and prophylactic treatment as appropriate.

Sharma P, Rakela J. Management of pre-liver transplantation patients–part 1. *Liver Transpl.* 2005;11:124–133. [PMID: 15666386]

Sharma P, Rakela J. Management of pre-liver transplantation patients–part 2. *Liver Transpl.* 2005;11:249–260. [PMID: 15719412]

CONTRAINDICATIONS

Contraindications to liver transplantation differ among the various liver transplant centers. Although certain absolute contraindications are observed (Table 50–4), some conditions that would be considered contraindications at one institution are not deemed so at others. These relative contraindications are also listed in Table 50–4. Many of these relative contraindications may be treated with multiorgan transplants in specialized centers.

TRANSPLANTATION PROCEDURES

Surgical options for transplantation have undergone tremendous changes since the first operation. Presently, the options include cadaveric and live donor transplantation. Cadaveric transplantation is further differentiated into complete or split liver transplantation.

Table 50–4. Contraindications to liver transplantation.

Absolute Contraindications	Relative Contraindications
Uncontrolled bacterial or fungal infections not involving hepatobiliary system	Age >70 y
Active non hepatobiliary malignancy (exception: neuroendocrine tumors)	Portal vein thrombosis
Advanced cardiopulmonary disease that is not correctable	Pulmonary hypertension
Active drug or alcohol abuse	Severe hypoxemia not due to hepatopulmonary syndrome
	Congenital cardiac anomalies
	Noncompliance with medical care
	Psychiatric conditions that impair patient's ability to give consent or be compliant with post-transplant care
	HIV infection
	Hepatocellular carcinoma with disease extent greater than criteria established by UNOS
	Cholangiocarcinoma

UNOS, United Network for Organ Sharing.

Table 50–5. Components of the liver donor evaluation.

Selection of donor
ABO compatible
Brain dead donor with satisfactory blood pressure and oxygenation
Liver size compatible with hepatic cavity of recipient
Factors affecting donor selection
Preexisting liver disease
Diabetes mellitus
Uncontrolled hypertension
Active malignancy, excluding brain tumors
Active bacterial, viral, or fungal infection
Ischemia from asystole or hypotension
Active alcohol or substance abuse
Morbid obesity

1. Donor Suitability & Procurement

Careful evaluation of the donor is required before considering procurement. Certain factors such as hemodynamic instability, advanced age, and hepatic steatosis have been associated with graft nonfunction or preservation injury. Macrovesicular steatosis in excess of 30% is associated with initial poor graft function, graft loss, and higher 3-month mortality rates. Microvesicular steatosis does not appear to affect graft function. Testing for HCV, HBV, and HIV is standard. If abnormal liver enzymes are found, a biopsy of the donor liver should be considered to ensure that advanced histopathologic changes are not present. In general, however, the presence of abnormal liver enzymes in the donor does not preclude liver transplantation. Table 50–5 summarizes the important components of the evaluation of the donor liver.

Verran D, Kusyk T, Painter D, et al. Clinical experience gained from the use of 120 steatotic donor livers for orthotopic liver transplantation. *Liver Transpl.* 2003;9:500–505. [PMID: 12740794]

2. Cadaveric Transplantation

Cadaveric or orthotropic liver transplantation is the most commonly used technique. After a suitable graft is identified, the potential candidate for transplantation is prepared for surgery. The technique involves removing the cirrhotic liver with careful dissection. Prior to surgery, a venovenous bypass is considered by some surgeons. The graft is then placed with anastomosis of the portal vein, hepatic artery, and common bile duct. Flow of bile during surgery is an indicator of a functioning graft.

Split liver transplantation involves the use of the graft by two separate recipients. Typically, the right lobe is used for an adult recipient and the left lobe is used for children. Although the principles of surgery remain the same, the technique is different and beyond the scope of this chapter.

3. Live Donor Transplantation

In general, the technique for live donor transplantation is the same as that for cadaveric transplantation; however, unlike cadaveric transplantation, there are considerable risks to the donor. These risks are considerable and include death. The evaluation includes a comprehensive workup of both the donor and recipient. In addition to the standard recipient evaluation and the preoperative evaluation of the donor, live donor transplantation requires a thorough psychosocial evaluation of the donor.

Live donor transplantation can reduce the waiting time for patients with cirrhosis. However, it is best used for candidates with relatively preserved hepatic function.

COMPLICATIONS

Complications from liver transplantation can occur early or late and can be related to technical problems involving the surgical procedure, medical sequelae, or transplantation itself. Most complications occurring immediately after transplantation are technical and are related to surgery.

1. Surgical Complications

A. Primary Graft Nonfunction

This complication is apparent during surgery. One of the first signs of graft function is the production of bile. The surgeon will note this during the surgery. Lack of bile production is consistent with primary graft nonfunction. This is a true emergency and most patients need to be listed for retransplantation. Supportive care and aggressive medical therapy for infectious and hemodynamic complications are needed.

B. Hepatic Artery Thrombosis

This complication usually occurs within the first few days after transplantation and complicates between 1.6% and 8.9% of procedures. Risk factors include technical complications during the surgical procedure, low donor size to recipient size ratio, immunologic factors, clotting abnormalities, smoking, and infection. Typically patients show lack of improvement in liver enzymes postoperatively. Additionally, the need for clotting factors does not decrease, and mental status changes may occur. Diagnosis usually requires imaging of the hepatic artery using Doppler ultrasound, MRI, or arteriogram. Thrombosis can be treated using interventional techniques, including thrombolysis, angioplasty, or stent placement. However, most patients require reoperation and reanastomosis. If these measures are not successful, the patient may need to be relisted for a second transplantation.

Pastacaldi S, Teixeira R, Montalto P, et al. Hepatic artery thrombosis after orthotopic liver transplantation: a review of nonsurgical causes. *Liver Transpl.* 2001;7:75–81. [PMID: 11172388]

2. Biliary Complications

Biliary complications after liver transplantation occur in up to 15–25% of patients. Biliary strictures and bile leaks are the most common biliary complications.

In the first few days to weeks after transplantation, anastomotic stricturing is common; its occurrence is suggested by abnormal liver enzymes. Abdominal imaging using ultrasound or CT scan is required to detect biliary dilation. Caution is required in interpreting abdominal imaging as biliary dilation may not be apparent after transplantation. Generally, these patients require endoscopic retrograde cholangiopancreatography or percutaneous transhepatic cholangiography. If a stricture or leak is found, then stent insertion can be considered. Surgical reanastomosis or conversion to Roux-en-Y is needed for cases not amenable to endoscopic or radiologic methods.

A second form of posttransplant biliary stricture is believed to be the result of ischemic and immunologic injury. Multiple strictures are found in the intrahepatic and extrahepatic biliary tree. Unless a dominant stricture is found, endoscopic, percutaneous, or surgical options are limited. Risk factors identified in a recent study included primary sclerosing cholangitis in the native liver, Rouxen-Y hepaticojejunostomy, use of a high-viscosity preservation solution, and postoperative CMV infection. Occurrence of sclerosing cholangitis and cirrhosis has been reported, sometimes resulting in retransplantation. Graft loss rates of up to 46% at 2 years posttransplantation have been reported.

Abdalian R, Heathcote EJ. Sclerosing cholangitis: a focus on secondary causes. *Hepatology.* 2006;44:1063–1074. [PMID: 17058222]

Park JS, Kim MH, Lee SK, et al. Efficacy of endoscopic and percutaneous treatments for biliary complications after cadaveric and living donor liver transplantation. *Gastrointest Endosc.* 2003;57: 78–85. [PMID: 12518136]

3. Medical Complications

A. Allograft Rejection

One of the most common complications after transplantation is allograft rejection. There are three forms of rejection: hyperacute, acute, and chronic.

1. Hyperacute rejection—Hyperacute rejection results from recipient presensitization to donor antigens. With improved donor and recipient antigen matching, its incidence has become very rare. This condition requires removal of the donor graft and a second transplantation. Patients are generally listed with highest priority for a graft.

2. Acute and chronic rejection—Acute rejection is encountered after transplantation in up to 60% of recipients. Episodes of acute rejection that occur within 3 months of transplant are generally not associated with an increased risk of graft failure or mortality. After transplantation, antigen-presenting cells (APCs) present donor HLA-antigens to the recipient CD4 T cells. APCs also release interleukin (IL)-1, which enhances activation of T cells in response to antigen. Activated T cells produce IL-2, which further recruits activated T cells (CD4, CD8) into the graft. CD8 T cells are the so-called cytotoxic cells and cause graft damage. IL-2 is also responsible for clonal T-cell proliferation. The severity of injury is related to the clonal expansion of cytotoxic lymphocytes.

The pathogenesis of chronic rejection is not entirely understood. Aberrant expression of HLA class II antigens on bile ducts is believed to have a role. Differences in donor and recipient class I antigens are also believed to be contributory.

B. Prevention of Rejection

For the graft to survive and function in the recipient, the recipient's immune system needs to be suppressed, particularly in the early posttransplant period. This is achieved by treatment of the various steps of rejection described above. A typical immunosuppression protocol is shown in Table 50–6. The protocol may vary among institutions but the principles remain the same. Corticosteroids are used for their potent anti-inflammatory effects in suppressing IL-1, IL-2, IL-6, tumor necrosis factor, and interferon-γ. Cyclosporine and tacrolimus are calcineurin inhibitors that suppress IL-2–dependent T-cell proliferation. Mycophenolate mofetil and azathioprine inhibit B-cell and T-cell proliferation by interfering with purine synthesis. Sirolimus is generally not used as a first-line immunosuppressant because of initial concerns of hepatic artery thrombosis and impaired wound healing. It appears to interrupt IL-2 receptor signaling pathways.

Table 50–7 lists the common side effects of the various immunosuppressant medications.

Table 50–7. Common side effects of immunosuppressants.

Drug	Side Effect
Azathioprine	Bone marrow suppression
Cyclosporine	Nephrotoxicity, hypertension, hypercholesterolemia, tremor, headache, gingival hyperplasia, hirsutism
Mycophenolate mofetil	Nausea, vomiting, diarrhea, bone marrow suppression, alopecia
Prednisone	Hyperglycemia, peptic ulcer disease, osteoporosis, bruising, cataracts, myopathy, depression, psychosis
Rapamune	Bone marrow suppression, electrolyte abnormalities, edema, hyperlipidemia
Tacrolimus	Nephrotoxicity, hypertension, alopecia, hypercholesterolemia, neurotoxicity (including tremor, seizure, headaches), diabetes, nausea, vomiting

Perry I, Neuberger J. Immunosuppression: towards a logical approach in liver transplantation. *Clin Exp Immunol.* 2005;139:2–10. [PMID: 15606606]

1. Acute rejection—Most patients with acute rejection present with abnormal liver enzymes. A pathway toward evaluating abnormal liver enzymes in the posttransplant setting is shown in Figure 50–3. To confirm rejection, a liver biopsy is needed. Histopathologic changes of rejection include mixed portal and lobular infiltrate, arteriolar and ductular injury in the form, and endothelialitis and ductopenia. The typical

Table 50–6. Sample transplant immunosuppression protocol.

Month	Cyclosporine Plus Tacrolimus (Therapeutic Range[a,b])	Mycophenolate Mofetil Plus Azathioprine	Prednisone
0–1	C: 300–350 mg/dL T: 12–15 mg/dL	M: 1 g orally twice daily A: 75–100 mg orally daily	Taper to 15 mg orally twice daily
1–3	Same	Same	Taper to 15 mg orally daily
3–6	Same	Same	Taper off
6–12	C: 200–300 mg/dL T: 8–12 mg/dL	Taper	Off
>12	C: 150–250 mg/dL T: 8–12 mg/dL	Off	Off

A, azathioprine; C, cyclosporine; M, mycophenolate mofetil; T, tacrolimus.
[a]Dose titrated to levels.
[b]Typical starting dose is cyclosporine, 6 mg/kg/day divided in twice-daily dosing; tacrolimus, 0.06 mg/kg/day divided in twice-daily dosing. Dose adjustment is based on therapeutic range.

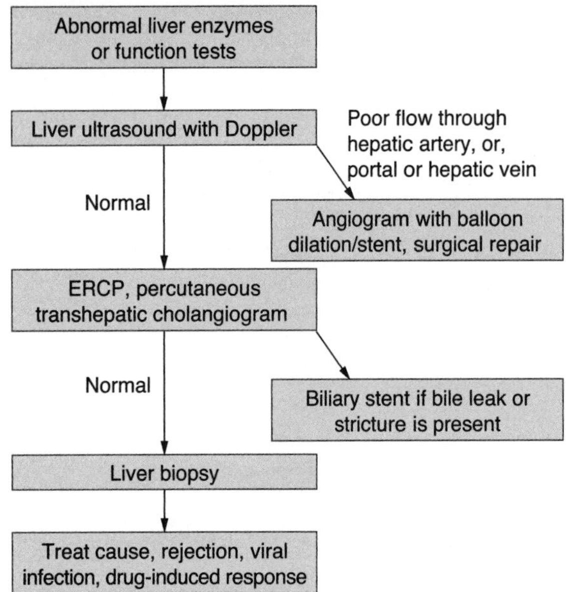

▲ **Figure 50–3.** Evaluation of abnormal liver enzymes or liver function tests after liver transplantation. ERCP, endoscopic retrograde cholangiopancreatography.

treatment includes pulse steroids and, if unsuccessful, the use of more potent immunosuppressant agents. These include OKT3, which blocks the CD3 receptor; Thymoglobulin, which causes nonselective depletion of lymphocytes; or daclizumab and basiliximab, which are chimeric IL-2 receptor–inhibiting monoclonal antibodies.

2. Chronic rejection—As in acute rejection, the diagnosis of chronic rejection requires a liver biopsy. Unfortunately, there are no effective therapies for chronic rejection and most patients will require retransplantation.

INFECTION & LIVER TRANSPLANTATION

Infectious risk among transplant patients is related to exposure to pathogens and the net state of immunosuppression. In addition to immunosuppression, disrupted integrity of the mucocutaneous and epithelial barriers, instrumentation, uremia, diabetes, and infections with immunomodulating viruses are among the factors that affect the infectious risk. The typical pattern of infection is shown in Figure 50–4.

Commonly used approaches against *Pneumocystis carinii* infection, CMV, and EBV are discussed later.

1. *Pneumocystis carinii*

Infection with *Pneumocystis carinii* pneumonia (PCP) is rare in the transplant setting. This is because prophylaxis against PCP is practiced by all transplant centers. In the absence of prophylaxis, the incidence of PCP is 10–12%. The standard regimen is to use single-strength trimethoprim–sulfamethoxazole (TMP-SMZ) daily for 4–12 months. Atovaquone can be considered in patients with insensitivity to TMP-SMZ. An additional benefit of TMP-SMZ is the decreased risk of toxoplasmosis, *Listeria monocytogenes,* and *Nocardia asteroides.*

2. Cytomegalovirus

CMV is the most important pathogen affecting patients after liver transplantation. The virus can be either acquired after transplantation from the donor or reactivated in the recipient by immunosuppression (Table 50–8). The severity of infection is affected by several factors, including the use of cytotoxic and antilymphocyte drugs, systemic infection, and inflammation. Cases of de novo infection and super-infection are generally associated with clinical disease. Up to 50% of recipients who are seronegative and receive a seropositive donor graft will develop infection. The risk for recipients who are CMV antibody positive is much less, and many transplant centers do not practice routine prophylaxis.

Diagnosis is obtained by demonstrating viremia (ie, CMV antigenemia, polymerase chain reaction amplification, or tissue biopsy). Clinical CMV infection can manifest itself in a number of different ways. The presentation can be in the form of leukopenia, thrombocytopenia, pneumonitis, gastroenteritis, pancreatitis, colitis, dermatitis, neuritis, or ophthalmitis.

In addition to its direct effect, CMV is also associated with an increased risk of acute and chronic rejection, post-transplantation lymphoproliferative disorder (PTLD), and recurrent HCV.

The treatment consists of intravenous gancicyclovir until clearance of virus is documented. Some transplant centers also consider the use of anti-CMV hyperimmune globulin for severe or recurrent disease. Patients intolerant to gancicyclovir can be treated with foscarnet.

The ideal regimen for prevention of CMV is not known, but the role of prophylaxis is generally well accepted. The intensity of immunosuppression may dictate the duration of prophylaxis. Prophylaxis should be started before reactivation and continued long after documenting negative CMV surveillance studies. The exact duration is not well known.

3. Posttransplantation Lymphoproliferative Disorder & Epstein-Barr Virus Infection

PTLD is a heterogeneous group of hematologic disorders of polyclonal or monoclonal lymphoid and nonlymphoid organs affecting nodal and particularly extranodal sites. It is a serious complication after transplantation and occurs in 1–3% of liver transplant recipients. Risk factors include severity of immunosuppression and use of antilymphocyte antibodies. The clinical presentation of PTLD is broad, ranging from symptoms suggestive of mononucleosis to

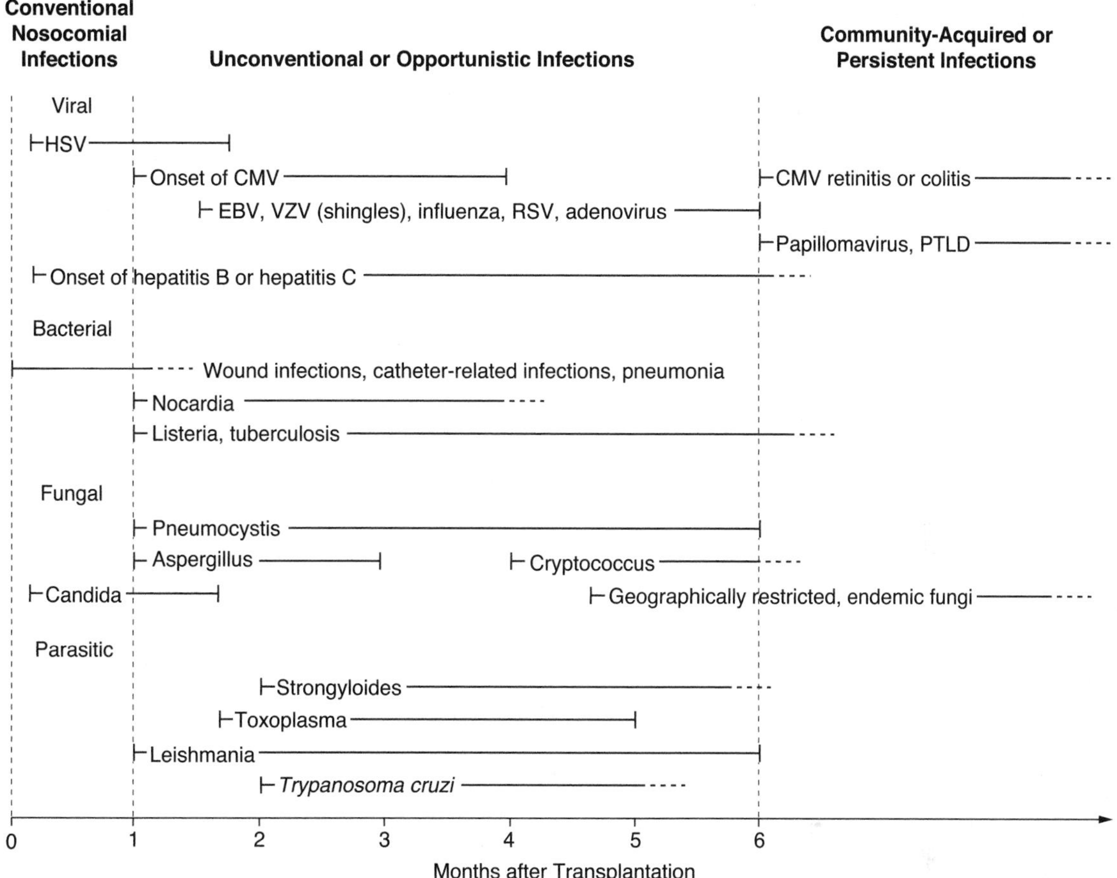

▲ **Figure 50–4.** Usual sequence of infections after organ transplantation. Exceptions to the usual sequence of infections after transplantation suggest the presence of unusual epidemiologic exposure or excessive immunosuppression. CMV, cytomegalovirus; EBV, Epstein-Barr virus; HSV, herpes simplex virus; PTLD, posttransplantation lymphoproliferative disease; RSV, respiratory syncytial virus; VZV, varicella-zoster virus. Zero indicates the time of transplantation. Solid lines indicate the most common period for the onset of infection; dotted lines and arrows indicate periods of continued risk at reduced levels. (Reproduced, with permission, from Rubin RH, Fishman JA. Infection in organ-transplant recipients. *N Engl J Med*. 1998;338:1743.)

Table 50–8. Antiviral prophylaxis for cytomegalovirus (CMV).

CMV Status	Risk	Prophylaxis
Donor negative/Recipient negative	Low	Valacyclovir
Donor negative/Recipient positive	Moderate	Valacyclovir
Donor positive/Recipient positive	Moderate	Valgancyclovir
Donor positive/Recipient negative	High	Valgancyclovir ± anti-CMV hyperimmune globulin (CytoGam)

those consistent with lymphoma or related to an affected organ. Extranodal involvement of the liver, brain, gastrointestinal tract, and bone marrow is common. In a recent study, 77% of patients with PTLD presented with extranodal disease.

PTLD has a close association with EBV, but not all patients with this condition are positive for EBV. The diagnosis requires histopathologic examination. The treatment generally consists of reducing immunosuppression, which may be effective in inducing a long complete response rate in 20–50%. Antiviral therapy in EBV–positive PTLD may also be considered. If this is unsuccessful, chemotherapy can be considered, although the ideal regimen remains uncertain.

Lim W, Russ GR, Coates PT. Review of Epstein-Barr virus and post-transplant lymphoproliferative disorder post-solid organ transplantation. *Nephrology (Carlton)*. 2006;11:355–366. [PMID: 16889577]

LONG-TERM MEDICAL CARE AFTER LIVER TRANSPLANTATION

Patients who undergo liver transplantation remain at risk of developing common medical problems seen in the general population.

1. Diabetes Mellitus

The incidence of posttransplant diabetes mellitus is between 4% and 20%. This risk may be related to the use of tacrolimus and cyclosporine. Prospective studies have shown a significant increased incidence of hyperglycemia after administration of these agents. The treatment includes diet, weight loss, oral hypoglycemic agents, and insulin.

Reuben A. Long-term management of the liver transplant patient: diabetes, hyperlipidemia, and obesity. *Liver Transpl.* 2001;7(Suppl 1):S13–21. [PMID: 11689772]

2. Hypertension

Hypertension is a common occurrence after transplantation likely to the result of age and the use of calcineurin inhibitors. Standard antihypertensive regimens are efficacious in patients posttransplantation. Nifedipine is the agent of choice, and β-blockers are second-line agents.

Galioto A, Angeli P, Guarda S, et al. Comparison between nifedipine and carvedilol in the treatment of de novo arterial hypertension after liver transplantation: preliminary results of a controlled clinical trial. *Transpl Proc.* 2005;37:1245–1247. [PMID: 15848684]

3. Hyperlipidemia

Hyperlipidemia is a common occurrence after liver transplantation, with an incidence of up to 50%. Weight loss and dietary changes are recommended; if these strategies are unsuccessful, treatment with a HMG CoA inhibitor is recommended.

Reuben A. Long-term management of the liver transplant patient: diabetes, hyperlipidemia, and obesity. *Liver Transpl.* 2001;7 (Suppl 1):S13–21. [PMID: 11689772]

4. Renal Insufficiency

In a landmark article by Ojo and colleagues, it was shown that the incidence of chronic renal failure after solid organ transplantation was 7–21% among non–renal transplant recipients. An increased risk of renal failure was associated with female sex, older age, hepatitis C, hypertension, diabetes mellitus, and posttransplant acute renal failure. The study also showed that patients who experienced chronic renal failure were at four times greater mortality risk.

Strategies to prevent renal failure are limited by the need to use a calcineurin inhibitor to prevent rejection. Sirolimus, a less nephrotoxic drug, has fallen out of favor as a first-line immunosuppressant because of concerns about hepatic artery thrombosis and impaired wound healing. However, in patients with mild renal insufficiency, transition from a calcineurin inhibitor to sirolimus can be considered when the risk of hepatic artery thrombosis is reduced, usually many months to years after transplantation.

Ojo AO, Held PJ, Port FK, et al. Chronic renal failure after a transplantation of a nonrenal organ. *N Engl J Med.* 2003; 349:931–940. [PMID: 12954741]

5. Osteoporosis

Pretransplant bone disease resulting from impaired vitamin D absorption in cholestatic liver disease, low calcium intake and activity, or use of diuretics and prednisone in autoimmune hepatitis is common. Inactivity after the transplant procedure and the use of high doses of steroids further accelerate bone loss. Consequently, posttransplant osteoporosis is a major cause of morbidity in patients undergoing transplantation. All patients should receive calcium and vitamin D supplementation after transplantation. A bone densitometry scan should be considered and bisphosphonates prescribed if osteoporosis is noted.

Guichelaar MM, Kendall R, Malinchoc M, et al. Bone mineral density before and after OLT: long-term follow-up and predictive factors. *Liver Transpl.* 2006;12:1390–1402. [PMID: 16933236]

6. Pregnancy

Pregnancy has occurred as soon as a few weeks after liver transplantation. Because transplantation is associated with an increased incidence of premature and low birth weight infants, pregnant patients should be managed by an obstetrician who specializes in high-risk pregnancy. To minimize the risk of rejection and graft failure, immunosuppression is continued. Table 50–9 lists the known teratogenicity and effects on fetal growth in pregnancy of various immunosuppressants.

7. Neurologic Conditions

Chronic headaches are noted with calcineurin inhibitors and may require modification in dosing. A tremor is often seen in calcineurin toxicity. Seizure disorder after transplantation has been reported.

Table 50–9. Pregnancy risk by FDA category for commonly used immunosuppressant medications after liver transplantation.

Drug	Uses	FDA Category
Corticosteroids	Maintenance, antirejection	
Prednisone, prednisolone		B
Methylprednisolone		B
Azathioprine	Maintenance	D
Imuran		
Cyclosporin A (CyA)	Maintenance	C
Novartis formulation		
Sandimmune		
Cyclosporine capsules	Maintenance	C
Generic microemulsion		
Formulation of cyclosporine		
Neoral		
Tacrolimus or FK506	Maintenance, antirejection	C
Prograf		
Mycophenolate mofetil	Maintenance	C
CellCept		
Sirolimus	Maintenance	C
Rescue agents used for treatment of rejection or induction		
Muromonab-CD3 (OKT-3)		C
Orthoclone OKT3		
Antithymocyte globulin		C
Atgam, ATG		
Antithymocyte globulin		C
Thymoglobulin		C

Data from Mastrobattista JM, Katz AR. Pregnancy after organ transplantation. *Obstet Gynecol Clin North Am.* 2004;31:14. Original data from Armenti VT, Radomski JS, Moritz MJ, et al. Report from the National Transplantation Pregnancy Resister (NTPR): Outcomes of pregnancy after transplantation. In: Cecka JM, Terasaki PI (editors). *Clinical Transplants* 2002. UCLA Immunogenetics Center, 2003:121–130; and Armenti VT, Moritz MJ, Davison JM. Renal transplantation and pregnancy. In: Gleicher N (editor). *Principles and Practice of Medical Therapy in Pregnancy*, 3rd ed. Appleton & Lange, 1998:1081–1091.

8. Psychiatric Conditions

Depression and anxiety are common after transplantation. Early identification and treatment may prevent substance abuse relapse posttransplantation. Various antidepressants have been shown to be effective in posttransplant patients.

Erim Y, Beckmann M, Valentin-Gamazo C, et al. Quality of life and psychiatric complications after adult living donor liver transplantation. *Liver Transpl.* 2006;12:1782–1790. [PMID: 17133566]

9. Malignancy

Malignancy is the second most common cause of late death in patients after transplantation and is closely associated with the long-term use of immunosuppressants. The incidence of cancer in patients who undergo transplant is between 4% and 16%. The incidences of PTLD, sarcomas, uterine cervical dysplasia, and skin cancers are clearly higher than in the general population. However, conclusive data for other forms of cancer are lacking. Risk factors for the development of posttransplant cancers include smoking, alcohol, and inflammatory bowel disease.

Overall, colon cancer is no more common in posttransplant patients than in the general population. However, patients with primary sclerosing cholangitis and ulcerative colitis who undergo transplantation have an incidence of colon cancer ranging between 5.3% and 13% after liver transplantation.

Table 50–10 outlines the recommended guidelines for screening in patients after liver transplantation.

Oo YG, Gunson BK, Lancashire RJ, et al. Incidence of cancers following orthotopic liver transplantation in a single center: comparison with national cancer incidence rates for England and Wales. *Transplantation.* 2005;80:759–764. [PMID: 16210962]

Table 50–10. Cancer screening after transplantation.

Cancer	Recommended Screening
Skin and lip	Monthly self examinations and annual physician examinations
Anogenital carcinoma	Annual physician examination of anogenital area
Kaposi sarcoma	Annual physician examination of skin, conjunctiva, and oropharyngeal mucosa
Posttransplantation lymphoproliferative disorder	Physician evaluation every 3 months
Cervical cancer	Annual Papanicolaou smear for all females >18 y and any female <18 y who is sexually active
Breast cancer	Mammography every 1–2 y
Colon cancer	Colonoscopy every 5 y
Prostate cancer	Annual prostate-specific antigen and digital rectal examination

Reproduced, with permission, from Kasiske BL, Varquez MA, Harmon WE, et al. Recommendations for the outpatient surveillance of renal transplant recipients. American Society of Transplantation. *J Am Soc Nephrol.* 2000;11:S1–S86.

Table 50–11. Recurrence and 5-year survival rates after liver transplantation.

Etiology of Disease	Recurrence Rate	Five-Year Survival	Five-Year Graft Survival
Hepatitis C	>90%	70%	57%
Hepatitis B	<5% with prophylaxis	79%	68%
Hepatocellular carcinoma	8-15%	52%	46%
Primary biliary cirrhosis	11-23%	86%	73%
Primary sclerosing cholangitis	9-47%	86%	73%
Autoimmune hepatitis	16-46%	77%	68%
Alcohol-induced cirrhosis	<5%	72%	65%
Nonalcoholic steatohepatitis	11-38%	73%	66%

Adapted, with permission, from Kotlyar DS, Campbell MS, Reddy KR. Recurrences of diseases following orthotopic liver transplantation. *Am J Gastroenterol.* 2006;101:1370–1378. [PMID: 16771963]

Trotter JF. Cancer surveillance following orthotopic liver transplantation. *Gastrointest Endosc Clin N Am.* 2001;11:199–214. [PMID: 11175982]

Vallejo GH, Romero CJ, de Vicente JC. Incidence and risk factors for cancer after liver transplantation. *Crit Rev Oncol Hematol.* 2005;56:87–99. [PMID: 15979889]

PROGNOSIS

Over the past decade the prognosis for patients who undergo liver transplantation has improved considerably. For certain conditions, such as amyloidosis, liver transplantation is a cure; for others, disease recurrence is a possibility. Recurrence of hepatitis C or hepatocellular cancer is associated with a guarded prognosis; other conditions, such as autoimmune hepatitis, primary biliary cirrhosis, and primary sclerosing cholangitis, have good 5-year survival rates (Table 50–11).

Most patients who undergo liver transplantation do not have liver-related morbidity but suffer from complications of long-standing immunosuppression.

Kotylar DS, Campbell MS, Reddy KR. Recurrence of diseases following orthotopic liver transplantation. *Am J Gastroenterol.* 2006;101:1370–1378. [PMID: 16771963]

1. Recurrent Hepatitis C

Recurrent hepatitis C is almost universal after transplantation. Older age of the donor, use of steroids, and rejection are predictors of worse prognosis. Due to the impact of steroids, many transplant centers limit the dose and duration of steroids in immunosuppression protocols. Steroid-free immunosuppressive protocols have been considered but remain controversial.

The treatment of recurrent hepatitis C is more difficult after transplantation. The use of immunosuppressant medications and comorbidities leave patients more susceptible to the side effects of interferon and ribavirin. Hematopoietic growth factor support is generally needed to continue treatment.

Dienstag JL, McHutchinson JG. American Gastroenterological Association technical review on the management of hepatitis C. *Gastroenterology.* 2006;130:231–264. [PMID: 16401486]

2. Recurrent Hepatitis B

Recurrent hepatitis B is uncommon after transplantation. The risk of recurrence is greatest among patients who are hepatitis B e antigen positive or have high viral loads at the time of transplantation.

Prophylactic therapy has become routine for most transplant centers after transplantation. Typically, patients receive hepatitis B immunoglobulin (HBIG) for up to 6 months or indefinitely after transplantation. Generally, hepatitis B surface antibody levels are followed and HBIG is transfused when levels fall below 500 IU/mL. The use of nucleotide and nucleoside analogs varies among centers. However, many programs now use a combination of HBIG and nucleotide or nucleoside analogs such as entecavir, lamivudine, and adefovir. Adefovir is used less commonly due to the small risk of nephrotoxicity. Lamivudine should generally be avoided because of a high rate of viral resistance.

Primary Biliary Cirrhosis

51

Daniel S. Pratt, MD

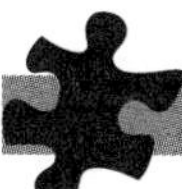

ESSENTIALS OF DIAGNOSIS

- Most patients with primary biliary cirrhosis (PBC) are asymptomatic at the time of diagnosis but eventually develop symptoms, including fatigue and pruritus.
- Consider PBC in any patient in whom liver enzymes are elevated in a cholestatic pattern; an isolated elevated alkaline phosphatase level always requires further evaluation.
- Antimitochondrial antibodies have 95% sensitivity for PBC and are central to the diagnosis.

General Considerations

Primary biliary cirrhosis (PBC) is a classical autoimmune disease. Although it is predominantly a disease of middle-aged woman, with a median age of diagnosis of approximately 50 years, 5–10% of patients are men, and the reported age range is 22–93 years. It is reported throughout the world, but with varying geographic incidence and prevalence; the highest reported incidence and prevalence is in northern Europe. Studies have suggested the incidence and prevalence are increasing worldwide. Antimitochondrial autoantibodies (AMAs) are found in 95% of patients with PBC. The targets of the autoantibodies are members of the family of the 2-oxo-acid dehydrogenase complexes, most particularly the E2 subunits of the pyruvate dehydrogenase complex (PDC-E2). The immunologic injury is marked by a T-cell–mediated destruction of the intrahepatic bile ducts. The only proven therapy for PBC is ursodeoxycholic acid (UDCA). Despite early diagnosis and treatment, most patients have an inexorable disease progression leading ultimately to cirrhosis and end-stage liver disease.

Kaplan MM, Gershwin ME. Primary biliary cirrhosis. *N Engl J Med.* 2005;353:1261–1273. [PMID: 16177252]

Lindor KD, Gershwin ME, Poupon R, Kaplan M, Bergasa NV, Heathcote EJ. Primary biliary cirrhosis. *Hepatology.* 2010;50: 291–306. [PMID: 19554543]

Pathogenesis (Figure 51–1)

A. Genetic Factors

There have been several studies indicating the role of genetics in determining the susceptibility to PBC. Particularly important observations include the following:

1. First-degree relatives of patients with PBC have a 4–6% prevalence of disease.
2. PBC has the highest reported concordance rate (62.5%) in monozygotic twins of any autoimmune disease.
3. The prevalence of AMAs in first-degree relatives of patients with PBC was 13.1% compared with 1% of controls.

A number of candidate genes have been implicated in PBC including CTLA4 and IL12A.

B. Environmental Factors

As with other autoimmune conditions, molecular mimicry is felt to be the mechanism for the initiation of autoimmunity. Several candidate environmental triggers have been suggested, including infectious agents (viruses and bacteria) and chemicals. These potential triggers have significant homology to human mitochondrial proteins, particularly PDC-E2. The role of transient environmental agents in the pathogenesis of PBC was supported by a recent study that demonstrated highly statisitically significant space-time clustering in 1015 cases of PBC in northeast England.

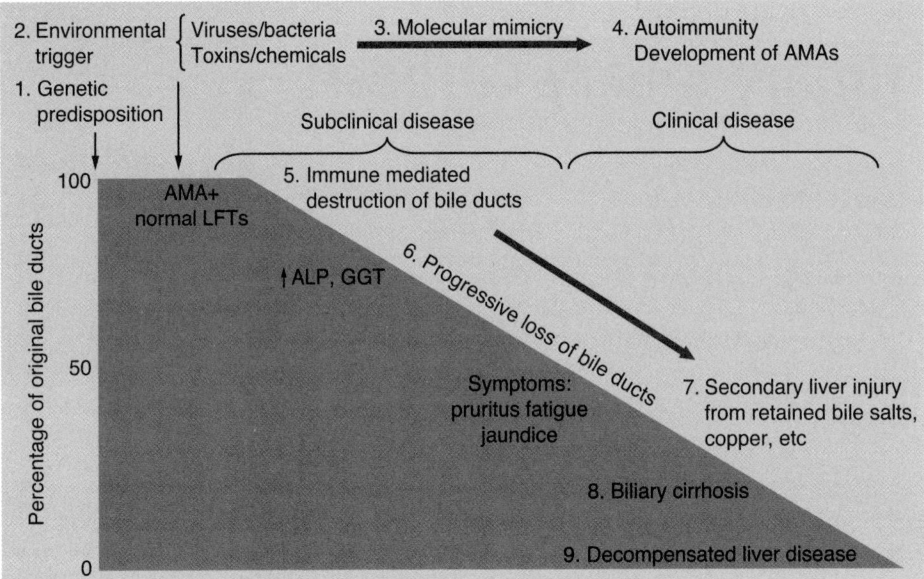

▲ **Figure 51–1.** Pathogenesis and natural history of primary biliary cirrhosis (PBC). It is believed that genetically susceptible patients if exposed to specific environmental triggers may develop autoimmunity through molecular mimicry, with the primary target of the resultant antimitochondrial antibodies being pyruvate dehydrogenase E2 complex (PDC-E2). Through an as yet undetermined process this leads to a persistent T-cell–mediated destruction of the intrahepatic bile ducts. Untreated, this destructive process eventually destroys a critical percentage of bile ducts and secondary injury from retained bile salts ensues. Injury progresses to biliary cirrhosis and eventually to decompensated liver disease. ALP, alkaline phosphatase; AMA, antimitochondrial antibody; GGT, γ-glutamyl transferase; LFTs, liver function tests.

C. Immunologic Factors

The T cells infiltrating the portal triads are specific for the PDC-E2 autoepitope. However, it is not clear why the immune attack has such specificity for the biliary epithelium when the target mitochondrial proteins are present in all nucleated cells. Studies have suggested that the mechanism of the metabolic processing of PDC-E2 in biliary epithelium results in the autoantigen remaining immunologically intact and available for presentation to antigen-presenting cells. In all other cell types the autoepitope is destroyed during apoptosis.

Lazaridis KN, Juran BD, Boe GM, et al. Increased prevalence of antimitochondrial antibodies in first-degree relatives of patients with primary biliary cirrhosis. *Hepatology.* 2007;46:785–782. [PMID: 17680647]

McNally RJQ, Ducker S, James OFW. Are transient environmental agents involved in the cause of primary biliary cirrhosis? Evidence from space-time clustering analysis. *Hepatology.* 2009;50:1169–1174. [PMID: 19711423]

Parés A, Rodés J. Natural history of primary biliary cirrhosis. *Clin Liver Dis.* 2003;7:779–794. [PMID: 14594131]

Selmi C, Mayo MJ, Bach N, et al. Primary biliary cirrhosis in monozygotic and dizygotic twins: genetics, epigenetics, and environment. *Gastroenterology.* 2004;127:485–492. [PMID: 15300581]

Clinical Findings

A. Symptoms and Signs

The common practice of checking serum liver enzyme tests as part of annual physical examinations has increased the percentage of patients with PBC who are asymptomatic at the time of diagnosis, raising it to more than 50%. Most patients will go on to develop symptoms over time. For those who are symptomatic, fatigue and pruritus are the most common complaints, each found in approximately 20% of patients. Both of these symptoms may be found even in early-stage disease. The fatigue can be severe enough to impair quality of life. The pruritus can be either local or diffuse, worse at night, exacerbated by heat, and profoundly distressing. Other symptoms seen less commonly are dry eyes and dry mouth (sicca symptoms), and unexplained right upper quadrant discomfort. Jaundice is a late finding and a poor prognostic sign as are other symptoms of hepatic decompensation, including fluid retention (ascites and peripheral edema), gastrointestinal bleeding, and encephalopathy.

The asymptomatic patient almost always lacks physical findings. Early-stage findings include skin hyperpigmentation, excoriations from itching, xanthelasmas, xanthomas, and hepatomegaly. Later stages are marked by findings of portal hypertension and hepatic decompensation: splenomegaly, caput medusa, ascites, spider nevi, palmar erythema, jaundice, proximal and temporal muscle wasting, and asterixis.

B. Laboratory Findings

The liver enzymes in patients with PBC are typically in a cholestatic pattern; that is, the alkaline phosphatase (ALP) is elevated out of proportion to the aminotransferases. An isolated elevated ALP level should first be evaluated to verify its biliary origin by obtaining values for γ-glutamyl transferase (GGT), 5′ nucleotidase, or fractionation of the ALP. The degree of ALP elevation does not correlate with disease severity; rare cases have been reported of patients with normal ALP diagnosed with early-stage PBC on the basis of positive AMAs and consistent histology.

The presence of autoantibodies, particularly antimitochondrial antibodies, is the hallmark of PBC. The AMA titer does not correlate with disease activity in patients with PBC. Also, the absence of AMAs does not rule out the diagnosis of PBC. There are well-described patients with "AMA-negative PBC" who have the typical clinical, biochemical, and histologic features of PBC. Other autoantibodies—most commonly antinuclear antibodies (ANAs)—are reported in PBC. Nuclear rim and nuclear-dot patterns of ANAs are highly specific for PBC. Serum immunoglobulin M levels are often elevated.

C. Histologic Findings

There are four histologic stages of PBC. Stage 1 is marked by the presence of the florid bile duct lesion (a bile duct at the center of a dense lymphocytic infiltrate). PBC is initially a ductocentric process; the inflammation does not extend beyond the portal tracts. Stage 2 is marked by loss of normal bile ducts, development of bile duct reduplication, and extension of the inflammation into the hepatic parenchyma. Stage 3 is marked by bridging fibrosis of the portal triads and progressive loss of bile ducts. Stage 4 is frank cirrhosis and end-stage liver disease. The presence of copper deposition is supportive of a cholestatic process.

The liver is not involved uniformly in PBC, a fact that increases the likelihood of sampling variability. All four stages of PBC may be seen in a single large biopsy. The convention is to report either the highest stage of disease or the range of stages. Although some have questioned the need for histologic staging in the diagnosis of PBC, it can both aid in determining prognosis and guiding treatment by providing baseline histologic findings against which treatment response can be assessed.

Treatment

A. Primary Therapy

UDCA is the only therapy approved by the U.S. Food and Drug Administration for the treatment of PBC. The mechanism of action of UDCA remains unknown. It is a choleretic agent. It has been shown to slow progression of disease in patients with early-stage disease and is highly effective as monotherapy in 25–30% of patients. As is seemingly true with all therapies used for PBC, UDCA is not as effective in advanced disease. There is clearly a point in the natural history of PBC where sufficient numbers of bile ducts are destroyed and the condition has passed the point of reversibility. The appropriate dosage of UDCA is 13–15 mg/kg/day split into two doses. It is well tolerated with the most common side effect being diarrhea.

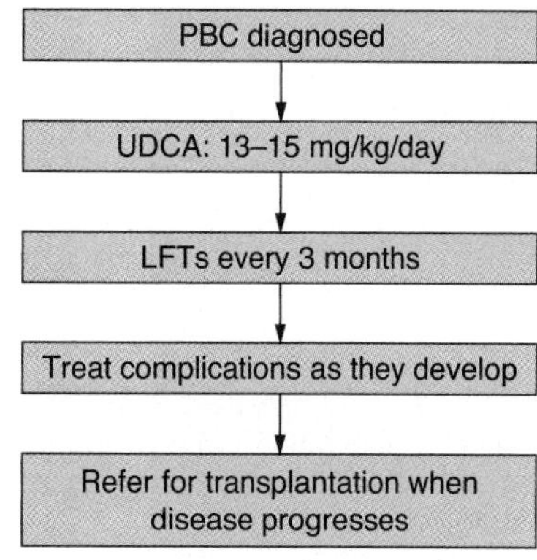

▲ **Figure 51–2.** Treatment of primary biliary cirrhosis (PBC). The most widely accepted algorithm is illustrated. Ursodeoxycholic acid (UDCA) is initiated and patients are then monitored for progression of disease and complications. The only other active intervention in this algorithm is referral of patients for transplantation when their liver disease has decompensated. LFTs, liver function tests.

Although many hepatologists do not recommend consideration of any therapy beyond UDCA (Figure 51–2), there is a growing consensus that it is important for the clinician to differentiate between patients who have responded to UDCA and those who have not; studies have shown that patients with a biochemical and histological response to UDCA have a better prognosis than those who do not respond. These data support a more aggressive approach to management in these selected patients who are at a higher risk of disease progression and in young patients with early-stage disease with the ultimate goal of improving outcomes (Figure 51–3). If patients have an incomplete biochemical or histologic response to UDCA, the use of alternative therapies including colchicine, methotrexate, and budesonide should be considered.

In contrast to some studies that failed to show a benefit of colchicine, several prospective double-blind trials found that colchicine improved biochemistry profiles, symptoms (pruritus), and histologic findings. A meta-analysis reported that colchicine delayed the need for transplantation and reduced the incidence of major complications.

Methotrexate has been shown in some studies to improve biochemical and histologic findings in patients with an

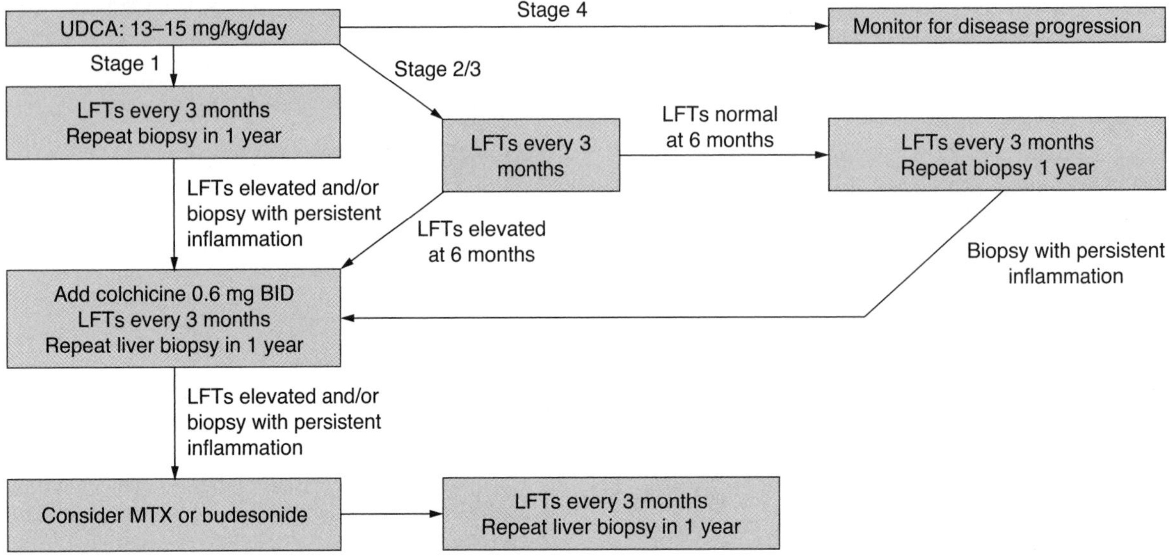

▲ **Figure 51–3.** Treatment of primary biliary cirrhosis (PBC): a stepwise approach. This algorithm highlights the use of the baseline histologic staging to direct treatment as well as monitor the response to therapy. It also reflects the reality that ursodeoxycholic acid (UDCA) monotherapy is effective in only a minority of patients and that there are subsets of patients who respond to colchicine, methotrexate (MTX), or budesonide, but there is no way to predict response. LFTs, liver function tests.

incomplete response to UDCA monotherapy. Other studies have failed to show any benefit of methotrexate, either alone or in combination with UDCA. One 10-year study suggested that patients with early-stage disease were most likely to benefit from methotrexate.

Short duration, randomized, placebo-controlled trials of budesonide have shown that it improves biochemical and histologic findings in PBC. Longer trials will be needed to assess the impact on survival and ensure osteopenia is not an issue. Budesonide is contraindicated in patients with cirrhosis.

Figure 51–3 highlights the stepwise approach for patients with stage 1–3 disease. This approach is based on the observation that clinical response to medical therapy varies greatly from patient to patient and that a significant percentage of patients will progress on UDCA monotherapy. In this approach, histology is a critical component in decision making, both in determining whether to add additional agents to UDCA and whether to continue those agents. The severity of the portal inflammation is typically the major deciding factor in determining whether to add additional therapies.

Liver transplantation is the only effective therapy for patients with end-stage PBC. These patients have post-transplant outcomes that exceed most other indications. Disease recurrence has been reported—30% at year 10 in one series—but it is exceedingly rare to lose a graft to recurrent disease.

Corpechot C, Abenavoli L, Rabahi N, et al. Biochemical response to ursodeoxycholic acid and longterm prognosis in primary biliary cirrhosis. *Hepatology.* 2008;48:871–877. [PMID: 18752324]

Corpechot C, Carrat F, Bahr A, et al. The effect of ursodeoxycholic acid therapy on the natural course of primary biliary cirrhosis. *Gastroenterology.* 2005;128:297–303. [PMID: 15685541]

Kuiper EM, Hansen BE, de Vries RA, et al. Improved prognosis of patients with primary biliary cirrhosis that have a biochemical response to ursodeoxycholic acid. *Gastroenterology.* 2009;136:1281–1287. [PMID: 19208346]

Lindor K. Ursodeoxycholic acid for the treatment of primary biliary cirrhosis. *N Engl J Med.* 2007;357:1524–1529. [PMID: 17928600]

B. Secondary Therapy

1. Pruritus—As with primary therapy, management of pruritus is most effective when one proceeds in a logical and stepwise fashion. Cholestyramine is effective in more than 90% of patients and should be the first-line agent. The starting dosage is typically 4 g, two to three times a day, and some improvement of symptoms is usually seen within 2–4 days. Tolerance can be an issue, with gastrointestinal side effects (unpleasant taste and constipation) being prominent. It is critical to educate patients regarding the need to separate the dosing of cholestyramine from other medications. The second-line agent for pruritus is rifampin; a dosage of 150 mg twice daily is well tolerated and has little risk of toxicity. Oral opioid receptor antagonists are a reasonable third-line agent. Sertraline, 75–100 mg a day was shown of benefit in one study of pruritus in patients with cholestatic hepatitis. Antihistamines have little role aside from use as a sleep aid. Plasmapheresis has been effective in truly refractory cases.

2. Fatigue—This symptom can be incapacitating, even in patients with early-stage disease. Modafinil has been shown to be effective in two small, uncontrolled pilot trials and in personal experience. Controlled trials are awaited. The dosage is 100–200 mg/day.

3. Osteoporosis—Approximately one third of patients with PBC develop osteoporosis, which can manifest before the onset of jaundice. Bone density should be checked every 2 years in patients with PBC and osteopenia managed aggressively. While benefit has not been proven, these patients should be on calcium (1500 mg a day) and vitamin D (1000 IU/day) supplementation. Alendronate has been shown to be beneficial in two trials and estrogen replacement in two studies of postmenopausal women; however, this benefit needs to be weighed against the increased risk of vascular disease and cancer.

4. Hyperlipidemia—Although serum lipids are often elevated in PBC, patients seemingly do not have an increased risk of atherosclerosis. This finding is explained partly by the presence of high levels of high-density lipoprotein and partly by the presence of a subfraction of low-density lipoproteins, called lipoprotein X, that has anti-atherogenic properties. Thus, it is rare that PBC patients require lipid-lowering agents. However, statin drugs can be used safely, if indicated, so long as standard monitoring for hepatotoxicity is performed.

5. Fat soluble vitamin deficiency—Deficiency of fat-soluble vitamins occurs in patients with PBC, particularly those with advanced stage disease. Vitamin A deficiency can occur in up to one third of patients and cases of night blindness have been reported. Fat-soluble vitamin levels should be checked every 2 years and supplemented as needed.

Primary Sclerosing Cholangitis

52

Norton J. Greenberger, MD
John R. Saltzman, MD

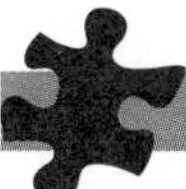

ESSENTIALS OF DIAGNOSIS

- Progressive inflammatory, sclerosing, and obliterative disease of the extrahepatic or intrahepatic bile ducts, or both.
- Disproportionate elevation of serum alkaline phosphatase (4–10 times normal) is seen in almost all patients.
- MRCP or ERCP shows multifocal stricturing of the intrahepatic and extrahepatic bile ducts.
- Small duct disease is diagnosed by liver biopsy.
- Liver biopsy findings that are highly specific include fibrous obliteration of small bile ducts with concentric replacement by connective tissue in an "onion skin" pattern.
- Patients have an 8–15% lifetime risk of developing cholangiocarcinoma, and it is often difficult to distinguish a dominant stricture from a cholangiocarcinoma.

General Considerations

Primary sclerosing cholangitis (PSC) is a disorder of unknown etiology that is characterized by a progressive, inflammatory, sclerosing, and obliterative process affecting medium-sized and large extrahepatic or intrahepatic bile ducts, or both. A vast majority of patients (prevalence rates range from 70% to 90%) have underling inflammatory bowel disease, especially ulcerative colitis. PSC has also been associated (although rarely) with multifocal fibrosclerosis syndromes such as retroperitoneal, mediastinal, and periureteral fibrosis. In retrospect, it appears that some of these latter cases actually represented patients with autoimmune pancreatitis and bile duct strictures masquerading as PSC.

The median survival of patients with PSC from time of diagnosis to death in several series has ranged from 9 to 12 years. Late in the course of the disease, complete biliary obstruction, secondary biliary cirrhosis, portal hypertension with bleeding varices, liver failure, and development of cholangiocarcinoma may occur.

Maggs JR, Chapman RW. Sclerosing cholangitis. *Curr Opin Gastroenterol.* 2007;23:310–316. [PMID: 17414848]

Clinical Findings

A. Symptoms and Signs

Patients with PSC are often asymptomatic at the time of diagnosis. The disorder is often suspected in patients with inflammatory bowel disease who have a persistent and otherwise unexplained abnormal elevation in serum alkaline phosphatase (ie, values at least two times the upper limit of normal), and with abnormal values persisting for longer than 6 months. Asymptomatic patients with persistent elevations of serum alkaline phosphatase are often screened for PSC, and many actually turn out to have the disease.

Symptomatic patients who have PSC often present with signs and symptoms of chronic biliary obstruction, right upper quadrant abdominal pain, pruritus, jaundice, and acute cholangitis. Fatigue and pruritus are common features at presentation.

B. Laboratory Findings

Liver tests usually demonstrate a cholestatic pattern, with serum alkaline phosphatase disproportionately elevated to levels 4–10 times normal and serum aminotransferase that is usually 300 IU/L or less. Serum albumin and globulin levels are usually normal except in patients with advanced disease. As noted later, in the discussion of differential diagnosis, the presence of positive tests for antinuclear antibodies or smooth muscle antibodies, or both, should raise the suspicion of PSC–autoimmune hepatitis (AIH) overlap syndrome.

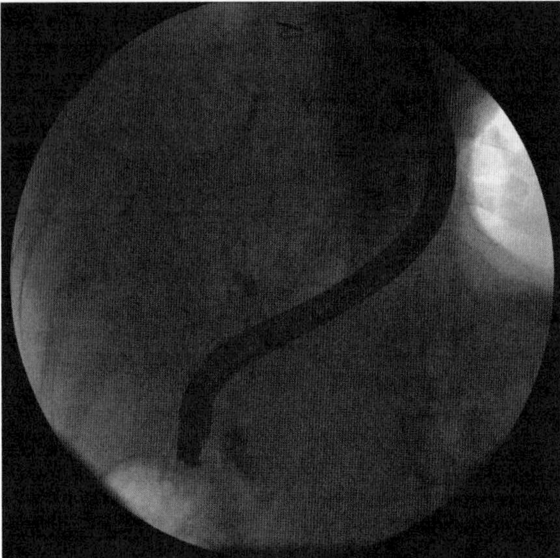

▲ **Figure 52–1.** Endoscopic retrograde cholangiopancreatogram demonstrating diffusely narrowed intrahepatic bile ducts and one beaded area.

C. Imaging Studies

The diagnosis of PSC is usually established by demonstration of the characteristic multifocal stricturing with normal and or dilated areas of intrahepatic or extrahepatic bile ducts, or both, on cholangiography. The typical appearance reveals narrowing and beading of the bile ducts (Figure 52–1). These abnormalities can be demonstrated by either magnetic resonance cholangiopancreatography (MRCP) or endoscopic retrograde cholangiopancreatography (ERCP). MRCP is currently preferred as it is a noninvasive procedure and does not carry the risk of either pancreatitis or cholangitis. The vast majority of patients (~85%) have both intrahepatic and extrahepatic bile duct strictures, approximately 10–20% have intrahepatic bile duct strictures alone, and 2–4% have extrahepatic biliary strictures alone.

It should be emphasized that patients with small duct PSC do not demonstrate cholangiographic abnormalities. In these patients, diagnosis is suspected on the basis of an elevated serum alkaline phosphatase level and established by a liver biopsy in conjunction with other clinical features.

D. Histologic Findings

Liver biopsy findings often support the diagnosis of PSC. The most characteristic histologic finding is fibrous obliteration of small bile ducts with concentric replacement by connective tissue in an "onion skin" pattern (Plate 96). More often, histologic abnormalities in PSC are nonspecific and may be similar to those seen in primary biliary cirrhosis.

PSC is frequently staged according to the histopathologic findings. In stage 1 disease, there is enlargement, mononuclear cell infiltration, and scarring in the portal triads. Stage 2 disease is characterized by fibrosis extending into the surrounding parenchyma, stage 3 by bridging fibrosis, and stage 4 by cirrhosis (Figure 52–2).

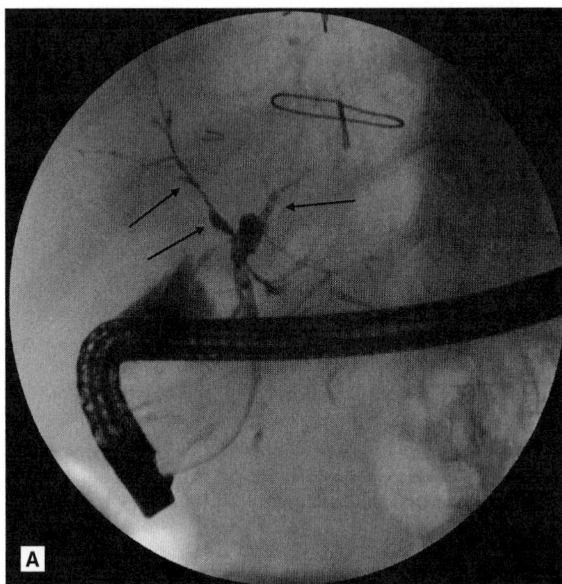

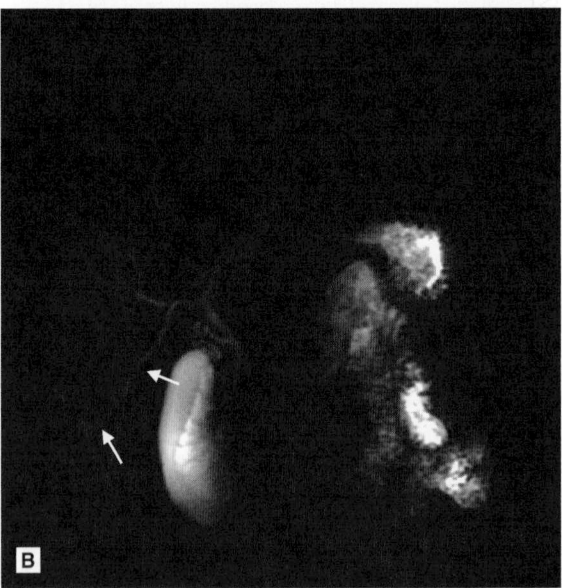

▲ **Figure 52-2.** Imaging findings. **A:** ERCP demonstrating stricturing and beading of the intrahepatic ducts (arrows denote stricturing). **B:** MRCP showing stricturing (arrows) of the biliary tree. (Used with permission from Dr. John R. Saltzman, Brigham and Women's Hospital.)

Differential Diagnosis

Four disorders need to be considered the differential diagnosis of patients presenting with a cholestatic picture: small duct PSC, autoimmune pancreatitis, PSC-AIH overlap syndrome, and acquired immunodeficiency syndrome (AIDS).

A. Small Duct Primary Sclerosing Cholangitis

Small duct PSC is defined by the presents of chronic cholestasis and hepatic histologic findings consistent with PSC but with normal findings on cholangiography. Small duct PSC is found in about 5% of patients with PSC, and represents an earlier stage of PSC associated with a significantly better long-term prognosis. However, such patients may progress to classic PSC or end-stage liver disease, or both, with consequent necessity of liver transplantation.

Angulo P, Maor-Kendler Y, Lindor KD. Small duct primary sclerosing cholangitis: a long-term follow-up. *Hepatology.* 2002; 35:1494–1500. [PMID: 12029635]

B. Autoimmune Pancreatitis (Immunoglobulin G_4 Associated Cholangitis and PSC)

Autoimmune pancreatitis (AIP) is characterized by focal or generalized pancreatic enlargement, pancreatic duct narrowing or strictures, elevated serum IgG_4 immunoglobulin levels (>140 mg/dL), and bile duct strictures similar to those present on PSC. Jaundice is present in 60% of cases. Pancreatic abnormalities are not found in 10% of cases that are appropriately termed IgG_4-associated cholangitis (IAC). Because patients with AIP frequently respond to corticosteroids, it is important to measure IgG_4 levels in all patients with possible PSC. See Chapter 27 for a detailed discussion of autoimmune pancreatitis.

C. Primary Sclerosing Cholangitis—Autoimmune Hepatitis Overlap Syndrome

Diagnosis of an overlap syndrome by use of a modified autoimmune hepatitis (AIH) score has been demonstrated in 8% of 113 PSC patients from the Netherlands, 1.4% of 211 PSC patients from the United States, and 17% of 41 PSC patients from Italy (see later).

Patients with PSC-AIH overlap syndrome have cholangiographic abnormalities characteristic of PSC but serologic features of AIH. The overlap syndrome should be suspected in patients diagnosed with PSC who have elevated circulating levels of antinuclear antibodies or smooth muscle antibodies (titer ≥ 1:40), elevated levels of immunoglobulin G, and evidence of severe interface hepatitis on liver biopsy. In addition, a liver biopsy sample may reveal bile duct abnormalities such as fibrosis and cholestasis. Abnormal cholangiography findings are present in the vast majority of cases, the exception being patients with small duct PSC. Further, cholestatic liver test abnormalities, such as a disproportionately elevated serum alkaline phosphatase level, are often present.

Reports have described patients with clinical features of AIH on presentation but with a subsequent diagnosis of PSC when immune suppression failed to achieve clinical remission. This is noted especially in patients with AIH and ulcerative colitis. If a disproportionately elevated serum alkaline phosphatase level is demonstrated in such patients, the clinician should have a heightened suspicion of PSC. This sequence has been described, in particular, in children, adolescents, and young adults. Finally, failure of a patient with AIH to respond to immunosuppressive therapy should raise the suspicion of an overlap syndrome, and especially the PSC-AIH overlap syndrome.

Floreani A, Rizzoto ER, Ferrera F, et al. Clinical course and outcome of autoimmune hepatitis/primary sclerosing cholangitis overlap syndrome. *Am J Gastroenterol.* 2005;100:1515–1522. [PMID: 15984974]

D. Acquired Immunodeficiency Syndrome

In patients with AIDS, cholangiopancreatography may demonstrate a broad range of biliary tract changes as well as pancreatic duct obstruction and occasionally pancreatitis. Biliary tract lesions in AIDS include cholangiopancreatographic changes similar to PSC. Such changes include (1) diffuse involvement of the intrahepatic bile ducts alone, (2) involvement of both intrahepatic and extrahepatic bile ducts, (3) ampullary stenosis, and (4) stricture of the intrapancreatic portion of the common bile duct.

Associated infectious organisms that have been demonstrated in this setting include *Cryptosporidium, Mycobacterium avium–intracellulare* complex, Cytomegalovirus, Microsporidia, and *Isospora.*

Treatment

A. Medical Therapy

In all patients with a new diagnosis of PSC and no previous history or symptoms of inflammatory bowel disease, a full colonoscopy with biopsies should be performed. Colon cancer risk is significantly increased in patients with *both* PSC and ulcerative or Crohn colitis. In such patients surveillance colonoscopy with biopsies should be carried out at one- to two-year intervals.

The term *hepatic osteodystrophy* encompasses both osteopenia (T score between 1 and 2.5) and osteoporosis (T scores beneath 2.5). The incidence of osteoporosis in PSC ranges between 4% and 10%. The incidence increases with age and with increasing duration of disease. Accordingly, hepatic osteodystrophy should be checked by bone density examinations to exclude osteopenia or osteoporosis in all newly diagnosed patients with PSC. Although no data are available on subsequent appropriate intervals it appears reasonable to screen for osteopenia at 2–3 year intervals after an initial evaluation.

PSC is a progressive, debilitating disease for which few treatment options are currently available. Although many classes of drugs have been studied, none has shown efficacy in slowing disease progression. A major focus of medical treatment, therefore, is on managing symptoms.

Pruritus is common in PSC patients and is often difficult to control; this is especially vexing when it causes nocturnal symptoms and interferes with sleep. Medications that have proved useful in some patients include bile salt–sequestering agents such as cholestyramine, as well as naltrexone and rifampin. One agent that may be helpful in promoting better sleep is doxepin.

Ursodeoxycholic acid (UDCA) is the most extensively evaluated treatment in patients with PSC. Doses of 10–15 mg/kg/day have not shown benefit, while doses of 20–30 mg/kg/day have shown modest improvement in liver biochemical tests. However, such treatment has not resulted in survival benefit or delay in the need for liver transplantation. The latest AASLD (American Association for the Study of Liver Disease) guidelines do not recommend UDCA for medical therapy.

Other agents that have been studied include corticosteroids, budesonide, cyclosporine, methotrexate, azathioprine and 6-mercaptopurine, penicillamine, tacrolimus, pentoxifylline, colchicine, cholestyramine, mycophenolate, and anti-TNF monoclonal antibodies. None of these therapies has consistently been shown to halt disease progression.

In patients with increases in serum bilirubin and/or worsening pruritus or progressive bile duct dilatation, it is appropriate to perform an ERCP to exclude a proximal dominant stricture. In patients with a dominant stricture, management with endoscopic dilatation with or without stenting is usually recommended. The percutaneous approach is reserved for patients with a proximal dominant stricture in whom an endoscopic approach failed. Importantly, brush cytology and/or endoscopic biopsy should be performed to exclude a superimposed malignancy prior to endoscopic therapy for a dominant stricture.

Immunoglobulin G_4–associated cholangitis (IAC) can mimic PSC. Approximately 60% of IAC patients treated with corticosteroids have resolution of strictures and normalization of liver enzymes. Thus, this seeming variant of PSC appears to be responsive to corticosteroids (see Chapter 27 for details).

Chapman R, Fevery J, Kalloo A, et al. Diagnosis and management of primary sclerosing cholangitis. *Hepatology.* 2010;51:660–678. [PMID: 20101749]

Ghazale A, Chari ST, Zang L, et al. Immunoglobulin G_4-associated cholangitis: clinical profile and response to therapy. *Gastroenterology.* 2008;134:706–715. [PMID: 18222442]

Smith T, Befeler AS. High-dose ursodeoxycholic acid for the treatment of primary sclerosing cholangitis. *Curr Gastroenterol Rep.* 2007;9:54–59. [PMID: 17335678]

B. Liver Transplantation

Liver transplantation is best choice for patients with advanced PSC; 5-year survival rates of approximately 85% and a 10-year survival rate of approximately 70% have been reported.

Course & Prognosis

PSC is usually a progressive disease that leads ultimately to biliary obstruction, secondary biliary cirrhosis, hepatic failure, portal hypertension with bleeding varices, and the development of cholangiocarcinoma. Several studies have identified variables that appear to predict progression of PSC; these include age at time of diagnosis, hepatomegaly, splenomegaly, serum alkaline phosphatase, histologic stage of the disease, and serum bilirubin levels. In particular, a serum bilirubin level of 3.0 mg/dL or higher usually portends ultimately irreversible disease. The Mayo risk score is a well-validated statistical model that identifies variables associated with prognosis and PSC. This score is valuable in assessing prognosis and determining the timing for liver transplantation.

Patients with PSC are at increased risk of developing cholelithiasis and choledocholithiasis. However, bacterial cholangitis can develop in patients with PSC without evidence of cholelithiasis or choledocholithiasis. The risk is increased after endoscopic manipulation of the extrahepatic biliary tree. However, cholangitis can also develop spontaneously with high-grade obstructing strictures. Patients with PSC who experience a decreased secretion of conjugated bile salts in the small intestine may develop steatorrhea as well as impaired absorption of fat-soluble vitamins A, D, E, and K. Metabolic bone disease is also a complication of advanced PSC, with radiologic evidence of osteopenia, especially in the lumbar spine, iliac crest, and femur.

Patients with PSC have an 8–15% lifetime risk of developing cholangiocarcinoma. Patients with coexisting inflammatory bowel disease and cirrhosis are at the highest risk. The annual risk of developing cholangiocarcinoma has been estimated to be 1.5%. On imaging studies, it is often difficult to distinguish a dominant stricture from a cholangiocarcinoma. Biliary brush cytology may facilitate the diagnosis; however, cytologic evaluation, along with computed tomographic or magnetic resonance imaging screening tests and serum tumor markers (carcinoembryonic antigen [CEA] or CA 19-9), is not uniformly helpful in ruling out a diagnosis of associated cholangiocarcinoma.

Two long-term studies have described the natural history of PSC. The first was a study of 305 patients of Swedish decent with PSC. One hundred thirty-four (44%) of the patients were asymptomatic at the time of diagnosis and 22 of the 134 (22%) became symptomatic during the median follow-up period of 63 months. The median survival rate from the time of diagnosis to death or liver transplantation was 12 years. The independent predictors influencing prognosis were age, serum bilirubin concentration, and liver histologic changes. Cholangiocarcinoma was found in 24 patients (8%). Inflammatory bowel disease was closely associated with PSC and had a prevalence of 81% in this study population.

A more recent study, which described the natural history of PSC patients and evaluated the prognostic significance of clinical, biochemical, and cholangiographic findings, afforded an opportunity to construct a prognostic model. Two hundred seventy-three German patients with PSC underwent a median follow-up of 76 months (range, 1–280). Median survival from the time of diagnosis to death or liver transplantation was 9.6 years. One hundred eight patients (39.6%) underwent liver transplantation, and 39 (14.3%) developed hepatic biliary malignancies. Age at diagnosis, low serum albumin, persistent bilirubin elevation longer than 3 months, hepatomegaly, splenomegaly, abdominal bile duct stenosis, and ductal changes at the time of diagnosis were found to be independent risk factors. In particular, persistent serum bilirubin elevations lasting longer than 3 months identified a novel risk factor correlating with a poor outcome.

Broomé U, Olsson R, Lööf L, et al. Natural history and prognostic factors in 305 patients with primary sclerosing cholangitis. *Gut.* 1996;38:610–615. [PMID: 870797]

Kim WR, Therneau TM, Wiesner RH, et al. A revised natural history model for primary sclerosing cholangitis. *Mayo Clin Proc.* 2000;75:689–694. [PMID: 10907383]

Tischendorf JJ, Hecker H, Krüger M, et al. Characterization, outcome and prognosis in 273 patients with primary sclerosing cholangitis. *Am J Gastroenterol.* 2007;102:107–114. [PMID: 17037993]

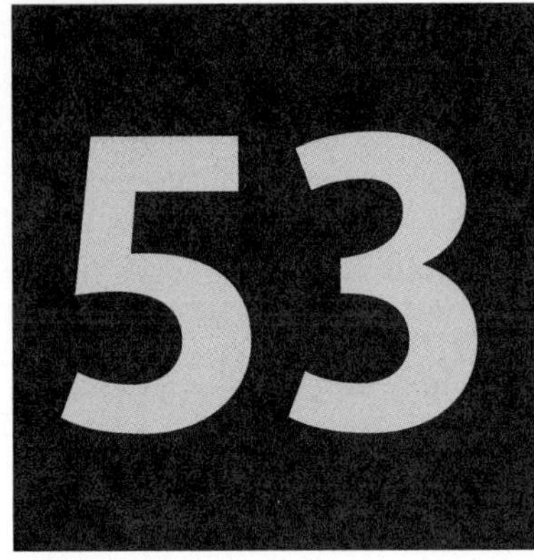

Gallstone Disease

Gustav Paumgartner, MD
Norton J. Greenberger, MD

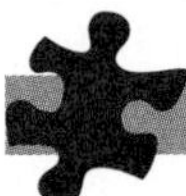

ESSENTIAL CONCEPTS

- Major risk factors for cholesterol gallstones include age >50 years, female sex, Mexican or Native American ethnicity, genetic predisposition, family history, pregnancy and parity, estrogens, obesity, and the metabolic syndrome.
- Gallstones are often found incidentally during abdominal ultrasonography, which has >95% sensitivity for cholesterol stones ≥1.5 mm.
- In ~80% of cases gallstones remain asymptomatic; in symptomatic patients, biliary colic is almost always present, often radiating to the right scapula or shoulder.
- Laparoscopic cholecystectomy is indicated in patients with symptomatic gallstones.
- Major complications of gallstone disease requiring treatment are acute cholecystitis, choledocholithiasis, obstructive jaundice, cholangitis, and pancreatitis.
- Acute cholangitis caused by an obstructing gallstone should be treated by endoscopic removal of the stone under antibiotic coverage as soon as possible.

General Considerations

Gallstone disease represents a considerable health problem in Western industrialized countries. With a prevalence of 10–15% in adults in the United States and in Europe, it is one of the most common digestive diseases. In the United States, it is the gastrointestinal disorder that, after gastroesophageal reflux disease, accounts for the second-highest costs. The clinical manifestations of gallstones include episodic abdominal pain, acute cholecystitis, obstructive jaundice, cholangitis, and pancreatitis.

In Western industrialized countries, >90% of gallstones consist mainly of cholesterol. Thus, in the majority of patients, cholelithiasis may be regarded as a disturbance of cholesterol disposal. A complex solubilizing system in bile is required to keep cholesterol in solution. If this system fails, or if its capacity is exceeded by hypersecretion of cholesterol into bile, cholesterol precipitates and gallstones may develop.

A. Epidemiology and Genetics

In the third National Health and Nutrition Examination Survey (NHANES III), a large epidemiologic survey that compiled data including gallbladder ultrasonography findings, the overall prevalence of gallstones in the United States was 7.9% in men and 16.6% in women, with a progressive increase after age 20 years. The prevalence was high in Mexican Americans (8.9% in men, 26.7% in women), intermediate for non-Hispanic whites (8.6% in men, 16.6% in women), and low for African Americans (5.3% in men, 13.9% in women). Overall prevalence rates in Europe, from large ultrasonic surveys in adults aged 30–69 years, are similar to those in the NHANES III study. The prevalence of gallstone disease is lower in Asians (ranging from 3% to 15%) and very low (<5%) in Africans. Certain ethnic groups are particularly susceptible; among Native Americans in the western United States, the prevalence of gallstones is over 75%.

Epidemiologic surveys and family clustering point to the critical role of genetics in determining susceptibility to gallstones. The genetic component in the pathogenesis of symptomatic gallstone disease in the Swedish population has been estimated to be about 25%. A single nucleotide polymorphism conferring an increased risk of gallstone formation has been identified in the hepatic cholesterol transporter ABCG5/G8 of patients with gallstones. In a recent genome-wide analysis of serum bilirubin levels, the uridine diphosphate-glucuronyltransferase 1A1 (*UGT1A1*) Gilbert syndrome gene variant was associated with gallstone disease and with the presence of bilirubin in gallstones in men. Since most gallstones associated with the *UGT1A1* variant were cholesterol stones, this finding points to the role of pigment particles in the pathogenesis of gallbladder stones, possibly as nucleation factors.

Although in the vast majority of patients, the predisposition to gallstones appears to be polygenic, rare forms of monogenic gallstone disease exist. Thus, a single gene defect, namely, a mutation in the gene encoding the canalicular phospholipid transporter (ABCB4) of the hepatocyte, has been identified by Rosmorduc and coworkers in a rare form of cholesterol cholelithiasis. This gene defect is associated with low phosphatidylcholine in bile and has been named *GBD1* (*gallbladder disease 1*) in the Online Mendelian Inheritance in Man (OMIM) database (http://www.ncbi.nlm.nih.gov/sites/entrez?db=OMIM). The extremely low phospholipid levels in the bile of these patients cause cholesterol precipitation.

B. Risk Factors

The prevalence of gallstones increases with age. It is about twice as high in women as in men. The gender difference at least partly results from endogenous estrogens, which increase biliary cholesterol secretion and cholesterol saturation of bile. Pregnancy increases the risk of gallstones because impaired gallbladder emptying, caused by progesterone, combines with the influence of estrogen, which increases cholesterol hypersecretion. In obese persons an overproduction of cholesterol causes cholesterol hypersecretion into bile and thus predisposes to gallstone formation. In many obese patients, cholesterol gallstones may be regarded as a component of the metabolic syndrome. (Table 53-1)

Attili AF, De Santis A, Capri R, et al. The natural history of gallstones: the GREPCO experience. The GREPCO Group. *Hepatology.* 1995;21:655–660. [PMID: 7875663]

Table 53–1. Major risk factors for cholesterol gallstones.

General
Increasing age
Female gender
Ethnicity
Family history
Diet
Overnutrition
High calorie
Low fiber
High refined carbohydrates
Lifestyle
Low-grade physical activity
Prolonged fasting
Rapid weight loss
Weight cycling
Pregnancy and parity
Oral contraceptives
Associated conditions
Obesity
Metabolic syndrome
Estrogen replacement therapy

Buch S, Schafmayer C, Volzke H, Seeger M, Miquel JF, Sookoian SC, Egberts JH, et al. Loci from a genome-wide analysis of bilirubin levels are associated with gallstone risk and composition. *Gastroenterology.* 2010;139:1942–1951. [PMID: 20837016]

Everhart JE, Khare M, Hill M, et al. Prevalence and ethnic differences in gallbladder disease in the United States. *Gastroenterology.* 1999;117:632–639. [PMID: 10464139]

Grünhage F, Acalovschi M, Tirziu S, et al. Increased gallstone risk in humans conferred by common variant of the hepatic ABC transporter for cholesterol. *Hepatology.* 2007;46:793–801. [PMID: 17626266]

Katsika D, Grjibovski A, Einarsson C, et al. Genetic and environmental influences on symptomatic gallstone disease: a Swedish study of 43,141 twin pairs. *Hepatology.* 2005;41:1138–1143. [PMID: 15747383]

Rosmorduc O, Hermelin B, Boelle PY, et al. ABCB4 gene mutation associated cholelithiasis in adults. *Gastroenterology.* 2003;125: 452–459. [PMID: 12891548]

Sandler RS, Everhart JE, Donowitz M, et al. The burden of selected digestive diseases in the United States. *Gastroenterology.* 2002;122:1500–1511. [PMID: 11984534]

Schafmayer C, Hartleb J, Tepel J, et al. Predictors of gallstone composition in 1025 symptomatic gallstones from Northern Germany. *BMC Gastroenterol.* 2006;6:36. [PMID: 17121681]

Pathogenesis

Gallstones classified as cholesterol stones contain more than 50% cholesterol with variable admixtures of calcium salts, bile pigments, proteins, and fatty acids. Cholesterol stones account for more than 90% of all gallstones in Western industrialized countries. Pigment stones are composed primarily of calcium bilirubinate; they contain less than 20% cholesterol.

A. Cholesterol Stones

Because cholesterol is practically insoluble in water, solubilizing lipids (bile acids and phospholipids) are required for its incorporation into bile. Biliary lipid secretion is regulated by ATP-binding cassette (ABC) transporters in the hepatocyte canalicular membrane. The bile salt export pump (BSEP; ABCB11) transports bile acids into the bile, the multidrug resistance p-glycoprotein 3 (MDR3; ABCB4) translocates phosphatidylcholine from the inner to the outer leaflet of the canalicular membrane, and the transporter ABCG5/G8 secretes cholesterol into the bile.

Cholesterol and phosphatidylcholine reach the bile as unilamellar vesicles and are subsequently converted into water-soluble mixed micelles by the bile acids (Figure 53–1). Supersaturation of bile with cholesterol is the thermodynamic requirement for the formation of cholesterol gallstones. It can result from secretion of cholesterol into bile that exceeds the solubilizing capacity of bile acids and phospholipids. If all cholesterol phosphatidyl vesicles cannot be converted into water-soluble mixed micelles, unstable cholesterol-rich

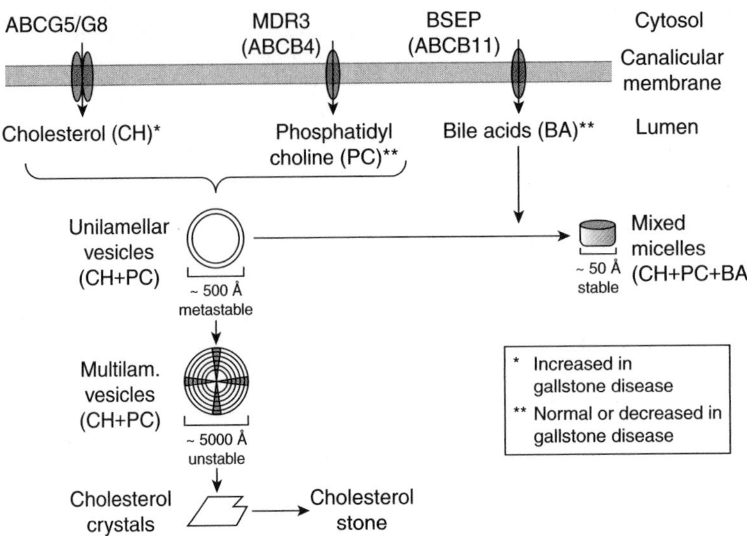

▲ **Figure 53–1.** Biliary secretion and solubilization of cholesterol. Cholesterol is secreted by the ABC-binding cassette (ABC) transporter ABCG5/G8, phosphatidylcholine by the multidrug resistance p-glycoprotein 3 (MDR3; ABCB4), and bile acids by the bile salt export pump (BSEP; ABCB11). Cholesterol and phosphatidylcholine reach the bile as metastable unilamellar vesicles, which are converted into water-soluble stable mixed micelles by the bile acids. If the secretion of cholesterol into bile exceeds the solubilizing capacity of bile acids and phospholipids, cholesterol-rich vesicles remain, which aggregate into large unstable multilamellar vesicles from which cholesterol crystals precipitate. These crystals may aggregate and form cholesterol stones. Recent evidence indicates that a variant in the hepatocanalicular cholesterol transporter gene *ABCG8* contributes to the risk of cholesterol gallstone formation (for details see text).

vesicles remain. The unstable vesicles aggregate into large multilamellar vesicles from which cholesterol crystals precipitate. These crystals—if not expelled from the gallbladder—become entrapped in gallbladder mucin gel, where they grow and agglomerate to form stones.

The pathogenesis of cholesterol hypersecretion is multifactorial, with genetic and environmental components.

1. Cholesterol supersaturation of bile—An excess of biliary cholesterol in relation to its carriers (phospholipids and bile acids) is a *sine qua non* condition for the formation of cholesterol gallstones. It may result from hypersecretion of cholesterol, hyposecretion of bile acids or phospholipids, or a combination of the two. Relative *cholesterol hypersecretion* is by far the most common cause of supersaturation of bile. It may result from increased synthesis of cholesterol, increased uptake by the liver of endogenous (via low-density lipoproteins) or exogenous (via chylomicrons) cholesterol, and increased hepatocanalicular transport of cholesterol. An inappropriately low rate of cholesterol 7α-hydroxylation, the rate-limiting step in the conversion of cholesterol to bile acids, can also increase cholesterol secretion into bile. This may occur in a rare genetic defect, but also with age. A defect in the ileum characterized by impaired absorption and increased fecal loss of bile acids, thus lowering the amount of bile acids in the enterohepatic circulation, may also play a role. Obese individuals secrete more cholesterol into bile because they ingest and synthesize more cholesterol. During weight loss, there is an increased excretion of cholesterol into bile, often combined with decreased gallbladder emptying.

2. Destabilization of bile—Supersaturation of bile is a prerequisite for stone formation, but alone it is not sufficient for lithogenesis. About 50% of adults have supersaturated bile at least at some times during the day, but only about 10–15% form stones. The majority of people with supersaturated bile do not have stones because the time required for cholesterol crystals to nucleate and to grow is longer than the time the bile spends in the gallbladder. The stability of phospholipid cholesterol vesicles depends on their cholesterol content and on the balance between inhibitors and promoters of cholesterol crystal formation. Normally, inhibitors of cholesterol crystal formation and growth appear to outweigh the promoters. The influence of promoting and inhibiting factors on the appearance of crystals in bile has been assessed by the "nucleation time" or crystal "observation time." It is much shorter in gallbladder bile from patients with cholesterol gallstones than in equally supersaturated gallbladder bile from normal subjects. A protein that promotes crystal nucleation or growth, or both, is gallbladder mucin. Gallbladder mucin, a mixture of high molecular weight mucus glycoproteins, is layered at the mucosal surface of the gallbladder wall, where it forms a viscous bed facilitating nucleation and aggregation of cholesterol crystals (Figure 53–2). Release of mucin and perhaps other glycoproteins from the gallbladder is stimulated by deoxycholic acid.

3. Stasis of bile in the gallbladder—If the gallbladder emptied all supersaturated bile completely before crystals had formed, stones would not be able to grow. Thus, prolonged retention of all or parts of the gallbladder contents seems to be another important prerequisite for lithogenesis. A high percentage of patients with gallstones exhibit abnormalities of gallbladder emptying. Studies of gallbladder motility using ultrasonography have shown that patients with gallstones have increased fasting and residual gallbladder volume and that fractional emptying of the gallbladder is decreased (Figure 53–3). The incidence of gallstones is increased in conditions associated with infrequent or impaired gallbladder emptying, such as fasting, parenteral nutrition, or pregnancy, and in patients using drugs that inhibit gallbladder motility. Gallbladder hypomotility during fasting results from lack of gallbladder stimulation. Consequently, the risk of stone formation during parenteral nutrition can be decreased by administration of cholecystokinin. During pregnancy, both the fasting volume and the residual volume of the gallbladder rise with serum progesterone, which inhibits smooth muscle contractility and impairs emptying.

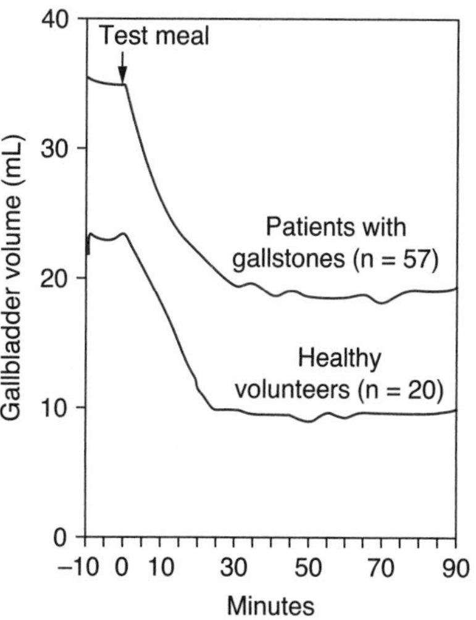

▲ **Figure 53–3.** Impaired gallbladder emptying after a test meal in patients with gallstones measured by ultrasonography. (Data from Paumgartner G, Pauletzki J, Sackmann M. Ursodeoxycholic acid treatment of cholesterol gallstone disease. *Scand J Gastroenterol Suppl.* 1994;204:27–31.)

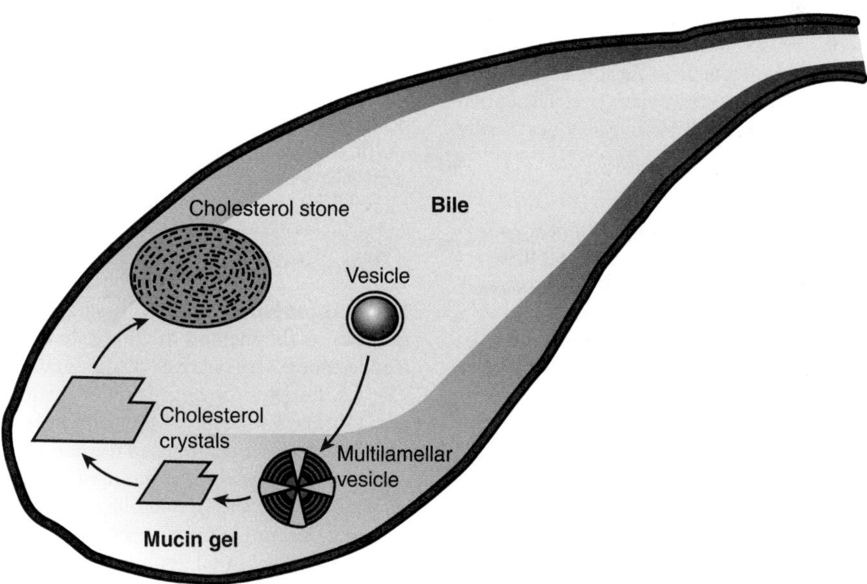

▲ **Figure 53–2.** Formation, growth, and aggregation of cholesterol crystals in the mucin gel layered at the mucosal surface of the gallbladder wall (for details see text).

Table 53–2. Major risk factors for pigment stones.

Associated conditions
Chronic hemolysis
Pernicious anemia
Liver cirrhosis
Cystic fibrosis
Chronic biliary tract infections
Biliary parasites
Ileal disease
Ileal resection or bypass
Demographic factors
Asia, rural setting

B. Pigment Stones

Pigment stones can be *black pigment stones,* which are composed of either pure calcium bilirubinate or polymer-like complexes containing mainly calcium and mucin glycoproteins. They are more common in patients who have chronic hemolytic states (with increased conjugated bilirubin in bile), liver cirrhosis, Gilbert syndrome, or cystic fibrosis (Table 53–2). Gallbladder stones in patients with ileal disease, ileal resection, or ileal bypass generally are also black pigment stones. Enterohepatic cycling of bilirubin contributes to their pathogenesis.

Brown pigment stones consist of calcium salts and unconjugated bilirubin with varying amounts of cholesterol and protein. They are caused by the presence of increased amounts of unconjugated, insoluble bilirubin in bile. Deconjugation of soluble conjugated bilirubin glucuronide may be caused by bacterial enzymes when bile is infected, but may also occur by spontaneous alkaline hydrolysis. Brown pigment stones are frequent in Asia, where there is a high prevalence of infection of the biliary tree. They often form in the bile ducts, whereas cholesterol gallstones usually originate in the gallbladder.

Grundy SM. Cholesterol gallstones: a fellow traveler with metabolic syndrome? *Am J Clin Nutr.* 2004;80:1–2. [PMID: 15213019]

Paumgartner G, Sauerbruch T. Gallstones: pathogenesis. *Lancet.* 1991;338:1117–1121. [PMID: 1682550]

Portincasa P, Moschetta A, Palasciano G. Cholesterol gallstone disease. *Lancet.* 2006;368:230–239. [PMID: 16844493]

Clinical Findings

A. Symptoms and Signs

Only 20–25% of persons with gallstones have symptoms that can be attributed to their stones. Not all symptoms in patients with gallstones are caused by the stones. Gallstones are often discovered incidentally during abdominal ultrasonography and remain asymptomatic in nearly 80% of cases. Unspecific gastrointestinal symptoms, such as belching, heartburn, and bloating in the absence of biliary pain should not be attributed to gallstones without considering other diagnoses (eg, reflux disease). The discovery of gallstones on imaging studies does not, therefore, mean that symptomatic gallstone disease is present.

The first symptom of gallstone disease almost always is biliary colic. Only in about 10% of patients is the first manifestation of gallstone disease cholecystitis, obstructive jaundice, or pancreatitis. Biliary colic results from obstruction of the cystic duct or common bile duct by a stone that, by distention of the viscus, causes visceral pain that usually is a severe, steady ache or fullness in the epigastrium or right upper quadrant of the abdomen, frequently radiating to the interscapular area, right scapula, or shoulder. Usually it begins quite suddenly and may persist for 15 minutes to 5 hours, subsiding gradually or rapidly. It is steady rather than intermittent as would be suggested by the word *colic,* which must be regarded as a misnomer, although in widespread use. The term *biliary pain* appears more appropriate. There may be concomitant nausea with or without vomiting. Nocturnal presentation awakening the patient is common. Many patients develop pain after eating, fatty foods often being the culprit. Some patients have pain unrelated to eating.

After the first manifestation of biliary pain, about 30% of patients do not have another episode, but the majority of patients suffer from further attacks of pain, and the rate of complications is 1–3% per year. By contrast, the rate of complications for a carrier of a gallstone that has never had a biliary colic is only 0.1–0.3% per year. If there are no further episodes of biliary colic within 5 years after the first attack, the natural history of the patient may be regarded as that of asymptomatic gallstone disease.

Symptomatic gallstone disease is called *uncomplicated* if it is characterized by episodes of biliary pain of less than 5 hours only. *Complicated gallstone disease* should be suspected if an episode of biliary pain persists beyond 5 hours and if clinical or laboratory findings of acute cholecystitis, acute biliary pancreatitis, biliary obstruction, or symptoms and signs of other complications develop.

B. Laboratory and Imaging Studies

1. Ultrasonography—Ultrasonography of the right upper quadrant is the method of choice for the diagnosis of gallbladder stones (see Figure 9–35). Its sensitivity is greater than 95% for the detection of gallstones 1.5 mm or more in diameter. Complete imaging of the gallbladder in various planes and in at least two positions of the patient is mandatory. The characteristic finding is a mobile echogenic focus with an acoustic shadow within the gallbladder lumen that moves in a gravity-dependent fashion with the patient's position. The gravity-dependent mobility of the echogenic foci allows differentiation from gallbladder polyps or carcinoma.

Ultrasonography also offers information about the size of the gallbladder, the presence of a thickened gallbladder wall, and pericholecystic fluid (signs of acute cholecystitis). Ultrasonography has high sensitivity (94%) and specificity (78%) for the diagnosis of acute cholecystitis.

Complications such as perforation into the abdominal cavity can be detected or excluded. Bile duct dilation may point toward bile duct obstruction. For the detection of bile duct stones, however, ultrasonography offers only low to moderate sensitivity (see below).

Functional ultrasonography provides additional information about gallbladder emptying and cystic duct patency.

2. Computed tomography (CT)—CT is occasionally useful for the detection or exclusion of gallstones, especially calcified stones, but it is less sensitive and more expensive than ultrasound and requires exposure to radiation. It is valuable for visualization of the biliary system in suspected biliary obstruction. It should be used if biliary pancreatitis or common bile duct stone obstruction is suspected.

3. Magnetic resonance imaging (MRI) and cholangiopancreatography (MRCP)—MRI is not recommended for screening for gallstones, but is useful for visualizing pancreatic ducts and bile ducts and has excellent sensitivity for bile duct or pancreatic duct dilations. Its sensitivity for detection of bile duct stones is approximately 85%. MRCP can be used as an alternative to ERCP to exclude bile duct stones in the preoperative screening of patients undergoing laparoscopic cholecystectomy if there is a low to intermediate level of suspicion for bile duct stones.

4. Endoscopic retrograde cholangiopancreatography (ERCP)—ERCP is not useful for detection of gallstones in the gallbladder but is the method of choice for the detection of bile duct stones. In contrast to MRI, it has both diagnostic and therapeutic value for visualization and extraction of bile duct stones.

5. Endoscopic ultrasound—This is the most sensitive method for the detection of ampullary stones.

6. Hepatobiliary scintigraphy—This test has no role in the detection of gallstones and a limited one in the diagnosis of cholecystitis. If acute cholecystitis with blockage of the cystic duct by a gallstone is suspected, cholecystoscintigraphy (HIDA scanning) has 95% sensitivity for detecting the cystic duct obstruction.

7. Oral cholecystography—This modality has been replaced by ultrasonography and is regarded as obsolete.

Kalimi R, Gecelter GR, Caplin D, et al. Diagnosis of acute cholecystitis: sensitivity of sonography, cholescintigraphy, and combined sonography-cholescintigraphy. *J Am Coll Surg.* 2001; 193:609–613. [PMID: 11768676]

Lammert F, Neubrand MW, Bittner R, et al. S3-guidelines for diagnosis and treatment of gallstones. German Society for Digestive and Metabolic Diseases and German Society for Surgery of the Alimentary Tract. *Z Gastroenterol.* 2007;45:971–1001. [PMID: 17874360]

Lowenfels AB, Lindström CG, Conway MJ, et al. Gallstones and risk of gallbladder cancer. *J Natl Cancer Inst.* 1985;75:77–80. [PMID: 3859698]

Rickes S, Treiber G, Mönkemüller K, et al. Impact of the operator's experience on value of high-resolution transabdominal ultrasound in the diagnosis of choledocholithiasis: a prospective comparison using endoscopic retrograde cholangiography as the gold standard. *Scand J Gastroenterol.* 2006;41:838–843. [PMID: 16785198]

Verma D, Kapadia A, Eisen GM, et al. EUS vs MRCP for detection of choledocholithiasis. *Gastrointest Endosc.* 2006;64:248–254. [PMID: 16860077]

Differential Diagnosis

The differential diagnosis of acute right upper quadrant abdominal pain should include duodenal ulcer disease, acute pancreatitis, appendicitis, duodenal obstruction, lower rib margin syndrome, right lower lobe pneumonia, mesenteric vascular ischemia, and gastroparesis. An ultrasound examination and, if necessary, a HIDA scan will help establish the diagnosis of acute cholecystitis.

Complications

A. Acute Cholecystitis

Acute cholecystitis is the most frequent complication of gallstone disease. In 90% of patients it is caused by a transient or permanent obstruction of the cystic duct by a stone. It represents an inflammatory response to mechanical, chemical, or bacterial causes. The increased intraluminal pressure and distention of the gallbladder result in ischemia of the mucosa and the wall of the gallbladder. Inflammatory agents, such as lysolecithin, and local tissue factors may be released. Bacterial inflammation playing a role in 50–85% of patients with acute cholecystitis, in general, is a secondary event occurring late in the course. The organisms most frequently isolated by culture of gallbladder bile in these patients include *Escherichia coli*, *Klebsiella* species, *Streptococcus* species, and *Clostridium* species.

Acute cholecystitis usually begins as an attack of biliary pain that progressively worsens. Most patients have previously experienced episodes of biliary pain. When cholecystitis develops, the pain, which initially is more diffuse, becomes localized in the right upper quadrant. Peritoneal signs of inflammation, such as increased pain with jarring or on deep inspiration, may become apparent. Nausea and vomiting are frequent.

Physical examination of patients with acute cholecystitis reveals right upper quadrant tenderness. Usually there is marked tenderness and inhibition of inspiration on deep palpation under the right subcostal margin (Murphy sign). An enlarged, tense gallbladder is palpable in about one third of patients, often associated with a stone in the neck of the gallbladder (see Figure 9–37).

Low-grade fever is usually present, but shaking chills or rigors may occur. Mild to moderate leucocytosis is common. Serum bilirubin and serum liver enzymes may be mildly elevated in some patients, but substantial elevations suggest bile duct obstruction concomitant with acute cholecystitis. They may also occur when edematous, inflammatory changes involve the bile ducts. Serum amylase levels usually are normal; if substantially elevated, they suggest pancreatitis.

Chronic cholecystitis is a chronic inflammation of the gallbladder wall that results from repeated attacks of acute and subacute cholecystitis or mechanical irritation of the gallbladder mucosa by gallstones. It may progress from asymptomatic to symptomatic.

In 10–30% of the patients with acute cholecystitis severe complications, such as gallbladder gangrene, empyema, or perforation, occur. Fistulization between gallbladder and bowel occur in less than 1% of all patients with gallstones. A biliodigestive fistula can manifest itself by ascending cholangitis or a bile acid malabsorption syndrome. In about 60% of cases, the fistulas are located between the gallbladder and the duodenum and remain asymptomatic. Passage of large stones through a fistula can cause gallstone ileus, especially in the terminal ileum. Aerobilia is an important sign of a biliodigestive fistula. Magnetic resonance cholangiography (MRC) may be valuable for diagnosis in this situation.

Mirizzi syndrome is a rare complication in which a gallstone becomes impacted in the neck of the gallbladder or cystic duct, causing compression of the common bile duct and obstructive jaundice.

B. Choledocholithiasis

Passage of gallstones into the common bile duct occurs in approximately 10–15% of patients with gallbladder stones. In up to 25% of elderly patients who undergo cholecystectomy, stones in the common duct are found. The large majority of them are cholesterol stones that originate in the gallbladder. Stones that primarily form in the bile ducts are usually pigment stones (see "Pathogenesis," earlier). An exception is the formation of cholesterol gallstones in the bile ducts of patients with an ABCB4 gene defect causing impaired biliary phospholipid secretion. Most patients with common bile duct stones present with biliary pain accompanied by abnormal liver tests with or without jaundice. Major complications of choledocholithiasis are obstructive jaundice, cholangitis, pancreatitis, and secondary biliary cirrhosis.

The presentation of acute obstruction of the common bile duct by a stone usually includes biliary pain, similar to the pain of cystic duct obstruction, and—if of sufficient duration—is followed by jaundice. Most patients with obstruction have elevated liver enzymes (alanine amino-transferase [ALT], aspartate aminotransferase [AST]) in the acute phase of obstruction. In the later course ALT and AST decrease toward normal even if the obstruction persists, whereas alkaline phosphatase rises, followed by bilirubin elevation and eventually jaundice.

Table 53–3. Criteria for simultaneous choledocholithiasis in patients with gallbladder stones.

High probability for simultaneous bile duct stones
Common bile duct dilated (>6–8 mm) + hyperbilirubinemia + elevated GGT, alkaline phosphatase and/or ALT
Common bile duct >10 mm in presence of gallbladder stones
Direct evidence of stone in bile ducts by ultrasound
Low probability for simultaneous bile duct stones
Common bile duct not dilated
GGT, alkaline phosphatase, and ALT within normal limits

ALT, alanine aminotransferase; GGT, γ-glutamyl transferase.

Transcutaneous abdominal ultrasonography has only moderate diagnostic accuracy for the detection or exclusion of bile duct stones. Sensitivities between 38% and 82% have been reported. If the diameter of the common bile duct is larger than 6 mm, a bile duct stone must be suspected (see Table 53–3). Determination of γ-glutamyl transferase (GGT), alkaline phosphatase, ALT, and serum bilirubin levels is mandatory for differential diagnosis in this situation.

If direct proof or exclusion of bile duct stones by ultrasonography is not possible, clinical symptoms and signs of biliary obstruction guide the planning of further diagnostic measures. If there is high suspicion of the presence of a bile duct stone, endoscopic retrograde cholangiography (ERC) is indicated because it permits simultaneous therapeutic intervention (endoscopic papillotomy and stone extraction). Its sensitivity and specificity for the detection of bile duct stones are greater than 90%. However, a general recommendation for exclusion of bile duct stones with ERC prior to laparoscopic cholecystectomy would expose too many patients to unnecessary risks of this diagnostic procedure, because the prevalence of bile duct stones in patients with gallbladder stones, depending on age, ranges between 5% and 15% only. If findings are questionable and bile duct stones are suspected, endosonography or MRC (see Figure 9–36) may be performed prior to ERC. Endosonography has the highest sensitivity for the detection of stones in the common duct. It is associated with lesser risks than the diagnostic ERC, especially for small (<5 mm) and ampullary stones. A recent meta-analysis of five randomized controlled studies including a total of 301 patients did not find a significant difference between endoscopic ultrasound and MRCP with regard to sensitivity (93% vs 85%) and specificity (96% vs 93%) for the diagnosis of bile duct stones.

C. Cholangitis

The characteristic presentation of cholangitis involves biliary pain, jaundice, and spiking fevers with chills (the Charcot triad). Leukocytosis is typical, and blood cultures are positive in about 75% of patients.

D. Biliary Pancreatitis

Biochemical evidence of pancreatic inflammation complicates acute cholecystitis in about 15% and choledocholithiasis in about 30% of patients. The common cause appears to be passage of stones through the common duct.

Treatment

A. Surgical Therapy

1. Asymptomatic gallstones—Treatment of persons with asymptomatic gallstones, with certain exceptions (see later discussion), is not recommended because the risks of biliary colic, complications, and gallbladder cancer are low. Sixty to 80% of persons with asymptomatic gallstones remain asymptomatic over follow-up periods of up to 25 years. The probability of developing symptoms within 5 years after diagnosis is 2–4% per year and decreases in the years thereafter to 1–2%. The yearly incidence of complications is about 0.1–0.3%. Treatment of patients with asymptomatic gallstones does not prolong life expectancy, because the risk of complications caused by the stones is counterbalanced by the operative risks. Finally, the costs of expectant management without prophylactic cholecystectomy until symptoms or complications occur are lower than those of an active approach. In countries with a low prevalence of gallbladder carcinoma, the slightly elevated risk of gallbladder carcinoma does not justify surgical intervention in patients with asymptomatic gallstones. Additionally, in diabetic patients, asymptomatic gallstones should be left alone.

Prophylactic cholecystectomy is, however, indicated for asymptomatic patients with an increased risk of gallbladder cancer (eg, patients with a so-called porcelain gallbladder; see Figure 9–38), patients with large stones (≥3 cm in diameter), or Native Americans, whose risk of cancer is 3–5%. It is important to distinguish between homogenous and patchy calcifications of the gallbladder wall. Especially with patchy calcification there seems to be a high (7%) risk of carcinoma.

Prophylactic cholecystectomy has been proposed for patients with small gallstones (≤5 mm in size) and preserved gallbladder motility, because they may have a high risk for acute pancreatitis. However, further studies are needed to support this recommendation. Some practitioners also consider prophylactic cholecystectomy in patients with a high risk of becoming symptomatic, such as children who will be exposed to the risks of the stones for a long time.

Patients with gallstones and gallbladder polyps larger than 1 cm should be cholecystectomized irrespective of symptoms. For polyps larger than 1 cm, the probability of neoplastic alteration is markedly increased and a carcinoma may be found in up to 50%. For polyps with a diameter of less than 1 cm, the risk is considerably lower, but in patients aged 50 years or older, cholecystectomy should be considered.

In patients with asymptomatic gallstones who undergo surgery for morbid obesity, prophylactic cholecystectomy should be considered, because they have a 10–15% risk of becoming symptomatic or developing complications after surgery for obesity. During large abdominal surgery (eg, surgery for obesity, extended bowel resections for Crohn disease, and radical gastrectomy with removal of lymph nodes), simultaneous cholecystectomy for asymptomatic stones may be performed.

Although asymptomatic patients in general should be managed expectantly, litholytic therapy may be considered if the stones appear to be ideal for dissolution by oral bile acid therapy with ursodeoxycholic acid (UDCA), psychosocial factors favor an active approach, or medical factors are present creating a high risk for surgery.

Miller K, Hell E, Lang B, et al. Gallstone formation prophylaxis after gastric restrictive procedures for weight loss: a randomized double-blind placebo-controlled trial. *Ann Surg.* 2003;238: 697–702. [PMID: 14578732]

2. Symptomatic gallstones—Patients with symptomatic gallstones should receive treatment. In addition to analgesic therapy, surgical or medical options must be offered. Elective laparoscopic cholecystectomy is the standard method of cholecystectomy in patients with symptomatic gallstones. It provides a permanent cure for nearly all patients. It is cost-effective if compared with open cholecystectomy. Today, more than 93% of all cholecystectomies are started by laparoscopy and only 4–7% have to be converted to open cholecystectomy. A meta-analysis of randomized studies comparing laparoscopic and open cholecystectomy shows identical complication rates for both methods, but on the average 3-day shorter hospital stays and 3-week shorter convalescences. This is reflected by the costs, which are 18% lower for laparoscopic than for open cholecystectomy. A historic comparison shows that complications (bile leakage, 0.4–1.5%; wound infection, 1.3–1.8%; pancreatitis, 0.3%; bleeding, 0.2–1.4%) are lower after laparoscopic than after open cholecystectomy. The rate of bile duct injuries is low and comparable for the two procedures, ranging from 0.2–0.6%.

In patients with liver cirrhosis (Child class A or B) and portal hypertension, laparoscopic cholecystectomy seems to be superior to open cholecystectomy. Laparoscopic cholecystectomy should not be performed if advanced gallbladder carcinoma is suspected.

3. Preoperative diagnostic studies—Preoperative ultrasonography must be performed not only for diagnosis of gall-bladder stones but also for detection of potential complications. Preoperative determination of liver enzymes (GGT, alkaline phosphatase, transaminases) and serum bilirubin is mandatory to assess the likelihood of simultaneous bile duct stones or preexisting liver disease. The likelihood of simultaneous bile duct stones is high if the diameter of the common bile duct is greater than 6–8 mm and GGT, alkaline phosphatase, or serum bilirubin value is elevated. It is low if the diameter of the common bile duct is normal and serum enzymes indicative of cholestasis are not elevated (Table 53–3). (See also "Complications," earlier.)

Lammert F, Neubrand MW, Bittner R, et al. S3-guidelines for diagnosis and treatment of gallstones. German Society for Digestive and Metabolic Diseases and German Society for Surgery of the Alimentary Tract. *Z Gastroenterol.* 2007;45:971–1001. [PMID: 17874360]

B. Nonsurgical Therapy

1. Oral bile acid dissolution—In selected patients who have symptomatic gallbladder stones without complications and have mild and infrequent episodes of biliary pain, stone dissolution with UDCA may be employed. The patient must, however, be informed about the high risk of recurrent stones. UDCA reduces cholesterol saturation of bile and also produces a lamellar liquid crystalline phase in bile that allows dispersion of cholesterol from stones by physical-chemical means. In carefully selected patients with radiolucent stones smaller than 5–10 mm in diameter in a functioning gallbladder, complete dissolution can be achieved with UDCA in about 50% of patients. In general, 6–18 months of therapy are required to achieve complete dissolution of stones 5–10 mm in diameter, as gallstone dissolution occurs at a mean rate of 0.7-mm decrease in diameter per month. For good results within a reasonable time period, this therapy should be limited to radiolucent stones smaller than 5 mm in diameter. The dose of UDCA should be 10–15 mg/kg/day. Stones larger than 15 mm in size rarely dissolve. Pigment stones are not responsive to UDCA therapy. Recurrence of stones in 30–50% of patients within 3–5 years after stone dissolution have reduced the role of gallstone dissolution to patients who want to avoid or are unfit for cholecystectomy. A report from Japan that UDCA may reduce the risk of biliary pain independently from dissolution of the stones has not been confirmed in a recent study, which could not demonstrate a decrease of the incidence of biliary symptoms in gallstone patients awaiting elective cholecystectomy.

2. Extracorporeal shock wave lithotripsy—Following the introduction of laparoscopic cholecystectomy, this nonsurgical therapeutic modality has been abandoned mainly because of high rates of stone recurrence (11–29% at 2 years, 60–80% at 10 years). Extracorporeal shock wave lithotripsy has maintained a limited role in the treatment of bile duct stones resistant to endoscopic extraction.

3. Medical prophylaxis of cholesterol gallstone disease—UDCA may prevent gallstone formation in obese patients during rapid weight loss. In patients who completed a 3-month, 520-kcal/day diet, UDCA at a dose of 600 mg/day proved highly effective in preventing gallstone formation; gallstones developed in only 3% of patients receiving UDCA compared with 28% receiving placebo. In a more recent study of stone prophylaxis by UDCA in obese patients treated by gastric banding, 500 mg/kg/day of UDCA reduced the risk of gallstone formation from 30% to 8% within a follow-up of 6 months. For prophylaxis of gallstone formation during rapid weight loss (>1.5 kg/week) a minimal dose of UDCA of 500 mg/kg/day is recommended until constant body weight is attained.

4. Symptomatic treatment of biliary colic—In general, combinations of analgesics with spasmolytic drugs are used for relief of pain. Paracetamol may be sufficient, but nonsteroidal antirheumatic drugs, such as diclofenac or indomethacin, may also be used in combination with *N*-butyl scopolamine. Often opiates such as pethidine or buprenorphine are required. Nitroglycerin may also be effective because it relaxes the sphincter of Oddi. The patient should be kept NPO (nothing by mouth). In case of vomiting, parenteral fluid and electrolyte replacement may be indicated.

Lammert F, Neubrand MW, Bittner R, et al. S3-guidelines for diagnosis and treatment of gallstones. German Society for Digestive and Metabolic Diseases and German Society for Surgery of the Alimentary Tract. *Z Gastroenterol.* 2007;45:971–1001. [PMID: 17874360]

May GR, Sutherland LR, Shaffer EA. Efficacy of bile acid therapy for gallstone dissolution: a meta-analysis of randomized trials. *Aliment Pharmacol Ther.* 1993;7:139–148. [PMID: 8485266]

Paumgartner G, Pauletzki J, Sackmann M. Ursodeoxycholic acid treatment of cholesterol gallstone disease. *Scand J Gastroenterol Suppl.* 1994;204:27–31. [PMID: 7824875]

Paumgartner G, Sauter GH. Extracorporeal shock wave lithotripsy of gallstones: 20th anniversary of the first treatment. *Eur J Gastroenterol Hepatol.* 2005;17:525–527. [PMID: 15827443]

Shiffman ML, Kaplan GD, Brinkman-Kaplan V, et al. Prophylaxis against gallstone formation with ursodeoxycholic acid in patients participating in a very-low-calorie diet program. *Ann Intern Med.* 1995;122:899–905. [PMID: 7755224]

C. Management of Complications

1. Cholecystitis—Patients with acute cholecystitis should undergo early elective laparoscopic cholecystectomy, ideally within 72 hours after diagnosis. Four randomized studies have compared early and late (>6 weeks after diagnosis) cholecystectomy in a total of 388 patients. A meta-analysis of these studies confirms the advantages of early elective laparoscopic cholecystectomy. Hospital stay for the late operation was 3 days longer, and 17.5% of the patients had to undergo emergency operation during the preoperative waiting period. Early operation did not increase the complication rate (13.1%) as compared with late cholecystectomy (17.8%). When laparoscopic cholecystectomy was performed for acute cholecystitis, the conversion rate ranged between 16.4% and 20.3%, being markedly higher than for elective operation of uncomplicated gallstone disease.

From admission until operation the patient should be kept NPO and intravenously hydrated with careful control of serum electrolytes. Administration of broad-spectrum antibiotics early in the course is recommended, because secondary infection often supervenes in what is initially a non-infectious process.

After conservative therapy, about 75% of patients with acute cholecystitis will recover, but about one third of them will be readmitted because of biliary pain or complications and about 20% will have a recurrence of cholecystitis within 1 year.

If a complication of cholecystitis, such as diffuse peritonitis with suspected perforation, gangrene, or empyema develops, an emergency operation should be performed within 24 hours. When the patient is prepared for surgery, it must be considered that the circulating blood volume is often reduced in patients with cholecystitis or cholangitis. Volume substitution with colloids or albumin solution may therefore be indicated to prevent renal complications. In patients older than 65 years or with markedly increased operative risk (American Society of Anesthesiologists [ASA] risk class ≥IV), percutaneous drainage of the gallbladder is feasible and associated with low mortality.

If, because of late diagnosis or other medical reasons (high operative risk), cholecystectomy cannot be performed within 1–5 days, it should be performed within 6 weeks after acute cholecystitis has subsided.

Johansson M, Thune A, Nelvin L, et al. Randomized clinical trial of open versus laparoscopic cholecystectomy in the treatment of acute cholecystitis. *Br J Surg.* 2005;92:44–49. [PMID: 15584058]

Macrì A, Scuderi G, Saladino E, et al. Acute gallstone cholecystitis in the elderly: treatment with emergency ultrasonographic percutaneous cholecystostomy and interval laparoscopic cholecystectomy. *Surg Endosc.* 2006;20:88–91. [PMID: 16333552]

Papi C, Catarci M, D'Ambrosio L, et al. Timing of cholecystectomy for acute calculous cholecystitis: a meta-analysis. *Am J Gastroenterol.* 2004;99:147–155. [PMID: 14687156]

2. Choledocholithiasis—Symptomatic bile duct stones should be removed. Data on the natural history of bile duct stones show that symptomatic bile duct stones will cause recurrent colic in more than 50% of the patients and complications in about 25%. Asymptomatic bile duct stones seem to be more benign than symptomatic bile duct stones. Although long-term prospective data are not available, short-term prospective and long-term retrospective studies indicate that less than half of the patients become symptomatic and more than 20% of the stones pass spontaneously. From these data it may be concluded that patients with asymptomatic bile duct stones may be treated, but that treatment is not necessary for every patient. Spontaneous passage of stones into the bowel appears to be common, especially when the stones are small. Examination of the feces after extracorporeal shock wave lithotripsy of gallbladder stones has shown that stone fragments up to 8 mm in diameter can pass the papilla spontaneously without severe symptoms.

Patients with symptomatic bile duct stones who have had cholecystectomy previously should undergo endoscopic papillotomy (EPT) and stone extraction. Patients with simultaneous gallbladder and bile duct stones should undergo so-called therapeutic splitting. In this technique, ERC is performed before or after cholecystectomy. If the probability of simultaneous choledocholithiasis is high, preoperative EPT and stone extraction is preferred in most hospitals. EPT and cholecystectomy should not be performed on the same day to exclude complications of EPT before surgery. If the probability of choledocholithiasis is low, preoperative ERC should not be the standard; rather—depending on availability—less-invasive procedures should be used. Both endosonography and MRC have high sensitivity and specificity for the detection of bile duct stones. If bile duct stones are found, preoperative EPT with stone removal should be performed. In centers with high expertise, laparoscopic cholecystectomy may be combined with laparoscopic revision of the common duct and removal of the stones.

If endoscopic transpapillary therapy is not possible or fails, percutaneous, transhepatic, or surgical therapy of choledocholithiasis may be employed. In high-risk patients the placement of an endoprosthesis may be considered for primary therapy.

After successful endoscopic or percutaneous removal of bile duct stones in patients with gallbladder stones, cholecystectomy should be performed. This recommendation is based on a study randomizing patients (>60 years of age) after endoscopic sphincterotomy and clearance of their bile duct stones to receive either expectant management or early laparoscopic cholecystectomy. Within a median follow-up of approximately 5 years, 24% of patients with the gallbladder left in situ returned with further biliary events (cholangitis, acute cholecystitis, biliary pain, and jaundice) as compared with only 7% (cholangitis, biliary pain) in the cholecystectomy group. Cholecystectomy should be performed early, preferably during the same hospital admission. A recent randomized study showed that recurrent biliary events occurred in 17 out of 47 patients (36.2%) whose laparoscopic cholecystectomy was delayed for 6–8 weeks, but only in 1 out of 49 patients who underwent early laparoscopic cholecystectomy within 72 hours after endoscopic sphincterotomy. Early laparoscopic cholecystectomy after sphincterotomy was safe and prevented the majority of biliary events in the period following sphincterotomy and removal of bile duct stones.

Lau JY, Leow CK, Fung TM, et al. Cholecystectomy or gallbladder in situ after endoscopic sphincterotomy and bile duct stone removal in Chinese patients. *Gastroenterology.* 2006;130:96–103. [PMID: 16401473]

Reinders JS, Goud A, Timmer R, et al. Early laparoscopic cholecystectomy improves outcomes after endoscopic sphincterotomy for choledochocystolithiasis. *Gastroenterology.* 2010;138:2315–2320. [PMID: 20206179]

Schiphorst AH, Besselink MG, Boerma D, et al. Timing of cholecystectomy after endoscopic sphincterotomy for common bile duct stones. *Surg Endosc.* 2008;22:2046–2050. [PMID: 18270768]

3. Cholangitis—Acute cholangitis caused by an obstructive gallstone should be treated as soon as possible (in septic patients, as an emergency procedure) by endoscopic removal of the stone. A randomized study has shown a significant advantage of the endoscopic versus the surgical approach with regard to complications and mortality. An accompanying systemic antibiotic therapy is indicated to prevent septic complications. If stone extraction fails, nasobiliary drainage or a biliary stent should be placed. Nasobiliary drainage and a biliary stent are equally effective, but nasobiliary drainage offers the advantage of bile sampling for microbiological tests and flushing the bile duct.

Lai EC, Mok FP, Tan ES, et al. Endoscopic biliary drainage for severe acute cholangitis. *N Engl J Med.* 1992;326:1582–1586. [PMID: 1584258]

4. Biliary pancreatitis—Management of biliary pancreatitis depends on its severity. Most cases of biliary pancreatitis are mild, resolve spontaneously, and may be managed expectantly. After resolution, patients with gallbladder or bile duct stones, or both, should undergo cholecystectomy and removal of bile duct stones prior to discharge from the hospital. If biliary pancreatitis is severe and is associated with choledocholithiasis and signs of cholestasis, ERC with papillotomy and stone extraction should be performed as soon as possible, in the presence of cholangitis within 24 hours.

Index

Note: Page numbers followed by *f* or *t* indicate figures or tables, respectively.